T0198179

EMERGENCY MEDICINE SECRETS

SEVENTH EDITION

EMERGENCY MEDICINE SECRETS

EDITORS:

KATHERINE M. BAKES, MD

JENNIE A. BUCHANAN, MD, FACEP, FACMT

MARIA E. MOREIRA, MD, FACEP

RICHARD BYYNY, MD, MSC, FACEP

PETER T. PONS, MD, FACEP

ELSEVIER

Elsevier

Philadelphia, PA

Elsevier
1600 John F. Kennedy Blvd.
Ste 1800
Philadelphia, PA 19103-2899

EMERGENCY MEDICINE SECRETS, SEVENTH EDITION

ISBN: 978-0-323-69473-5

Notice

Practitioners and researchers must always rely on their own experience and knowledge in evaluating and using any information, methods, compounds or experiments described herein. Because of rapid advances in the medical sciences, in particular, independent verification of diagnoses and drug dosages should be made. To the fullest extent of the law, no responsibility is assumed by Elsevier, authors, editors or contributors for any injury and/or damage to persons or property as a matter of products liability, negligence or otherwise, or from any use or operation of any methods, products, instructions, or ideas contained in the material herein.

Previous editions copyrighted 2016, 2011, 2006, 2003, 1999, and 1993

Library of Congress Control Number: 2020936198

Content Strategist: Marybeth Thiel
Content Development Specialist: Sara Watkins
Publishing Services Manager: Deepthi Unni
Project Manager: Radjan Lourde Selvanadin
Design Direction: Bridget Hoette

Printed in India

Last digit is the print number: 9 8 7 6 5 4 3 2

Working together to grow libraries in developing countries

www.elsevier.com • www.bookaid.org

To Peter Bakes, my prince and the love of my life. Without you, there is nothing. With you, we have built a life of love, laughter, and support. I am forever grateful that God brought us together, and I love you more with each passing day.
Katherine M. Bakes

To Tyler Kennedy, my husband, who has allowed me to reach for my dreams while raising two amazing kids and to my Mom, Helen Buchanan, whose love, tenacity, support, and belief shaped me into the person I am.
Jennie A. Buchanan

To my husband Mark Hafley and my three children (Nicolas, Gabriela, and Natalia) for their support, encouragement, and patience. I could not have asked for a better husband or better children in life's journey. To my parents, Carmen and Jose, for serving as amazing role models for friendship, leadership, compassion, and hard work through my life. I miss them every day.
Maria E. Moreira

To my wife, Jen Byyny, who has persisted through all of the stages of my career in medicine and has been an enduring source of support, and to my parents, Jo and Dick Byyny, who have shown me the value of honesty, integrity, and hard work. I would not be who I am or where I am without you. Thank you.
Richard Byyny

To my wife, Kathy, whose love, support, and remarkable patience make every day worthwhile; to my parents John and Cecelia who always supported my choice of career; and to my emergency medicine mentors, Peter Rosen and Vince Markovchick, whose leadership and guidance lead me down pathways I never considered.
Peter T. Pons

EDITORS

Katie Bakes, MD
Medical Director
Pre-Health Programs
Denver Health Medical Center
Director, At-Risk Intervention and Mentoring (AIM)
Denver Health Medical Center
Professor
Department of Emergency Medicine and Pediatrics
University of Colorado School of Medicine
Aurora, Colorado

Jennie A. Buchanan, MD, FACEP, FACMT
Associate Program Director Denver Health Residency in
   Emergency Medicine
SANE Physician Advisor Denver Health & Hospital
   Authority
Uncompahgre College Advisor University of Colorado
   School of Medicine
Longitudinal Curriculum Liaison Emergency Medicine at
   Denver Health & Hospital Authority
Rocky Mountain Poison & Drug Safety Staff Toxicologist
Associate Professor Department of Emergency Medicine
   University of Colorado School of Medicine
Denver Health & Hospital Authority Department
   of Emergency Medicine
Denver, Colorado

Maria E. Moreira, MD, FACEP
Medical Director of Continuing Education & Simulation
Denver Health & Hospital Authority Office of Education
Denver, Colorado
Director of Professional Development & Wellbeing
Denver Health & Hospital Authority Department
   of Emergency Medicine
Denver, Colorado
Associate Professor of Emergency Medicine
University of Colorado School of Medicine
Aurora, Colorado

Richard Byyny, MD, MSc, FACEP
Denver, Colorado

Peter T. Pons, MD, FACEP
Professor Emeritus
Department of Emergency Medicine
University of Colorado School of Medicine
Denver Health and Hospital Authority
Denver, Colorado

CONTRIBUTORS

Jean Abbott, MD, MH
Professor Emerita, Emergency Medicine
CU Anschutz Medical Campus
Faculty, Master of Science in Palliative Care,
  CU Anschutz
Center for Bioethics and Humanities, CU Anschutz
Aurora, Colorado

Daniel Adams, MD
Clinical Instructor, Emergency Medicine
NYU Langone Health and NYC Health + Hospitals/
  Bellevue
New York, New York

Forrest Andersen, MD
Emergency Physician
Piedmont Atlanta Hospital
Atlanta, Georgia

Arian Anderson, MD
Denver Health Residency in Emergency Medicine
Denver, Colorado

Darryl Auston, MD, PhD
Chair, Department of Surgery
Director, Orthopedic Trauma
North Suburban Medical Center
Thornton, Colorado

Anthony W. Bacon, MD
Visiting Professor
Department of Surgery
University of Utah
Salt Lake City, Utah

Jenelle Badulak, MD
Assistant Professor
Department of Emergency Medicine
Division of Pulmonary, Critical Care and Sleep Medicine
University of Washington
Seattle, Washington

Keith Baker, MD
Departments of Emergency Medicine and Medical
  Toxicology
Core Faculty, Emergency Medicine Residency Program
Clinical Assistant Professor of Emergency Medicine
  (Adjunct)
Lewis Katz School of Medicine at Temple University
St. Luke's University Health Network
Bethlehem, Pennsylvania
Division of Medical Toxicology
Department of Emergency Medicine
Volunteer Attending, Medical Toxicology Fellowship
  Program
Denver Health and Hospital Authority
Denver, Colorado

Whitney Barrett, MD
Associate Professor
Emergency Medicine
University of New Mexico School of Medicine
Albuquerque, New Mexico

Vik Bebarta, MD
Vice Chair, Strategy and Growth
Director, Center for COMBAT Research
Director, TRIAD Research Colorado
Professor, Emergency Medicine and Medical Toxicology,
  Pharmacology
University of Colorado School of Medicine
Aurora, Colorado
Colonel, USAF Reserve IMA
Senior Leader
Office of the Chief Scientist, 59MDW, JBSA
San Antonio, Texas

Daniel Berman, MD
Emergency Medicine Physician
Beth Israel Deaconess Medical Center
Boston, Massachusetts

Maxwell Blodgett, MD
Resident Physician
Harvard Affiliated Emergency Medicine Residency
  at Beth Israel Deaconess Medical Center
Boston, Massachusetts

Barbara K. Blok, MD
Associate Program Director
Denver Health Residency in Emergency Medicine
Associate Professor
Department of Emergency Medicine
University of Colorado School of Medicine
Aurora, Colorado

Dowin Boatright, MD
Assistant Professor
Department of Emergency Medicine
Yale School of Medicine
New Haven, Connecticut

Caitlin F. Bonney, MD
Attending Medical Toxicologist
Northern New England Poison Center
Attending Emergency Physician
Maine Medical Center
Portland, Oregon

Thomas L. Bostwick, MD, FACEP, AMO, USPHS/USCG CAPT. (ret)
Section Chief of Emergency Department
Phoenix VA Health Care System
Assistant Professor, Affiliate Faculty Emergency Medicine
Creighton University, SOM
Clinical Assistant Professor
Department of Emergency Medicine
University of Arizona, Phoenix Campus
Associate Professor of Medicine
University of Arizona College of Medicine
Tucson, Arizona

Nick Brandehoff, MD
Assistant Clinical Professor
University of Colorado School of Medicine
Aurora, Colorado

Julia Aogaichi Brant, MD
Instructor of Pediatrics/Pediatric Emergency Medicine Fellow
Children's Hospital Colorado
Aurora, Colorado

Andrew Brookens, MD
Nephrologist
Altitude Kidney Health/Rocky Mountain Kidney Care
Denver, Colorado

Dr. Tom Califf, MD
Emergency Physician
Aurora, Colorado

Alexa Camarena-Michel, MD
Medical Toxicology Fellow, Emergency Medicine Physician
Rocky Mountain Poison and Drug Safety
Denver Health and Hospital Authority
Denver, Colorado

Stephen V. Cantrill, MD, FACEP
Emergency Physician and Consultant
Denver Health Medical Center
Denver, Colorado

Mitchell Jay Cohen, MD
Professor of Surgery
University of Colorado School of Medicine
Aurora, Colorado

James Dazhe Cao, MD, FACEP, FACMT
Assistant Professor of Emergency Medicine
Division Chief of Medical Toxicology
UT Southwestern Medical Center
Dallas, Texas

Lilia Cervantes, MD
Associate Professor
Department of Medicine
Denver Health
Denver, Colorado

Edward W. Cetaruk, MD, FACMT
Assistant Clinical Professor of Medicine
University of Colorado Denver
Anschutz Medical Campus
Aurora, Colorado
Department of Emergency Medicine & Section of Medical Toxicology and Pharmacology
Toxicology Associates, L.L.C.
Littleton, Colorado

Ryan Chuang, MD
Emergency Physician
Medical Toxicologist
Clinical Associate Professor
Calgary, Canada

Jeremy Collado, MD
Chief Resident
Denver Health Medical Center
Denver, Colorado

Christopher B. Colwell, MD, FACEP
Chief of Emergency Medicine
Zuckerberg San Francisco General Hospital and Trauma Center
Professor and Vice Chair
Department of Emergency Medicine
UCSF School of Medicine
San Francisco, California

Ashley Curry, MD
Psychiatrist
Psychiatric Emergency Services
Denver Health and Hospital Authority
Denver, Colorado

Tracy Cushing, MD, MPH
Associate Professor of Emergency Medicine
University of Colorado School of Medicine
Aurora, Colorado

Daniel F. Danzl, MD, MAAEM, FACEP
Professor and Emeritus Chair
Department of Emergency Medicine
University of Louisville School of Medicine
Louisville, Kentucky

Chris Davis, MD, MBA
Associate Professor of Emergency Medicine
University of Colorado School of Medicine
Aurora, Colorado

Hillary E. Davis, MD, PhD
Department of Emergency Medicine
University of Tennessee Medical Center
Knoxville, Tennessee

Nadia Markovchick Dearstyne, MD
Physician
St Joseph Hospital
Denver, California

H. Evan Dingle, MD
Attending Physician
Emergency Medicine
Lexington Medical Center
West Columbia, South Carolina

Jeff Druck, MD
Co-Director, Office of Professional Excellence
Assistant Dean for Student Affairs
Office of Student Life
Professor, Department of Emergency Medicine
School of Medicine University of Colorado
Aurora, Colorado

Nicole Dubosh, MD
Assistant Professor of Emergency Medicine Harvard
    Medical School
Director of Undergraduate Medical Education Director
Medical Education Fellowship Beth Israel Deaconess
    Medical Center
Boston, Massachusetts

Joshua Easter, MD, MSc
Associate Professor of Emergency Medicine
University of Virginia
Charlottesville, Virginia

Morgan Eutermoser, MD
Emergency Medicine Physician
Medical Director
Denver Health NurseLine
Denver Health Medical Center
Denver, Colorado

Christopher M.B. Fernandes, MD
Professor of Emergency Medicine (retired)
Western University
London, Ontario, Canada

Henrik Galust, MD, PGY-3
Denver Health
Denver, Colorado

Shamai A. Grossman, MD, MS
Associate Professor of Medicine and Emergency
    Medicine
Harvard Medical School
Vice Chair for Health Care Quality
Director of Observation Medicine
Department of Emergency Medicine
Beth Israel Deaconess Medical Center
Boston, Massachusetts

Sasha Gubser, MD, MPH
Clinical Instructor of Pediatrics
University of Colorado School of Medicine
Denver Health and Hospital Authority
Denver, Colorado

Alexander Warren Dalton Guillaume, MD
Emergency Medicine Physician
Loma Linda University Medical Center
Loma Linda, California

Mindi Guptill, MD, FACEP
Associate Professor
Loma Linda University Health
Loma Linda, California

Matthew M. Hall, MD
Attending Physician
Department of Emergency Medicine
Providence Regional Medical Center
Washington State University School of Medicine
Everett, Washington

Laurie Seidel Halmo, MD
Assistant Professor of Pediatrics
Sections of Hospital Medicine and Medical Toxicology
University of Colorado School of Medicine
Aurora, Colorado

Jason Haukoos, MD, MSc
Professor of Emergency Medicine, Epidemiology,
    and Clinical Sciences
University of Colorado School of Medicine
Colorado School of Public Health
University of Colorado Denver
Director of Emergency Medicine Research
Department of Emergency Medicine
Denver Health Medical Center
Denver, Colorado

James D. Haycock, MD
Emergency Medicine Physician
St. David's North Austin Medical Center
Austin, Texas

Paul Hinchey, MD, MBA, FACEP, FAEMS
Chief Strategy Officer
Boulder Community Health
Boulder, Colorado

Martin Huecker, MD
Associate Professor, Research Director
Dept of Emergency Medicine
UofL School of Medicine
Louisville, Kentucky

Kyros Ipaktchi, MD, FACS
Chief of Hand Microvascular Surgery
Denver Health Medical Center
Department of Orthopedics
Denver, Colorado

Janetta L. Iwanicki, MD
Attending Physician
Medical Toxicology
Rocky Mountain Poison & Drug Safety
Emergency Medicine, Denver Health Medical Center
Denver, Colorado
Assistant Professor
Department of Emergency Medicine
University of Colorado School of Medicine
Aurora, Colorado

Zachary J. Jarou, MD, MBA
Emergency Physician
St. Joseph Mercy Health System
Adjunct Professor
University of Michigan
Ann Arbor, MI

Nicholas Jouriles, MD
Professor & Chair, Emergency Medicine
Northeast Ohio Medical University, Rootstown and Vice
 Chair Faculty Development, Emergency Medicine
Summa Health
Akron, Ohio

Patrick Y. Joynt, MD MA
Pediatric Emergency Medicine Fellow
Children's Hospital Colorado
Aurora, Colorado

Bonnie Kaplan, MD, MA
Residency Program Director
Denver Health Medical Center
Assistant Professor
University of Colorado School of Medicine
Denver, Colorado

Juliana Karp, MD
Attending Emergency Department Physician
Lakeland Regional Health
Lakeland, Florida

C. Ryan Keay, MD, FACEP
Emergency Department Medical Director
North Sound Emergency Medicine
Providence Regional Medical Center Everett
Everett, Washington

Danya Khoujah, MBBS, MEHP, FACEP, FAAEM
Attending Physician
Department of Emergency Medicine
MedStar Franklin Square Medical Center
Volunteer Adjunct Assistant Professor
Department of Emergency Medicine
University of Maryland School of Medicine
Baltimore, Maryland

Renee A. King, MD, MPH
Emergency Medicine Director
Miners Colfax Medical Center
Raton, New Mexico

Robert Klemisch, MD
Critical Care Fellow
Washington University School of Medicine
St. Louis, Missouri

Patricia Klingenbjerg, MD
Emergency Medicine Physician
US Acute Care Solutions
Denver, Colorado

John G. Knight, MD
Deputy Chair
Emergency Medicine Dept.
Madigan Army Medical Center, Joint Base
Lewis McCord, Washingon

Kelly J. Ko, PhD
Director
Data Governance and Interoperability
Sharp HealthCare
San Diego, California

Joshua Kolikof, MD
Emergency Medicine Chief Resident
Beth Israel Deaconess Medical Center
Boston, Massachusetts

Daniel Lapidus, MD
Emergency Medicine Physician
Windham Hospital
Willimantic, Connecticut

Paul Leccese, MD
Denver Health Medical Center
Denver, Colorado

Eric Legome, MD, FACEP
Professor and Chair
Department of Emergency Medicine
Mount Sinai West & Mount Sinai St. Luke's Hospitals
Vice Chair, Academic Affairs
Dept. of Emergency Medicine
Icahn Mount Sinai School of Medicine
New York, New York

Adriane E. Lesser, MS
Associate Director, Clinical Research
West Health Institute
La Jolla, California

Benjamin Li, MD
Clinical Research Fellow
Denver Health Medical Center
Denver, Colorado

Daniel M. Lindberg, MD
Associate Professor of Emergency Medicine | Pediatrics
University of Colorado – Anschutz Medical Campus
Aurora, Colorado

Erin Lindsay, MD
Attending Physician
St. Anthony's Hospital
Lakewood, Colorado

Louis J. Ling, MD
Professor of Emergency Medicine
Hennepin County Medical Center
University of Minnesota Medical School
Minneapolis, Minnesota

Rodolfo Loureiro, MD
Emergency Medicine Physician
St. Joseph Hospital
Tampa, Florida

Avery MacKenzie, MD
Emergency Medicine Physician
Montrose Memorial Hospital
Montrose, Colorado

Elizabeth N. Malik, MD
Resident Physician
Denver Health Emergency Medicine Residency
Denver, Colorado

Vincent J. Markovchick, MD
Staff Physician
Professor Emeritus of Emergency Medicine
University of Colorado School of Medicine,
    Denver Health
Denver, Colorado

Kent McCann, MD
Emergency Medicine Resident
Baystate Medical Center
Springfield, Massachusetts

Taylor McCormick, MD, MSc
Assistant Professor of Emergency Medicine
Denver Health and the University of Colorado
    School of Medicine
Denver, Colorado

Chelsea McCullough, MD, MPH
Emergency Medicine Physician
Chinle Comprehensive Healthcare Facility,
    Indian Health Services
Chinle, Arizona

Rick A. McPheeters, DO, FAAEM
Professor and Vice Chair of Emergency Medicine, UCLA
Chief of Emergency Medicine, Kern Medical
Bakersfield, California

Michelle Metz, BSN, RN, SANE-A, CEN
Forensic Nurse Program Manager
Denver Health Medical Center
Denver, Colorado

James C. Mitchiner, MD, MPH, FACEP
Attending Physician
Emergency Department
St. Joseph Mercy Chelsea Hospital
Chelsea, Michigan
Clinical Assistant Professor of Emergency Medicine
University of Michigan Medical School
Ann Arbor, Michigan

Lori A. Montagna, MD
Attending Physician
Emergency Medicine, US Acute Care Solutions,
    Mountain North
Pediatric Medical Director, Flight for Life Colorado
Attending Physician
Emergency Medicine, Denver Health Medical Center
Denver, Colorado

Ernest E. Moore, MD
Ernest E. Moore Shock Trauma Center at Denver Health
Distinguished Professor of Surgery
University of Colorado
Denver, Colorado

Sean Morell, MD
Assistant Professor
University of Arkansas for Medical Sciences
Little Rock, Arkansas

Alexander Morton, MD
Assistant Professor of Surgery – University
    of Colorado School of Medicine
General and Bariatric Surgery – Denver Health
Denver, Colorado

Ryan A. Murphy, MD
Emergency Medicine Physician
CarePoint Health
Sky Ridge Medical Center
Lone Tree, CO

Jacob Nacht, MD
Staff Physician
Denver Health Medical Center
Assistant Professor
University of Colorado School of Medicine
Denver, Colorado

Monica Noori, MD
Department of Emergency Medicine
Denver Health Medical Center
Denver, Colorado

Donald Norris, MD, FACEP
Core Faculty
Summa Health System, USACS North & West
Canton, Ohio

Travis D. Olives, MD, MPH Med
Faculty Physician
Department of Emergency Medicine
Hennepin Healthcare
Minneapolis, Minnesota
Associate Medical Director
Minnesota Poison Control System
Minneapolis, Minnesota

Melissa Parsons, MD, FACEP
Assistant Professor
University of Florida College of Medicine – Jacksonville
Jacksonville, Florida

Ryan Pedigo, MD, MHPE
Associate Residency Program Director
Department of Emergency Medicine
Harbor-UCLA Medical Center
Torrance, California

Blake Phillips, DMD
Oral and Maxillofacial Surgeon
Private Practice, Buck and Phillips Oral Surgery
Birmingham, Alabama

K. Barry Platnick, MD
Trauma and Acute Care Surgeon/Surgical Intensivist
(Trauma Medical Director at the time of the writing
    but not currently)
Ernest E. Moore
Shock Trauma Center at Denver Health
Denver, Colorado

John Rague, MD
Emergency Medicine Attending, Medical Toxicology
  Fellow
Denver Health and Hospital Authority
Rocky Mountain Poison and Drug Safety
Denver, Colorado

Lara D. Rappaport, MD
Associate Professor of Emergency Medicine
Pediatric Emergency Department and Urgent Care
  Denver Health
Associate Medical Director of Denver Health Paramedic
  Division
EMS Fellowship Director Denver Health
Denver, Colorado

David Richards, MD, FACEP
Associate Professor of Emergency Medicine
University of Colorado School of Medicine
Denver, Colorado

Kristine Knuti Rodrigues, MD, MPH
Assistant Professor of Pediatrics
Denver Health Pediatric Emergency Department
  and Urgent Care and University of Colorado
  School of Medicine
Denver, Colorado

Jedd Roe, MD, MBA, FACEP
Medical Director
UF Health Jacksonville – North
Professor & Assistant Chair
Program Development and Community Operations
Department of Emergency Medicine
University of Florida College of Medicine – Jacksonville
Jacksonville, Florida

Genie E. Roosevelt, MD, MPH
Professor of Emergency Medicine
Denver Health Hospital and Authority
Denver, Colorado

Carlo L. Rosen, MD
Associate Professor
Harvard Medical School
Program Director and Vice Chair for Education
Associate Director of Graduate Medical Education
Beth Israel Deaconess Medical Center
Harvard Affiliated Emergency Medicine Residency
West CC-2, One Deaconess Road
Boston, Massachusetts

Sarah E. Rowan, MD
Associate Director of HIV and Viral Hepatitis Prevention
Denver Public Health, Denver Health and Hospital
  Authority
Associate Professor of Medicine
University of Colorado School of Medicine
Denver, Colorado

Regina Royan, MD, MPH
Emergency Medicine Resident
University of Chicago
Chicago, Illinois

Dr. Kari Sampsel, MD, MSc, FRCPC, DipForSci
Attending Staff Physician
Medical Director – Sexual Assault and Partner Abuse
  Care Program
Department of Emergency Medicine
The Ottawa Hospital
Ottawa, Canada

Jeffrey Sankoff, MD
Assistant Medical Director, Emergency Department
Denver Health Medical Center
Denver, Colorado
Associate Professor
Department of Emergency Medicine
University of Colorado School of Medicine
Aurora, Colorado

Jonathan Schimmel, MD
Assistant Professor of Emergency Medicine
Mount Sinai Hospital Icahn School of Medicine
New York, New York

Andrew Schmidt, DO, MPH
Assistant Professor
Department of Emergency Medicine
University of Florida – Jacksonville
Jacksonville, Florida

Sarah Tolford Selby, DO, FACEP
Assistant Professor
Department of Emergency Medicine
Lead Emergency Physician of Oncologic Emergencies
The Ohio State University Wexner Medical Center
Columbus, Ohio

Marshall Sheide, DO, PGY-3
University of Texas – San Antonio
San Antonio, Texas

Lee Shockley, MD, MBA
Retired Emergency Physician
Denver, Colorado

Scott A. Simpson, MD, MPH
Psychiatric Emergency Services
Denver Health Medical Center
Denver, Colorado

Corey M. Slovis, MD
Professor of Emergency Medicine and Medicine
Chairman Emeritus
Department of Emergency Medicine
Vanderbilt University Medical Center
Medical Director
Metro Nashville Fire Dept. and Nashville International
  Airport
Nashville, Tennessee

Jeffrey R. SooHoo, MD
Associate Professor of Ophthalmology
Sue Anschutz-Rodgers Eye Center
Assistant Dean of Admissions
University of Colorado School of Medicine
Aurora, Colorado

Philip F. Stahel, MD, FACS
Professor of Orthopedics and Neurosurgery
Rocky Vista University
College of Osteopathic Medicine
Parker, Colorado

W. Gannon Sungar, DO
Staff Physician, Denver Health Medical Center
Assistant Professor, Department of Emergency Medicine
University of Colorado School of Medicine
Denver, Colorado

Jamal Taha, Doctor of Medicine (MD), Master of Healthcare Administration (MHA)
Emergency Medicine Senior Associate Physician
Grady Memorial Hospital
Emory University School of Medicine
Atlanta, Georgia

Taku Taira, MD
Clinical Assistant Professor
LAC+USC Department of Emergency Medicine
Los Angeles, California

Rakesh Talati, MD, MBA
Chair of Emergency Medicine
Baystate Franklin Medical Center
Greenfield, Massachusetts

Molly E.W. Thiessen, MD, FACEP
Emergency Ultrasound Fellowship Director
Staff Physician, Denver Health Medical Center
Denver, Colorado
Associate Professor, Department of Emergency Medicine
University of Colorado School of Medicine
Aurora, Colorado

Gunjan Tiyyagura, MD
Associate Professor of Pediatrics and Emergency
  Medicine
Yale University School of Medicine
New Haven, Connecticut

Spencer Tomberg, MD, MS
Emergency Medicine and Sports Medicine Physician
Departments of Emergency Medicine and Orthopedics
  at Denver Health Medical Center
Denver, Colorado

Ronald R. Townsend, MD
Associate Professor of Radiology
Colorado University
Denver Colorado

Kyle W. Trecartin, MD
Emergency Physician and Associate Director of
  Emergency Medicine
Beth Israel Hospital Plymouth
Plymouth, Massachusetts

Stacy A. Trent, MD, MPH
Department of Emergency Medicine
Denver Health Medical Center
Denver, California

Shawn M. Varney, MD, FACEP, FAACT, FACMT
Professor of Emergency Medicine
Medical Director
South Texas Poison Center
University of Texas Health – San Antonio
San Antonio, Texas

Christopher Vercollone, MD
Attending Physician
Cape Cod Hospital
Hyannis, Massachusetts

Deborah Vinton, MD
Systems Medical Director for Emergency Medicine and
  Hospitalist Medicine
TeamHealth
Richmond, Virginia

George Sam Wang, MD
Associated Professor of Pediatrics
University of Colorado Anschutz Medical Campus
Children's Hospital Colorado
Aurora, Colorado

Brooke Watson, BSN CPEN
Clinical Nurse Educator
Denver Health Medical Center
Denver, Colorado

Jean McFall Wheeler Hoffman, MD
Assistant Professor Emergency Medicine & Anesthesia
Vanderbilt University Medical Center
Nashville, Tennessee

Andrew M. White, MD, PhD
Associate Professor
Pediatric Neurology
University of Colorado
Denver Health Medical Center
Denver, Colorado

James D. Whitledge, MD
Department of Emergency Medicine
Beth Israel Deaconess Medical Center
Boston, Massachusetts

Daniel A. Willner, MD, MPH
Assistant Professor of Emergency Medicine
University of Colorado School of Medicine
Aurora, Colorado

Sophia Zabadayev, MD, MS
Resident Physician
UT Health San Antonio
San Antonio, Texas

David Young, MD, MS
Assistant Professor
University of Colorado School of Medicine
Aurora, Colorado

PREFACE

This book is for all students and practitioners of emergency medicine, both novice and experienced. Because emergency medicine continues to mature as a specialty and our daily practice of it continues to evolve, we have reorganized some of the chapters and added appropriate content to reflect these changes. With difficulty we have also selected the Top 100 Secrets from more than 300 submitted by the chapter authors and editors. We hope that this book continues to be a concise, valuable, and enjoyable method of imparting information and knowledge. Knowing some of the most important questions about a particular presentation or problem is the first step to obtaining the answers needed at the patient's bedside. However, medicine being both an art and a science is nothing if not humbling, and knowledge alone does not treat all that ails. Listen to your patients and make them feel heard. Treat them all with the care and empathy you would wish for any member of your family. Getting to the correct diagnosis can be and is invigorating, but positively impacting a life confirms our calling.

Katherine M. Bakes, MD
Jennie A. Buchanan, MD, FACEP, FACMT
Maria E. Moreira, MD, FACEP
Richard Byyny, MD, MSc, FACEP
Peter T. Pons, MD, FACEP

ACKNOWLEDGMENTS

Collectively, the editors would like to thank Carol Lucas for her tireless and exacting work to bring this text together. We are immensely grateful to you for your hard work and wonderful spirit. You are family.

We would also like to thank the contributors of all previous editions and this current edition for their work in the field of emergency medicine and for their contributions to *Emergency Medicine Secrets*.

Last but certainly not least, we thank our mentors and heroes – Dr. Vince Markovchick, Dr. Steve Cantrill, and Dr. Peter Pons – GIANTS of emergency medicine. They solidified emergency medicine's position in health care, created a storied residency at Denver General, and spent tireless hours building and defending our specialty, all while supporting those of us following after them. Like so many others, we are honored to stand on their shoulders. We would like to take this opportunity to recognize the impact on innumerable clinicians who benefited from their enormous wealth of knowledge and the countless individuals healed by their wisdom and gracious hearts. They have taught us the privilege of taking care of patients during their most vulnerable moments. They have collectively elevated our field in ways we can never repay. We have been fortunate to call them colleagues and friends. We are humbled by the impact of these great men, and we hope that we will do them proud in continuing to champion their belief that every patient deserves exceptional, empathetic, evidence-based emergency care. This book, and the field we have dedicated our lives to, would not have been possible without each one of them. Thank you.

CONTENTS

3   NONTRAUMATIC ILLNESS

4   CENTRAL NERVOUS SYSTEM

5   RESPIRATORY SYSTEM

6   CARDIOVASCULAR SYSTEM

14 Toxicologic Emergencies

15 Gynecology And Ostetrics

16 Trauma

17   BEHAVIORAL EMERGENCIES

18   EMS AND DISASTER MANAGEMENT

TOP 100 SECRETS

1. Emergency treatment of preeclampsia includes:
   - Magnesium sulfate for patients who present with preeclampsia with severe features.
   - For patients with sustained systolic blood pressure (SBP) >160 mmHg or diastolic blood pressure (DBP) >110 mmHg, antihypertensives should be used in consultation with an obstetrician.
   - Administer corticosteroids to patients between 24 and 34 weeks' gestation to enhance fetal lung maturity.

2. A woman does NOT have to be pregnant to have preeclampsia or eclampsia. Twenty percent of cases occur in the postpartum period, when the most common presenting symptoms include headache, shortness of breath, blurry vision, nausea or vomiting, edema, or epigastric pain.

3. Button or disc batteries that are retained in the esophagus require emergent removal. Even for just a few minutes, button batteries can cause significant burns and erosions through the entire esophageal wall, leading to potentially massive bleeding, perforation, fistula formation, mediastinitis, and death.

4. With overdoses of drugs that cause sodium channel blockade, give sodium bicarbonate for the treatment of dysrhythmias or prolongation of the QRS duration. If the QRS duration does not narrow after administration of sodium bicarbonate, give a second bolus. Hyperventilation should be initiated to induce a serum pH of 7.5–7.55. Hypertonic saline can also be administered in a dose of 200 mL of 7.5% solution or 400 mL of a 3% solution. In addition to sodium bicarbonate, patients with cardiovascular toxicity often require fluids and vasopressors for hypotension, benzodiazepines for seizures, and endotracheal intubation for altered mental status.

5. Through stimulation of the cerebral respiratory center, salicylate overdose causes an acute respiratory alkalosis, without hypoxia. If the patient is hypoxic, coingestion of a sedative or salicylate-induced noncardiogenic pulmonary edema should be considered. Within 12–24 hours after ingestion, the acid-base status in an untreated patient shifts toward an anion-gap metabolic acidosis as a result of accumulation of lactic acid and ketoacids. A mixed respiratory alkalosis and metabolic acidosis typically is seen in adults. In patients with respiratory acidosis, concomitant ingestion of a central nervous system (CNS) depressant should be suspected. Metabolic acidosis is the predominant acid-base disturbance in children, patients who ingest massive amounts of salicylates, hemodynamically unstable patients, and patients of all ages who have chronic salicylate toxicity.

6. Standard indications for hemodialysis in salicylate poisonings include persistent, refractory metabolic acidosis (arterial pH < 7.10), renal failure with oliguria, cardiopulmonary dysfunction (e.g., pulmonary edema, dysrhythmias, cardiac arrest), CNS deterioration (e.g., seizures, coma, cerebral edema), and a serum salicylate level greater than 100 mg/dL at 6 hours post-ingestion in the acute setting. Because ingestion of more than 300 mg/kg predicts severe toxicity, a nephrologist should be consulted early in anticipation of the possible need for dialysis.

7. The acetaminophen nomogram can only be used with an accurate estimate of the time of ingestion. Treat patients with a credible history of acetaminophen exposure and unknown ingestion time by checking a single acetaminophen level and liver enzymes; if the acetaminophen level is >20 µg/mL or hepatic transaminases are elevated, treat with N-acetylcysteine (NAC) for 12 hours and then repeat the laboratory tests. If acetaminophen is undetectable and liver function has improved, NAC can be halted; otherwise, continue NAC and contact the regional Poison Control Center (1-800-222-1222).

8. The Glasgow-Blatchford score (GBS) is a risk stratification tool applied to patients with acute non-variceal upper gastrointestinal (GI) bleeding. The GBS is calculated by totaling points assigned for laboratory and clinical risk markers (Table 36.1). A score >0 is 99.6% sensitive in predicting high-risk patients who will require clinical interventions, including blood transfusion, endoscopy, or surgery. Low-risk patients with a score of 0 are candidates for outpatient management.

9. Peritoneal fluid criteria for SBP are:
   - Neutrophil count >250 cells/mm^3
   - Positive Gram stain
   - Positive culture result (gold standard)

10. Autonomic dysreflexia/hyperreflexia is an abnormality of the autonomic nervous system seen in patients with long-standing cervical or high thoracic spinal cord lesions (e.g., patients with quadriplegia and high paraplegia). It is caused primarily by unchecked reflex sympathetic discharge secondary to visceral or somatic stimuli below the level of the spinal injury. This potentially life-threatening syndrome includes severe paroxysmal hypertension, diaphoresis, tachycardia or bradycardia, anxiety, headache, and flushing. Uncontrolled, it may result in seizures and coma. Morbidity has resulted from cerebrovascular events, subarachnoid hemorrhage, and respiratory arrest. One of the most common precipitating stimuli is overdistention of the bladder from a plugged or kinked catheter; therefore always evaluate catheter patency in this population.

11. The inappropriate excretion of salt and water after relief of urinary obstruction is called postobstruction diuresis. Patients with abnormal renal function or chronic urinary retention are most susceptible. A physiologic diuresis is normal, because the kidneys excrete the overload of solute and volume retained while the urinary system is obstructed. If urine output persists at high levels, significant fluid and electrolyte abnormalities may develop. Patients who exhibit a continuous diuresis after clinical euvolemia is reached often require hospitalization for hemodynamic monitoring and fluid and electrolyte repletion.

12. BRASH stands for **b**radycardia, **r**enal failure, **A**V nodal blockers, **s**hock, and **h**yperkalemia. These patients present with bradycardia and hyperkalemia in the setting of renal failure, acidosis, and typically, the use of an AV nodal blocking agent such as a β-blocker or calcium channel blocker. In BRASH, renal failure causes hyperkalemia and accumulation of the patient's nodal blocking agent, both of which worsen bradycardia. In a dangerous cycle, bradycardia then leads to shock, further worsening renal perfusion, and so on.

13. In hyponatremia, there has been much debate over how rapidly Na$^+$ should be corrected, ranging from 0.5 to 2.0 mEq/L/h. In most patients, if serum Na$^+$ is <120 mEq/L, serum Na$^+$ should be corrected slowly, rising by no more than 0.5 mEq/h. This approach avoids the possible development of central pontine myelinolysis (which is also called osmotic demyelinating syndrome by some purists), a catastrophic neurologic illness seen with too-rapid Na$^+$ correction: coma, flaccid paralysis, and usually death.

14. Treatment of hyperkalemia is based on the presence or absence of electrocardiogram (ECG) changes, serum levels, and the patient's underlying renal function. If the patient has life-threatening ECG changes of hyperkalemia (widening QRS complex, a sine wave–like rhythm or bradycardia/heart block), 10% calcium chloride should be given (10 mL, preferably through a central line) to temporarily stabilize the myocardial cell membranes. Although calcium is relatively fast-acting, its effect lasts only 30–60 minutes, requiring additional measures to lower K$^+$ levels. However, most patients with hyperkalemia will not have QRS widening, and only require K$^+$ moved intracellularly, and then removed from the body.

15. Kidney stones reaching the distal ureter are more likely to pass than those impacting proximally. Stones 2–4 mm pass 95% of the time; stones 4–6 mm pass 50% of the time, and stones >6 mm pass 10% of the time. When estimating stone size, the x-ray image is magnified; the actual size is 80% of what is measured on the films.

16. Two potentially reversible entities should be considered in a patient with renal failure and cardiac arrest:
    - *Hyperkalemia.* When a patient suffers an arrest from whatever cause, respiratory and metabolic acidosis and the efflux of potassium from cells can be expected to produce hyperkalemia secondarily. In the patient who already may have a tendency toward hyperkalemia, this further increase could cause the patient to be refractory to standard advanced cardiac life support (ACLS) interventions. Patients with chronic kidney disease (CKD) who are in cardiac arrest should receive intravenous (IV) calcium if they do not respond immediately to the first round of ACLS measures.

- *Acute pericardial tamponade.* Cardiac arrest may result from the accumulation of pericardial fluid or spontaneous bleeding into the pericardial sac, and patients with uremia are more susceptible. Patients with tamponade tend to display refractory hypotension, pulseless electrical activity, or both. Bedside ultrasound may be diagnostic, and emergency pericardiocentesis may be life-saving.

17. Patients with metformin-associated lactic acidosis (MALA) have a very high lactate and a low pH, out of proportion to clinical presentation. Chronic toxicity usually arises from patients who develop renal failure for some reason and continue to take therapeutic doses of their metformin. Because metformin is cleared by the kidneys, it starts to accumulate, resulting in a severe lactic acidosis. The mechanism for the lactic acidosis is unknown. The treatment is emergent dialysis for patients with renal failure and a severe acidosis.

18. In primary adrenal insufficiency, hyperkalemia may be present from lack of aldosterone as well as cortisol deficiency. Hyponatremia may be present from lack of aldosterone and the syndrome of inappropriate secretion of antidiuretic hormone (SIADH). Cortisol is one of the counter-regulatory hormones that increase liver glucose production with fasting. In the setting of adrenal insufficiency, hypoglycemia may develop if the patient has not eaten. Anemia and an increase in eosinophils may be seen. Rarely, adrenal insufficiency causes hypercalcemia.

19. In alcoholic ketoacidosis (AKA), patients are in a redox state that favors the formation of lactate from pyruvate. Dextrose-containing fluids reduce fatty acid oxidation (thus limiting acetoacetate generation) and provide another source of adenosine triphosphate (ATP), shifting the nicotinamide adenine dinucleotide/reduced nicotinamide adenine dinucleotide (NAD^+/NADH) ratio to reduce lactate generation.

20. Isopropyl or rubbing alcohol is metabolized in the liver to acetone, which results in measurable ketonemia in the serum. Acetone is excreted by the kidney, resulting in ketonuria, and is exhaled through the lungs, giving the breath an acetone aroma. Because acetone is not acidic, isopropyl alcohol poisoning does not cause metabolic acidosis and is far less toxic than either methanol or ethylene glycol, although it may still result in depressed mental status, gastritis, or gastrointestinal bleeding.

21. Clinical manifestations of ethylene glycol and methanol overdose are often delayed 6–12 hours, causing symptoms only once sufficient quantities of the toxic metabolites accumulate. The delay in symptoms is even greater with concurrent ethanol intoxication, because ethanol stops or slows the rate of methanol and ethylene glycol metabolism.

22. Ventilation and oxygenation remain an essential component of adult cardiopulmonary resuscitation (CPR). While various ventilation and oxygenation strategies have been studied for many years, there is still incomplete evidence regarding optimal: type of delivery used (i.e., passive oxygen insufflation, bag mask ventilation (BVM), advanced airway placement); timing of advanced airway placement in relation to other interventions; or type of advanced airway device used (supraglottic airway [SGA] vs. endotracheal tube [ETT]). What is known to improve survival in adults experiencing nontraumatic out-of-hospital cardiac arrest (OHCA) is early high-quality CPR (and for VF/pVT – defibrillation). Therefore the tasks and timing of ventilation and oxygenation need to be integrated in a way that minimizes interruptions or quality of chest compressions.

23. Even when performed by experts, CPR provides only approximately 30% of normal blood flow to the brain and 10%–20% of normal blood flow to the heart. Blood flow to the heart occurs during the relaxation phase of CPR, whereas blood flow to the brain occurs during the compression phase of CPR. This is the foundation for the American Heart Association's recommended CPR "duty cycle" of 50% (the proportion of the compression/decompression cycle spent in compression).

24. Targeted temperature management (TTM) refers to induced core hypothermia (32°C–36°C) and active temperature control (i.e., prevention of hyperthermia) for approximately 24 hours in comatose OHCA survivors. Two landmark studies published in the early 2000s showed this intervention to be highly efficacious for improving neurologic function, and a study published in 2013 showed similar results to the original studies but no advantage of cooling to 33°C versus 36°C.

25. Passive apneic oxygenation is a technique for preventing hypoxia during rapid-sequence intubation (RSI), where a nasal cannula with high-flow oxygen is placed on the patient during

the preoxygenation phase of RSI and left in place throughout the intubation attempt. Studies have shown that despite apnea during paralysis, passive oxygenation can greatly extend the time it takes for a patient to become critically hypoxic. To prevent harm, care should be taken with pediatric patients, as appropriate flow rates are based on size.

26. The lack of a gag reflex is an unreliable marker for airway collapse, as up to 25% of the population lacks a gag reflex at baseline. Also, the presence of a gag reflex does not guarantee the ability to protect the airway.

27. Serum lactate concentration rises as cells convert to anaerobic metabolism and, thus, is commonly used as a marker to assess the extent of systemic hypoperfusion and tissue hypoxia. An elevated serum lactate concentration is an early marker of systemic hypoperfusion and often precedes overt changes in a patient's vital signs. Higher serum lactate concentrations are associated with higher morbidity and mortality, and a lactate concentration >4 mEq/L has been used to define those with the highest mortality rates. A decrease in serial serum lactate measurements, or lactate clearance, indicates effective shock resuscitation.

28. The systemic inflammatory response syndrome (SIRS) is classically defined by two or more of the following: temperature >38°C or <36°C, heart rate >90 beats per minute (bpm), respiratory rate >20 breaths per minute, or partial pressure of carbon dioxide <32 mmHg, serum white blood cell count >12,000 mm^3 or <4000 mm^3 or >10% band forms. The SIRS response contributes to distributive shock, as inflammation causes reduced systemic vascular resistance and increased capillary permeability. This definition, although standardized, is not specific for defining serious illness or shock. Although most commonly described in the context of sepsis, a systemic inflammatory response may result from a variety of noninfectious insults, including trauma, burns, pancreatitis, or overdose.

29. An intrauterine pregnancy (IUP) may be detectable as early as 4 weeks' gestational age by transvaginal ultrasound (6 weeks using transabdominal ultrasound). The discriminatory zone is the level of β-human chorionic gonadotropin (β-HCG) at which one would expect to see evidence of an IUP by ultrasound. Although this depends on the institution where the patient is being seen, it is typically at a β-HCG level of 1000–2000 mIU/mL by transvaginal ultrasound and 5000 mIU/mL by transabdominal ultrasound. A gestational sac is seen at approximately 4–5 weeks' gestational age, and cardiac activity can be measured as early as 6 weeks' gestational age.

30. A combination of ultrasound evaluations can be used to differentiate the etiology of shock in emergency department (ED) patients. There are multiple protocols used to perform resuscitative ultrasound. However, most include the following: a subcostal cardiac view to evaluate for pericardial effusion and tamponade; an inferior vena cava (IVC) view looking for greater than 50% collapse with inspiration, indicating low intravascular volume; a parasternal long-axis cardiac view to estimate overall left ventricular function; a parasternal short-axis view to evaluate right ventricular enlargement; an apical four-chamber cardiac view to estimate overall function and evaluate relative chamber size (right vs. left); a view of the hepatorenal recess to evaluate for free intraperitoneal fluid; a view of the pelvis and retrovesical area to evaluate for free intraperitoneal fluid; lung views bilaterally in the second intracostal space to rule out pneumothoraces; and finally, a view of the abdominal aorta to evaluate for aneurysm. Use of this systematic, goal-directed protocol in patients in the ED, who have undifferentiated nontraumatic hypotension, allows physicians to narrow their differential diagnosis sooner and gives them a more accurate impression of the class of shock and final diagnosis.

31. The confidence interval is the expected range of results in the study population. A 95% confidence interval means that if you repeated the study 100 times, the result would fall within the 95% confidence interval 95 of the 100 times. The confidence interval is a measure of precision, where a narrower interval is considered more precise and is associated with larger sample sizes. Confidence intervals provide more detail than P values, as they not only demonstrate statistical significance, but also help determine clinical significance. The wider the confidence interval, the more likely the study results are not clinically meaningful. Look at the upper and lower boundaries of the confidence interval and determine whether both values still would hold clinical significance. If only the upper boundary value would have significance, there may not be broad clinical benefit.

32. Clinical signs of child abuse (abdominal bruising or tenderness) are very specific, but not sensitive for identifying abdominal injuries. We recommend obtaining aspartate transaminase (AST) and alanine

transaminase (ALT) for all children with concern for physical abuse and a significant injury (like a long-bone fracture), and abdominal computed tomography (CT) for those with AST or ALT >80 IU/L, or for those with abdominal bruising, tenderness, distention, or with a report of abusive abdominal trauma. The yield of CT using this protocol is >20%, and outweighs the risk from radiation. AST and ALT normalize over hours or days, regardless of whether an injury is present, so rechecking these tests is not a good alternative. Ultrasound has limited sensitivity and should not be used in place of CT.

33. What is the sensitivity of noncontrast CT of the head for subarachnoid hemorrhage (SAH)?
    There have been several studies that have shown that a negative CT completed within 6 hours of symptom onset has a 100% sensitivity to rule out SAH and that no further testing needs to be performed. However, the literature is consistent in demonstrating a decreasing sensitivity of head CT from headache onset time. A reasonable estimate is 95% within 24 hours, 80% at 48 hours, 70% at 72 hours, and 50% at 5 days.

34. Alteplase (also called tissue plasminogen activator [tPA]) is the only thrombolytic currently approved by the US Food and Drug Administration (FDA) for acute stroke. In 1995, the National Institute of Neurological Disorders and Stroke (NINDS) trial showed that tPA improved functional outcome (modified Rankin scale) at 3 months, if given within 3 hours of symptom onset, with a number needed to treat (NNT) of 6. In 2008, ECASS III showed similarly improved functional outcome within the 3- to 4.5-hour timeframe (NNT = 14). In all the stroke literature thus far, there has never been shown to be a mortality benefit for systemic administration of tPA in patients with suspected stroke. Recently, the PRISMS trial demonstrated that for patients with a National Institutes of Health Stroke Scale (NIHSS) <5, there was no benefit of tPA over aspirin alone.

35. The primary risk of tPA is systemic bleeding, particularly intracerebral hemorrhage (ICH). For the NINDS trial, ICH with tPA was 6.4% versus 0.6% for the non-treatment group, or a number needed to harm (NNH) of 17. For ECASS III, ICH occurred in 7.9% of the receiving tPA versus 3.5% in the placebo arm, absolute risk difference of 4.4% and NNH of 23. The SITS-ISTR has shown a similar rate of about 2% ICH in their extended time window of 4.5 hours since last normal. The factors that appear associated with increased risk of hemorrhage are older age, brain edema or mass effect on CT, and higher baseline stroke severity. Angioedema may occur in 1%–5% of patients.

36. The most common error in the management of meningitis is delaying administration of antibiotics until the lumbar puncture (LP) is done. If there is a clinical suspicion of bacterial meningitis, antibiotics should be administered promptly. Intravenous antibiotics given <2 hours before the LP (and ideally after blood and urine cultures are obtained) will not affect the results of the cerebrospinal fluid (CSF) analysis.

37. Compared with that of younger patients, elderly patients with acute abdominal pain have mortality rates that are six to eight times higher, with two times the surgery rates. Elderly patients have decreased pain perception and are more likely to have normal vital signs with significant intraabdominal pathology; 80% of older patients with a perforated ulcer do not have rigidity. In one study, 30% of older adults who had surgical abdominal pain did not show signs of either a fever or leukocytosis. These factors cause delays in diagnosis, higher perforation rates, and higher mortality rates in the elderly. Keep a broad differential diagnosis and consider the common disorders such as appendicitis and cholecystitis, but also diseases specific to older patients, such as diverticulitis, volvulus, mesenteric ischemia, abdominal aortic aneurysm, and carcinomas.

38. Children with simple febrile seizures should be evaluated and treated based on fever alone, because the concomitant presentation of the seizure does not increase the risk of serious bacterial illnesses above baseline.

39. There are several important differences between the adult and the pediatric airway that make airway problems more serious in children. The child's tongue is large and is the most common cause of airway obstruction in the obtunded child. The narrowest portion of the pediatric airway is at the cricoid ring, making obstruction with subglottic pathology more likely than in adults. The small size of the pediatric airway (approximately one-third the diameter of an adult's at birth) means that small changes in diameter cause significant increases in resistance. (Resistance is inversely related to the fourth power of the radius.) Higher oxygen consumption in children contributes to more rapid decrease in arterial oxygen levels after airway obstruction.

40. In children with croup, aerosolized epinephrine decreases airway obstruction. It is indicated for children with stridor at rest or increased work of breathing (e.g., tachypnea, retractions). Racemic epinephrine (0.5 mL of a 2.25% solution) is used most commonly, but L-epinephrine alone (5 mL of a 1:1000 solution to maximum of 5 mL) is equivalent. Maximal effect is seen within 30 minutes, with potential to return to increased work of breathing and stridor at rest within 3 hours. Patients with unlabored breathing and without resting stridor after 3 hours can be safely discharged home.

41. In children, maintenance fluids per hour are calculated based on weight in kilograms using the 4-2-1 rule: 4 mL/kg for the first 1–10 kg, an additional 2 mL/kg for the next 11–20 kg, and 1 mL/kg for every additional kg. For example, a 32-kg child should receive (4 mL/kg × 10 kg) + (2 mL/kg × 10 kg) + (1 mL/kg × 12 kg) = 72 mL/h of maintenance fluids.

42. Bilious emesis in a neonate could represent malrotation with midgut volvulus. Congenital malrotation of the midgut predisposes the bowel to twisting on itself, leading to bowel obstruction and vascular compromise, with bowel necrosis of the entire involved segment developing in as little as 2 hours. All neonates with bilious emesis, irrespective of their appearance, require emergent pediatric surgical consultation.

43. For a typical Kawasaki's disease diagnosis, in addition to having a fever for 5 days, children must display four of the five following features described by the CRASH mnemonic:
    - **C**onjunctivitis: bilateral, nonexudative, bulbar conjunctival injection
    - **R**ash: polymorphous, generalized rash
    - **A**denopathy: cervical node >1.5 cm
    - **S**trawberry tongue: pharyngeal erythema, or red and cracked lips
    - **H**ands and feet: erythema and swelling

44. The combination of a fever and petechiae in a child can arise with several emergent diseases, including meningococcemia, disseminated intravascular coagulation (DIC), Rocky Mountain spotted fever, pneumococcal bacteremia, or leukemia. A complete blood count (CBC), C-reactive protein (CRP), coagulation studies, and blood culture should be obtained on nearly all children with fever and petechiae. Well-appearing patients with normal laboratory values can be discharged with close follow-up. Children with a single petechial lesion or petechiae distributed only above the nipple after coughing or vomiting are less likely to have serious bacterial infections and do not require testing if they are well appearing.

45. Ketamine, a dissociative agent causing a trancelike cataleptic state, is a commonly used medication for pediatric procedural sedation and analgesia (PSA). It provides strong sedation, analgesia, and amnesia while maintaining cardiovascular stability and protective airway reflexes. Ketamine onset is within a few minutes IV and 5–10 minutes intramuscularly (IM). Ketamine can increase salivation; however, coadministration with an antisialagogue, such as atropine, is no longer recommended because it does not decrease adverse respiratory events. Recovery agitation or emergence phenomenon consisting of vivid dreams, hallucinations, or delirium may occur. Coadministration of midazolam has not been shown to reduce its occurrence, but can be used to treat severe emergence phenomenon that occurs in 1.4% of patients. These patients are typically older or have a history of psychiatric illness. Ondansetron has been shown to reduce recovery emesis associated with ketamine that occurs in approximately 8% of patients. Ketamine, although protective of airway reflexes, is associated with such airway or respiratory complications as oxygen desaturation or airway obstruction in 2.8%, transient apnea in 0.8%, and transient laryngospasm in 0.8%.

46. To determine ETT size in children between the ages of 1 and 8 years, the simple formula (age/4) + 4 can be used for uncuffed tube sizes, and (age/4) + 3.5 for cuffed tubes. More and more evidence suggests that cuffed tubes are preferred to prevent air leaks that can require risky tube changes and limit effective ventilation (particularly in children requiring high ventilator pressures). Cuff pressures must be checked with a manometer and should not exceed 20 cmH$_2$O, as even 30 minutes of higher pressures can lead to permanent airway injury.

47. The cricothyroid membrane is too small for an open cricothyrotomy in children under ~10 years old; needle cricothyrotomy is recommended for infants and children after failed endotracheal intubation, failed supraglottic airway placement, and ineffective bag-valve mask ventilation. This is a temporizing measure to provide some oxygenation while awaiting definitive operative intervention; ventilation is passive through the mouth, and not effectively provided through needle cricothyrotomy.

48. In neonatal resuscitation, compressions should be started if the heart rate is <60 bpm. The compressor should stand at the head of the warmer and the person delivering positive pressure ventilation (PPV) should stand to the side. Compressions should be delivered by encircling the baby's chest with the hands and placing thumbs side by side or on top of each other in the center of the sternum at the nipple line. Compress approximately one-third the anterior-posterior diameter of the chest at a rate of 90 compressions per minute. Coordinate compressions with ventilations by repeating out loud "one-and-two-and-three-and-breath." Allow recoil of the chest during the "ands." Increase the fraction of inspired oxygen (FiO$_2$) to 100% after the infant is intubated and compressions initiated. Recheck the heart rate using a cardiac monitor every 60 seconds, and stop compressions if the heart rate reaches 60 bpm. If the heart rate does not improve, prepare for umbilical vein catheter placement and epinephrine.

49. A prior history of suicide attempt is the single greatest predictive factor of suicide. Patients who continue to express suicidal ideation after an attempt are especially at risk for a subsequent attempt. Previous suicide attempts should always be inquired about, as these patients are 100 times more likely to die from suicide than the general public. The risk of completed suicide is much higher in the first year after an attempt, particularly for people >45 years of age.

50. If a patient has an afferent pupillary defect (APD; Marcus Gunn pupil), it confirms damage to the retina or optic nerve. To perform the swinging flashlight test, shine a light toward the normal eye, and after several seconds swing it to the other eye. After a brief pupillary constriction in the abnormal eye, the redilation in response to light reflects afferent deprivation; this response may only be appreciated in a dark room.

51. In a patient on a ventilator with acutely worsening oxygenation or ventilation, first remove the patient from the ventilator and provide manual ventilation to the patient by using a bag ventilatory device. The **DOPE** mnemonic taught in pediatric life support can be helpful in remembering the remainder of the approach:
    - **D**isplacement. Confirm that the ETT is in the proper place by using some combination of auscultation, measurement of CO$_2$ exchange, radiography, and direct visualization.
    - **O**bstruction. Confirm that the ETT is patent by passing a suction catheter down the lumen. Sometimes an ETT can become kinked simply as a result of patient positioning.
    - **P**atient. Consider various causes within the patient. First and foremost is the possibility of secretions obstructing large bronchi. Vigorous suctioning may remedy this situation. Next, consider pneumothorax. Confirm that there is no evidence of barotrauma, usually by a combination of physical examination and a chest radiograph.
    - **E**quipment. Confirm that the ventilator circuit and ventilator itself are functioning properly.

52. Massive transfusion is defined as the transfusion of 10 units of red cells in 24 hours or more than three units over an hour in a patient with ongoing blood loss. A massive transfusion protocol (MTP) is the delivery of a prespecified ratio of blood and blood products (platelets and fresh frozen plasma). Blood that is universally compatible is Type O (Rh− should be reserved for childbearing-aged females; otherwise, use Rh+). Blood should be transfused in a 1:1:1 ratio (1 unit of blood, 1 unit of platelets, and 1 unit of fresh frozen plasma, infused at the same time if possible). In practice, a cooler for trauma may contain six units of packed red blood cells (PRBCs), 4–6 units of thawed plasma, and six units of pooled platelets, or one apheresis unit. Tranexamic acid (TXA) is an antifibrinolytic agent often transfused with MTP, as it may decrease mortality when given within 3 hours of injury. MTP is activated, based on obvious severe hemorrhage, or a combination of factors that predict the need for significant blood transfusion. While clinical judgment may be used, objective scoring systems may be best to activate the protocol. The ABC scale is a scoring system that gives points for penetrating mechanism, hypotension, tachycardia, and a positive focused assessment with sonography for trauma (FAST). Scoring ≥2 predicts increasing likelihood to require the protocol. Using the shock index (HR/SBP) ≥1 is also common.

53. Cardiovascular collapse may occur during intubation in patients that are elderly, hypotensive, or hemorrhaging. In these high-risk patients, consider lower dose induction agents, ketamine instead of opioids or etomidate, blood prior to intubation (when safe), and push-dose peri-intubation pressors.

54. If a patient sustains trauma to the orbit resulting in a retrobulbar hematoma, the buildup of pressure behind the globe can lead to ischemia of the optic nerve and retina, and permanent blindness

in as little as 90 minutes after injury. The ocular compartment syndrome can present as proptosis, impaired extraocular movement, decreased vision, and increased intraocular pressure; retrobulbar hematoma can by confirmed by CT scan. In order to prevent optic nerve or retinal ischemia, a lateral canthotomy is performed by incising the lateral canthal ligaments of the orbit to relieve intraocular pressure, in conjunction with emergent ophthalmology consultation.

55. Blunt cerebrovascular injury (BCVI) to the carotid or vertebral artery is found in nearly 0.5% of all blunt craniomaxillary facial trauma patients, and may cause significant morbidity if left untreated. These injuries may initially be silent, without focal neurologic deficits noted. Computed tomography angiography (CTA) should be performed in patients suspected of having a BCVI based on signs or symptoms, or focal neurologic deficits. High-risk patients that should be screened include those with a Le Fort II or III fractures, mandibular fractures, certain cervical spine fracture patterns (subluxation, fractures extending into the transverse foramen, vertebral body fractures of C1, C2, or C3), basilar skull fracture with carotid canal involvement, traumatic brain injury with Glasgow Coma Scale (GCS) scores <6, near-hangings with anoxic brain injury, or seat belt sign of the neck.

56. All patients with nasal trauma and suspicion of a nasal fracture require inspection of the nasal septum for a septal hematoma. This is a collection of blood between the mucoperichondrium and the cartilage of the septum. It appears as a grapelike swelling over the nasal septum. If left undrained, it may result in septal abscess, necrosis of the nasal cartilage, and permanent saddle nose deformity. If a septal hematoma is identified, incision and drainage, with suction and irrigation, is indicated in the ED. This is followed by nasal packing (similar to epistaxis), antistaphylococcal antibiotics (prophylaxis for toxic shock syndrome), and urgent follow-up.

57. Alkali burns (fertilizers, drain cleaners, airbag propellants, cement and plaster components, and some detergents) are more dangerous than acid burns, quickly penetrating ocular tissues through liquefactive necrosis. Acid burns (car batteries, refrigerants, and pool cleaners) cause coagulation necrosis, with depth of penetration limited by eschar formation. Following irrigation, perform a slit lamp and fluorescein examination, evaluating for extent of corneal damage and perforation. If perforation is excluded, measure intraocular pressure, as pressures can spike following chemical injuries. Obtain emergent consultation for severe exposures (pH <2 or >12), severe injuries (corneal perforation or ischemia), or elevated intraocular pressure.

58. Entrapment of the inferior rectus muscle stimulates the oculocardiac reflex, vagal stimulation from ciliary ganglion via the trigeminal nerve, which can cause severe sinus bradycardia, heart block, hemodynamic collapse, asystole, and death. The reflex is exacerbated by strain on the entrapped inferior rectus muscle. Having the patient look down can relieve some of this stimulus. Atropine may be effective in cases of oculocardiac reflex–induced bradycardia. In severe cases, emergent operative intervention is indicated to release the entrapped muscle.

59. Any hemodynamically unstable patient with ongoing chest hemorrhage should be emergently taken to the operating room. In the hemodynamically stable patient having sustained blunt trauma, immediate drainage of 1500 mL of blood with ongoing bleeding is an indication for operative intervention. For penetrating trauma, surgical intervention is indicated after immediate drainage of 1000 mL of blood with ongoing bleeding. Finally, drainage greater than 200 mL/h of gross blood for more than 2 hours is an indication for exploration, mechanism of injury notwithstanding.

60. An ECG should be performed on any patient with suspected blunt cardiac injury (BCI). The most common ECG findings after BCI are sinus tachycardia or premature contractions. ECG alone does not rule out BCI. However, a normal ECG combined with a normal troponin has a negative predictive value of 100%. If an ECG shows a new dysrhythmia, new heart block, or ischemic changes, the patient should be admitted for continuous cardiac monitoring. Echocardiography (ECHO) should be performed on any symptomatic patient or any patient with any ischemic changes on ECG, new dysrhythmias, or hypotension.

61. Neurogenic shock occurs after cervical or high thoracic injuries cause impairment of sympathetic stimulation to the heart and peripheral vasculature. Signs and symptoms include vasodilatation resulting in flushing, warm extremities, hypotension, and bradycardia (i.e., absence of compensatory tachycardia). Neurogenic shock is treated with volume resuscitation and peripheral vasoconstrictors, such as dopamine or norepinephrine.

62. In pregnant patients with abdominal trauma, any viable (>23–24 weeks' gestation) fetus requires continuous electronic fetal monitoring (EFM). EFM is recommended even for patients without external evidence of trauma, because it has been well documented that these patients are at risk of placental abruption. Current guidelines suggest that these patients be observed for a minimum of 4 hours with a cardiotocograph. If any abnormalities are discovered, including contractions, amniotic membrane rupture, vaginal bleeding, serious maternal injury, significant abdominal pain, and concerning fetal HR variability, the patient should be hospitalized and monitored for 24 hours.

63. Children with neck pain, midline bony tenderness, decreased range of motion, torticollis, altered mental status (GCS score <14), focal neurologic abnormality, predisposing conditions, or transient spinal cord symptoms should have their cervical spine imaged. Plain radiographs (anteroposterior [AP], lateral, and odontoid views) are preferred for most patients. Patients with abnormal plain radiographs or concerning physical examination findings should undergo CT or MRI, and often require both.

64. Asymptomatic microscopic hematuria in adults is not a sensitive predictor of significant urologic injuries in patients with blunt trauma mechanisms, and the amount of blood in the urine does not correlate with the severity of injury. The relatively low incidence of positive studies requiring surgery does not justify an extensive radiographic evaluation. Repeat urinalysis is justified, with advanced imaging for persisting hematuria.

65. It is difficult to predict which burn patients will develop laryngeal edema and airway obstruction. Concerning history includes an enclosed space burn. Additionally, there is an increased risk with larger burns, typically greater than 40%. Physical examination findings suggestive of airway injury include soot around the mouth or nares, hoarseness or stridor, facial burns, or carbonaceous sputum. Since not all patients with carbonaceous sputum, oral or nasal soot, and/or facial burns have significant inhalation injury, clinical judgment must be used to decide on the need for intubation. Stridor, increased work of breathing, and hypoxemia are more reliable indicators of significant inhalational injury. However, decreased oxygen saturation occurs late in patients with significant airway injury. Patients who present with facial burns from smoking on oxygen have a low risk of significant inhalation injury, and normally have a baseline oxygen requirement.

66. To transport amputated body parts:
    - Remove gross contamination with saline irrigation.
    - Wrap the part in a saline-moistened (not soaked) sterile gauze.
    - Place the wrapped part into a sealed plastic bag or container.
    - Place the bag or container into an ice water bath.
    - Never put the amputated part directly onto ice or immerse it in disinfection solution.

67. The ankle-brachial index (ABI) is calculated by dividing the Doppler systolic arterial pressure measured in the injured leg by the pressure measured in an uninjured arm. An ABI value >0.9 is considered normal. The ABI measurement may be inaccurate in patients with risk factors for peripheral arterial disease, such as diabetes and hypertension. Vessel calcification in the elderly can also increase the risk of a false-positive result. An ABI <0.9 should trigger further diagnostic workup or surgical exploration in the operating room.

68. Fractures involving the physeal zone may result in growth disturbance, and parents must be informed accordingly. About 80% of these injuries are Salter-Harris types I and II, both of which have a low complication rate. Salter-Harris types III, IV, and V injuries have a worse prognosis. Displaced Salter-Harris types III and IV fractures may require open reduction to restore the normal anatomic physeal relationship. The five types of fracture according to the Salter-Harris classification are (Fig. 93.5):
    - Type I: physeal separation; this may appear as a widening of the radiolucent area representing the growth plate.
    - Type II: fracture traverses the physis and exits on the metaphyseal side.
    - Type III: fracture traverses the physis and exits on the epiphyseal side.
    - Type IV: fracture traverses through epiphysis, physis, and metaphysis.
    - Type V: physeal crush injury; this may be difficult to determine on plain radiographs.

69. The tumor lysis syndrome (TLS) is characterized by hyperkalemia, hyperphosphatemia, hypocalcemia, and hyperuricemia. TLS is commonly seen in cancer patients with a large tumor burden,

such as leukemia or lymphoma. Additional risk factors include baseline kidney injury and dehydration. Although it can occur spontaneously, it is more common in the week following treatment. Treatment is targeted at reversing metabolic abnormalities. Those with significant kidney injury may require dialysis.

70. The pulmonary embolism rule-out criteria (PERC) is used in patients with a low gestalt clinical suspicion for pulmonary embolus (PE). If all criteria are met, the patient has a less than 2% risk of PE, and further workup is not indicated. Patients with clinical suspicion who do not meet all criteria may require further evaluation. In patients with moderate or high clinical suspicion for PE, the PERC rule does not exclude PE.

71. D-dimer, a degradation product of cross-linked fibrin, is found in increased levels of the circulation of patients with acute venous thromboembolism (VTE). There are different assays available for measuring D-dimer with different sensitivities and specificities, including enzyme-linked immunosorbent assay (ELISA), rapid ELISA, turbidimetric assay and whole-blood agglutination D-dimer assay. Different tests can report results as either fibrin equivalent units or D-dimer units. Older latex agglutination tests cannot be used in these algorithms because of poor negative predictive values. Although useful in ruling out VTE disease in select populations, owing to a lack of specificity, D-dimer has not proven useful at ruling in the diagnosis.

72. In patients older than 50 years, with low to low-moderate pretest probability for VTE, PE can be ruled out with an age-adjusted D-dimer. For D-dimer assays using fibrin equivalent units, use a cut-off of age $\times$ 10 µg/L. For assays using D-dimer units, use age $\times$ 5 µg/L.

73. Platelet transfusion should be delayed in idiopathic thrombocytopenic purpura (ITP) and thrombotic thrombocytopenic purpura (TTP) to avoid disease-specific complications and alloimmunization. It is more commonly indicated for primary bone marrow problems. Each bag of random donor platelets raises the platelet count ~5000/mL. They are usually ordered six at a time.
   • Platelet count >50,000/mL – hemorrhage unlikely.
   • Platelet count 10,000–50,000/mL – variable risk of bleeding with trauma, ulcer, and invasive procedures. Choosing when to transfuse at these levels is not an exact science.
   • Platelet count <10,000 – platelet transfusion is indicated because there is a significant risk of spontaneous hemorrhage.

74. Incomplete cord syndromes are as follows:
   • Anterior cord syndrome results in loss of function in the anterior two-thirds of the spinal cord from damage to the corticospinal and spinothalamic pathways. Findings include loss of voluntary motor function as well as pain and temperature sensation below the level of the injury, with preservation of the posterior column functions of proprioception, pressure, and vibration. The key issue is the potential reversibility of this lesion if a compressing hematoma or disk fragment can be removed. This condition requires immediate neurosurgical evaluation.
   • Central cord syndrome results from injury to the central portion of the spinal cord. Because more proximal innervation is placed centrally within the cord, this lesion results in greater involvement of the upper extremities than of the lower extremities. Bowel or bladder control is usually preserved. The mechanism of injury is hyperextension of a cervical spine with a cord space narrowed by congenital variation, degenerative spurring, or hypertrophic ligaments. This syndrome can occur without actual fracture or ligamentous disruption.
   • Brown-Séquard syndrome is an injury to a hemisection of the spinal cord, usually from penetrating trauma. Contralateral sensation of pain and temperature is lost, and motor and posterior column functions are absent on the side of the injury.
   • Cauda equina syndrome is an injury to the lumbar, sacral, and coccygeal nerve roots, causing a peripheral nerve injury. There can be motor and sensory loss in the lower extremities, bowel and bladder dysfunction, and loss of pain sensation at the perineum (saddle anesthesia).

75. Typical synovial fluid counts in septic arthritis are >50,000 white blood cells (WBCs)/mm³, with predominantly polymorphonuclear neutrophilic (PMN) WBCs, and a Gram stain positive for bacteria. However, some patients with septic arthritis have synovial fluid counts <50,000 cells/mm³, particularly those with prosthetic joints. Synovial fluid lactate levels >10 mmol/L are highly suggestive of septic arthritis, whereas levels lactate levels <4.3 mmol/L make septic arthritis very unlikely.

76. The rash of erythema multiforme is morbilliform and usually on the palms and soles, resulting from viral/bacterial infections or medications. Erythema migrans is a bull's-eye rash that usually expands (rather than migrates), and is a common manifestation of early Lyme disease. Erythema marginatum, part of the Jones' criteria for diagnosis of rheumatic fever, is an evanescent, nonpruritic rash that typically involves the trunk and extremities while sparing the face. Erythema nodosum (EN) is an acute inflammatory reaction leading to appearance of red, painful, tender nodules on the lower legs; etiologies are diverse and often idiopathic.

77. The mainstay of therapy for nerve agents is atropine, combined with decontamination, pralidoxime, and benzodiazepines (for seizure).

78. The most appropriate course of action for a patient with both a radiation exposure and associated major trauma or medical issues is to care for life-threatening trauma or medical problems first; these life threats always take precedence over management of the radiologic exposure.

79. Infection causes the vast majority of fevers, but the following other causes are included in the differential diagnosis:
    - Neoplastic diseases (e.g., leukemia, lymphoma, or solid tumors)
    - Autoimmune disease (e.g., giant cell arteritis, polyarteritis nodosa, systemic lupus erythematosus, or rheumatoid arthritis)
    - Endocrine disorders (e.g., thyroid storm)
    - CNS lesions (e.g., stroke, intracranial bleed, or trauma)
    - Illicit drug use (e.g., cocaine, 3,4-methylenedioxymethamphetamine [MDMA, ecstasy], or other methamphetamines)
    - Withdrawal syndromes (e.g., delirium tremens or benzodiazepine withdrawal)

80. Life-threatening causes of acute chest pain include:
    - Acute coronary syndrome (ACS; unstable angina and myocardial infarction)
    - Pulmonary embolism (PE)
    - Pneumothorax
    - Aortic dissection
    - Pericarditis
    - Myocarditis
    - Cardiac tamponade
    - Mediastinitis/esophageal rupture
    - Trauma

81. The American College of Cardiology Foundation/American Heart Association (ACCF/AHA) guidelines suggest that the most important factor in predicting acute coronary syndrome in a patient with chest pain is the history of present illness, rather than cardiac risk. Classic risk factors for cardiac ischemia have had very limited utility in the ED setting when trying to determine the immediate risk of ACS. Nevertheless, various clinical decision rules have been developed to generate a risk profile for coronary ischemia in patients presenting with chest pain. The **HEART** score is perhaps the most useful to date: **H**istory, **E**CG, **A**ge, **R**isk factors, and **T**roponin. The low-risk cohort was associated with 0.99% risk of an adverse cardiac event in a retrospective study and 1.7% in a prospective study. When combined with a repeat troponin 3 hours later to form the HEART pathway, the HEART score can identify patients in a low-risk cohort who may be safely discharged with outpatient follow-up. Clinical decision rules are no substitute for physician judgment. Clinical gestalt can help identify cases that would otherwise be missed by clinical decision rules.

82. Factors associated with failure to diagnose acute myocardial infarction (MI) (1%–2% of ED chest pain patients) include:
    - Young age group
    - Non-White race
    - Failure to obtain an accurate history
    - Incorrect interpretation of the ECG
    - Failure to recognize atypical presentations
    - Hesitance to admit patients with vague symptoms
    - Reliance on laboratory assays, such as cardiac enzymes
    - Insufficient experience or training

83. Improvement in headache with sumatriptan or ketorolac does not mean that the diagnosis is migraine. Because the final common pathway for most pain in the head is limited, and vasogenic inflammation probably plays a role, the response to any analgesic or antimigraine medication is of no etiologic significance. This includes triptans, which have been documented to improve the headaches of patients with SAH and cervical artery dissections.

84. Cardiac causes of syncope comprise the riskiest group of patients and include ACS, PE, physical aortic outflow obstructions (e.g., hypertrophic obstructive cardiomyopathy (HOCUM), aortic steno-sis, or atrial myxoma), slow rhythms such as sick sinus syndrome, and tachyarrhythmias. Brugada syndrome, preexcitation, arrythmogenic right ventricular dysplasia (ARVD), and long QT syndrome can precipitate lethal dysrhythmias.

85. Suspect necrotizing fasciitis in patients with severe pain and tenderness that is out of proportion to the degree of visible cellulitis. Feel for crepitus, sometimes also appreciated on plain radiographs. Outline the area of visible infection to monitor for rapidly expanding signs of infection. CT or MRI can help evaluate the extent of the disease. Patients may appear septic, but this can occur later in the course of the disease.

86. Involvement of at least two of the following are needed to diagnose anaphylaxis:
    - Cutaneous manifestations (urticaria or rash)
    - Mucous membrane involvement (angioedema)
    - Upper respiratory tract involvement (edema and hypersecretion)
    - Lower respiratory tract involvement (bronchoconstriction)
    - GI symptoms (nausea, vomiting, or abdominal cramping)
    - Cardiovascular system effects (tachycardia, hypotension, and cardiovascular collapse)
    Hypotension in a patient who is exposed to a known allergen is adequate to make the diagnosis of anaphylaxis.

87. Initial treatment for life-threatening anaphylaxis includes:
    - Upper airway obstruction with stridor and edema is treated with high-flow nebulized oxygen, racemic epinephrine, and IV epinephrine. If airway obstruction is severe or increases, perform endotracheal intubation or cricothyroidotomy.
    - Acute bronchospasm is treated with epinephrine. Mild to moderate wheezing in patients with normal blood pressure may be treated with 0.01 mg/kg of 1:1000 epinephrine administered IM. If the patient is in severe respiratory distress or has a silent chest, administer IV epinephrine via a drip infusion: 1 mg of epinephrine in 250 mL of dextrose 5% in water (D5W) at an initial rate of 1 µg/min, with titration to desired effect. Bronchospasm refractory to epinephrine may respond to a nebulized β-agonist, such as albuterol or metaproterenol.
    - Cardiovascular collapse presenting with hypotension is treated with a constant infusion of epi-nephrine, titrating the rate to attain a systolic blood pressure of 100 mmHg or mean arterial pressure of 80 mmHg.
    - For patients in full cardiac arrest, administer 1:10,000 epinephrine, 1 mg slow IV push, or 2.0–2.5 mg epinephrine diluted in 10 mL NS via an ETT. Immediate endotracheal intubation or cricothyroidotomy should be performed as needed to secure the airway.

88. While early goal-directed therapy (EGDT) as a protocol-driven strategy is no longer recommended by the Surviving Sepsis Campaign guidelines, the general principles still apply. For example, multiple studies have shown an association between early antibiotics and improved outcomes. However, it is essential to note that source control often requires more than just appropriate anti-microbial coverage, and may require procedural intervention in some cases. Other studies have shown an association of adherence to the 3-hour sepsis "bundle" with improved outcomes.

89. Sepsis is now defined as a life-threatening organ dysfunction caused by a dysregulated host response to infection. There are two working definitions for the diagnosis of sepsis in clinical use. The first, and older definition, is the combination of SIRS criteria with suspicion for an infectious source. The second, recommended by the Surviving Sepsis Campaign, and published in 2016, is two out of the three qSOFA (quick sequential organ failure assessment) criteria (see Chapter 50).

90. Empiric antibiotics should NOT be used in well-appearing immunocompetent patients with infec-tious diarrhea. The treatment of certain bacterial pathogens with antibiotics may decrease duration

of symptoms by one day. However, the benefits are typically outweighed by risk of increasing antibiotic resistance and risk of hemolytic-uremic syndrome (HUS) with antibiotic-induced lysis of Shiga toxin–producing *Escherichia coli* (STEC)-releasing endotoxins. Empiric antibiotics may be considered in the following patient populations:
- Infants <3 months old with suspected bacterial source.
- Ill-appearing patients with dysentery.
- Patients who have travelled internationally with fever or sepsis.

Antimicrobial choice: First-line treatment is a single oral dose of ciprofloxacin 2 g or 3-day regimen of ciprofloxacin 500 mg twice daily. Alternative regimen (for children and pregnant women) is azithromycin 1 g (5–10 mg/kg) orally, as a single dose. In areas where amebiasis and giardiasis are endemic, consider metronidazole 500–750 mg orally three times daily for 10 days for amebiasis or 250 mg orally three times daily for 5 days for giardiasis (Fig. 53.1).

91. For treatment of acute pulmonary edema, follow the ABCs (airway, breathing, and circulation). In severe hypoxia, airway and breathing may be compromised, requiring intubation. The use of noninvasive mask continuous or bilevel positive airway pressure (CPAP/BiPAP) has decreased the need for intubation in patients with pulmonary edema; however, this has not significantly affected in-hospital mortality. Intubation may also be avoided with prompt medical treatment (see later). Patient symptoms can be dynamic, requiring frequent reevaluations for further medical management. Administer oxygen to maintain sufficient oxygen saturation (>90%), either by nasal cannula or nonrebreather mask, CPAP, or BiPAP. Continuously monitor oxygen saturation with pulse oximetry.

92. Drug therapy for acute pulmonary edema is aimed at decreasing preload. Nitrates are first-line drugs and are useful in the form of sublingual nitroglycerin (NTG) or an IV NTG drip. NTG is predominantly a venodilator, reducing preload. However, NTG also dilates coronary arteries, and may be especially helpful in the setting of coronary artery disease. Diuretics should only be administered to patients with signs of obvious fluid overload (e.g., peripheral edema, elevated jugular venous distention). When indicated, furosemide is given as a 40-mg IV bolus (larger amounts if the patient is already taking diuretic medication, although high-dose diuretics are associated with worse outcomes). Initially, within 5–15 minutes of the injection, venodilation occurs, although this is of limited clinical benefit in the setting of nitrates. This action is followed within 30 minutes by diuresis.

93. The most common presenting symptom in patients with acute ischemic heart disease is chest pain. Typically, ischemic pain is described as heaviness, pressure, tightness, or squeezing. It is less commonly described as sharp or aching. Usually the pain lasts minutes, as opposed to seconds or hours. Patients may describe their pain as indigestion, which can lead to the misdiagnosis of reflux esophagitis. Although precordial discomfort is most common, it may be felt anywhere on the chest, the right or left shoulder or arm, the throat or jaw, or the upper abdomen. The pain often radiates to one of these locations as well. Less commonly, patients may simply have pain in other more unusual locations (e.g., left ear or upper back). Associated symptoms include dyspnea, nausea, vomiting, diaphoresis, lightheadedness or syncope, palpitations, or malaise. Diaphoresis and vomiting, in particular, increase the likelihood of ACS. One-third of patients may not experience pain and just present with associated symptoms – in this case, it is termed an anginal equivalent or atypical angina. The most common symptom is shortness of breath. This is more common in the elderly, women, and patients with diabetes.

94. ST elevation caused by infarction may display one or more of the following:
- *Morphology.* Convex upward ST elevation ("tombstone" morphology) is highly predictive of injury. However, the morphology may also be concave upward or horizontal.
- *Reciprocal changes.* The presence of ST depression in another area of the ECG is highly predictive of injury, but is not always present.
- ST elevation caused by injury is dynamic; serial ECGs usually show changes over time.

95. Hypertensive emergency is characterized by severely elevated blood pressure (BP; typically >220/120 mmHg) with acute end-organ (brain, heart, kidneys) damage. The absolute BP is not a criterion. The terms "malignant hypertension (HTN)" and "accelerated HTN" are used in the International Classification of Diseases, 10th edition (ICD-10). Examples include:
- Hypertensive encephalopathy
- Ischemic and hemorrhagic stroke

- Subarachnoid hemorrhage (SAH)
- Acute myocardial infarction (AMI)
- Decompensated congestive heart failure (CHF) with pulmonary edema
- Aortic dissection
- Preeclampsia/eclampsia
- Acute kidney injury (AKI): a controversial topic that requires special consideration, as isolated elevations in creatinine may reflect chronic kidney disease (CKD) rather than an acute process.

96. Most patients with abdominal aortic aneurysms (AAAs) are asymptomatic, and the aneurysm is found incidentally. Patients with symptoms of acutely expanding AAA may have gradually increasing abdominal pain, low back pain, or flank pain radiating to the groin. It is often described as dull, throbbing, or colicky.
    - 3% of men >50 years old have an occult AAA.
    - 75% of aneurysms are >5 cm and can be palpated.
    - 5%–10% of patients with an AAA have an abdominal bruit.

97. Patients with thoracic aortic dissections experience a sudden onset (85%) of severe chest pain with radiation to the jaw, neck, or back in the intrascapular region. Clinical patterns include:
    - Pain is most severe at onset and is often described as sharp, ripping, or tearing in quality.
    - Pain starts in one region and moves to another (abdomen to chest or chest to abdomen).
    - The patient may have nausea, vomiting, diaphoresis, lightheadedness, and apprehension or a sense of impending doom.
    - Syncope can also be the presenting complaint, and in some cases may be the only symptom.
    - Proximal dissections may cause aortic regurgitation and pericardial effusion with tamponade (16%).
    - Occlusion of aortic branches may cause AMI (coronary artery involvement); stroke (carotid or vertebral artery involvement); or paresthesias and arm pain (subclavian artery involvement), which may be suggested by unequal BPs or pulses.
    - Spinal artery occlusion can cause neurologic compromise.
    - Hoarseness may result from recurrent laryngeal nerve compression.
    - Chest pain unrelieved by large doses of narcotic analgesics should raise the concern for this diagnosis.

98. In general, if the patient is hemodynamically unstable, a specific dysrhythmia does not usually need to be diagnosed prior to treatment. In the unstable patient with a dysrhythmia, a general rule of thumb is to provide electricity (perform electrical cardioversion) if the heart rate is fast, and if the heart rate is slow, pace the patient with a pacemaker.

99. Differentiate ventricular tachycardia (VT) from supraventricular tachycardia (SVT) with aberrancy based on findings on the 12-lead ECG. In unstable patients, assume that the rhythm is VT and treat accordingly whenever there is any question. Treating SVT with aberrancy as if it were VT is less problematic than treating VT as if it were SVT with aberrancy. Any of these findings on the 12-lead ECG strongly suggest VT:
    - Atrioventricular (AV) dissociation
    - Fusion or capture beats
    - Left- or right-axis deviation
    - QRS width of >140 msec
    - Concordance of QRS complexes
    - Monophasic or biphasic QRS in lead V1
    - RS or QS in lead V6
    - History of coronary artery disease or CHF
    - Evidence of AV dissociation on physical examination (cannon A waves)

100. A job won't make you happy. You can find someone miserable and someone joyful in any profession. Be kind, listen with intention, work hard toward something meaningful, stay curious, respect wisdom, be humble, laugh often, and love easily. Emergency medicine affords us the unique opportunity to share in patients' most profound moments, teaching us that, in the end, happiness is more about gratitude and human connection. Relish the privilege.

DECISION MAKING IN EMERGENCY MEDICINE

Nadia Markovchick Dearstyne, MD and Vincent J. Markovchick, MD, FAAEM

1. **Is there anything unique about emergency medicine?**
   Although there is significant crossover between emergency medicine and all other clinical specialties, emergency medicine approaches to patient care and the decision-making processes are unique. Emergency medicine physicians must be knowledgeable about all aspects of medical care, with an emphasis on identifying and treating acute life threats.

2. **Describe the conventional method of evaluating a patient.**
   A comprehensive history, physical examination including vital signs, routine laboratory diagnostic studies, special diagnostic procedures, and the formulation of a problem-oriented medical record and rational course of therapy constitute the ideal approach to patient care, because it is so comprehensive.

3. **Why is the conventional methodology not ideal for use in the ED?**
   Even though in retrospect only 10% to 20% of patients presenting to an ED truly have emergent problems, it must be presumed that every patient who comes to an ED has an emergent condition. Therefore the first and most important question that must be answered is, "What is the life threat?" The conventional approach does not ensure an expeditious answer to this question. Time constraints, multitasking, and limited resources also impede the use of conventional methodology in the ED.

4. **How do I identify the patient with a life-threatening condition?**
   Three components are necessary to quickly identify the patient with a life-threatening condition:
   1. A chief complaint and a brief, focused history relevant to the chief complaint
   2. A complete and accurate set of vital signs in the field and in the ED
   3. A rapid, focused physical examination that includes visualization, auscultation, palpation, and observation

5. **What is so important about the chief complaint?**
   The chief complaint, which sometimes cannot be obtained directly from the patient but must be obtained from family members, observers, emergency medical technicians (EMTs), or others at the scene, will immediately help categorize the general type of problem (e.g., cardiac, traumatic, respiratory, or psychiatric).

6. **Why are vital signs important?**
   Vital signs are the most reliable objective data that are immediately available to ED personnel, provided they are accurately taken and critically interpreted. Vital signs and the chief complaint, when used as triage tools, will identify the majority of patients with life-threatening conditions. Familiarity with normal vital signs for all age groups is essential.

7. **What are the determinants of (normal) vital signs?**
   Age, underlying physical condition, medical problems (e.g., hypertension), and current medications (e.g., β-blockers) are important considerations in determining normal vital signs for a given patient. For example, a well-conditioned, young athlete who has just sustained major trauma and arrives with a resting supine pulse of 80 beats per minute may have significant blood loss because the normal pulse is probably in the range of 40 to 50 beats per minute.

8. **What is the most inaccurate vital sign taken in the field and ED?**
   In the field the most common inaccurate vital sign is the respiratory rate, because it is sometimes estimated rather than counted. In the ED, the temperature may be inaccurate if a temporal or tympanic thermometer was used or if the patient was hyperventilating or mouth breathing when the oral temperature was taken. When either fever or hypothermia is suspected, measure a rectal temperature.

9. **Why do I need to compare field vital signs with ED vital signs?**
   Most prehospital care systems with a level of care beyond basic transport also provide therapy to patients. Because this therapy usually makes positive changes in the patient's condition, the patient may look deceptively well on arrival in the ED. For example, a 20-year-old woman is found in the field with acute onset of left lower quadrant abdominal pain. She is cool, clammy and diaphoretic, with a pulse of 116 beats per minute and blood pressure of 78 palpable. She receives 1000 mL of intravenous (IV) fluid on route to the ED. She may arrive with

normal vital signs and no skin changes. If one does not read and pay attention to the EMT's description of the patient and the initial vital signs, the presumption may be made that this is a stable patient.

10. **When are normal vital signs abnormal?**
This is when the vital signs, although in the normal range, are inconsistent with the patient's chief complaint and overall clinical appearance. For example, a 20-year old man with severe asthma who presents with hours of dyspnea and poor air movement may have a "normal" respiratory rate of 14 breaths per minute. For this patient one would expect a respiratory rate of 20 to 30 breaths per minute, and thus a respiratory rate of 14 is abnormal, indicating fatigue and impending respiratory failure. This is a classic example of when "normal" is abnormal.

11. **Why do I need to visualize, auscultate, and touch the patient?**
In many instances these measures help to identify the life threat (e.g., Is it the upper airway, lower airway, or circulation?). Touching the skin is important to determine whether shock is associated with vasoconstriction (i.e., hypovolemic or cardiogenic) or with vasodilatation (i.e., septic, neurogenic, or anaphylactic). Auscultation will identify life threats associated with the lower airway (e.g., bronchoconstriction, tension pneumothorax).

12. **Once I have identified the life threat, what do I do?**
Stop immediately and intervene to reverse the life threat. For example, if the initial encounter with the patient identifies upper-airway obstruction, take whatever measures are necessary to alleviate upper-airway obstruction such as suctioning, positioning, or intubating the patient. If the problem is hemorrhage, volume restoration and hemorrhage control are indicated.

13. **I have identified and stabilized or ruled out an immediate life threat in the patient. What else is unique about the approach to this patient in the ED?**
The differential diagnosis formulated in the ED must begin with the most serious condition possible to explain the patient's presenting symptoms and be continued from there. An example is a 60-year-old man who exhibits nausea, vomiting, and epigastric pain. Instead of assuming the condition is caused by a gastrointestinal disorder, an acute myocardial infarction (MI) must first be considered and appropriate steps must be taken to stabilize the patient (i.e., start an IV, initiate oxygen [O_2], and place a cardiac monitor). Then, rule out an MI, aortic dissection, or surgical or other acute abdominal pathology, by completing an adequate history and physical examination, an electrocardiogram (ECG), and appropriate laboratory studies.

14. **Why does formulating a differential diagnosis sometimes lead to problems?**
The natural tendency in formulating a differential diagnosis is to think of the most common or statistically most probable condition to explain the patient's initial presentation. This approach may overlook the most serious, albeit sometimes a very uncommon, problem. Therefore the practice of emergency medicine involves some degree of healthy paranoia to consider the most serious conditions compatible with the patient's presenting symptoms. Through a logical process of elimination, first rule in or out the life threats before gravitating to the more likely diagnoses.

15. **Is a diagnosis always possible or necessary in the ED?**
No. Patients should be informed of goals in the ED. Sometimes, the most important thing is to know that they don't have a life-threatening condition. It may take days, weeks, or months for a final diagnosis to be made. It is unreasonable to expect that every patient should or must have a diagnosis made in the ED.

16. **If I cannot make the diagnosis, what do I do?**
It is the role of the ED physician to rule out and stabilize serious or life-threatening conditions, not to always arrive at a definitive diagnosis. For example, a patient who comes to the ED with abdominal pain; who has had an appropriate history, physical examination, and diagnostic studies; and who in your best judgment does not have a life-threatening or acute surgical problem should be so informed. The discharge diagnosis would be abdominal pain of unknown etiology. This avoids the trap of labeling the patient with a benign diagnosis such as gastroenteritis or gastritis that is not supported by the medical record. More important, it avoids giving the patient the impression that there is a totally benign process occurring and will help to avoid the medical (and legal) problem of the patient returning 1 or 2 days later with something more serious, such as a ruptured appendix.

17. **What is the most important question to ask a patient who comes to the ED with a chronic, persistent, or recurrent condition?**
"What's different now?" This question should be asked of all patients who have a chronic condition that has resulted in a visit to the ED. The classic example is migraine headache. The patient with a chronic, recurrent migraine headache who is not asked this question may on this occasion have had an acute subarachnoid bleed. Such a patient may not volunteer that this headache is different from the pattern of chronic migraines unless asked.

18. **How do I decide if the patient needs hospitalization?**
The medical condition is the first obvious factor to consider. Beyond this, ask yourself the following questions: Is there a medical need that can be fulfilled only by hospitalization, or can the patient be safely observed in the outpatient setting? For example, does the patient need oxygen therapy or cardiac monitoring? Can patients who

have sustained head trauma adhere to head trauma precautions, or do they require in-patient care because of homelessness or living alone? The patient's ability to pay for services should not determine disposition decisions.

19. **If the patient does not need admission, how do I arrange a satisfactory disposition?**
All patients should be instructed to follow up or return to the ED for new or worsening symptoms. Failure to do so constitutes patient abandonment. Specific verbal and written follow-up instructions should be given to all patients.

20. **What is the most important thing to document in the ED discharge instructions?**
All follow-up instructions must include specific mention of the most serious potential complications of the patient's condition. For example, a patient who is being discharged home with the diagnosis of a probable herniated L4-5 intervertebral disk should be instructed to return immediately if any bowel or bladder dysfunction develops. This takes into account the most serious complication of a herniated lumbar disk, which is a central midline disk herniation (i.e., cauda equina syndrome) with bowel or bladder dysfunction, an acute neurosurgical emergency.

21. **What three questions should always be asked (and answered) before a patient is discharged from the ED?**
    1. Why did the patient come to the ED?
    2. Have all specific concerns or fears been addressed?
    3. Have I made the patient feel better?
Generally, most patients come to the ED because of pain, somatic or psychological, and a reasonable expectation is that this pain will be acknowledged and appropriately treated. If such pain cannot be alleviated, a thorough explanation should be given to the patient regarding the reasons why analgesics cannot be provided. Reassurance is sometimes all that is needed to relieve anxiety about serious medical conditions.

22. **Why is the previous question and answer one of the most important in this chapter?**
Attention to treating and alleviating a patient's pain will dramatically reduce subsequent complaints concerning care in the ED and remove one of the significant risk factors for initiation of a malpractice suit. It may also decrease the likelihood of an unnecessary return visit to the ED. It is also how you would want to be treated.

23. **What about the chart?**
The chart must reflect the answers to the preceding questions in this chapter. It need not list the entire differential diagnosis, but one should be able to ascertain from reading the chart that the more serious diagnoses were indeed considered. It also must contain appropriate follow-up instructions.

24. **What role do clinical decision rules have in decision making in the ED?**
Evidence-based clinical decision rules (such as pulmonary embolism rule-out criteria [PERC]) should be followed unless specific circumstance makes deviation from the rule in the best interest of the patient. In such cases, document the reasoning for deviation.

25. **What is the role of shared decision making in the ED?**
Shared decision making can be useful in a day and age of access to too much information via the Internet. It is important to get agreement from the patient as to their course of treatment. This can be accomplished by explaining the reasons that a particular study does or does not need to be done. The patient can then feel more comfortable with the decisions made.

KEY POINTS: DECISION MAKING IN EMERGENCY MEDICINE

1. Stabilize the patient before performing diagnostic procedures.
2. Always consider the most serious possible cause of the patient's signs and symptoms.
3. Always inquire about a patient's social situation before ED discharge.
4. Remember to focus on alleviating the patient's somatic or psychological pain.

BIBILIOGRAPHY

Hess EP, Grudzen CR, et al. Shared decision-making in the emergency department: respecting patient autonomy when seconds count. *Acad Emerg Med.* 2015;22(7):856–864. doi:10.1111/acem.12703.
Pines JM. Profiles in patient safety: confirmation bias in emergency medicine. *Acad Emerg Med.* 2006;13(1):90–94.
Zink BJ. The biology of emergency medicine: what have 30 years meant for Rosen's original concepts? *Acad Emerg Med.* 2011;18(3): 301–304. doi:10.1111/j.1553-2712.2011.01011.x.

CHAPTER 2

ADULT CARDIAC ARREST

Ryan Murphy, MD and Jason Haukoos, MD, MSc

1. **What is cardiac arrest and what is its incidence?**
   Cardiac arrest is defined by the triad of unconsciousness, apnea, and pulselessness.
   In 2017, incidence of EMS–assessed out-of-hospital cardiac arrest (OHCA) in people of any age was 111 per 100,000 population, based on extrapolation from the Resuscitation Outcomes Consortium.

2. **What are the most common causes of nontraumatic OHCA in adults?**
   The most common etiology of nontraumatic OHCA in adults is coronary heart disease (CHD). Other causes include respiratory failure, sepsis, circulatory obstruction, hypovolemia, electrolyte disturbances (most commonly hyperkalemia), drug toxicity, electrocution, and hypothermia.

3. **What are the four initial rhythms seen in cardiac arrest? Which is most common?**
   The four initial rhythms are ventricular fibrillation (VF), pulseless ventricular tachycardia (pVT), pulseless electrical activity (PEA), or asystole. These rhythms are generally categorized as shockable (VF, pVT) or nonshockable (PEA, asystole). As most arrests are initially unmonitored, the prevalence of each initial rhythm is unknown. The 2019 American Heart Association (AHA) Heart Disease Statistic Update reported that initial recorded cardiac rhythm was shockable in 19% of EMS-treated OHCAs in 2017. Underlying CHD accounts for the majority of VF arrests. PEA and asystole can be due to various underlying causes but is also commonly the result of prolonged or untreated VF/pVT.

4. **What are the "H's and T's" of treating cardiac arrest?**
   A mnemonic is used to remember reversible causes of cardiac arrest (especially in patients with initial rhythms of PEA or asystole). H's and T's: **h**ypovolemia, **h**ypoxia, **h**ydrogen ion (acidosis), **h**ypo/**h**yperkalemia, **h**ypothermia, **t**ension pneumothorax, **t**amponade, **t**oxins, **t**hrombosis (cardiac or pulmonary).

5. **Why are the ABCs of cardiac arrest better represented as CAB?**
   In 2010, the AHA recommended the basic life-support sequence for all *adult* patients experiencing cardiac arrest be changed from airway-breathing-chest compressions (ABC) to chest compressions, airway, and breathing (CAB). (See Chapter 69 for details related to management of pediatric cardiac arrest.) All rescuers (regardless of training) are recommended to initiate chest compressions before giving rescue breaths. In nontraumatic adult OHCA, oxygen delivery to the heart and brain during the *first few minutes* of cardiopulmonary resuscitation (CPR) is limited by blood flow, rather than by arterial oxygen content. This sequence change was recommended to prioritize the early initiation of chest compressions, which are often delayed when opening the airway and rescue breaths are prioritized.

6. **Is ventilation and oxygenation still important during adult CPR?**
   Yes, ventilation and oxygenation remains an essential component of adult CPR. While various ventilation and oxygenation strategies have been studied for many years, there is still incomplete evidence regarding optimal procedures: type of delivery used (i.e., passive oxygen insufflation, bag mask ventilation [BVM], advanced airway placement); timing of advanced airway placement in relation to other interventions; or type of advanced airway device used (supraglottic airway [SGA] vs. endotracheal tube [ETT]). What is known to improve survival in adults experiencing nontraumatic OHCA is early high-quality CPR (and, for VF/pVT, defibrillation). Therefore the tasks and timing of ventilation and oxygenation need to be integrated in a way that minimizes interruptions or quality of chest compressions.

7. **How should a healthcare provider perform cardiopulmonary resuscitation (CPR) on an adult as described by the AHA?**
   Simultaneously check for pulse (<10 seconds allowed for pulse check) while checking to see if patient is not breathing or having only agonal respirations.
   1. If the arrest occurs in the:
      a. out-of-hospital setting → call 911 (activate EMS)
      b. in-hospital setting → activate the hospital's cardiac arrest team
   2. Begin high-quality CPR for 2 minutes
      a. Chest compression technique guidelines for adults in ALL settings:
         i. compression rate = 100–120 compressions per minute
         ii. adequate depth of at least 2 inches (5 cm), while avoiding excessive compression depths >2.4 inches (6 cm)

      iii. allow full chest wall recoil (avoid leaning on chest between compressions)

      iv. minimize interruptions (goal of compression fraction, defined as the time performing compressions divided by total time, as high as possible, with a target of at least 60%)

    b. Ventilation guidelines:

      i. Prior to advanced airway:

        1. recommended compressions:ventilation ratio of 30:2 (via mouth-to-mouth/mouth-to-mask if lone rescuer, BVM if two or more trained rescuers present)

      ii. If advanced airway (SGA or ETT): one ventilation every 6 seconds (10 ventilations per minute) with continuous chest compressions

        1. ideal timing of advanced airway unclear, but it should NOT delay initial CPR and should not cause significant ($>$10 seconds) interruption in chest compressions

      iii. When supplementary oxygen is available, use the maximal feasible inspired oxygen concentration during CPR

  3. Use automatic external defibrillator (AED) as soon as ready and defibrillate if indicated (i.e., VF/pVT)

    a. If **lone rescuer** and AED is **not nearby or easily accessible**:

      i. begin cycle of 30 chest compressions and two breaths until help arrives, then have additional rescuer obtain AED

    b. if **lone rescuer** and AED is **nearby or easily accessible**:

      i. immediately obtain AED, attach defibrillator/monitor, then perform compressions/rescue breaths

    c. If two or more trained rescuers are present:

      i. one rescuer begins CPR while other rescuers obtain the AED and other emergency equipment

      ii. defibrillate as soon as ready, if indicated

  4. Obtain IV/intraosseous (IO) access, give epinephrine (1 mg IV/IO push every 3–5 minutes)

  5. Every 2 minutes, check rhythm/pulse (aim for a $<$10 second pause in compressions) and consider additional medications/advanced airway/capnography depending on suspected etiology of arrest.

8. Explain the mechanism of blood flow during CPR.

Two basic models explain the mechanism of blood flow during CPR. In the cardiac pump model, the heart is squeezed between the sternum and the spine. Chest compressions mimic systole, and the atrioventricular valves close normally, ensuring unidirectional, antegrade flow. During the relaxation phase (diastole), intracardiac pressures fall, the valves open, and blood is drawn into the heart from the lungs and vena cava. In the thoracic pump model, the heart is considered a passive conduit. Chest compressions result in uniformly increased pressures throughout the thorax. Forward blood flow is achieved selectively in the arterial system, because the stiff-walled arteries resist collapse and retrograde flow is prevented in the great veins by one-way valves. Chest recoil results in increased negative intrathoracic pressures, which improve ventricular filling and coronary blood flow. These mechanisms have been substantiated in animal models, and both likely contribute to blood flow during CPR.

9. Is blood flow to the brain and heart adequate during CPR?

Even when performed by experts, CPR provides only approximately 30% of normal blood flow to the brain and 10% to 20% of normal blood flow to the heart. Blood flow to the heart occurs during the relaxation phase of CPR, whereas blood flow to the brain occurs during the compression phase of CPR. This is the foundation for the AHA's recommended CPR "duty cycle" of 50% (the proportion of the compression/decompression cycle spent in compression).

10. What is coronary perfusion pressure (CPP)? What is the association between CPP, CPR, and return of spontaneous circulation (ROSC)?

CPP is defined as the aortic pressure minus the right atrial pressure during diastole.

    Better CPR produces better CPPs and higher CPPs are directly correlated with higher rates of ROSC. This emphasizes the importance of performing high-quality CPR with an ultimate emphasis on optimizing CPP.

11. What is capnography and how can it be used during resuscitation?

Capnography involves measurement of the partial pressure of carbon dioxide in exhaled gases (including quantitative end-tidal carbon dioxide [EtCO$_2$] values and display of the capnogram, a real-time CO$_2$ waveform). During periods of acutely decreased cardiac output, such as with cardiac arrest with performance of CPR, EtCO$_2$ levels may reflect acute changes in cardiac output. Animal studies have confirmed that EtCO$_2$ detected during CPR correlates with CPP, while clinical studies have demonstrated correlation between EtCO$_2$ levels and ROSC and survival after cardiac arrest. EtCO$_2$ levels $<$10 mmHg are strongly predictive of poor cardiac arrest outcomes, whereas elevated EtCO$_2$ levels suggest possible good outcomes. While no absolute value or relative change in EtCO$_2$ is perfectly predictive, use of capnography to guide chest compression quality and ROSC is useful.

12. Describe hands-off CPR.

Hands-off CPR refers to lifting the hands off the chest wall during decompression to maximize chest recoil. Incomplete chest wall recoil, commonly observed in human studies, has been shown to impede forward blood flow in animal models and is probably detrimental in humans

13. **Discuss the role of vasopressors (epinephrine and vasopressin) during treatment of cardiac arrest.**
    The immediate goal of vasopressor pharmacologic therapy is to improve CPP, and thus myocardial blood flow, which is associated with ROSC. Epinephrine is an adrenergic agonist that increases systemic vascular resistance, thus improving CPP by augmenting the diastolic aortic:right atrial gradient. Epinephrine (1 mg IV/IO push every 3–5 minutes) is the only vasopressor currently included in the AHA Advanced Cardiac Life Support (ACLS) algorithm. If the rhythm is shockable, there is insufficient evidence regarding optimal timing of epinephrine in relation to defibrillation, but in nonshockable rhythms, epinephrine can be administered as soon as feasible after the onset of arrest.

14. **Why is vasopressin no longer included in AHA ACLS guidelines?**
    Vasopressin is a nonadrenergic agonist that acts directly on V_1 receptors and had been included in prior guidelines as an adjunct to epinephrine. Vasopressin was removed from the AHA ACLS algorithm in the interest of simplicity, as more recent evidence did not show an added benefit to administering either vasopressin alone or in combination with epinephrine, compared with epinephrine alone.

15. **What are the appropriate routes of drug administration?**
    IV administration is the preferred route of drug therapy when treating cardiac arrest. A central venous catheter is ideal, although placement should not supersede other resuscitation efforts (e.g., chest compression). Use of a peripheral venous catheter results in a slightly delayed medication onset of action, although the peak drug effect is similar to that for the central route. An IO line may also be used and should take precedence over other approaches, including intramuscular or endotracheal routes. All drugs used for resuscitation can be given in conventional doses using IO access. Intracardiac administration should be reserved for cases of open cardiac massage.

16. **I thought IO cannulation was only used as a last resort. What's the deal?**
    IO cannulation provides a quick, effective, and safe means to access a noncollapsible venous plexus, either in the proximal tibia, proximal humerus, or sternum. (The sternum should be avoided as an IO site in cardiac arrest, because it interferes with chest compressions.) It can be used in all age groups and allows for effective fluid resuscitation, drug delivery, and blood sampling for laboratory evaluation. In fact, the IO functions similar to that of a central line in terms of rapid access to the patient's central circulation.

17. **What are the initial key treatment principles when managing patients with a shockable rhythm (VF/pVT)?**
    Adult patients treated by EMS with a shockable rhythm have a much higher probability of surviving to hospital discharge than patients with nonshockable presenting rhythms (according to CARES Registry 2017, 29% and 6%, respectively). Rapid identification and immediate defibrillation of VF/pVT as soon as the AED is available and ready (in addition to high-quality CPR) is the only rhythm-specific therapy proven to increase survival to hospital discharge and should not be delayed for other ACLS measures. While the AED is being retrieved and applied, high-quality uninterrupted CPR should be immediately initiated and resumed after rapid defibrillation. Recommended shock energy levels for defibrillation on biphasic monitors (preferred and most common) is based on the manufacturer recommendation (initial dose 120–200 J), or if unknown, use maximum available. If only monophasic defibrillator available, 360 J is recommended. If there are no signs of ROSC, continue down the ACLS algorithm, including additional shocks and consideration of antiarrhythmics.

18. **What is the optimal placement of electrode pads used for defibrillation?**
    For ease of placement, the anterolateral pad position is recommended. However, for ventricular dysrhythmias, there is no efficacy difference between this position and the three others (anteroposterior, anterior–left infrascapular, or anterior–right infrascapular).

19. **Should you administer one shock at a time or a sequence of shocks (also referred to as stacked shocking)?**
    No study has shown survival benefit with stacked shocks. If one shock fails to eliminate VF/pVT, the incremental benefit of another shock is low, and resumption of CPR is likely to confer greater value than another immediate shock.

20. **Discuss the role of antiarrhythmics in shock refractory VF/pVT and the updated 2018 AHA focused guideline regarding addition of lidocaine to the choices of antiarrhythmic.**
    The primary objective of antiarrhythmics is to facilitate successful defibrillation and reduce risk of recurrent dysrhythmia. While early CPR and defibrillation are the only therapies associated with improved long-term survival in patients with VF/pVT, antidysrhythmics (2015 AHA guidelines included amiodarone) have been associated with increased rates of ROSC and survival to hospital admission. In 2018, the AHA updated the 2015 recommendations for antidysrhythmics for adult VF/pVT to include consideration of amiodarone (first dose, 300 mg IV/IO bolus; second dose, 150 mg IV/IO bolus) OR lidocaine (first dose, 1.0–1.5 mg/kg IV/IO; second dose, 0.5–0.75 mg/kg), class Ib antidysrhythmic, for VF/pVT that is unresponsive to defibrillation. The addition of lidocaine was based on the most recent randomized controlled trial (RCT) to date which found that lidocaine had comparable efficacy to amiodarone. The optimal sequence of administration of antidysrhythmic drugs during resuscitation or timing of drug administration in relation to shock delivery is still not known.

21. **Should I routinely administer magnesium in adults with shock refractory VF/pVT?**
No. The recent AHA guidelines recommend against the routine use of magnesium in patients with shock-refractory VF/pVT. However, magnesium should be considered for torsades de pointes.

22. **What about esmolol for refractory VF? I've heard there may be compelling evidence to support its use in this situation.**
Esmolol is a Class II antidysrhythmic and has been hypothesized to abort refractory VF. Evidence for its use in this setting comes from two small observational studies. The first, a retrospective study published in 2014, originates from a single center in the United States and compares six patients who received esmolol (loading dose 500 mcg/kg, infusion 0–100 mcg/kg/min) after usual ACLS care (including at least three defibrillation attempts, 3 mg epinephrine, and 300 mg amiodarone) with 19 patients who received otherwise usual ACLS care but without esmolol. In the esmolol group, 50% ($n = 3$) were discharged from the hospital with good neurologic function as compared with only 11% ($n = 2$) in the nonesmolol group. The second study, a retrospective pre-post study performed in Korea and published in 2016, included a similar small number of patients with refractory VF and used the same dose of esmolol, again after usual ACLS care. Sustained ROSC was significantly more common in the esmolol group compared with the nonesmolol group (56% [$n = 9$] vs. 16% [$n = 4$]), and improved rates of survival with good neurologic function (19% [$n = 3$] vs. 8% [$n = 2$]). Based on this current limited evidence, esmolol may be considered in patients with refractory VF.

23. **Should I routinely administer sodium bicarbonate during resuscitation?**
Similarly, sodium bicarbonate is not recommended as routine therapy in the setting of cardiac arrest. A no- or low-flow state causes progressive respiratory and metabolic acidosis as a result of accumulation of carbon dioxide and lactate, respectively. Neither state can be corrected without adequate oxygenation, ventilation, and tissue perfusion. At present, no clinical data support the routine use of sodium bicarbonate, except in cases of hyperkalemia, tricyclic antidepressant overdose, or preexisting metabolic acidosis.

24. **Should I routinely administer calcium during resuscitation?**
Calcium is also not recommended as routine therapy in the setting of cardiac arrest. Although no data exist to support its routine use, it may be beneficial in the setting of hyperkalemia (most often seen in chronic renal failure/dialysis patients), hypocalcemia, or calcium channel blocker toxicity.

25. **How should asystole be treated?**
Identify and treat the underlying cause. Confirm the absence of cardiac activity in more than one electrocardiogram lead. Check for loose or disconnected cables and monitor leads. Finally, increase the amplitude to detect occult, fine VF.

26. **Is defibrillation or electrical pacing useful for asystole?**
Defibrillation is reserved for cases in which differentiation between asystole and fine VF is difficult. In these ambiguous situations, defibrillation should be employed after administration of epinephrine. Electrical pacing is occasionally attempted for asystole, but rarely effective in restoring pulses and is not recommended.

27. **What should I do after ROSC?**
Once ROSC is achieved, the vulnerable and highly tenuous postresuscitation period begins. This period is marked by a profound systemic inflammatory response syndrome resulting from whole-body ischemia and reperfusion. Patients often experience hemodynamic instability, multiple-organ dysfunction, and subsequent death (hours to days later). Prompt recognition and treatment of the inciting event and meticulous intensive care unit support are required to provide patients with the best probability for survival. In addition, early aggressive percutaneous coronary intervention and targeted temperature management (TTM) should be performed to improve survival and neurologic recovery, respectively.

28. **What is TTM?**
TTM refers to induced core hypothermia (32°C–36°C) and active temperature control (i.e., prevention of hyperthermia) for approximately 24 hours in comatose out-of-hospital cardiac arrest survivors. Two landmark studies published in the early 2000s showed this intervention to be highly efficacious for improving neurologic function, and a more recent study, published in 2013, showed similar results to the original studies, but no advantage of cooling to 33°C versus 36°C.

29. **How much time do I have to reach the target temperature and should I perform this in the ED?**
Although not known for sure, it is thought the sooner TTM is initiated the better. If possible, this intervention should be initiated in the ED.

30. **What's the best approach to cooling for TTM?**
Surface cooling and catheter-based cooling are the two approaches used for TTM. While both work to obtain hypothermic core temperatures, catheter-based cooling is probably superior in maintaining a constant core temperature while also preventing excessive hypothermia.

31. **When may prehospital resuscitation efforts be terminated?**
According to the most recent AHA ACLS guidelines, prehospital resuscitation can be discontinued in the out-of-hospital setting by EMS authorities when a valid no-CPR order is presented to the rescuers or when a patient is

deemed nonsurvivable after an adequate trial of basic life support and ACLS, including successful endotracheal intubation, achievement of IV/IO access, and administration of appropriate medications, and determination of a persistent asystolic or agonal rhythm, as well as when no reversible cause for the arrest is identified.

32. Can capnography be used *in isolation* to predict when to terminate a prolonged resuscitation?

No! While multiple prospective observational studies have found that survival is very unlikely in intubated patients if their $EtCO_2$ is ≤ 10 mmHg after 20 minutes of CPR, these studies are limited (observational and relatively small) and low $EtCO_2$ values in real clinical scenarios are difficult to interpret in isolation. Low $EtCO_2$ values may reflect inadequate cardiac output, but the low value could be confounded due to bronchospasm, obstruction of the endotracheal tube (due to mucus plugging, kinking or alveolar fluid), hyperventilation, and airway leak. Thus the 2015 AHA updated recommendations state:

> In intubated patients, failure to achieve an $EtCO_2$ of greater than 10 mmHg by waveform capnography after 20 minutes of CPR may be considered as one component of a multimodal approach to decide when to end resuscitative efforts, but it should not be used *in isolation*.

33. What are other reversible causes and immediate treatments of cardiopulmonary arrest?
- Hyperkalemia: calcium chloride (preferred over calcium gluconate), sodium bicarbonate, insulin and glucose, and nebulized albuterol.
- Anaphylaxis: intravascular volume expansion (using crystalloid) and epinephrine.
- Cardiac tamponade: pericardiocentesis or pericardiotomy.
- Tension pneumothorax: thoracic decompression.
- Hypovolemia: intravascular volume expansion using crystalloid solutions. In the setting of trauma, blood products should be given judiciously and concomitantly with crystalloid. Always consider using a level I infuser when large volumes are required over a short period of time.
- Torsades de pointes: defibrillation, magnesium sulfate, isoproterenol, or overdrive pacing.
- Toxic cardiopulmonary arrest:
  - Carbon monoxide poisoning occurs after prolonged exposure to smoke and inhalation of exhaust from incomplete combustion. High-flow and hyperbaric oxygen and management of acidosis are the cornerstones of treatment.
  - Cyanide poisoning occurs after intentional ingestion or after exposure to fire involving synthetic materials. The antidote for this includes hydroxycobalamin, which combines with cyanide to form cyanocobalamin (vitamin B_{12}). Sodium nitrite and sodium thiosulfate are considered second-line therapy for cyanide toxicity.
  - Tricyclic antidepressants act as type Ia antidysrhythmic agents and cause cardiac conduction slowing, ventricular dysrhythmias, hypotension, and seizures. Vigorous serum alkalinization with sodium bicarbonate and seizure control are required.
- Primary asphyxia: in addition to anaphylaxis, obstructive asphyxia may occur after foreign body aspiration, inflammatory conditions of the hypopharynx (e.g., epiglottitis or retropharyngeal abscess), or neck trauma. The latter results in edema or hematoma formation, subcutaneous emphysema, or laryngeal or tracheal disruption. Treatment includes establishment of a patent airway via endotracheal intubation or by cricothyrotomy and assisted ventilation with 100% oxygen.

34. What are the indications for open-chest cardiac massage?

The primary indication for open-chest cardiac massage is traumatic arrest. However, several other non–trauma-related indications include hypothermia, pulmonary embolism, cardiac tamponade, abdominal hemorrhage, third-trimester pregnancy, and patients with chest wall deformities that prevent adequate chest compressions.

35. What percentage of adult out-of-hospital cardiac arrest patients survive to hospital discharge?

Ten percent, according to national epidemiologic data from 2017.

KEY POINTS: MANAGEMENT OF CARDIAC ARREST

CPR and defibrillation are the most important components to the initial management of the cardiac arrest patient.
1. Treat VF with immediate defibrillation if the arrest is witnessed on monitor and AED ready; treat with CPR and then defibrillation if the arrest is unwitnessed or if need to obtain/apply AED.
2. If the arrest is caused by PEA, remember its common reversible causes (i.e., hypovolemia, hypoxia, cardiac tamponade, tension pneumothorax, hypothermia, massive pulmonary embolism, drug toxicity, electrolyte disturbances, acidemia, or myocardial infarction) and treat them appropriately.
3. If the arrest is the result of asystole, remember to exclude fine VF.
4. Quality of CPR should be continuously monitored.

Websites
American Heart Association: www.americanheart.org/

BIBILIOGRAPHY

Aufderheide TP, Pirallo RG, Yannopoulos D, et al. Incomplete chest wall decompression: a clinical evaluation of CPR performance by EMS personnel and assessment of alternative manual chest compression-decompression techniques. *Resuscitation.* 2005;64:353–362.

Driver BE, Debaty G, Plummer DW, et al. Use of esmolol after failure of standard cardiopulmonary resuscitation to treat patients with refractory ventricular fibrillation. *Resuscitation.* 2014;85:1337–1341.

Kudenchuk PJ, Brown SP, Daya M, et al. Amiodarone, lidocaine, or placebo in out-of-hospital cardiac arrest. *N Engl J Med.* 2016;374: 1711–1722.

Layek A, Maitra S, Pal S, et al. Efficacy of vasopressin during cardio-pulmonary resuscitation in adult patients: a meta-analysis. *Resuscitation.* 2014;85:855–863.

Lemkes JS, Janssens GN, van der Hoeven NW, et al. Coronary angiography after cardiac arrest without ST-segment elevation. *N Engl J Med.* 2019;380:1397–1407.

Link MS, Berkow LC, Kudenchuck PJ, et al. Part 7: adult advanced cardiovascular life support: 2015 American Heart Association guidelines update for cardiopulmonary resuscitation and emergency cardiovascular care. *Circulation.* 2015;132:s444–s464.

Nielsen N, Wetterslev J, Cronbert T, et al. Targeted temperature management at 33°C versus 36°C after cardiac arrest. *N Engl J Med.* 2013;369:197–206.

Paradis NA, Martin GB, Rivers EP, et al. Coronary perfusion pressure and the return of spontaneous circulation in human cardiopulmonary resuscitation. *JAMA.* 1990;263:1106–1113.

Perkins GD, Ji C, Deakin CD, et al. A randomized trial of epinephrine in out-of-hospital cardiac arrest. *N Engl J Med.* 2018;379:711–721.

Wik L, Hansen TB, Fylling F, et al. Delaying defibrillation to give basic cardiopulmonary resuscitation to patients with out-of-hospital ventricular fibrillation: a randomized trial. *JAMA.* 2003;289:1389–1395.

CHAPTER 3

AIRWAY MANAGEMENT

Jeremy Collado, MD and W. Gannon Sungar, DO

1. **Which ED patients need airway assessment?**
Emergency physicians are masters of the airway and every patient in the ED should have their airway assessed.

2. **What are the different mechanisms of respiratory failure?**
Respiration consists of oxygenation and ventilation. Patients can experience respiratory failure by four main mechanisms:
   - **Loss of airway protective reflexes** – often due to a nonrespiratory cause (e.g., trauma, toxicologic), resulting in collapse of the airway anatomy and loss of airway patency.
   - **Hypoxemia** – failure of oxygenation, manifested by cyanosis and/or low readings on pulse oximetry.
   - **Hypercapnia** – failure of ventilation, leading to elevated pCO_2 levels that results in acidosis and altered mental status.
   - **Mixed** – failure of both oxygenation and ventilation.

3. **How do I assess a patient's respiratory status?**
If patients are able to speak clearly, they have an intact airway. Lacking this, signs of airway collapse include sonorous respirations, pooling of secretions, and inability to swallow. Assessment of oxygenation and ventilation is achieved by looking at the patient's skin color, work of breathing, respiratory rate, and mental status.

4. **Does a lack of a gag reflex mean my patient can't protect their airway?**
No, the lack of a gag reflex is an unreliable marker for airway collapse, as up to 25% of the population lacks a gag reflex at baseline. Also, the presence of a gag reflex does not imply ability to protect the airway.

5. **What is a definitive airway?**
A definitive airway is defined as a cuffed endotracheal (ET) tube inflated below the level of the vocal cords.

6. **What is the most common cause of airway obstruction?**
The tongue is the most common cause of airway obstruction, as it blocks the airway far more commonly than do foreign bodies or edema. With decreasing levels of consciousness, the supporting muscles in the floor of the mouth lose tone and the tongue falls posteriorly, obstructing the oropharynx.

7. **How can I initially assist a patient in respiratory failure?**
Patients with airway collapse may benefit from an airway maneuver or airway stenting, including:
   - **Head tilt/chin lift** – lift the chin cephalad and anterior, creating slight extension of the head.
   - **Jaw thrust** – lift anteriorly at the bilateral mandibular angles, moving the tongue off of the posterior oropharynx.
   - **Artificial airway** – a nasopharyngeal airway (NPA) or an oropharyngeal airway (OPA) can be placed in the naris or mouth, respectively, to stent the tongue off of the posterior oropharynx and maintain upper airway patency.
   - **Bag valve mask (BVM)** – after using one or more of the airway maneuvers above to establish airway patency, BVM can be used to support oxygenation and ventilation.

8. **How do I predict patients who will be difficult to assist with a BVM?**
The MOANS mnemonic can be a useful tool for predicting difficulty in using a BVM.
   - **M** – Mask seal – things that could impair mask seal may include beard, vomitus, blood, facial trauma, anatomic abnormalities, or incorrect mask size.
   - **O** – Obesity/obstruction, including oropharyngeal swelling or masses will also cause difficulty in using a BVM.
   - **A** – Age >55 years old.
   - **N** – No teeth – while edentulousness may make intubation easier, it makes using a BVM more difficult as the soft tissue collapses onto itself.
   - **S** – Stiff lungs – pathology such as chronic obstructive pulmonary disease (COPD), asthma, chest trauma, etc., can impair easy movement of air in and out of the lungs.

9. **What is rapid sequence intubation (RSI)?**
RSI is a method of facilitating ET intubation by inducing unconsciousness and paralysis. Because patients requiring emergent airway management are at risk for aspiration, the airway must be secured as quickly as possible, ideally, after a period of preoxygenation followed by induction of unconsciousness, paralysis, and then intubation. Preferably, preoxygenation is performed without positive pressure ventilation to avoid insufflating the stomach.

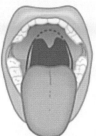 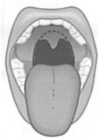 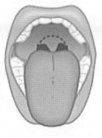 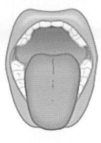

Class I: Soft palate, uvula, fauces, pillars visible

Class II: Soft palate, uvula, fauces visible

Class III: Soft palate, base of uvula visible

Class IV: Only hard palate visible

No difficulty **No difficulty** **Moderate difficulty** **Severe difficulty**

Fig. 3.1 Mallampati score. *(From Brown CA, Walls RM. Airway. In: Walls RM, Hockberger RS, Gausche-Hill M, eds. Emergency Medicine Concepts and Clinical Practice. 9th ed. Philadelphia: Elsevier; 2018:5.)*

10. **How do I assess for a difficult intubation?**
    The LEMON mnemonic is a helpful reminder of factors associated with a difficult intubation:
    - L – Look externally to assess for facial trauma, blood in the airway, etc.
    - E – Evaluate using the 3-3-2 rule to predict difficult airway anatomy.
      - Patients who cannot open their mouth to fit three fingers between their central incisors may have limited mouth opening necessary for direct laryngoscopy.
      - A hyomental distance (hyoid to tip of chin) fewer than three finger breadths predicts a more difficult anterior larynx.
      - Fewer than two finger breadths from hyoid to the thyroid cartilage predicts a short neck and a cephalad larynx.
    - M – The Mallampati score (Fig. 3.1) is a measure of baseline airway patency and is a good predictor of ease of laryngoscopy.
      - Class I – complete visualization of the uvula and the tonsillar pillars
      - Class II – visualization of the entire uvula
      - Class III – visualization of only the base of the uvula
      - Class IV – limited to visualization of the hard palate only
    - O – Obstruction – evaluate for visualized foreign bodies and stridor.
    - N – Neck mobility – decreased neck mobility due to kyphosis, c-collar, etc., may limit manipulation techniques that can aid in direct laryngoscopy.

11. **What basic equipment is necessary for ET intubation?**
    - **Laryngoscope** – Direct and video (see later). There are two common direct laryngoscope blades, specifically:
      - **Macintosh** (curved blade), which is placed anterior to the epiglottis, into the vallecula, acting to lever the epiglottis off of the cords using the median glossoepiglottic fold.
      - **Miller** (straight blade), which is used to lift the underside of the epiglottis anteriorly, revealing the cords underneath. Miller blades are more commonly used in pediatric intubations where the epiglottis tends to be floppier.
    - **Suction** – A Yankauer suction catheter should be available to help remove saliva, blood, or emesis from the airway, enhancing the view of the cords.
    - **ET tube** – Adult males are generally able to accommodate a 7.5–9.0-mm ET tube, whereas women are generally intubated with a 7.0–8.0-mm tube.
    - **Syringe** – A 10 mL syringe is needed to inflate the ET tube cuff.
    - **Stylet** – A flexible, metal probe that is inserted into and used to shape the ET tube for intubation.
    - **Gum elastic bougie** – A bougie is a semirigid introducer with a flexed tip that is frequently used for difficult intubations with incomplete visualization of the larynx. Lacking direct visualization, a bougie can be passed under the epiglottis and tracheal insertion can be confirmed as the flexed tip of the bougie bounces along the tracheal rings. An ET tube is then inserted into the trachea over the bougie. A bougie can also be used with clear, direct visualization of the airway anatomy. Although not standard of practice, recent data suggest an improvement in first-pass intubation success rate in patients with difficult airways using a bougie first approach.

12. **What is a video laryngoscope and what types are there?**
    A video laryngoscope is a laryngoscope blade with a camera embedded at its tip that displays images on a screen most commonly placed at the patient's bedside. There are multiple companies that produce video laryngoscopes, many of which have several interchangeable blade shapes, from a traditional Macintosh blade to more

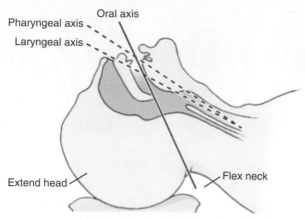

Fig. 3.2 Sniffing position. *(From Driver BE, Reardon RF. Tracheal intubation. In: Roberts JR, Hedges JR, eds. Clinical Procedures in Emergency Medicine. 7th ed. Philadelphia: Elsevier; 2019:71.)*

angulated blades. The systems with traditional blades often have the advantage of being able to be used both for direct as well as video laryngoscopy, depending on user preference and need.

13. **What are the steps (7 P's) to RSI?**
    - **Preparation** – As with all procedures, preparation is the key to success. With every RSI attempt, equipment should be checked, medications should be planned in advance, and a back-up plan should be in place should the attempt fail.
    - **Positioning** – The sniffing position (Fig. 3.2), with the neck flexed relative to the torso, the head extended, and the ear canal aligned horizontally with the sternal notch optimally aligns the oral, pharyngeal, and laryngeal axes for direct laryngoscopy. Sometimes pillows, blankets, soft ramps, and bed positioning are used to achieve the sniffing position, especially in obese patients.
    - **Preoxygenation** – Adequate preoxygenation maximizes the time available to perform the intubation before desaturation occurs by replacing alveolar nitrogen with oxygen (nitrogen washout). Proper preoxygenation can be achieved with 3–5 minutes of normal ventilation with a nonrebreather mask or with eight vital capacity breaths at 100% fraction of inspired oxygen (FiO_2).
    - **Pretreatment** – Laryngoscopy is a strong stimulus that can activate both the sympathetic and parasympathetic nervous systems. However, routine pretreatment with any medication other than a sedative and a paralytic has not been shown to improve outcomes. Atropine may be considered in children less than 12 months old to prevent bradycardia. Patients with head injuries may benefit from fentanyl and/or lidocaine to decrease the transient increase in intracranial pressure during intubation. Nebulized albuterol may help prevent laryngospasm in patients with reactive airway disease.
    - **Paralyze** (and sedate with induction) – Induction medication should be immediately followed by administration of the paralytic (Table 3.1).
    - **Pass the tube** – The tube should be visualized passing through the cords.
    - **Postintubation management** – Immediately following intubation and confirmation of tube placement, the patient should be sedated, most commonly with propofol or a combination of an opioid and benzodiazepine.

14. **What is passive apneic oxygenation?**
    Passive apneic oxygenation is a technique for preventing hypoxia during RSI, where a nasal cannula with high-flow oxygen is placed on the patient during the preoxygenation phase of RSI and left in place throughout the intubation attempt. Studies have shown that despite apnea during paralysis, passive oxygenation can greatly extend the time it takes for a patient to become critically hypoxic. Care should be taken with pediatric patients, as appropriate flow rates in order to prevent harm are based on size.

15. **What medications are used for RSI?**
    Table 3.1 describes the pretreatment, induction, and paralytic medications frequently used for RSI.

16. **What are the contraindications to using succinylcholine?**
    Because succinylcholine causes muscle depolarization and release of intracellular potassium, potentially life-threatening hyperkalemia can occur in certain high-risk populations. Succinylcholine is contraindicated in patients at risk for baseline hyperkalemia, including end-stage renal disease, severe acidosis, patients with major burns or crush injuries in the past 3–5 days (NOT ACUTELY), and any condition causing upregulation of acetylcholine receptors at the neuromuscular junction, including neuromuscular disease, stroke, and spinal injury.

Table 3.1 Common Medications for Rapid Sequence Intubation

	Pretreatment				Induction			Paralytic	
	ATROPINE	**LIDOCAINE**	**FENTANYL**	**ETOMIDATE**	**KETAMINE**	**MIDAZOLAM**	**PROPOFOL**	**SUCCINYL-CHOLINE**	**ROCURONIUM**
Class	Anticholinergic	Amino amide	Opioid analgesic	Imidazole derivative	PCP derivative	Benzodiazepine	GABA agonist	Depolarizing agent	Nondepolarizing agent
Dose	0.02 mg/kg	1.5–2 mg/kg	2–5 mcg/kg	0.3 mg/kg	1–2 mg/kg	0.1–0.3 mg/kg	1.5–3 mg/kg	1.5 mg/kg	1.2 mg/kg
Administration	3–5 min before intubation			Immediately before paralytic				Onset: 45–60 sec Duration: 5–9 min	Onset: 45–60 sec Duration: 20–75 min
Effect/benefit	Blunts bradycardic response to increased vagal tone from laryngoscopy Decreases bronchorrhea	Blunts elevation in ICP associated with laryngoscopy	Decreases sympathetic response to intubation ↑ICP, tachycardia, hypertension)	Hemodynamically neutral Decreases ICP	Bronchodilator (good for RAD) Preserves respiratory drive (awake intubation) Nystagmus May elevate ICP/IOP	Anticonvulsant effect Decreases ICP	Decreases ICP Decreased airway resistance Rapid on/off	Fasciculations Hyperkalemia Increased ICP, IOP	Nondepolarizing so no fasciculations or risk of hyperkalemia May increase HR, BP, CO
Notes	Not routinely recommended except before a second dose of succinylcholine in young children Max dose 1 mg	No longer routinely used for patients with suspected head trauma	Use in patients at risk for decompensation with sympathetic surge (aortic dissection, ICH, etc.)	Proposed adrenal suppression, but not clinically relevant with single dose used for RSI	Adverse effects: • Bronchorrhea • Laryngospasm • Cardiac depressant • Tachycardia • Hypertension • Emergence phenomenon	Adverse effects: • Negative inotrope • Hypotension	Adverse effects: • Hypotension • Pain on infusion • Anaphylaxis with soy/egg allergy	Life-threatening hyperkalemia in burns, crush injury, neuromuscular disease, and acidosis Malignant hyperthermia	Prolonged duration may delay neurologic examination in trauma patients

BP, Blood pressure; CO, cardiac output; GABA, γ-aminobutyric acid; HR, heart rate; ICH, intracranial hemorrhage; ICP, intracranial pressure; IOP, intraocular pressure; PCP, phencyclidine; RAD, reactive airway disease; RSI, rapid sequence intubation.

17. **How deep do I advance an ET tube?**
    A traditional rule is that an ET tube should be placed at a depth equal to three times the tube size in centimeters (e.g., an 8.0-mm tube should be placed 24 cm at the teeth). Due to airway anatomy, deeper tube placement will usually end up in the right mainstem bronchus.

18. **How do I confirm ET tube placement?**
    ET tube placement is best confirmed by direct visualization of the tube passing through the vocal cords. Signs of correct tracheal tube placement include condensation in the tube, bilateral breath sounds with bagging, absence of breath sounds over the epigastrium, and color change on colorimetric capnometry. Continuous waveform end-tidal CO_2 (capnography) is the most reliable method for confirming and monitoring correct ET tube placement. If continuous waveform is not available, a colorimetric end-tidal CO_2 detector should be used. Chest x-ray is valuable for confirming appropriate depth of tube placement, but should not be relied upon to confirm ET placement due to the time it takes to complete.

19. **What are the contraindications to RSI?**
    RSI is contraindicated in any patient where securing of the airway is predicted to be difficult. Anticipation of a difficult airway based on anatomic features (foreign body, allergic reaction, airway infections, malignancies) or traumatic anatomic distortion (massive facial trauma, facial burns) is a relative contraindication to RSI. Difficult airway must be considered in the context of the environment, skill of the operator, and available equipment.

20. **What are the steps to awake fiberoptic intubation?**
    Awake fiberoptic intubation is an excellent option for patients with some respiratory effort in whom RSI is contraindicated, most commonly due to airway obstruction. Patients can be placed in the upright position, the oropharynx is anesthetized with nebulized or topical anesthetic spray, and patients are given moderate sedation, often with ketamine, maintaining their respiratory drive. A flexible fiberoptic scope already threaded through an ET tube is then maneuvered into the oropharynx via a nasal or oral approach and passed through the cords under direct visualization, at which point the ET tube is advanced.

21. **What is delayed sequence intubation (DSI)?**
    DSI can be used in patients with hypoxia refractory to traditional preoxygenation techniques. DSI is the use of ketamine for procedural sedation with the procedure being preoxygenation. Patients are given 1–2 mg/kg of ketamine and then bag valve mask ventilated or placed on a noninvasive ventilator until their oxygenation can be maximized, at which point standard RSI is performed.

22. **What is an extraglottic airway device (EAD)?**
    An EAD is a device that is placed without direct visualization above or posterior to the larynx, typically blocking off the esophagus, allowing ventilation and oxygenation. There are various types with differing pros and cons, including prevention of aspiration, ability to intubate through the device, and poor seal, to name a few. These are good rescue devices for patients who are difficult to bag valve mask or as a temporizing method after failed ET intubation.

23. **What is a laryngeal mask airway (LMA)?**
    An LMA is a type of EAD that has an oval mask with a cuffed rim that is inserted into the oropharynx. It is intended to create a seal directly over the larynx, allowing ventilation and oxygenation. An intubating LMA is an LMA with a rigid channel through which an ET tube can be directed through the cords. LMAs are considered the rescue device of choice in a cannot-intubate/cannot-ventilate scenario.

24. **What is a King airway? What is a Combitube?**
    Both the Combitube and the King airway (Fig. 3.3) are types of EADs that are most frequently used by prehospital providers.
    - **King airway** – The King LT is a single-lumen tube with a small distal balloon and a larger proximal balloon that is inserted blindly into the mouth with the intention of placing the tip in the esophagus. The two balloons are then inflated, blocking the esophagus and oropharynx, and isolating the supraglottic space. Ventilation is achieved through a side port between the two balloons.
    - **Combitube** – The Combitube is a dual-lumen tube that is blindly inserted into either the esophagus (95% of the time) or the trachea (remaining 5%). If the tip is placed in the esophagus, the oropharyngeal and esophageal balloons can be inflated, and the patient can be ventilated through a side port of the longer lumen, similar to the King LT. If the tip of the tube is placed in the trachea, the patient can be ventilated through the distal tip using the shorter lumen.

25. **What are the indications for a surgical airway?**
    Cricothyrotomy is the surgical airway of choice in the ED for patients with a failed airway. A failed airway is failure to intubate, ventilate, and oxygenate by other means. A cricothyrotomy is performed by making a vertical

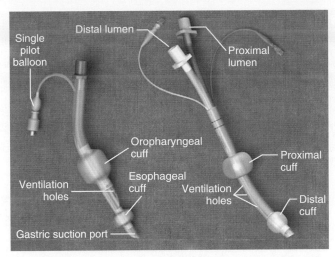

Fig. 3.3 King LT *(left)* and Combitube *(right)*. *(From: Driver BF, Reardon RF. Basic airway management and decision making. In: Roberts JR, Hedges JR, eds. Clinical Procedures in Emergency Medicine. 7th ed. Philadelphia: Elsevier; 2019:59.)*

| Table 3.2 Laryngoscope Blade Sizes for Pediatric Intubations ||
AGE	**LARYNGOSCOPE BLADE SIZE**
Premature infant	0
Full-term infant	1
Older children	2
Adults	3–4

incision over the cricothyroid membrane, palpating down to and making a horizontal incision through the membrane and inserting an ET tube.

26. **What factors make pediatric airway interventions more difficult?**
Direct laryngoscopy can be more challenging in the pediatric patient due to anatomic differences, including a relatively large occiput causing neck flexion, a more superior and anterior larynx, a relatively larger tongue, and an epiglottis that is shorter and more difficult to manipulate. Additionally, pediatric patients have higher relative oxygen consumption and lower residual capacity and, therefore, become hypoxic much more quickly than adult patients.

27. **How do I know what equipment size to use for pediatric airway interventions?**
Laryngoscope sizes can be seen in Table 3.2. Cuffed ET tubes are now recommended for pediatrics. Both cuffed and uncuffed ET tube size can be estimated using tools such as a Broselow-Luten tape, the age-based Handtevy system, or with the following formula:

$$\text{Cuffed ET tube size} = (\text{Age}/4) + 3.5$$

28. **What is the surgical airway option for pediatric patients?**
Because of anatomic differences in children, including a smaller or absent cricothyroid membrane and an immature larynx, surgical cricothyrotomy is contraindicated in children less than 5–12 years (cutoff age is controversial). The surgical airway of choice in pediatric patients is transtracheal jet ventilation, in which a large-bore needle is inserted through the cricothyroid membrane and high-flow oxygen is delivered. This is only a temporizing measure, as hypoventilation with this device quickly leads to hypercarbia.

KEY POINTS: AIRWAY MANAGEMENT

1. Approach every airway with a clear plan in place for initial intervention as well as a complete set of back-up plans should your initial attempt be unsuccessful.
2. Preoxygenation with 100% FiO_2 for 5 minutes or eight vital-capacity breaths as well as passive apneic oxygenation are critical steps to prevent oxygen desaturation during RSI.
3. Never paralyze a patient unless you are certain that they can be ventilated using a bag valve mask or an extraglottic rescue device.
4. Succinylcholine is contraindicated in patients at risk for baseline hyperkalemia or an exaggerated potassium shift, including end-stage renal disease, severe acidosis, neuromuscular disease, and delayed presentations of burn or crush injuries.
5. Many video laryngoscope systems can be used for both direct and video laryngoscopy without changing blades. They are therefore preferred by many as the first choice for RSI in the ED.

BIBLIOGRAPHY

Brown CA, Walls RM. Airway. In: Walls RM, Hockberger RS, Gausche-Hill M, eds. *Emergency Medicine Concepts and Clinical Practice.* 9th ed. Philadelphia: Elsevier; 2018:3–24.

Carlson JN, Brown CA. Does the use of video laryngoscopy improve intubation outcomes? *Ann Emerg Med.* 2014;64(2):165–166.

Driver BE, Reardon RF. Basic airway management and decision making. In: Roberts JR, Hedges JR, eds. *Clinical Procedures in Emergency Medicine.* 7th ed. Philadelphia: Elsevier; 2019:39–61.

Driver BE, Reardon RF. Tracheal intubation. In: Roberts JR, Hedges JR, eds. *Clinical Procedures in Emergency Medicine.* 7th ed. Philadelphia: Elsevier; 2019:62–110.

Herbert RB, Thomas D. Cricothyrotomy and percutaneous translaryngeal ventilation. In: Roberts JR, Hedges JR, eds. *Clinical Procedures in Emergency Medicine.* 7th ed. Philadelphia: Elsevier; 2019:127–141.

Schwartz RB, McCollum D. Pharmacologic adjuncts to intubation. In: Roberts JR, Hedges JR, eds. *Clinical Procedures in Emergency Medicine.* 7th ed. Philadelphia: Elsevier; 2019:111–126.

Sharma B, Sahai C, Sood J. Extraglottic airway devices: technology update. *Med Devices (Auckl).* 2017;10:189–205.

CHAPTER 4

SHOCK

Chelsea McCullough, MD, MPH and Jason Haukoos, MD, MSc

1. **Define shock.**
   Shock is a clinical syndrome characterized by widespread inadequate oxygenation and supply of nutrients to tissues and organs, resulting in cellular dysfunction.

2. **How common is shock?**
   Although the prevalence is not precisely known, it is thought that shock constitutes approximately 1% of all ED visits.

3. **What is the overall mortality rate of patients who develop shock?**
   The mortality rate exceeds 20% for patients across all categories of shock.

4. **List the five categories of shock and provide examples of each.**
   1. Hypovolemic: hemorrhagic, including trauma, gastrointestinal bleeding, ruptured ectopic pregnancy, and ruptured abdominal aortic aneurysm; nonhemorrhagic, including vomiting, diarrhea, diabetic ketoacidosis, and insensible losses, especially among those at extremes of ages.
   2. Cardiogenic: acute myocardial infarction, cardiomyopathy, dysrhythmias, and valvular dysfunction.
   3. Distributive: sepsis, anaphylaxis, pancreatitis, and neurogenic processes secondary to spinal cord injury
   4. Obstructive: pulmonary embolism, cardiac tamponade, and tension pneumothorax.
   5. Toxic/metabolic: carbon monoxide, cyanide, β-blocker, calcium channel blocker, adrenal insufficiency, and thyroid storm.

5. **How do I identify a patient in shock?**
   Shock is a clinical syndrome that reflects hypoperfusion of vital organs. The successful treatment of these patients with a high risk of mortality is predicated on early recognition and treatment. These patients generally appear ill and possess a pattern of signs and symptoms that aid in the identification of shock. A brief focused history and targeted physical examination will help determine whether shock is present and its underlying cause. Some signs and symptoms may vary, depending on the category of shock. Examples of end-organ symptoms and signs include the following:
   - Central nervous system: Altered mental status
   - Cardiovascular: Tachycardia, bradycardia (neurogenic shock), hypotension, and weak rapid pulses
   - Pulmonary: tachypnea and hyperpnea
   - Renal: decreased urine output
   - Skin: delayed capillary refill; cool and mottled skin in hypovolemic or cardiogenic shock; warm and moist skin in distributive shock.

6. **How should urine output be used during the resuscitation of a patient in shock?**
   Urine output is an excellent indicator of end-organ perfusion, assuming the patient has normal renal function at baseline. A normal urine output is more than 1 mL/kg/h, a reduced urine output ranges from 0.5 to 1 mL/kg/h, and a severely reduced urine output is less than 0.5 mL/kg/h. During resuscitation, therapy should include improving or normalizing urine output.

7. **Describe compensated and decompensated shock.**
   Shock initiates a sequence of stress responses intended to preserve perfusion to vital organs. Compensated shock occurs soon after the onset of shock and is marked by the maintenance of tissue perfusion pressures. Such patients typically have evidence of a stress response (e.g., tachycardia and tachypnea), but also have a normal or high blood pressure and normal or mildly elevated serum lactate concentrations. If left untreated, compensated shock may progress to decompensated shock, which is characterized by profound global tissue hypoperfusion, elevated serum lactate concentration, and hypotension.

8. **What is the initial management of a patient who is experiencing shock?**
   Management of all critically ill patients begins with rapid assessment of a patient's airway, breathing, and circulation (ABCs). All patients thought to be in shock should be placed on cardiopulmonary monitoring, have their intravascular volume depleted, and receive treatment for the precipitating cause (e.g., antibiotics in septic shock).

Type of fluid may vary based on the type of shock (i.e., normal saline or Ringer's lactate for distributive shock; blood products for hemorrhagic shock). *One exception to this is cardiogenic shock, in which rapid fluid administration may be detrimental and cause worsening shock.*

9. **What type of intravenous (IV) access should be utilized for rapid fluid administration in the treatment of shock?**
From Poiseuille's equation, resistance of any vessel is a function of both length and diameter. As vessel length increases or diameter decreases, resistance increases. Following this logic, a short and wide catheter is best to administer fluids quickly. Large-bore peripheral IV catheters (14 or 16 gauge) and centrally placed cordis catheters (6–8.5 French) have lower resistance than triple lumen central venous catheter lines (typically 7 French, but consisting of three smaller lumens), and therefore are most appropriate for shock resuscitation.

10. **How useful are vital signs in assessing and treating someone in shock?**
A complete set of vital signs are crucial. Heart rate, respiratory rate, blood pressure, and pulse oximetry should be monitored closely in patients with confirmed or suspected shock. Physiologic compensation and decompensation (see Question 7) are commonly reflected in a patient's vital signs. Additionally, improvement or normalization of abnormal vital signs is one indicator of a patient's response to resuscitation.

11. **If a patient has normal vital signs, should I be reassured?**
No. A patient's heart rate and blood pressure could be "normal" in the setting of severe illness, but may deviate significantly from a patient's baseline. In the setting of shock, heart rate and blood pressure values correlate poorly with cardiac output, and often do not reflect the severity of systemic hypoperfusion.

12. **Are there other signs or laboratory tests that are helpful in assessing an acutely ill patient?**
Yes. Besides vital signs and components of the physical examination (e.g., level of consciousness, capillary refill, and urinary output), serum lactate concentrations are helpful in the diagnosis and management of shock.

13. **What is "early goal-directed therapy?"**
Goal-directed therapy, specifically introduced for septic shock, refers to the practice of resuscitating patients to defined physiologic end points that indicate systemic tissue perfusion and vital organ function have been restored. Previously, other markers of intravascular volume and perfusion, such as central venous pressure (CVP), and central venous oxygen saturation ($ScvO_2$) or mixed venous oxygen saturation (SvO_2), had been utilized in an early goal-directed approach. More recent studies have shown that resuscitation based on serum lactate values can guide the management of shock as well as these other clinical indicators, furthermore reducing the number of invasive procedures needed for central hemodynamic monitoring.

14. **How should I use and interpret serum lactate concentration?**
Serum lactate rises as cells convert to anaerobic metabolism and thus is commonly used as a marker to assess the extent of systemic hypoperfusion and tissue hypoxia. An elevated serum lactate is an early marker of systemic hypoperfusion and often precedes overt changes in a patient's vital signs. Higher serum lactate concentrations are associated with higher morbidity and mortality, and a lactate concentration greater than 4 mEq/L has been used to define those with the highest mortality rates. A decrease in serial serum lactate measurements, or *lactate clearance,* indicates effective shock resuscitation.

15. **What is the lactate clearance index, and how can it be used during resuscitation of a patient in shock?**
The lactate clearance index refers to measurements of serum lactate at two or more times during the course of the resuscitation. If after 1 hour of resuscitative efforts the serum lactate concentration has not decreased by 50%, additional steps should be undertaken to improve systemic perfusion.

16. **What is the shock index and how is it helpful?**
Shock index (SI) equals heart rate divided by systolic blood pressure. Normal values are 0.5–0.7, with values exceeding 0.9 associated with hypoperfusion. Studies in both medical and trauma patients show elevated SI values as being associated with increased levels of mortality and in-hospital resource utilization (hospital length of stay, intensive care unit days, and blood product use).

17. **List the primary resuscitation goals in patients who are experiencing shock.**
- Optimize oxygenation and ventilation.
- Improve vital organ perfusion.
- Treat the underlying cause of shock.

18. **What is the Trendelenburg position? What purpose does it serve?**
A patient in the Trendelenburg position is in a supine, approximately 45-degree, head-down position. The purposes of this position have been reported to include improving blood pressure, redistributing circulating blood volume, facilitating the placement of central lines, and improving the sensitivity of abdominal ultrasound for intraabdominal fluid. Although commonly used for the purpose of improving hemodynamic parameters, several studies have not demonstrated its utility in significantly improving blood pressure or redistribution of blood volume.

19. **Define systemic inflammatory response syndrome (SIRS).**
    SIRS is classically defined by two or more of the following:
    - Temperature greater than 38°C or less than 36°C
    - Heart rate greater than 90 beats per minute
    - Respiratory rate greater than 20 breaths per minute or partial pressure of carbon dioxide less than 32 mmHg
    - Serum white blood cell count greater than 12,000 mm^3 or less than 4000 mm^3 or greater than 10% band forms

    The SIRS response contributes to distributive shock, as inflammation causes reduced systemic vascular resistance and increased capillary permeability. This definition, although standardized, is not specific for defining serious illness or shock. Although most commonly described in the context of sepsis, a systemic inflammatory response may result from a variety of noninfectious insults, including trauma, burns, pancreatitis, or overdose.

20. **Define sepsis, severe sepsis, and septic shock, and discuss their specific therapies.**
    See Chapter 50.

21. **What are the roles of vasopressor and ionotropic medications in shock?**
    Administration of vasopressors results in increased systemic vascular resistance to augment blood pressure. Inotropic agents work to increase cardiac contractility, resulting in increased cardiac output. Some of these medications also increase heart rate, an effect known as chronotropy. Vasopressors can be given as a continuous infusion or a "push dose" when needed for temporary hemodynamic support. The term "push dose" indicates that the medication is given as a one time or repeated bolus. The selection of vasopressor or ionotropic medication depends on the underlying pathophysiology of the patient's shock.

22. **Name several vasopressor and ionotropic medications, their uses, and their mechanisms of action.**
    Table 4.1.

Table 4.1 Vasoactive Agents

AGENT	RECEPTOR	MAIN EFFECT	PRIMARY USE	SIDE EFFECTS AND OTHER NOTES
Epinephrine	α_1, α_2, β_1, β_2	Vasoconstriction, ionotropy and chronotropy, and bronchodilation	Hypotension, anaphylaxis and severe asthma	α Effects predominate at high doses
Norepinephrine	$\alpha^1 > \alpha^2 > \beta^1$	Vasoconstriction and ionotropy	Hypotension; first line for septic shock	Used in most types of shock
Phenylephrine	$\alpha^1 > \alpha^2$	Vasoconstriction	Hypotension, frequently used as "push dose" vasopressor	May cause reflex bradycardia
Vasopressin	V_1	Vasoconstriction	Refractory hypotension	Not used as first-line vasopressor
Dopamine	$D_1 = D_2 > \beta$ $> \alpha$	Ionotropy, chronotropy, vasoconstriction	Unstable bradycardia, hypotension, cardiogenic shock	β Effects predominate at lower doses, α effects at higher doses; may cause tachy-dysrhythmias
Dobutamine	$\beta_1 > \beta_2$, α	Ionotropy > chronotropy, mild vasodilatation	Cardiogenic and obstructive shock	Mild changes in heart rate

Receptor functions (*not a complete list of all receptor functions):
α_1, Vascular smooth muscle contraction; α_2, decreased sympathetic outflow (central); β_1, heart rate and cardiac contractility; β_2, vascular smooth muscle dilation, bronchodilation; D_1, renal, mesenteric, and cerebral smooth muscle vasodilatation; D_2, modifies transmitter release (central); V_1, vascular smooth muscle contraction.

23. **How do I dose common vasopressor and ionotropic medications?**
    Table 4.2.

Table 4.2 Vasoactive Agent Dosing	
AGENT	**DOSE**
Epinephrine	Continuous infusion: 0.05–2 mcg/kg/min Push dose: 5–20 mcg every 1–5 min (see No. 25)
Norepinephrine	Continuous infusion: 0.01–3 mcg/kg/min
Phenylephrine	Continuous infusion: 0.5–6 mcg/kg/min Push dose: 50–200 mcg every 1–5 min
Vasopressin	Continuous infusion: fixed rate of 0.04 U/min
Dopamine	Continuous infusion: 2–50 mcg/kg/min 2–10 mcg/kg/min for β effects >10 mcg/kg/min for α effects
Dobutamine	Continuous infusion: 2–40 mcg/kg/min

24. **Can vasopressors be given through a peripheral IV line?**
Administration of vasopressors through peripheral IV lines, as compared with central venous lines, may result in slightly more local tissue necrosis and extravasation events, especially when using distal lines for prolonged periods of time (i.e., >24 hours). However, due to the importance of not delaying vasopressor therapy, some institutions allow vasopressor administration via well-functioning peripheral lines for up to 24 hours.

25. **How do I make "push dose epinephrine"?**
"Cardiac epinephrine," also known as "code dose epi," consists of 1 mg of 1:10,000 epinephrine in a 10 mL ampule. Obtain a 10 mL saline syringe and push out 1 mL, leaving 9 mL of saline. Add 1 mL cardiac epinephrine (100 mcg) to create a solution of 10 mcg/mL inside the 10 mL syringe. "Push dose epinephrine" can be given to a hypotensive patient at a rate of 5–20 mcg (0.5–2 mL) every 1–5 minutes.

26. **Is there a preferred first-line vasopressor for shock?**
The choice of vasopressor may vary depending on the type of shock, but the most commonly used vasopressor is norepinephrine. Studies have shown improved rates of mortality as well as decreased incidence of arrhythmic events with norepinephrine when compared with dopamine. Some types of shock may benefit from the added ionotropic or chronotropic effects of epinephrine, such as some cardiogenic and neurogenic shock.

27. **How do I treat shock resulting from anaphylaxis?**
See Chapter 21.

28. **How do I treat cardiogenic shock?**
The treatment of cardiogenic shock should focus on improving myocardial contractility and overall pump function. Provide oxygen and ventilatory support, including the judicious use of noninvasive positive-pressure ventilation when pulmonary edema is present. Initiate inotropic support using dobutamine or dopamine, and identify the precipitating cause of cardiogenic shock and administer the appropriate treatment (e.g., thrombolysis or percutaneous coronary intervention in the setting of cardiogenic shock secondary to acute coronary syndrome). Consider intra-aortic balloon counter-pulsation, extracorporeal membrane oxygenation (ECMO), or cardiopulmonary bypass for patients with refractory shock.

29. **How do I treat shock caused by pulmonary embolism (PE)?**
Massive PE causes obstructive shock by reducing the cross-sectional area of the pulmonary outflow tract, thus causing right ventricular dilation, increased right-sided heart pressures, and ventricular septal bowing with decreased left ventricular filling, all of which result in hemodynamic compromise. Treatment includes optimizing oxygenation and ventilation, hemodynamic support using IV fluids and vasoactive agents, and use of thrombolytics or surgical embolectomy in the setting of refractory shock.

30. **In the above situation, aren't IV fluids dangerous?**
Traditional teaching is to increase right ventricular preload via IV fluid administration to "overcome" the obstructive shock state. Right ventricular preload can be measured using the CVP when this type of invasive monitoring is available. However, too much fluid may exacerbate right ventricular dilation, resulting in worsening right ventricular wall stress and decreased contractility, leading to further hemodynamic deterioration. Cautious use of IV fluids is recommended, keeping in mind that if a patient deteriorates while receiving a fluid bolus, it may be due to overly aggressive fluid administration. Excessive fluid administration leading to worsening cardiac output is a concern in both shock secondary to PE and cardiogenic shock. Early use of vasopressors, such as epinephrine or norepinephrine, is important in the setting of refractory shock.

31. **How do I treat shock resulting from cardiac tamponade?**

    As always, optimize oxygenation and ventilation, and then administer IV fluids to maintain elevated filling pressures. However, the principal therapies for cardiac tamponade are pericardiocentesis or pericardiotomy to relieve the source of the obstruction.

32. **What is neurogenic shock and how is it treated?**

    Neurogenic shock is a form of distributive shock resulting from spinal cord injury, in which sympathetic tone is lost. As a result of the loss of sympathetic innervation to the heart and vasculature, patients experiencing neurogenic shock are commonly hypotensive with either a normal or low heart rate. Administer IV fluids to normalize intravascular volume, and if hypotension persists, administer a vasopressor agent: IV phenylephrine (0.15–0.75 mcg/kg/min) is considered the classic first-line agent.

33. **How is ECMO used in the treatment of shock?**

    ECMO relies on a machine to function as an out-of-body lung that both oxygenates blood and removes carbon dioxide. It is used in the treatment of acute severe respiratory or cardiac failure that is refractory to usual treatment and will likely result in death if ECMO is not initiated. These conditions must be reversible, such that the use of ECMO is a temporary bridge to recovery. The two most common types of ECMO are venovenous (VV) and venoarterial (VA). In VV, the most common, blood is drained from a central vein and oxygenated prior to being returned proximal to the right atrium. This type of ECMO is utilized for severe respiratory failure without cardiac dysfunction: pneumonia, ARDS, smoke inhalation, status asthmaticus, airway obstruction, drowning, bridge to lung transplant, and pulmonary contusion. VA ECMO is utilized for cardiac failure with or without respiratory failure. Blood is drained from a central vein, oxygenated, and then returned to the aorta. VA ECMO is useful for multiple types of shock: obstructive shock secondary to massive PE; nonischemic cardiogenic shock, including cardiac arrest, distributive shock secondary to sepsis or anaphylaxis; and shock related to drug overdose.

KEY POINTS: SHOCK

1. *Shock* is defined as a clinical syndrome characterized by widespread inadequate oxygenation and supply of nutrients to tissues and organs, resulting in cellular dysfunction.
2. The five categories of shock are hypovolemic, cardiogenic, distributive, obstructive, and toxic/metabolic.
3. Serum lactate is a commonly used marker to assess the extent of systemic hypoperfusion and the response to resuscitation.
4. The primary resuscitation goals in patients suffering from shock are to optimize oxygenation and ventilation, improve hemodynamic support, and treat the underlying cause.

BIBLIOGRAPHY

De Backer D, Aldecoa C, Njimi H, et al. Dopamine versus norepinephrine in the treatment of septic shock: a meta-analysis. *Crit Care Med.* 2012;40(3):725–730.

Gaieski DF, Band RA, Abella BS, et al. Early goal-directed hemodynamic optimization combined with therapeutic hypothermia in comatose survivors of out-of-hospital cardiac arrest. *Resuscitation.* 2009;80:418–424.

Jones AE, Shapiro NI, Trzeciak S, et al. Lactate clearance vs central oxygen saturation as goals of early sepsis therapy: a randomized clinical trial. *JAMA.* 2010;303:739–746.

Liao MM, Lezotte D, Lowenstein SR, et al. Sensitivity of systemic inflammatory response syndrome for critical illness among ED patients. *Am J Emerg Med.* 2014;32:1319–1325.

Nguyen HB, Rivers EP, Knoblich BP, et al. Early lactate clearance is associated with improved outcome in severe sepsis and septic shock. *Crit Care Med.* 2004;32:1637–1642.

Rivers EP, Nguyen B, Havstad S, et al. Early goal-directed therapy in the treatment of severe sepsis and septic shock. *N Engl J Med.* 2001;345:1368–1377.

Shapiro NI, Howell MD, Talmor D, et al. Serum lactate as a predictor of mortality in emergency department patients with infection. *Ann Emerg Med.* 2005;45:524–528.

Yealy DM, Kellum JA, Huang DT, et al. A randomized trial of protocol-based care for early septic shock. *N Engl J Med.* 2014;370: 1683–1693.

CHAPTER 5

EMERGENCY ULTRASOUND

Julia Aogaichi Brant, MD and Molly E.W. Thiessen, MD

1. **What is ED ultrasound all about?**

   An ultrasound probe in the hands of the clinician has historically been considered the stethoscope of the twenty-first century. Extending beyond this definition, the technology of ultrasound is now an integral part of the evaluation and management of patients in the ED.

2. **Why should ultrasound be performed in the ED?**

   Focused ultrasound examinations performed by ED physicians allow for more timely, less invasive, and safer evaluations of patients. The etiology of undifferentiated hypotension or shortness of breath can be quickly determined and treatment initiated within minutes of ED arrival. Ectopic pregnancy and biliary colic may be evaluated rapidly, intraabdominal traumatic hemorrhage may be diagnosed without the invasiveness of diagnostic peritoneal lavage or the delay of a computed tomography (CT) scan, and patients with major trauma or suspected abdominal aortic aneurysm (AAA) may be evaluated quickly in the safety of the ED. The most recent American College of Emergency Physicians (ACEP) ultrasound guidelines add echocardiography, soft-tissue, bowel, musculoskeletal, urinary tract, thoracic, ocular, and deep venous thrombosis (DVT) ultrasound to core emergency ultrasound modalities. Their use in the ED can assist in rapid diagnosis of a variety of conditions. Additionally, ultrasound for procedural guidance, including line placement, nerve blocks, and lumbar punctures (LPs), has been shown to improve the safety of these emergency procedures.

3. **How does emergency ultrasound differ from ultrasound performed by the radiology department?**

   Emergency ultrasound is meant to be a focused, goal-directed examination with the intent of answering a specific clinical question that will direct immediate care at the bedside. Specific findings, such as the presence of intraperitoneal fluid in blunt abdominal trauma; intrauterine pregnancy (IUP) in suspected ectopic pregnancy; gallstones, wall thickness, or a sonographic Murphy sign in right upper quadrant pain; aortic dilation in suspected AAA; and pericardial fluid in patients with possible pericardial tamponade are used to make real-time patient care decisions in the ED. In contrast, an ultrasound performed by a radiologist is more comprehensive in that all structures viewed are evaluated.

4. **How about some basic ultrasonography physics?**

   Ultrasound images are generated as sound waves at various frequencies (MHz) that reflect off tissue interfaces. The higher the ultrasound frequency, the greater the resolution, but at the expense of reduced tissue penetration. Dense tissues, such as bone or gallstones, appear bright because most of the ultrasound energy is absorbed or reflected. Solid organs, such as the liver or spleen, show a gray scale of tissue architecture. All of the ultrasound energy passes through fluid or blood, leaving a black (anechoic) area on the screen. Ultrasound energy does not propagate well through air. Thus lung, hollow viscous structures, and air trapped within soft tissues or bowel are difficult to visualize. In general, abdominal and cardiac examinations utilize a 3.5- to 5-MHz probe, transvaginal ultrasound examinations a 7.5- to 10-MHz probe, and vascular or soft-tissue studies a 10- to 12-MHz specialized probe.

5. **Describe the basics of the trauma ultrasound examination.**

   The trauma ultrasound examination (also known as *focused assessment with sonography for trauma [FAST]*) is done rapidly at the patient's bedside during the secondary survey. The primary goal is to detect free intraperitoneal fluid, which appears as anechoic areas within the peritoneal cavity. Sites in the abdomen that are evaluated are the potential spaces that occur at dependent sites within the peritoneal cavity. These include the hepatorenal recess or Morison's pouch (Fig. 5.1), the splenorenal recess, the retrovesicular recess (pouch of Douglas in females), and both pericolic gutters. Oblique views of the right and left chest are obtained to search for hemothorax, and a subxiphoid or left parasternal cardiac image is obtained to locate pericardial effusion (Fig. 5.2).

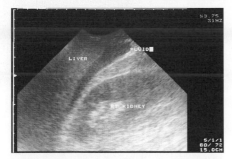

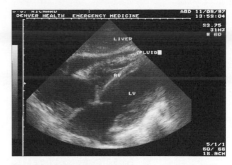

Fig. 5.1 View of the Morison pouch showing intraperitoneal fluid. *RT,* Right.

Fig. 5.2 Subxiphoid cardiac view shows a pericardial effusion. *LV,* Left ventricle; *RV,* right ventricle.

6. **Where is the best place to look for intraperitoneal fluid?**
   The sonographic examination should include all sites previously mentioned. The sensitivity increases from approximately 51% if only Morison's pouch is viewed to almost 90% if all are used.

7. **How does ultrasound compare with traditional means of evaluating the traumatic abdomen?**
   Physical examination is only 50% to 60% sensitive for detecting abdominal injuries after blunt trauma. Diagnostic peritoneal lavage is 95% sensitive but is not specific, resulting in unnecessary laparotomies. CT is sensitive for detecting abdominal injuries (>95%) but is costly, time consuming, and requires the patient to leave the ED. Prospective studies of ultrasound showed an 85%–96% sensitivity and upwards of 98% specificity for the detection of hemoperitoneum, with sensitivity approaching 100% in patients who were hypotensive from an abdominal source. The accuracy of ultrasound to detect the underlying parenchymal lesion varies widely.

8. **How should I use ultrasound in my evaluation of patients with blunt trauma?**
   Consider patient scenarios based on the following vital signs and ultrasound findings:
   • Stable vital signs, negative ultrasound
   • Stable vital signs, positive ultrasound
   • Unstable vital signs, negative ultrasound
   • Unstable vital signs, positive ultrasound

KEY POINTS: PRIMARY CHARACTERISTICS OF THE EMERGENCY ULTRASOUND EXAMINATION

1. Performed for a defined indication
2. Focused, not complete
3. Easily learned and quickly performed
4. Directed toward one or two easily recognizable findings
5. Directly impacts clinical decision making
6. Performed at the bedside

Patients with stable vital signs and a negative ultrasound who have no other significant injuries, have normal mental status, and are not intoxicated can be managed with observation, serial physical examinations, and serial ultrasound studies. Patients with stable vital signs and a positive ultrasound warrant an abdominal CT scan. If the vital signs are unstable and ultrasound is negative or indeterminate, other sources of hypotension should be considered, and if intraabdominal injury is not excluded, a bedside diagnostic peritoneal lavage can be performed. If the vital signs are unstable and the ultrasound is positive for free fluid, the patient should directly undergo a laparotomy.

9. **Can I determine how much intraperitoneal fluid is present based on the ultrasound image?**
   No; conflicting data exist. No study has yet shown an accurate means of quantifying the amount of intraperitoneal fluid that is present based on its sonographic appearance.

10. **What are some of the pitfalls I may encounter during a trauma ultrasound examination of the abdomen?**
    Although relatively rare, one of the more concerning aspects of emergency ultrasound is the false-negative study. In terms of abdominal trauma, clotted blood is the finding that mimics a negative study the closest. An example of clotted blood found in the Morison pouch is shown in Fig. 5.3. This image was initially interpreted to be liver parenchyma because of a similar echogenic pattern. False-positive findings that simulate hemoperitoneum can occur in the setting of ascites, urine from a ruptured bladder, bowel contents from bowel perforation, perinephric

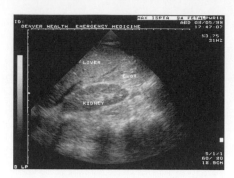

Fig. 5.3 Clotted blood in the Morison pouch.

fat, fluid from a vetriculoperitoneal (VP) shunt, and a fluid-filled stomach or bowel. Serial ultrasounds may identify free intraperitoneal fluid that was not present on initial ultrasound.

11. **What is extended focused assessment with sonography for trauma (EFAST)?**
    EFAST incorporates use of thoracic ultrasound into a standard FAST examination to detect pneumothorax. In most cases, a high-frequency linear transducer is applied to the anterior chest wall in the midclavicular line at the level of the second intercostal space, and the clinician is looking for the absence of normal lung "sliding" and lack of comet-tail artifact, indicating pneumothorax. Additional views are often obtained in the midaxillary line, and alternative probes may be used. EFAST has been found to be more sensitive than chest radiography for the detection of occult pneumothoraces in patients experiencing trauma (69% vs. 37%), although both have a very high specificity (99% for EFAST and 98% for chest radiography).

KEY POINTS: ELEMENTS OF THE EFAST EXAMINATION

1. Hepatorenal recess or Morison pouch image (see Fig. 5.1) to search for hemoperitoneum, with additional oblique view of the right chest to search for hemothorax
2. Splenorenal recess image to search for hemoperitoneum, with additional oblique view of the left chest to search for hemothorax
3. Retrovesicular recess image (pouch of Douglas in females) to search for hemoperitoneum
4. Images of both pericolic gutters to search for hemoperitoneum
5. Subxiphoid or left parasternal cardiac image to search for pericardial effusion
6. Bilateral anterior chest wall images to evaluate for pneumothorax

---

12. **What are the sonographic appearances of the gallbladder and related structures?**
    The gallbladder is cystic, so the sonographic appearance is a pear-shaped structure that is anechoic. Surrounding this anechoic area is a ring of midechogenicity that corresponds to the gallbladder wall. Normally it is less than 4 mm wide, but it can be thicker immediately after eating (when contracted), or if in an edematous state, such as liver failure, ascites, congestive heart failure, renal disease, or AIDS. The wall should be measured from outer wall to inner wall on the most anterior portion of the scan (that closest to the probe). Stones are typically circular in nature, can be of any size, and are bright, or hyperechoic, on their proximal side. Ultrasound does not penetrate stones, so distal to the stone there is a shadow (Fig. 5.4). This also is called the *headlight sign,* signifying the presence of a calcified gallstone. Polyps or folds in the gallbladder can sometimes be confused for stones, but they lack shadowing. Sludge is a collection of the precipitants of bile that collects in layers within the gallbladder and appears sonographically as mildly echogenic material without any shadowing.

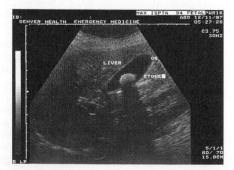

Fig. 5.4 Long-axis view of the gall bladder shows a gallstone. The gallstone is represented by an echogenic proximal surface and distal attenuation shadow. *GB,* Gall bladder.

13. **What findings are suggestive of acute cholecystitis?**
The primary findings of the emergency gallbladder ultrasound are the presence of gallstones and a sonographic Murphy sign (defined as maximal tenderness over an ultrasound-detected gallbladder). The presence of these primary findings has a 92% positive predictive value and a 95% negative predictive value for the presence of cholecystitis. Other findings, such as wall thickening (>4 mm), ductal dilation (>5 mm, increasing 0.04 mm/year over age 50 years), pericholecystic fluid, sludge, and an emphysematous gallbladder, are considered secondary findings and are less reliably seen. Ultrasound is insensitive at detecting choledocholithiasis.

14. **What are the indications for pelvic ultrasonography in the ED?**
Ultrasonography is the imaging study of choice for evaluating abdominal pain or bleeding in patients in the first or second trimester of pregnancy. The goal of ED ultrasound is to establish the presence of an IUP, so as to effectively rule out an ectopic pregnancy. Ruptured ectopic pregnancy is the second leading cause of maternal mortality, and the number one cause of maternal mortality during the first trimester.

15. **How early can an IUP be detected using ultrasound? What value of β-human chorionic gonadotropin (HCG) does this correspond to?**
An IUP may be detectable as early as 4 weeks' gestational age by transvaginal ultrasound (6 weeks using trans-abdominal ultrasound). The discriminatory zone is the level of β-HCG at which one would expect to see evidence of an IUP by ultrasound. Although this depends on the institution where the patient is being seen, it is typically at a β-HCG level of 1000–2000 mIU/mL by transvaginal ultrasound and 5000 mIU/mL by transabdominal ultrasound. A gestational sac is seen at approximately 4–5 weeks' gestational age, and cardiac activity can be measured as early as 6 weeks' gestational age. A transabdominal scan should be the first approach to identifying an IUP, followed by a transvaginal scan if unable to visualize an intrauterine pregnancy as evidenced by a yolk.

16. **How sensitive is ultrasound for the evaluation of ectopic pregnancy?**
Transvaginal ultrasound has a sensitivity of 67% and specificity of 92% for true IUP. But how does this translate into identifying ectopic pregnancy in the ED? Studies have shown that 75%–80% of pregnant patients have a diagnostic ultrasound (i.e., either an IUP or a demonstrable ectopic pregnancy). In the remaining 20% of patients with nondiagnostic ultrasounds, nearly one-fourth have ectopic pregnancies. Patients with a β-HCG level above the discriminatory zone without evidence of an IUP on ultrasound are at particularly high risk of an ectopic pregnancy, even in the absence of a visualized ectopic pregnancy at the time of ED examination. This increased risk of ectopic pregnancy among patients with nondiagnostic ultrasounds warrants obstetric-gynecologic consultation in the ED.

17. **Describe the pitfalls in pelvic ultrasonography.**
For emergency physicians the goal of pelvic ultrasonography is to determine whether an IUP is present. It is not clear how well emergency physicians evaluate the adnexa, pelvic free fluid, or ovaries. Cornual pregnancies may be mistaken for an IUP, with an attendant risk of rupture and hemorrhage. The question of heterotopic pregnancies (i.e., simultaneous IUP and ectopic pregnancy) must also be considered. In populations without risk factors for ectopic pregnancy, the risk of a heterotopic gestation is approximately 1 in 30,000 pregnancies. The incidence increases markedly, however, in patients with preexisting pelvic inflammatory disease or scarring and is greatest for patients receiving medical fertility assistance, in whom the incidence is estimated to be 1 in 100 to 1 in 900 pregnancies, depending on the type of assistance. Thus a comprehensive pelvic ultrasound performed by a certified sonographer must be performed in these patients, irrespective of an IUP identified on bedside ultrasound. A pseudosac can be seen in 20% of ectopic pregnancies. It consists of a single-ringed structure in the endometrial cavity, formed in response to the β-HCG produced by the abnormal pregnancy, and is easily mistaken for a true gestational sac, which consists of two concentric rings. Transvaginal ultrasound is sensitive enough to detect fluid or blood within the endometrial cavity, which should raise suspicion that it is not a true gestational sac.

18. **How can emergency ultrasound help in the management of abdominal complaints?**
In addition to trauma, emergency ultrasound can rapidly identify a number of bowel emergencies. Acute appendicitis can be identified by emergency ultrasound, resulting in a decrease in time to diagnosis and less exposure to CT radiation. The sensitivity and specificity of emergency ultrasound for appendicitis is 60%–96% and 68%–98%, respectively. Small bowel obstruction and ileus can also be evaluated with emergency ultrasound, and is more sensitive and specific than x-ray. Ultrasound can rapidly determine the presence of a suspected hernia, and aid in real-time reduction. In pediatrics, emergency providers have shown 100% sensitivity and 100% specificity in identifying pyloric stenosis. Additionally, emergency ultrasound can rapidly diagnose intussusception in children, reducing complications such as bowel perforation from delayed diagnosis.

19. **What other abdominal structures can be evaluated by emergency ultrasound?**
Evaluation of the abdominal aorta can be useful in elderly patients who have a pulsatile abdominal mass, nontraumatic abdominal pain, flank pain, hypotension of unknown cause, or unexplained pulseless electrical activity. AAA is manifested by aortic diameter greater than 3 cm, with most symptomatic aneurysms being greater than 5 cm (Fig. 5.5). Studies by emergency physicians showed sensitivity of 99% and a specificity of 99% for the detection of AAA. Ultrasound-determined aortic diameter has shown a 90% correlation to pathologic specimens, and use of emergency ultrasound has been shown to result in decreased length of stay (average, 50 minutes) and time to treatment for AAA.

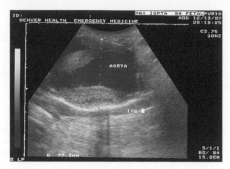

Fig. 5.5 Long-axis view of a 7.75-cm diameter abdominal aortic aneurysm. *IVC,* Inferior vena cava.

20. **What is the significance of increased aortic diameter?**
    Longitudinal studies have shown that patients with AAA have an increase in aortic diameter of approximately 0.5 cm/year. Patients with an aortic diameter of greater than 5 cm have a 25% chance of rupture within 5 years, with larger aneurysms having a greater chance of rupture. Patients who have aneurysms that rupture have a mortality rate of greater than 80%, so ultrasound is an important tool in the detection of AAA.

21. **Describe the uses of cardiac ultrasonography in the ED.**
    These are primary indications for cardiac ultrasonography in the ED (see Table 5.1):
    • It may be used during the trauma examination to detect pericardial effusions in patients thought to have mechanisms of injury or clinical presentations consistent with pericardial tamponade or cardiac rupture.
    • It may be used for detection of nontraumatic pericardial effusions (i.e., malignancy, uremic, rheumatologic).
    • It may be used for the detection of right ventricular strain as seen in the setting of a pulmonary embolus or pulmonary hypertension.
    • Another important indication includes the evaluation of patients experiencing cardiac arrest. Contractility can be assessed in patients with cardiac arrest when there is a question of pulseless electrical activity. When there is no evidence of cardiac contractility and other reversible causes of pulseless electrical activity have been ruled out, strong consideration should be given to terminating the resuscitation.
    • Emergent echocardiography can be used for assessing undifferentiated hypotension.
    • Some physicians are utilizing transesophageal echocardiography to guide resuscitation in the setting of cardiac arrest.

Table 5.1 Emergency Ultrasound Core Application	
CORE APPLICATIONS	
Abdominal	**Musculoskeletal**
Aortic	Abscess incision and drainage
Biliary	Fracture evaluation
Urinary tract	Nerve block
Bowel	**Ocular**
Pelvic	Retinal detachment
Intrauterine pregnancy	Vitreous hemorrhage
Trauma	Ocular trauma
Focused abdominal sonography for trauma	Increased intracranial pressure
Cardiac	**Procedural**
Emergent echocardiography	Pericardiocentesis
Pericardial effusion	Thoracentesis
Tamponade	Foreign body and detection and removal
Contractility	Arthrocentesis
Deep Venous Thrombosis Evaluation	Pacemaker placement
Thoracic	Central line placement
Pleural effusion	Lumbar puncture
Pneumothorax	
Airway	

Updated from American College of Emergency Physicians (ACEP): ACEP Emergency Ultrasound Guidelines, 2016.

22. **How can ultrasound be used in the ED to evaluate patients with undifferentiated hypotension?**
    A combination of ultrasound evaluations can be used to differentiate the etiology of shock in ED patients. There are multiple protocols used to perform resuscitative ultrasound. However, most include the following: a subcostal cardiac view to evaluate for pericardial effusion and tamponade; an inferior vena cava (IVC) view looking for greater than 50% collapse with inspiration, indicating low intravascular volume; a parasternal long-axis cardiac view to estimate overall left ventricular function; a parasternal short-axis view to evaluate right ventricular enlargement; an apical four-chamber cardiac view to estimate overall function and evaluate relative chamber size (right vs. left); a view of the hepatorenal recess to evaluate for free intraperitoneal fluid; a view of the pelvis and retrovesical area to evaluate for free intraperitoneal fluid; lung views bilaterally in the second intracostal space to rule out pneumothoraces; and, finally, a view of the abdominal aorta to evaluate for aneurysm. Use of this systematic, goal-directed protocol in patients in the ED who have undifferentiated nontraumatic hypotension allows physicians to narrow their differential diagnosis sooner and gives them a more accurate impression of the class of shock and final diagnosis (Table 5.2).

Table 5.2 Use of Ultrasound for Undifferentiated Shock

	CARDIAC VIEWS	IVC VIEW	ABDOMINAL VIEWS
Hypovolemia caused by abdominal injury	Hyperdynamic	>50% collapse with inspiration	+ Free fluid
Hypovolemia without injury	Hyperdynamic	>50% collapse with inspiration	− Free fluid
Tamponade	+ Pericardial effusion on subcostal cardiac view	No collapse	
AAA	Hyperdynamic (depending on patient's underlying cardiac function)	± collapse depending on presence of abdominal free fluid	+ AAA, ± free fluid
Cardiogenic shock	Globally hypodynamic or regional wall-motion abnormalities on parasternal long-axis and apical four-chamber cardiac views	No collapse	− Free fluid
Pulmonary embolism	Right heart strain on parasternal long-axis and apical four-chamber cardiac views	No collapse	− Free fluid

AAA, Abdominal aortic aneurysm; *IVC,* inferior vena cava.

23. **What is the role of ultrasound in the evaluation of patients with suspected renal colic?**
    Emergency ultrasound for renal colic has been recently studied in a large, randomized population. Patients who received emergency ultrasound for renal colic initially, over CT scan, had a significantly lower radiation exposure, without significant missed high-risk diagnoses, adverse events, hospitalizations, or return ED visits. When possible, emergency ultrasound should be the first diagnostic study for renal colic, with further imaging with CT based on patient presentation and clinician judgment.

24. **How is lower extremity venous ultrasound performed in the ED to diagnose DVT?**
    A linear transducer with a high frequency range is used. The examination should start proximally with the vein in a transverse plane just below the inguinal ligament where the common femoral vein can be visualized. Compression followed by no compression should occur in 1-cm increments until the femoral vein dives into the adductor canal. Next, the popliteal region is visualized again in 1-cm increments. An examination is considered to be negative when complete compression occurs to the point that the anterior and posterior walls of the vein touch. In a positive study, the vessel walls will not touch; the clot echogenicity can vary greatly from echogenic to nonechogenic. A 2018 study shows the sensitivity and specificity of ED DVT studies as high as 93% and 90%, respectively. For accurate diagnosis of DVT, additional components, such as pretest probability and the D-dimer assay, may need to be considered.

25. **How can soft-tissue/musculoskeletal ultrasound be utilized in the ED?**
    The most common way to use ultrasound for this modality in the ED is for assessment of abscess in the setting of cellulitis. Ultrasound has been shown to be 98% sensitive and 88% specific for suspected abscess (vs. needle aspiration). It has been shown to change management in 56% of patients with cellulitis. It is also effective in

reducing rate of abscess drainage failure from 17% to 3%, reducing the need for additional procedures. Emergency ultrasound is also expanding to include fracture detection, tendon injuries, and joint effusions.

26. **What are some procedural uses for ultrasound in the ED?**
Emergency ultrasound for LPs is especially useful for patients with difficult landmarks secondary to obesity or spinal curvature. The curvilinear probe is used to identify lumbar spinous processes, the sacrum, and the L4-5 interspace, and the intersection marked with a sterile pen. LP success rates improve from 76% to 96% using this method of ultrasound guidance for landmarks., decreasing the need for multiple attempts, length of ED stay, and need for irradiation under fluoroscopy. Another use of ultrasound in the ED is for nerve blocks to provide anesthetic for complex laceration repairs or foreign body removals, as well as for pain control fractures at low risk of compartment syndrome. Nerve blocks can reduce opioid use in the department while waiting for the appropriate surgical intervention. Ultrasound has been shown to dramatically reduce the complications associated with nerve blocks.

27. **How can emergency ultrasound be used for eye complaints?**
In the ED, many patients present with ocular complaints. Ocular ultrasound can be used to determine true ocular emergencies from those that could suffice with outpatient follow-up. Emergent ocular conditions that can be diagnosed by emergency ultrasound include foreign body, lens dislocation, retina detachment, vitreous detachment, and vitreous hemorrhage. The optic nerve sheath diameter can be measured on ultrasound as a noninvasive way to estimate intracranial pressure (ICP) in critically ill patients. The sensitivity and specificity of increased optic nerve sheath diameter for elevated ICP is 88% and 93%, respectively. Additionally, in patients who have significant eyelid edema, emergency ultrasound can be used to identify pupillary response and extraocular movements.

28. **What is the utility of emergency ultrasound in airway management?**
Emergency ultrasound can be used to confirm endotracheal (ET) tube placement in the trachea, or inappropriately in the esophagus, with gentle manipulation to demonstrate movement.

29. **What are some future applications for emergency ultrasound?**
Uses for emergency ultrasound continue to rapidly expand. This is clearly demonstrated in the 2016 ACEP clinical practice guidelines for ultrasound that expand upon core applications. For instance, one of the fastest-growing applications is to guide invasive procedures. This is not confined to vascular access, which is already widely done by many trained ancillary staff members in the ED, but is also applicable to other procedures like central lines, fracture identification and reduction, placement of an intravenous pacer wire, and suprapubic bladder aspiration. Transesophageal ECHO (TEE) is now being used in some EDs to guide resuscitation, although its use is still controversial. Emergency ultrasound is tremendously useful in the evaluation of patients in cardiac arrest, with undifferentiated hypotension or shock, testicular or ovarian torsion, and lung pathology.

30. **Has the political environment changed with respect to emergency physicians using ultrasound?**
Ultrasound use by emergency physicians has evolved from a novelty experience to something that is taught across all levels of medical education. Many medical schools are incorporating clinical ultrasound into their basic science curriculum. The availability of handheld devices has made it easy to bring ultrasound into almost every setting, including those that are more remote and resource limited. As such, it is recommended by ACEP to be taught in all residency programs early in training, is a required element of the recently instated Accreditation Council for Graduate Medical Education (ACGME) milestones, and is tested on emergency medicine specialty boards and the national in-service examinations. There are now more than 100 emergency ultrasound fellowships across the country, and ultrasound is widely used in clinical practice. As such, the question is no longer whether or not ultrasound will be used by emergency physicians, but rather how it can or should be used for optimal care of patients in the ED.

BIBLIOGRAPHY

Policy Statement, Ultrasound Guidelines: Emergency, Point-of-Care, and Clinical Ultrasound Guidelines in Medicine, American College of Emergency Physicians, approved by Board of Directors June, 2016, https://www.acep.org/globalassets/new-pdfs/policy-statements/ultrasound-guidelines—emergency-point-of-care-and-clinical-ultrasound-guidelines-in-medicine.pdf. Accessed April 10, 2020.
Bloom BA, Gibbons RC. Focused Assessment with Sonography for Trauma (FAST) [Updated 2018 Oct 27]. In: *StatPearls* [Internet]. Treasure Island, FL: StatPearls Publishing; 2018 Jan.
Evans DP, Tozer J, Joyce M, et al. Comparison of ultrasound-guided and landmark-based lumbar punctures in inexperienced resident physicians. *J Ultrasound Med*. 2019;38:613–620.
Gaspari RJ, Sanseverino A, Gleeson T. Abscess incision and drainage with or without ultrasonography: a randomized controlled trial. *Ann Emerg Med*. 2019;73(1):1–7.
Pedraza García J, Valle Alonso J, Ceballos García P, et al. Comparison of the accuracy of emergency department–performed Point-of-Care-Ultrasound (POCUS) in the diagnosis of lower-extremity deep vein thrombosis. *J Emerg Med*. 2018;54(5):656–664.
Sivitz AB, Tejani C, Cohen SG. Evaluation of hypertrophic pyloric stenosis by pediatric emergency physician sonography. *Acad Emerg Med*. 2013;20(7):646–651.
Smith-Bindman R, Aubin C, Bailitz J, et al. Ultrasonography versus computed tomography for suspected nephrolithiasis. *N Engl J Med*. 2014;371(12):1100–1110.
Zenobii MF, Accogli E, Domanico A, et al. Update on bedside ultrasound (US) diagnosis of acute cholecystitis (AC). *Intern Emerg Med*. 2016;11(2):261–264.
Zieleskiewicz L, Fresco R, Duclos G, et al. Integrating extended focused assessment with sonography for trauma (eFAST) in the initial assessment of severe trauma: impact on the management of 756 patients. *Injury*. 2018;49(10):1774–1780.

CHAPTER 6

GERIATRIC EMERGENCY MEDICINE

Kathleen Davenport, MD, Adriane Lesser, MS, and Kelly Ko, PhD

1. **Why dedicate a chapter to geriatric emergency medicine?**

   In 2015, there were 46 million adults aged 65 and older in the United States, a number that is expected to double by 2060, when this age bracket will account for nearly a quarter of all Americans. ED encounters associated with this age group are also increasing, from about 16 million in 2001 to over 21 million in 2015. Furthermore, older adults account for up to 46% of all ED visits resulting in admission, as well as the majority of potentially avoidable admissions. Geriatric patients have unique medical and social characteristics, and diseases often present atypically in this population. They often have multiple medical comorbidities, take multiple medications, and experience complex physiologic changes. Not surprisingly, geriatric patients stay in the ED longer and require more diagnostic studies than younger patients. Additionally, cognitive impairment is not uncommon in older adult patients, and so a careful assessment of the patient's psychosocial environment is essential before making decisions about disposition.

2. **What is a geriatric ED?**

   Geriatric EDs (GEDs) are EDs with specialized workflows and processes to address the unique needs of older patients, with an emphasis on improving outcomes (including reducing unnecessary hospitalizations and ED revisits). Senior-specific risk screenings may be conducted by a trained nurse, and specialized assessment, treatment, disposition, and follow-up processes are provided by an interdisciplinary team, which could include staff from pharmacy, geriatrics, physical therapy, psychiatry, social work, and other relevant areas. GEDs may also have physical design enhancements such as nonskid floors, as well as walkers and visual and hearing aids for patients in need. The American College of Emergency Physicians (ACEP) launched a national GED accreditation program in 2018.

3. **What are common geriatric conditions, and how can the ED respond?**

   Frailty, delirium and cognitive decline, functional impairments, falls, and polypharmacy are among the most common geriatric conditions. In addition, access to adequate social supports and services can also present challenges to geriatric patients presenting to the ED. When warranted, brief risk screenings can be conducted to assess general risk, functional capacity, mobility/fall risk, mentation (e.g., depression, agitation, dementia, and delirium), nutrition, potentially inappropriate medications, and elder abuse, among others.

4. **What important physiologic or normal changes often occur with aging?**
   - Neurologic: Loss of brain mass, decreased efficiency of the blood–brain barrier, decreased response to temperature changes and change in autonomic system function
   - Body composition: Decreased lean body weight and bone mass, increase in adipose tissue with redistribution, decreased total body water
   - Cardiovascular: Decreased cardiac output, decreased maximal heart rate of the sinus node, reduction in baroreflex-mediated cardioacceleration with increased systolic blood pressure and increased afterload
   - Pulmonary: Decreased vital capacity, decreased functional reserve, and decreased cilia movement
   - Musculoskeletal: Decreased skeletal muscle, leading to loss of muscle strength and mass, deterioration of cartilage, decreased bone mineralization, and loss of height
   - Head, eye, ear, nose, and throat (HEENT): Impaired hearing (loss of ability to hear high-frequency sounds); vision (presbyopia or difficulty seeing close up); smell ability diminishes; taste changes with decreased ability to taste salt
   - Renal: Decreased renal function due to decrease in the number of glomeruli and decreased blood flow; decreased ability to concentrate urine
   - Immune system: Decreased T cells and cellular immunity; decreased number of circulating antibodies
   - Dermatologic: Impaired thermoregulation due to decreased sweat glands, atrophy of skin, reduced elasticity

5. **Don't older patients always have abnormal laboratory values?**

   No. Most laboratory values in geriatric patients do not require different reference ranges from traditional adult values, and the fact that the patient is elderly does not justify an abnormal laboratory value. There are, however, some exceptions in patients older than age 65:
   - Elevated serum alkaline phosphatase (may be 2.5 times greater than the normal)
   - Elevated fasting blood glucose (range 135–150 mg/dL)

- Elevated erythrocyte sedimentation rate (40 mm/h)
- Decreased hemoglobin (11.0 g/dL in women or 11.5 g/dL in men)
- Elevated blood urea nitrogen (28–35 mg/dL)
- Decreased creatinine clearance (even with a normal creatinine) due to decreased glomerular filtration rate (GFR)

6. **How can prehospital personnel facilitate the care of older patients?**
   Older patients account for more than one third of emergency medical services (EMS) transports to the ED. Prehospital providers can obtain information from family or health care workers at the scene regarding the patient's social and physical environment, his or her baseline functional and mental status, and reason for EMS activation. EMS personnel should obtain lists of medications the patient is using and any documentation regarding living wills or advance directives (see Chapter 7).

7. **Why is a fall considered a serious threat to the older patient?**
   Ten to fifteen percent of geriatric falls result in serious injury, and 50% of patients who require hospitalization die within 1 year of their fall. Falls are the main cause of ED admissions for elderly patients (15%–30%). Falls may result from either physiologic or environmental factors. Physiologic factors include muscle weakness, gait and balance disorders, visual impairment, cognitive impairment, postural hypotension, and syncope. Environmental factors include dark hallways, loose rugs, and low-lying tables. Nearly 6% of falls result in fractures. Falls may also be the chief symptom of other pathologies, such as acute myocardial infarction (AMI), sepsis, medication toxicity, acute abdominal pathology, and elder abuse. Use of psychotropic medications, such as benzodiazepines, narcotics, and other sedatives, are associated with an increased risk of falls in the elderly.

8. **Should I be concerned about atypical presentations of AMI in older patients?**
   Yes; 80% of deaths caused by ischemic heart disease are in patients >65 years. Atypical presentations are the norm for AMI in the elderly. Chest pain and diaphoresis are less likely; dyspnea is the most common chief complaint in patients >80 years of age presenting with an AMI. Diagnosis is made even harder by the fact that 50% of patients with an AMI had no evidence of ischemia or infarct on their presenting electrocardiograms (ECGs). The ECG is often nondiagnostic in older adults because of preexisting conduction system disease (e.g., left bundle-branch block), presence of a ventricular pacemaker, prior infarct, left ventricular hypertrophy, metabolic abnormalities, or drug effects (e.g., hypokalemia, digoxin), and the high prevalence of non–ST-segment elevation myocardial infarction (NSTEMI). The atypical presentations of AMI in older patients can be remembered by the mnemonic *GRANDFATHERS:*
   General malaise
   Refers to a gastrointestinal complaint
   Altered mental status
   Neurologic deficits
   Dyspnea
   Falls or Flu symptoms
   Atypical chest pain
   Trouble walking
   Hypotension
   Exhaustion
   Reverse in functional status
   Syncope or presyncope

9. **What is the significance of fever in older patients?**
   Infection, especially from pneumonia, influenza, and bacteremia, are among the top 10 causes of death in older adults. Aging is associated with a decreased response to pyrogens, lower basal body temperature, changes in thermal homeostasis, and a decreased production and conservation of heat, which all lead to a blunted fever response. Tachycardia is also less likely, given that older patients have a lower maximum heart rate and decreased catecholamine response. This is especially true for seniors living in long-term care facilities. The Practice Guidelines Committee of the Infectious Diseases of America recommend a clinical evaluation for residents in skilled nursing facilities with single oral temperature over 100°F (37.8°C), or persistent oral temperature of over 99°F (37.2°C). If an older patient has a fever, that is a significant finding and a concerning warning sign for a serious bacterial infection.

10. **Speaking of infections, how do infectious pathologies present in older patients?**
    Immune system function decreases as we age due to altered macrophage function, compromised mucocutaneous defenses, and diminished cytokine production and T-cell function. Other comorbidities such as renal dysfunction, diabetes, congestive heart failure, chronic lung disease, and malnutrition further exacerbate the weakened immune defense mechanisms. The most common conditions are pneumonia (25%), urinary tract infection (22%), and sepsis/bacteremia (18%). Infectious presentations are often atypical in the elderly. Falls, delirium, decreased appetite, and failure to thrive may be the only clinical manifestations of otherwise serious infections. For example, a potentially serious infection, such as acute cholecystitis, may present without pain (5%), without fever (56%), and without leukocytosis (41%). Similarly, appendicitis presents with classic symptoms in only 20% of geriatric cases, with fever in less than half of these patients.

11. **Why is it important to know the current medications of older patients?**

Adverse drug-related events and polypharmacy (i.e., use of multiple medicines) are a significant cause of morbidity, including iatrogenic illness, in older patients. The average older person takes more than four prescription drugs daily, an amount that is even higher for institutionalized patients. Adverse reactions to medications are directly proportional to the number of medications being taken. Recent data suggest that three medication classes caused 48% of all ED visits for adverse drug effects in patients >65 years: oral anticoagulant or antiplatelet agents (warfarin, aspirin, and clopidogrel), antidiabetic agents (insulin, metformin, glyburide, and glipizide), and agents with a narrow therapeutic index (digoxin and phenytoin).

12. **What presenting complaints should lead me to suspect that the patient is experiencing an adverse reaction to medications?**

- Falls – even if the patient describes a trip and fall, an adverse reaction from a high-risk medication may have caused the altered balance
- Altered level of consciousness
- Weakness
- Dizziness or lightheadedness
- Syncope

13. **Do older patients tolerate trauma very well?**

No. Geriatric patients have different mechanisms of injury, with falls making up a large proportion of severe trauma. The number of comorbidities and the use of anticoagulants generally are higher in the geriatric population, and this appears to contribute directly to poorer outcomes related to trauma. Trauma in older patients is often undertriaged, leading to delay in care and missed injuries. Whereas geriatric patients make up only 18.6% of the trauma population, they account for 28% of trauma deaths in the United States and consume approximately one-third of health care dollars spent on trauma.

14. **Should I be reassured if a geriatric victim of trauma has normal vital signs with apparently minor injuries?**

No. Vital signs in older patients may remain normal until acute deterioration occurs. Geriatric patients have a blunted tachycardic response to injury and may be on medications to further blunt an increase in heart rate. A "normal" blood pressure of 120/80 mmHg may represent relative hypotension in the elderly patient with hypertension. Additionally, the elderly patient's diminished cardiovascular reserve, increased susceptibility to fractures, and the presence of comorbid conditions such as coronary artery disease can result in significant morbidity, even with injuries that appear to be minor. Older patients also have the highest trauma mortality rate of any age group, and normal vital signs or a low injury severity score should never put the physician at ease. Furthermore, ~11% of older patients experience abuse and may present with "minor trauma."

15. **Which presentations in geriatric trauma are associated with an extremely high mortality rate?**

- Major automobile accidents in drivers over 75 have the highest mortality of any age group (>50% mortality)
- Pedestrian struck (>25% mortality)
- Falls – which are the main cause of death in geriatric trauma
- Presenting systolic blood pressure <130 mmHg
- Acidosis (pH <7.35)
- Multiple fractures – especially rib fractures (12% mortality for >1 rib fracture); hip and pelvic fractures (1-year mortality rate of 30%)
- Head injury (67% of unconscious older trauma patients die)

16. **Can procedural sedation be performed safely in the geriatric patient?**

Yes. Procedural sedation can be performed safely, but with age, there are changes in the distribution, metabolism, absorption, and elimination of medications. Elderly patients also have increased central nervous system sensitivity to analgesic and sedative medications. A rule of thumb in older patients is to start low and go slow with medications.

17. **Should I resuscitate an older patient who is in cardiac arrest?**

Yes. Resuscitation studies document no difference in the percentage of successful outcomes across the age spectrum, and elderly patients who survive are no more likely to sustain irreversible brain injury than younger patients, making high-quality cardiopulmonary resuscitation (CPR) even more important. Unless there is a well-defined advance directive, there should be no discrimination based on age in resuscitating elderly patients in cardiac arrest.

18. **How does my approach to acute abdominal pain change in older patients?**

Compared with that of younger patients, elderly patients' mortality rates are six to eight times higher and surgery rates are doubled. Elderly patients have decreased pain perception and are more likely to have normal vital signs in the face of significant intraabdominal pathology; 80% of older patients with a perforated ulcer do not have rigidity. In one study, 30% of older adults who had surgical abdominal pain did not show signs of either a fever

Table 6.1 Differentiation Between Delirium and Dementia

DELIRIUM	DEMENTIA
Acute in onset	Insidious in onset
Decreased level of consciousness	Clear consciousness
Waxes and wanes	Progressive decline
Reversible cause	Usually irreversible cause
Irregular sleep-wake pattern	Regular sleep-wake pattern

or leukocytosis. These factors cause delays in diagnosis, higher perforation rates, and higher mortality rates in the elderly. Keep a broad differential diagnosis and consider the common disorders such as appendicitis and cholecystitis, but also diseases specific to older patients, such as diverticulitis, volvulus, mesenteric ischemia, abdominal aortic aneurysm, and carcinomas. Abdominal pain in the elderly may also be the presenting symptom of a cardiac event.

19. **Which is more concerning in the acute setting, dementia or delirium?**
Delirium is more concerning in the acute setting, as it is considered a medical emergency and is associated with a higher mortality rate following ED visits. The older patient may already have dementia, which is a chronic condition, but a sudden change in mental status may represent an acute organic process, such as infection or an adverse reaction to a medication.

20. **How do I differentiate between delirium and dementia?**
See Table 6.1.

21. **What are the four types of elder abuse?**
Elder abuse prevalence in the United States is estimated at 11%. It is often underdiagnosed and occurs as one or more of the following types:
    • *Physical abuse.* Use of force that results in bodily injury or pain (e.g., hitting, biting, slapping, sexual assault, burns, or unreasonable restraint [physical, chemical]).
    • *Psychological abuse.* Verbal and nonverbal threats made with the intent of causing emotional pain or injury (most common form – about 35% of elder abuse).
    • *Financial/material exploitation.* Illegal or improper use of an older adult's resources for monetary or personal profit.
    • *Neglect.* Failure of the caretaker to provide the services necessary to avoid physical harm, mental anguish, or mental illness. This neglect can be intentional or unintentional.

22. **What red flags in an older patient's history should alert the physician to the possibility of elder abuse?**
    • Delay in presentation with injury
    • Vague or implausible explanation for injury
    • Repetitive injuries
    • Missed appointments and noncompliance with medications
    • No caregiver accompanying an impaired patient to the ED

23. **What red flags in the physical examination of an older patient should alert the physician to the possibility of elder abuse?**
    • Subdued, oversedated, or withdrawn behavior
    • Fear or hesitancy to talk
    • Unkempt appearance or poor nutrition
    • Multiple or unexplained bruises, abrasions, or lacerations
    • Burns, bites, or pressure sores
    • Occult fracture
    • Fecal impaction

24. **What special concerns are there in discharging older patients?**
    • *Cognitive function.* Does the patient understand the discharge instructions? Can the patient safely live independently and self-administer medications?
    • *Physical function.* Can the patient perform the activities of daily living (e.g., bathing, dressing, and feeding)? Does the patient require an assistance device such as a walker or wheelchair?
    • *Physical environment.* Can the patient safely return with his or her current cognitive or functional status? Did the current environment contribute to the ED presentation? For example, are there fall risk reduction changes that could be made in the home such as handrails in the bathroom and decluttering walkways?

- *Social environment.* Will the caregiver or spouse be able to care for the patient? Is health care supervision available?
- *Resources.* Is a telephone available? Is money available for medicine or follow-up appointments? Is there transportation to get to a follow-up appointment or to pick up prescriptions?

KEY POINTS: PRINCIPLES OF GERIATRIC EMERGENCY MEDICINE

1. The geriatric age group ($>$65 years) is a rapidly growing segment of the population, and their numbers are expected to double nationwide by 2060.
2. Older patients have unique physiologic changes and comorbidities, and unique medical and social characteristics that hold implications for providing quality care.
3. Falls in older patients are a serious problem and may be the result of environmental or physiologic causes. Consider a fall as the initial presentation of a more serious disease and an opportunity to implement fall-reduction strategies and avoid a recurrent fall.
4. Atypical presentations of serious disease are more common in older patients.

BIBLIOGRAPHY

American College of Emergency Physicians, American Geriatrics Society, Emergency Nurses Association; Society for Academic Emergency Medicine; Geriatric Emergency Department Guidelines Task Force. Geriatric emergency department guidelines. *Ann Emerg Med.* 2014;63(5):e7–e25.

Han JH, Wilber ST. Altered mental status in older patients in the emergency department. *Clin Geriatr Med.* 2013;29(1):101–136.

Kahn JH, Magauran BG, Olshaker JS, eds. *Geriatric Emergency Medicine: Principles and Practice.* Cambridge, UK: Cambridge University Press; 2014.

Kodadek LM, Selvarajah S, Velopulos CG, et al. Undertriage of older trauma patients: is this a national phenomenon? *J Surg Res.* 2015;199(1):220–229.

Mather M, Jacobsen LA, Pollard KM. Aging in the United States. *Popul Bull.* 2015;70(2).

Rui P, Kang K. *National Hospital Ambulatory Medical Care Survey: 2015 Emergency Department Summary Tables.* Centers for Disease Control National Center for Health Statistics; 2016.

Shankar KN, Liu SW, Ganz DA. Trends and characteristics of emergency department visits for fall-related injuries in older adults, 2003–2010. *Western J Emerg Med.* 2017;18(5):785–793.

Vognar L, Gibbs LM. Care of the victim. *Clin Geriatr Med.* 2014;30(4):869–880.

Vollbrecht M, Biese K, Hastings SN, et al. Systems-based practice to improve care within and beyond the emergency department. *Clin Geriatr Med.* 2018;34(3):399–413.

Williams BA, Chang A, Ahalt C, et al., eds. *Current Diagnosis and Treatment: Geriatrics.* 2nd ed. New York, NY: McGraw-Hill; 2014.

CHAPTER 7

PALLIATIVE CARE AND ADVANCE DIRECTIVES

Jean Abbott, MD, MH and K. Barry Platnick, MD

PALLIATIVE CARE

1. **What is palliative care (PC) medicine?**
   PC medicine focuses on relieving the stresses of serious and complex medical illnesses. The goal is to improve quality of life and prevent suffering by addressing the physical, intellectual, emotional, social, and spiritual needs of patients and families. PC's interdisciplinary approach provides comprehensive support, and can also supplement potentially curative or life-extending treatments.

2. **What is the difference between PC and hospice?**
   PC is the general term for medical care, focusing on comfort and symptom management – that is, quality of life – for patients whose serious illnesses are not curable. Hospice in the United States is an interdisciplinary service covered by major insurances, including Medicare, for patients who are no longer pursuing life-prolonging therapies, and whose predicted life expectancy is 6 months or less. Hospice teams include nurses, physicians, aides, social workers, chaplains, and trained volunteers dedicated to addressing medical, spiritual, and psychosocial needs near the end of life.

3. **How does emergency medicine fit in with the specialty of PC and hospice?**
   The American Board of Emergency Medicine (ABEM) was one of 10 boards that sponsored the newly established subspecialty of Hospice and Palliative Care Medicine in 2006. This sponsorship recognizes that emergency physicians (EPs) need PC skills for those patients who need medical management but may wish to avoid burdensome or invasive interventions near the end of life. EPs can do a fellowship in PC after residency or take continuing medical education offerings in the field. Resources and essential tools for emergency medicine (EM) physicians are available through the National Center to Advance Palliative Care at https://www.capc.org/toolkits/integrating-palliative-care-practices-in-the-emergency-department/.

4. **What are the core PC skills that emergency physicians need to know?**
   PC skills for EPs are listed in Box 7.1. Although PC specialists may be available in some acute care hospitals, these core competencies should be part of initial emergency medicine care. Many treatments can be considered to be palliative interventions if their purpose is to improve quality of life and reduce suffering. ED management of patients focusing on palliative interventions may include fluid resuscitation, administering pain- and symptom-directed medications, starting antibiotics, or even some surgical interventions. Invasive diagnostics and treatment interventions must be assessed for their burdens, benefits, and overall congruence with the patient's goals and values.

5. **Why would a hospice patient call 911? Shouldn't they be calling their hospice provider?**
   Hospice patients and their families call emergency medical services (EMS) when they are overwhelmed with symptoms such as pain, fatigue, or trouble breathing. Despite hospices' commitment to provide comprehensive care, patients and families may become afraid and overwhelmed. The ED can serve an important role in providing an opportunity to assess and relieve acute symptoms. In nonemergent situations, the family's first call should be to the hospice nurse or agency, to allow the hospice to provide initial interventions. While an ED visit will be covered if families can't access their hospice provider, hospital admission requires discussion with the hospice to assure that the admission is necessary and is covered by Medicare or other payers. An ED visit may also alert the hospice that the patient and family are not getting the support they need or may need more intensive home or inpatient hospice care. Ultimately, the call to EMS should be respected; EMS providers should be trained in evaluation and management of these patients.

Box 7.1 Core Palliative Skills for Emergency Medicine Physicians
Establishing goals of care Assessing prognosis and trajectory of illness Understanding advance directives Delivering bad news and death disclosure Symptom assessment and management Management of pain Spiritual, psychologic, and social needs assessment Recognizing and managing last hours of life

6. What is an advance directive?

The term "advance directive" (AD) refers to one of a number of documents that establishes a patient's wishes or designates a surrogate to make medical decisions if the patient lacks capacity (Table 7.1). The most common forms of ADs are the living will (LW), cardiopulmonary resuscitation (CPR) directive, and medical durable power of attorney (MDPOA). State-specific forms exist, as does the legal recognized *Five Wishes* form (https://fivewishes.org).

Table 7.1 Advance Directives

ADVANCE DIRECTIVE TYPE	DEFINITION	PROS	CONS	COMMENTS
State DNAR, DNR, or no-CPR directives	State-based forms valid in out-of-hospital setting documenting no CPR in the event of cardiac arrest	To be honored by EMS and all facilities	Does not instruct on how much to intervene on other pre-death care, such as dialysis, transfusions, and intubation for respiratory distress	Valid across settings; only effective in cardiopulmonary arrest
Living will	Patient determines whether to continue to support when lacking DMC and in terminal or persistent vegetative state	Must be honored unless an MDPOA is given express authority to override	Only in effect when patient in terminal condition or PVS as determined by two doctors	Very narrow, inflexible
MDPOA	Agent appointed by patient to make decisions when patient lacks capacity, temporarily or permanently	Broad range of authority to respond to situation at hand according to patient values	Patient must have shared values with agent; only for health care decisions	Standard power of attorney cannot make medical decisions; patient can fire agent; the most adaptable way for patient wishes to be expressed
POLST-type form	Legal state-based orders (not directives) signed by patient (or representative) and health care provider to determine treatment wishes near the end of life	Orders are to be fully honored by all providers in all settings	Intended only for patients with end-stage serious illness or frailty	Broader scope than CPR directives; wishes for intensity of treatments can be expressed
Proxy decision maker for health care	Surrogate assigned to make decisions when patient lacks capacity but hasn't designated an agent (MDPOA); selected according to state's laws	Speaks for patient to provide consent or refusal for interventions	Family and friends may disagree, causing significant stress; proxy cannot withhold artificial hydration or nutrition in most instances	Less freedom than MDPOA appointed by patient for medical decisions
Five Wishes	Privately produced legally accepted document by patient to express preferences for medical treatment, predeath and postdeath wishes	Opportunity to express wide range of perideath wishes	Procedure-based medical wishes; not very useful as guide in clinical care in most situations	Wishes are intended to be followed but may be overridden by MDPOA or proxies

CPR, Cardiopulmonary resuscitation; *DMC*, decision-making capacity; *DNAR*, do not attempt resuscitation; *DNR*, do not resuscitate; *EMS*, emergency medical services; *MDPOA*, medical durable power of attorney; *POLST*, Physician Orders for Life-Sustaining Treatment; *PVS*, persistent vegetative state.

Modified from Ballentine *J. Summary/Comparison of Advance Directives and Surrogate Health Care Decision Making Processes for Colorado.* Colorado Advance Directives Consortium; 2017. Available at http://coloradoadvancedirectives.com/wp-content/uploads/2014/07/ADcompare-05.171.pdf. Accessed February 9, 2019.

7. **What are the new advance directive forms called Physician Orders for Life-Sustaining Treatment (POLST)?**

POLST paradigm forms, which are authorized in almost all states, are orders based on a patient's current medical status to be honored by EMS providers, physicians, and nurses. They include resuscitation preferences as well as a broader range of interventions like intubation, intensive care unit (ICU) admission, or preference for "comfort" care. These forms differ from standard advance directives in that they are signed by providers and patients or their representatives. They are legally protected orders to be followed in the whole range of inpatient, EMS, and outpatient settings. In the ED, physicians should confirm the continued validity with the patient if he or she has decisional capacity or with a surrogate if one is available. If that is not possible, valid POLST documents should be honored while the patient's comfort is ensured.

8. **How should advance directives be used when they are available to the EP in the ED?**

The most important use for ADs in any setting is to understand what level of care is aligned with the patient's wishes and goals when they can't. For the patient who arrives with documentation such as a CPR directive or a POLST form, or who is accompanied by a surrogate decision maker, this may prevent unwanted resuscitative measures. Alternatively, it may guide the ED in providing care that may seem aggressive but is consistent with the patient's wishes. This highlights the need to determine the patient's capacity for medical decision making as well as understanding of surrogate decision makers.

If there are no ADs, the patient lacks decision-making capacity, and the patient requires life-saving measures, physicians should err on the side of life-prolonging measures. The patient, family members, and physicians can have further discussions once the patient is stabilized in the ED or hospital about how they would like to proceed if it becomes apparent that this was inconsistent with the patient's wishes. Treatments can always be withdrawn in a comfortable and controlled manner when the patient's wishes and situation are understood more fully.

9. **How do I determine a patient's medical decision-making capacity (DMC) and what surrogate decision makers should I use if my patient lacks DMC?**

A patient with decisional capacity has the right to consent or refuse treatments, even those that could be life sustaining. The four elements for determining capacity are the ability to communicate, understand, appreciate, and reason. This means that the patient can manipulate information and communicate the treatment options he or she faces, the likely consequences of those choices, and the reason for his or her choice. If the patient lacks DMC, the EP should use any written ADs and identify the person who can speak for the patient, that is a surrogate decision maker. There are two types of surrogates: the person assigned as agent with MDPOA is appointed by the patient when they had capacity and has full authority to make decisions on behalf of the patient. The "proxy" is typically a person who assumes the role of surrogate decision maker if the patient hasn't previously assigned an agent. That person will vary according to state law. Pertinent documents signed by the patient when they had DMC generally supersede decisions made by an agent or proxy, though the documents often don't cover the exact situation people find themselves in near the end of life.

10. **What happens when patients or family members of patients change their goals of care while in the ED?**

Patients may revoke or change their wishes or ADs at any time, and patient goals often evolve during the course of illness. This can be confusing for the EP and requires a conversation with the patient and loved ones to explore reasons to either follow prior wishes or implement modified goals of care moving forward. The EP needs to reassure loved ones that care focusing on comfort is not abandonment and that the ED is always committed to aggressively managing symptoms and to honoring the patient's goals.

11. **How should I introduce PC or hospice and who should I call when I encounter a patient who might benefit from an assessment by them?**

In assessing patients with severe chronic diseases, the EM physician may think that a PC consultation would be useful, as our own Choosing Wisely recommendations suggest. Helpful conversation starters could include:
- How can we best help you today?
- Given the situation in which you find yourself, what are you hoping for? or
- I understand you are at a point where your primary goal is quality and comfort in the time you have remaining. What would help you most?

There are often temporizing less-invasive treatments that can stabilize the patient and allow time for conversation. Phrases that are *not* helpful and should be avoided include:
- Do you want us to do everything we can?
- There is nothing more that we can do for you.
- Do you realize you will die if I don't (intubate [or other procedure]) you?

If a hospital has a PC consult service available, an ED consultation might result in a plan better aligned with the patient's wishes and may better manage spiritual, physical, and social suffering for the patient and for family and friends. If the patient is enrolled in a hospice, a PC consult may help by notifying the providing organization and assessing whether home-based disposition is possible. If patients have not heard of palliative care or have misconceptions, the ED physician can "plant the seed" for the patient, loved ones, and admitting team that this is an important call to be considered once the patient is admitted.

12. **When is it appropriate to withhold resuscitation in a patient who comes to the ED?**
American College of Emergency Physicians (ACEP) policy emphasizes the need to take patient preferences into account when deciding whether to initiate or continue resuscitation. Indications for not attempting resuscitation include direct discussion with the patient, valid "do not attempt resuscitation" (DNAR), POLST, or "no CPR" orders, or a request from a patient's MDPOA to not attempt resuscitation. Unofficial documentation may be taken into consideration but is only advisory. Neither hospice nor PC services require patients to decline attempted resuscitation.

13. **Withdrawing or stopping resuscitation feels worse than not starting. Which is more ethical?**
Both withdrawing and withholding unwanted treatments, when consistent with the patient's wishes, can be ethically correct. In the ED, complete information about a patient's prior wishes is often unknown. Initiating resuscitative measures to stabilize a patient buys time and errs on the side of survival. If definitive information through a CPR directive, POLST paradigm form requesting no resuscitation, or direction from the patient's MDPOA become clear in the ED, withdrawing unwanted interventions is indicated and ethically appropriate.

14. **What are best practices for delivering bad news?**
One of the core competencies for EM providers is the skillful delivery of bad news, whether in an acute trauma situation, making a new diagnosis of a potentially life-limiting disease, or caring for a patient at the end of life. There are several well-studied approaches that the EM physician can learn and use to improve their ability to be clear and compassionate when these difficult times arise. Prior to having the conversation, it is critical to have the correct data (right patient, history, labs, and other studies). Several approaches applicable to EM providers have been described, including the GRIEV_ING, Best Case-Worst Case, SPIKES, and ABCDE. All of these methods are helpful in the acute and stressful ED environment, and encourage listening, educating, and supporting patients, survivors, and ED staff.

KEY POINTS

1. PC is comprehensive treatment of patients with serious illnesses, often in parallel with life-extending treatments.
2. End-of-life care is an important responsibility and core competency of EM physicians.
3. Identification of ADs or discussion with an MDPOA or authorized proxy is critical to delivering respectful care to the patient who lacks capacity in the ED.
4. Delivering difficult news is a learnable skill that allows respectful care of the patient, family, and friends.
5. Withdrawing unwanted emergent interventions is ethically equivalent or superior to withholding treatments when patient wishes become clear.
6. Treatment wishes of a patient or loved ones should be honored when they are known and valid, even including refusal of life-saving interventions that are burdensome or unwanted to the patient.
7. Aggressive symptom management is appropriate in all patients, including those in hospice.

BIBLIOGRAPHY

Abbott J. The POLST paradox: opportunities and challenges with honoring patient wishes in the ED. *Annals Emerg Med.* 2018;73(3): 294–301. Available at: https://www.sciencedirect.com/science/article/pii/S0196064418313751. Accessed February 9, 2019.
American College of Emergency Physicians. *Ten Things Physicians and Patients Should Question. The "Choosing Wisely" Campaign.* Available at: http://www.choosingwisely.org/societies/american-college-of-emergency-physicians/. Accessed October 2, 2019.
Berkey FJ, Wiedemer JP, Vithalani ND. Delivering bad or life-altering news. *Am Fam Physician.* 2018;90:99–104.
Bernacki RE, Block SD. Communication about serious illness care goals: a review and synthesis of best practices. *JAMA Intern Med.* 2014;174:1994–2003.
Kruser JM, Nabozny MJ, Steffens NM, et al. "Best Case/Worst Case": qualitative evaluation of a novel communication tool for difficult in-the-moment surgical decisions. *J Am Geriatr Soc.* 2015;63:1805–1811.
Lamba S, Bryczkowski S, Tyree L, et al. Death disclosure and delivery of difficult news in trauma #305. Fast facts and concepts. *J Palliat Med.* 2016;19:566–567.
Lamba S, Quest T, Weissman DE. Palliative care consultation in the emergency department #298. Fast facts and concepts. *J Palliat Med.* 2016;19:108–109.
Policy Statement. Ethical Issues of Resuscitation. American College of Emergency Physicians; 2015. Available at https://www.acep.org/patient-care/policy-statements/ethical-issues-of-resuscitation/#sm.00004mhe2gagjee8y3u1qvx4d1ro6. Accessed September 2, 2019.
Shoenberger JM, Yeghiazarian S, Rios C, et al. Death notification in the emergency department: survivors and physicians. *West J Emerg Med.* 2013;14:181–185.
Siegel M, Bigelow S. Palliative care symptom management in the emergency department: the ABC's of symptom management for the emergency physician. *J Emerg Med.* 2018;54:25–32.
Wang D. Beyond code status: palliative care begins in the emergency department. *Ann Emerg Med.* 2017;69:437–443.

CHAPTER 8

RESEARCH METHODS AND HOW TO CRITICALLY REVIEW EMERGENCY MEDICINE LITERATURE

Stacy Trent, MD, MPH and Jason Haukoos, MD, MSc

1. **Can I skip this chapter if I don't plan to do research?**
   No! Weighing medical literature carefully and incorporating it into clinical practice are important for all physicians.

2. **Why should I read medical journals?**
   - To learn the clinical features and management of diseases seen in practice
   - To determine whether a new or existing diagnostic test or treatment would be beneficial for your patients
   - To stay abreast of recent medical developments and evolving issues

3. **What is an experiment?**
   A research study that includes an intervention (e.g., a treatment or protocol that is introduced and controlled by the investigators) and that includes patient-level randomization.

4. **What is a quasi-experiment?**
   A research study that includes an intervention but that does not include patient-level randomization. Common examples of quasi-experiments include before-after studies, time-series studies, and cluster randomized trials.

5. **Are there other study designs?**
   Yes. Experiments and quasi-experiments include interventions as commonalities; observational study designs, on the other hand, do not include investigator-initiated interventions.

6. **Which study design is the best and why?**
   The best study design is a randomized controlled trial (experiment). Randomization is the most powerful research design feature and it is used to allocate patients to interventions while limiting confounding, by balancing both measured and unmeasured characteristics between groups. If done well, study groups should be well balanced, with the only difference being whether they received or did not receive the intervention. This allows investigators to estimate the independent effect of the intervention and to estimate a causal relationship between the intervention and the outcome.

7. **What other study designs should I be familiar with?**
   - *Cohort studies.* They divide groups by exposure status and either prospectively or retrospectively observe the groups over time to determine who develops the disease. Traditionally, these studies are used to calculate the relative risks of various exposures.
   - *Case-control studies.* They retrospectively compare cases (individuals with the disease) with controls (individuals without the disease) to determine the associations between exposures and disease. These study designs are most commonly used with rare diseases but, like all retrospective designs, are subject to recall bias.
   - *Cross-sectional studies.* Exposure and disease are collected at the same time; survey studies commonly use this design, although it is subject to temporal and recall biases.
   - *Case series.* They report characteristics of patients with a particular disease and can be valuable when looking at new or rare diseases or outcomes (e.g., HIV was first reported in the United States as a case series of *Pneumocystis* pneumonia published in the *New England Journal of Medicine*).

8. **What is concealed allocation?**
   Concealed allocation is an important clinical trial design feature where the individual screening and enrolling patients in a randomized study does not know the sequence in which study group allocation will occur. True randomization cannot occur without concealment, which prevents both selection bias and confounding.

9. **What is blinding and why is it important?**
   Blinding is an important research design feature used in clinical trials where patients, physicians, investigators, and anyone else involved in the study are unaware of whether patients are assigned to the experimental or control groups. This helps eliminate potential biases related to how patients are treated in the trial or how variables (including outcomes) are measured.

10. **What is a hypothesis?**
    A specific, clear, and testable statement about the possible effect of an intervention on an outcome of a study.

11. **Do sample size and power matter?**
    Power is the probability that the study will detect a treatment effect between the two experimental groups. The smaller the effect size, the larger the sample size required. Many studies do not have a large enough sample size to detect a statistically significant difference and may report negative results when a significant difference may have been detected; this is referred to as a type 2 error. Without adequate power, the study results may be inconclusive. (Conversely, type 1 errors occur when a difference between groups *is* found, but *does not* really exist: e.g., a false-positive result.)

12. **What does number needed to treat mean?**
    This is the number of patients who would have to receive the treatment for just one patient to benefit from the treatment. For example, if the number needed to treat (NNT) is 100, then 100 patients would need to have the treatment for one person to benefit from it. A lower number is obviously better, but if the benefit is preventing mortality, a larger value may be acceptable. You can calculate the number needed to treat by dividing 1 by the absolute risk reduction proportion (e.g., for a 5% difference in mortality between two different treatments, NNT $= 1/0.05 = 20$).

13. **What should I look for when evaluating a chart review study?**
    - Trained chart abstractors
    - Explicit criteria for case selection and exclusion
    - Defined study variables
    - Standardized abstraction forms for data collection
    - Periodic meetings among researchers to resolve abstraction disputes
    - Monitored performance of abstractors
    - Blinded chart reviewers
    - Measures of interrater agreement

14. **What does a *P* value refer to?**
    A *P* value reflects the probability that the results of a study or the differences between study subsets occurred by chance. The most commonly used value, $P < 0.05$, means that there is less than a 5% probability that the study results occurred by chance. This is considered statistically significant but may not be clinically significant. A decrease by 1 minute in overall ED length of stay may be statistically significant ($P < 0.05$), but is unlikely to be clinically relevant for physicians or patients.

15. **How do I interpret confidence intervals?**
    A confidence interval is the expected range of results in the study population. A 95% confidence interval means that if you repeated the study 100 times, the result would fall within the 95% confidence interval 95 of the 100 times. The confidence interval is a measure of precision where a narrower interval is considered more precise and is associated with larger sample sizes. Confidence intervals provide more detail than *P* values, as they not only demonstrate statistical significance but also help determine clinical significance. The wider the confidence interval, the more likely the study results are not clinically meaningful. Look at the upper and lower boundaries of the confidence interval and determine whether both values still would hold clinical significance. If only the upper boundary value would have significance, there may not be broad clinical benefit.

16. **Does it matter who sponsors a study?**
    Yes. Any direct involvement in a study by a sponsor, particularly one with a financial interest in the outcomes of the research (e.g., pharmaceutical industry), has the potential to influence the study and thus represents a potential conflict of interest. Ideally, sponsors should not have input into study design, data collection, or reporting the results. Unfortunately, many research studies do not adhere to these standards. Disclosure of financial support is important and should alert the reader that there is the potential for bias. Industry-sponsored studies may provide valuable information, but must be reviewed carefully and, ideally, independently confirmed.

17. **Should I read reviews on clinical topics?**
    Probably, but this depends on several factors, such as:
    - Are you looking for basic knowledge or understanding of a disease process? If so, a clinical review may be sufficient and can provide the foundation for you to continue your reading on the topic.
    - Are you looking for the latest information? Clinical reviews may be outdated by the time of publication because the literature on which they are based was written before the review.
    - Is it a narrative or systematic review? In narrative reviews, the author selects the articles to include in the review and summarizes the topic based in part on the author's experience. In a systematic review, the author identifies articles through a search and includes or excludes the articles based on predefined criteria and summarizes the topic based on strength of the evidence from the included articles.

18. **How should I interpret blog posts or other online reviews of clinical medicine?**
    Although these reviews are often written by emergency medicine clinicians, these online posts do not usually go through peer review. These posts may have useful information but should be interpreted with caution unless clear citations of rigorous research studies are included.

Disease

		Present	Absent
Exposure/ test results	Positive	A	B
	Negative	C	D

Fig. 8.1 Disease versus exposure grid.

19. What are some statistical terms (besides *P* value and 95% confidence intervals) that I should be familiar with?
    - *Relative risk.* A measure of association that estimates the risk of developing a disease after an exposure when compared with individuals without an exposure (Fig. 8.1): $A/(A + B) \div C/(C + D)$.
    - *Odds ratio.* A measure of association that estimates the odds of developing a disease after an exposure when compared with those without an exposure: $(AD)/(BC)$.
    - *Sensitivity.* The proportion of individuals with the disease who have a positive test result: $A/(A + C)$.
    - *Specificity.* The proportion of individuals without the disease who have a negative test result: $D/(B + D)$.
    - *Positive predictive value.* The proportion of individuals with a positive test result who actually have the disease: $A/(A + B)$.
    - *Negative predictive value.* The proportion of individuals with a negative test result who do not have the disease: $D/(C + D)$.
    - *Likelihood ratio (LR).* The likelihood that a given test result would be expected in an individual with the disease compared with the likelihood that the same results would be expected in an individual without the disease: positive LR = sensitivity/1 − specificity; negative LR = 1 − sensitivity/specificity.

KEY POINTS

1. Randomized controlled trials are the best studies, but other studies may also be valid.
2. A $P < 0.05$ is statistically significant.
3. A smaller confidence interval is better.
4. Sponsorship may influence how results are presented.

BIBLIOGRAPHY

Barratt A, Wyer PC, Hatala R, et al. Tips for learners of evidence-based medicine. 1. Relative risk reduction, absolute risk reduction, and number needed to treat. *CMAJ.* 2004;171:353–358.
Davidoff F, DeAngelis CD, Drazen JM, et al. Sponsorship, authorship, and accountability. *JAMA.* 2001;286:1232–1234.
Gallagher EJ. P < 0.05: threshold for decerebrate genuflection. *Acad Emerg Med.* 1999;6:1084–1087.
Jones JB. Research fundamentals: statistical considerations in research design: a simple person's approach. *Acad Emerg Med.* 2000;7:194–199.

CHAPTER 9

EVIDENCE-BASED RATIONAL USE OF DIAGNOSTIC IMAGING

*Ronald R. Townsend, MD, MS, FACR, Nishant Mehta, MD,
and Stephen V. Cantrill, MD, FACEP*

1. **What does evidence-based rational use of imaging mean?**
   Evidence-based imaging is the application of evidence-based medicine methodology to decisions regarding the use of diagnostic imaging or interventional image-guided procedures. A rational decision is made regarding use of imaging in a particular clinical situation based upon knowledge of the results of published research on the use of imaging for the problem at hand, the clinical expertise of the provider(s), and the patient's values and preferences. Such an analysis may lead to a decision to perform a specific imaging study or no study at all. Use of evidence-based imaging is motivated by desires to provide optimal quality patient care, and to avoid costs and radiation exposure associated with examinations that will not benefit the patient.

2. **Describe the evidence-based approach.**
   The evidence-based medicine approach incorporates five steps in the determination of a specific patient scenario.
   1. Ask an answerable question.
   2. Search the literature for current best evidence.
   3. Appraise the retrieved evidence.
   4. Apply the findings.
   5. Evaluate your success with the process.
   Crucial to this process are narrow definitions of the question, complete retrieval of current literature, and critical analysis of the validity and relevance of the available research.

3. **How is the evidence used by the clinician?**
   The clinician must decide what, if any, imaging is appropriate based on integration of the details of the patient's history, symptoms, and signs with the available evidence. The unique nature of a given patient's case may make an examination inappropriate, even if its use is generally supported by evidence.

4. **How can I apply evidence-based imaging in my clinical practice?**
   Although education regarding use of evidence-based medicine (and its application to imaging) in medical schools, residencies, and postgraduate settings is increasing, most practitioners are overwhelmed by the concept of doing a complete analysis themselves. Fortunately there are many resources available to aid the physician in determining what the evidence suggests will be useful imaging for some common clinical problems.

   Many specialty societies have developed guidelines or appropriateness criteria that include analyses of application of imaging in many emergency situations (e.g., American College of Radiology [ACR] Appropriateness Criteria). These range from opinion papers (not evidence-based) to true attempts at rigorous evidence-based analysis. Consulting the radiologist is always an option.

5. **Are clinical prediction rules helpful?**
   Evidence-based clinical prediction rules are widely available, validated tools to guide emergency imaging for many scenarios. They typically define specific history, physical findings, or laboratory parameters that accurately predict the utility or lack of utility of specific imaging.

6. **Is radiation exposure from x-rays and computed tomography (CT) dangerous when used for patients in the ED?**
   When evidence-based imaging is performed, the benefit of the diagnostic information obtained will generally far outweigh any small risk associated with radiation exposure. For example, a victim of major trauma should not be denied a CT and the potential of image-directed life-saving treatment, even if she may be pregnant.

   However, as of 2007, medical radiation is the largest source of exposure to the US population, surpassing background radiation. The medically related radiation exposure of the US population has increased substantially in recent years, related primarily to increased use of newer diagnostic studies (especially CT, interventional procedures, and nuclear medicine). Diagnostic radiographs *(plain films)* have relatively low associated radiation, so there is less risk. Some examples of average adult effective dose for some imaging procedures are given in Table 9.1. Newer CT scanning technology may facilitate obtaining diagnostic images with significantly lower radiation doses for many examinations, which helps minimize risk (see Table 9.1).

Table 9.1 Adult Effective Doses for Imaging Procedures

EXAMINATION	AVERAGE EFFECTIVE DOSE (mSv)	RANGE OF VALUES REPORTED (mSv)[a]
PA chest radiograph	0.02	0.007–0.05
Pelvis radiograph	0.6	0.2–1.2
Head CT	2	0.9–4
Chest CT for pulmonary embolism	15	13–40
Abdomen CT	8	3.5–25
Pelvis CT	6	3.3–10
IR-pelvic vein embolization	60	44–78
Background (annual)	3	Geographic variation

[a]CT doses may be below the lower ends of these ranges for some examinations performed with recently available dose-reduction technologies.

CT, Computed tomography; IR, interventional radiology; mSv, millisieverts (1 mSv = 100 mrem); PA, posteroanterior.
From Mettler FA, Huda W, Yoshizumi TT, et al. Effective doses in radiology and diagnostic nuclear medicine: a catalog. *Radiology.* 2008;248:254–263.

Dose-reduction strategies in CT have now become standard practice. Dose is aimed to be "as low as reasonably achievable" (ALARA) while preserving diagnostic image quality to answer the clinical question. CT radiation dose is proportional to fixed tube current (mA) and tube potential (kV) but inversely proportional to gantry rotation time. CT technologists/operators should be trained to modulate the mA according to patient body habitus based on technique charts, in addition to selecting the lowest possible kV to preserve image contrast and increasing gantry rotation time to reduce motion artifact and blurring. Nearly all CT systems now employ automatic exposure control that automatically adjusts mA in real time in response to output at the CT detector, thereby resulting in dose reduction.

7. **Which patients are at highest risk from imaging-related radiation exposure?**
Young patients and those who receive many CT scans are at highest risk. The primary concern related to significant patient radiation exposure is risk of development of neoplasm. The lifetime risk is highest for children. The patients placed at highest risk as a result of medical imaging are those who receive multiple high-dose examinations (e.g., CT of multiple body parts), especially when done repeatedly over months to years. Before ordering any examinations, it is prudent to carefully review the imaging history of a patient who often comes to the ED with recurrent problems such as chest pain, abdominal pain, or renal colic.

KEY POINTS: RISKS OF IMAGE-RELATED RADIATION

1. Risk–benefit analysis clearly favors the performance of evidence-based imaging in the ED.
2. Patients who receive multiple high-dose imaging examinations (especially CT) are at highest risk of long-term consequences.
3. Young patients are at higher risk than older patients.

8. **What question should be asked when ordering diagnostic imaging studies in young patients?**
Is there an evidence-based imaging approach that can address the patient's need without the use of ionizing radiation? This often involves use of ultrasound or magnetic resonance imaging (MRI). Consultation with a radiologist can be very helpful with planning imaging.

9. **What else should be considered when ordering diagnostic imaging?**
Unnecessary imaging contributes to the high cost of health care that ultimately is a burden to society. A CT of the chest, abdomen, and pelvis, for example, may result in charges of more than $5000. For the individual patient, an incidental finding at imaging may result in wasted time and money to work up the finding, which most often proves not significant. There is the potential for substantial morbidity or even mortality if this leads to biopsy or surgery. This may be viewed as unavoidable if the initial imaging was clearly indicated, but it could be tragic if it was not.

10. **Should a cervical spine (C-spine) CT be obtained in all trauma patients?**
No. The National Emergency X-Radiography Utilization Study (NEXUS) criteria and Canadian C-Spine Rule define patients in whom no imaging is necessary (see Chapter 84). There is no clear evidence to favor one over the

other, and there are not enough data to confirm validity in children. In patients who are at high risk of cervical spine injury, CT is more sensitive and specific than plain radiography.

11. **Which patients should get a cervical spine CT without cervical spine radiography?**
    A validated rule (referred to as the *Harborview high-risk cervical spine criteria*) defines a subgroup of patients who meet NEXUS or Canadian C-Spine Rule criteria and who may be effectively managed with CT as the initial cervical spine imaging. This includes adults with any one of these parameters (who would typically be getting head CT contemporaneously):
    - Injury mechanism parameters
      - High-speed (>35 mph combined impact) motor vehicle accident (MVA)
      - Crash with death at scene of MVA
      - Fall from height >10 feet
    - Clinical parameters
      - Significant closed head injury (or intracranial hemorrhage seen on CT)
      - Neurologic symptoms or signs referred to the cervical spine
      - Pelvic or multiple extremity fractures

12. **Which patients with chest pain should get a CT to exclude pulmonary embolism?**
    A clinical prediction rule can be used to distinguish patients who may benefit from imaging for possible pulmonary embolism from those unlikely to have embolism (see Chapter 30).

13. **When should patients with clinical suspicion of kidney stones get a noncontrast CT of the abdomen and pelvis (CT-KUB)?**
    CT has the highest sensitivity and specificity of all imaging modalities for ureterolithiasis. It can facilitate management decisions by accurately assessing stone size, number of stones, and the degree of collecting system dilation. However, many patients with prior CT documentation of urinary stone disease come to the ED on multiple occasions, and it may not be necessary or prudent to perform a CT-KUB at each visit. Those patients with a clear diagnosis, normal renal function, noninfected urine, and effectively treated pain are unlikely to require repeat imaging.

14. **What imaging other than CT-KUB should be considered for patients who often come to the ED with symptomatic urinary stone disease?**
    Many patients with recurrent urinary calculi may be managed with symptomatic treatment. If any imaging is necessary to facilitate management, ultrasound may provide the necessary information. Ultrasound may detect hydronephrosis as a sign of obstruction. The low sensitivity of ultrasound for ureteral calculi limits its utility in the initial evaluation of patients with possible stone disease.

15. **Is CT or MRI ever appropriate to evaluate extremity trauma?**
    In the vast majority of clinical situations, the presence or absence of fracture in an extremity is accurately determined by physical examination with or without plain radiography. Evidence-based rules defining which trauma patients need radiography are well validated for some body parts (e.g., Ottawa ankle, foot, and knee rules).

    Some patients may have persistent symptoms but no radiographic confirmation of fracture. The appropriate imaging approach to these patients depends on the anatomic site involved and specific symptoms and signs. In some situations, additional radiographic views (e.g., obliques) may define an injury. Many of these situations are uncommon enough that strong evidence to guide practice is limited. For many non–weight-bearing bones, persistent clinical suspicion of nondisplaced fracture can be addressed with 10-day follow-up radiography, at which time a healing fracture may become evident.

    In a patient who is unable to ambulate, additional imaging may be necessary, particularly with suspected hip fractures. CT, MRI, and bone scan can diagnose radiographically occult hip fracture. CT with multiplanar reconstructions is most useful to diagnose subtle cortical disruption, but MRI has the advantage of better assessing soft tissue (e.g., cartilage).

    There is strong evidence to support the use of MRI in assessing soft-tissue injuries in the knee, but this is rarely required during an ED visit. Emergent CT to further define some fractures may be needed to plan treatment. This is most common for fractures of the hindfoot and midfoot and intraarticular fractures about the knee, ankle, or elbow. When clinical findings lead to suspicion of vascular injury associated with extremity fracture or fracture-dislocation, catheter angiography or CT angiography may be appropriate.

16. **Does the evidence support use of CT or plain films for facial fracture imaging?**
    CT (especially thin-section multidetector CT with multiplanar reconstruction) has higher sensitivity and specificity than plain radiography in diagnosis of many types of facial fractures. Complex facial fractures are almost all managed based on CT findings. In general practice, most practitioners use CT as the initial and only examination in evaluating patients with definite fractures clinically and those felt to have high probability of fractures. (The exception is nasal bone fractures, which usually require no imaging for diagnosis or treatment.)

17. What are the indications for emergent MRI for patients in the ED?

MRI is usually the best examination for patients with acute atraumatic myelopathy, who may be at risk for progressive neurologic deficit related to spinal cord compression by tumor, abscess, or hematoma. The urgency of the examination cannot be completely defined by evidence but requires clinical judgment.

Acute focal neurologic deficits referable to intracranial pathology often require emergent imaging. Either CT or MRI (either examination often requiring contrast) may be supported by evidence in some circumstances. Patient-specific factors (e.g., history, details of deficit, time course) and local imaging equipment capability/availability may be important factors in deciding on CT or MRI. Consultation with the radiologist should be considered.

Evidence supports use of contrast-enhanced CT in patients with clinical suspicion of aortic dissection. MRI with or without contrast may also be used. However, intravenous (IV) contrast administration may be contraindicated in patients with severe allergy or acute renal failure. Transesophageal ultrasound is an alternative where available.

18. What imaging should be done when appendicitis is suspected clinically?

No imaging should be done if management will not be changed (e.g., the surgeon is clinically convinced the patient has appendicitis). CT of the abdomen and pelvis has the best accuracy in diagnosis of appendicitis, and differentiating it from other causes of right lower quadrant pain. Use of oral or rectal contrast for the examination is largely a matter of institutional experience or preference. IV contrast has been used in most studies evaluating CT for appendicitis, but accuracy is similar in other studies without it. Use of IV contrast may improve definition of associated abscess or other pathology causing right lower quadrant pain.

Compression ultrasound is less sensitive than CT for appendicitis but avoids radiation exposure in pregnant or other high-risk patients, including children. MRI may be useful to accurately diagnose appendicitis in pregnant patients, based on relatively small published studies. MRI offers advantages over CT, including elimination of the potential harmful effect of radiation on the fetus and related parental anxiety. It does not require contrast material, thus avoiding potential side effects.

19. What imaging should be performed for a clinical diagnosis of acute pancreatitis?

With a patient's first diagnosis of acute pancreatitis, ultrasound is appropriate to evaluate for gallstones as a possible cause of the pancreatitis. If biliary dilation is identified on that examination, further evaluation may be required. CT with IV contrast is most useful to evaluate complications of pancreatitis (e.g., necrosis, pseudocyst), but is usually not appropriate at the time of initial diagnosis in the ED.

20. What imaging should be performed to evaluate a palpable abdominal or pelvic mass?

The patient's demographics (e.g., gender, age) and location of the palpable mass affect imaging choice.

A palpable pelvic mass in a woman, most often related to uterine or ovarian pathology, is best evaluated with pelvic ultrasound (transabdominal and transvaginal), including Doppler.

A pulsatile midline abdominal mass in an older adult may be well evaluated with ultrasound of the abdominal aorta to identify any aneurysm and determine its size and extent. If ultrasound is technically limited (e.g., patient is obese), CT can be used to evaluate for aneurysm or another cause of the mass. In a patient with acute symptoms suspicious for aneurysm rupture, the patient's condition should determine whether imaging is advisable before intervention, but ultrasound cannot accurately determine the presence or absence of blood leaking from an aneurysm. CT with IV contrast is best for that assessment.

In an adult, a palpable abdominal mass not clearly related to any organ by examination is best evaluated by CT. There is a paucity of data comparing imaging approaches for abdominal masses, however. When a palpable mass may be an enlarged organ (e.g., liver or spleen), ultrasound may confirm that diagnosis without requiring use of ionizing radiation.

In an infant, palpable masses often relate to kidneys or the biliary tree, with the best initial evaluation being ultrasound.

21. What is appropriate evidence-based imaging for right upper quadrant pain?

Abdominal ultrasound is highly accurate in the diagnosis of cholelithiasis and should be the first imaging study when that is the primary question. Ultrasound and clinical or laboratory parameters together allow accurate diagnosis of acute cholecystitis in most patients without additional imaging. In problematic cases (especially possible acalculous cholecystitis), cholescintigraphy (nuclear medicine examination of the gallbladder) may be useful to diagnose acute cholecystitis, but it is not often required for management of patients in the ED. Cholescintigraphy does have a higher sensitivity than ultrasound in the diagnosis of acute cholecystitis. One advantage of ultrasound is its ability to identify nonbiliary causes of right upper quadrant pain in these patients (e.g., disease in the liver or right kidney).

KEY POINTS: EVIDENCE-BASED IMAGING

1. Base imaging choices on patient symptoms and signs. Avoid "shotgun imaging."
2. Only perform imaging studies that will affect patient management. Abdominal radiographs are generally wasteful if CT or ultrasound will be performed regardless of findings on the radiograph.

22. **What imaging should be done for suspected small bowel obstruction?**
Abdominal radiographs have limited sensitivity for detection of small bowel obstruction and limited ability to determine the cause of any obstruction present. If management decisions are not to be made based on results of the radiographs, they should not be obtained (e.g., if the patient will undergo CT and be managed based on results of the CT whether the radiographs are positive or negative). CT of the abdomen and pelvis with IV (but not oral or rectal) contrast will best define presence of obstruction, its cause, and any evidence of secondary compromise of bowel. Ultrasound can also identify findings of small bowel obstruction, but it is not as sensitive as CT.

23. **What is appropriate evidence-based imaging for left lower quadrant pain?**
When diverticulitis is the primary clinical concern, CT of the abdomen and pelvis with IV and oral (with or without rectal) contrast best defines the presence and extent of diverticulitis. It defines presence or absence of complications, such as perforation or abscess formation, which are important in patient management. Other conditions that can mimic diverticulitis clinically (e.g., epiploic appendagitis) can be diagnosed with CT. Compression ultrasound can be used for diagnosis of diverticulitis, but it appears to be less accurate than CT.

24. **What imaging is appropriate for suspected abdominal abscess?**
CT of the abdomen and pelvis with IV and enteric (oral or rectal) contrast can effectively evaluate for abdominal abscess in patients with abdominal pain and fever or other history, symptoms, and signs causing suspicion of abscess. If there are localizing symptoms and signs, a targeted ultrasound may be effective (e.g., clinical question of pericholecystic abscess or question of abdominal wall abscess along a surgical wound), but there is little data comparing alternative imaging approaches in this context. For possible pelvic abscess related to infections of gynecologic origin, transabdominal and transvaginal pelvic ultrasound with Doppler should be considered.

25. **When is imaging appropriate for patients with scrotal pain?**
When the cause of acute scrotal pain is not evident clinically, scrotal ultrasound with Doppler evaluation of testicular blood flow is the most accurate examination in diagnosing testicular torsion and distinguishing torsion from other pathologies. It should be performed emergently to optimize the chance of testicular salvage if torsion is present (see Chapter 39).

26. **Should a head CT be performed in all trauma patients?**
No. Many patients will not benefit from a head CT. History, symptoms, and signs can be used to identify patients at significant risk of intracranial injury post trauma (see Chapter 85). The New Orleans Criteria for patients with a minor head injury and a Glasgow Coma Scale score of 15 limits CT to patients with one of seven findings: headache, vomiting, age >60 years, drug or alcohol intoxication, deficits in short-term memory, physical evidence of trauma above the clavicles, or seizure.

27. **How about a head CT for trauma patients who are receiving anticoagulants?**
Data indicate that trauma patients who are receiving anticoagulants are at greater risk to develop a traumatic brain injury and that when it occurs, the injury will be more severe with a higher fatality rate. For this reason, the threshold for obtaining a head CT on such a patient should be very low. These patients may also require closer monitoring and potential repeat head CTs because of the possible development of a delayed acute subdural hematoma.

28. **Should patients with closed head injury routinely receive a CT of the abdomen and pelvis at the time of head CT (pan CT or whole body CT)?**
The clinical threshold for obtaining a CT of the abdomen and pelvis from trauma patients with head injuries is reduced at many centers. Whole body CT (WBCT) facilitates detection of occult injuries, but drawbacks include increased radiation exposure and detection of incidental findings. The REACT-2 study, a prospective, randomized controlled trial with intention to treat analysis comparing WBCT with selective trauma imaging, showed a decreased time to diagnosis and length of stay in the ED with WBCT, but no significant difference in mortality. WBCT may be beneficial in polytrauma patients with abnormal mental status, hemodynamic instability, or suspected critical injury. Selective trauma imaging may be utilized in patients who can provide an appropriate history and physical examination.

29. **Should imaging be repeated when a patient is transferred from another institution?**
This is usually unnecessary and will contribute to increased costs, excessive radiation exposure, and delays in care. Electronic transmission of images may facilitate image review at the receiving institution, even before the patient arrives. The presence or absence of need for any additional imaging to direct patient management can be determined after that review and examination of the patient. The concept that prior patient evaluation (imaging or otherwise) should be reviewed before embarking on additional diagnostic testing is crucial to avoiding waste in medicine.

Websites
ACR Appropriateness Criteria: www.acr.org/Clinical-Resources/ACR-Appropriateness-Criteria; accessed
March 11, 2019.
Harborview High-risk Cervical Spine Criteria: www.ajronline.org/doi/pdf/10.2214/ajr.174.3.1740713; accessed
March 11, 2019.
NEXUS Criteria: www.aafp.org/afp/20060515/poc.html; accessed March 11, 2019.

BIBLIOGRAPHY

Fesmire FM, Brown MD, Espinosa JA, et al. Critical issues in the evaluation and management of adult patients presenting to the emergency
department with suspected pulmonary embolism. *Ann Emerg Med.* 2011;57:628–652.
Jagoda AS, Bazarian JJ, Bruns JJ Jr, et al. Clinical policy: neuroimaging and decision making in adult mild traumatic brain injury in the
acute setting. *Ann Emerg Med.* 2008;52:714–748.
Long B, April MD, Koyfman A. The reign of the "pan-scan": whole body CT vs. selective imaging in trauma. *emDOCS.* 2017;June.
McCollough CH, Primak AN, Braun N, et al. Strategies for reducing radiation dose in CT. *Radiol Clin North Am.* 2009;47(1):27–40.
Medina LS, Blakemore CC. *Evidence-Based Imaging: Optimizing Imaging in Patient Care.* New York: Springer; 2006:1–569.
Mettler FA, Huda W, Yoshizumi TT, et al. Effective doses in radiology and diagnostic nuclear medicine: a catalog. *Radiology.*
2008;248:254–263.

CHAPTER 10

EMTALA, THE JOINT COMMISSION, AND HIPAA

Kyle Trecartin, MD

EMERGENCY MEDICAL TREATMENT AND LABOR ACT

1. **What is the Emergency Medical Treatment and Labor Act (EMTALA)?**
   In 1986, Congress enacted EMTALA as part of the Consolidated Omnibus Reconciliation Act (COBRA) to ensure public access to emergency services regardless of ability to pay. It was intended to prevent the dumping of patients; that is, the inappropriate transfer or discharge of uninsured patients in an unstable condition solely for the economic benefit of the treating hospital. If an emergency medical condition is found to exist, the hospital and the treating physician must use all of the resources normally available to them in stabilizing the emergency medical condition (EMC) before that patient can be discharged or transferred to another facility. Failure to comply with EMTALA can mean criminal sanctions, stiff financial penalties, and exclusion from participating in governmental programs such as Medicare and Medicaid.

2. **What is an Emergency Medical Condition (EMC)?**
   An EMC includes any medical condition (including psychiatric disturbances or symptoms of substance abuse) that without immediate medical attention might result in the patient's loss of life, a serious impairment of bodily function, serious dysfunction of any body organ or part, severe pain, or, in the case of a woman in active labor, the death or disability of the woman or unborn child.

3. **Why was EMTALA enacted?**
   For much of the twentieth century, private hospitals were under no obligation to offer emergency care to the uninsured. Consequently, indigent or undesirable patients were often denied such care and forced either to seek care elsewhere or go without any assistance whatsoever. To mitigate the situation, in 1946 Congress enacted the Hill–Burton Act, requiring any hospital receiving federal funds for construction or other expenses to open its doors to all people residing within its territorial area. The statute lacked any real means of enforcement, which led to poor compliance.
   Over the course of the 1960s and 1970s, the number of civil legal actions taken against hospitals that denied emergent medical treatment to indigent patients grew dramatically. Ultimately, Congress enacted EMTALA in 1986. Many amendments over the years have sharpened the focus and increased both the scope and the enforcement powers of the statute.

4. **Are hospitals or individual physicians subject to penalties for EMTALA violations?**
   Most provisions of EMTALA apply to hospitals. However, there are a few provisions that apply to physicians. When the law was originally enacted, a hospital that had more than 100 beds, or a physician working in such a hospital, could have been fined up to $50,000 per violation and a hospital with fewer than 100 beds, or a physician working in such a hospital, could have been fined up to $25,000. Since September 2016, these maximum penalties have been increased annually to adjust for inflation. As of 2018, the maximum fines are $106,965 for hospitals with >100 beds and $53,484 for hospitals with <100 beds.

5. **Will my malpractice insurance cover me for an EMTALA violation?**
   Malpractice insurers generally will not cover monetary sanctions imposed for an infraction of the statute. As a result, the EMTALA penalties amount to a major out-of-pocket expense for the practitioner. Another important difference is that EMTALA is not intended to police standards of medical care per se, but rather to ensure that every patient is treated equally without regard to ability to pay. The patient does not have to suffer damages or have a poor outcome, nor does a practitioner have to commit negligence for a physician or a hospital to be cited for an EMTALA violation. If a patient has a poor outcome from treatment and alleges malpractice in the state courts, EMTALA is invoked only if it can be proven that the care was substantially different from what the hospital would provide to any other patient with similar complaints and circumstances.

6. **Does EMTALA apply when a patient in need comes to any part of a hospital's campus, even if it is not an ED?**
   Yes. If an individual seeks care anywhere on hospital property, an EMTALA obligation on the part of the hospital may be triggered if the individual requests examination or treatment for an EMC or if a prudent layperson would believe that the individual is suffering from an EMC. The term *hospital property* means the entire main hospital

campus; this includes the parking lot, sidewalk, driveway, hospital departments, and any buildings owned by the hospital that are within 250 yards of the hospital. The patient must be moved to a dedicated ED within the hospital to receive an appropriate MSE.

7. **What is a dedicated ED?**
A hospital location is designated as a dedicated ED if it meets any one of three criteria: (1) it is licensed by the state to function as an ED; (2) it holds itself out to the public as a place providing care for emergent medical conditions on an urgent basis without requiring a previously scheduled appointment; or (3) if a representative sample of its patient population seen over the previous year demonstrated that at least one third of all outpatient visits were for urgent patient complaints that did not require a previously scheduled appointment. More recently, freestanding EDs have grown in number and are further categorized as hospital outpatient departments (HOPDs) or independent freestanding emergency departments (IFSEDs). HOPDs are owned and operated by medical centers or hospital systems, which means they operate under the same Centers for Medicare and Medicaid Services (CMS) rules and regulations as the hospital or medical center. IFSEDs are not recognized as EDs by Medicare and therefore do not have the same federal regulations.

8. **Is a hospital obligated under EMTALA to medically screen and stabilize any patient seeking care in an ambulance it owns and operates?**
No, as long as the hospital-owned ambulance operates under community-wide emergency medical services (EMS) protocols or EMS protocols mandated by state law that direct the ambulance to transport patients to the closest appropriate facility.

9. **How does EMTALA describe a proper MSE?**
An MSE is not an isolated event. It is an ongoing process, conducted by qualified medical personnel (QMP), that typically begins with triage but can involve a wide spectrum of actions, ranging from a brief history and physical examination, performance of diagnostic studies and procedures, or evaluation by any on-call consultant normally available to the dedicated ED. Triage helps prioritize the order in which individuals will be seen by QMP. The MSE must be appropriate to the individual's presenting signs and symptoms, as well as the capability and capacity of the hospital. The complex reality is that an adequate MSE can range from a quick history and physical to confirm the presence of an upper respiratory tract infection to a complex workup involving multiple tests, diagnostic procedures, consultations from specialists, and hospital admission for further evaluation and treatment.

10. **Who can perform the MSE?**
EMTALA states simply that a QMP must perform the MSE. A nurse or midlevel provider may perform the MSE if the hospital's governing board sets forth in the bylaws or hospital rules and regulations that they are qualified to perform screenings for the hospital. The QMP must have in their personnel files a job description for this role, qualifications, competencies, and a formal designation to perform an MSE.

11. **When has the MSE been satisfactorily completed under EMTALA?**
An individual is considered stabilized if the treating physician or designated QMP attending to the individual in the ED has determined, with reasonable clinical confidence, that the EMC has been resolved. Once the EMC is resolved, the individual may be discharged home with follow-up care instructions, admitted for ongoing care, or transferred to another facility. Patients in need of psychiatric care are considered stable when they are protected and prevented from injuring or harming themselves or others. EMTALA ceases to apply once the hospital admits an individual as an inpatient. Importantly, that cessation applies to patients formally admitted to the hospital but who may be boarded in the ED awaiting an inpatient bed.

12. **Is it an EMTALA violation if the patient decides to leave against medical advice before the MSE is complete?**
It depends on when during the triage and evaluation process that the patient decides to refuse care, and on his or her capacity to make medical decisions. If, during the course of the MSE, a patient refuses further evaluation and treatment after discussion of the potential risks of such a decision, the patient is considered to have withdrawn the initial request for evaluation, and EMTALA no longer applies. The burden of proof falls on the hospital and the treating physician, however, to demonstrate that no coercion was used to dissuade the patient from consenting to further treatment with suggestions or statements that the continued care could be prohibitively expensive. Proper documentation is essential. The medical record should reflect that screening, examination, or treatment were offered by the hospital before the patient's refusal.

A more difficult situation arises when a patient is triaged to the waiting room and then decides to leave before being formally evaluated in the ED. On the surface, this situation can be interpreted as the patient withdrawing the initial request for medical evaluation. EMTALA and the courts have focused considerable attention on the potential for inequity in triage practices, with the uninsured or undesirable patient being subjected to long waiting times in the hopes that he or she will simply leave. In such situations, the hospital must be able to prove that no different standard of triage was used and that a reasonable effort was made to call the patient back to the ED to address the initial complaint.

13. **What is meant by transfer under EMTALA?**

    EMTALA defines *transfer* as the movement of a patient away from the hospital, not simply as the act of transporting a patient to another hospital. By this definition, even a patient sent home from the ED is considered to have been transferred under the statute. If such a patient is subsequently found to have been discharged in an unstable condition, claim of an EMTALA violation could be made.

14. **When does EMTALA say it is OK to transfer a patient?**

    If a patient is deemed stable (i.e., an EMC is no longer present, and no significant medical deterioration is likely during or after the transfer), a transfer can proceed without the statute being applicable. EMTALA applies only to the transfer of patients in unstable conditions. Patients who are unstable can be transferred under the following conditions:
    - The patient requests the transfer. In that case, an informed request for the transfer must be signed by the patient, and it is important for the hospital and the treating physician to document that a discussion of cost did not enter into the patient's decision to ask for a transfer.
    - A patient in an unstable condition needs to be moved because the initial facility lacks the capability or the resources to treat the emergent condition adequately. This might occur when a patient who has multiple traumatic injuries comes to a small rural ED and requires transfer to a level 1 trauma center to receive proper care. Similarly, a patient with a complicated hand injury who comes to an ED with no hand specialist on call may need to be transferred to a facility capable of providing that service. The expected benefits of the transfer outweigh the risks of the transfer.

15. **List the requirements for transferring a patient who is unstable.**
    - A physician must certify that the benefits of the transfer outweigh the risks and that, when possible, this has been discussed with the patient or responsible party.
    - Every effort must be made to minimize the risk involved in the transfer in terms of proper treatment before the patient's departure.
    - The receiving facility has accepted the patient and has the capacity and capability to treat the EMC.
    - The receiving facility has been provided with all medical records related to the patient's emergency condition.
    - The transfer is conducted with qualified personnel and proper transportation, including the use of necessary and medically appropriate life-support measures.

16. **Can an on-call consultant refuse to see a patient who is unstable?**

    No. If an on-call physician fails or refuses to respond or come to the hospital in a timely fashion (i.e., within a reasonable time under the circumstances or within the time frame established by the hospital's medical staff bylaws), the hospital and the on-call physician may be in violation of EMTALA. If the on-call physician does not respond, the emergency medicine physician treating the patient must decide at what point it is appropriate to transfer the patient to a facility with the capability of treating the EMC. In this circumstance, the emergency medicine physician transfers the patient without personally violating EMTALA. Each hospital must have written policies and procedures in place to respond to situations in which a particular specialty is not available or the on-call physician does not respond, and the emergency physician must document on the transfer form the name and address of the consultant who failed to treat the patient.

17. **How is the hospital's on-call list determined?**

    Hospitals have flexibility in determining on-call coverage for their hospitals. However, they must ensure that they are providing sufficient on-call resources to meet the needs of their community. Hospitals must maintain a list of physicians who are on call to stabilize an individual with an EMC after the initial MSE. A hospital must have written policies and procedures that clearly delineate the responsibilities of on-call physicians to respond, examine, and treat patients with an EMC.

18. **Can a hospital refuse to accept a transfer under EMTALA?**

    A receiving hospital cannot refuse an appropriate transfer from a referring hospital within the boundaries of the United States if they have the capacity and capability to treat the patient.

19. **If I receive an inappropriate transfer at my hospital, do I have an obligation to report an EMTALA violation?**

    EMTALA states that any hospital that receives an inappropriate transfer must report the suspected EMTALA violation within 72 hours or face penalties. This is, however, an obligation of the hospital, not of an individual physician.

KEY POINTS: REQUIREMENTS WHEN TRANSFERRING A PATIENT WHO IS UNSTABLE

1. Physician certifies that benefits of transfer outweigh the risks.
2. The transfer is coordinated, and risks are minimized before transfer.
3. The receiving facility has accepted the patient and has the capacity and capability to treat him or her.
4. Medical records related to the EMC are copied and sent with the patient (including diagnostic imaging).
5. The transfer is accomplished with qualified personnel and appropriate equipment.

THE JOINT COMMISSION

20. What is The Joint Commission?

The Joint Commission is an independent, not-for-profit organization that evaluates and accredits health care organizations and programs. The origins of The Joint Commission date to 1917, when the American College of Surgeons (ACS) developed the *Minimum Standards for Hospitals* in an effort to establish basic national standards to be met by every hospital operating in the United States. The following year, the ACS began on-site inspections to ensure that hospitals met the minimum requirements. Decades later, the ACS, the American College of Physicians (ACP), the American Hospital Association (AHA), the American Medical Association (AMA), and the Canadian Medical Association joined to create The Joint Commission on Accreditation of Hospitals (JCAH), dedicated to further defining a set of standards recommended as essential to the safe and effective delivery of health care by hospitals throughout the United States.

In 1965, Congress empowered JCAH by linking hospital eligibility to participate in the Medicare program with accreditation by JCAH. The CMS deems qualified, private organizations with the authority to evaluate health care organizations' compliance with Medicare regulations in addition to their own established standards. Over the years, the standards changed to represent optimal achievable levels of quality and safety, rather than minimum essential levels of quality. As the scope of the organization expanded to include accreditation of clinical laboratories, ambulatory care centers, home health networks, and managed care organizations, the organization changed its name to *The Joint Commission on Accreditation of Healthcare Organizations (JCAHO)* and, finally, to *The Joint Commission* on January 1, 2007. The mission of The Joint Commission is to continuously improve health care for the public, in collaboration with other stakeholders, by evaluating health care organizations and inspiring them to excel in providing safe and effective care of the highest quality and value. Currently, The Joint Commission evaluates and accredits more than 20,500 health care organizations and programs in the United States.

21. What are the standards and performance measurements that The Joint Commission requires?

The Joint Commission collaborates with health care experts, research and quality organizations, providers, performance improvement experts, purchasers, and consumers to develop hospital accreditation standards that focus on an organization's ability to provide safe and high-quality care in a safe environment. The *Comprehensive Accreditation Manual* includes standards and performance in such areas as emergency management, patient care, medication management, infection prevention, the record of care, leadership, medical staff, and the National Patient Safety Goals (NPSG).

The NPSG became effective in 2003 and were established to help organizations address specific areas of concern in patient safety. The NPSG highlight problematic areas in health care and focus on system-wide solutions to improve safety and prevent adverse patient outcomes. Annual review and update of the goals is overseen by an expert panel that has hands-on experience addressing patient safety issues in a variety of health care settings. The NPSG often relate to media-grabbing issues, such as hospital-acquired infections, patient suicide in a hospital, and wrong-site surgery. Examples of the NPSG include improving the accuracy of patient identification, standardization of communication during hand-offs, medication safety, and reduction of health care associated infections. The NPSG continue to evolve and require greater attention and more resources. They are increasingly important for patient safety and are an important focus of the accreditation process.

22. How is compliance with the standards evaluated and enforced?

The Joint Commission conducts unannounced, on-site surveys that occur 18 to 36 months after the previous unannounced survey. Surveyors are trained and certified in quality-related performance improvement. Their responsibility is to evaluate the hospital's performance and actual care processes using the tracer methodology. The tracer methodology evaluates the patient experience, using the patient's record as a roadmap to move backward from the patient's current hospital location to their point of access into the hospital. In addition to observing and evaluating the direct care provided to patients, the surveyors scrutinize operational systems that cross all boundaries in the hospital and influence the safety and quality of patient care. Chart review; interviews with staff, patients, and families; observation of the processes of care; compliance with the NPSG; and system tracers are central features of the survey.

To earn and maintain Joint Commission accreditation, a hospital must maintain continuous compliance with Joint Commission requirements. In the current, complex health care environment, hospitals are required to meet a variety of accrediting, regulatory, and licensing requirements. The burden is significant and requires organizational commitment. Whenever feasible, hospitals should embed best practice into daily work to ensure compliance. In an effort to improve operational systems, standard work, computerized provider order entry, hand-held personal digital assistants, bar-coded patient bracelets, computerized decision support, and electronic medical records are tools that should be considered to promote patient safety and quality of care.

23. What is a sentinel event?

A *sentinel event* is defined by The Joint Commission as "an unexpected occurrence involving death or serious physical or psychological injury or the risk thereof." A sentinel event requires immediate attention, investigation, and response. Not all sentinel events occur as a result of a medical error. An appropriate response to a sentinel event is to conduct a timely, credible, and thorough root cause analysis (RCA). An RCA is a process determined by the organization that facilitates the evaluation and identification of the fundamental reason for variation in performance that led to the occurrence of a sentinel event. The outcome of an RCA should be an action plan designed to implement improvements and reduce risk.

24. **How do The Joint Commission standards influence the practice of emergency medicine?**
As the pressures of increasing patient volume, overcrowding, patient boarding, increasing complexity, and limited resources mount, so do the challenges to maintain safe, high-quality patient care in the ED setting. Assessment and treatment of pain, emergency preparedness, infection control and prevention, safe medication use, procedural sedation, monitoring restraint use, patient rights, staffing, staff competency, ED security, health care literacy, and standardized communication are all areas of focus for The Joint Commission in the ED.

Since 2005, there has been additional focus on patient flow and overcrowding in the ED. The Joint Commission requires that hospital leadership manage patient flow throughout the hospital to minimize ED overcrowding and minimize delays in care delivery. Since January 2014, hospitals have been required to set goals for managing patients who are boarded in the ED. Leadership must plan, measure, and guide processes to improve patient-flow processes and must have plans in place to care for admitted patients in the ED.

HEALTH INSURANCE PORTABILITY AND ACCOUNTABILITY ACT

25. **What is Health Insurance Portability and Accountability Act (HIPAA)?**
HIPAA was enacted by Congress in 1996 in order to protect individuals from the unauthorized or inappropriate use of their personal health information. The act's privacy regulations went into full force on April 14, 2004. HIPAA applies to all covered entities, public or private, that create, store, or transmit health information pertaining to specific individuals. This includes information in oral, written, or electronic form. HIPAA not only details when and how personal health data may be accessed and shared but also delineates standard transaction formats and data code sets that must be used in transferring such information.

26. **What prompted the enactment of such a statute?**
Patient privacy and the confidentiality of the physician–patient relationship have been recognized as fundamental ethical and moral obligations in medicine since the time of Hippocrates. With the rise of informatics and the evolution of medical care, individual patient information is now often shared among numerous practitioners, quality assurance auditors, billing coders, and third-party payers. As a result, the potential for unauthorized or inappropriate access to patients' personal information has escalated exponentially. HIPAA is intended to delineate the manner in which personal health data can be accessed, by whom, and for what reason.

27. **What is protected health information (PHI)?**
PHI is all information pertaining to an individual's medical or psychiatric status, treatment, or payment for health-related services. PHI is linked to specific patients by individually identifiable health information, which HIPAA defines as the person's name; specific contact information; place of residence by geographic subdivision smaller than the state; Social Security, medical record, or specific account numbers; photographs; biometric identifiers such as fingerprints or voice recognition; or any other unique identifier characteristic or code.

28. **What is the difference between the use and the disclosure of PHI?**
HIPAA defines use of PHI as the sharing, employment, application, utilization, examination, or analysis of PHI within the covered entity that maintains the PHI. In general, use of PHI within the covered entity for treatment, payment, and normal health care operations without the individual's consent is permissible under HIPAA. The sharing of PHI among physicians, nurses, or other health care providers involved in the direct care of a patient is considered use and is not restricted under HIPAA. Disclosure is the release of PHI to entities outside of the covered entity, such as the press, law enforcement, or marketers. PHI disclosure is much more restricted under HIPAA.

29. **According to HIPAA, when is it okay to disclose PHI?**
PHI may be disclosed without patient consent to other care providers as necessary to deliver medical or mental health treatment.

There are other circumstances under which it is appropriate to disclose PHI, but a hospital HIPAA authority should be consulted before disclosure. The 12 PHI exceptions allowed or required are:
1. Public health activities
2. Requirement by law
3. Victims of abuse, neglect, or domestic violence
4. Health oversight activities

5. Judicial and administrative proceedings
6. Law enforcement purposes
7. Decedents
8. Organ donation
9. Research
10. Serious threat to health or safety
11. Essential government functions
12. Workers' compensation

30. **How is the statute enforced, and what are the penalties for a HIPAA violation?**
    The OCR oversees enforcement of HIPAA privacy standards. Individuals may lodge HIPAA grievances with the covered entity or the federal government. Penalties for an established violation include potential monetary fines and jail sentences for the offender(s). Inadvertent violations carry a $100 fine, not to exceed $25,000 per year. If the violation occurred with the knowledge of the offender, punishment can include fines up to $50,000 and up to 1 year in prison. If the violation was committed knowingly and with false pretenses, potential penalties include fines up to $100,000 and a maximum of 5 years in prison. Violation with the intent to sell or profit from PHI disclosure carries a fine of up to $250,000 and up to 10 years in prison.

31. **What steps should be taken to prevent disclosure of PHI in the ED?**
    Maintaining patient privacy is problematic in a busy, crowded ED. Patients and visitors often overhear discussions pertaining to individuals unknown to them in the normal operation of the department. Such inadvertent disclosures are permissible under HIPAA, provided that the department has taken steps in good faith to minimize the likelihood of their occurrence. Examples of such measures include:
    - Conducting patient interviews and examinations in individual examining rooms when possible
    - Posting signs reminding staff members of the importance of maintaining patient privacy
    - Removing easily identifiable patient information on electronic tracking boards and computer screens
    - Documenting staff training with regard to HIPAA issues

KEY POINTS: BASIC HIPAA COMPLIANCE IN THE ED

1. Perform interviews and examinations in private areas whenever possible.
2. Remove patient identifiers from highly visible areas.
3. Document staff training with regard to HIPAA requirements.

Websites
The Joint Commission Sentinel Event Policy and Procedure: www.jointcommission.org?SentinelEvents/
    policyandprocedure; accessed January 30, 2015.
Journey through the History of the Joint Commission: www.jointcommission.org/AboutUs/joint_
    commission_history.htm.
Privacy Rule: www.hhs.gov/ocr/privacy/; accessed January 30, 2015.

RISK MANAGEMENT

32. **What is risk management?**
    Risk management is the effort to identify (and, when possible, improve or rectify) situations that place a service provider in jeopardy. Good risk management not only deals with situations as they arise (e.g., dealing appropriately with a patient's complaint about care) but also anticipates health delivery problems before they occur (e.g., establishing in advance the procedures for dealing with a patient who wishes to leave against medical advice).

33. **Why are emergency physicians at high risk for malpractice lawsuits?**
    The primary reasons are the lack of an established physician–patient relationship and lack of communication. The patient often feels little rapport with a physician unknown to the patient before the visit to the ED. The visit is usually not at the patient's wish, occurring at an unscheduled time and in a situation in which the patient is under stress and sometimes pain. All of these factors may contribute to feelings of anger and hostility, laying the groundwork for feelings of dissatisfaction about the provided care. Another major reason is that in emergency medicine, the decisions are often irrevocable. If a mistake or misjudgment is made on a patient who is admitted to the hospital, a second chance to correct the error usually exists because the patient is still accessible. In patients wrongly discharged from the ED, sometimes no such second chance exists.

34. What must be proved in a malpractice case?
- Duty to treat. Was there an obligation for the physician in question to treat the patient? In emergency medicine, this answer is almost always yes. By working in an ED, an emergency physician automatically assumes the duty to treat any patient coming to the ED and requesting care. The EMTALA statute mandates an MSE on all patients coming to the ED.
- Actual negligence. Was the care provided actually negligent? This often involves showing (to the jury's satisfaction) that the care provided fell below what is to be considered the standard of care. This point is the one most often contested by the opposing sides in a malpractice suit. Negligence may result from acts of commission or omission.
- Damages. Did the patient suffer actual damages? This can include the nebulous pain and suffering.
- Proximate cause. Did the negligence cause the damages? It must be shown to the jury's satisfaction that the alleged damages were truly the result of the alleged negligent care.

35. Give some examples of patients who place a provider at high risk for a malpractice suit.
- The hostile or belligerent patient. These patients are difficult to deal with and sometimes get less than complete or careless evaluation. Intoxicated patients represent a significant subgroup of this class of patients. Demanding patients also fall into this class.
- The patient with a problem that may be a potential life threat. With these patients, the challenge is to discover and address the life threat (see Chapter 1). Inappropriately discharging these patients often results in a risk management issue.
- The returning patient. The patient who returns unscheduled to the ED should raise a red flag. What problem is being missed? These patients deserve extra care in reevaluation and the need for additional, diagnostic workup should be carefully considered. The threshold for admitting an unscheduled, returning patient should be low.
- The private patient. Patients may be sent to the ED by a private physician for diagnostic studies or treatment but not to be seen and evaluated by the emergency physician. In general, any patient in the ED becomes the responsibility of the emergency physician. If something goes wrong with the care of these patients, the emergency physician also may be held liable. It is advisable to have very clear established policies concerning private patients in the ED. These patients should be seen by the emergency physician on duty if the patient so requests, if there is a delay in the arrival of the private physician, or if their triage category so warrants.

KEY POINTS: RISK MANAGEMENT

1. Treat every patient as you would want a family member to be treated.
2. Always address the potential life threats, based on the patient's condition.
3. Review nursing records for congruency and document if there is a discrepancy.
4. Communicate clearly with patients, families, and staff.

36. What clinical problems tend to get emergency physicians into malpractice difficulty?
There is regional variation in clinical problems that tend to cause malpractice problems for emergency physicians, but the following entities are generally major causes:
- Acute coronary syndromes
- Meningitis/sepsis (especially in young children)
- Missed fractures (including spine and pelvis)
- Appendicitis
- Stroke management
- Retained foreign bodies
- Aortic aneurysms
- Tendon/nerve injuries associated with wounds
- Intracranial hemorrhage (subdural, epidural, and subarachnoid hemorrhages)
- Wound infections

37. What is the most common error emergency physicians make with regard to their malpractice insurance policy?
The most common error is failure to read carefully and understand the conditions of the policy. Particular areas of misunderstanding include what is or is not covered, what are the settlement options, and what are the "tail" requirements to provide coverage for past patient encounters when the current policy is no longer in force.

38. What common deficiencies in the medical record exacerbate malpractice problems for emergency physicians?
The following documentation flaws can cause issues when defending a malpractice case:
- An illegible record. Think about how the record will look when it is enlarged to 4 feet $\times$ 4 feet by the plaintiff's attorney to show to the jury. Electronic, dictated, or typed records avoid this problem.

- Not addressing the chief complaint or nurses' and paramedics' notes. Make sure your evaluation addresses why the patient came to the ED and what others observed and documented about the patient.
- Not addressing abnormal vital signs. As a rule, patients must not be discharged from the ED with abnormal vital signs. Whenever this is done, the record must contain a discussion of why the physician is taking this action.
- An incomplete recorded history. As with all other parts of the medical record, an attempt will be made to convince the jury that *not recorded* equals *not done.* The history must include information concerning all potential serious problems consistent with the patient's presenting condition. Significant negatives should be recorded as well.
- Labeling the patient with a diagnosis that cannot be substantiated by the rest of the record. This not only may cause difficulty if the physician's guess is wrong but also leads to premature closure on the part of the next physician to treat the patient, removing the slim chance of correcting the diagnostic error if the patient returns to the ED because of no improvement.
- Inadequate documentation of the patient's course in the ED with inadequate attention to the patient's condition at discharge. Often the patient's condition may improve dramatically while in the ED, justifying discharge, but this fact is not reflected in the record. If this case becomes a malpractice problem, it appears that the patient was discharged in the original (unimproved) condition.
- Inadequate discharge (follow-up, aftercare) instructions. The greatest risk in dealing with patients is being wrong in judgment. The best insurance is careful and complete patient discharge instructions that include when and where to seek follow-up care and under what conditions to return to the ED. It is striking how little effort is put into this component of the record. After completing your evaluation and treatment of a patient, ask yourself, "What if I am wrong, and what is the worst possible complication that can occur?" Address these possibilities completely in your discharge instructions, and document them carefully in the record.

39. What systems problems often lead to lawsuits?
Systems problems are not under the emergency physician's control but can still cause difficulty. Such problems include:
- Inadequate follow-up review on radiology rereads of radiographs
- Inadequate follow-up review of cardiology rereads of electrocardiograms (ECGs)
- Inadequate follow-up review of delayed clinical laboratory results (e.g., cultures)
- Poor availability of previous medical records
- Inadequate handling of patient complaints (your chance to possibly head off a malpractice suit)
- Inadequate physician and ED staffing patterns (leading to prolonged patient waits and subsequent patient hostility)

40. When a patient refuses care, what are the two criteria that must be present?
If a patient desires to leave the ED against medical advice, the patient must meet the following conditions:
- Have medical decision-making capacity
- Understand the possible untoward sequelae that could result from refusal of care

All patients have the right to refuse care if these two criteria are met. Common sense (and most risk managers) would tell you to err on the side of treating the patient if there is any doubt as to competence.

41. What clinical problem-solving approach is most helpful in avoiding lawsuits?
When dealing with any patient, make sure you address the life threats: major problems that could exist, given this presentation for this patient. The safe approach is to assume the presence of these life threats, then set about to disprove them.

42. How can writing admission orders for patients cause problems for the emergency physician?
In many situations, writing admission orders for patients has made the emergency physician liable for untoward events occurring to the patient in the hospital before he or she is seen by the private physician. There is often significant peer pressure for the emergency physician to write such orders. This practice is potentially dangerous and must be discouraged.

43. What physician behaviors may help avoid lawsuits?
- Be courteous and kind to the patient and to the patient's family.
- Take time to communicate with the patient. It takes only seconds to tell the patient what is going on, what the results of diagnostic studies are, and what you are thinking concerning his or her case. Make sure all patient questions and concerns are addressed.
- Dress neatly.
- Explain and apologize for inordinate delays in patient care.
- Avoid writing admission orders when possible.
- Make sure the medical record accurately reflects the care provided and the thought processes behind the care.

44. **What are the criteria for reporting a physician to the National Practitioner Data Bank (NPDB)?**
The NPDB was established by the federal government in 1989 to track potential problem physicians. The criteria for reporting a physician to the NPDB are as follows:
- Payment made for a claim or judgment against a physician
- Action taken by a state medical licensing board against a physician
- Disciplinary action lasting more than 30 days taken against a physician by a group or institution.

A hospital must query the NPDB about any physician applying for staff privileges and at the time of reappointment of a physician to the medical staff.

45. **How can clinical policies (evidence-based practice guidelines) decrease malpractice risk for the emergency physician?**
Many groups and organizations are developing evidence-based practice guidelines. If it can be shown that a physician's care was consistent with these guidelines, it may help to show the appropriateness of the care and the lack of negligence.

46. **How can clinical policies potentially increase malpractice risk for emergency physicians?**
Malpractice risk can be increased by applicable evidence-based practice guidelines if the emergency physician is not aware of them or if he or she chooses not to follow these guidelines without carefully documenting the reasons for not doing so.

47. **Does emergency medicine residency training decrease my malpractice risk?**
One study revealed emergency medicine residency-trained physicians had significantly less malpractice indemnity than non–emergency medicine residency-trained physicians. This difference was not because of differences in the average indemnity but was a result of significantly fewer closed claims against emergency medicine residency-trained physicians with indemnity paid. This resulted in a cost per physician-year of malpractice coverage for non–emergency medicine residency-trained physicians that was more than twice that of emergency medicine residency-trained physicians.

Websites
Center for Medicare and Medicaid Services: www.cms.hhs.gov; accessed January 30, 2015.
National Quality Forum: www.qualityforum.org; accessed January 30, 2015.

BIBLIOGRAPHY

Branney SW, Pons PT, Markovchick VJ, et al. Malpractice occurrence in emergency medicine: does residency training make a difference? *J Emerg Med.* 2000;19:99–105.
Cantrill SV, Karas S. *Cost-Effective Diagnostic Testing in Emergency Medicine: Guidelines for Appropriate Utilization of Clinical Laboratory Radiology Studies.* 2nd ed. Dallas: American College of Emergency Physicians; 2000:2–5, 25–26.
Centers for Medicare and Medicaid Services revisions to appendix v, Emergency Medical Treatment and Labor Act Interpretive Guidelines § 489.24(d)(1)(i) 5/29/09.
Freestanding Emergency Departments: An Information Paper. July 2013. Available at www.acep.org. Accessed December 10, 2014.
Health and Human Services Department. *Annual Civil Monetary Penalties Inflation Adjustment.* Available at: https://www.federalregister.gov/documents/2018/10/11/2018-22005/annual-civil-monetary-penalties-inflation-adjustment.

CHAPTER 11

EMERGENCY MEDICINE OBSERVATION MEDICINE

Rodolfo Loureiro, MD and Matthew M. Hall, MD

1. What is observation?

The term "observation" encompasses three concepts: it is a family of billing codes, a service, and a location. The family of billing codes describes physician services that the Center for Medicare and Medicare Services (CMS) describes as follows:

> *Observation care is a well-defined set of specific, clinically appropriate services, which include ongoing short-term treatment, assessment, and reassessment before a decision can be made regarding whether patients will require further treatment as hospital inpatients, or if they are able to be discharged from the hospital. Observation services are commonly ordered for patients who present to the ED and who then require a significant period of treatment or monitoring in order to make a decision concerning their admission or discharge.*

Hospital observation *services* require documentation of medical necessity and a physician order for the service. *Observation service* is considered an outpatient service and can be delivered by any specialty. This has implications on billing, especially for Medicare patients, and is principally a billing decision based upon length to stay and complexity of care.* In terms of *location*, observation care can occur in a traditional ED treatment space or bed but it is not tied to a specific site of care. The name of the location is based on the conditions treated or institutional preference (e.g., ED observation unit [EDOU], clinical decision unit [CDU], short-stay unit, chest pain unit, or rapid diagnosis and treatment unit). Although these units are sometimes called *23-hour units,* patients may be kept in observation >48 hours.

2. Which patients are appropriate for observation services? Which are not?

Observation units are appropriate for two categories of patients. For one category there remains a diagnostic uncertainly and more evaluation is needed to determine if inpatient services are warranted (e.g., abdominal pain, chest pain). A second category is patients with selected diagnosed conditions who require a therapeutic intervention to prevent an inpatient hospital admission (e.g., acute asthma exacerbation, cellulitis). In contrast, patients with instability, those without a clear endpoint in care, or those with significant comorbidities may not be the best candidates for observation.

3. How common are EDOUs?

The number of EDOUs has grown since the turn of the century. According to a 2003 survey, 19% of US hospitals reported having EDOUs, with another 12% planning a unit. A subsequent analysis of 2007 National Hospital Ambulatory Medical Care Survey data indicated that the percent of US hospitals with an EDOU had increased to 36%, with more than half administratively managed by the ED. Internationally, emergency observation services have been reported in several countries and continents, including Canada, Britain, throughout Europe, Australia, India, China, Singapore, and South America.

4. What are some typical diagnoses that are appropriate for ED observation?

ED diagnoses may include low-risk chest pain to be evaluated for acute coronary ischemia; mild asthma/chronic obstructive pulmonary disease (COPD)/reactive airway disease exacerbation; syncope; transient ischemic attack (TIA); deep vein thrombosis; acute-onset atrial fibrillation; abdominal pain; acute congestive heart failure; head injury; uncomplicated pyelonephritis; cellulitis/soft-tissue infections; upper gastrointestinal (GI) bleeding; abdominal trauma; toxicology/drug overdose; pneumonia; dehydration/vomiting/diarrhea; social services management; physical therapy evaluation/rehab screening; renal colic/kidney stones; extremity pain/injury and intractable back pain; vertigo/ear, nose, and throat (ENT) problems; blood product transfusions; alcohol intoxication; and intractable headache. In some hospitals, patients who present with a primary psychiatric complaint can also be placed in ED observation after being medically cleared while a psychiatric bed search is in progress.

5. Can EDOUs provide services to pediatric patients?

Nearly one third of all ED visits are pediatric patients, of which an estimated 4% of patients are admitted to observation units nationally.

6. What are some common pediatric conditions of patients admitted to an EDOU?

Pediatric conditions include asthma/reactive airway disease, dehydration, gastroenteritis, pneumonia, abdominal pain, seizures, fever, bronchiolitis, croup, poisonings/ingestions, and trauma.

7. How does care provided in an EDOU compare with inpatient care for the same conditions?

A number of prospective randomized controlled studies have shown that patients with chest pain, TIA, syncope, and cellulitis who were managed in an EDOU had shorter lengths of stay, lower costs, comparable or better clinical outcomes, and improved patient satisfaction compared with similar patients admitted to an inpatient hospital unit.

8. **I have heard that time is an important factor for observation. Why is it important and how is it calculated?**
   Medicare and some insurance carriers (payers) require that a patient be admitted to observation status for at least 8 hours in order for the provider to be reimbursed for services. Observation time begins when an "admit to observation" order is written and ends with the time of final patient disposition.

9. **Does the time of ED services count toward observation time?**
   No. In most circumstances, the ED group is providing both the emergency medicine and observation care services. Most payers limit payment to only one type of service emergency medicine or observation care.

10. **Does observation care have to occur in an observation unit?**
    No. Observation services can be performed and billed while the patient is in a typical ED bed anywhere in the department. However, the best practice endorsed by the American College of Emergency Physicians (ACEP) is a dedicated observation area with committed staff and resources.

11. **What is the advantage of ED observation medicine to hospitals?**
    Studies have shown that EDOUs can provide high-quality care that is more efficient financially with shorter lengths of stay than inpatient care. One study also found that opening an EDOU decreased ambulance diversion and patients who left without being seen. By decreasing the number of short-stay admissions that are placed into hospital beds, EDOUs also help to increase the acuity case mix of hospitals, assuming there is sustained demand for hospital and ED services.

12. **What is the difference between observation and inpatient services?**
    For Medicare patients the difference is one of cost. Outpatient services, including ED and observation services, require more out-of-pocket costs be covered by beneficiaries (covered only by Medicare Part B) versus inpatient admission (covered by Medicare Parts A and B). It is the intensity of service and the anticipated time (i.e., length of stay) that drive the decision about inpatient versus observation status. It is important to remember that a patient "admitted" to the inpatient service may still be billed as an "observation" visit. Per a note from the CMS to beneficiaries:
    The decision for inpatient hospital admission is a complex medical decision based on your doctor's judgment and your need for medically necessary hospital care. An inpatient admission is generally appropriate when you're expected to need 2 or more midnights of medically necessary hospital care, but your doctor must order such admission and the hospital must formally admit you in order for you to become an inpatient.

13. **What is the difference between ED and non-ED (hospital-based) observation services?**
    From a billing perspective there is no significant difference; the same family of current procedural terminology (CPT) codes is used. However, EDOUs ideally care for patients who have a high likelihood of discharge (approximately 70%) within 24 hours. These patients tend to be those without significant comorbid conditions and those who have a complaint or condition that can follow a straightforward care pathway.

14. **Are observation visits limited to only 24 hours?**
    No. CPT codes (99224-6) describe services that extend longer than 1 calendar day. However, according to CMS:

    In the majority of cases, the decision whether to discharge a patient from the hospital following resolution of the reason for the observation care or to admit the patient as an inpatient can be made in less than 48 hours, usually in less than 24 hours. In only rare and exceptional cases do reasonable and necessary outpatient observation services span more than 48 hours.

    Similarly, the ACEP urges providers to aim for most observation stays not to last >24 hours.

15. **What is required to bill for observation services?**
    To bill for observation services the patient must require observation to determine whether inpatient hospitalization is required. In addition, there must be a medical observation record containing a timed and dated physician's admit-to-observation order. The observation record should describe the patient care delivered while the patient was in the observation unit with physician and nurse progress notes. This record must be supplemental to any ED encounter note.

16. **I heard that there is some recent controversy about Medicare patients admitted for observation care. What is the issue?**
    Because observation status is considered an outpatient status, these charges are not covered by Medicare Part A (which covers hospital charges). Instead, these services are billed under Medicare Part B, which requires beneficiaries to pay 20% of the cost (with no cap on the total expenditures) and also requires that they pay out of pocket for medications received during their stay. Beneficiaries who have Medicare Part D prescription drug coverage may be reimbursed for their medications depending on their type of Medicare coverage. Additionally, Medicare will only cover skilled nursing facility care with a qualifying stay of at least 3 days in a row. Observation care does not count toward this requirement.

KEY POINTS

1. Observation services are not tied to a specific site of care and are commonly ordered for patients who present to the ED and require a significant period of treatment or monitoring to make the decision on admission or discharge.
2. Billing for observation services requires documentation of medical necessity and a physician order. The decision for observation versus inpatient services requires complex medical decision making, based on medical necessity, and can impact patient co-pay responsibilities.
3. Observation services can be used for both pediatric and adult patients that require an extended period of time for therapeutic or evaluation purposes.
4. ED observation units can provide high-quality care that is more efficient financially, with shorter lengths of stay, than inpatient care.
5. ED observation units are most appropriate for patients without significant comorbid conditions who have straightforward care pathways (e.g., TIA), and for whom discharge is highly likely after the observation period.

BIBLIOGRAPHY

Are you a hospital inpatient or outpatient? If you have Medicare – ask! Centers for Medicare and Medicaid Services website. May 2014. Available at www.medicare.gov/Pubs/pdf/11435.pdf. Accessed September 1, 2019.

Emergency Department Observation Services. *ACEP Policy Statement.* May 2008. Available at www.acep.org/Clinical—Practice-Management/Emergency-Department-Observation-Services/. Accessed September 1, 2019.

Feng Z, Wright B, Mor V. Sharp rise in Medicare enrollees being held in hospitals for observation raises concerns about causes and consequences. *Health Affairs.* 2012;31(6):1251–1259.

Medicare Benefit Policy Manual. *Chapter 6 – Hospital Services Covered Under Part B. 20.6 – Outpatient Observation Services.* Available at www.cms.gov/Regulations-and-Guidance/Guidance/Manuals/downloads/bp102c06.pdf. Accessed September 2, 2019.

Nahab F, Leach G, Kingston C, et al. Impact of an emergency department observation unit transient ischemic attack protocol on length of stay and cost. *J Stroke Cerebrovasc Dis.* 2012;21(8):673–678.

Ross MA, Aurora T, Graff LG, et al. *State of the Art: Observation Units in the Emergency Department.* May 2011. Policy Resource and Education Paper. From American College of Emergency Physicians. Available at http://www.acep.org/workarea/DownloadAsset.aspx?id=82396. Accessed September 1, 2019.

Sun BC, McCreath H, Liang LJ, et al. Randomized clinical trial of an emergency department observation syncope protocol versus routine inpatient admission. *Ann Emerg Med.* 2014;64(2):167–175.

Venkatesh AK, Geisler BP, Gibson Chambers JJ, et al. Use of observation care in US emergency departments, 2001 to 2008. *PLoS One.* 2011;6(9):e24326.

Volz KA, Canham L, Kaplan E, et al. Identifying patients with cellulitis who are likely to require inpatient admission after a stay in an ED observation unit. *Am J Emerg Med.* 2013;31(2):360–364.

Wiler JL, Ginde AA. 440: National study of emergency department observation services. *Ann Emerg Med.* 2010;56:S142.

CHAPTER 12

PERFORMANCE EVALUATION AND IMPROVEMENT IN EMERGENCY MEDICINE

Stephen V. Cantrill, MD, FACEP

1. **Why should I care about my performance in my delivery of health care?**

   Physicians have the obvious moral obligation to provide high-quality care at a reasonable cost, resulting in the best possible outcome for their patients. Unfortunately, there is a paucity of data supporting the routine achievement of this laudable goal, in spite of ever-increasing expenditures on health care. This has led to an increasing interest in performance measurement and reporting by health care institutions, governmental and nongovernmental agencies, medical societies, and certifying boards. This has led to the development of the National Quality Strategy (NQS), which is a guiding document for federal efforts to encourage and promote a high-value and high-quality health care system.

2. **What are the broad aims specified in the NQS?**
   - Better care through improved quality
   - Improved health of people and communities
   - More affordable care

3. **What are the priorities outlined by the NQS?**
   - Making care safer by reducing harm caused in the delivery of care
   - Ensuring that each person and family are engaged as partners in their care
   - Promoting effective communication and coordination of care
   - Promoting the most effective prevention and treatment practices for the leading causes of mortality, starting with cardiovascular disease
   - Working with communities to promote wide use of best practices to enable healthy living
   - Making quality care more affordable for individuals, families, employers, and governments by developing and spreading new health care delivery models

4. **How will this impact me and my practice?**

   The Centers for Medicare and Medicaid Services (CMS) has stated that it will support the NQS through quality measurement and reporting programs, payment incentives, and rule making that will stress effectiveness of care, coordination of care, safety of care, improved patient experience, healthy communities, and improved affordability of care. These efforts will include performance measures targeted for emergency care providers and their institutions, with a direct impact on reimbursement.

5. **Aside from CMS, who are the other major players in performance measures and performance measurement?**

   There are several. The National Quality Forum (NQF) is a nonprofit, nongovernmental organization created in 1999 by the federal government, along with public and private-sector leaders, to encourage performance improvement and endorse national consensus measures for evaluating and publicly reporting provider and institutional performance. CMS is obligated to promulgate any performance measures approved by NQF. Another important player is the Physician Consortium for Performance Improvement (PCPI), initially established by the American Medical Association. PCPI's mission is to align patient-centered care, performance measurement, and quality improvement. PCPI has historically developed more than 250 clinical performance measures covering all specialties. These have been used in national reporting and quality improvement programs. The Agency for Healthcare Research and Quality (AHRQ) is also active in this area. It is an agency within the Department of Health and Human Services that is dedicated to research in improving the safety and quality of care. The American Board of Medical Specialties (ABMS) and most specialty boards, including the American Board of Emergency Medicine (ABEM), are also involved in this area from the point of view of maintenance of physician certification (MOC).

6. **What recent legislative activity has occurred in this area?**

   In April 2015, the Medicare Access and CHIP Reauthorization Act of 2015 (MACRA) was signed into law. This legislation established the CMS Quality Payment Program (QPP), which involves value-based reimbursement for care to Medicare patients. This program encompasses two paths to systemic improvement: the Merit-Based Incentive Payment System (MIPS) and the Advanced Alternative Payment Models (APM). These programs will provide incentive payments (or penalties) for performance (or lack of same) in the areas of care costs, care quality (e.g., reporting on performance measures), advancing care information (e.g., use of an electronic health record), and improvement activities (e.g., increased shared decision making, improved patient safety, increased care coordination, and increasing access).

7. **What has changed in performance measures in emergency medicine?**
Many of the old measures have been "topped out," meaning that CMS feels there is no more to gain from these measures and they have been retired. A major change is that CMS is moving away from claims-based measures (based on patient billing information) and towards reporting via a Qualified Clinical Data Registry (QCDR). Such a registry is not limited to just Medicare patient data but can apply to all payers. Also, the QCDR mechanism is more flexible in that it can include a wider range of performance measures, facilitating compliance with CMS performance measure requirements.

8. **How about QCDRs in emergency medicine?**
Any group can attempt to set up a QCDR, but it must meet with CMS's approval. To facilitate performance measure reporting in emergency medicine, the American College of Emergency Physicians (ACEP) has developed a CMS-approved QCDR, named CEDR (Clinical Emergency Data Registry). This registry currently offers a choice of 44 quality measures and 30 improvement activities to fulfill QPP/MIPS quality reporting requirements.

9. **How many measures do I need to report to satisfy the QPP/MIPS requirement?**
Currently, six measures need to be reported, with one of them being an outcome measure.

10. **What are some of the problems with performance measure development?**
Performance measure creation is a surprisingly difficult process. Several issues have come to light, including lack of good evidence for the measure (e.g., blood cultures in all admitted pneumonia patients), limitations of using only claims-based data when much information is only in the corpus of the patient's record, and assuming that a performance measure for one practice location (e.g., a private office) would be valid in another (e.g., an ED).

11. **How is cost of care playing into performance measures?**
There are several measures applicable to emergency medicine that deal with the efficiency or cost of care domain. That is, are we, as physicians, ordering ancillary studies that are not indicated? Many of these performance measures address evidence-based criteria for computed tomography (CT) or magnetic resonance imaging (MRI). Other important aspects of the efficiency domain are total cost per beneficiary and Medicare spending per beneficiary.

12. **What developments have there been in the area of addressing rising health care costs?**
One recent development has been the establishment of the *Choosing Wisely* campaign. This is an attempt to address the issues of low-yield testing and therapeutics. It was started in 2012 by the American Board of Internal Medicine Foundation and aims to publicize and engage clinicians and patients to discuss these issues of testing and treatment to determine what is appropriate care for each patient. As of March 2019, 77 specialty societies, including the ACEP, have subscribed to this program.

13. **What are the Choosing Wisely recommendations from ACEP?**
ACEP's 10 recommendations for the *Choosing Wisely* campaign are (http://www.choosingwisely.org/clinician-lists/):
1. Avoid CT of the head in ED patients with minor head injury who are at low risk based on validated decision rules. Minor head injury is a common reason for visiting an ED. The majority of minor head injuries do not lead to skull fractures or bleeding in the brain, which would need to be diagnosed by a CT scan.
2. Avoid placing indwelling urinary catheters in the ED for either urine output monitoring in stable patients who can urinate on their own, or for patient or staff convenience. These catheters are used to assist when patients cannot urinate, to monitor how much they urinate, or for patient comfort.
3. Do not delay available palliative and hospice care services in the ED for patients likely to benefit. This is medical care that provides comfort and relief for patients who have chronic or incurable diseases. Early referral from the ED to hospice or palliative care services can benefit patients, resulting in both improved quality and quantity of life.
4. Avoid wound cultures in ED patients with uncomplicated skin and soft-tissue abscesses after successful incision and drainage and with adequate medical follow-up care.
5. Avoid instituting intravenous (IV) fluids before doing a trial of oral hydration in uncomplicated ED cases of mild to moderate dehydration in children. Many patients who come to the ED with dehydration require fluids. To avoid pain and potential complications, it is preferable to give these fluids by mouth instead of the use of an IV.
6. Avoid CT of the head in asymptomatic adult patients in the ED with syncope, insignificant trauma, and a normal neurologic evaluation. Syncope (passing out or fainting) or near syncope (lightheadedness or almost passing out) is a common reason for visiting an ED, and most of those visits are not serious. Many tests may be ordered to identify the cause of the problem. However, these tests should not be routinely ordered, and the decision to order them should be guided by information obtained from the patient's history or physical examination.
7. Avoid CT pulmonary angiography in ED patients with a low pretest probability of pulmonary embolism and either a negative pulmonary embolism rule-out criteria (PERC) result or a negative D-dimer. Advances in medical technology have increased the ability to diagnose even small blood clots in the lung. Now, the most commonly used test is known as a *CT pulmonary angiogram (CTPA)*. However,

disadvantages of the CTPA include patient exposure to radiation, the use of dye in the veins that can damage kidneys, and high cost.

8. Avoid lumbar spine imaging in the ED for adults with atraumatic back pain unless the patient has severe or progressive neurologic deficits or is suspected of having a serious underlying condition, such as vertebral infection or cancer with bony metastasis. Low back pain without trauma is a common presenting complaint in the ED. Most of the time, such pain is caused by conditions such as a muscle strain or a bulging disc that cannot be identified on plain film or CT scan.

9. Avoid prescribing antibiotics in the ED for uncomplicated sinusitis. Sinusitis is a common reason for patients to visit the ED. Most patients with acute sinusitis do not require antibiotic treatment, because 98% of acute sinusitis cases are caused by a viral infection and resolve in 10–14 days without treatment.

10. Avoid ordering CT of the abdomen and pelvis in young, otherwise healthy, ED patients with known history of ureterolithiasis who have symptoms consistent with uncomplicated kidney stones. Many patients in the ED who are younger than 50 years and who have symptoms of recurrent kidney stones do not need a CT scan unless these symptoms persist or worsen, there is a fever, or there is a history of severe obstruction with previous stones.

14. **Are there Choosing Wisely recommendations from other specialties that apply to emergency medicine?**
Yes. A modified Delphi technique has been used to evaluate all 412 *Choosing Wisely* recommendations in terms of their relevancy to emergency medicine. Thirty-eight recommendations from other specialties were identified as being relevant to our specialty. Here are a few of interest:
- Avoid prescribing antibiotics for upper respiratory infections (Infectious Diseases Society of America).
- Do not prescribe antibiotics for otitis media in children ages 2–12 years with nonsevere symptoms where the observation option is reasonable (American Academy of Family Physicians).
- Neuroimaging (CT, MRI) is not necessary for a child with a simple febrile seizure (American Academy of Pediatrics).

15. **These are recommendations for use of specific studies. Is there an overarching philosophy that I can use to guide me in appropriately ordering diagnostic studies?**
Yes. Before ordering any study, ask, "How useful will this test be in establishing a diagnosis or assisting in treatment?" Also, try to avoid ordering diagnostic studies for the wrong reasons, such as intellectual curiosity, defensive medicine, unrealistic patient expectations, or peer (consultant) pressure.

16. **Should I order tests to "cover" myself?**
No, good medicine is good law. The criteria for ordering studies should be strictly based on medical concerns, not based on the physician's notion of what would be helpful to have in a court of law. Laboratory or radiographic studies should not be used as a substitute for a proper history and physical examination.

17. **How much can be saved with no compromise in patient care?**
The costs of medical testing in the ED can be contained by careful, thoughtful ordering without sacrificing patient care. In a multicenter study of 20 hospital EDs (both teaching and nonteaching), an ancillary educational program was developed to address the appropriate use of diagnostic studies. Seventeen tests or groups of tests or studies were targeted, with a 12.5% decrease in targeted test charges. No decrease in quality of care could be shown.

KEY POINTS

1. CMS, in its quality and performance reporting programs, is taking guidance from the NQS.
2. MACRA, MIPS, APMs, and QCDRs will all play a major role in our future practice of emergency medicine.
3. The *Choosing Wisely* campaign, in which emergency medicine participates, is an attempt to address the issues of low-yield testing and therapeutics.

Websites
CMS Quality Payment Program (includes Alternate Payment Models [APM] and Merit-Based Incentive Payment System [MIPS]): www.qpp.cms.gov; accessed May 3, 2019.
Choosing Wisely: www.choosingwisely.org; accessed May 3, 2019.
ACEP, quality and MIPS related: www.acep.org/quality; accessed May 3, 2019.
ACEP, qualified clinical data registry related: www.acep.org/administration/quality/cedr/cedr-home/; accessed May 3, 2019.

BIBILIOGRAPHY

ACEP Now. *ACEP Joins Choosing Wisely Campaign.* Available at www.acepnow.com/article/acep-joins-choosing-wisely-campaign/. Accessed May 3, 2019.

ACEP Now. *ACEP Releases Second Choosing Wisely List of Tests, Procedures Emergency Physicians Should Question.* Available at www.acepnow.com/article/acep-releases-second-choosing-wisely-list-tests-procedures-emergency-physicians-question/. Accessed May 3, 2019.

Lin MP, Nguyen T, Probst MA, et al. Emergency physician knowledge, attitudes, and behavior regarding ACEP's Choosing Wisely recommendations: a survey study. *Acad Emerg Med.* 2017;24:668–675.

Maughan BC, Rabin E, Cantrill SV. A broader view of quality: Choosing Wisely recommendations from other specialties with high relevance to emergency care. *Ann Emerg Med.* 2018;72:246–253.

Radecki RP. *Choosing Wisely Recommendations from Medical Specialties Beyond Emergency Medicine.* Available at www.acepnow.com/article/choosing-wisely-recommendations-medical-specialties-beyond-emergency-medicine/. Accessed May 3, 2019.

Schuur JD, Carney DP, Lyn ET, et al. A top five list for emergency medicine. *JAMA Intern Med.* 2014;174:509–515.

Schuur JD, Hsia RY, Burstin H, et al. Quality measurement in the emergency department: past and future. *Health Aff (Millwood).* 2013;32:2129–2138.

US Department of Health and Human Services. *2011 Report to Congress: National Strategy for Quality Improvement in Health Care.* Available at www.ahrq.gov/workingforquality/nqs/nqs2011annlrpt.htm. Accessed May 3, 2019.

Venkatesh AK, Goodrich K. Emergency care and the National Quality Strategy: highlights from the Centers for Medicare & Medicaid Services. *Ann Emerg Med.* 2015;65:396–399.

Welch SJ, Asplin BR, Stone-Griffith S, et al. Emergency department operational metrics, measures and definitions: results of the second Performance Measures and Benchmarking Summit. *Ann Emerg Med.* 2011;58:33–40.

PROFESSIONALISM AND SOCIAL MEDIA APPLICATIONS

Zachary Jarou, MD and Regina Royan, MD, MPH

CHAPTER 13

1. **What is social media?**
   - Social media is the creation, curation, consumption, and discussion of user-generated content through mobile and web technologies. The advent of social media has disrupted traditional means of communication and transformed the way that people communicate with one another in the twenty-first century.
   - While the Internet was initially prototyped by the US Department of Defense in the late 1960s, it would be another three decades before the Internet and social media were accessible to the general public. In 1989, Tim Berners-Lee invented the World Wide Web, the "www. dot com" system of hyperlinks, accessed by browsers, to help solve the problem of how to keep track of complex evolving systems like the Internet. Facebook was founded in 2004. What started as a crazy idea by a group of friends in a Harvard dorm room has since grown into the world's largest social media platform, linking 30% of the world's population (Fig. 13.1).

2. **What does social media have to do with emergency medicine (EM)?**
   Emergency physicians are lifelong learners and team members. The use of social media allows for better connectivity and can offer health professionals many benefits (e.g., asynchronous learning, mentorship, tools for advocacy, and promoting diversity). Social media allows you to stay up to date with new literature that may change the way you practice medicine, increasing the speed of knowledge translation (Box 13.1). You can be part of the many communities within EM and beyond.

3. **What is #FOAMed?**
   #FOAMed is a hashtag. FOAM is a movement – a global, crowd-sourced, collaborative network of medical educational communities and resources developed to augment traditional learning. Coined by Australian emergency physician Dr. Mike Cadogan over a pint of Guinness in Dublin, Ireland at the 2012 International Conference on Emergency Medicine, FOAM stands for Free, Open-Access Medical Education.

4. **What is a hashtag?**
   - A hashtag is a way of labeling or categorizing a social media post. Using the hashtag #FOAMed indicates that your post is open access medical education. The hashtag #EMconf indicates that a post is from a weekly education conference at an EM residency program. The hashtag #TipsForNewDocs has significant activity every July when new interns start residency.
   - Hashtags can also be used to identify online communities, such as #MedTwitter, #MedEd, #WomenInMedicine, or EM subspecialty content, such as #POCUS or #WildernessMed.
   - Most EM conferences also have a hashtag which makes it easy to follow conference news, and connect with conference presenters – even if you aren't there! (Table 13.1)

5. **Why should I trust #FOAMed? Is it peer reviewed?**
   Throughout medical school, you've learned about the importance of practicing evidence-based medicine. Changing your medical practice based solely on a single tweet or a blog post is never a good idea, but tweets and blog posts can bring attention to new, cutting-edge primary literature that you may not have otherwise been exposed to. Some #FOAMed creators have implemented traditional prepublication peer review processes used by medical journals. Additionally, once an idea has been shared on social media, it can be discussed, critiqued, challenged, or built upon by a community of learners, educators, and researchers – a form of postpublication peer review.

6. **I'm overwhelmed by the number of #FOAMed resources and I'm unsure of the quality of each resource. How do I know which resources to trust?**
   Since the early 2000s, there has been an exponential explosion of #FOAMed blogs and podcasts. Unfortunately, learners have limited time and do not always review references. To make life easier, Academic Life in Emergency Medicine (ALiEM), a blog and #FOAMed community, created both the Social Media Index (SMi), a tool to rate the overall quality of a #FOAMed website, and AIR (Approved Instructional Resource) scores. The top three #FOAMed resources according to ALiEM's SMi are (1) LifeInTheFastLane.com, (2) EMCrit.org, and (3) ALiEM.com. ALiEM's AIR modules are curated collections of #FOAMed content, each focused on a different educational topic, and completion of each module can be used to earn credit for asynchronous conference credit if approved by your residency program director.

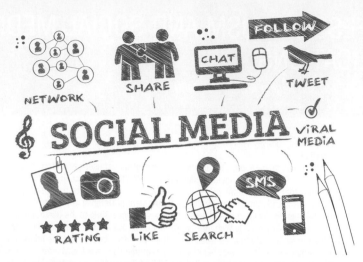

Fig. 13.1 Popular social media. *(From: Chapter 1 – Social media in society. In: Smith D, ed. Growing Your Library Career with Social Media. Elsevier; 2018. Figure.1.1.)*

Box 13.1 Knowledge Translation: Be Cutting Edge Sooner

If you want to know we practiced medicine **5 years ago**, read a **textbook**.
If you want to know we practiced medicine **2 years ago**, read a **journal**.
If you want to know we practiced medicine **now**, go to a (good) **conference**.
If you want to know we practiced medicine in the **future**, listen in the hallways and use **social media**.

Courtesy Joe Lex, MD, FAAEM, FACEP (Temple University).

Table 13.1 Emergency Medicine Conference Hashtags

CONFERENCE	HASHTAGS[a]
American College of Emergency Physicians (ACEP) Scientific Assembly	#ACEP20
Council of Residency Directors in Emergency Medicine Annual Meeting	CORDAA20
Society for Academic Emergency Medicine Annual Meeting	#SAEM20
ACEP Leadership and Advocacy Conference	#LAC20
FemInEM Idea Exchange (FIX)	#FIX20
American Academy of Emergency Medicine Scientific Assembly	#AAEM20
Rocky Mountain Winter Conference on Emergency Medicine	#RMWC20

[a]Note: numbers in hashtag change with each calendar year.

---

7. **Many #FOAMed resources seem to focus on "cutting edge" topics. Are there resources available to master core content in EM?**
   There are those who believe that textbooks, as we currently know them, are dead (or will be in the near future). One thing that textbooks do an excellent job of, however, is organizing content into a framework, which is

something that learners will not necessarily be able to construct on their own if jumping from resource to resource. There are also a few #FOAMed resources that specialize in teaching core content, including:

- **CanadiEM's CRACKCast** (Core Rosen's and Clinical Knowledge Podcast) is a series of podcasts covering each and every chapter of Rosen's *Emergency Medicine* textbook. [Website: CanadiEM.org/CRACKCast // Twitter: @ WeAreCanadiEM @CRACK_cast]
- **CoreEM** is the official blog and podcast of the NYU/Bellevue EM residency program, and features core content, procedure videos, and journal article reviews. [Website: CoreEM.net // Twitter: @Core_EM]
- **EM BASIC: Your Boot Camp Guide to Emergency Medicine** is a chief complaint-based podcast designed to teach the important history questions to ask, physical exam findings to look for, the workup, treatment, and disposition for commonly encountered patient presentations. [Website: EMBasic.org]
- **FOAMcast** is a mashup of both cutting-edge topics paired with core content from everyone's favorite imaginary EM textbook, Rosenalli's (Rosen's + Tintinalli's). [Website: FOAMcast.org // Twitter: @FOAMpodcast]

8. What is a personal learning network?

In addition to the education content produced by "branded" content creators, there are also opportunities to use social media to directly connect with subject-matter experts from across the country and around the world. A personal learning network is composed of the connections you make with those who share the same interests as you. Creating this network is a dynamic process and you can tailor the content that shows up in your social media feed by following and unfollowing accounts who create and curate content that enhances your learning. You can directly connect with leading EM researchers, residency faculty from across the country, faculty from other specialty areas, and your physician-in-training peers! Engaging in health care social media is a great way to stand out from the crowd, brand yourself, and develop a niche within your specialty. EM is a small community and you may end up making virtual acquaintances that end up being your new friends or mentors when you meet them at an EM conference.

9. How do you become a #FOAMed content creator?

Some tips for creating your own content include:

- Post a de-identified clinical image with a teaching point, or build off another's teaching point with additional clinical pearls.
- Highlight your scholarly projects by uploading your e-posters to Twitter, sparking a conversation with similarly interested folks who might be future collaborators.
- Make your presentations count twice, post them to SlideShare and tweet out the link.

10. What does it mean to be "professional" when using social media?

If there were an award for the most succinct, yet comprehensive, policy on social media professionalism, it would undoubtedly go to Dr. Farris Timimi, Medical Director of the Mayo Clinic's Social Media Network. His simple 12 word policy is: "Don't Lie, Don't Pry. Don't Cheat, Can't Delete. Don't Steal, Don't Reveal." (Table 13.2)

Table 13.2 Rules for Social Media Professionalism	
Don't Lie	A good rule for life in general, but especially important for social media. Anything posted on the Internet is easily searchable. #MedTwitter is a small community and being found out to be a liar isn't the type of content you want to go viral.
Don't Pry	Do not use social media to seek out personal health care data or potentially identifiable protected health information.
Don't Cheat	It's well known that "cheaters never prosper," and this is equally true on social media, where things are more likely to be discovered and exposed.
Can't Delete	While most social media platforms will allow you to delete posts, they may not really be gone. Others take screenshots and multiple websites regularly create backups of publicly posted content. Once you post something, assume it's going to be out there forever.
Don't Steal	Give credit where credit is due. It's the right thing to do, and you would want to be recognized if others were to share content that you created. Plus, it's as easy as tagging the original author or including a link to the original content that inspired the post.
Don't Reveal	This is probably the area where people face the most difficulty. Obviously, you don't want to reveal proprietary or confidential information about your patients or colleagues in a public forum. However, even when you have consent, you must be careful to follow any institution-specific guidelines and ensure that your posts are compliant with HIPAA. (See the question later in this chapter to learn how to ensure that your posts are HIPAA compliant.)

HIPAA, Health Insurance Portability and Accountability Act.

Box 13.2 Best Practices for Sharing Medical Cases on Social Media

1. Don't post anything that you wouldn't want your patient, their family, or your grandma to see. If in doubt, don't post it.
2. Make the learning point, not the patient, the focus of your post. You don't need to include specific ages or say where or when you encountered the real-world or hypothetical patient that inspired your educational pearl. Dates and locations are technically considered patient identifiers. Many educators will delay sharing cases for weeks, months, or even years.
3. Do not share photos with any patient body part (including identifiable radiology) without consent from your patients. Look at photos carefully for incidental items where patients could identify their clothes, belongings, or other personal information.
4. If posting photographs, ensure that there aren't any accidental protected health information photobombs in the background such as departmental track boards.

11. **Should I use an anonymous account or my real name?**
    This depends on what you hope to gain from your social media use. If you are looking for an authentic experience – to gain mentorship, interact with leaders in your field, promote your research, or engage in academic discussions – then you should also be authentic and post using your real name and accurate credentials. But don't forget, that every time you share a picture, retweet another account, or vent about your work day, these too are signed with your name.

12. **Should I change my name on social media accounts when applying for residency?**
    Many medical schools advise that you should change your name on personal social media accounts as you enter interview season. This advice may stem from a heightened concern that the content displayed by an applicant on social media may be unflattering or detrimental. On the flip side, there is a rapidly growing academic movement to incorporate digital and social media scholarship criteria for academic advancement through the creation of social media portfolios. What's most important is making sure that your online presence (pictures, posts, etc.) is not something that could reflect poorly on you in the first place. If you have a professionally focused account, this should not need to be changed, and can even be a great way to get advice and engage with programs before and after the interview!

13. **What are the rules regarding the Health Insurance Portability and Accountability Act (HIPAA) and sharing on social media?**
    The HIPAA of 1996 defines regulatory standards for the security and privacy of protected health information (PHI). What might be allowed by HIPAA may not be allowed by your institution. To stay informed, be careful to review your medical school or residency program's policy on social media (Box 13.2).

14. **What do I do if someone from the media contacts me through social media?**
    Occasionally, members of the media may ask to use pictures or reference your social media posts. If you are an employee of a hospital and the post has anything to do with patient care or your position as a student/trainee/employee, you should reach out to your institution's public relations team. These folks are well-equipped to give advice to make sure that you aren't breaking any rules and can also help you navigate interviews or statements with the media.

KEY POINTS

1. The Internet has revolutionized the way that humans communicate with one another. Social media is a powerful tool for knowledge translation and is changing the way that medical education is delivered.
2. Social media is a platform for building a personal learning network. By connecting with like-minded people who share your daily experience, and subject-matter experts from around the world, you can learn new things and participate in online communities.
3. The professionalism of your online interactions should reflect the level of professionalism you would exhibit in face-to-face interactions.

KEY POINTS

1. Don't avoid social media because you're stressed out about the technology, or because you don't think you have anything to contribute. Podcasts, blogs, RSS readers, and Twitter are made to be easy. It's okay to start out as a pure content consumer. Like things. Share things. Engage in conversations.
2. Professionalism: "Don't Lie, Don't Pry. Don't Cheat, Can't Delete. Don't Steal, Don't Reveal." (Dr. Farris Timimi, Mayo Clinic).
3. The things you like, follow, or interact with on social media are used to customize the content delivered to you based on what an algorithm thinks you'll want to see. Determine the purpose of your social media presence on each platform, and optimize it for what you're there to do. Are you there to follow friends, family, news, politics, sports, or are you there to stay up to date with the latest and greatest, cutting-edge medical education? Seeing too much of something? Unfollow it. Don't be afraid to expose yourself to new, different, or challenging thoughts and ideas; you don't want to end up in an online echo chamber.

BIBILIOGRAPHY

Cabrera D, Bryan S, Vartabedian BS, et al. More than likes and tweets: creating social media portfolios for academic promotion and tenure. *J Grad Med Educ.* 2017;9(4):421–425.

Joshi N. *Introducing #EMConf Twitter Hashtag.* August 12, 2013. Academic life in emergency medicine. Available at: https://www.aliem.com/2013/08/emconf-hashtag/. Accessed March 6, 2019.

Lewis JD, Fane KE, Ingraham AM, et al. Expanding opportunities for professional development: utilization of Twitter by early career women in academic medicine and science. *JMIR Med Educ.* 2018;4(2):e11140. doi:10.2196/11140.

Mallin M, Schlein S, Doctor S, et al. A survey of the current utilization of asynchronous education among emergency medicine residents in the United States. *Acad Med.* 2014;89(4):598–601.

Mishori R, Singh L, Lin KW, et al. #Diversity: conversations on Twitter about women and black men in medicine. *J Am Board Fam Med.* 2019;32(1):28–36. doi:10.3122/jabfm.2019.01.180175.

Pearson D, Cooney R, Bond MC. Recommendations from the Council of Residency Directors (CORD) Social Media Committee on the role of social media in residency education and strategies on implementation. *West J Emerg Med.* 2015;16(4):510–515.

Ranney ML, Betz ME, Dark C. #ThisIsOurLane – firearm safety as health care's highway. *N Engl J Med.* 2019;380(5):405–407. doi:10.1056/NEJMp1815462.

Rashid MA, McKechnie D, Gill D. What advice is given to newly qualified doctors on Twitter? An analysis of #TipsForNewDocs tweets. *Med Educ.* 2018;52:747–756. doi:10.1111/medu.13589.

Scott KR, Hsu CH, Johnson NJ, et al. Integration of social media in emergency medicine residency curriculum. *Ann Emerg Med.* 2014;64(4):396–404.

Shillcutt SK, Silver JK. Social media and advancement of women physicians. *N Engl J Med.* 2018;378(24):2342–2345. doi:10.1056/NEJMms1801980.

CHAPTER 14

ALTERED MENTAL STATUS AND COMA

Thomas L. Bostwick, MD, FACEP

1. What is coma? What terms should be used to describe altered sensorium?
Coma is a depressed mental state in which verbal and physical stimuli cannot elicit useful responses. Other terms, such as *lethargic, stuporous,* or *obtunded,* mean different things to different observers and should be avoided. You may be *alert but confused* as you read this chapter. It is best to describe the mental functions the patient can perform (e.g., the patient is oriented to person, place, and time, and can count backward from 10).

2. What causes coma?
Mental alertness is maintained by the cerebral hemispheres in conjunction with the reticular activating system. Coma can be produced by diffuse disease of both cerebral hemispheres (usually a metabolic problem), disease in the brain stem that damages the reticular activating system, or a structural central nervous system (CNS) lesion that compresses the reticular activating system. Fewer than 30% of patients have a structural cause for coma.

3. How can I remember the causes of coma and altered mental status?
The mnemonic TIPS and vowels can be used; that is, TIPS and AEIOU.
TIPS

       Trauma, **t**emperature
       Infection (CNS and systemic)
       Psychiatric
       Space-occupying lesions, **s**troke, **s**ubarachnoid hemorrhage, **s**hock
VOWELS

       Alcohol and other drugs
       Epilepsy, **e**lectrolytes, **e**ncephalopathy
       Insulin (hypoglycemia, diabetes, diabetic ketoacidosis [DKA])
       Oxygen (lack of), **o**piates
       Uremia

4. What important historical facts should be obtained from the patient with altered mental status or coma?
Since a comatose patient cannot give any history, you should carefully question prehospital personnel and attempt to contact any eye witnesses, including the patient's friends and family.
       Questions should include:
- Onset of symptoms (acute or gradual and timing)
- Recent neurologic symptoms (e.g., headache, seizure, or focal neurologic abnormalities)
- Drug or alcohol abuse
- Recent trauma
- Prior psychiatric problems
- Past medical history (e.g., neurologic disorders, diabetes, renal failure, cancer, or liver failure)
       If you are having trouble getting historical information, search the patient's belongings for pill bottles, check for a medical alert bracelet, check the patient's wallet for telephone numbers or names of friends, consider accessing their phone, if possible, and review previous medical records.

5. How can I perform a brief, directed physical examination on a patient with altered consciousness?
The goal of the physical examination is to differentiate structural focal CNS problems from diffuse metabolic processes. Pay special attention to vital signs, general appearance, mental status, eye findings, and the motor examination. Vital signs and eye findings are discussed elsewhere in this chapter.
       The general appearance should be noted before examining the patient. Are there signs of trauma? Is there symmetry of spontaneous movements?
       Motor examination is done to determine the symmetry of motor tone or strength and response of deep tendon reflexes. It is also critical to completely undress patients and thoroughly examine their skin for signs of infection, rashes, track marks, etc.

6. How do I evaluate the patient's mental status?
Mental status can be assessed quickly. Ask three sets of progressively more difficult questions.
1. Orientation to person, place, and time
2. Count backward from 10 (if done correctly, ask for serial 3's or 7's)

3. More difficult questions would include: recent recall of three unrelated objects or asking a question the patient has to think about, such as, "Who is the Vice President?" Asking who the president is in general is too easy, as most Americans know.

7. **What is the Glasgow Coma Scale?**
The Glasgow Coma Scale is a simple scoring system used in patients to describe the level of consciousness. It is useful for standardizing assessments among multiple observers and for monitoring changes in the patient's mental status. The score is determined by eliciting the best response obtained from the patient in three categories (Table 14.1). It is, however, not able to reliably detect subtle alterations of consciousness or focal neurologic deficits.

8. **How important is measuring the temperature of the patient who is comatose?**
Vital signs often provide clues to the cause of coma. A core (e.g., rectal) temperature should be obtained. An elevated temperature should lead you to investigate the possibility of infection (such as meningitis or sepsis), heat stroke, or hyperthyroidism. Hypothermia can result from environmental exposure, hypoglycemia, sepsis, hypothyroidism or, rarely, addisonian crisis. Do not assume that an abnormal temperature has a neurologic cause until you eliminate other causes.

9. **What is the significance of other vital signs?**
   - Check the cardiac monitor. Bradycardia or arrhythmias can alter cerebral perfusion and cause altered sensorium. Additionally, bradycardia can be seen with hypothyroidism or with increased intracranial pressure (ICP). Tachycardia can be seen with sympathomimetic agents, anticholinergic poisoning, hyperthyroidism, and sepsis.
   - Carefully count respirations. Tachypnea may indicate the presence of hypoxemia, salicylates, or a metabolic acidosis. Diminished respiratory efforts may indicate opioids and may require naloxone or assisted ventilation.
   - Check the blood pressure. Do not assume that hypotension has a cause related to the CNS. Look for hypovolemia or sepsis as a cause for hypotension. Hypertension may be a result of increased intracranial pressure, sympathomimetic intoxication, eclampsia, or hyperthyroidism. Uncontrolled hypertension also may cause encephalopathy and coma.
   - Do not forget to measure oxygen saturation.

10. **What is the Cushing reflex?**
The Cushing reflex is an alteration of vital signs (increased blood pressure and decreased pulse) secondary to increased ICP.

11. **Define decorticate and decerebrate posturing.**
Posturing may be seen with noxious stimulation in a patient who is comatose with severe brain injury.
   - Decorticate posturing is hyperextension of the legs with flexion of the arms at the elbows. Decorticate posturing results from damage to the descending motor pathways above the central midbrain.

Table 14.1 Glasgow Coma Scale		
OBSERVATION		**POINTS**
Eye opening	Spontaneous	4
	To verbal command	3
	To pain	2
	No response	1
Best motor response	Obeys	6
	Localizes pain	5
	Flexion withdrawal	4
	Decorticate posture	3
	Decerebrate posture	2
	No response	1
Best verbal response	Oriented or converses	5
	Confused conversation	4
	Inappropriate words	3
	Incomprehensible sounds	2
	No response	1
Total points		3–15

- Decerebrate posturing is hyperextension of the upper and lower extremities; this has a worse prognosis. Decerebrate posturing reflects damage to the midbrain and upper pons.

  If you have trouble remembering which position is which, think of the upper extremities in flexion with the hands over the heart *(cor)* in de-*cor*-ticate posturing or by "pulling a cord toward you." Additionally, decerebrate has more "e's," like *extension* of the patient's arms and legs.

12. **What information can be obtained from the eye examination of the patient who is comatose?**
The eyes should be examined for position and reactivity. When the eyelids are opened, note the position of the eyes. If the eyes flutter upward, exposing only the sclera, suspect psychogenic coma. If the eyes exhibit bilateral roving movements that cross the midline, the brain stem is intact. Pupil reactivity is relatively resistant to metabolic insult and usually is preserved in a metabolic coma. Pupil reactivity may be subtle, necessitating use of a bright light in a dark room. Fundoscopic examination may reveal increased ICP and hemorrhages.

13. **I want to impress the attending physicians. Do you have any tips on physical examination that will let me assume my rightful position as star student?**
   - If a confused patient is suspected of being postictal, look in the mouth. A tongue laceration supports the diagnosis of a seizure.
   - Put on gloves and inspect the scalp. Occult trauma is often overlooked, and you may find a laceration or dried blood. An old scar on the scalp may tip you off to a posttraumatic seizure disorder. Check for shunt ports in the temporal region of the scalp.
   - Do not be fooled by a positive blink test in a patient with suspected psychogenic coma. When you rapidly flick your hand at a patient who is comatose and has open eyes, air movement may stimulate a corneal reflex in a patient who is truly comatose.
   - Do not be misled by the odor of alcohol. Alcohol has almost no detectable odor, which is why alcoholics drink vodka at work. Other spirited liquors such as brandy have a strong odor. Furthermore, the executive who is comatose and smells drunk may have had a sudden subarachnoid hemorrhage and spilled brandy on his or her shirt.
   - Make sure that the patient is completely undressed so that occult injuries are not missed.

14. **Which diagnostic tests should be obtained in the patient with a significantly altered level of consciousness?**
Every patient should have a bedside blood glucose level. If alcohol intoxication is suspected, determine the alcohol level. If the pupils are constricted or if narcotic ingestion is suspected, naloxone should be given. If opioids, hypoglycemia, or alcohol intoxication is not found to be the cause of the patient's confusion, a complete blood count, electrolytes, creatinine, and blood urea nitrogen should be obtained. Toxicologic screens may be done in a patient with a suspected ingestion, but they are expensive, do not reliably detect every ingested substance, and a positive test does not preclude the possibility of another cause for alteration in consciousness. In suspected self-injury, consider sending acetaminophen and salicylate levels. Liver function tests (albumin, international normalized ratio [INR]), calcium level, carboxyhemoglobin level, creatine phosphokinase (CPK), and thyroid function studies may be helpful in selected patients. In cases of suspected sepsis, urinalysis can help localize the source to the urine as can a chest radiograph.

15. **Which radiologic studies should be obtained in the patient who is comatose?**
Computed tomography (CT) of the cervical spine should be obtained in any patient who is comatose with trauma to the face or head. A chest radiograph may be helpful if hypoxemia, pulmonary infection, or aspiration is suspected.

16. **When should I order a CT scan of the head?**
A head CT is not indicated in every patient who is comatose. A good history, a physical examination, and a few simple laboratory tests are adequate in many cases seen in the ED because drug and alcohol abuse are common. If a structural lesion is suspected (e.g., focal neurologic finding, head trauma, history of cancer), a non–contrast-enhanced CT scan should be ordered immediately. If the condition of a patient with a suspected metabolic coma worsens or does not improve after a brief period of observation, a CT scan should be obtained.

17. **When should a lumbar puncture (LP) be done?**
The indications and timing of LP depend on the following two questions (Fig. 14.1):
   1. Is CNS infection suspected? Rapid treatment with antibiotics should not be delayed while waiting to perform the LP.
   2. Is there a suspicion of a structural lesion causing increased ICP? Perform head imaging before LP.

18. **I have made the diagnosis of coma. What are my initial treatment priorities?**
Emergency medicine requires simultaneous assessment and treatment. A brilliant diagnosis is useless in a dead patient. Start with the ABCs – airway, breathing, and circulation – and the cervical spine. Intubate patients with apnea or labored respirations, patients who are likely to aspirate, and any patient who is thought to have increased ICP. Maintain cervical spine precautions until the possibility of trauma has been excluded. Hypotension should be corrected so that cerebral perfusion pressure is maintained.

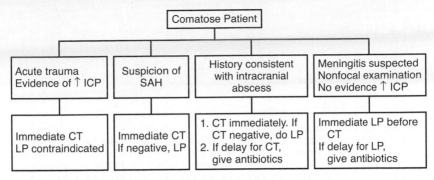

Fig. 14.1 Timing and indications for lumbar puncture. *CT,* Computed tomography; *ICP,* intracranial pressure; *LP,* lumbar puncture; *SAH,* subarachnoid hemorrhage.

KEY POINTS: ALTERED MENTAL STATUS AND COMA

1. The goal of physical examination is to differentiate structural from metabolic causes.
2. Focus on vital signs, mental status, and motor examination.
3. Obtain a rapid blood glucose test for every patient who is comatose.

---

19. I've addressed the ABCs. What do I do next?

Obtain a rapid blood glucose test; if the glucose is low, treat the patient with dextrose 50% in water ($D_{50}W$). It is better to do a rapid blood glucose determination rather than to give glucose empirically. If opioid use is suspected, give naloxone titrated to correct respiratory depression. Thiamine may be administered to patients who are malnourished or those with a history of alcohol abuse. Antibiotic administration should be considered in all patients who are febrile with coma of unknown etiology. Intubation should be performed in patients who are hypoxic, hypercapneic, and those not protecting their airways. Avoiding hypotension and hypoxia is essential to optimize favorable outcomes.

20. I think my patient is faking it. How can I tell if this is psychogenic coma?

First, be careful. Even astute clinicians have underestimated patients. If the patient actually is faking, be grateful. A patient in psychogenic coma is better than one who is angry and combative. Approach the patient incorrectly, and you can awaken the patient to a hostile alert state.

- Do a careful neurologic examination. Open the eyelids. If the eyes deviate upward and only the sclera show (Bell phenomenon), you should suspect psychogenic coma. When the eyelids are opened in a patient with true coma, the lids close slowly and incompletely. It is difficult to mimic this movement.
- Lift the arm and drop it toward the face; if the face is avoided, this is most likely psychogenic coma. If this does not work, you may want to check some simple laboratory tests, including a bedside glucose.
- If the patient remains comatose, irritating but nonpainful stimuli, such as tickling the feet with a cotton swab, may elicit a response. Remember that this is not a test of wills between you and the patient. There is no indication for repetitive painful stimulation because it can make the patient angry and ruin attempts at therapeutic intervention.

21. My patient has a history of seizures. Is there any special diagnosis I should consider?

Consider nonconvulsive status epilepticus. The patient may be having seizures with little or no motor findings. Check carefully for any subtle rhythmic jerking of the eyes, facial musculature, or fingers. An electroencephalograph (EEG) may be required to make the diagnosis of nonconvulsive status.

22. What is locked-in syndrome?

Patients with locked-in syndrome are quadriplegic and cannot speak because damage has occurred to their motor tracts, but they remain completely awake and alert. Some of these patients retain the ability of limited eye movements.

BIBILIOGRAPHY

Charles L, Clay S. Depressed consciousness and coma. In: *Rosen's Emergency Medicine: Concepts and Clinical Practice.* 9th ed. Mosby; 2018:123–131.
Koita J, Riggio S, Jagoda A. The mental status examination in emergency practice. *Emerg Med Clin North Am.* 2010;28:439–451.
Odiari EA, Sekhon N, Han JY, et al. Stablizing and managing patients with altered mental status and delirium. *Emerg Med Clin North Am.* 2015;33(4):753–764.

CHAPTER 15

FEVER

James D. Haycock, DO and Lori A. Montagna, MD

1. **What temperature constitutes a fever?**

   The literature defines fever as a core temperature above the normal range. However, the upper limit of normal typically varies between 38°C (100.4°F) and 38.3°C (100.9°F), depending on the source and the clinical context. Not all patients mount the same febrile response. A temperature of 38.0°C is considered a neonatal fever, whereas a neutropenic fever is defined as a single reading ≥38.3°C or two consecutive hourly readings ≥38.0°C. In high-risk patients, low-grade temperature elevations should be approached thoughtfully and with caution. Clinicians should consider fever, even when one is not measured on initial vital sign assessment, in patients at the extremes of age, those who are immunocompromised, and those with comorbid conditions such as diabetes, cancer, sickle cell disease, chronic alcoholism, and intravenous drug abuse.

2. **How does the body produce a fever?**

   Core body temperature is regulated by the anterior hypothalamus, and a fever is caused by elevation of the hypothalamic set point. Inflamed tissue or infecting organisms release pyrogens, which, in turn, activate prostaglandin E_2 (PGE$_2$). PGE$_2$ stimulates the hypothalamus to increase its thermoregulatory set point. The body responds with heat conservation and thermogenesis (e.g., by utilizing vasoconstriction, increasing muscle tone, initiating a shivering response, and increasing basal metabolic rate) to elevate the core temperature. The hypothalamus can also counter-regulate metabolic heat production with the body's systems of heat dissipation (e.g., by stimulating sweating and increasing ventilation).

3. **What is the difference between a fever and hyperthermia?**

   In contrast to fever, hyperthermia results in an elevated temperature without alteration of the hypothalamic set point. This uncontrolled failure of thermoregulation occurs when the body absorbs or produces more heat than it releases. Some examples of hyperthermia include heat stroke, thyroid storm, burns, and toxidromes such as neuroleptic malignant syndrome, serotonin syndrome, and malignant hyperthermia. It is important to distinguish between fever and hyperthermia, because the latter can be rapidly fatal and does not typically respond to antipyretics. The distinction is often made based on the history and the events immediately preceding the elevated temperature (e.g., heat exposure, medication use, and illicit drug exposure). Rapid cooling measures are imperative in cases of severe hyperthermia.

4. **What is hyperpyrexia?**

   Any temperature greater than 41.5°C (106.7°F) constitutes hyperpyrexia, which can be caused by either fever or hyperthermia. Fever-induced hyperpyrexia can be caused by severe infections, but more commonly it is caused by central nervous system (CNS) lesions such as intracranial hemorrhages. Hyperthermia-related hyperpyrexia may be caused by many of the etiologies listed in Question 3. Regardless of the cause, rapid action must be taken to cool the body to prevent neuronal damage.

5. **Are all methods of measuring temperature equivalent?**

   The most accurate body temperatures are core body temperatures, measured through invasive techniques, such as placing an intrabladder probe or a pulmonary artery catheter, the latter of which is considered the gold standard. Of less-invasive measurements, rectal temperatures are the most accurate representation of core body temperature. Oral, axillary, temporal, and tympanic temperature measurements are less sensitive and, thus, absence of temperature elevation when measured by these methods does not exclude fever. Additionally, there is no reliable correction factor for these alternative modalities. However, rectal temperatures are generally considered to be 0.4°C–0.6°C (0.7°F–1.0°F) higher than oral readings. When an accurate temperature measurement is crucial to the patient's care, a rectal temperature or a more-invasive measurement (such as a temperature-sensing Foley catheter) is necessary.

6. **How do I address a patient with a subjective fever at home who is afebrile in the ED?**

   This situation is most commonly encountered in pediatrics. Parental palpation overestimates the presence of a fever, and parents are more likely to be accurate when they report that their baby is afebrile. Palpable fevers should be taken seriously, and an appropriate assessment of the patient should be made to determine need for further infectious evaluation. It is also important to obtain a history of any recent antipyretic use which may mask a fever in the ED.

7. **Does the degree of fever indicate the severity of the infection?**

   In general, no. Before the *Haemophilus influenzae vaccine* in the early 1990s and the pneumococcal vaccine in the early 2000s, there were specific temperature thresholds that were associated with a greater likelihood of serious bacterial illness (SBI) in children. But, subsequently, the prevalence of these organisms as human pathogens has dramatically decreased. Another example in which the height of fever is associated with a higher rate of infection is that of pediatric urinary tract infection (UTI). Temperatures of greater than 39°C are more frequently associated with UTI in children less than 2 years of age. With the exception of neonates, it is generally recognized that clinical appearance is a stronger predictor of SBI than the degree of fever.

8. **What are the causes of fever?**
   Infection causes the vast majority of fevers, but the following other causes must also be included in the differential diagnosis:
   - Neoplastic diseases (e.g., leukemia, lymphoma, or solid tumors)
   - Autoimmune disease (e.g., giant cell arteritis, polyarteritis nodosa, systemic lupus erythematosus, or rheumatoid arthritis)
   - Endocrine disorders (e.g., thyroid storm)
   - CNS lesions (e.g., stroke, intracranial bleed, or trauma)
   - Illicit drug use (e.g., cocaine, 3,4-methylenedioxymethamphetamine [MDMA, ecstasy], or other methamphetamines)
   - Withdrawal syndromes (e.g., delirium tremens or benzodiazepine withdrawal)

9. **Which medications can cause fevers?**
   Any medication is capable of producing a drug fever; however, antibiotics cause one third of cases (Table 15.1). The fever usually begins 7 to 10 days after initiation of drug therapy. Associated findings include chills (53%), myalgias (25%), eosinophilia (22%), and rash (18%). Drug fever is a diagnosis of exclusion.

10. **What are some key elements of the history and physical examination in patients with fever?**
    Pay particular attention to associated symptoms (e.g., cough, dysuria, diarrhea, abdominal pain, or headache), duration of fever, response to antipyretics, exposure to ill contacts, risk factors for immunocompromise, travel history, and comorbid conditions. Perform a thorough physical examination when the patient is undressed and gowned. Consider sites of occult infection, such as the ears, nose, sinuses, feet, rectum, and genitals. Look closely at the skin for evidence of petechiae, purpura, cellulitis, or other concerning rashes.

11. **What is the best way to reduce a fever?**
    Acetaminophen and nonsteroidal anti-inflammator drugs (NSAIDs), such as ibuprofen, are the most commonly used antipyretics. Both reduce the production of PGE_2. However, ibuprofen has been shown to be more effective than acetaminophen, and ibuprofen has the added benefit of its anti-inflammatory effects. Caution should be taken to avoid ibuprofen in patients those with decreased renal function and in those less than 6 months of age. Other NSAIDs and aspirin are also options. However, aspirin is not recommended in children due to the association with Reye syndrome. There are newer anticytokine agents (interleukin 1 [IL-1] blockers), such as anakinra or canakinumab, which are used for patients with autoimmune and chronic inflammatory conditions to reduce fevers. Complementary methods, such as undressing and cool bathing, generally do not significantly lower body temperature. If the temperature is greater than 41.5°C (106.7°F), rapid cooling measures should be initiated for hyperpyrexia (see Chapter 60).

12. **What is the relationship between fever and tachycardia?**
    The pulse should increase by eight beats per minute for each 1°C (1.8°F) increase in temperature (Liebermeister's rule). A pulse–temperature dissociation occurs when the patient has a fever but a heart rate that is lower than would be expected for the degree of fever (Faget's sign). This dissociation can occur with typhoid, malaria, legionnaires' disease, yellow fever, tularemia, brucellosis, and mycoplasma infections. Tachycardia that is out of proportion to the degree of fever is common in early septic shock. Tachypnea out of proportion to fever is characteristic of etiologies affecting gas exchange, such as with pneumonia or severe metabolic acidosis seen in severe sepsis.

13. **Do all patients with sepsis have a fever?**
    No. Just as not all fevers are caused by infection, not all patients with infection have a fever. Remember that systemic inflammatory response syndrome (SIRS) criteria include a temperature greater than 38°C (100.4°F) *or* less than 36°C (96.8°F). Therefore, hypothermia can also be a sign of sepsis. Additionally, patients may be normothermic.

14. **Should everyone with a fever get antibiotics?**
    Absolutely not. Antibiotic use should be based on the patient's specific presentation and diagnosis after completing an appropriate history, physical examination, and directed testing. Consider immediate antibiotics for patients who appear toxic or who have a suspected severe bacterial infection, as well as those in the high-risk groups previously mentioned.

15. **What is a neutropenic fever?**
    Neutropenia is defined as an absolute neutrophil count (ANC) of fewer than 500 cells/mm^3 or an ANC that is expected to decrease to fewer than 500 cells/mm^3 within the next 48 hours (see Chapter 45). A neutropenic fever is a single oral temperature ≥38.3°C (101°F) or a temperature ≥38°C (100.4°F) sustained over 1 hour. In general,

Table 15.1 Drugs Commonly Associated With Drug Fevers	
Antibiotics Penicillins	**CNS Acting Drugs** Phenytoin
Cephalosporins	Phenobarbital
Isoniazid	Carbamazepine
Nitrofurantoin	Thioridazine
Rifampin	**Nonsteroidal Anti-inflammatory Drugs** Ibuprofen
Sulfonamides	
Minocycline	Salicylates
Antineoplastic Drugs Bleomycin	**Other** Cimetidine
Streptozocin	Iodides
Cardiac Drugs Procainamide	Allopurinol
	Prostaglandin E_2
Quinidine	Interferon

CNS, Central nervous system.

rectal temperatures should be avoided in neutropenic patients. Theoretically, a rectal temperature (or examination, for that matter) increases the risk of a local or systemic infection by translocating bacteria across the rectal mucosa.

16. **What is a fever of unknown origin (FUO)?**
    The classic 1961 definition by Petersdorf et al. described an FUO as a temperature greater than 38.3°C (100.9°F) documented on several occasions over more than *3 weeks* and an uncertain diagnosis after 1 week of inpatient evaluation. Modern modifications on the definition exclude immunocompromised patients and advocate for an outpatient workup with certain obligatory tests, including laboratory tests plus chest and abdominal imaging. When identified, the most common causes of FUO are occult infection, neoplastic disease, and noninfectious inflammatory disease. But in many cases, a source for the fever is never found.

17. **Is there anything unique about fever in the elderly?**
    Elderly patients with fever are more likely to have a serious bacterial or viral illness compared with younger patients. However, 20%–30% of elderly patients with a serious infection may exhibit a blunted or absent febrile response. These factors, as well as atypical presentations for infections in the elderly, may delay diagnoses. Unlike the young, the source for an FUO can be found in the majority of cases (87%–95%). The elderly patient with FUO is more likely to have an occult infection. Tuberculosis, abscesses, and endocarditis occur more commonly in older patients. They are also more likely to have autoimmune disease, such as temporal arteritis and polymyalgia rheumatica, as well as malignancies, compared with their younger counterparts.

18. **How long do typical febrile illnesses last?**
    In most cases, the fever resolves within 3–7 days. An acute fever is defined as a fever lasting less than 7 days.

19. **Is a fever a friend or foe?**
    This question has been controversial for centuries. Although fever, per se, is self-limited and rarely serious, it is often considered by patients, parents, and doctors to be a sign of severe illness. More research is proving, however, that fever may be beneficial in fighting some infections. Higher temperatures increase the activity of neutrophils and lymphocytes, and decrease the levels of serum iron, a substrate that many bacteria need to reproduce. Fever enhances immunologic processes, including increasing the activity of IL-1, T-helper cells, and cytolytic T cells, as well as stimulating the synthesis of B cells and immunoglobulin.

20. **Does fever reduction affect outcome from an infection-related illness?**
    There is no significant clinical evidence that antipyretics affect common infections or that fever facilitates faster recovery. As such, the appropriate treatment of fever and its symptoms with routine antipyretics does no harm. They improve patient comfort and can decrease metabolic demands in patients with limited reserve.

21. **Many physicians recommend alternating or combined acetaminophen and ibuprofen for fevers. Is this effective?**

    A recent Cochrane review has shown that there is some evidence that both alternating and combined antipyretic therapy may be more effective than monotherapy at reducing temperatures in children. However, there is no clear evidence as to whether dual therapy improves patient comfort, and overall, there is insufficient evidence to know whether dual therapy is beneficial. Many experts have expressed concern over inappropriate dosing and dosing intervals by caretakers, given the more complex management of alternating or combined therapy.

22. **Should antipyretics be given to prevent febrile seizures?**

    There is no evidence that antipyretics prevent febrile seizures, but it is reasonable to instruct caretakers to initiate antipyretics when fever is discovered.

KEY POINTS: FEVER

1. Increased body temperature may be indicative of either a fever or hyperthermia from another cause.
2. Of the readily available methods, rectal temperatures are the most accurate representation of core body temperature.
3. The degree of temperature elevation is not predictive of serious illness in adults.

BIBILIOGRAPHY

Dinarello CA, Porat R. Fever and hyperthermia. In: Longo DL, Fauci AS, et al., eds. *Harrison's Principles of Internal Medicine.* 18th ed. New York: McGraw-Hill; 2012.

Dinarello CA, Simon A, van der Meer JW. Treating inflammation by blocking interleukin-1 in a broad spectrum of diseases. *Nat Rev Drug Discov.* 2012;11:633.

Freifeld AG, Bow EJ, Sepkowitz KA, et al. Clinical practice guideline for the use of antimicrobial agents in neutropenic patients with cancer: 2010 update by the Infectious Diseases Society of America. *Clin Infect Dis.* 2011;52:e56–e93.

High KP, Bradley SF, Gravenstein S, et al. Clinical practice guideline for the evaluation of fever and infection in older adult residents of long-term care facilities: 2008 update by the Infectious Diseases Society of America. *Clin Infect Dis.* 2009;2:149–171.

Niven DJ, Gaudet JE, Laupland KB, et al. Accuracy of peripheral thermometers for estimating temperature: a systematic review and meta-analysis. *Ann Intern Med.* 2015;163:768.

Offringa M, Newton R, Cozijnsen MA, et al. Prophylactic drug management for febrile seizures in children. *Cochrane Database Syst Rev.* 2012;2:CD003031.

O'Grady NP, Barie PS, Bartlett JG, et al. Guidelines for evaluation of new fever in critically ill adult patients: 2008 update from the American College of Critical Care Medicine and the Infectious Diseases Society of America. *Crit Care Med.* 2008;36:1330–1349.

Wong T, Stang AS, Ganshorn H, et al. Combined and alternating paracetamol and ibuprofen therapy for febrile children. *Cochrane Database Syst Rev.* 2013;(10):CD009572.

CHAPTER 16

CHEST PAIN

Maxwell Blodgett, MD, Daniel Lapidus, MD and Shamai A. Grossman, MD, MS

1. **Why is the cause of chest pain often difficult to determine in the ED?** (Fig. 16.1)
   - Numerous disease processes in a variety of organs may result in chest pain.
   - More than one disease process may be present.
   - The causes of acute chest pain can often be a dynamic process.
   - The severity of the pain is often unrelated to the potential life threat of its source.
   - The location of the pain as perceived by the patient may not correspond with the pain's source.
   - Reproducible chest pain can have a cardiac etiology.
   - Physical findings, laboratory assays, and radiologic studies are often nondiagnostic in the ED.

2. **What life-threatening causes of acute chest pain must be considered first when evaluating a patient in the ED?**
   - Acute coronary syndrome (ACS) (unstable angina and myocardial infarction [MI])
   - Pulmonary embolism (PE)
   - Pneumothorax
   - Aortic dissection
   - Pericarditis
   - Myocarditis
   - Cardiac tamponade
   - Mediastinitis/esophageal rupture
   - Trauma

3. **What are examples of other conditions that may present with chest pain?**
   - Cardiac
     - Stable angina
     - Valvular heart disease
   - Pulmonary
     - Pneumonia
     - Pleurisy
   - Gastrointestinal (GI)
     - Gastroesophageal reflux disease (GERD)
     - Esophageal spasm
     - Peptic ulcer disease
     - Cholecystitis
     - Pancreatitis
   - Hematologic
     - Symptomatic anemia
     - Sickle cell anemia
   - Cutaneous
     - Herpes zoster
   - Psychiatric
     - Anxiety
   - Anatomic
     - Thoracic outlet syndrome
   - Musculoskeletal pain
   - Toxicologic
   - Vasoactive drug use

4. **Why is the location of chest pain not diagnostic of its cause?**
   Somatic fibers from the dermis are numerous and enter the spinal cord at a single level, resulting in sharp, localized pain. Visceral afferent fibers from the thorax and upper abdomen are less numerous. They enter the spinal cord at multiple levels, resulting in a pain that is dull, aching, and poorly localized. Connections between the visceral and somatic fibers may result in the visceral pain being perceived as originating from somatic locations, including not only the chest but also the shoulder, arm, neck, jaw, abdomen, or back. In a classic example, the myocardium, which is innervated by the T1-4 roots, refers pain during infarction to the arm and shoulder.

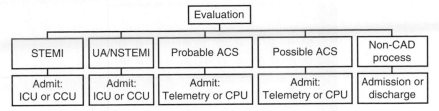

Fig. 16.1 Evaluation of chest pain. *ACS,* Acute coronary syndrome; *CAD,* coronary artery disease; *CCU,* coronary care unit; *CPU,* chest pain observation unit; *ICU,* intensive care unit; *NSTEMI,* non–ST-segment elevation myocardial infarction; *STEMI,* ST-segment elevation myocardial infarction, *UA,* unstable angina.

5. **What is the best initial approach to patients with chest pain?**
   All patients with acute chest pain should be approached with the assumption that a life-threatening cause is present. With few exceptions, once patient stability is established, intravenous (IV) access, pulse oximetry, and cardiac monitoring should be initiated before any diagnostic studies are initiated.

6. **How do I initially evaluate the patient with chest pain?**
   An accurate history is the most important component of the evaluation. This history can be used to direct a physical examination and further studies.
   - Factors to be considered include onset, character and quality, severity, location, pattern of radiation, duration of pain, and associated symptoms.
   - Precipitating factors (such as exertion, movement, or inspiration) and relieving factors (such as rest or body position) may provide clues to the origin of the pain (Table 16.1).
   - Relief of chest pain with nitroglycerin or a GI cocktail is not useful in distinguishing between cardiac and noncardiac causes of chest pain.

7. **What are the major risk factors associated with ischemic heart disease, PE, and aortic dissection?**
   See Chapters 32 and 33.

8. **Is knowing risk factors for cardiac ischemia useful in the ED?**
   The American College of Cardiology Foundation/American Heart Association (ACCF/AHA) guidelines suggest that the most important factor in predicting ACS in a patient with chest pain is the history of present illness, rather than cardiac risk factors. Classic risk factors for cardiac ischemia have had limited utility in the ED setting when trying to determine the immediate risk of ACS.
   Nevertheless, various clinical decision rules have been developed to generate a risk profile for coronary ischemia in patients presenting with chest pain. The HEART score is perhaps the most useful to date (Table 16.2). The name of this validated score is an acronym for the five elements it comprises: **H**istory, **E**lectrocardiograph (ECG), **A**ge, **R**isk factors, and **T**roponin. The low risk cohort was associated with 0.99% risk of adverse cardiac event in a retrospective study and 1.7% in prospective study. When combined with a repeat troponin 3 hours later to form the HEART pathway, the HEART score can identify patients in a low-risk cohort who may be safely discharged with outpatient follow-up. Clinical decision rules are no substitute for physician judgment. Clinical gestalt can help identify cases that would otherwise be missed by clinical decision rules.

9. **Are there any useful clinical prediction rules for stratifying patients with suspected PE according to their level of risk?**
   Yes, see Chapter 29.

10. **Is radiation of chest pain significant?**
    Radiating chest pain is suggestive but not diagnostic of cardiac ischemia. Visceral pain (including that caused by cardiac, aortic, esophageal, gastric, and pulmonary processes) may present with radiation of pain to the neck, shoulder, or arm. Chest pain that radiates to the arms specifically increases the likelihood of acute MI. Interestingly, although "typical" cardiac chest pain is traditionally taught as radiating to the left arm, recent evidence has suggested that referred chest pain to the right arm may be found more frequently than the classically described left arm radiation.

11. **How does the patient's appearance correlate with the origin of chest pain?**
    - Catastrophic illnesses often result in anxiety, diaphoresis, and an ill appearance.
    - Splinting may be caused by PE, pleurisy/pleural irritation, pneumothorax, pneumonia, or musculoskeletal chest pain.
    - Patients with cardiac ischemia may have a wide range of presentations, from appearing comfortable to the classic diaphoretic patient with a fist clenched over his or her sternum (Levine's sign).

Table 16.1 Classic Patterns of Chest Pain

ETIOLOGY	QUALITY	LOCATION	RADIATION	DURATION	ASSOCIATED SYMPTOMS	ONSET
Myocardial infarction	Visceral	Retrosternal	Neck, jaw, shoulder, arm	>15 min	Nausea, vomiting, diaphoresis, dyspnea	Variable
Angina	Visceral	Retrosternal	Neck, jaw, shoulder, arm	5–15 min	Nausea, diaphoresis, dyspnea	Gradual
Aortic dissection	Severe, tearing	Retrosternal	Interscapular	Constant	Nausea, dyspnea, diaphoresis	Sudden
Pulmonary embolism	Pleuritic	Lateral		Constant	Dyspnea, apprehension	Sudden
Pneumothorax	Pleuritic	Lateral	Neck, back	Constant	Dyspnea	Sudden
Pericarditis	Sharp, stabbing	Retrosternal	Neck, back, shoulder, arm	Constant	Dyspnea, dysphagia	Variable
Esophageal rupture	Boring	Retrosternal, epigastric	Posterior thorax	Constant	Diaphoresis, dyspnea (late)	Sudden
Esophagitis	Aching, boring	Retrosternal	Interscapular	Minutes to hours	Dysphagia	Variable
Esophageal spasm	Visceral	Retrosternal	Interscapular	Minutes to hours	Dysphagia	Variable
Musculoskeletal	Sharp, aching, superficial	Localized		Variable	Dyspnea	Variable

Table 16.2 HEART Score

Heart Score	Points		
	0 POINTS	1 POINTS	2 POINTS
History[1]	Slightly suspicious	Moderately suspicious	Highly suspicious
Electrocardiograph	Normal	Non-specific repolarization disturbance[2]	Significant ST deviation[3]
Age (years)	<45	45–64	≥65
Risk factors[4]	No known risk factors	1–2 risk factors	≥3 risk factors or history of atherosclerotic disease
Initial troponin[5]	≤ normal limit	1–3 × normal limit	>3 × normal limit

Low risk (0–3 points), intermediate risk (4–6 points), and high risk (≥7 points).
1. For example: retrosternal pain, pressure, radiation to jaw/left shoulder/arms, duration 5–15 minutes, initiated by exercise/cold/emotion, perspiration, nausea/vomiting, reaction on nitrates within minutes, patient recognizes symptoms. Low-risk features of chest pain include well localized, sharp, non-exertional, no diaphoresis, no nausea or vomiting, and reproducible with palpation.
2. Left bundle branch block (LBBB), typical changes suggesting left ventricular hypertrophy (LVH), repolarization disorders suggesting digoxin, unchanged known repolarization disorders.
3. Significant ST-segment deviation without LBBB, LVH, or digoxin.
4. Hypertension, hypercholesterolemia, diabetes, obesity (body mass index [BMI] >30 kg/m^2), smoking (current, or smoking cessation ≤3 months), positive family history (parent or sibling with cardiovascular disease [CVD] before age 65).
5. Use local assays and corresponding cutoffs.
Data from Amsterdam EA, Wenger NK, Brindis RG, et al. 2014 AHA/ACC guideline for the management of patients with non–ST-elevation acute coronary syndromes: a report of the American College of Cardiology/American Heart Association Task Force on Practice Guidelines. *J Am Coll Cardiol* 2014;64(24):e139–e228; Goodacre SW, Angelini K, Arnold J, et al. Clinical predictors of acute coronary syndromes in patients with undifferentiated chest pain. *QJM.* 2003;96:893–898; Goodacre S, Locker T, Morris F, et al. How useful are clinical features in the diagnosis of acute, undifferentiated chest pain? *Acad Emerg Med.* 2002;9:203–208.

- The Kussmaul sign is a paradoxic filling of the neck veins during inspiration, suggesting a right ventricular infarction, PE, or pericardial effusion with tamponade.

12. **How are vital signs helpful?**
    - A blood pressure difference of more than 20 mmHg between the upper extremities, or a loss or reduction of lower extremity pulses, is suggestive of an aortic dissection.
    - Hypotension is an ominous but nonspecific sign commonly indicative of a more serious pathologic condition. This may be cardiogenic (as may occur in MI) or obstructive (as in PE, tension pneumothorax, or pericardial tamponade), or hemorrhagic (free rupture of an aortic dissection), or distributive (sepsis from pneumonia or mediastinitis).
    - The presence of tachycardia should raise the suspicion of serious abnormality, with severe pain or anxiety as diagnoses of exclusion.
    - Tachypnea may be caused by a PE, pneumonia, or pneumothorax, or may be secondary to pain or metabolic derangement.
    - An elevated temperature usually indicates an infectious or inflammatory process, such as pericarditis or pneumonia.
    - Hypoxia is a sensitive but nonspecific marker of ominous pathologic findings. It can be caused by a variety of cardiopulmonary pathologies and should be treated with supplemental oxygen or positive pressure ventilation as clinically indicated. It is important to re-evaluate the patient's clinical appearance and laboratory results, if indicated, after implementing new forms of supplemental oxygen.

13. **Which physical examination findings may help differentiate the causes of acute chest pain?**
    Isolated physical findings are rarely diagnostic of the origin of chest pain, but when used in context with the history they may be extremely valuable. Palpation may reveal localized tenderness and reproduce musculoskeletal pain and this finding has a negative likelihood ratio of ACS of 0.10. However, 5%–10% of patients with ACS have chest tenderness. Cardiac auscultation may reveal a new murmur of aortic insufficiency suggestive of aortic dissection or a new murmur of mitral regurgitation secondary to papillary muscle dysfunction from ACS. A third or fourth heart sound increases the likelihood of ACS. Asymmetric pulses or neurologic deficits may indicate aortic dissection into the subclavian or carotid arteries, respectively. A pericardial friction rub is associated with pericarditis. Distant heart sounds and distended neck veins may indicate pericardial tamponade. Pneumopericardium from an esophageal or bronchial rupture can result in a crunching sound timed with the cardiac rhythm and is best heard in left lateral decubitus called *Hamman's sign* or *Hamman's crunch.* Decreased breath sounds, localized subcutaneous emphysema, or hyperresonance may indicate a pneumothorax. Localized rales suggest pneumonia as the cause of the chest pain. Patients with unilateral leg swelling, pitting edema of one leg, tenderness over the deep venous system, or calf swelling may be related to a deep vein thrombosis (DVT) and resultant PE.

14. **How is the ECG helpful in the evaluation of chest pain?**
    The ECG is an excellent rapid-screening assessment that can provide many clues, which are often diagnostic, to the source of chest pain.
    - The ECG findings most often associated with ACS are ST segment elevation, ST segment depression, inverted T waves, and new bundle branch blocks. However, the initial ECG may be normal in 20%–50% of patients in the ED who are later diagnosed as having had an acute MI.
    - ST-elevation MI (STEMI) should be diagnosed by evaluating both an ECG and the patient's clinical presentation (see Chapter 31). STEMI mimics, such as aortic dissection and pericarditis, should be considered but have unique presentations and risk factors.
    - In pericarditis, the initial ECG changes may consist of diffuse ST elevation with depression of the PR segment. Tachycardia and low voltages are seen with tamponade. Rarely, electrical alternans may be seen in a severe pericardial effusion or tamponade.
    - As a result of improved imaging technology, pulmonary emboli are more commonly diagnosed in patients with normal ECGs. Common ECG abnormalities associated with acute PE are sinus tachycardia (44%) and new T-wave inversions (33%) and T-wave flattening (30%), both most commonly in inferior leads. Right heart strain secondary to a PE may also result in peaked P waves, right-axis deviation, or a prominent S wave in lead I; a Q wave in lead III; and a new T-wave inversion in lead III (S1 Q3 T3 pattern); however, the S1 Q3 T3 pattern is neither sensitive nor specific.
    - Comparison with previous ECGs is critical when possible.

15. **What abnormalities may appear on the chest radiograph in diseases causing chest pain?**
    The chest radiographs of patients with chest pain are often normal but may provide a rapid diagnosis of several conditions, such as the following:
    - Pneumothorax can often show a visceral pleural line on upright films or deep sulcus sign on supine films. If tension is present, the mediastinum will be shifted away from the side of pneumothorax.
    - Aortic dissection may show a widened mediastinum, depression of the left main stem bronchus, loss of the paratracheal stripe, a 4- to 5-mm or greater separation between the calcified intima and the lateral edge of the aortic knob, apical capping (usually on the left), deviation of the esophagus or trachea to the right, or loss of aortic pulmonic window.
    - A PE usually has a normal chest x-ray but occasionally will show nonspecific signs, such as atelectasis or an elevated hemidiaphragm. Rare PE signs include a Hampton hump, a wedge-shaped, pleural-based infiltrate representing an area of infarction, and the Westermark sign, which is an absence of pulmonary vascular markings distal to a proximal embolism.
    - Pneumonia typically produces one or more areas of pulmonary consolidation, a pleural effusion, or cavitation.
    - Esophageal rupture is classically associated with subcutaneous emphysema, pneumomediastinum, a left-sided pleural effusion, or a left-sided pneumothorax.

16. **Are cardiac enzymes useful in the evaluation of chest pain in the ED?**
    Yes. See Chapter 31.

17. **Is bedside ultrasound useful in identifying the cause of emergency chest pain?**
    The use of bedside ultrasound is becoming standard practice in the evaluation of patients with chest pain, particularly when they present *in extremis*. Multiple studies have demonstrated that with proper training, emergency physicians (EPs) can become quite adept at using bedside ultrasound to answer focused clinical questions. Bedside ultrasound can rapidly and accurately elucidate multiple sequelae of conditions causing emergent chest pain, including pericardial effusion, pleural fluid, pneumothorax, and gross cardiac dysfunction. More advanced users may detect more subtle findings, such as tamponade, contractility abnormalities in MI, pneumonia, pulmonary edema, enlarged aortic root, and right heart strain in PE. In many circumstances, these studies are more accurate and rapid than plain radiographs. Although such findings are important supplements to clinical care, it is important to realize the limitations of such studies, including user variability (in both acquisition and interpretation of ultrasounds), image quality of bedside ultrasound machines, and factors that may confound imaging. Important uses of ultrasound in the diagnosis of chest pain include the following:
    - Pulmonary: Lung sliding between the visceral and parietal pleura visualized in real time and the presence of the "sandy shore" sign on M-mode are both reassuring against a pneumothorax; pleural effusions, whether transudative/exudative or hemorrhagic, can be visualized above the diaphragm.
    - Cardiac: Pericardial effusions and right ventricular collapse, when concerned for tamponade, can be identified by the EP; left ventricular ejection fraction can be approximated by the EP using end-point septal separation, which visualizes the distal aspect of the mitral leaflet and its proximity on end systole to the interventricular septum. Signs of right ventricular strain include McConnell sign (akinesia of the mid-free wall of the right ventricle [RV], septal bowing towards the left ventricle [LV] during systole, and RV dilatation are all concerning for acute PE).

18. **Are there any other useful diagnostic imaging studies to help determine the cause of chest pain?**
    - Aortic dissection may be diagnosed by chest computed tomography (CT) scan with IV contrast or a transesophageal echocardiogram.

- A suspected PE may be confirmed by CT pulmonary angiography or ventilation-perfusion scan.
- Esophageal rupture may be diagnosed by an esophagogram with a water-soluble contrast material.

19. **What special considerations must be taken into account when evaluating chest pain in patients who are geriatric, have diabetes, or are female?**
    - Although the sources of chest pain in the elderly do not differ significantly from the general population, their presenting symptoms are often atypical. Instead of chest pain, ischemic heart disease may manifest as sudden progressive dyspnea, abdominal or epigastric fullness, extreme fatigue, confusion, or syncope.
    - Patients with diabetes mellitus may have altered pain perception, resulting in an atypical presentation similar to that of the elderly. The risk of coronary heart disease in women increases with menopause.
    - Women with ischemic heart disease show atypical symptom patterns more often than men. This is likely because of the higher prevalence of less common causes of ischemia, such as vasospastic and microvascular angina.

20. **Is provocative stress testing useful in the emergent assessment of chest pain?**
    The current standard of care suggests that it is not only important to rule out an ongoing cardiac emergency but also to stratify patients for risk of an imminent major adverse cardiac event. Stress testing is an important tool for this purpose. Stress testing is a noninvasive tool to screen patients with emergent chest pain for intervenable coronary vascular lesions that may predispose them to future adverse cardiac events. It is important to note that stress testing is not appropriate in patients with a very low pretest probability for disease, because stress testing is more likely to evoke a false-positive result than a true-positive result and therefore will not change management and may lead to unnecessary use of valuable ED resources. On the other hand, stress testing in a patient with an extremely high pretest probability for a coronary vascular lesion can also result in false negatives and should be done in conjunction with cardiology. Clinical decision rules, such as the HEART score, can help identify appropriate candidates for stress testing. Imaging stress testing, such as stress echocardiography and myocardial perfusion studies, may produce lower false-positive and false-negative rates. Not all stress testing must be performed emergently. If patients are reliable, are at low risk for an intervenable coronary lesion, and have access to good follow-up care, it may be reasonable to administer stress tests to them as outpatients.

21. **Approximately 1%–2% of patients with chest pain caused by acute MI are discharged to home. What factors have been associated with failure to make the diagnosis?**
    - Young age group
    - Non-White race
    - Failure to obtain an accurate history
    - Incorrect interpretation of the ECG
    - Failure to recognize atypical presentations
    - Hesitance to admit patients with vague symptoms
    - Over-reliance on laboratory assays, such as cardiac enzymes
    - Insufficient experience or training

KEY POINTS: CHEST PAIN

1. The primary goal of the evaluation of acute chest pain is the inclusion or exclusion of a life-threatening disease process.
2. A normal ECG on initial presentation does not exclude ACS.
3. Twenty-five percent of patients ultimately diagnosed with ACS do not have a primary complaint of chest pain.
4. Relief of chest pain by nitroglycerin or antacids is not diagnostic for either cardiac or noncardiac disease.
5. Chest pain in patients who are elderly or have diabetes is more commonly an emergent illness than in the general population, but often presents in atypical fashion because of underlying neuropathy.

WEBSITES
American Heart Association: www.americanheart.org; accessed January 14, 2015.

ACKNOWLEDGMENTS

Special thanks to Lee S. Jacobson, MD, PhD and Eric Wong, MD, who contributed to previous versions of this chapter.

BIBILIOGRAPHY

Amsterdam EA, Wenger NK, Brindis RG, et al. 2014 AHA/ACC guideline for the management of patients with non–ST-elevation acute coronary syndromes: a report of the American College of Cardiology/American Heart Association Task Force on Practice Guidelines. *J Am Coll Cardiol.* 2014;64(24):e139–e228.

Backus BE, Six AJ, Kelder JC, et al. A prospective validation of the HEART score for chest pain patients at the emergency department. *Int J Cardiol.* 2013;168(3):2153–2158.

Co I, Eilbert W, Chiganos T. New electrocardiographic changes in patients diagnosed with pulmonary embolism. *J Emerg Med.* 2017;52(3):280–285.

Farsi D, Hajsadeghi S, Hajighanbari MJ, et al. Focused cardiac ultrasound (FOCUS) by emergency medicine residents in patients with suspected cardiovascular diseases. *J Ultrasound.* 2017;20(2):133–138.

Gibler WB, Cannon CP, Blomkalns AL, et al. Practical implementation of the guidelines for unstable angina/non–ST-segment elevation myocardial infarction in the ED. *Circulation.* 2005;111:2699–2710.

Goodacre SW, Angelini K, Arnold J, et al. Clinical predictors of acute coronary syndromes in patients with undifferentiated chest pain. *QJM.* 2003;96:893–898.

Goodacre S, Locker T, Morris F, et al. How useful are clinical features in the diagnosis of acute, undifferentiated chest pain? *Acad Emerg Med.* 2002;9:203–208.

Hamilton GC, Malone S, Janz TG. Chest pain. In: Hamilton GC, Sanders AB, Strange GR, et al., eds. *Emergency Medicine: An Approach to Clinical Problem-Solving.* 2nd ed. Philadelphia, PA: Saunders; 2003:131–153.

Hwang JQ, Kimberly HH, Liteplo AS, et al. An evidence-based approach to emergency ultrasound. *Emerg Med Pract.* 2011;13:1–27.

Ioannidis JP, Salem D, Chew PW, et al. Accuracy of imaging technologies in the diagnosis of acute cardiac ischemia in the emergency department. *Ann Emerg Med.* 2001;37:471–477.

Jneid H, Anderson JL, Wright RS, et al. 2012 ACCF/AHA focused update of the guideline for the management of patients with unstable angina/non–ST-elevation myocardial infarction (updating the 2007 guideline and replacing the 2011 focused update). *Circulation.* 2012;126:875–910.

Jones ID, Slovis CM. Emergency department evaluation for the chest pain patient. *Emerg Med Clin North Am.* 2001;19:269–282.

Lee PY, Alexander KP, Hammill BG, et al. Representation of elderly persons and women in published randomized trials of acute coronary syndromes. *JAMA.* 2001;286:708–713.

Lee TH, Goldman L. Evaluation of the patient with acute chest pain. *N Engl J Med.* 2000;342:1187–1195.

Lichtenstein D. Lung ultrasound in the critically ill. *Curr Opin Crit Care.* 2014;20(3):315–322.

Mahler SA, Miller CD, Hollander JE, et al. Identifying patients for early discharge: performance of decision rules among patients with acute chest pain. *Int J Cardiol.* 2013;168:795–802.

Mahler SA, Riley RF, Hiestand BC, et al. The HEART Pathway randomized trial: identifying emergency department patients with acute chest pain for early discharge. *Circ Cardiovasc Qual Outcomes.* 2015;8(2):195–203.

Marx JA, Hockberger RS, Walls RM, et al., eds. *Rosen's Emergency Medicine: Concepts and Clinical Practice.* 8th ed. St. Louis, MO: Brown; 2013:214–222.

McConnell MV, Solomon SD, Rayan ME, et al. Regional right ventricular dysfunction detected by echocardiography in acute pulmonary embolism. *Am J Cardiol.* 1996;78:469–473.

Panju AA, Hemmelgarn BR, Guyatt GH, et al. The rational clinical examination: is this patient having a myocardial infarction? *JAMA.* 1998;280:1256–1263.

Pope JH, Aufderheide TP, Ruthazer R, et al. Missed diagnosis of acute cardiac ischemia in the emergency department. *N Engl J Med.* 2000;342:1163–1170.

Ringstrom E, Freedman J. Approach to undifferentiated chest pain in the emergency department: a review of recent medical literature and published practice guidelines. *Mt Sinai J Med.* 2006;73:499–505.

Savonitto S, Ardissino D, Grauger CB, et al. Prognostic value of the admission electrocardiogram in acute coronary syndromes. *JAMA.* 1999;281:707–713.

Six AJ, Backus BE, Kelder JC. Chest pain in the emergency room: value of the HEART score. *Neth Heart J.* 2008;16(6):191–196.

Smith SW, Whitman W. Acute coronary syndromes: acute myocardial infarction and ischemia. In: Chan TC, Brady WJ, Harrigan RA, et al., eds. *ECG in Emergency Medicine and Acute Care.* Philadelphia, PA: Elsevier; 2005:151–172.

Steele R, McNaughton T, McConahy M, et al. Chest pain in emergency department patients: if the pain is relieved by nitroglycerin, is it more likely to be cardiac chest pain? *CJEM.* 2006;8:164–169.

Swap CJ, Nagurney JT. Value and limitations of chest pain history in evaluation of patients with suspected acute coronary syndromes. *JAMA.* 2005;294:2623–2629.

Turnipseed SD, Trythall WS, Diercks DB, et al. Frequency of acute coronary syndrome in patients with normal electrocardiogram performed during presence or absence of chest pain. *Acad Emerg Med.* 2009;16:495–499.

CHAPTER 17

ABDOMINAL PAIN, NAUSEA, AND VOMITING

Rick A. McPheeters, DO, FAAEM and Juliana Karp, MD

ABDOMINAL PAIN

1. **What is the difference between visceral and somatic pain? How is this of practical importance?**
   Evolving patterns of pain commonly reveal the source and give an idea of the extent to which the process has advanced. Early, the patient may describe a deep-seated, dull pain (visceral pain) emanating from hollow viscera or the capsule of solid organs. This pain is poorly localized but generally falls somewhere along the midline of the abdomen. Later, as inflammation progresses to the parietal peritoneum, the pain becomes better localized, lateralized over the involved organ, sharper in intensity (somatic or parietal pain), and constant. Visceral pain that is superseded by somatic pain often signals the need for surgical intervention.

2. **What is the difference between localized and generalized peritonitis?**
   As the peritoneum adjacent to a diseased organ becomes inflamed, palpation or any abdominal movement causes stretching of the sensitized peritoneum and, consequently, pain localized at that site (localized peritonitis). If irritating material (e.g., pus, blood, or gastric contents) spills into the peritoneal cavity, the entire peritoneal surface may become sensitive to stretch or motion, and any movement or palpation may provoke pain at any or all points within the abdominal cavity (generalized peritonitis).

KEY POINTS: MESENTERIC ISCHEMIA

1. Abdominal pain is out of proportion to physical findings.
2. Diffuse abdominal tenderness, rebound, and rigidity are ominous signs.
3. Definitive diagnosis is by mesenteric arteriography or surgical exploration.

---

3. **Which tests for peritoneal irritation are best?**
   Rebound tenderness during the physical examination is the traditional finding for peritonitis. In a patient with likely generalized peritonitis (e.g., obvious distress, excruciating pain every time the ambulance hits a bump), the standard tests for rebound tenderness are unnecessarily harsh. Asking the patient to cough generally supplies adequate peritoneal motion to give a positive test. When in every respect the examination is normal, highly sensitive and repeatable tests for peritoneal irritation are the heel-drop jarring (Markle) and hop tests. Among patients with appendicitis, these tests have sensitivities of ~70%–75%, and generally outperform the standard rebound test.

4. **Why is it important to establish the temporal relationship of pain to vomiting?**
   Generally, pain preceding vomiting is suggestive of a surgical process, whereas vomiting before onset of pain is more typical of a nonsurgical condition (negative likelihood ratio 0.02). Epigastric pain that is relieved by vomiting suggests intragastric pathology or gastric outlet obstruction.

5. **What is the relationship of peritoneal inflammation to loss of appetite?**
   Anorexia, nausea, and vomiting are directly proportional to the severity and extent of peritoneal irritation. The presence of appetite, however, does not rule out a surgically significant inflammatory process, such as appendicitis. A retrocecal appendicitis with limited peritoneal irritation may be associated with minimal gastrointestinal (GI) upset, and one third of all patients with acute appendicitis do not report anorexia as an initial symptom.

6. **Discuss the pitfalls of evaluating elderly patients with acute abdominal pain.**
   Advanced age may and often does blunt the manifestations of acute abdominal disease. Pain may be less severe; fever often is less pronounced, and signs of peritoneal inflammation, such as muscular guarding and rebound tenderness, may be diminished or absent. Elevation of the white blood cell (WBC) count is also less sensitive. Approximately two thirds of patients over 65 years of age with abdominal pain have a surgical cause. Cholecystitis, intestinal obstruction, and appendicitis are the most common causes for acute surgical abdomen in the elderly. Because of atypical clinical presentations, additional tests (such as lipase, liver function studies, alkaline phosphatase, and lactic acid) and the liberal use of ultrasound and computed tomography (CT) scans is prudent in this age group.

7. **What other factors should be sought in the history that may alter significantly the presenting symptoms of patients with abdominal pain?**
   Symptoms and physical findings in patients with schizophrenia and diabetes may be muted significantly. The use of immunomodulating medications (such as steroids) or antibiotics may alter signs and laboratory results.

KEY POINTS: APPENDICITIS

1. The most sensitive findings are right lower quadrant tenderness, nausea, and anorexia.
2. Clinical scoring systems are useful for risk stratification, but not for excluding the diagnosis.
3. Advanced imaging (predominantly CT) has had the greatest impact on lowering the negative laparotomy rate.

8. **What is the significance of obstipation?**
   Obstipation is the inability to pass either stool or flatus for more than 8 hours despite a perceived need, and is highly suggestive of intestinal obstruction.

9. **What vital sign is associated most closely with the degree of peritonitis?**
   Tachycardia is virtually universal with advancing peritonitis. The initial pulse is less important than serial observations. An unexplained rise in pulse may be an early clue that surgical exploration is indicated. However, this response may be blunted or absent in elderly patients, or in those taking medications such as β-blockers.

10. **Does the duration of abdominal pain help in categorizing cause?**
    Severe abdominal pain persisting for 6 or more hours is likely to be caused by surgically correctable problems. Patients with pain lasting longer than 48 hours have a significantly lower incidence of surgical disease than patients with pain of shorter duration.

11. **Name the two most commonly missed surgical causes of abdominal pain.**
    Appendicitis and acute intestinal obstruction

12. **Is there a place for narcotic analgesics in the management of acute abdominal pain of uncertain cause?**
    Yes. It is humane to alleviate the patient's suffering. Historically, it was suggested that narcotics should be avoided until a firm diagnosis is established, for fear of masking vital symptoms or physical findings. However, it is now well understood that although pain control with opioids may alter the physical examination findings, opioids do not increase management errors. In fact, the evaluation of acute abdominal disease may be facilitated by pain medications when severe pain prevents full patient cooperation.

13. **Which are the most useful preliminary laboratory tests to order?**
    A complete blood count with differential and urinalysis are generally recommended. The initial hematocrit level helps to determine whether there is antecedent anemia. An elevated WBC count suggests significant pathologic findings but is not sensitive or specific. Elevated urinary specific gravity reflects dehydration, and an increased urinary bilirubin level in the absence of urobilinogen points toward obstruction of the common bile duct. Pyuria, hematuria, and a positive dipstick for glucose and ketones may point toward urinary infection, kidney stones, or diabetic ketoacidosis, respectively. For patients with epigastric or right upper quadrant pain, lipase and liver function studies are advised. Any woman with childbearing capability should receive a pregnancy test. Serum electrolyte, glucose, blood urea nitrogen, and creatinine tests are indicated if there is clinical dehydration or other reason to suspect abnormality such as renal failure, diabetes, or a metabolic acidosis. C-reactive protein can be useful in discerning the probability of cholecystitis and appendicitis. In patients suspected of mesenteric ischemia or concomitant sepsis, a serum lactate level may be helpful in risk stratification.

14. **Are plain radiographs always indicated in the initial evaluation of suspected small bowel obstruction?**
    No. Abdominal CT has been shown to be significantly superior to plain films both in its diagnostic accuracy and in determining the level and cause of the obstruction. Exceptions include unavailable CT, expected delay in obtaining CT scans, or the patient is *in extremis*.

15. **Is oral contrast necessary when performing CT scans for suspected appendicitis?**
    No. In the ED, patients with acute abdominal pain and suspected appendicitis, oral contrast does not improve the diagnostic accuracy of CT and only delays the time to diagnosis.

16. **Do all patients with uncomplicated appendicitis require surgery?**
    No. However, current data suggest that recurrent appendicitis can be as high as 39% at 5 years in those patients treated with antibiotics alone.

17. **A 7-year-old child comes to the ED with acute abdominal pain and a history of several similar bouts over the past 5 months. Physical examination is unremarkable. What is the most likely cause?**
    In children older than 5 years, abdominal pain that is intermittent and of more than 3 months' duration is functional in more than 95% of cases, especially in the absence of objective findings, such as fever, delayed growth patterns, anemia, GI bleeding, or lateralizing pain and tenderness.

18. **A patient with severe abdominal pain is found to be suffering from DKA. How do I decide whether the abdominal pain is a manifestation of the DKA or whether a surgical condition has precipitated the DKA?**
Patients with DKA often come to the ED with severe abdominal pain. Although the precise mechanism of abdominal pain and ileus in patients with DKA is not well understood, ketonemia, hypovolemia, hypotension, and a total-body potassium deficit probably contribute. An acute surgical lesion may initiate DKA; nevertheless, most patients with DKA have no such pathologic findings. Abdominal symptoms characteristically resolve as medical treatment restores the patient to biochemical homeostasis. Treatment of the DKA must precede any surgical intervention because of the extremely high intraoperative mortality among patients whose conditions are not stabilized. If symptoms persist despite adequate correction of DKA, then an underlying reason for surgery becomes more likely.

19. **Is a rectal examination necessary in the patient with suspected acute appendicitis?**
No. However, it may help in assessing for alternative causes of abdominal pain (e.g., prostatitis or GI bleed) and therefore reducing the length of the differential diagnosis.

20. **Is there a reliable laboratory test that will either rule in or rule out appendicitis?**
No. In a recent systematic review of both traditional (e.g., WBC) and novel (e.g., interleukin 6 [IL-6]) biomarkers, none performed sufficiently at diagnosing appendicitis in isolation.

NAUSEA AND VOMITING

21. **Vomiting? Do I really need to read this section when there are so many more interesting topics in this book?**
Yes. One of the most common and harmful mistakes made in the ED is assuming that nausea and vomiting are the result of gastroenteritis without thinking of and ruling out more serious causes. In addition, vomiting is one of the most common presenting complaints in the ED.

22. **What causes vomiting?**
The act of vomiting is highly complex and involves a vomiting center in the medulla. This center may be excited in four ways:
   1. Via vagal and sympathetic afferent nerves from the peritoneum; GI, biliary, and genitourinary tracts; pelvic organs; heart; pharynx; head; and vestibular apparatus
   2. By impulses converging at the nucleus tractus solitarius in the medulla
   3. Via the chemoreceptor trigger zone located in the floor of the fourth ventricle
   4. Via the vestibular or vestibulocerebellar system (motion sickness and some medication-induced emesis)

23. **Can vomiting itself lead to potential complications?**
Yes. Some of these are life threatening.
   - Esophageal perforation or Mallory–Weiss tear
   - Severe dehydration
   - Metabolic alkalosis
   - Severe electrolyte depletion (particularly sodium, potassium, and chloride ions)
   - Pulmonary aspiration
   - Esophageal or gastric bleeding

24. **List the common causes of vomiting.**
See Table 17.1.

Table 17.1 Common Causes of Vomiting

	GASTROINTESTINAL	NONGASTROINTESTINAL
Functional	Gastroparesis, irritable bowel syndrome, cyclic vomiting syndrome	Normal pregnancy, hyperemesis gravidarum
Infectious/inflammatory	Gastroenteritis, hepatitis, appendicitis, cholecystitis, pancreatitis	Pneumonia, meningitis, sepsis
Mechanical	Small bowel obstruction, ileus, gastric outlet obstruction	Renal calculi, ovarian torsion, testicular torsion
Medication side effects	NSAID-induced gastritis, drug-induced pancreatitis (valproic acid, ACE inhibitors, metformin, statins, and many others)	Digoxin, theophylline, aspirin, iron, opiates, antibiotics, chemotherapy, radiation therapy
Neurologic/psychiatric	N/A	Increased intracranial pressure, vestibular disorders, bulimia nervosa and binge-eating disorders
Toxicologic/metabolic	Alcoholic gastritis and pancreatitis, acetaminophen-induced hepatitis, chronic cannabis use (cannabis hyperemesis syndrome)	Diabetic ketoacidosis, uremia, hypercalcemia

ACE, Angiotensin-converting enzyme; *N/A,* not applicable; *NSAID,* nonsteroidal anti-inflammatory drug.

25. Are there different GI causes of vomiting in children?
Yes, particularly during the first year of life. These include GI atresia, malrotation, volvulus, Hirschsprung disease, gastroesophageal reflux, pyloric stenosis, intussusception, and inguinal hernia (see Chapter 65).

26. Can the character of the vomit help me make a diagnosis?
Yes it can, especially GI disorders. In acute gastritis, vomit is usually stomach contents mixed with a little bile. In biliary or ureteral colic, the vomit is usually bilious. In sympathetic shock (acute torsion of abdominal or pelvic organ), it is common for the patient to retch often, but vomit only a little. In intestinal obstruction, the character of vomit varies – first gastric contents, then bilious material, with progression to brown feculent material that is pathognomonic of distal small or large bowel obstruction.

27. What else do I need to ask the patient?
- Ask about associated signs and symptoms, such as pain, fever, jaundice, and bowel habits. Think of hepatitis or biliary obstruction with jaundice. Remember that gastroenteritis is uncommon without diarrhea.
- Discuss the relationship of vomiting to meals. Vomiting that occurs soon after a meal is common with gastric outlet obstruction from peptic ulcer disease. Vomiting after a fatty meal is common with cholecystitis. Vomiting of food eaten more than 6 hours earlier is seen with gastric retention.
- Consider causes other than GI for vomiting. Ask about medications and possible drug use, headache and other neurologic symptoms, last menstrual period and possibility of pregnancy. Think about myocardial ischemia! Nausea or vomiting may be the only complaint of a patient with an acute myocardial infarction, particularly in women, patients with diabetes, or the elderly.

28. What do I look for during the physical examination?
Physical examination is helpful but can be unreliable. Look for signs of dehydration, particularly in children. Check for bowel sounds, which are increased in gastroenteritis and absent or high-pitched and "tinkling" with obstruction, or often absent with serious abdominal infections. Abdominal tenderness may be present in a variety of disorders, but a rigid abdomen suggests peritonitis, a surgical emergency. Women of childbearing age with vomiting and abdominal or pelvic pain require a pregnancy test. Perform a neurologic examination if there are any associated symptoms, such as headache or vertigo.

29. Are laboratory tests indicated?
This question must be answered on an individual basis. In general, tests should be ordered based on the history and physical examination. Patients with diabetes, immunosuppression, and at the extremes of age can have serious pathology presenting as vomiting. Be careful with these patients.

30. When should I order radiographs?
This decision is made on a case by case basis. However, flat plate radiographs of the abdomen are not useful in most patients. Upright abdominal radiography is usually nonspecific, but may show free air with perforation of an abdominal viscus, dilated bowel with obstruction, or air fluid levels with obstruction or ileus. A chest film can be useful in cases of protracted vomiting, to rule out aspiration or pneumomediastinum. Pneumonia may cause vomiting with abdominal pain and few respiratory symptoms.

KEY POINTS: DIAGNOSIS OF THE VOMITING PATIENT

1. Always consider etiologies other than GI disorders.
2. Take a thorough history, especially in immunocompromised patients or those at extremes of age.
3. Consider accidental ingestions in children and medication side effects or toxicities in adults.
4. Laboratory testing and radiographs are seldom useful in gastroenteritis but may be helpful to identify other causes of vomiting.

31 How should I treat the vomiting patient?

- Always remember to protect the airway. Patients with altered mental status should be placed on their sides to prevent aspiration. Intubate the patient early if necessary.
- IV fluids usually are indicated for rehydration. In some patients, especially children, oral rehydration may be preferred.
- Nasogastric suction can be therapeutic and diagnostic and may be indicated when there is a small bowel obstruction.
- Medications to relieve nausea and vomiting must be used judiciously, especially in patients with altered mental status, hypotension, or uncertain diagnosis. Additionally, almost all of these medications cause QT prolongation, which, in conjunction with electrolyte abnormalities, can lead to life-threatening dysrhythmias.
- Determine and, if possible, treat the underlying cause for the vomiting.

32. What medications should I use?

See Table 17.2.

33. Controversy

The use of ondansetron in pregnancy, particularly in the first trimester, remains controversial. The most recent evidence indicates that it is probably safe, but should be third or fourth line. A large database review found a small increased incidence of congenital heart defects and cleft lip and palate. Judicious use in pregnancy is recommended. Currently, the American College of Obstetrics and Gynecology recommends pyridoxine and doxylamine as first-line agents followed by prochlorperazine or metoclopramide

Table 17.2 Common Antiemetic Medications

GENERIC NAME	TRADE NAME	INDICATION	DOSAGE
Prochlorperazine	Compazine	Nausea, vomiting, anxiety	10 mg PO, IM, or IV qid, 25 mg PR bid (black box warning: elderly patients with dementia-related psychosis[a])
Doxylamine + pyridoxine[a]	Diclegis	Nausea and vomiting of pregnancy	Dosage varies, 2–4 tabs in divided doses qid
Dimenhydrinate	Dramamine	Nausea, motion sickness	50–100 mg PO, IM, or IV qid
Aprepitant	Emend	Nausea and vomiting, with chemotherapy	125 mg PO on day 1, 80 mg PO on days 2 and 3
Phosphorated carbohydrate	Emetrol	Nausea and vomiting	15–30 mL q 15 min (not to exceed 5 doses)
Droperidol	Inapsine	Nausea and vomiting	0.625–2.5 mg IV or 2.5 IM (black box warning: QT prolongation[a])
Granisetron	Kytril, Sancuso, Sustol	Nausea and vomiting with chemotherapy	10 mg/kg IV or 1 mg PO bid (only on day of chemotherapy); also comes in patch
Dronabinol	Marinol	Refractory nausea and vomiting with chemotherapy	Dosage varies
Promethazine	Phenergan	Nausea, vomiting, motion sickness, anxiety	12.5–25 mg PO, PR, or IV qid (black box warning: children younger than 2 years, respiratory depression); (IV use concern for severe tissue injury, gangrene[a])

Continued on following page

Table 17.2 Common Antiemetic Medications *(Continued)*

GENERIC NAME	TRADE NAME	INDICATION	DOSAGE
Metoclopramide	Reglan	Nausea, vomiting, gastro-esophageal reflux, gastroparesis	5–10 mg PO or IV dosage varies (black box warning: tardive dyskinesia[a])
Chlorpromazine	Thorazine	Nausea, vomiting, anxiety	10–25 mg PO qid or 25 mg IM qid (black box warning: elderly patients with dementia-related psychosis[b])
Trimethobenzamide	Tigan	Nausea and vomiting	300 mg PO tid or qid, 200 mg IM tid or qid
Scopolamine	Transderm Scop	Nausea, vomiting, motion sickness	1 patch every 3 days
Doxylamine[a]	Unisom	Nausea and vomiting due to pregnancy	12.5 mg PO bid or qid; often used in combination with pyridoxine (Unisom may contain diphenhydramine instead of doxylamine)
Hydroxyzine pamoate	Vistaril	Nausea, vomiting, anxiety	25–100 mg PO or IM tid or qid
Ondansetron	Zofran	Nausea and vomiting	4–8 mg PO, IV, or IM; also comes in ODT form (black box warning: avoid in long QT prolongation), controversial in pregnancy, data unclear

[a]From www.uptodate.com. Accessed February 1, 2019.
[b]Still not done.
bid, Twice a day; *IM,* intramuscularly; *IV,* intravenously; *ODT,* orally disintegrating tablet; *PO,* per os (by mouth); *PR,* per rectum; *qid,* four times a day; *tid,* three times a day.

34. **What about cyclic vomiting syndromes?**
    Cyclic vomiting syndrome and cannabis hyperemesis syndrome are becoming more frequently diagnosed. The etiology of cyclic vomiting syndrome is unclear, but there is an association with migraines. Cannabis hyperemesis syndrome is associated with both acute and chronic marijuana use. These conditions may be associated and can be difficult to diagnose. Many ED visits may occur before a diagnosis is made. Keep these on your mental list. Frequent hot showers or topical capsaicin cream can be helpful in cannabis hyperemesis syndrome. Ondansetron, benzodiazepines, and haloperidol may also be helpful.

WEBSITES

www.uptodate.com (search cyclic vomiting syndrome, cannabis hyperemesis syndrome, vomiting in pregnancy, nausea and vomiting); accessed February 1, 2019.

BIBILIOGRAPHY

Abdominal Pain

Abdominal pain in elderly persons. http://emedicine.medscape.com/article/776663-overview. Accessed February 1, 2019.
Acharya A, Markar SR, Ni M, et al. Biomarkers of acute appendicitis: systematic review and cost-benefit trade-off analysis. *Surg Endosc.* 2017;31:1022–1031.
Appendicitis. http://emedicine.medscape.com/article/773895-overview. Accessed February 1, 2019.
Jackson K, Taylor D, Judkins S. Emergency department abdominal X-rays have a poor diagnostic yield and their usefulness is questionable. *Emerg Med.* 2011;28:745–749.
Manterola C, Vial M, Moraga J, et al. Analgesia in patients with acute abdominal pain. *Cochrane Database Syst Rev.* 2011;(1):CD005660.

Nausea and Vomiting

Huybrechts KF, Hernández-Díaz S, Straub L, et al. Association of maternal first trimester ondensetron use with cardiac malformations and oral clefts in offspring. *JAMA.* 2018;320:2429–2437.
Koren G, Hankins GD, Clark S, et al. Effectiveness of doxylamine-pyridoxine for morning sickness. *Am J Obstet Gynecol.* 2016;214:664–666.
Richards JR. Cannabinoid hyperemesis pathophysiology and treatment in the emergency department. *J Emerg Med.* 2018;54:354–363.

CHAPTER 18

HEADACHE

Christopher Vercollone, MD and Nicole M. Dubosh, MD

1. **How common are headaches, and what percentage of patients in the ED have headache as a chief complaint?**
   Nearly everyone has a headache at some point in their lives; about 12% of the general population has migraines. While most patients do not seek medical care, approximately 2% of all ED visits are for headaches, with a female predominance (62%). Of those who come to the ED with headache, only about 5% will have a serious cause.

2. **When someone has a headache, what exactly is it that hurts?**
   The brain, the pia and arachnoid mater, the skull, and the choroid plexus are not the source of headache pain. The structures in the head that are pain sensitive include the scalp; skin; vessels; scalp muscles; parts of the dura mater; dural arteries; intracerebral arteries; cranial nerves V, VI, and VII; and the cervical nerves. Irritation, inflammation, distention, or traction of any of these may result in a headache.

3. **Name the most common headaches for which patients seek treatment.**
   Muscle contraction (tension) and vascular (migraine) headaches are by far the most common, even in an acuity-skewed ED population. These are often referred to as *primary headache disorders*. Although painful, these disorders do not have life-threatening sequelae. There are a number of *cannot miss* causes of headache that, although less common, are crucial for emergency physicians to diagnose correctly.

4. **What causes of headache are cannot miss?**
   True emergencies, or *cannot miss* causes of headache, are conditions that threaten life, limb, brain, or eye, and are treatable (Table 18.1). Headaches that are true emergencies include:
   - Subarachnoid hemorrhage (SAH)
   - Subdural or epidural hematoma
   - Intraparenchymal hemorrhage
   - Ischemic cerebrovascular accident
   - Dissection of a carotid or vertebral artery
   - Pre-eclampsia
   - Hypertensive encephalopathy
   - Brain tumor
   - Giant cell arteritis (temporal arteritis) and other vasculitides
   - Central nervous system infections (meningitis and abscess)
   - Idiopathic intracranial hypertension (also known as pseudotumor cerebri)
   - Cerebral venous sinus thrombosis (CVST)
   - Angle-closure glaucoma
   - Spontaneous intracranial hypotension

5. **What are some clinical clues to distinguish primary headaches from cannot miss headaches?**
   By definition, tension and migraine headaches are recurrent, requiring at least 5–10 episodes; these episodes are usually similar to one another in any individual patient. Therefore, any first severe headache can never be definitively diagnosed as a tension or migraine headache. A headache that is described as a *first* or *worst* headache, or even substantially different from prior headaches, requires careful evaluation. A sudden, severe-onset episode, commonly described as "The worst headache I have ever had," is classic for an SAH. Likewise, any headache associated with new focal neurologic signs should be investigated. An associated fever requires evaluation for infection, tumor, or drug use. A careful history and physical examination is usually the diagnostic element that helps decide which headaches warrant further evaluation.

6. **Why are age and context important in the history of a patient with a headache?**
   Migraines most commonly begin before age 30. Tension-type headaches usually begin before age 50. Headaches that begin after age 55 are much more likely to have a serious cause, such as a mass lesion, giant cell arteritis, or cerebrovascular disease. Headaches occurring in the peripartum period may be caused by cortical vein or CVST, or pre-eclampsia. In general, if a patient has a long history of previous similar attacks, a serious cause is less likely. If a patient reports numerous identical attacks treated at home, it is important to understand why this particular episode led to an ED visit.

Table 18.1 Red Flags in Patients With Headaches

HEADACHE CHARACTERISTICS	DIFFERENTIAL DIAGNOSIS	POSSIBLE WORKUP (BEYOND HISTORY AND PHYSICAL EXAMINATION)
Headache begins after age 50	Mass lesion, temporal arteritis, stroke	ESR, CRP, neuroimaging
Sudden onset of headache	SAH, pituitary apoplexy, hemorrhage into a mass lesion or vascular malformation, mass lesion (especially posterior fossa), vascular dissection and CVST	Neuroimaging, LP if CT is negative
Headaches increasing in frequency and severity	Mass lesion, subdural hematoma, medication overuse	Neuroimaging
New-onset headache in patient who has risk factors for HIV, cancer	Meningitis (chronic or carcinomatous), brain abscess (including toxoplasmosis), metastasis	Neuroimaging, LP if neuroimaging is negative
Headache with fever, meningismus, rash, or altered mentation	Meningitis, encephalitis, Lyme disease, systemic infection, collagen vascular disease	Neuroimaging, LP, serology
Focal neurologic symptoms or signs of disease (other than typical aura)	Mass lesion, vascular malformation, stroke	Neuroimaging
Papilledema	Mass lesion, idiopathic intracranial hypertension, meningitis	Neuroimaging, LP
Headache that worsens with standing up	Spontaneous intracranial hypotension, postdural puncture headache (if following an LP)	For the former: LP with opening pressure; MRI
Headache with ocular or visual symptoms	Pseudotumor cerebri, acute narrow angle glaucoma, temporal arteritis	LP for pseudotumor, tonometry for glaucoma, ESR, and biopsy for arteritis
Headache after head trauma	Intracranial hemorrhage, subdural hematoma, epidural hematomas, posttraumatic headache	Neuroimaging of brain and possibly cervical spine

CT, Computed tomography; *CVST,* cerebral venous sinus thrombosis; *ESR,* erythrocyte sedimentation rate; *HIV,* human immunodeficiency virus; *LP,* lumbar puncture; *MRI,* magnetic resonance imaging; *SAH,* subarachnoid hemorrhage.

7. **What questions in the history are most important to ask in evaluating a patient with a headache?**
   - Do you get headaches often? Have you ever needed to go to an ED for one? Is this current headache the same as prior ones that you have had? If not, how does it differ? These questions are aimed at assessing the quality of pain.
   - How bad is this headache? Have you had headaches this severe in the past? These questions assess the severity.
   - How long did it take from when the headache began to when it reached maximal intensity? If sudden, what were you doing at the time it began? These questions consider the onset.
   - What symptoms accompany the headache? Did you vomit? Was there any fainting, seizure, photophobia, or double vision? Did you have these same associated symptoms with prior episodes or not (for patients with a prior history of headache)? These associated symptoms can suggest secondary causes. For example, a patient with migraines, who has never had photophobia or vomiting with prior episodes and now does, should undergo further evaluation. On the other hand, if this headache is similar to prior episodes, it is most likely the result of that same etiologic cause.
   - Have you had any recent head trauma? Note that this includes even minor trauma for elderly patients, who are more susceptible to chronic or delayed-presentation subdural hematomas.
   - What treatment have you used at home, and was it helpful? This can also help if a headache has responded in the past as it does for the current visit. But be careful; see Question 14.
   - Do you take any blood thinners? Patients on anticoagulants (e.g., warfarin or rivaroxaban) are more likely to have an intracranial hemorrhage.

8. **Does the physical examination add any information?**
   The history often leads to the correct diagnosis or at least a short list of possible diagnoses. The physical findings may support or refute those diagnoses or change the likelihood of various possibilities. Fever may reflect infection. Hypertension may be a sign that there is increased intracranial pressure, or simply be caused by the headache or anxiety of an ED visit. Abnormal temperature, pulse, or respiration may be caused by infection or toxins.
   - Palpate the temporal arteries, sinuses, temporomandibular joints, and the scalp for tenderness.
   - Examine the fundi for papilledema and spontaneous venous pulsations.
   - Check for nuchal rigidity and photophobia.
   - Perform a detailed neurologic examination including cranial nerves, strength, sensation, pronator drift, finger to nose, and gait.

9. **How common are headaches in children?**
   As with adults, headaches are also common in children, with nearly 60% having headaches at some point. The history and physical examination are paramount in sorting out who needs a workup and who does not. Treatment can start with acetaminophen or ibuprofen. Children can have dangerous secondary headaches caused by primary tumors, meningitis, and hydrocephalus.

10. **How do I treat tension headaches?**
    If the diagnosis is secure, treatment starts with reassurance and education. Because these headaches are usually chronic, they should be treated with nonaddictive analgesics. The overuse or prolonged use, of over-the-counter analgesics should be avoided because these can lead to "medication overuse headaches." Biofeedback and acupuncture may be beneficial. All patients with this diagnosis should be screened for mood disorders, because depression is a common cause of tension headaches.

11. **What are migraine headaches?**
    A migraine is a specific type of headache. Migraines tend to be familial and affect women twice as often as men. The underlying pathophysiologic cause is thought to be vasogenic inflammation. The first headache usually occurs in an individual in the teens or twenties. Headaches typically are described as unilateral, severe, and throbbing, and are commonly associated with photophobia and nausea. Variations on all of the symptoms occur, but each patient tends to experience a similar constellation of symptoms with each headache. Patients who experience an aura will often have positive symptoms (e.g., scotoma [flashing lights or zig-zag patterns in vision], tingling of the face or arm, or shaking of a limb) as opposed to negative symptoms (e.g., absence of vision, anesthesia, or absence of movement of a limb), which are more common with brain ischemia or infarction. However, occasionally, patients with migraine will have weakness. Patients will often use the word *migraine* to describe any severe headache, so if a patient says they have a history of migraines, get more details about their duration, frequency, and what workup has been done in order to make sure that their headaches are truly migraines.

12. **How do I treat a migraine headache?**
    Patients who are unable to control their headache at home often come to the ED for better pain control or supportive therapy. Often, first-line therapy is intravenous (IV) Reglan (metoclopramide) or Compazine (prochlorperazine), both shown to be highly effective. However, the choice of treatment is based on case presentation, prior medications used, time elapsed since onset, the patient's prior response to therapy, existence of comorbid conditions, and severity of the current attack. Narcotics should be used only as a last resort (Table 18.2).

13. **How are cluster headaches different from migraines? How are they treated?**
    These are nonfamilial headaches predominantly affecting men. Excruciating, unilateral pain lasting 30–90 minutes occurs multiple times a day for weeks, followed by a pain-free interval. During the attacks, autonomic signs of rhinorrhea and lacrimation commonly occur ipsilateral to the headache. Attacks may be induced by smoking or alcohol. First-line treatments are oxygen (via nonrebreather for at least 15 minutes) and subcutaneous triptans. Other treatments include corticosteroids, calcium channel blockers, lithium, intranasal lidocaine, and methysergide.

14. **If a headache patient improves or the pain completely resolves with sumatriptan or ketorolac, does that mean that the diagnosis is migraine (or some other primary headache cause)?**
    The answer to this question is an emphatic *no*. Because the final common pathway for most pain in the head is limited, and vasogenic inflammation probably plays a role, the response to any analgesic or antimigraine medication is of no etiologic significance. This includes triptans, which have been documented to improve the headaches of patients with SAH and cervical artery dissections.

15. **What is the sensitivity of a noncontrast, head computed tomography (CT) for detection of an SAH?**
    With advances in imaging technology, approximately 90%–95% of SAHs are detected on CT scans. In neurologically intact patients, this number approaches 100% if the CT scan is performed within 6 hours of headache onset and is interpreted by an attending radiologist. A helpful rule is 95% in 24 hours, 80% at 48 hours, 70% at 72 hours, and 50% at 5 days. Incorporating shared decision making with the patient, if the CT is not completed within 6 hours of onset, a lumbar puncture (LP) is recommended.

Table 18.2 Selected Medications for Acute Migraine Attacks

MEDICATION	DOSAGE AND ROUTE[a]	COMMENTS
Mild to Moderate		
Acetaminophen	500–1000 mg	Avoid in patients with liver disease
Aspirin	325–1000 mg	Avoid in patients with ICH concern, GI upset
Ibuprofen	400–800 mg	GI upset
Naproxen	275–550 mg	GI upset
Indomethacin	50 mg PO/PR	
Moderate to Severe		
Dihydroergotamine	1 mg IV or IM	May be repeated in 1 hour but not if triptans used already Contraindicated in HTN, PVD, CAD, and pregnancy
Sumatriptan	6 mg SQ	May be repeated in 1 hour but not if ergots used already Contraindicated in HTN, PVD, CAD, and pregnancy
Metoclopramide	10 mg IV or IM	Sedation and dystonic reaction
Prochlorperazine	10 mg IV or IM	Sedation and dystonic reaction
Ketorolac	30–60 mg IM or 15–30 mg IV	GI upset Caution in elderly and patients at risk for renal failure
Morphine	0.1 mg/kg	Opioids should be used as last resort
Hydromorphone	0.5–2 mg IV (note: 1 mg hydromorphone = 8–10 mg of morphine)	Opioids should be used as last resort
Butorphanol	2 mg IV	Opioids less efficacious than other medications
Refractory Attack, Status Migrainosus		
Dihydroergotamine	1 mg IV	Use in conjunction with antiemetic
Dexamethasone	10–25 mg IV	A single IV administration decreases migraine recurrence

[a]Assumes average-size adult patient.

CAD, Coronary artery disease; *GI*, gastrointestinal; *HTN*, hypertension; *ICH*, intracranial hypertension; *IM*, intramuscularly; *IV*, intravenously; *PVD*, peripheral vascular disease; *SQ*, subcutaneously.

16. What are the cerebrospinal fluid (CSF) findings in an SAH?

As with CT, the findings on LP evolve with time. Even in the first hours after SAH, large numbers of red blood cells (RBCs) are found in the lumbar theca. Over days, these numbers fall with the circulation of CSF and the breakdown of the RBCs and hemoglobin. This leads to the finding of xanthochromia (see below). Thus RBCs are nearly always present early. Measuring the opening pressure can be helpful and is often elevated in SAH.

17. How do I differentiate between a traumatic tap and SAH?

Xanthochromia, the yellow color of CSF that occurs from hemoglobin catabolism, is almost always present if blood has been in the CSF for 12 hours or longer, and confirms an intracranial bleed. However, >90% of laboratories use visual inspection alone, which can be inaccurate and insensitive. Clearing of RBCs from the first to the last tube collected is commonly used and is helpful. However, unless the last tube contains no cells, SAH is still a possibility. An elevated opening pressure is suggestive of an SAH and not a traumatic tap. As with CT, you must factor in the timing of the LP from onset of the headache in interpreting the LP results.

18. If the CT and LP are both normal, do I need to pursue the diagnosis of SAH with some form of angiography?

The data strongly support, and American College of Emergency Physicians (ACEP) clinical policy recommends, stopping the workup for SAH if both tests are negative. However, there are other causes of acute, severe, sudden-onset headache associated with a normal CT and LP. These include the following (Table 18.3):

- Expanding aneurysm
- Pituitary apoplexy
- Cervical artery dissections
- CVST
- Posterior reversible encephalopathy syndrome (PRES; related to eclampsia).
- Acute stroke (especially posterior fossa).

19. What is a blood patch?

One third of patients experience headaches after a diagnostic LP or spinal anesthesia. This is the result of a persistent CSF leak from the dural hole that results in low CSF pressure, dilation of intracranial vessels, and traction on intracranial contents. This postdural puncture headache is worse when the patient sits or stands up and improves with lying down. Using a small-caliber LP needle, maintaining the bevel parallel with the dural fibers, reinsertion of the stylet prior to withdrawing the needle from the dural space, and using a needle with a noncutting tip can decrease the incidence of postdural puncture headache. Treatment includes fluids, caffeine, and analgesia. If conservative methods fail, blood is drawn from the patient and injected into the soft tissue at the site of the LP, the so-called blood patch. In most institutions, this is performed by an anesthesiologist.

20. What is a sentinel bleed?

Up to 50% of patients with aneurysmal SAH will have experienced a warning or sentinel hemorrhage before their catastrophic bleed. These small hemorrhages occur days to months before the major event. These events are still characterized by abrupt onset of severe, unusual headache and, if worked up with CT and LP, should be diagnosable in the vast majority of cases. Unfortunately, these episodes are often not worked up and are misdiagnosed as migraine, sinusitis, or tension-type headache, and the patients are discharged from medical care.

21. What specific entities must be considered in patients with a headache and a history of cancer or immunosuppression?

In a patient with a history of cancer, consider brain metastases or infections related to immunosuppression. In patients who are HIV positive, especially if they have low CD4 counts, opportunistic infections, such as cryptococcal meningitis or toxoplasmosis, brain abscess, and primary lymphoma of the central nervous system, should be considered.

Table 18.3 Differential Diagnosis and Workup for Acute, Severe Headache

PATHOLOGIC PROCESS	CLINICAL CHARACTERISTICS	WORKUP
Subarachnoid hemorrhage	Headache worst of life Headache abrupt, effort related Normal neurologic examination to focal deficit or coma	CT followed by LP if >6 hours after onset
Cervical artery dissections	History of trauma, Marfan syndrome, collagen disorders Headache is ipsilateral Carotid: neck or head pain, Horner syndrome, stroke Vertebral: occipitonuchal pain and posterior circulation stroke	Magnetic resonance or CT angiography Vascular ultrasound and conventional angiography
Intracerebral hemorrhage	History of hypertension History of brain tumor Severe headache with signs of elevated intracranial pressure and depressed mental status	CT
Cerebral venous thrombosis (superior sagittal sinus or transverse sinus)	Postpartum, hypercoagulable states, and abrupt, dull, constant headache Sixth nerve palsy, seizures Signs of raised intracranial pressure	MRI, magnetic resonance venography, or conventional angiography; CT angiography shows promise
Pituitary apoplexy	Abrupt severe headache, progressive visual loss with subsequent signs of pituitary insufficiency	CT or MRI with coronal views of the pituitary

CT, Computed tomography; *LP*, lumbar puncture; *MRI*, magnetic resonance imaging.

22. **What special diagnostic considerations must be given to a patient with AIDS and headache?**
    Headache is a common complaint among patients with AIDS, occurring in 11%–55% of patients, and may occur in many AIDS-related conditions. Acute lymphocytic meningitis can be seen at the time of acute HIV infections, sometimes associated with fever, lymphadenopathy, sore throat, and myalgias. Cryptococcal meningitis is a common cause of headache in patients who have AIDS, occurring in 10% of patients. Unlike patients with bacterial meningitis, patients with cryptococcal meningitis can have an indolent course and may have no fever or meningismus. *Toxoplasma gondii* produces multiple brain abscesses and bilateral, persistent headaches. The diagnosis of toxoplasmosis is made by CT, magnetic resonance imaging (MRI), or brain biopsy. Other central nervous system lesions include B-cell lymphoma and progressive multifocal leukoencephalopathy. Patients who have HIV and who come to the ED with persistent headache usually require neuroimaging, and, if imaging is normal, an LP.

23. **What specific diagnosis should be considered in older patients with a new-onset headache and general malaise or other systemic symptoms?**
    Temporal arteritis is a systemic arterial vasculitis that is rare before age 50 and dramatically increases in incidence afterward. It is more common in females. Also known as *giant cell arteritis,* temporal arteritis should be considered in any patient older than age 50 who has a new-onset headache or a change in an established pattern of headache. It is associated with localized scalp tenderness (anywhere in the scalp), malaise, myalgias, arthralgias, polymyalgia rheumatica, low-grade fevers, or other constitutional symptoms. Jaw claudication, if present, is strongly suggestive of the disorder. Erythrocyte sedimentation rate (ESR) is usually greater than 50 mm/h, and biopsy is required to establish the diagnosis; however, in certain cases, only the C-reactive protein (CRP) will be elevated. Untreated temporal arteritis can result in blindness or stroke. Treatment should be initiated in the ED, based on the clinical presumption and results of the ESR, and not delayed by biopsy. The initial doses of prednisone range from 40 to 60 mg daily. Finally, because primary headaches start less commonly after the age of 50, many of the other serious etiologies become more common in this age group, and therefore neuroimaging is often warranted.

24. **Which toxin may bring in entire families complaining of headache?**
    Carbon monoxide poisoning. See Chapter 74.

25. **Does sinusitis commonly cause headache? If a CT scan shows sinusitis, is that the likely cause of a patient's headache?**
    Patients will often use the term *sinus headache* just as inaccurately as they use the term *migraine*. When sinusitis causes headache, there are generally other symptoms and signs of sinusitis (e.g., nasal congestion, fever, boggy nasal mucosae), and the pain is generally unilateral. Tenderness over a sinus is nonspecific and may be a function of how hard one is pressing. CT findings of chronic sinusitis, such as mucosal thickening, retention cysts, or ostial narrowing, should never be considered the cause of a patient's acute headache.

26. **What rapidly progressive infectious entity presents with headache, fever, and altered mental status?**
    Herpes simplex encephalitis, the most common form of sporadic encephalitis and occurring with an incidence of 10 cases/million in neonates to 6 cases/million in adults, is a necrotizing, hemorrhagic infection that results in brain destruction that mandates early aggressive treatment with IV acyclovir. LP with CSF polymerase chain reaction (PCR) and gadolinium-enhanced MRI are the diagnostic methods of choice. On imaging, there is a predilection for temporal lobe involvement. Other causes of viral encephalitis (e.g., West Nile, eastern equine) have no treatment.

27. **What is idiopathic intracranial hypertension, and what is the complication if not treated appropriately?**
    Also known as *benign intracranial hypertension* or *pseudotumor cerebri*, this entity is related to an increase in intracranial pressure of unknown cause, and presents classically in obese young women with recurrent headaches that are constant or intermittent. The headaches may present with bilateral papilledema and loss of spontaneous retinal venous pulsations. Transient pulsatile tinnitus and visual symptoms are common. Occasionally, sixth nerve palsy is found. Sixth nerve palsy has no localizing value; it has longest intracranial course and is thus sensitive to pressure and inflammation. Brain imaging should be done to rule out a mass lesion and, if negative, LP is done; this not only is diagnostic but also commonly therapeutic. High opening pressure (25–40 cmH$_2$O) and a suggestive clinical scenario are diagnostic. Without treatment, there is a risk of visual loss. Treatment is with serial LPs, acetazolamide, and diuretics such as furosemide. Optic nerve fenestration is indicated in refractory cases. It is important to consider the diagnosis of CVST, because these two entities can mimic one another.

28. **Which cranial nerves pass through the cavernous sinus?**
    Cranial nerves III, IV, V$_{1-2}$, and VI. Cavernous sinus disease may present as only a retro-orbital headache. Any combination of involvement of the nerves passing through the cavernous sinus is suggestive of the diagnosis, however, and warrants further evaluation. Invasion by tumor, vascular disease such as aneurysm or carotid cavernous sinus fistula, and clot (either bland or infection related) are the more common causes. Patients with other CVSTs will often experience isolated headache, seizure, and elevated intracranial pressure.

29. In the pregnant (or recently postpartum) woman, are there particular causes of headache that I should worry about?

Pregnant women can get any kind of headache that nonpregnant women can get; however, some headache disorders that occur more commonly or exclusively in this situation are CVST, eclampsia, pituitary apoplexy, SAH, and PRES. Added to this list in the postpartum patient who has had an epidural anesthetic are postdural puncture headache and the additional complication of a postpuncture subdural hematoma. As for imaging, MRI eliminates radiation, but you should get the tests that are needed, trying to balance radiation exposure with the need for an accurate and rapid diagnosis.

30. Is high blood pressure causing my patient's headache?

One potential mistake is to diagnose hypertensive urgency in patients with headache who have high blood pressure. Coexistent headache and hypertension can occur for several reasons. The most probable is that pain and anxiety are elevating the blood pressure. A second reason is that the underlying cause of the headache is also causing some degree of raised intracranial pressure, with the body reactively raising the arterial blood pressure to preserve cerebral perfusion pressure. If hypertension is causing hypertensive encephalopathy, the patient should also have papilledema. In this situation, lower the systolic blood pressure about 25% below the peak, using rapidly acting, titratable agents. In patients with acute ischemic stroke and headache, one should be cautious about pharmacologically treating high blood pressure, as high blood pressure may be the result of brain autoregulation needed to maintain cerebral perfusion.

31. When should I be concerned about a brain tumor?

Isolated headache is not often caused by a brain tumor. One half to two thirds of all patients with brain tumors have headache, but only 38% of brain tumor patients without a previous headache history develop headaches as the result of the tumor. The pain characteristics are not specific, and the classic early morning headache is not pathognomonic. Localization (other than neck pain with posterior fossa tumors) does not usually occur. One risk for patients with brain tumors is to have a headache that is different from their previous headaches. Therefore, a careful history and physical examination are most important in deciding which patients need a workup for a tumor, as they are for any other secondary cause of headache.

KEY POINTS: HEADACHE

1. A response to analgesics does not exclude life-threatening causes of headache.
2. CT scanners may miss 5%–10% of SAHs, but the sensitivity markedly improves if the imaging is performed within 6 hours of headache onset. LP is needed if SAH is a major diagnostic concern after 6 hours of onset.
3. Patients who are HIV positive with headache should have a CT head scan with contrast or MRI to exclude opportunistic infections, including toxoplasmosis, followed by an LP if the imaging is negative.
4. A careful history and physical examination, including neurologic examination, will identify most patients who need further evaluation.

BIBLIOGRAPHY

Chu KH, Howell TF, Keijzers G, et al. Acute headache presentations to the emergency department: a statewide cross-sectional study. *Acad Emerg Med.* 2017;24:53–62.

Dubosh NM, Bellolio MF, Rabinstein AA, et al. Sensitivity of early brain computed tomography to exclude aneurysmal subarachnoid hemorrhage: a systematic review and meta-analysis. *Stroke.* 2016;47:750–755.

Edlow JA, Panagos PD, Godwin SA, et al. Clinical policy: critical issues in the evaluation and management of adult patients presenting to the emergency department with acute headache. *Ann Emerg Med.* 2008;52:407–436.

Friedman BW. Managing migraine. *Ann Emerg Med.* 2017;69:202–207.

Kirby S, Purdy RA. Headaches and brain tumors. *Neurol Clin.* 2014;32:423–432.

Marmura MJ, Silberstein SD, Schwedt TJ. The acute treatment of migraine in adults: the American Headache Society evidence assessment of migraine pharmacotherapies. *Headache.* 2015;55:3–20.

Modi S, Mahajan A, Dharaiya D, et al. Burden of herpes simplex virus encephalitis in the United States. *J Neurol.* 2017;264:1204–1208.

Pope JV, Edlow JA. Favorable response to analgesics does not predict a benign etiology of headache. *Headache.* 2008;48:944–950.

The International Classification of Headache Disorders, 3rd edition (beta version). *Cephalalgia.* 2013;33:629–808.

CHAPTER 19

SYNCOPE, VERTIGO, AND DIZZINESS

Elizabeth N. Malik, MD and Katherine M. Bakes, MD

KEY POINTS: CAUSES OF DIZZINESS

1. Serious (cerebellar and brainstem infarction or ischemia, central tumor, arrhythmia, low-flow states)
2. Benign (benign paroxysmal positional vertigo (BPPV) vestibular neuritis, labyrinthitis, vestibular migraine, Meniere disease)

1. **Do I need to be concerned by a complaint of dizziness?**
   Yes. Approximately 5% of patients who come to the ED with dizziness will have a serious neurologic condition, such as ischemic stroke, intracranial hemorrhage, brain neoplasm, demyelinating disease, or cerebral infection. Risk factors for serious neurologic etiologies include age $\geq$60 years, risk factors for stroke (e.g., atrial fibrillation, hypertension, and diabetes), chief complaint of imbalance, and any focal neurologic abnormality (other than nystagmus).

2. **How do I approach the vague and ill-defined complaint of dizziness?**
   It is critical to start your history with open-ended questions! Patients should be allowed to describe their symptoms without prompting, so you can understand what they mean by *dizzy*. *Dizzy* can describe the sensation of vertigo (the illusion of motion), lightheadedness (presyncope or syncope), or disequilibrium (imbalance). Although these descriptions cannot accurately distinguish between benign and serious causes, the evaluation for each is different and requires an accurate understanding of the patient's symptomatology.

3. **How does the vestibular system work?**
   The vestibular system, located in the temporal bone, is made up of a semimembranous labyrinth that is filled with fluid (endolymph) and contains the utricle, the saccule, and the three semicircular canals. The utricle and saccule respond to gravitational forces and linear movement, whereas the semicircular canals, oriented in the three planes of space, respond to rotational movements. Otoliths rest on the hair cells of the utricle and the saccule. The mass of the otoliths is needed to stimulate the hair cells in response to gravitational pull. When the head turns, endolymph bends and stimulates the hair cells within the semicircular canals. Impulses from the hair cells are then sent to the brain via the eighth cranial nerve. The nucleus of the eighth cranial nerve then interconnects with other cranial nerves, the cerebellum, and the sensory and motor tracts to coordinate visual and motor responses.

4. **What is the difference between central versus peripheral vertigo?**
   This is an anatomic distinction. Peripheral vertigo is caused by a dysfunction of the inner ear or vestibular nerve, whereas central vertigo is from etiologies of the brain or brain stem. BPPV, vestibular neuritis, and Meniere disease are common causes of peripheral vertigo, whereas vertebrobasilar ischemia, multiple sclerosis, cerebellar infarction/hemorrhage, and basilar migraine are some causes of central vertigo.

5. **What are the common characteristics of peripheral vertigo?**
   Deafness (unilateral, best detected with the Weber test)
   Ringing in the ears (tinnitus)
   Fatigable on repeated testing (central suppressive mechanisms still function)
   Latency after Dix-Hallpike maneuver
   Intense symptoms (with head movement to one side)
   Positional in nature
   The mnemonic *DR FLIP* reminds you that the Epley maneuver, which flips the patient, helps BPPV.

6. **What are the characteristics of central vertigo?**
   - Focal neurologic deficits (including cranial nerves)
   - Vertical or rotary nystagmus (not seen in peripheral vertigo)
   - Non-fatigable nystagmus (nystagmus which persists with lateral gaze)
   - Ataxia (with gait impairment and not only with head turning)

7. **What are the key points for the main causes of peripheral vertigo?**
   See Table 19.1.

Table 19.1 Key Points for the Main Causes of Peripheral Vertigo

Benign Paroxysmal Positional Vertigo
Most common cause (50%)
Hearing not affected
Recurrent; <1-minute paroxysms elicited with head turning and asymptomatic between
Result of otolith dislodgement into a semicircular canal
Responds to Epley maneuver or half-somersault maneuver

Vestibular Neuritis
Less common cause (20%)
Probable viral etiology
Positive asymmetric head thrust test
Associated with tinnitus
May respond to steroids

Meniere Disease
Less common cause (10%)
Less acute onset (hours) and can last for weeks at a time
Associated with hearing loss, tinnitus
Caused by swelling of the semimembranous labyrinth (vestibular and cochlear components)
Responds to diuretics or fluid restriction
Can lead to permanent hearing loss

8. **What should be included in the physical examination of a patient with vertigo?**
   Examine the eyes for ocular palsies (central etiology) and document the presence and characteristics of nystagmus. Examine the ears for foreign bodies, infection, perforation, cholesteatomas, and unilateral hearing loss – the Weber and Rinne tests should be used for an objective and sensitive assessment. Perform a full neurologic examination, including cranial nerves, gait, cerebellar function, and a HINTS examination.

9. **What is a HINTS examination?**
   The HINTS examination is composed of three bedside physical examination maneuvers, the **H**ead **I**mpulse test, **N**ystagmus, and **T**est of **S**kew, which can identify a posterior circulation stroke more accurately than an MRI in the first 48 hours from symptom onset. The absence of concerning findings in all three tests strongly suggests a peripheral problem. However, if any maneuver has a worrying finding, you should consider central etiologies of the dizziness.

10. **What is a head impulse test?**
    This maneuver is a way to test the vestibulo-ocular reflex (VOR), which is not dependent on the brain stem or cerebellum, and may point to a peripheral cause of dizziness. The examiner stands in front of the patient, holds the patient's head in both hands, and instructs the patient to look at the examiner's nose. With the patient's eyes open, the head is rapidly turned 30 degrees to one side. Normally, the eyes continue to fix on the examiner's nose, demonstrating an intact VOR. If there is a unilateral vestibular lesion, such as vestibular neuritis, the eyes don't stay fixed on the target and saccade (i.e., drift) back to refocus on the examiner's nose. A normal head impulse test in a patient with dizziness can be concerning for a central process, because this examination tests a peripheral reflex. A patient with a central process, like a stroke or tumor, will have a *normal* VOR and therefore a *normal* head impulse test, which is a worrisome finding. Unfortunately, a patient without any dizziness at all will also have an intact VOR and a normal head impulse test, so think carefully when to use this examination.

11. **What is the test of skew?**
    The test of skew evaluates the patient's eye movements (when fixed on a target) while the examiner alternates covering of each eye every 2–3 seconds. Small vertical corrections should not occur, and suggest a central etiology of vertigo when present.

12. **What does nystagmus mean in the workup of vertigo?**
    Horizontal or rotary nystagmus can be found in peripheral or central etiologies, and thus does not exclude brain or brain stem pathologic abnormality. Vertical, changing-direction, and nonsuppressible nystagmus are pathognomonic for a central etiology. Because the brain's central suppressive mechanisms are intact, patients with peripheral etiologies will be able to suppress their nystagmus (and the sensation of vertigo) by visually fixating on a stationary object. Suspect a central etiology in patients who have very active nystagmus and prefer to keep their eyes closed.

13. **What is the Dix-Hallpike maneuver?**
    This diagnostic maneuver tests only for BPPV. It involves moving the patient rapidly from a sitting position with the head turned 45 degrees to one side, to a supine position with the head hanging down at 30-degrees' extension.

A positive test is when you see nystagmus, often toward the effected inner ear, which is characteristically associated with a delay of a few seconds as the dislodged otoliths move through endolymph. In BPPV, this maneuver should fatigue the symptoms of vertigo on repetition due to intact central suppressive mechanisms. Be cautious because in patients with vertebrobasilar insufficiency, hyperextending the neck can stimulate symptoms and give a false-positive Dix-Hallpike.

14. **What is the Epley maneuver?**
The Epley maneuver treats BPPV and is utilized to physically move otoliths, most commonly in the posterior semicircular canal, into the utricle. It is successful about 75% of the time on the first attempt and up to 98% after two attempts. See Fig. 19.1 on how to perform this maneuver. It is important to allow adequate time for the otoliths to settle between each change in position. Because of the natural fatigability of symptoms as above, the patient's sensations cannot be relied on to guide the time spent in each position. Thus the examiner should note the time it takes for both symptoms and nystagmus to abate during the Dix-Hallpike maneuver and apply that time to each position of the Epley maneuver. An alternative to the Epley maneuver is called the half-somersault maneuver which has been shown to be superior to the Epley in some research.

15. **How do I treat peripheral and central vertigo?**
   - Meniere disease is treated with diuretics or salt/fluid restriction.
   - BPPV is treated by the Epley maneuver or half-somersault maneuver.
   - Nonspecific vestibular suppressants include the following:
     - Anticholinergics (e.g., scopolamine transdermal)
     - Antihistamines (meclizine 25 mg orally [per os; PO] every 6 hours as needed for vertigo and diphenhydramine 25–50 mg PO every 4–6 hours)
     - Benzodiazepines (diazepam 5–10 mg PO every 6 hours)
   - Peripheral vertigo not amenable to repositioning maneuvers is best monitored by an ear, nose, and throat (ENT) physician, who can do more specialized vestibular testing to localize the lesion.
   - Central vertigo requires evaluation by a neurologist or neurosurgeon. Magnetic resonance imaging (MRI) to evaluate the posterior fossa and brainstem is recommended.

KEY POINTS: CAUSES OF SYNCOPE

1. HEAD (**h**ypoxemia, **e**pilepsy, **a**nxiety, **d**ysfunctional brain)
2. HEART (**h**eart attack, **e**mbolism of pulmonary artery, **a**ortic obstruction, **r**hythm disturbance, **t**achydysrhythmia)
3. VESSELS (**v**asovagal, **e**ctopic pregnancy, **s**ituational, **s**ubclavian steal, **E**NT, **l**ow **s**ystemic vascular resistance, **s**ensitive carotid sinus)

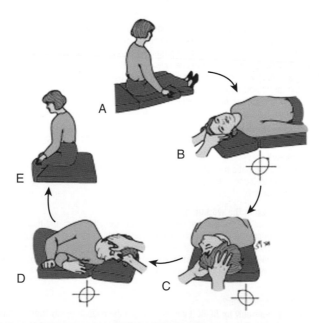

Fig. 19.1 Epley maneuver.

16. What is syncope?
Syncope is sudden temporary loss of consciousness with the inability to maintain postural tone. It is a symptom, not a disease, with a wide variety of benign and life-threatening causes. Seizures may mimic syncope.

17. Discuss the causes of syncope as related to the head.
Diffuse cerebral malfunction from lack of vital nutrients, such as oxygen (hypoxemia) or sugar (hypoglycemia), is often correctable but easily overlooked. Seizures don't cause, but can mimic, syncope. Vertebrobasilar insufficiency and subarachnoid hemorrhage (SAH) indicate a dysfunctional brain.

18. Discuss the cardiovascular causes of syncope.
Cardiac causes of syncope comprise the riskiest group of patients and include acute coronary syndrome (ACS), pulmonary embolism, physical aortic outflow obstructions (e.g., hypertrophic obstructive cardiomyopathy [HOCM], aortic stenosis, or atrial myxoma), slow rhythms such as sick sinus syndrome, and tachyarrhythmias. Brugada syndrome, preexcitation, arrhythmogenic right ventricular dysplasia (ARVD), and long QT syndrome can precipitate lethal dysrhythmias.

19. What are the vascular causes of syncope?
Vascular causes include:
- The common faint (vasovagal)
- Hypovolemia
- Situational faints (e.g., micturition, defecation, cough, or Valsalva maneuver)
- Subclavian steal
- ENT causes (e.g., glossopharyngeal and trigeminal neuralgia)
- Low systemic vascular resistance (from medications and autonomic insufficiency)
- Carotid sinus sensitivity (only accounting for 4% of syncope cases)

20. Summarize the initial concerns when evaluating a patient with syncope.
Most patients with syncope rapidly return to a normal mental status and have stable vital signs once they are recumbent. However, there are treatment priorities:
- Obtain vital signs and evaluate and treat for immediate life threats.
- Check a bedside glucose level and consider naloxone for any patient with persistent altered mental status.
- Oxygen, intravenous access, and cardiac and blood pressure monitoring should be initiated on patients who have abnormal vital signs, a persistent altered level of consciousness, chest pain, dyspnea, abdominal pain, or a significant history of cardiac disease.
- Assess for any trauma secondary to fall. Elderly patients are more likely to suffer head trauma secondary to syncope, and this may be a greater life threat initially than the cause of the syncope, particularly if the patient is taking anticoagulants.

21. I've ruled out the immediate life threats. Now what do I do?
Obtain a detailed history, perform a thorough physical examination, and obtain an electrocardiogram (ECG). Then do a risk assessment to determine whether further testing or admission is indicated.

22. What components of the history are most important?
The most important historical clue is the patient's recollection of the events just before the syncope. An abrupt onset of loss of consciousness with a brief (<5 seconds) prodrome is indicative of a cardiac etiology, particularly if the patient did not have time to protect himself or herself from injuries (e.g., facial trauma). Similarly, syncope associated with exercise, or while the patient was reclining or recumbent, is associated with cardiac obstructive causes or arrhythmias. Patients who have vasovagal syncope often have premonitory symptoms of dizziness, yawning, nausea, and diaphoresis, and the event is during a period of some psychosocial stress. Clues to hypovolemia include thirst, postural dizziness, decreased oral intake, vomiting, diarrhea, frequent urination, melena, or unusually heavy vaginal bleeding. Syncope after micturition, cough, head turning, defecation, swallowing, or meals suggests situational syncope. Note any previous episodes of syncope, syncope associated with upper extremity exertion (e.g., subclavian steal syndrome), and the presence of cardiac risk factors. A family history of sudden death may suggest HOCM, Brugada, preexcitation, ARVD, or long QT syndromes. Many medications and medication interactions can cause syncope, so determine all of the patient's current medications and recent medication changes, especially when treating the elderly.

23. How do I know it was not a seizure?
Victims of arrhythmias and vasovagal faints often exhibit myoclonic jerks that may mimic a seizure. Recovery from syncope is usually rapid if the patient is allowed to become recumbent, whereas a patient who has had a generalized seizure awakens slowly with prolonged confusion or postictal state. Both may have trauma. Lateral tongue biting has been shown to be specific but insensitive for a seizure. Loss of bladder control also can increase the posttest probability of the episode being a seizure.

24. **What is a directed physical examination?**

Be a detective, using head, heart, and vessels as a guide. The patient with syncope from abrupt effort or exercise syncope may have aortic stenosis or hypertrophic cardiomyopathy. Look for narrow pulse pressure, systolic murmur, or change in murmur with the Valsalva maneuver. The presence of physical signs of congestive heart failure (CHF) places the patient at high risk. Examine the head carefully for trauma. Examine the neck for bruits. Perform a complete neurologic examination, looking for focal neurologic signs. Check blood pressure in both arms, looking for subclavian steal. Consider occult blood loss. Finally, think about autonomic insufficiency by searching for signs of toxins, infection, or neurologic disease such as Parkinson's or Guillain-Barré syndrome.

25. **What tests are needed to assist in diagnosis?**

Other than a urine pregnancy test in females, a detailed history, physical examination, and ECG are the foundation and usually sufficient in young, otherwise healthy, patients. A patient who has returned to normal mental status is unlikely to have hypoglycemia as the cause of syncope. If anemia is suspected on clinical examination (pale skin and pale conjunctivae), a bedside hematocrit or hemoglobin test is indicated. The addition of a specific confirmatory test (e.g., echocardiography) is recommended for suspected cardiomyopathy.

26. **Who needs an ECG? What am I looking for?**

Almost all patients with syncope should have an ECG because it is not invasive and may be diagnostic. Check for markers of cardiac disease, such as ischemia, infarction, and conduction abnormalities. Look for specific patterns associated with HOCM (dagger Q waves), Brugada (coved-type or saddle-back RSR), ARVD (epsilon wave), preexcitation (delta wave), or prolonged QT. Left ventricular hypertrophy may be a clue to aortic stenosis, hypertension, or cardiomyopathy.

27. **Who should receive further testing?**

Patients with CHF, age greater than 65 years, abnormal ECG, and unexplained syncope who have suspected heart disease should be admitted and evaluated for ACS. Echocardiography, exercise treadmill testing, Holter ECG monitoring, and electrophysiologic studies may be useful during the inpatient stay.

28. **What factors help to assign a patient to a high-risk or low-risk group?**

Physician gestalt plays a large role, although admittedly this takes time and experience to develop. Studies attempting to determine highly sensitive risk factors have had mixed results but do help identify risk factors for serious conditions; see Table 19.2. The San Francisco syncope rule predicted short-term adverse events in patients with the following signs: abnormal ECG result, shortness of breath, systolic blood pressure less than 90 mmHg, hematocrit level less than 30%, and CHF by history or examination. Unfortunately, this rule was found to have only 75% sensitivity on external validation. The Boston syncope rule has demonstrated excellent sensitivity, but still requires external validation. The rule recommends admission for any patient with ACS, conduction disease, worrisome cardiac history (e.g., dysrhythmia, pacemaker), valvular heart disease, family history of sudden death or conduction abnormality, volume depletion (e.g., gastrointestinal bleed, hematocrit <30%), persistent abnormal vital signs in the ED, or a primary central nervous system etiology.

29. **What are the odds of determining the cause of a syncopal episode?**

Despite extensive and expensive ED workups, no cause is found in about 50% of cases. This should be discussed with the patient so that there are no unrealistic expectations.

ACKNOWLEDGMENT

The editors and author of this chapter would like to acknowledge and thank Dr. William F. Young, Jr., for his previous contributions to this chapter.

Table 19.2 Syncope at High Risk for Cardiac Etiology

HISTORICAL	EMERGENCY DEPARTMENT EVALUATION
Age >65 years	Abnormal vital signs
Cardiovascular disease history (especially heart failure)	Systolic blood pressure <90 mmHg
Lack of prodrome	Evidence of congestive heart failure
Exertional	Abnormal electrocardiogram
Chest pain or palpitations with event	Hematocrit <30%
Family history of sudden death	

Bibliography

Bakes KM, Faragher J, Markovchick VJ, et al. The Denver Seizure Score: anion gap metabolic acidosis predicts generalized seizure. *Am J Emerg Med.* 2011;29:1097–1102.

Casani AP, Dallan I, Cerchiai N, et al. Cerebellar infarctions mimicking acute peripheral vertigo: how to avoid misdiagnosis? *Otolaryngology.* 2013;148:475–481.

Chan Y. Differential diagnosis of dizziness. *Curr Opin Otolaryngol Head Neck Surg.* 2009;17:200–203.

Edlow J. Diagnosing patients with acute-onset persistent dizziness. *Ann Emerg Med.* 2018;71:625–631.

Edlow JA, Newman-Toker D. Using the physical examination to diagnose patients with acute dizziness and vertigo. *J Emerg Med.* 2016;50(4):617–628.

Gold DR, Morris L, Schubert MC, et al. Repositioning maneuvers for benign paroxysmal positional vertigo. *Curr Treat Options Neurol.* 2014;16:307.

Grossman SA, Bar J, Fischer C, et al. Reducing admissions utilizing the Boston syncope criteria. *J Emerg Med.* 2012;42:345–352.

Kattah JC, Talkad AV, Wang DZ, et al. HINTS to diagnose stroke in the acute vestibular syndrome: three step bedside oculomotor examination more sensitive than early MRI diffusion-weighted imaging. *Stroke.* 2009;40(11):3504–3510.

Navi BB, Kamel H, Shah MP, et al. Rate and predictors of serious neurologic causes of dizziness in the emergency department. *Mayo Clin Proc.* 2012;87:1080–1088.

Ozono Y, Kitahara T, Fukushima M, et al. Differential diagnosis of vertigo and dizziness in the emergency department. *Acta Otolaryngol.* 2014;134:140–145.

Post RE, Dickerson, LM. Dizziness: a diagnostic approach. *Am Fam Physician.* 2010;82(4):361–368.

CHAPTER 20

SEIZURES

Shawn M. Varney, MD, FACEP, FACMT and Marshall Sheide, DO

1. **What is a seizure?**
   A seizure is an episode of abnormal brain function caused by excessive and aberrant neuronal discharge and may manifest in a broad spectrum of ways. In addition to tonic-clonic muscle activity (*tonic* refers to muscle stiffening; *clonic* refers to muscle jerking), generalized seizures may also manifest as staring episodes, lip smacking or other minor motor activity, or complete disruption of muscle tone (drop attacks). Generalized seizures are often followed by a postictal phase characterized by confusion or lethargy. This phase usually lasts for 5–15 minutes, although it may last longer.
   The recognition and appropriate management of seizures are critically important, because prolonged, excessive electrical activity in the brain directly causes neuronal destruction, especially in the hippocampus.

2. **How are seizures classified?**
   Seizures are usually divided into two groups: generalized and focal (Table 20.1). Generalized seizures affect a large portion of the brain tissue, whereas focal seizures involve a specific part of the brain. Focal seizures, whether simple (consciousness unaffected) or complex (impairment of consciousness), may result in bizarre manifestations, including hallucinations, memory disturbance, visceral symptoms (abdominal symptoms), and perceptual distortions, and may be misdiagnosed as a psychiatric problem.

3. **Name some causes of seizures?**
   Primary seizures are recurrent episodes of abnormal electrical brain activity without a recognized underlying cause and are classically referred to as *epilepsy*. Secondary seizures (also called *provoked seizures*) usually have a nonneurologic underlying condition. Table 20.2 lists the most common etiologies for secondary seizures.

4. **What is included in the differential diagnosis of seizure?**
   Anything that can cause a sudden disturbance of neurologic function may be mistaken for a seizure. Common seizure mimics include syncope, myoclonic jerks, hyperventilation syndrome, migraines, movement disorders, narcolepsy, and psychologic disorders. *Pseudoseizure,* also known as psychogenic nonepileptiform seizure, is a special category and is discussed later (see Question 16).

5. **When taking a patient history, which findings suggest a seizure?**
   Important elements to include when taking a history are history of a seizure disorder or brain neoplasm, a preceding aura (warning symptoms and signs of an imminent seizure, such as an odor), known precipitants (strong emotions, flashing lights, stress, lack of sleep), and circumstances surrounding the event (compliance with medication regimen, drug/alcohol use or withdrawal, head trauma, infection).

6. **What are the most important aspects of the physical examination in a seizure patient?**
   Neurologic examination (most important). Focal neurologic findings may indicate a focal cerebral lesion (e.g., tumor, abscess, or cerebral contusion) or focal paresis after seizure (Todd paralysis). Evaluation of the cranial nerves and the fundi can reveal increased intracranial pressure.
   Secondary injuries. A complete head-to-toe examination may reveal trauma from the seizure. Physical findings associated with seizures include tongue biting, bowel or bladder incontinence, and a postictal state of confusion or somnolence.
   Differential examination signs. Additionally, examine the skin (meningococcemia or stigmata of liver failure), head (recent trauma), and neck (nuchal rigidity may indicate meningitis or subarachnoid hemorrhage).

7. **What should my priorities be in managing a patient who is actively experiencing a seizure?**
   Clinical priorities are airway, breathing, and circulation (ABCs). Suction oral secretions to prevent aspiration and position the patient on his or her side. Give supplemental oxygen to treat the increased oxygen demand and impaired respiratory physiology caused by the generalized muscle activity. Supplemental ventilation (bag-valve-mask) is rarely needed. Do not place objects into the patient's mouth that might be bitten off (including fingers). A jaw thrust or nasopharyngeal airway may assist in maintaining a patent airway and improve ventilation. Note the patient's blood pressure, pulse, and capillary refill. Gently restrain the patient or place a blanket or sheet under the head to help the patient avoid self-harm. Diagnostic priorities should focus on likely reversible causes of seizures, such as hypoglycemia, metabolic disturbances, and potential toxicologic exposures.

8. **Which medications are first in the management of seizures?**
   Intravenous (IV) or intramuscular (IM) benzodiazepines are the first-line therapy for the seizing patient. Midazolam (IM 10 mg for >40 kg, 5 mg for <40 kg; or IV 5 mg >40 kg, 2 mg <40 kg) has been shown to be the most

Table 20.1 Classification of Seizures

Type

Generalized
Tonic-clonic (grand mal)
Absence (petit mal)
Atonic (drop attacks)
Myoclonic (extremely brief, <0.1 second)
Tonic (muscle stiffening)
Clonic (repeating muscle jerking, 2–3/seconds)

Partial or Focal
Simple partial
Complex partial
Partial with secondary generalization

Table 20.2 Etiologies of Secondary (Provoked) Seizures

CATEGORY	EXAMPLE
Drugs/toxins (multiple)	Anticholinergics/antihistamines Anticonvulsants (carbamazepine, valproic acid) Antidepressants (bupropion, tricyclics) Camphor CO, CN, hydrogen sulfide, azides GHB Gyromitra (mushroom), hydrazine Iron Isoniazid Lidocaine Lithium Opioids (meperidine, propoxyphene, tramadol) Organophosphates/carbamates Salicylates Sympathomimetics (amphetamines and derivatives, cocaine) Synthetic cannabinoids Theophylline
Central nervous system lesions	Hypertensive encephalopathy Intracranial hemorrhage Mass lesions Structural Trauma (recent and remote) Vascular lesions
Infectious diseases	Cerebral abscess Cerebral parasitosis Encephalitis HIV Meningitis
Metabolic	Fever ("febrile seizures") Hepatic encephalopathy High anion-gap acidosis Hypocalcemia Hypoglycemia, hyperglycemia Hypomagnesemia Hyponatremia, hypernatremia Hypothyroidism, hyperthyroidism Uremia
Other	Eclampsia Subtherapeutic antiepileptic drug levels Withdrawal (barbiturates, ethanol, sedative-hypnotics)

CO, Carbon monoxide; *CN,* cyanide; *GHB,* γ-hydroxybutyric acid; *HIV,* human immunodeficiency virus.

effective choice for aborting seizures, although lorazepam (2–4 mg IV), and diazepam (5–10 mg IV) are also considered appropriate first-choice medications. Midazolam may be administered IM, IV, or intranasally (IN). Lorazepam is a popular choice because of its longer duration of action. However, it may have a slightly slower onset of action compared with diazepam, which can also be administered by the intraosseous, IN, and rectal routes, but is not recommended for IM use because of uneven uptake.

Once the seizure has ceased, anticonvulsants are used to prevent recurrence. Levetiracetam, phenytoin/fosphenytoin, and valproic acid are appropriate choices for postseizure anticonvulsants. They may also be administered as second-line therapy if the benzodiazepines are unable to abort the seizure. Levetiracetam is commonly used due to its low side-effect profile, equal efficacy with phenytoin, and better safety profile in pregnancy. Although phenytoin and fosphenytoin are often used, they are not always successful, may cause cardiovascular compromise when rapidly infused, and are not effective for toxin-induced seizures. Table 20.3 shows the medications with their dosage and route of administration.

9. **What is status epilepticus? How is it managed?**
When seizures last >5 minutes despite acute pharmacologic intervention, or recur so frequently that normal mentation does not resume between the seizures, it is called *status epilepticus*. Immediate seizure-abortive intervention with benzodiazepines is indicated along with simultaneous attention to the ABCs, screening for underlying causes, and immediate treatment of life-threatening etiologies. Table 20.4 gives an algorithm for managing the patient with status epilepticus.

Table 20.3 Anticonvulsants

DRUG	ADULT DOSAGE
Levetiracetam	Status: 40–60 mg/kg with maximum of 4500 mg in single dose at 100 mg/min over 15 min IV. Prophylactic dose: 20 mg/kg with maximum of 1500 mg daily
Phenytoin	20 mg/kg at a maximum rate of 50 mg/min
Fosphenytoin	15–20 mg PE/kg IV at 100–150 mg PE/min; may be given IM
Valproic acid	20–40 mg/kg IV over 1 hr
Phenobarbital	20 mg/kg IV at 50 mg/min; may be given IM; may repeat dose in 10 min
Pentobarbital	5 mg/kg IV at 25 mg/min, then titrate to EEG; intubation required

EEG, Electroencephalogram; *IM,* intramuscularly; *IV,* intravenously; *PE,* phenytoin sodium equivalents.

Table 20.4 Proposed Guidelines for Management of the Patient with Status Epilepticus

TIME FRAME	MEASURES
0–5 min	Establish/maintain airway IV/oxygen/monitor Dextrose, 0.5 g/kg IV, if indicated Consider thiamine, 100 mg IV
5–20 min	Lorazepam, given at 2 mg/min, 0.1 mg/kg IV up to 4 mg per dose, may repeat in 5 min (*or* diazepam, 0.15 mg/kg IV up to 10 mg per dose, may repeat in 5 min; *or* midazolam 0.2 mg/kg up to 10 mg IM or 0.2 mg/kg IV load, followed by infusion of 0.05–0.2 mg/kg/h)
20–40 min	Levetiracetam, 40–60 mg/kg with maximum of 4500 mg in single dose at 100 mg/min over 15 min IV Phenytoin, 20 mg/kg IV at 50 mg/min (to 30 mg/kg if seizures continue); *or* fosphenytoin, 20 mg/kg PE IV at 150 mg/min Valproate, 20–40 mg/kg IV at 3–6 mg/kg/min; may give additional 20 mg/kg after 10 min
40+ min	or General anesthesia with midazolam, 0.2 mg/kg initial infusion at 2 mg/min, then continuous infusion of 0.05–2 mg/kg/h Propofol, 2 mg/kg IV, then 5 mg/kg/h; may repeat 2 mg/kg in 5 min Phenobarbital, up to 20 mg/kg IV at 50 mg/min; may repeat in 10 min Pentobarbital, 5–15 mg/kg at 50 mg/min, then 0.5–5 mg/kg/h[a]

[a]By this time a critical care physician would be involved.
IV, Intravenous; *IM,* intramuscular; *PE,* phenytoin sodium equivalents.

10. **What ancillary testing should I do in the patient with a history of seizures?**
Extensive ancillary testing is reserved for the patient with new-onset seizure. For a patient with a history of seizures who has an unprovoked attack, measuring appropriate serum anticonvulsant levels may be all that is required. The decision to proceed with further testing depends on the patient's history and physical findings. There are no perfect tests with definitive thresholds to determine whether a major motor seizure occurred, but some test options are creatine phosphokinase (stays elevated up to 24 hours), anion gap (elevated if done within 1 hour), or prolactin (elevated if drawn within 20 minutes of seizure and compared with a 6-hour level).

11. **And if the patient does not have a history of seizures?**
Routine screening laboratory tests in a patient with new-onset seizure who has returned to baseline have low yield, but it is reasonable to check serum electrolytes (sodium, calcium, magnesium), glucose, renal and liver function, toxicology screen, and complete blood count. A pregnancy test for women of childbearing years may affect the choice of antiepileptic therapy or disposition. An electrocardiogram may rule out seizure mimics. The routine use of lumbar puncture in patients with new-onset seizures is not indicated.

12. **What imaging studies are indicated?**
In the patient with a first-time seizure, emergent noncontrast head computed tomography (CT) is recommended when suspecting a structural lesion (intracranial bleeds, masses, large strokes, or trauma). This includes patients with new focal deficits, persistent altered mental status, fever, recent head trauma, persistent headache, history of cancer, or presence of a coagulopathy or platelet disorder; patients receiving anticoagulation therapy; patients who are immunosuppressed or HIV positive; and patients who had a partial seizure. In addition, patients with a history of seizures who have a new or different seizure pattern should undergo imaging studies.

13. **What should be the disposition of the patient who has a seizure?**
Patients who come to the emergency department (ED) with any of the following should be considered for hospital admission for evaluation and therapy: persistent altered mental status, central nervous system (CNS) infection, new focal abnormality, new intracranial lesion, underlying correctable medical problem (e.g., hypoxia, hypoglycemia, hyponatremia, dysrhythmia, and uncontrollable alcohol withdrawal), traumatic or spontaneous intracranial hemorrhage, status epilepticus, and eclampsia. In the patient with a history of seizures who has a simple seizure and a subtherapeutic anticonvulsant level, correct the level before discharge. Patients with new-onset seizures who have normal workups in the ED and are medically stable may be discharged.

14. **Outline appropriate discharge instructions?**
Arrange follow-up consultation with the patient's primary care physician or a consulting neurologist. Inform the patient of the possibility of another seizure and instruct him or her to avoid working with hazardous machines, driving, and performing other activities that may result in serious injury if another seizure occurs. Many states have mandatory reporting laws to the Department of Motor Vehicles if the patient has a driver's license.

15. **Should I start antiepileptic medication before discharge in the patient with a new seizure?**
In general, no, but this decision is best made in consultation with the patient's primary care physician or neurologist. Most patients with a single new-onset seizure, who can be discharged, do not need to be prescribed anticonvulsants until seen in a follow-up visit, and after further testing (i.e., electroencephalogram [EEG]).

16. **What is a psychogenic nonepileptic seizure (PNES) or a "pseudoseizure?"**
PNES are functional events that may mimic seizures in their motor activity or behavior but are *not* caused by abnormal electrical discharges in the brain. In general, patients with PNES have underlying anxiety, depression, or personality disorders. PNESs may be difficult to diagnose in the ED. Asynchronous extremity movements, forward thrusting movement of the pelvis, and eyes deviated toward the ground regardless of the head position and side-to-side head movements are consistent with PNES. Simultaneous video and EEG monitoring can help to differentiate a true seizure from a PNES. Treatment includes suggesting to the patient that the seizure will stop soon or attempting to distract the patient during the seizure activity. Exercise caution in diagnosing PNES, as up to 50% of patients with PNES also have epilepsy. And although PNES may not represent a neurologic emergency, patients are often struggling emotionally and need appropriate resources for identifiable stressors.

17. **Name some etiologies of seizures that generally do not respond to the usual medications and name the antidote (adult doses).**
    - *Eclampsia.* Magnesium sulfate 6 g IV over 15 minutes, then 2 g/h or 10 mg IM split in 2 separate doses. Consider this etiology in women between 20 weeks' gestation and 6 weeks' postpartum.
    - *Hypoglycemia.* Dextrose 0.5–1 g/kg IV
    - *Hyponatremia.* 3% hypertonic saline 100–200 mL over 1 hour
    - *Isoniazid (INH) ingestion.* Pyridoxine (vitamin B_6) 5 g IV given over 10 minutes, or 1 g for each gram of INH ingested.

18. **What are simple febrile seizures?**
See Chapter 63.

KEY POINTS: SECRETS FOR SEIZURES

1. Regardless of the agent chosen, the primary goal is to stop the seizure as rapidly as possible.
2. Always check a blood glucose level early in the resuscitation of a seizure patient.
3. Drugs of choice for status epilepticus include benzodiazepines (first-line therapy), followed by levetiracetam, phenytoin/fosphenytoin, or valproic acid, and finally propofol or barbiturates.
4. Obtain images for seizure patients with focal neurologic deficits, persistent altered mental status, fever, recent trauma, persistent headache, history of cancer, history of anticoagulation, HIV (AIDS), and when timely follow-up care cannot be ensured.

BIBILIOGRAPHY

Beghi M, Negrini PB, Perin C, et al. Psychogenic non-epileptic seizures: so-called psychiatric comorbidity and underlying defense mechanisms. *Neuropsychiatr Dis Treat.* 2015;11:2519–2527.
Brophy GM, Bell R, Claassen J, et al. Guidelines for the evaluation and management of status epilepticus. *Neurocrit Care.* 2012;17:3–23.
Glauser T, Shinnar S, Gloss D, et al. Evidence-based guideline: treatment of convulsive status epilepticus in children and adults: report of the Guideline Committee of the American Epilepsy Society. *Epilepsy Curr.* 2016;16(1):48–61.
Huff JS, Melnick ER, Tomaszewski CA, et al. Clinical policy: critical issues in the evaluation and management of adult patients presenting to the emergency department with seizures. *Ann Emerg Med.* 2014;63:437–447.e15.
Schachter SC. Evaluation of the first seizure in adults. In: Pedley TA, Waltham MA, eds. *UpToDate.* UpToDate; 2014. Accessed January 4, 2019.
Teran F, Harper-Kirksey K, Jagoda A. Clinical decision making in seizures and status epilepticus. *Emerg Med Pract.* 2015;17(1):1–24; quiz 24–25.

CHAPTER 21

ANAPHYLAXIS

Nadia S. Markovchick Dearstyne, MD and Vincent J. Markovchick, MD, FAAEM

1. **What is anaphylaxis?**

   Anaphylaxis is a serious allergic reaction usually mediated by immunoglobulin E (IgE), rapid in onset, and may cause death after exposure to an allergen in a previously sensitized individual within minutes to hours of allergen exposure. Anaphylaxis includes the acute onset, after allergen exposure, with one of the following clinical presentations: (1) skin/mucosal reaction, with respiratory tract involvement or hypotension; (2) involvement of two organ systems (i.e., respiratory tract, skin, persistent gastrointestinal symptoms); or (3) hypotension alone, thought to be related to known allergen.

2. **What is an anaphylactoid reaction?**

   An anaphylactoid reaction is a potentially fatal syndrome clinically similar to anaphylaxis but is not an IgE-mediated response, and may follow a single first-time exposure to certain agents, such as radiopaque contrast media, salicylates, and opiates.

3. **Name the most common causes of anaphylaxis.**

   Anaphylaxis is caused by ingestion, inhalation, or parenteral injection of antigens that sensitize predisposed individuals. Common antigens include:
   - drugs (e.g., penicillin)
   - foods (e.g., shellfish, nuts, or egg whites)
   - insect stings (hymenoptera) and bites (snakes)
   - diagnostic agents (ionic contrast media)
   - physical and environmental agents (e.g., latex, exercise, and cold)

   Idiopathic anaphylaxis is a diagnosis of exclusion that is made when no cause is identified.

4. **How do I make the diagnosis clinically?**

   Involvement of at least two* of the following must be present:
   - Cutaneous manifestations (urticaria or rash)
   - Mucous membranes (angioedema)
   - Upper respiratory tract (edema and hypersecretion)
   - Lower respiratory tract (bronchoconstriction)
   - Gastrointestinal symptoms (nausea, vomiting, or abdominal cramping)
   - Cardiovascular system (tachycardia, hypotension and cardiovascular collapse)

   * Note that hypotension in a patient who is exposed to a known allergen is adequate to make the diagnosis.

5. **What are the most common signs and symptoms?**

   The clinical presentation ranges from mild to life-threatening conditions. Mild manifestations include urticaria and dermal angioedema. Life-threatening manifestations involve the respiratory and cardiovascular systems. Respiratory signs and symptoms include acute upper airway obstruction presenting with stridor, or lower airway manifestations of bronchospasm with diffuse wheezing. Cardiovascular collapse presents in the form of syncope, hypotension, tachycardia, and dysrhythmias.

6. **What is the role of diagnostic studies?**

   There is no immediate role for diagnostic studies in the ED, because diagnosis and treatment is based solely on the clinical presentation. However, if there is a question about the diagnosis, serum tryptase and plasma and urine histamine levels may be elevated for up to 6 hours after an allergic reaction but have no role in the ED setting. These tests are sometimes used in the postmortem setting to determine the cause of death. There is a role for skin testing either before administration of an antigen or in follow-up referral to determine the exact allergens involved.

7. **What is the differential diagnosis?**

   Conditions include hereditary angioedema (HAE), septic and cardiogenic shock, asthma, croup and epiglottitis, vasovagal syncope, and any acute cardiovascular or respiratory collapse of unclear origin.

8. **What is the most common form of anaphylaxis, and how is it treated?**

   Urticaria, either simple or confluent, is the most benign and the most common clinical manifestation. However, skin signs maybe absent in 20% of cases. This is thought to be the result of a capillary leak mediated by histamine release. It may be treated by the administration of antihistamines (oral, intramuscular [IM], or intravenous [IV]), or if no contraindications, IM epinephrine.

9. **What is HAE? How is it related to anaphylaxis?**
   Hereditary angioedema is edema of subcutaneous tissue, most often involving the face, tongue, lips, larynx, gastrointestinal tract, and the male genitals. When this occurs with urticaria, it is likely an allergic reaction. If angioedema occurs without urticaria, it may be HAE.

10. **How does the treatment of HAE differ from that of anaphylaxis?**
    HAE is a genetic condition, usually presenting first in adolescence, involving a deficiency or absence of C1 ester-ase inhibitors. In adults, the condition can present as an acquired C1 esterase deficiency. Angiotensin-converting enzyme (ACE) inhibitors have been implicated as a trigger. Regardless of the cause, HAE is not IgE mediated; antihistamines and steroids are not as effective as in anaphylaxis. Because the initial diagnosis of C1 esterase deficiency is often unknown at the time of examination in the ED, treat the patient as if he or she were having an allergic reaction. If there is minimal or no response to therapy, consider IV fresh frozen plasma (FFP), which contains C1 esterase inhibitor, or C1 esterase inhibitor concentrate.

11. **Should I treat HAE and drug-induced angioedema in the same way?**
    In known C1 esterase deficiency (HAE), C1 esterase concentrate is the treatment of choice. FFP may be used, but does carry the risk of transmission of bloodborne illness and transfusion-related acute lung injury (TRALI). Ecal-lantide is a recombinant protein that inhibits plasma kallikrein. Icatibant is a synthetic bradykinin antagonist. Both are approved for HAE. Tranexamic acid (TXA) has been used in patients with ACE inhibitor–induced angioedema but is shown to be ineffective in HAE.

12. **Summarize the initial treatment for life-threatening forms of anaphylaxis.**
    - Upper airway obstruction with stridor and edema is treated with high-flow nebulized oxygen, racemic epi-nephrine, and IV epinephrine. If airway obstruction is severe or increases, perform endotracheal intubation or cricothyroidotomy.
    - Acute bronchospasm is treated with epinephrine. Mild to moderate wheezing in patients with normal blood pressure may be treated with 0.01 mg/kg of 1:1000 epinephrine administered IM. If the patient is in severe respiratory distress or has a silent chest, administer IV epinephrine via a drip infusion: 1 mg of epinephrine in 250 mL of dextrose 5% in water (D5W) at an initial rate of 1 mcg/min, with titration to desired effect. Broncho-spasm refractory to epinephrine may respond to a nebulized β-agonist, such as albuterol or metaproterenol.
    - Cardiovascular collapse presenting with hypotension is treated with a constant infusion of epinephrine, titrating the rate to attain a systolic blood pressure of 100 mmHg or mean arterial pressure of 80 mmHg.
    - For patients in full cardiac arrest, administer 1:10,000 epinephrine, 1 mg slow IV push, or 2–2.5 mg epinephrine diluted in 10 mL normal saline (NS) via endotracheal tube. Immediate endotracheal intubation or cricothyroidotomy should be performed as needed to secure the airway.

13. **What is the role of a "dirty" epi drip in the treatment of anaphylaxis?**
    The role of a dirty epi drip is to stabilize a patient prior to starting a patient on an epinephrine drip prepared by pharmacy.

14. **How do I prepare a "dirty" epi drip?**
    - Step 1: get 1 mg code cart epinephrine. It does not matter if it is 1:1000 or 1:10,000 as the dose of 1 mg of epinephrine is the same.
    - Step 2: inject 1 mg of epinephrine into 1 L NS
    - Step 3: run the epinephrine NS mixture wide open. This will administer 20–30 mL/min (or 20–30 mcg/min) of epinephrine if run through an 18 G IV.
    - Step 4: titrate to blood pressure in the normal systolic range using the IV roller or a pressure bag.

15. **Can I push code cart epinephrine IV instead of administering IM epi in a patient with anaphylaxis?**
    Never push code cart epinephrine IV in a patient with a pulse. This is likely to result in supraventricular tachycar-dia (SVT), ventricular tachycardia (VT), or severe hypertension. Use a dirty epi drip instead and administer 0.01 mg/kg epi up to a max of 0.5 mg IM epi while setting up your dirty epi drip.

KEY POINTS: ANAPHYLAXIS

1. Life-threatening target organs are the upper airway mucosa, bronchiole smooth muscle, and the cardiovascular system.
2. Hypotension is the indication for IV epinephrine.
3. Administer IV epinephrine as a drip, not as a bolus, in the non–cardiac arrest situation.

16. **What are the adjuncts to initial epinephrine and airway management?**
    If intubation is unsuccessful and cricothyroidotomy is contraindicated, percutaneous transtracheal jet ventilation via needle cricothyroidotomy should be considered, especially in small children. IV diphenhydramine (1 mg/kg up to 50 mg) should be given to all patients. Simultaneous administration of an H_2 blocker, such as cimetidine,

300 mg IV, may be helpful. Aerosolized bronchodilators are useful if bronchospasm is present. Glucagon, 50–150 mcg/kg IV over 1 minute followed by 1–5 mg/h IV infusion may be helpful in patients resistant to epinephrine who are on long-term β-adrenergic blocking agents, such as propranolol. Corticosteroids have limited benefit because of the delayed (4–6 hours) onset of action, but may be beneficial in patients with prolonged bronchospasm or hypotension.

17. **What are the potential complications of IV epinephrine administration?**
When epinephrine 1:10,000 is administered via IV push in patients who have an obtainable blood pressure or pulse, there is significant potential for overtreatment and the potentiation of hypertension, tachycardia (SVT or VT), ischemic chest pain, acute myocardial infarction, and ventricular dysrhythmias. Extreme care must be exercised in elderly patients and in patients with underlying coronary artery disease. IV epinephrine should be administered by a controlled titratable drip infusion with continuous monitoring of cardiac rhythm and blood pressure.

18. **What is biphasic anaphylaxis? How common is it?**
Biphasic anaphylaxis is a recurrence of the symptoms of anaphylaxis after the initial symptoms resolve. This may occur anywhere from several hours to as long as 72 hours later. This may be caused by persistence of the allergen or immune mediators relative to the duration of the therapy. The reported incidence is between 1% and 23% of all anaphylactic reactions. Some risk factors that may make biphasic anaphylaxis more likely are as follows:
- A history of biphasic anaphylaxis
- Delays in onset of initial symptoms, in initial treatment, or in resolution of symptoms with proper therapy
- Severe reactions involving hypotension or laryngeal edema
- Patients taking β-blockers
- Patients exposed to ingested allergens

19. **Is there a role for prophylactic treatment in anaphylaxis? How is this performed?**
When the potential benefits of treatment or diagnosis outweigh the risks (e.g., administration of antivenom for life-threatening or limb-threatening snake bites, or patients with neurosyphilis requiring penicillin), informed consent should be obtained if the patient is competent. Pretreat with IV diphenhydramine and corticosteroids, and prepare an IV epinephrine infusion drip. The patient should be in an intensive care unit (ICU) setting with continuous monitoring of blood pressure, cardiac rhythm, and oxygen saturation; have full intubation and cricothyroidotomy equipment at the bedside. Under the supervision of a physician capable of immediately administering IV epinephrine and managing the airway, administration of the antigen (e.g., the antivenom) should be started. Nonionic contrast medium for diagnostic imaging studies should be given to patients with a history of anaphylaxis to ionic contrast material.

20. **What about steroids?**
The usual practice has been to administer steroids and send the patient home on burst dose steroids. However, multiple recent studies have shown no significant decrease in the rate of return ED visits or biphasic reactions. Corticosteroids have an onset of action of approximately 4–6 hours after administration, and they have limited to no benefit in the initial acute treatment of anaphylaxis. A single dose of hydrocortisone (250–1000 mg IV) or methylprednisolone (125–250 mg IV) may be administered, knowing that the benefit, if any, will be delayed.

21. **What is the disposition of a patient who initially responds to treatment?**
Although most patients become asymptomatic after early treatment, all patients with true anaphylactic reactions should be admitted to either an ED or hospital observation unit for a minimum of 4 hours after last administration of epinephrine. Patients who experience rebound or continue to have life-threatening symptoms (e.g., bronchospasm, hypotension, or upper airway obstruction) should be admitted.

22. **What follow-up instructions are given to patients treated for anaphylaxis?**
Patients who have had a moderate to severe anaphylactic reaction (anything other than isolated urticaria) should be prescribed epinephrine (i.e., the EpiPen; youth <30 kg should receive the EpiPen "junior"), and educated in the self-administration of epinephrine into the muscles of the thigh with an autoinjector at the first sign of anaphylactic symptoms. Self-administration of oral diphenhydramine is indicated to treat mild reactions, such as urticaria, and should be taken concomitant with the administration of IM epinephrine.

23. **Are there special considerations for treating anaphylaxis in pregnancy?**
Anaphylaxis in pregnancy is geared toward treating the mother and the treatment algorithm should be the same. Remember to think about alternate diagnoses, such as hemorrhage or amniotic fluid embolism, as the cause of hypotension in the postpartum period.

Bibiliography

Campbell RL, Kelso JM, et al. Anaphylaxis: emergency treatment. *UpToDate.com*. 2019.

Chipps BE. Update in pediatric anaphylaxis: a systematic review. *Clin Pediatr (Phila)*. 2013;52:451–461.

Cuniowski PA, Hunter CJ. Would you recognize this patient's biphasic anaphylaxis? *Emerg Med*. 2009;41:30–34.

Coralic Z, Pharm D. The dirty epi drip: IV epinephrine when you need it. *Aliem.com*. June 27, 2013.

Dhami S, Panesar SS, Roberts G, et al. Management of anaphylaxis: a systematic review. *Allergy*. 2013;69:168–175.

Hassen GW, Kalantari H, Parraga M, et al. Fresh frozen plasma for progressive and refractory angiotensin converting enzyme inhibitor induced angioedema. *J Emerg Med*. 2013;44:764–772.

Schatz M, Dombrowski MP, et al. Anaphylaxis in pregnant and breastfeeding women. *UpToDate.com*. 2019.

CHAPTER 22

LOW BACK PAIN

Omid Adibnazari, MD and Ryan A. Pedigo, MD

1. **Can I skip this chapter?**

   Not if you anticipate a career that involves caring for adults. Low back pain (LBP) is the most common musculo-skeletal complaint leading to an emergency department (ED) visit. The vast majority (up to 85%) of individuals will have LBP at some point in their lives. One in four adults report having LBP in the past 3 months. It is the second most common cause of disability among adults in the United States, causing an estimated 149 million lost work days per year. The cost of diagnosis, treatment, disability, lost productivity, and litigation as a result of LBP is estimated to be $100–$200 billion annually.

2. **What are the common causes of LBP?**

   Idiopathic back pain is also referred to as *musculoskeletal back pain, acute lumbosacral sprain, lumbago,* and other similar terms. Importantly, there is no specific identifiable anatomic injury when patients have these diagnoses. Although most patients will feel better within 4 weeks, the majority will also have a recurrence within 1 year. Patients with idiopathic LBP have asymmetric pain in the paraspinal muscles of the lumbar spine that is worse with activity.

   Lumbar disk herniation is LBP that often radiates down the leg in the dermatome served by the affected nerve. Herniations that occur at L4-5 or L5-S1 cause pain that radiates down the lateral and posterior aspects of the leg, respectively, termed *sciatica*. These account for >90% of the cases of radiculopathy. Nerve root impinge-ment can also be a result of other etiologies, such as spinal stenosis or more life-threatening etiologies such as malignancy or abscess. The challenge in emergency medicine is finding the three or four patients out of 100 who have emergent causes of LBP and treating them aggressively, while preventing excessive imaging and testing in patients who do not have features indicative of a serious cause of their pain.

3. **What are the emergent causes of LBP?**

   Although almost all causes of acute back pain are self-limited and benign, there are a few life-threatening diagno-ses that should always be considered and ruled out by a thorough history and physical examination (Table 22.1).

   Epidural abscess (or other spinal infection such as vertebral osteomyelitis or discitis) should be considered in high-risk patients with back pain and fever. Risk factors include immunocompromised states (e.g., HIV/AIDS, alcoholism, diabetes), older age (most commonly ages 60–70 years), intravenous drug use, and recent spinal surgery. Emergent contrast-enhanced magnetic resonance imaging (MRI) is the diagnostic test of choice.

   Ruptured abdominal aortic aneurysm (AAA) should be considered in older individuals who have LBP and risk factors for atherosclerosis. A contained AAA rupture can cause significant back pain and be a sentinel event to a fatal rupture. AAA is defined as an aortic diameter over 3 cm, with the risk of rupture increasing with size. ED point-of-care ultrasound can quickly and accurately evaluate for this diagnosis.

   Cauda equina or conus medullaris syndrome occurs when there is compression of the cauda equina or conus, typically around the L1 area in adults. This is usually from a herniated disk but can be caused by anything that impinges on the distal spinal canal (e.g., metastatic disease, epidural abscess, hematomas). The classic presentation is severe LBP, associated saddle anesthesia, bilateral lower extremity weakness, and urinary inconti-nence/retention. The most sensitive finding is urinary retention, so a postvoid residual (PVR) test should be checked in individuals for whom the diagnosis is considered (with either urinary catheterization or ultrasound). A PVR over 100 mL is abnormal, and anything over 300 mL is markedly abnormal. The negative predictive value of a normal PVR for ruling out cauda equina syndrome is nearly 100%. Emergent noncontrast MRI is the diagnostic test of choice for herniated discs. Add contrast if concern for epidural abscess or metastatic disease.

   Spinal fracture should be considered in individuals who have a history of antecedent blunt trauma before the onset of pain. There should be a low threshold to image (with radiography or computed tomography [CT]) patients who have LBP after significant blunt trauma. In individuals with risk factors for osteoporosis (e.g., elderly, bedridden, chronic corticosteroid use), the risk of a fracture is much higher. There is a 10-fold increase in fracture risk among patients taking chronic corticosteroids.

   Malignancy should be suspected in individuals with LBP who have known cancer or experience worsening back pain that lasts longer than 4 weeks, often is worse at night, does not respond to routine analgesics, and is associated with recent weight loss. Further testing to identify the primary site of malignancy should be under-taken; malignancies that commonly metastasize to bone include prostate, breast, kidney, thyroid, and lung (Pb KTL, or "lead kettle").

Table 22.1 Differential Diagnosis of Low Back Pain

MECHANICAL SPINE DISORDERS	NONMECHANICAL SPINE DISORDERS	VISCERAL DISEASE
Lumbar strain	Malignancy	Abdominal aortic aneurysm
Degenerative disk/facet disease	Multiple myeloma	Psoas abscess
Herniated disk	Metastatic cancer	Pelvic organs
Spinal stenosis	Spinal column or cord cancer	PID
Spondylolysis	Lymphoma	Prostatitis
Spondylolisthesis	Infection	Renal disease
Congenital spinal disease	Septic discitis	Pyelonephritis
Traumatic fracture	Osteomyelitis	Nephrolithiasis
Osteoporotic compression fracture	Epidural abscess	Gastrointestinal disorders
	Inflammatory arthritis	Pancreatitis
		Penetrating ulcer
		Cholecystitis

PID, Pelvic inflammatory disease.

KEY POINTS: HIGH-RISK CAUSES OF LOW BACK PAIN

1. Abdominal aortic aneurysm (AAA)
2. Cauda equina syndrome
3. Lumbar disk herniation with severe neurologic compromise
4. Spinal malignancy
5. Spinal infection (e.g., vertebral osteomyelitis, epidural abscess, discitis)

4. **How should I focus my history?**
   The following historical features, termed *red flag features,* should be investigated routinely to assess for an emergent cause in patients presenting with LBP (Table 22.2):
   - A history of recent trauma should raise concern for spinal fractures.
   - A history of malignancy or symptoms consistent with malignancy (e.g., pain at night, persistent chronic worsening pain, and unexplained weight loss) makes metastatic disease more likely.
   - Immunocompromised patients (e.g., diabetes, HIV/AIDS, chronic steroid use, intravenous drug use) and those with fever are at risk for epidural abscesses.
   - Elderly patients and those taking steroids for chronic conditions are at higher risk for fractures, even with minor trauma.
   - Neurologic symptoms, such as urinary retention, saddle anesthesia, or bilateral leg numbness or weakness, cause concern for cauda equina syndrome.

Table 22.2 Red Flag Features of Low Back Pain

RED FLAG FEATURES	POSSIBLE CAUSE	IMAGING
Age >50 years	Fracture, malignancy	LS spine radiography
Trauma	Fracture	LS spine radiography
Fever, intravenous drug use, recent infection, lumbar spinal surgery in past year	Infection	MRI
Unexplained weight loss, history of cancer	Metastases	LS spine radiography
Urinary retention, motor deficits at multiple levels, fecal incontinence, saddle anesthesia	Cauda equina syndrome	MRI
Progressive motor weakness	Myelopathy	MRI
Failure to improve after 1 month	Fracture, malignancy	LS spine radiography
Immunosuppression or steroid use	Fracture, infection	LS spine radiography, MRI, or CT
Midline spinal tenderness	Fracture, infection, malignancy	LS spine radiography

CT, Computed tomography; *LS,* lumbosacral; *MRI,* magnetic resonance imaging.

Additional features that should be assessed:

- Radiation of pain suggests radiculopathy from a disk herniation or mass lesion impinging on a nerve root. Pain radiating below the knee is more consistent with radiculopathy.
- Aggravation of pain in the back and calves with walking (termed *pseudoclaudication*) and alleviation of pain with bending forward suggests spinal stenosis. Pseudoclaudication can be distinguished from claudication caused by peripheral vascular disease by the alleviation with bending forward (which widens the spinal canal and relieves stenosis) and from the duration of pain after rest, which is typically longer (e.g., 15 minutes with spinal stenosis versus 5 minutes with vascular disease).

5. **How should I focus my physical examination?**

All patients with LBP should receive a complete neurologic examination with a particular focus on lower extremity strength, sensation, and reflexes (Table 22.3). Mechanical spine disorders, with the exception of herniated lumbar disks or severe spondylolisthesis, should not compromise neurologic function. Red flag features of the physical examination include fever, midline spinal tenderness, and significant neurologic deficits, including saddle anesthesia (see Table 22.2). A straight leg raise (SLR) test should be performed to assess for sciatica, but a positive result is not necessarily a red flag sign. An abdominal examination is important to assess for visceral disease and AAA. Rectal tone and sensation should be assessed if there is any concern for cord compression.

6. **What does it mean when a patient with LBP also has leg pain?**

Patients with LBP and leg pain (termed *sciatica*) may have one of two syndromes:

- Referred pain is caused by inflammation of the sciatic nerve. It is usually dull and poorly localized, does not radiate distal to the knee, and is not associated with a positive SLR test or neurologic impairment.
- Radicular pain is usually caused by nerve root impingement from a herniated lumbar disk or the narrowing of a vertebral foramen from spinal stenosis, but it may also occur with epidural metastases or abscesses in high-risk patients. It is sharp and well localized, commonly (but not always) radiates distal to the knee, usually is associated with a positive SLR test, and may be associated with neurologic impairment.

7. **How do I perform an SLR test? How do I interpret the results?**

To perform an SLR test, have the patient lie supine while you slowly raise the involved leg (flexing the hip while keeping the knee extended) until the patient complains of discomfort. A positive SLR test occurs when leg elevation results in pain that radiates down the involved leg past the knee usually occurring at 30–60 degrees of flexion (Lasègue's sign). Merely evoking pain confined to the low back or hamstrings does not count as a positive test. The SLR test is 91% sensitive but only 26% specific for a herniated disk; a crossed SLR test, in which raising the uninvolved leg evokes pain radiating down the involved leg, is only 29% sensitive but 88% specific for disk herniation. Dorsiflexion of the foot at the point of pain should worsen the pain, and plantar flexion should alleviate it.

8. **What imaging or laboratory testing should be routinely performed?**

None. In the absence of any red flag features (see Table 22.2), imaging is estimated to change clinical decision making only once for every 2500 studies performed. Despite popular belief, studies have shown that routine imaging does not improve patient reassurance or decrease anxiety, but it does increase patient radiation exposure, ED length of stay, and health care costs. Patients often come to the ED expecting imaging, so explaining early on that imaging is unnecessary for uncomplicated back pain, and only increases cost and radiation exposure, is important to ensure that they understand why imaging is not being performed.

If concerning features are present, appropriate laboratory tests and imaging should be ordered. When spinal infection or malignancy is suspected, an erythrocyte sedimentation rate (ESR) and C-reactive protein (CRP) should be obtained. An elevated ESR (usually greater than 60–80 mm/h) or CRP should lead to further investigation with a spinal MRI. If malignancy is suspected, either CT or MRI may be appropriate. An MRI should be obtained emergently in patients whenever there is evidence of acute neurologic compromise (e.g., loss of bowel or bladder function, motor weakness, or sensory changes).

9. **What should I know about children who come to the ED with back pain?**

Back pain is rare in children. LBP that interferes with activities previously enjoyed by a child may be indicative of a serious underlying pathologic condition. Spondylolysis and spondylolisthesis resulting from sports are the most

Table 22.3 Clinical Features of Lumbar Disk Herniation

DISK	L4	L5	S1-2
Pain	Front of leg	Side of leg	Back of leg
Weakness	Knee extension	Great toe dorsiflexion	Foot plantar flexion
Sensory loss	Knee and medial foot	Side of calf, web of great toe	Back of calf and lateral foot
Reflex loss	Knee jerk	None	Ankle jerk

common causes of LBP in children (see Question 10). Scoliosis does not usually cause back pain, but conditions that cause scoliosis (e.g., cancer, fracture, limb length discrepancy, infection, or tumors) may cause pain. Although every attempt should be made to limit gonadal radiation in pediatric patients, children with LBP that is not clearly mechanical in nature should be imaged. An ESR or CRP may prove helpful when infection or malignancy is suspected.

10. **Is there a difference between spondylosis, spondylolysis, and spondylolisthesis?**
    Yes. The terminology is confusing. The prefix *spondylo-* means *vertebrae.*
    - *Spondylosis* is a nonspecific term for degenerative spine disease.
    - *Spondylolysis* implies severe degeneration with a resulting fracture of the pars interarticularis, which is the portion of the lateral mass of the vertebrae between the superior and inferior articular processes.
    - When spondylolysis occurs bilaterally, anterior slippage of one vertebral body on another can occur, termed *spondylolisthesis.* Severe spondylolisthesis can cause neurologic impairment.

11. **How should patients with LBP be treated in the ED?**
    There is no need to await definitive diagnosis before providing pain relief. Oral or parenteral nonsteroidal anti-inflammatory drugs (NSAIDs) and application of superficial heat are first-line agents. Parenteral narcotics may be necessary to provide adequate analgesia in patients with severe discomfort.

12. **When should patients be hospitalized for treatment?**
    Patients with LBP may require hospitalization to expedite evaluation and treatment when an emergent cause of LBP (e.g., epidural abscess, cauda equina) is suspected or when patients experience severe pain requiring continued administration of parenteral analgesics.

13. **How should patients with musculoskeletal LBP be treated as outpatients?**
    Bed rest is not recommended for patients with acute LBP in the absence of acute disc herniation associated with severe pain. In general, patients who remain active recuperate faster and experience less disability than those who rest in bed. Most patients benefit from oral NSAIDs, but some require opioids to produce adequate analgesia during the first few days. Sedatives and muscle relaxants should not be used as adjuncts in treating LBP, given a recent randomized trial showing that the addition of diazepam to NSAIDs did not improve outcomes.

14. **What aftercare instructions should I give my patients?**
    Patients with suspected disk disease and patients with symptoms that do not improve within 1–2 weeks should be seen by a physician for follow-up evaluation. All patients should be instructed to return immediately if they develop worsening symptoms, or if they develop any of the red flag features previously mentioned.

15. **What happens to patients with LBP when they leave the ED?**
    The prognosis for patients experiencing a first episode of idiopathic or mechanical LBP is good: 70% are better by 1 week, 80% by 2 weeks, and 90% by 1 month. Most studies comparing medical management, chiropractic manipulation, and other treatment modalities rarely find significant differences in long-term outcome, because almost everyone gets better no matter what they do. Patients who do not improve with conservative management may have significant underlying medical disorders (e.g., inflammatory disorders, malignancy, infections, or disk disease) that were not apparent at the time of initial evaluation; alternatively, they may suffer from psychiatric disorders, drug dependence, or job dissatisfaction, which can increase their likelihood of developing chronic, disabling back pain. However, recurrence rates are also high, and patients should be educated that this is likely to be a continuing problem for them in the future. Performing exercises that strengthen the abdominal and back muscles (after the acute pain has subsided), avoiding activities that twist and torque the back, and maintaining good cardiovascular health may decrease the incidence and severity of LBP recurrences.

BIBILIOGRAPHY

Borenstein D. Mechanical back pain: a rheumatologist's view. *Nat Rev Rheumatol.* 2013;9:643–653.
Chou R, Qaseem A, Owens DK, et al. Diagnostic imaging for low back pain. *Ann Intern Med.* 2011;154:181–189.
Cohen SP, Argoff CE, Carragee EJ. Management of low back pain. *BMJ.* 2009;338:100–106.
Friedman BW, Irizarry E, Solorzano C, et al. Diazepam is no better than placebo when added to naproxen for acute low back pain. *Ann Emerg Med.* 2017;70:169–176.
Miller SM. Low back pain: pharmacologic management. *Prim Care.* 2012;39:499–510.
Patrick N, Emanski E, Knaub MA. Acute and chronic low back pain. *Med Clin North Am.* 2014;98:777–789.
Qaseem A, Wilt TJ, McLean RM, et al. Noninvasive treatments for acute, subacute, and chronic low back pain: a clinical practice guideline from the American College of Physicians. *Ann Intern Med.* 2017;166:514–530.
Srinivas SV, Deyo RA, Berger ZD. Application of "less is more" to low back pain. *Arch Intern Med.* 2012;172:1016–1020.
Verhagen AP, Downie A, Popal N, et al. Red flags presented in current low back pain guidelines: a review. *Eur Spine J.* 2016;25: 2788–2802.

NONTRAUMATIC OCULAR EMERGENCIES

Martin R. Huecker, MD and Daniel F. Danzl, MD

CHAPTER 23

1. What are some tricks to evaluate the red eye?

Always document near ± distance visual acuity in each eye independently. Topical application of anesthetic drops should decrease or eradicate pain secondary to an abrasion or conjunctivitis (not so with iritis or glaucoma). Redness at the corneal–scleral junction (perilimbic flush) suggests iritis or glaucoma. Shining a light into the normal eye should make the opposite eye hurt if the patient has iritis (because of consensual movement of the inflamed affected contralateral iris). In addition to the consensual pupillary reflex test, a positive accommodative test, which is simply pain precipitated by accommodation, is suggestive of ciliary spasm.

2. What typical findings help with the differential diagnosis of the red eye?

See Table 23.1.

3. What is conjunctivitis?

Conjunctivitis is inflammation of the bulbar and palpebral conjunctivae. Viral conjunctivitis is usually bilateral with clear tearing and may be associated with an upper respiratory infection (URI). A preauricular lymph node suggests epidemic keratoconjunctivitis (adenovirus). Two common viral pathogens are herpes simplex, with dendritic ulcers, and herpes zoster, with involvement of the fifth cranial nerve. Ocular zoster is suggested by involvement of the nasociliary branch of V_1, manifested by lesions on the tip of the nose (Hutchinson sign) (Fig. 23.1).

Bacterial conjunctivitis initially may be unilateral with purulent drainage. Always consider an undiagnosed foreign body with unilateral conjunctivitis. *Chlamydia* or gonococcus should be considered in neonates or adults with sexually transmitted diseases. Allergies may cause papillae under the lids, chemosis, and itching.

4. How is conjunctivitis treated?

Commonly agents include polymyxin B sulfate/trimethoprim drops (or erythromycin 0.5% ointment). Reserve the topical fluoroquinolones for severe infections and for contact lens wearers who are at risk for *Pseudomonas*. Avoid neomycin because hypersensitivity reactions are common.

5. What is endophthalmitis?

Endophthalmitis is infection or inflammation within the globe. It usually is seen as a collection of pus in the anterior chamber (hypopyon) that resembles a dependent meniscus similar to the blood collection in a hyphema. Antecedent causes include corneal ulcers, direct inoculation, or hematogenous spread, and conjunctivitis with organisms capable of penetrating the cornea (e.g., *Neisseria gonorrhoeae, Corynebacterium species, Listeria monocytogenes, Listeria,* and *Haemophilus aegyptius*).

6. What is the difference between periorbital and orbital cellulitis?

Periorbital (preseptal) cellulitis is soft-tissue infection of eye structures anterior to the tarsal plate, usually localized to the eyelids and conjunctivae. Orbital cellulitis is a more serious infection involving posterior eye structures. Both tend to be unilateral. Orbital cellulitis is most often the result of direct spread from ethmoid sinusitis or pansinusitis, whereas periorbital cellulitis often follows trauma, bites, or foreign body.

7. How do I differentiate clinically between periorbital and orbital cellulitis?

The two may be difficult to distinguish clinically, especially in children. Periorbital (preseptal) cellulitis tends to cause local eyelid symptoms and occasionally ocular discharge, and may be associated with fever or leukocytosis. Visual acuity and pupillary reflexes are normal.

Orbital (postseptal) cellulitis may present with all of the previous symptoms plus exophthalmos, fever, and pain with extraocular movements. Decreased visual acuity, loss of sensation over the ophthalmic and maxillary branches of the trigeminal nerve in V_1 and V_2 (divisions of cranial nerve V), and increased intraocular pressure are uncommon findings. Contrast computed tomography (CT) scanning of the orbit is liberally indicated with periorbital swelling when there is a possibility of postseptal infection.

Table 23.1 Differential Diagnosis of the Red Eye

	CONJUNCTIVITIS	ACUTE IRITIS	ANGLE-CLOSURE GLAUCOMA
Incidence	Extremely common	Common	Uncommon
Discharge	Moderate to copious	Reflex epiphora	None
Vision	Normal	Slightly blurred	Very blurred (haloes)
Pain	Gritty	Moderate	Severe
Conjunctival injection	Diffuse with limbic sparing	Perilimbic	Perilimbic
Cornea	Clear	Keratotic precipitates	Steamy or hazy
Pupil size	Normal	Constricted or dilated	Fixed and dilated
Pupillary light response	Normal	Poor and painful (+ consensual photophobia)	Poor or none if fixed
Intraocular pressure	Normal	Normal	Elevated

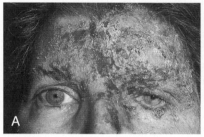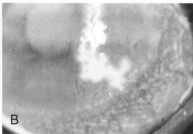

Fig. 23.1 (A) Ocular zoster, suggested by involvement of the nasociliary branch of V_1, manifested by lesions on the tip of the nose (Hutchinson sign). (B) Classic herpes simplex dendrite staining brightly with fluorescein. (A, From Kanski JJ. *Clinical Ophthalmology: A Synopsis*. New York: Butterworth-Heinemann; 2004. B, From Reeves SW, et al. Corneal infections. In: Vander JF, ed. *Ophthalmology Secrets*. 3rd ed. St. Louis: Elsevier Mosby; 2007:97, Fig. 8–11.)

8. **What is the common clinical presentation of cavernous sinus thrombosis?**
Patients often progress from fever, headache, and chemosis to ophthalmoplegia, exophthalmos (sclera visible above and below the cornea), and altered level of consciousness. The mnemonic *POTOMAC* can be used to remember the following structures traversing the cavernous sinus:
Pituitary
Ophthalmic branch of the trigeminal nerve (V_1)
Trochlear nerve (IV)
Oculomotor nerve (III)
Maxillary branch of the trigeminal nerve (V_2)
Abducens nerve (VI)
Carotid artery
    In thrombosis, paralysis of cranial nerves III, IV, and VI is usually noted. Magnetic resonance imaging (MRI) is indicated.

9. **Describe the clinical presentation of iritis.**
Patients often exhibit perilimbic injection or "flush," ciliary spasm, and a constricted miotic pupil. A consensual photophobia can be a clue to iritis as the etiology of unilateral injection, versus conjunctivitis, which only cause direct photophobia. Because both may exhibit photophobia, bilateral iritis can be misdiagnosed as conjunctivitis. Perform a slit lamp examination of the anterior chamber for cells, flare, and for keratic precipitates (white cells) on the back of the cornea.

10. **How is iritis treated?**
Iritis is treated with systemic analgesics and a topical cycloplegic, not simply a mydriatic, to paralyze accommodation and dilate the iris. This prevents adhesions between the iris and the lens (posterior synechiae). Consider steroids in consultation with an ophthalmologist.

11. **What is acute angle-closure glaucoma?**
Glaucoma is optic nerve damage from increased intraocular pressure. In a patient with a narrow anterior cham-ber angle, pupillary dilation or mydriasis (e.g., from reduced illumination) causes the thickened iris to abut the lens, preventing adequate aqueous humor drainage through the pupil. Once the pressure rises high enough, the outflow tract (Schlemm's canal) is also narrowed, preventing drainage and quickly elevating globe pressures (Fig. 23.2). The rapid elevation of intraocular pressure causes a hazy cornea, ciliary flush, firm globe, and optic nerve damage if not treated promptly. The diagnosis may be delayed by the misleading systemic complaints of nausea, vomiting, and headache.

12. **How is acute angle-closure glaucoma treated?**
Acute angle-closure glaucoma is treated with intravenous mannitol or glycerol to decrease intraocular pressure by osmotic diuresis, topical miotics (i.e., 2% pilocarpine or 0.5% timolol) to decrease pupil size and increase aqueous outflow, and acetazolamide intravenously to decrease aqueous production. Topical sympathomimetics, such as apraclonidine, also reduce aqueous humor production. Emergent ophthalmologic consultation is indicated. Defini-tive management involves creating a hole or bypass tract through the iris for drainage (laser iridotomy).

13. **What is a subconjunctival hemorrhage?**
Subconjunctival hemorrhage occurs when a blood vessel ruptures under the conjunctiva. Without trauma, it often results from a Valsalva maneuver associated with coughing or vomiting. Reassure the patient that vision will not be affected and that the blood will be absorbed over 10–14 days. Patients taking anticoagulant medication should have their international normalized ratio (INR) measured. In the setting of trauma, in a patient with 360 subconjunctival hemorrhage, consider globe rupture.

14. **What are some common diseases of the cornea?**
Diseases of the cornea include pterygium, pinguecula, and ulcerations. A pterygium is a wedge of conjunctival fi-brovascular tissue that extends over the cornea, unlike a pinguecula, which does not pass the corneal edge. Both of these are benign conditions and can be electively excised. Ulcerations are often surrounded by a cloudy white cornea. Emergent ophthalmologic recommendations often include a topical fluoroquinolone, such as moxifloxacin.

15. **What are some of the unique issues regarding ophthalmologic pharmacology?**
Topical agents may have systemic effects, so exercise caution when prescribing β-blockers, vasoconstrictors, and anticholinergics. Ointments have a longer duration of action, but blur vision. Generally, wait 10 minutes before instilling different drops.
     Diagnostic medications include stains, such as fluorescein, that help identify corneal and conjunctival abnor-malities, and topical anesthetics, which historically are not recommended as outpatient therapy. However, consensus is evolving regarding short-course therapy for uncomplicated corneal abrasions. Nonsteroidal anti-inflammatory drugs (NSAIDs), such as ketorolac or diclofenac, are useful for pain relief. Topical corticosteroids should generally be used only after consultation with an ophthalmologist.
     Miotic eye drop bottles have green tops, and mydriatic/cycloplegic agents have red tops.
     Some patients will have a pupil that is dilated as a result of taking a medication. If 1% pilocarpine fails to constrict the pupil, it is pharmacologically blocked, most commonly by phenylephrine, a scopolamine patch

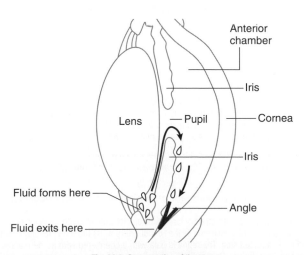

Fig. 23.2 Cross section of the eye.

(if it has been handled), or aerosolized anticholinergics/β-agonists. Other causes of a unilateral dilated pupil include posttraumatic mydriasis, third nerve palsy, or a normal variant.

16. **Name some of the considerations involving pupil dilation.**
Phenylephrine (2.5%) is a direct sympathomimetic and mydriatic agent. Dilation may last 4 hours, and patients with a shallow anterior chamber may develop acute glaucoma after leaving the ED. Pharmacologic pupillary dilation is rarely required in the ED. A panoptic ophthalmoscope provides a five times larger view of the undilated fundus. For short-term cycloplegia, consider tropicamide (1–6 hours) or 2%–5% homatropine (1–2 days); never use atropine (1–3 weeks).

17. **What does the presence of an afferent pupillary defect (APD), also known as a Marcus Gunn pupil, indicate?**
If the patient has an APD, it confirms damage to the retina or optic nerve. To perform the swinging flashlight test, shine a light toward the normal eye, and after several seconds swing it to the other eye. After a brief pupillary constriction in the abnormal eye, the redilation in response to light reflects afferent deprivation; this response may only be appreciated in a dark room.

KEY POINTS: COMMON CAUSES OF AN APD

1. Central retinal artery occlusion
2. Central retinal vein occlusion
3. Optic neuritis
4. Retrobulbar neuritis
5. Retinal detachment
6. Ischemic optic neuropathy (traumatic or nontraumatic)

18. **In a patient with anisocoria, how does one determine which pupil is abnormal?**
Begin the examination in a darkened room; if there is more anisocoria in the light, the large pupil is failing to constrict and is abnormal. More anisocoria that develops going into the dark indicates that the miotic pupil is failing to dilate. Never just assume that the larger pupil is abnormal.

KEY POINTS: COMMON CAUSES OF ANISOCORIA

1. Horner syndrome
2. Argyll-Robertson pupil
3. Adie pupil
4. Posttraumatic or medication-induced mydriasis
5. Third nerve palsy

19. **What are common causes of a miotic pupil?**
The two most common causes of a miotic pupil are Horner syndrome and an Argyll-Robertson pupil. The clinical manifestations of Horner syndrome include ptosis, miosis, and anhidrosis (in a cold ED, check for dilated conjunctival vessels). Bronchogenic carcinoma, stroke, and brachial plexus pathology may present with Horner syndrome.
The Argyll-Robertson pupil is miotic and irregular, and displays light-near dissociation. The pupil constricts to accommodation but not to light. This finding is common with diabetes and syphilis. A common testing error is to hold and shine a penlight directly in front of the eye, which can cause the pupil to constrict from accommodation, not light.

20. **Is there another cause of light-near dissociation?**
The only other cause is Adie pupil, which results from idiopathic parasympathetic denervation in the ciliary ganglion in the eye. The patient is often a young female with a mydriatic pupil that accommodates but does not react to light. Herpes zoster is another cause of Adie pupil. There are no diseases that cause a pupil to react to light but fail to accommodate.

21. **What are some common causes of nontraumatic loss of vision?**
See Table 23.2.

22. **Describe the presentation and treatment of central retinal artery occlusion and central retinal vein occlusion.**
Both occur in middle-age patients with atherosclerosis, or elderly patients with hypertension, and present as sudden painless loss of vision. Embolic occlusion of the retinal artery or its branches results in a dilated nonreactive pupil with an APD on the affected side. The retina is pale with a cherry-red spot at the macula (macular blood supply is from the choroidal circulation). Occasionally, amaurosis fugax precedes central retinal artery occlusion. The funduscopic examination of an ischemic central retinal vein occlusion is described as a *blood and thunder fundus,*

Table 23.2 Common Causes of Nontraumatic Loss of Vision

Transient monocular
Amaurosis fugax
Temporal arteritis
Migraine
Persistent monocular or binocular
Central retinal artery occlusion
Central retinal vein occlusion
Retinal detachment or hemorrhage
Vitreous or macular hemorrhage
Optic or retrobulbar neuritis
Macular degeneration
Acute binocular
Vertebral basilar insufficiency
Cerebrovascular disease
Toxins (e.g., methanol, salicylates, quinine)
Hysteria
Malingering

Table 23.3 Optic Neuritis Versus Papilledema

	OPTIC NEURITIS	PAPILLEDEMA
Pupil reactivity	Slow	Normal
Visual acuity	Decreased	Normal
Ocular pain	Present	Absent
Usual localization	Unilateral	Bilateral
Fundus	Blurred disc margins	Blurred disc margins

because of the presence of multiple large hemorrhages. Efforts to decrease intraocular pressure and dilate retinal vessels by increasing the partial pressure of carbon dioxide (pCO_2) (e.g., using a paper bag or carbogen) and globe massage have not been shown to alter the natural history of the disease. Prognosis for both entities is poor.

23. **What are other causes of sudden painless monocular loss of vision?**
Suspect vitreous hemorrhage in diabetic patients with an obscured red reflex and retinal details. Nontraumatic retinal detachments are more common in patients with significant myopia. Patients often see flashing lights or a falling curtain. Most commonly, patients report dark floating spots or floaters, which reflect vitreous separations and not a retinal detachment. Bedside ultrasound is increasingly being used to diagnose retinal detachment in the ED.

24. **How do optic neuritis and papilledema differ?**
Although these two processes appear similar on funduscopic examination, optic neuritis involves focal demyelination of the optic nerve, resulting in a hyperemic nerve head developing over hours to days. The average age of onset is in the 30s, and there is a 40% association with current or future diagnosis of multiple sclerosis.
Papilledema is swelling of the optic disc caused by increased intracranial pressure. It is usually bilateral but may be asymmetric and may be the result of brain abscess or tumor, intracranial bleeding, meningitis or encephalitis, hydrocephalus, severe hypertension, or pseudotumor cerebri. The earliest sign of papilledema is the loss of spontaneous venous pulsations normally present in 75% of patients. When difficult to appreciate, they can be elicited with ipsilateral jugular compression (Table 23.3). Bedside ocular ultrasonography can facilitate the diagnosis of vitreous hemorrhage, a detached retina, and increased intracranial pressure (nerve sheath diameter).

25. **What are a couple of tricks to prove that a patient can see?**
Induce nystagmus by spinning an opticokinetic drum, or simply hold a mirror in front of the eyes and slowly move it; tracking requires vision.

BIBILIOGRAPHY

Bagheri N, Wajda B, eds. *The Wills Eye Manual: Office and Emergency Room Diagnosis and Treatment of Eye Disease.* 7th ed. Philadelphia: Wolters Kluwer; 2017.

Channa R, Zafar SN, Canner JK, et al. Epidemiology of eye-related emergency department visits. *JAMA Ophthalmol.* 2016;134(3): 312–319.

Huff JS, Austin EW. Neuro-ophthalmology in emergency medicine. *Emerg Med Clin North Am.* 2016;34(4):967–986.

Kilker BA, Holst JM, Hoffmann B. Bedside ocular ultrasound in the emergency department. *Eur J Emerg Med.* 2014;21(4):246–253.

Stagg BC, Shah MM, Talwar N, et al. Factors affecting visits to the emergency department for urgent and nonurgent ocular conditions. *Ophthalmology.* 2017;124(5):720–729. doi:10.1016/j.ophtha.2016.12.039.

Waldman N, Densie IK, Herbison P. Topical tetracaine used for 24 hours is safe and rated highly effective by patients for the treatment of pain caused by corneal abrasions: a double-blind, randomized clinical trial. *Acad Emerg Med.* 2014;21:374–382.

CHAPTER 24

NONTRAUMATIC EAR, NOSE, AND THROAT EMERGENCIES

Dowin Boatright, MD, MBA

EPISTAXIS

1. **What are the most common causes of epistaxis?**

   Nosebleeds usually occur spontaneously. Common causes include dry nasal mucosa, infection (most commonly viral or bacterial rhinitis), nose picking, and direct blows to the nose. Less common causes are foreign bodies, tumors, coagulopathies, use of anticoagulant drugs (aspirin, clopidogrel, warfarin), and exposure to toxic or caustic materials (i.e., cocaine).

2. **Does hypertension cause epistaxis?**

   Not acutely. However, patients with chronic hypertension develop atherosclerosis, making blood vessels relatively fragile and more prone to bleeding.

3. **Does bleeding originate from any one particular source?**

   Approximately 90% of nosebleeds are anterior bleeds originating from Kiesselbach plexus (Little area), a vascular network on the anterior-inferior portion of the septum. The blood supply is from the external carotid system. Posterior bleeds arise from a branch of the sphenopalatine artery, tend to be more severe, are more difficult to control, and usually occur in patients over 50 years of age.

4. **What are the important components of the history?**
   - Prior nosebleed episodes
   - Excessive alcohol use or bleeding dyscrasias
   - Trauma or nose picking
   - Side where bleeding started
   - Recent sinus infections or surgeries
   - Warfarin, clopidogrel, direct thrombin inhibitor, or aspirin use

5. **Summarize the key points to successful management of nosebleeds.**
   - Assemble necessary equipment and supplies for treatment (Table 24.1).
   - Quickly assess airway, breathing, and circulation while obtaining the history.
   - Have the patient firmly pinch the nose, compressing the septum, or place a nasal clamp with firm pressure on the septum.
   - Wear disposable gloves, mask, and eye protection.

6. **How do I treat epistaxis?**
   - Remove existing clots – have patient blow their nose or directly remove with suction, and a water-moistened cotton swab.
   - Site identification – apply a pledget soaked with topical anesthetic plus a vasoconstrictor (e.g., lidocaine 4% and phenylephrine) for 5–10 minutes. Look for bleeding site after removal of pledget.
   - Bleeding control options:
     - Silver nitrate or electrocautery, if the source is in the Kiesselbach plexus and less than 1 cm^2.
     - Absorbable gelatin sponge (Gelfoam), absorbable cellulose (Surgicel), or similar substance moistened with a vasoconstrictor applied to the bleeding site.
     - 500 mg of tranexamic acid dissolved in 5 mL of saline and applied topically to the nasal mucosa.
     - Anterior nasal packing – insert a dry Merocel sponge or nasal tampon coated with antibiotic ointment horizontally back into the nostril, along the floor of the nasal cavity. Once in place, moisten the packing with saline or phenylephrine until it expands within the nasal cavity. If no continued bleeding is noted in the posterior pharynx after the vasoconstrictor wears off (about 30 minutes), discharge is appropriate.

7. **Any pearls about treatment with silver nitrate?**
   - Silver nitrate is helpful for slow minimal bleeding, not for brisk bleeding.
   - Hold silver nitrate to the septum for only 5–10 seconds. Only use on one side of the septum. Cauterizing too long or both sides of the septum can lead to perforation or permanent damage to the blood supply of the region.

Table 24.1 Supplies for the Treatment of Nosebleeds

EXAMINATION	STABILIZATION	TREATMENT
Protective garb	Bayonet forceps	Silver nitrate cautery sticks
Head lamp or light	Cotton pledgets	Electrocautery (if available)
Nasal speculum	Lidocaine 4%	Gelfoam (or similar material)
Cotton swabs	Epinephrine 1:1000	Merocel sponge or nasal tampon
Fraser tip suction	Tetracaine 0.5%	1/2-inch petroleum-impregnated gauze
Emesis basin	Oxymetazoline (Afrin)	Antibiotic ointment
4 × 4 gauze	0.25% phenylephrine (Neo-Synephrine)	Foley catheter or commercial balloon
		Rolled 4 × 4 gauze with silk suture

From Lucente F, Har-El G, eds. *Essentials of Otolaryngology*, 4th ed. New York: Lippincott Williams & Wilkins; 1999; Kucik CJ, Clenney T. Management of epistaxis. *Am Fam Physician.* 2005;7:305–311.

8. **What are the important discharge instructions?**
   - Leave packing in place for 2–3 days.
   - Take prophylactic antistaphylococcal antibiotics (cephalexin or trimethoprim-sulfamethoxazole) while packing is in place to prevent sinusitis (due to disruption of sinus drainage) or toxic shock syndrome.
   - Epistaxis failing to respond to direct pressure for 10 minutes should be seen in the ED.
   - Regular application of petroleum jelly or antibiotic ointment and use of room humidifiers may prevent bleeding from desiccated nasal mucosa.

9. **How do I diagnose posterior epistaxis?**
   Consider a posterior bleed, when anterior packing fails. Posterior packing is accomplished with rolled 4 × 4-inch gauze, a Foley catheter (French 16 or 18), or other balloon products. Pass a catheter through the nose into the oropharynx. Fill the balloon with 10–15 mL of saline and pull gently but firmly, wedging the balloon in the posterior nasal cavity. Clamp the catheter in position with an umbilical clamp placed just outside the nose. Gauze between the nose and the clamp prevents pressure necrosis of the nose.

10. **Do I discharge a patient home with a posterior pack?**
    No. Admission and otolaryngology (ear, nose, and throat [ENT]) consultation is required. Posterior packing stimulates the nasopulmonary reflex, which can lead to hypoxia and apnea. Place the patient on supplemental oxygen and continuous pulse oximetry. About 10% of posterior bleeds are not controlled by posterior packing.

KEY POINTS: DIAGNOSIS AND MANAGEMENT OF POSTERIOR EPISTAXIS

1. When anterior packing fails to control epistaxis, suspect a posterior bleed originating from the sphenopalatine artery.
2. Treatment consists of ENT consultation, posterior nasal packing, and hospital admission to monitor for hypoxia and apnea.

11. **When should I consult ENT?**
    Consult ENT when bleeding cannot be controlled, raising suspicion for a posterior bleed. Treatment options include endoscopic cauterization, ligation of the sphenopalatine artery, embolization, or septal surgery. Recurring anterior epistaxis warrants an outpatient ENT referral.

12. **What is the role of interventional radiology (IR)?**
    When epistaxis is refractory to packing, surgical ligation or arterial embolization may be required. IR techniques are typically targeted at embolizing the sphenopalatine artery. Severe epistaxis from the ethmoidal system may be better treated with surgical ligation.

13. **What about laboratory studies?**
    Labs are typically unnecessary. Patients taking warfarin or hemodynamically unstable should have a complete blood count, coagulation studies, and a type and screen.

FOREIGN BODIES

14. How should I remove a foreign body from the ear?
    - Kill insects – instill 2% lidocaine, mineral oil, or EMLA in the canal.
    - Removal techniques:
        - Intact tympanic membrane – direct irrigation (mixture of water and isopropyl alcohol evaporates faster and causes less swelling of organic matter) behind foreign body to force it out.
        - Direct instrumentation with alligator forceps, right-angle probe, tissue forceps, Adson forceps, Fogarty biliary catheter, ear curette, Water-Pik, skin hook, and day hook.
        - Suction.
        - Cyanoacrylate glue – place at end of cotton swab or balloon-tipped catheter, hold to object for 60 seconds, and then remove. Use an aural speculum to guide the swab, preventing adherence to the external auditory structures.

15. What symptoms do patients with nasal foreign bodies show?
    Unless foreign body is reported, the chief complaint is that of unilateral, malodorous nasal discharge. The discharge may be mucoid or serosanguineous but is classically purulent.

16. Is there any special trick to removing foreign bodies from the nose?
    Any of the following techniques can be used:
    - Pass a small Foley catheter (or commercially available Katz extractor) into the superior affected nasal cavity. Once past the foreign body, insufflate the balloon and pull out the device, retrieving the foreign body with it.
    - Spray a 50/50 mixture of topical vasoconstrictor (reduces congestion) and 4% lidocaine (provides anesthesia) into the involved nostril using an atomizer or spray bottle. Nebulized epinephrine can also be used. Subsequently, have the patient occlude the unaffected nostril and blow forcefully to expel the object.
    - Positive-pressure insufflation can be provided by delivering a quick breath through a face mask connected to an Ambu Bag while the unaffected nostril is occluded. Alternatively, a caregiver can provide positive pressure in direct mouth-to-mouth fashion.
    - Suction, forceps, and cyanoacrylate glue can be used, as described above for ear foreign bodies.

17. "Something is stuck in my throat." How is this patient managed?
    Immediately address possible airway compromise. Ability to talk is a good sign. Ask the patient about the nature of the foreign body, duration of the sensation, the ability to swallow liquids or solids, and the perceived location of the object. Patient estimates of location are often accurate. Direct visualization can identify sharp objects (i.e., fish bones) that may become impaled in the posterior pharynx or the base of the tongue. Indirect or fiberoptic laryngoscopy, in conjunction with local anesthesia (e.g., nebulized lidocaine), may help localize objects stuck in the vallecula, epiglottis, or pyriform sinus.

18. If the physical examination does not reveal the foreign body, what should be done next?
    Obtain soft-tissue lateral radiographs of the neck or chest radiographs. Large, sharp, angulated objects tend to lodge in the esophagus. If radiographs do not localize the foreign body, perform an esophagram under fluoroscopy using a water-soluble contrast agent like meglumine diatrizoate (Gastrografin). Avoid barium because it interferes with visualization during endoscopy. Esophagoscopy should be considered in patients with persistent symptoms or when the diagnosis is unclear.

19. If I can see a foreign body, how do I remove it?
    Apply a topical spray anesthetic (i.e., topical benzocaine or nebulized 4% lidocaine). Remove visualized objects with bayonet forceps or a Kelly clamp. Smooth objects, such as coins, in the esophagus for fewer than 24 hours, can be removed by placing the patient in the Trendelenburg position (head down), passing a Foley catheter beyond the object, expanding the balloon, and withdrawing the catheter. This procedure is best performed by experienced radiologists using fluoroscopy. Pharmacologic treatments for passage of esophageal foreign bodies are variably effective. Sublingual nitroglycerin or intravenous (IV) glucagon (0.5–2 mg) can be used to relax the lower esophageal sphincter to relieve a distal obstruction, such as a food bolus. Glucagon can elicit vomiting and has been associated with esophageal perforation in this setting. Benzodiazepines may also be effective. Never use papain-containing agents; they dissolve meat and, owing to gas formation, are associated with esophageal perforation. Sharp objects should be removed endoscopically.

KEY POINTS: ESOPHAGEAL FOREIGN BODIES

1. In the patient with the sensation of an esophageal foreign body, consider esophagoscopy for persistent symptoms or uncertain diagnosis.
2. Because glucagon commonly elicits vomiting, it may cause esophageal perforation.

20. **Any other pearls?**
    Eighty to ninety percent of gastrointestinal (GI) tract foreign bodies pass without significant problems, 10%–20% require endoscopy for removal, and only 1% require surgical removal. These latter objects tend to be sharp or long (>6.5 cm) and are among the 1% that cause perforation. Disk or button batteries are prone to leakage and need to be removed immediately if in the esophagus. Otherwise, in asymptomatic patients, the location in the GI system should be monitored with serial radiography until elimination is confirmed.

KEY POINTS: NATURAL HISTORY OF GI FOREIGN BODIES

1. Of foreign bodies, 80%–90% pass through the GI tract without significant problems.
2. The following often require removal: sharp or long (>6.5 cm) objects, disk or button batteries, and items that have not migrated on serial radiographs.

SINUSITIS

21. **What is sinusitis? What are the common causes?**
    Sinusitis is an inflammation of the paranasal sinuses (maxillary, ethmoid, frontal, and sphenoid sinuses). It is the consequence of ostia occlusion, most commonly caused by local mucosal swelling secondary to a viral upper respiratory infection. Allergies, trauma, mechanical obstruction from tumors, foreign bodies, or abnormal anatomy may also cause occlusion that leads to bacterial overgrowth and excess mucus production. Of all viral upper respiratory infections, 0.5%–5% are complicated by bacterial rhinosinusitis. When symptoms are present for less than 3 weeks, the process is characterized as acute.

22. **How do I make the diagnosis?**
    The four most helpful signs and symptoms of bacterial rhinosinusitis are purulent nasal discharge, upper tooth or facial pain (especially unilateral), maxillary sinus tenderness (unilateral), and a worsening of symptoms after initial improvement. The physical examination is often unrewarding. Anterior rhinoscopy with a headlamp and nasal speculum may reveal the presence of pus, foreign bodies, masses, or anatomic abnormalities.

23. **Which other diagnostic studies should I pursue?**
    Plain films and computed tomography (CT) are not recommended initially but may be used for recurrent or chronic conditions. A single Water view is as sensitive as a full sinus series. Findings may include mucosal thickening (>6 mm), air-fluid levels, and opacification. For uncomplicated sinusitis, CT is not specific. However, CT can diagnose facial or intracranial involvement. Nasal endoscopy, an excellent modality for identifying disease, is typically done nonemergently by an otolaryngologist.

24. **How is sinusitis treated?**
    Approximately 65% of cases in adults and children will resolve spontaneously. Most patients with a viral upper respiratory infection improve within 7 days. Reserve antibiotic use for patients who meet the clinical criteria described previously, and for those with persistent symptoms for more than 7 days. The most likely organisms are *Streptococcus pneumoniae*, nontypable *Haemophilus influenzae*, *Moraxella catarrhalis*, other *Streptococcus* species, and anaerobes.
    Antibiotic options for adults include amoxicillin, trimethoprim-sulfamethoxazole, amoxicillin-clavulanate, doxycycline, or azithromycin; for children, consider amoxicillin, amoxicillin-clavulanate, cefpodoxime, or cefuroxime. Optimal treatment duration remains unclear; a 10-day course is most often used. The use of vasoconstrictor sprays, such as phenylephrine (Neo-Synephrine) or oxymetazoline (Afrin), for symptomatic relief should not be used longer than 3 days because of the propensity for rebound edema. Avoid antihistamines because they are implicated in mucosal crusting and blockage of the ostia. Daily nasal saline irrigation and nasal topical steroids should be encouraged before antibiotics are prescribed.

25. **Which patients need referral and admission? What are the complications?**
    Referral to an otolaryngologist is reasonable without improvement after two complete courses of antibiotics. Complications arising during therapy can be classified as local, orbital, and intracranial.
    - Local – mucoceles, osteomyelitis
    - Orbital (most common, especially in children) – cellulitis, abscess
    - Intracranial – cavernous sinus thrombosis (from direct spread of infection through valveless veins; heralded by toxic appearance, high fever, cranial nerve palsies, retinal engorgement, bilateral chemosis and proptosis), meningitis, subdural empyema, brain abscess
      Patients with sinusitis showing evidence of orbital or central nervous system involvement are treated as having medical emergencies. The majority of these complications are diagnosed by CT.

26. **Any other pearls?**
    Check a glucose level in a sick patient with sinusitis. *Mucor* in diabetic patients and *Aspergillus* in immunocompromised patients can be life threatening. These patients require hospital admission and specialist consultation.

EPIGLOTTITIS

27. **List the signs and symptoms of epiglottitis in adults.**
Symptoms
- Sore throat (100%)
- Odynophagia/dysphagia (76%)
- Fever (88%)
- Shortness of breath (78%)
- Anterior neck pain
- Hoarseness or muffled ("hot potato") voice
Signs
- Lymphadenopathy
- Drooling
- Respiratory distress
- Extreme pain with palpation of the larynx

28. **What is the thumbprint sign?**
It is a finding on lateral neck radiographs caused by the presence of an edematous epiglottis. Lateral neck films are only 38% sensitive and 76% specific.

29. **Name the most common organisms identified in adult epiglottitis.**
The most common organisms are *H. influenzae* and β-hemolytic streptococci. However, in most cases, no organism is found, pointing to a viral cause. With the introduction of the *H. influenzae* type B (Hib) vaccine in children, the reservoir for *H. influenzae* has decreased dramatically so that epiglottitis is now seen more often in adults.

30. **How do I manage epiglottitis? What signs and symptoms indicate the need for airway intervention?**
Start antibiotics (second- or third-generation cephalosporin such as cefotetan or cefoxitin) immediately. Use of steroids is controversial and not shown to provide benefit. While there is concern about rebound edema with racemic epinephrine, there are few data to support this. Patients with symptomatic respiratory distress, stridor, drooling, shorter duration of symptoms, and *H. influenzae* bacteremia are at increased risk for airway obstruction. Observe patients with a respiratory rate of less than 20 breaths per minute and no respiratory distress in an intensive care unit (ICU). In patients with a respiratory rate greater than 30 breaths per minute, moderate to severe respiratory distress, partial pressure of carbon dioxide (pCO_2) of greater than 45 mmHg, or cyanosis, consider immediate active airway intervention.

31. **How is the definitive diagnosis of epiglottitis made?**
In adults, definitive diagnosis is with direct laryngoscopy, visualizing the inflamed or edematous epiglottis. In children, this approach is controversial. Some believe any attempt at visualizing the inflamed epiglottis should take place in a controlled setting (i.e., the operating room). Others believe it is appropriate to depress the tongue using a tongue depressor or laryngoscope blade to visualize the epiglottis of a child sitting in the parent's lap. Visualization should only be done by someone experienced in the management of pediatric airways.

OTITIS EXTERNA

32. **How does otitis externa present?**
The classic finding is pain with manipulation of the external ear. Cardinal symptoms include itching, pain, and tenderness to palpation. Common signs are erythema and edema of the auditory canal, with crusting, pus, or weeping secretions. Predisposing factors for otitis externa (swimmer's ear) are excessive moisture in the ear canal and trauma (typically from overzealous cleaning).

33. **What bacteria are usually responsible?**
    Pseudomonas aeruginosa and *Staphylococcus aureus.*

34. **How is it treated?**
    Goals include avoiding precipitants and eradicating infection. To treat infection, place 2% acetic acid (for drying) combined with hydrocortisone (for inflammation) in the ear canal. Alternatively, topical antibiotic drops (otic suspension of polymyxin B, neomycin sulfate, and hydrocortisone [Cortisporin]) can be used. If the tympanic membrane is ruptured, ofloxacin otic, ciprofloxacin eye drops, or ciprodex can be used. If the external ear canal is extremely inflamed and narrowed, place a wick to ensure drainage and instillation of medication. Topical ciprofloxacin, a second-generation fluoroquinolone antibiotic, also has demonstrated efficacy in the treatment of otitis externa. Ciprofloxacin has an excellent safety profile without evidence of ototoxicity. Additionally, the combination of ciprofloxacin with fluocinolone, a corticosteroid, has been shown to be more effective in the treatment of otitis externa than ciprofloxacin alone or Cortisporin with fluocinolone. If otitis media coexists, add systemic antibiotics.

35. **What is malignant otitis externa?**
    It is a potentially lethal extension of infection of the external ear canal into the mastoid or temporal bone, most commonly caused by *P. aeruginosa* in patients with diabetes or other immunocompromised states. The mortality rate approaches 50%. Consider this diagnosis when, despite adequate treatment, headache and otalgia persist. CT or magnetic resonance imaging (MRI) confirms the diagnosis. Treatment includes admission, IV antipseudomonal antibiotics, and, potentially, surgical debridement.

PERITONSILLAR ABSCESS

36. **State the typical signs and symptoms of peritonsillar abscess (quinsy).**
    • Symptoms: fever, unilateral sore throat, odynophagia, trismus, and occasionally referred otalgia. Patients typically have had pharyngitis with recent antibiotic treatment. Smokers, males, and those with periodontal disease are at increased risk.
    • Signs: limited mouth opening (usually cannot open more than 2.5 cm), drooling, muffled "hot potato" voice, and rancid breath. The oropharynx is erythematous with a deeper redness over the affected area. There is tense swelling of the anterior pillar and soft palate. Subsequently, the tonsil is pushed downward and toward the midline. The uvula may be either shifted away from or lying flat against the affected side.

37. **What are the treatment options for a peritonsillar abscess?**
    Needle aspiration followed by antibiotics is the treatment of choice and is successful in 85%–95% of patients. Position the patient with the head resting against the bed or dental chair. Visualize the tonsils with the aid of a tongue depressor or laryngoscope (which provides its own light source). Apply topical anesthetic using lidocaine or the combination of benzocaine, butamben, and tetracaine hydrochloride (Cetacaine). Cut a needle cover to provide a guard for an 18-gauge needle, exposing no more than 1 cm of the needle. Insert the guarded needle at the most fluctuant portion of the abscess. An endocavitary ultrasound probe can help identify the location of the abscess. If trismus prevents the use of intraoral ultrasound, submandibular ultrasound or video laryngoscopy can be used to improve visualization. The physician should not penetrate deeper than 1 cm and stay medial to avoid the more lateral-positioned carotid artery. A positive aspiration is achieved if 1 mL or more of pus is obtained. If needle aspiration fails, consult ENT for possible incision and drainage. Administration of 10 mg IV dexamethasone may decrease pain at 24 hours and allow quicker return to normal activities and dietary intake.

38. **Describe the presentation of a retropharyngeal abscess.**
    Symptoms include fever, odynophagia, and neck pain out of proportion to oropharyngeal findings. Patients are ill appearing and may hold the neck in slight extension. Patients may also resist neck movement, mimicking meningitis.

39. **Why is this diagnosis so concerning?**
    The retropharyngeal space of the neck involves three fascial layers between the paraspinal muscles and the pharynx. Infections and abscesses located here have the potential to cause airway compromise and offer a path of direct extension into the mediastinum.

KEY POINTS: OTHER HEAD AND NECK SOFT-TISSUE INFECTIONS

1. Evaluate the patient with respiratory compromise and suspected epiglottitis in a controlled environment, with someone skilled at performing emergent nonsurgical and surgical airway procedures.
2. Malignant otitis externa is caused most commonly by *P. aeruginosa* and occurs in patients with diabetes and immunocompromised states. The mortality rate can be greater than 50%.
3. Infections and abscesses in the retropharyngeal space can lead to airway compromise and direct extension into the mediastinum.

40. **What organisms are found in retropharyngeal and peritonsillar abscesses?**
Anaerobes, group A streptococci *(Streptococcus pyogenes)*, *S. aureus*, and *H. influenzae.*

41. **How is a retropharyngeal abscess diagnosed and treated?**
Definitive diagnosis is with CT. A soft-tissue lateral neck radiograph may show an increase in soft-tissue density, best seen with the neck in slight extension. Have advanced airway management equipment at the bedside while an emergent ENT consultation is obtained. Start IV antibiotics. Definitive treatment requires incision and drainage. The patient should be admitted to the ICU or taken directly to the operating room. Mediastinal extension mandates the involvement of a cardiothoracic surgeon.

ACUTE MASTOIDITIS

42. **What is mastoiditis?**
Mastoiditis is a suppurative infection of the mastoid air cells occurring when the thin, bony septae between air cells are destroyed by bacteria. In acute mastoiditis, symptoms are present for less than 1 month.

43. **How do I make the diagnosis?**
Acute mastoiditis is characterized by ear pain, erythema, and swelling over the mastoid, with displacement of the auricle. Eighty percent have an associated acute otitis media. Laboratory results, including white blood cell (WBC) count, erythrocyte sedimentation rate (ESR), and C-reactive protein (CRP) level, may be elevated but have low utility in making the diagnosis. Imaging of the temporal bone helps define the stage of mastoiditis, which ultimately guides treatment. Contrast-enhanced CT of the temporal bone is the preferred imaging modality.

44. **What are the complications?**
Complications include facial nerve palsy, hearing loss, labyrinthitis, osteomyelitis, neck abscess, meningitis, venous sinus thrombosis, and epidural empyema.

45. **How do I treat mastoiditis?**
Administer IV antibiotics (e.g., ceftriaxone or cefotaxime) covering against *S. pneumoniae, S. pyogenes,* and *S. aureus.* Antipseudomonal coverage is required with history of recurrent otitis media or recent antibiotic therapy. If there is evidence of complications, an ENT specialist should be consulted for possible tympanostomy tube placement and mastoidectomy.

ACKNOWLEDGMENT

The editors gratefully acknowledge the contributions of Christopher Davis, MD, Danielle Raeburn, MD, and Katherine Bakes, MD, authors of this chapter in previous editions.

BIBILIOGRAPHY

Goddard JC, Reiter ER. Inpatient management of epistaxis: outcomes and cost. *Otolaryngol Head Neck Surg.* 2005;132:707–712.
Hur K, Zhou S, Kysh L. Adjunct steroids in the treatment of peritonsillar abscess: a systematic review. *Laryngoscope.* 2018;128(1):72–77.
Loock JW. A randomized trial comparing intraoral ultrasound to landmark-based needle aspiration in patients with suspected peritonsillar abscess. *Clin Otolaryngol.* 2013;3:235–237.
Lorente J, Sabater F, Rivas MP, et al. Ciprofloxacin plus fluocinolone acetonide versus ciprofloxacin alone in the treatment of diffuse otitis externa. *J Laryngol Otol.* 2014;128:591–598.
Rehrer M, Mantuani D, Nagdev A. Identification of peritonsillar abscess by transcutaneous cervical ultrasound. *Am J Emerg Med.* 2013;31(1):267.e1–e3.
Shargorodsky J, Bleier BS, Holbrook EH, et al. Outcomes analysis in epistaxis management: development of a therapeutic algorithm. *Otolaryngol Head Neck Surg.* 2013;149:390–398.
Zahed R, Moharamzadeh P, Alizadeharasi S, et al. A new and rapid method for epistaxis treatment using injectable form of tranexamic acid topically: a randomized controlled trial. *Am J Emerg Med.* 2013;31:1389–1392.

CHAPTER 25

DENTAL AND ORAL SURGICAL EMERGENCIES

Blake Phillips, DMD and Mark J. Glasgow, DDS

1. **For what conditions should I emergently consult the dental team versus the oral surgery team? Which other conditions require urgent follow-up care (24–48 hours)?**
   See Table 25.1.

2. **What are the important anatomic structures of the orofacial region?**
   Important structures coursing through the orofacial region include the cranial nerves, major and minor salivary glands and their ducts, muscles of mastication and facial expression, and numerous blood vessels and lymph nodes. Teeth may be present in various states of repair, depending on the patient's age and history of oral hygiene and dental restorations. Healthy gingiva and mucosa should appear pink in color without edema, erythema, or bleeding, although patients with dark complexion may have splotchy areas of dark pigmentation. The submandibular and sublingual glands should be palpable on the floor of the mouth and submandibular region.

3. **How are teeth numbered?**
   Different tooth numbering systems exist, including the Universal, Palmer, and ISO systems. In the United States, the Universal system is the most common numbering method (Figs. 25.1 and 25.2), but the ISO system is commonly used as well. When communicating with consulting services or other facilities, it is helpful to clarify which tooth is being discussed (e.g., tooth 11, the upper left canine).

4. **How should I examine the orofacial region?**
   Use bright lighting. Palpate the neck for any masses or lymphadenopathy. Perform a standard cranial nerve examination. Look for facial asymmetry or injury. Examine the lips, inner cheeks, and gums. Dentures and orthodontic retainers should be removed. Retract the upper and lower lips until taut to expose the depths of the maxillary and mandibular vestibules. Use a tongue depressor to evaluate the lingual vestibules, floor of the mouth, and ventral surface of the tongue. Inspect the soft and hard palate, as well as the tonsils, uvula, and oropharynx. The uvula and soft palate should rise symmetrically. Palpate the teeth, mandible, and maxilla for mobility and pain. Gingival lacerations or bruising may be signs of underlying fractures or dental trauma. Retract the cheeks and ask the patient to bite his or her teeth together to evaluate the dental occlusion.

5. **How do you examine the temporomandibular joint (TMJ)?**
   Palpate the TMJ approximately 1 cm anterior to the tragus. Ask the patient to open and close their mouth to rule out trismus and assess any clicking, popping, or crepitus. Normal mouth opening ranges from about 40 to 60 mm, measured between the incisal edges of the central incisors. Watch for deviation of the mandible on opening or closing. Ask the patient to move the mandible as far left and right as possible. Palpate the masseter and temporalis muscles to check for myofascial pain or trigger points.

6. **How do I assess open TMJ lock?**
   Open and closed TMJ locks are typically caused by articular disc dislocation. You must first determine whether the condition is acute or chronic, because some patients have limited function for months or years. Imaging the joints with plain film radiographs or computed tomography (CT) scan can evaluate the condition of the mandibular condyle and glenoid fossa, which is especially useful when ankylosis is suspected. Magnetic resonance imaging (MRI) is useful for evaluating the articular disc and its movement during opening and closing movements. In the acute setting, open lock is typically caused by condylar dislocation anterior to the articular eminence. If the dislocation is unilateral, the patient's chin will be deviated away from the affected side.

7. **How do you treat open TMJ lock?**
   Treatment of open lock may require local anesthesia or deep sedation dependent on the technique used for reduction. In the intraoral technique, the physician's thumbs are placed over the posterior mandibular teeth or posterior alveolar ridge, with fingers beneath the inferior border of the mandible. Gauze padding is used to prevent trauma to the thumbs from sharp teeth. Pressure is placed downward and backward on the posterior teeth with upward pressure underneath the patient's chin. Other techniques include the syringe technique and the extraoral technique (see Chapter 83). After reduction, mouth opening should be limited for 2–4 weeks with either an elastic head wrap or Ivy loops with maxillomandibular elastics. Soft diet, nonsteroidal anti-inflammatory drugs (NSAIDs), and warm compresses are encouraged. Recurrent open lock may require surgical intervention.

Table 25.1 Guidelines for Managing Oral and Facial Consultations

EMERGENT DENTAL CONSULTATION[a]	EMERGENCY ORAL SURGERY CONSULTATION	URGENT DENTAL OR ORAL SURGERY FOLLOW-UP CARE
Fractured, avulsed, or luxated teeth	Uncontrollable bleeding from the oral cavity, face, head, or neck	Parotid or other salivary gland swelling
Alveolar housing fractures	Open facial fractures including frontal sinus, orbital, zygomatic, maxillary, nasal, and mandibular fractures	Lost or fractured dental restorations or dentures
Infections within the oral cavity		Chronic dental conditions such as gingivitis, periodontitis, exposed bone, or soft-tissue lesions
Refractory pain or bleeding from surgery site or dental extraction		
Gingival lacerations	Cellulitis or abscesses involving the oral cavity, face, head, and neck (e.g., Ludwig's angina)	TMJ pain, clicking, or popping
Failed reduction of an open or closed lock of the TMJ	Noma	Loose or broken dental implant
	Facial lacerations involving facial nerves, uncontrolled arterial bleeding, muscles of mastication and facial expression, the parotid, or submandibular, sublingual or calivary glands	ANUG
		Sexually transmitted diseases of the oral cavity
	Disease processes that require a surgical airway	Natal or neonatal teeth

[a]Severe or unusual conditions should be elevated directly to the oral surgery service.
ANUG, Acute necrotizing ulcerative gingivitis; *TMJ*, temporomandibular joint.

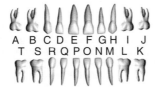

Fig. 25.1 Primary teeth, Universal numbering system.

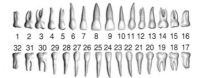

Fig. 25.2 Permanent teeth, Universal numbering system.

8. **How do I examine the parotid gland and parotid duct?**
   Visually inspect for asymmetry, swelling, erythema, and cutaneous fistulas. Palpate the parotid gland for masses, crepitus, pain, fluctuance, and asymmetry. Verify cranial nerve VII function. Locate the Stensen duct inside the cheek, adjacent to the second maxillary molar, and dry the area with gauze. While gently retracting the cheek, palpate the parotid gland from posterior to anterior, and you should see clear saliva emerge from the duct. Blood is a sign of injury, whereas pus is a sign of sialadenitis. To determine whether the duct has been lacerated, cannulate the Stensen duct with a flexible intravenous (IV) catheter; then gently inject up to 1 mL of sterile milk, propofol, or methylene blue. If the liquid emerges from the site of laceration, the duct has been compromised.

9. **What are some causes of parotid swelling?**
   - Bacterial or viral infection (e.g., paramyxovirus, Epstein-Barr virus, cytomegalovirus)
   - Salivary gland tumors
   - HIV parotitis
   - Trauma (edema, hematoma, or sialocele)
   - Salivary stones
   - Autoimmune diseases (e.g., Sjögren syndrome)
   - Sarcoidosis
   - Granulomatosis with polyangiitis (formerly known as Wegener granulomatosis)
   - Chronic recurrent parotitis
   - Pneumoparotid (from wind instruments, coughing, or dental work)
   - Kimura disease
   - Lymphoma
   - Radiation sialadenitis
   - Polycystic disease

10. **Which sensory nerves innervate the orofacial structures, and how can they be anesthetized?**
The maxillary and mandibular branches of the trigeminal nerve (cranial nerves V2 and V3) provide sensation of the teeth, gingiva, mucosa, anterior two thirds of the tongue, and the skin of the midface and lower face. The glossopharyngeal nerve (cranial nerve IX) provides sensation for the posterior two thirds of the tongue, tonsils, and pharynx. Local infiltration can be used to anesthetize most of the orofacial structures; however, nerve blocks are useful for anesthetizing large areas and for distancing the anesthetic administration from the site of injury or infection. Most of the terminal nerve branches of cranial nerves V2 and V3 can be blocked, including the nasopalatine nerve, greater and lesser palatine nerves, inferior alveolar nerve, lingual nerve, long buccal nerve, mental nerve, and the posterior/middle/anterior superior alveolar nerves.

11. **How are dental injuries treated?**
For all tooth injuries, instruct the patient to eat a soft diet for 2 weeks and to follow up with a dentist as soon as possible. The dentist will monitor the tooth vitality and radiographic appearance over time for evidence of pulpitis, necrosis, resorption, and ankylosis. Contaminated wounds and avulsed teeth that are reimplanted should be treated with tetanus prophylaxis. Reposition and reimplant teeth with the appropriate local anesthetic. Obtain a panoramic radiograph unless a CT scan is indicated. Fractured teeth may require root canal therapy and dental restorations as an outpatient.

12. **What is a dental concussion and how is it treated?**
Dental concussions occur when an impact to a tooth does not result in displacement or mobility of the tooth, but the periodontal ligament may be injured and the tooth's vitality may be compromised. The tooth may be sensitive to palpation or percussion. No immediate treatment is required.

13. **What is a subluxation, and how is it treated?**
Subluxation occurs when an injured tooth is mobile but without displacement from its original position. Bleeding from the gingival sulcus is a common finding. Depending on the degree of mobility, a splint can be applied to stabilize the tooth for 1–2 weeks or the tooth can be left untreated.

14. **What is luxation of a tooth, and how is it treated?**
Luxation occurs when a tooth is displaced in a buccal or lingual direction. Alveolar housing or root fractures are likely. Rinse the socket and exposed root surface with sterile saline; then grasp the tooth with gauze and reposition it back into the socket. Reducing the tooth may require pulling the tooth slightly out of the socket in order to redirect the root apex around the fractured bone. Splint the tooth for 4–6 weeks to stabilize the tooth and the alveolar housing fracture. Immediate extraction is indicated only for those teeth deemed hopeless or considered an aspiration risk.

15. **What is intrusion of a tooth, and how is it treated?**
Intrusion is the displacement of the tooth into the socket. Intruded teeth will often spontaneously erupt over time, depending on the depth to which they were intruded and the developmental stage of the root apex. When primary teeth are intruded, they require early extraction if the developing permanent tooth bud is disrupted. Otherwise, no immediate treatment is required. The patient's dentist will decide between spontaneous eruption versus orthodontic or surgical repositioning.

16. **What is extrusion of a tooth and how is it treated?**
Extrusion is the displacement of a tooth partially out of its socket. Rinse the exposed root surface with sterile saline and press back into the socket. Stabilize the tooth with a splint for 1–2 weeks.

17. **How is an avulsed tooth treated by emergency medical services (EMS) on scene?**
Avulsion, or complete displacement of a tooth out of its socket, requires rinsing the tooth and reimplanting it into the socket. Handle the tooth only by the crown, avoiding contact with the root surface. If the tooth is not reimplanted at the scene, possible transport media, in preferential order, include Hanks balanced salt solution, milk, sterile saline, or saliva. Avoid placing the tooth into tap water, juice, or soda. Primary teeth should not be reimplanted. Teeth reimplanted within the first 30 minutes have the best prognosis; any tooth out of the socket for more than 2 hours has a poor prognosis and should not be reimplanted.

18. **How should I treat avulsion of a tooth in the emergency department (ED)?**
Examine the tooth for evidence of root or crown fracture. If the tooth is intact and has been out of the socket for less than 60 minutes, rinse the tooth and its socket with sterile saline. Use manual pressure to reimplant the tooth and splint it for 1–2 weeks. If the tooth has been out of the socket for more than 60 minutes, gently remove any attached soft tissue with gauze, reimplant the tooth into the socket, and then splint it for 2–4 weeks. Administer antibiotics for 1 week: doxycycline twice daily if the patient is 12 years of age or older, and penicillin VK four times a day if the patient is younger than age 12. If the tooth or a portion of the tooth was not found at the scene, consider a chest radiograph to rule out aspiration. Teeth may also be swallowed or displaced into the nasal cavity, maxillary sinus, tongue, or lips.

19. **What are the tooth fracture classifications, and how are they treated?**
    - *Ellis class 1.* Fracture is through enamel only, and no immediate treatment is needed (Fig. 25.3).
    - *Ellis class 2.* Fracture is through enamel and dentin, and there is no exposed pulp. If the patient complains of sensitivity, apply a dental sealant or glass ionomer.
    - *Ellis class 3.* Fracture is through enamel and dentin with exposed pulp. Apply calcium hydroxide to the exposed pulp and dentin.
    - *Ellis class 4.* Fracture is through the tooth root. Splint the tooth for 1–2 weeks if the fracture is in the middle or apical third of the root. The tooth will need extraction if the fracture is in the coronal third.

20. **What are the signs of maxillary and mandibular fractures?**
    - Mobility
    - Crepitus
    - Gingival lacerations
    - Bleeding from the gingival sulcus
    - Ecchymosis
    - Open bite
    - Cross bite
    - Premature tooth contact
    - Step-off deformity between teeth
    - Trismus
    - Paresthesia or anesthesia
    - Pain to palpation
        Studies show the ability to bite into and crack a wooden tongue depressor has a negative predictive value greater than 90% for mandible fractures and a positive predictive value around 65%.

21. **What imaging should be ordered for known or suspected facial fractures?**
    Panoramic radiographs are often adequate for simple, isolated mandible fractures. A plain-film mandible series (includes Towne view, anteroposterior view, and right and left lateral oblique views) can help visualize displaced segments. CT scans are indicated for complex fractures of the mandible or suspected fractures of the midface, orbits, skull, or cervical spine. CT angiography (CTA) should be considered for patients at risk for a cerebrovascular injury based on the mechanism and clinical findings.

22. **What is an alveolar housing fracture?**
    An alveolar housing fracture is a fracture through the alveolar bone of the mandible or maxilla that surrounds and supports the teeth, often associated with tooth luxation or fracture. Signs include gingival lacerations, ecchymosis, and mobility of the alveolus. When multiple teeth are displaced and mobile *en bloc,* there is a high likelihood of an alveolar housing fracture. Consider panoramic radiography or CT of the face. Irrigate gingival lacerations and exposed bone with sterile saline. Manually reduce the displaced alveolus and any luxated teeth; then splint the affected teeth for 4–6 weeks. Some fractures may require open reduction internal fixation or maxillomandibular fixation. Repair gingival lacerations with 3-0 or 4-0 chromic gut or Vicryl sutures. Nondisplaced fractures may not require any surgical treatment. Instruct patients to avoid chewing with the affected segment for 6 weeks.

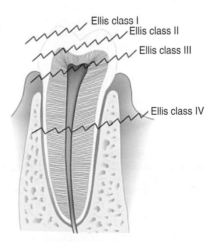

Ellis class I
Ellis class II
Ellis class III
Ellis class IV

Fig. 25.3 Ellis classifications of dental fractures.

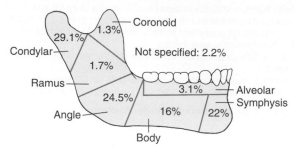

Fig. 25.4 Anatomic distribution of mandibular fracture sites. (From Hupp JR, Ellis E, Tucker MR. *Contemporary Oral and Maxillofacial Surgery.* 5th ed. St. Louis: Elsevier Mosby; 2008:499, Fig. 24-11.)

23. How are mandible fractures classified?

Mandible fractures are classified by anatomic location, including symphysis, parasymphysis, body, ramus, coronoid process, subcondylar, condylar neck, condylar head, and alveolar housing (Fig. 25.4). They are further described by the fracture pattern as simple, linear, nondisplaced, displaced, mobile, nonmobile, greenstick, comminuted, pathologic, monocortical, or bicortical.

24. Which fractures require antibiotics?

Open fractures of the maxilla and mandible require antibiotics. Open fractures include any fracture that communicates through a laceration of the skin, mucosa, or gingiva, as well as any fracture that extends through the socket of an erupted tooth. Prescribe penicillin VK 500 mg four times a day for 1 week, or clindamycin 300 mg four times a day for patients allergic to penicillin. Prescribe children weight-based doses of amoxicillin or clindamycin.

25. How are odontogenic abscesses treated?

Incision and drainage with removal of the offending tooth or root canal therapy are the desired treatments. In the ED, the incision and drainage may be performed at bedside if the abscess is in an accessible location, with the patient discharged to home on antibiotics and a follow-up appointment for extraction or root canal. Severe or deep space infections may require drainage in the operating room.

26. Which spaces are typically involved with infections of odontogenic origin?

Infections originating from the maxillary teeth typically perforate through the thin buccal plate to the maxillary canine and buccal spaces, but they may also involve the palate, the preseptal space around the eye, the infratemporal space, the parapharyngeal space, or paratonsillar spaces. Infections originating from the mandibular teeth spread to the buccal and sublingual spaces, extending into the submental, submandibular, sublingual, and masticator spaces. Severe infections may spread to the parapharyngeal, retropharyngeal, pretracheal, or prevertebral spaces, and down to the mediastinum.

27. What are the indications for admitting odontogenic infections?

Indications include impending airway compromise, sepsis, dehydration, inability to tolerate foods or liquids by mouth, uncontrolled pain, and deep space involvement.

28. What is alveolar osteitis?

Alveolar osteitis, or dry socket, is delayed healing and inflammation of the bony tooth socket after dental extraction. The condition is likely caused by fibrinolytic lysis and subsequent premature loss of the blood clot. Symptoms typically develop 3–4 days after the extraction and include pain, foul taste, and foul smell. Mandibular third molar sockets are most commonly affected. The condition is not associated with infectious signs such as erythema, fever, swelling, or purulence.

29. How is alveolar osteitis treated?

No antibiotics are indicated, and treatment is palliative. The socket should first be irrigated with sterile saline to dislodge any food debris. Do not curette the socket. Medicated dressings containing eugenol can be placed into the socket for temporary relief. Nonresorbable dressings must be replaced every 2 days until symptoms improve. The condition is usually self-limited to about 2 weeks with or without treatment.

30. What is Ludwig's angina?

Ludwig's angina is cellulitis with or without abscess formation of the submental, submandibular, and sublingual spaces bilaterally. Signs and symptoms may include:
- severe swelling
- erythema extending down to the chest
- elevated and/or protrusive tongue

- "hot potato" voice
- dysphagia
- dysphonia
- dyspnea
- crepitus
- "tripoding"
- stridor
- inability to tolerate secretions
- airway deviation or collapse on CT

    Treatment includes securing the airway, emergent incision and drainage of all involved spaces, extraction of the offending tooth, and antibiotics.

31. What is Lemierre syndrome?

Lemierre syndrome is septic thrombophlebitis of the internal jugular vein, usually resulting from paratonsillar or lateral pharyngeal infection. The resulting septic emboli may cause cavernous sinus thrombosis or travel to the heart, lungs, liver, bone, and joints.

32. What are some causes of gingival bleeding and potential treatments?

Bleeding is caused by:
- trauma
- periodontal disease
- postoperative wound
- thrombocytopenia
- vitamin deficiency
- blood dyscrasias
- leukemia

    First-line treatment of intraoral bleeding is direct gauze pressure and exploration to determine the source. Extraction sockets can be sutured with or without topical agents such as Gelfoam, Surgicel, and topical thrombin. Other treatments include electrocautery or chemical cautery, vessel ligation, vitamin K, tranexamic acid, and transfusion with fresh frozen plasma or platelets. Interventional radiology can be used for angiography and embolization of intractable or deep space hemorrhaging.

33. Describe the process for closing perioral and intraoral lacerations.

Close lacerations only after manipulating alveolar fractures or displaced teeth to avoid disrupting the wound closure.
- Anesthetize the area with local anesthesia, typically 1% or 2% lidocaine with 1:100,000 epinephrine.
- Use pulse irrigation and a soft brush or gauze to remove debris. Perform conservative surgical debridement with a scalpel or scissors to remove devitalized tissue and foreign bodies, but keep tissue removal to a minimum because of the prolific vascularity of the face and mouth.
- Achieve hemostasis with manual pressure, electrocautery, silver nitrate, or vessel ligation.
- Explore the wound to its depth to determine the complexity of the laceration and to inspect the underlying bone for fractures. Remove foreign bodies, such as tooth fragments and gravel.
- Close wounds in layers from inside to outside (e.g., from deep to superficial and from intraoral to extraoral). Lacerations of the gingiva and mucosa can usually be closed as a single layer with resorbable sutures such as 3-0 or 4-0 Vicryl or chromic gut. Small lacerations up to about 1 cm in the mucosa, gingiva, and tongue do not require closure.
- Irrigate full thickness lip or cheek lacerations again after mucosal closure.
- Take care to reapproximate the vermillion border of the lips to avoid a noticeable step-off.
- 5-0 or 6-0 nonresorbable, monofilament sutures should be used for skin closure, including the "dry" mucosa of the lips.
- Remove skin sutures 5–7 days after placement.

34. How do I close a wound if tissue has been avulsed?

In general, these types of wounds are beyond the expertise of most emergency medicine physicians, and they should be referred to an oral or plastic surgeon.

35. How do you treat animal bites to the orofacial region?

Irrigate all wounds with copious sterile saline under pressure. Because of the high vascularity of the face, small puncture wounds can be left to heal secondarily or closed primarily to reduce the risk of scarring. Larger lacerations and tissue avulsions should be repaired as described in Questions 33 and 34. Determine the type of animal bite and rabies status. Rabies vaccination should be considered for wild bats, raccoons, skunks, and unknown dogs. Administer tetanus vaccine or immune globulin as indicated. The need for antibiotic prophylaxis for dog bites is controversial, because only 5% will otherwise become infected. When given, antibiotics should cover *Pasteurella multocida* (amoxicillin with clavulanic acid; for patients allergic to penicillin, cefuroxime or doxycycline). Unlike dog bites, all cat bites should be given antibiotic prophylaxis, because 80% will otherwise become infected. Infecting organisms include *P. multocida, Bartonella henselae,* and *Clostridium tetani.* Water fowl, reptiles, amphibians, and mammals each carry a unique flora of bacteria and viruses and should be treated appropriately. Human bites are at risk for *Pseudomonas* and *Streptococcus* infection, as well as viruses such as HIV, hepatitis B, and hepatitis C. Animal hoof injuries may contaminate the wound with pathogens from the ground or barnyard, such as *Escherichia coli, Clostridium,* and *Staphylococcus.*

36. **What is acute necrotizing ulcerative gingivitis (ANUG)?**
ANUG is an interdental gingival necrosis that is rapid in onset and presents with gingival pain, bleeding, and halitosis. It is often caused by fusiform bacteria and spirochetes. Antibiotics (penicillin and metronidazole) should be administered, and in severe cases, dental consultation in the ED for possible surgical debridement.

37. **What is noma and how is it treated?**
Noma (Greek for "devour"), or cancrum oris, is an opportunistic, polymicrobial infection that causes destruction of the lips, cheeks, mucus membranes, and facial bones. ANUG is thought to be a precursor of noma. Caused by bacterial infection, noma is found primarily in patients with malnutrition, dehydration, immunocompromise, poor oral hygiene, and unsanitary living conditions. The disease typically progresses rapidly and without pain, but its effects are disfiguring, debilitating, and permanent. Treatment involves surgical debridement, nutrition, and empiric penicillin treatment.

38. **Patients taking bisphosphonate medications are at risk of developing what intraoral condition?**
Medication-related osteonecrosis of the jaws (MRONJ), defined as any area of exposed maxillary or mandibular bone that has persisted for more than 8 weeks in patients with a history of bisphosphonate use without a history of radiation to the area. IV bisphosphonates (e.g., zolendronate, pamidronate, ibandronate) carry the highest risk, but oral (PO) bisphosphonates (e.g., alendronate, risedronate) and antiresorptive medications such as denosumab have also been implicated. The exposed bone may develop spontaneously or after trauma to the oral mucosa or gingiva (including tooth extraction). Initial treatment includes analgesics and antibacterial mouth rinse, but as the lesion progresses, drug holiday, debridement, antibiotic therapy, and surgical resection may be required. Avoiding intraoral trauma in patients with a history of these medications is the best method of prevention.

KEY POINTS

1. Press downward and backward on the posterior teeth with upward pressure underneath the patient's chin to reduce open temporomandibular joint (TMJ) lock.
2. To determine if the parotid duct has been lacerated, cannulate the Stensen duct with a flexible IV catheter; then gently inject up to 1 mL of sterile milk, propofol, or methylene blue.
3. When primary teeth are intruded, they require early extraction if the developing permanent tooth bud is disrupted; otherwise, no immediate treatment is required.
4. If an avulsed permanent tooth is not reimplanted at the scene, possible transport media, in preferential order, include Hanks balanced salt solution, milk, sterile saline, or saliva.
5. Studies show the ability to bite into and crack a wooden tongue depressor has a negative predictive value greater than 90% for mandible fractures and a positive predictive value around 65%.
6. Ludwig's angina is cellulitis with or without abscess formation of the submental, submandibular, and sublingual spaces bilaterally.

ACKNOWLEDGMENT

The editors and author of this chapter would like to acknowledge and thank Drs. Richard D. Zallen, Colin T. Galbraith, and Valerie Byrnside for their previous contributions to this chapter.

BIBILIOGRAPHY

Andreasen JO. *The dental trauma guide.* Available at www.dentaltraumaguide.org. Accessed November 16, 2015.
Bagheri SC, Bell RB, Khan HA. *Current Therapy in Oral and Maxillofacial Surgery.* St. Louis, MO: Elsevier Saunders; 2012:108–1091.
Burlew CC, Biffl WL, Moore EE, et al. Blunt cerebrovascular injuries: redefining screening criteria in the era of noninvasive diagnosis. *J Trauma Acute Care Surg.* 2012;72:330–337.
Caputo ND, Raja A, Shields C, et al. Re-evaluating the diagnostic accuracy of the tongue blade test: still useful as a screening tool for mandibular fractures? *J Emerg Med.* 2013;45:8–12.
Hammel JM, Fischel J. Dental emergencies. *Emerg Med Clin N Am.* 2019;37:81–93.
Malamed SF. *Handbook of Local Anesthesia.* 6th ed. St. Louis: Elsevier Mosby; 2012.
Ruggiero SL, Dodson TB, Fantasia J, et al. American Association of Oral and Maxillofacial Surgeons position paper on medication-related osteonecrosis of the jaw – 2014 update. *J Oral Maxillofac Surg.* 2014;72:1938–1956.

TRANSIENT ISCHEMIC ATTACK AND CEREBROVASCULAR ACCIDENT

CHAPTER 26

Arian Anderson, MD and Richard Byyny, MD, MSc, FACEP

1. **What is a cerebrovascular accident (CVA) or stroke?**
   Stroke is a sudden spontaneous impairment of blood flow to a region of the brain, caused by either vascular occlusion or rupture. This interruption in tissue perfusion can lead to neuron cell dysfunction and death. Stroke is the third most common cause of mortality in the United States and the leading cause of adult disability.

2. **What are the two major types of acute stroke?**
   There are two major classes of stroke: ischemic and hemorrhagic. Ischemic stroke causes 90% of all CVAs in the United States, and hemorrhagic stroke accounts for the remaining 10%. Unfortunately, the quality, timing, and duration of neurologic dysfunction on clinical evaluation does not indicate which type of stroke the patient is experiencing. Rapid evaluation with a noncontrast computed tomography (CT) scan of the head is critical to differentiating between the two as each is managed very differently.

3. **What are some of the potential mimics of acute stroke?**
   Disorders that mimic stroke include:
   - postictal Todd's paralysis
   - hypoglycemia
   - complex migraine
   - conversion disorder
   - bell palsy
   - acute spinal cord compression
   - brain tumor
   - systemic infection
   - multiple sclerosis

4. **What are the types of hemorrhagic stroke?**
   These can be classified as either intracerebral hemorrhage (ICH) or intraparenchymal hemorrhage (IPH), which causes ~70% of hemorrhagic strokes, or subarachnoid hemorrhage (SAH), which is responsible for the remaining 30% of hemorrhagic strokes.

5. **What are the causes of ICH?**
   The most common etiologies of non-traumatic ICH are hypertension, anticoagulants, bleeding disorders, amyloid angiopathy, illicit drug use (usually sympathomimetics), and vascular malformations.

6. **What is the most common cause of atraumatic SAH?**
   Cerebral aneurysms are the most common cause of SAH, accounting for ~80%. These aneurysms develop over time; therefore they are more common with aging. SAH may also be caused by arteriovenous malformations and vertebral artery dissection. A small proportion are caused by perimesencephalic hemorrhage, a type of bleeding that does not have a known source and almost universally has a benign course.

7. **What historical factors are typical for SAH?**
   The most well-described complaint is that of a "thunderclap'" headache or sudden onset of the "worst headache of my life." Up to 15% of patients with sudden onset of the worst headaches of their lives have SAH. However, patients with SAH can have seizure, syncope, depressed mental status, or even focal neurologic deficits. It is helpful to ask for the timing between headache onset and maximal intensity. The rule which has been most robustly validated is the Ottawa SAH Rule (Table 26.1). While this rule had 100% sensitivity, it had only 14% specificity.

8. **What is the sensitivity of noncontrast CT of the head for SAH?**
   There have been several studies that have shown that a negative CT completed within 6 hours of symptom onset has a 100% sensitivity to rule out SAH and that no further testing needs to be performed. It is important to note that the literature is consistent in demonstrating a decreasing sensitivity of head CT from headache onset time. A reasonable estimate is 95% within 24 hours, 80% at 48 hours, 70% at 72 hours, and 50% at 5 days.

Table 26.1 Ottawa Subarachnoid Hemorrhage Rule

Age >40 years

Neck pain and stiffness

Witnessed loss of consciousness

Onset during exertion

Thunderclap headache (instantly peaking pain)

Limited neck flexion on examination

Inclusion Criteria
Age ≥15 years
New, severe nontraumatic headache
Maximum intensity within 1 hour

Exclusion Criteria
New neurologic deficit
Previous aneurysm
Known brain tumor
History of recurrent headaches

9. **If the noncontrast head CT is negative and outside of 6 hours from headache onset, what is the next step in a caring for patient with suspected SAH?**
The literature is evolving with regard to the answer to this question; however, most experts still recommend a lumbar puncture outside of 6 hours from headache onset. The reasoning is based upon the fact that the noncontrast head CT lacks 100% sensitivity, and the risk for missing even one patient with SAH could be catastrophic. The absence of aneurysms on CT angiography could reduce the risk of aneurysmal bleeding and effectively rule out SAH; however, this practice has yet to be prospectively validated. Additionally, in patients over 50, up to 5% will have an incidental aneurysm, creating a false-positive test.

10. **What should I do to treat the patient who is taking anticoagulant drugs and who has hemorrhagic stroke?**
Approximately 13% of patients with hemorrhagic stroke will be on oral anticoagulants. In general, for patients taking traditional vitamin K antagonists, it has been recommended to reverse the effects of the medication completely by using both vitamin K and fresh frozen plasma (FFP). More recently, plasma-derived factor concentrates (prothrombin complex concentrates [PCCs]) have been introduced. They have been shown to more rapidly normalize an abnormal international normalized ratio (INR); however, no mortality or morbidity benefit has been found to date. For patients with specific defects, such as hemophilia, the factor deficiency should be completely reversed, and those patients with thrombocytopenia should receive platelets. For patients on antiplatelet agents such as aspirin or clopidogrel, transfusion of platelets has been shown to *worsen* outcomes based upon the PATCH trial.

11. **What about patients taking novel/direct oral anticoagulants (NOACs/DOACs)?**
Pharmaceutical manufacturers have released direct thrombin inhibitors and direct factor Xa inhibitors called NOACs or DOACs, which are gaining popularity due to their ease of use and their lower risk for bleeding, when compared with more traditional agents like warfarin. Typical studies of coagulation, such as the partial thromboplastin time/prothrombin time (PTT/PT) and INR, often do not accurately reflect the degree of anticoagulation in these patients. Options can include reversal with PCCs, dialyzing off the drug, and specific reversal agents (idarucizumab, andexanet). Some institutions may use thromboelastography-guided management or alternative therapies, such as tranexamic acid (TXA). Because this is an evolving area of treatment, it is wise to use a team-based approach to management, which may include neurosurgeons, hematologists, pharmacy, and the blood bank.

KEY POINTS: MANAGEMENT OF ICH

1. Reverse any anticoagulants.
2. Administer antiepileptic drugs.
3. Control mean arterial pressure (MAP).
4. Position the head of the bed.
5. Control intracranial pressure (ICP).

12. **What are the causes of ischemic stroke?**
    - Thrombotic
      - Atherosclerosis
      - Vasculitis
      - Small vessel disease
    - Embolic
      - Atrial fibrillation
      - Mechanical heart valve
      - Low cardiac ejection fraction
      - Endocarditis
      - Atrial septal defects
      - Cervical artery dissection (i.e., carotid or vertebral arteries)

13. **What is a transient ischemic attack (TIA)?**
    The classic definition of TIA has been based on time (i.e., <24 hours of symptoms), although most TIAs will re-solve within 1 hour. However, up to 67% of classic TIAs will have evidence of acute ischemic lesions on diffusion-weighted magnetic resonance imaging (MRI). Because no time cut-off point can reliably determine whether underlying ischemic infarction has occurred, in 2009, the American Heart Association and American Stroke Association (AHA/ASA) transitioned to a tissue-based description of TIA: transient symptoms with lack of tissue injury confirmed by neuroimaging.

14. **Why should I be concerned about a TIA?**
    TIAs are associated with a high risk of early acute stroke (up to 10% within the first 2 days).

15. **Do patients with suspected TIA have to be admitted to the hospital?**
    Although many hospitals admit patients with TIA, there are an increasing number that use ED-based observation units or outpatient-based TIA clinics to rapidly perform the necessary diagnostic studies and initiate care.

16. **How do I differentiate between TIA and stroke?**
    TIA and stroke in the acute setting can be identical in clinical presentation, as both will have acute neurologic deficits. MRI can differentiate between the two; however, in the emergent setting, both should be managed as a possible acute stroke.

17. **How do I approach a patient with acute stroke symptoms?**
    As with all patients who have acute conditions, airway, breathing, and circulation (ABCs); intravenous (IV) access; and monitoring are the important first steps. Always remember to check a blood glucose level. History is critical to stroke assessment and should include time of symptom onset, evidence of preceding seizure, anticoagulation use, and potential associated trauma. A complete neurologic examination is essential. Perform the National Institutes of Health Stroke Scale (NIHSS), which is a standardized approach to calculate stroke severity. Abnormal blood pressures (BPs) are important to recognize; however, immediate reductions are unnecessary and should not distract the provider from other aspects of the patient's care. The next stages of care will depend on whether the stroke is hemorrhagic or ischemic and is determined by CT. Many hospitals have dedicated stroke protocols and stroke teams; a "stroke alert" may mobilize resources.

18. **Why is the time of onset an important historical factor for an acute stroke?**
    A common adage is "time is brain," meaning that reducing the time it takes to return blood flow to the tissue is critical to minimizing long-term tissue injury and disability. Symptom onset is critical to determine eligibility for thrombolytic therapy and must be documented for every patient. Unless the symptom onset is clearly witnessed or known by the patient, the time when the patient was last seen to be normal is used. If the patient awakens from sleep with stroke-like symptoms, then the last time the patient was awake and normal is considered the time of onset. If the patient is unable to communicate effectively, use alternative sources of history such as prehospital personnel, witnesses, or family members.

19. **What laboratory tests should be performed on patients with suspected CVA?**
    The first is that of a bedside glucose test. A basic metabolic panel can help assess for electrolyte derangements, and a complete blood count can be helpful to evaluate the platelet count in patients with hemorrhagic stroke. Studies of coagulation can help guide or exclude patients from therapy in both hemorrhagic and ischemic stroke. Electrocardiogram (ECG) and troponin can evaluate cardiac etiologies (e.g., atrial fibrillation).

20. **What imaging test should be performed on patients with suspected CVA?**
    The most important early imaging test is noncontrast CT scan of the head. This helps with one of the first branch points of therapy, which is distinguishing hemorrhagic from ischemic stroke. Some hospitals use emergent or rapid MRI to evaluate patients with possible stroke.

21. **What role do prehospital personnel play in patients with suspected stroke?**
    Besides stabilization (ABCs), prehospital personnel are tasked with early recognition of potential acute stroke. The AHA recommends that hospitals have systems in place to streamline evaluation, communication, and transport to

the receiving hospital. This allows early activation of the acute stroke team and preparation of CT/MRI, which can save precious minutes and maximize the number of patients seen within the time window for thrombolytic therapy.

22. **What is the importance of the NIHSS?**
The NIHSS is the most commonly used objective measure of acute stroke severity. It ranges from 0 to 42, involves 13 questions, and uses standardized pictures, sentences, and words.

23. **What is the appropriate time frame from symptom onset to administration of systemic thrombolytics?**
This is sometimes called the *thrombolytic window.* Initial literature suggested that the maximum window was 3 hours. More recent studies such as the European Cooperative Acute Stroke Study (ECASS) III in 2008 and the SITS-ISTR trial extended the window for systemic thrombolytics from 3 to 4.5 hours, showing similar functional benefit and risk of ICH in this extended window. The most important thing to remember is that functional outcome and risk of adverse event is time dependent and thrombolytic therapy should be initiated as soon as possible in qualifying patients.

KEY POINTS: RAPID TREATMENT GOALS OF ISCHEMIC STROKE WITH TISSUE PLASMINOGEN ACTIVATOR

1. Door to physician ≤10 minutes
2. Door to stroke team ≤15 minutes
3. Door to CT initiation ≤25 minutes
4. Door to CT interpretation ≤45 minutes
5. Door to drug (≥80% compliance) ≤60 minutes
6. Door to stroke unit admission ≤3 hours

24. **What is the evidence for tissue plasminogen activator (tPA) in acute ischemic stroke?**
Alteplase (also called *tPA*) is the only thrombolytic currently approved by the US Food and Drug Administration (FDA) for acute stroke. In 1995, the National Institute of Neurological Disorders and Stroke (NINDS) trial showed that tPA improved functional outcome (modified Rankin scale) at 3 months, if given within 3 hours of symptom onset, with a number needed to treat (NNT) of 6. In 2008, ECASS III showed similarly improved functional outcome within the 3- to 4.5-hour time frame (NNT=14). In all the stroke literature thus far, there has never been shown to be a mortality benefit for systemic administration of tPA in patients with suspected stroke. Recently, the PRISMS trial demonstrated that for patients with a NIHSS <5, that there was no benefit of tPA over aspirin alone.

25. **What is the risk of tPA?**
The primary risk of tPA is systemic bleeding, particularly ICH. For the NINDS trial, ICH with tPA was 6.4% versus 0.6% for the nontreatment group or a number needed to harm (NNH) of 17. For ECASS III, ICH with tPA was 2.4% versus 0.2%, or NNH of 45 (7.9% vs. 3.5%, or NNH of 23). The SITS-ISTR has shown a similar rate of about 2% ICH in their extended time window of 4.5 hours since last normal. The factors that appear associated with increased risk of hemorrhage are older age, brain edema or mass effect on CT, and higher baseline stroke severity. Angioedema may occur in 1%–5% of patients.

26. **What about a patient that wakes up with stroke symptoms?**
Approximately 20% of patients presenting with stroke either wake up with a neurologic deficit or have an unknown last normal and thus are outside the thrombolytic window and not candidates for tPA. There have been, however, several studies over the last few years that have attempted to use two types of MRI modalities (DWI and FLAIR) to compare area of infarct versus area of dead tissue with the goal of determining which patients may have salvageable tissue and benefit from IV thrombolytics regardless of the last time they were normal. The WAKE-UP trial randomized this patient population to tPA versus normal treatment, and showed improvement in functional outcomes; however, this study was underpowered and had an increase in ICH in the tPA group. Nonetheless, using advanced imaging modalities may be the future of determining thrombolytic candidates rather than time of last known normal.

27. **What are the indications and contraindications for tPA?**
The indications and contraindications are presented in Table 26.2. It is important to note that the NINDS trial, the ECASS III trial, and the AHA guidelines all vary slightly in their inclusion and exclusion criteria; thus, follow institutional stroke protocols.

28. **Why is there controversy with tPA for acute ischemic stroke?**
The controversy is multifactorial. Critics of tPA are concerned that most studies evaluating tPA in ischemic stroke show an increase risk of ICH and associated complications without a mortality benefit. Additionally, there has been

Table 26.2 Inclusion and Exclusion Criteria for Tissue Plasminogen Activator

NINDS INCLUSION CRITERIA	NINDS EXCLUSION CRITERIA	ECASS III EXCLUSION CRITERIA 3- TO 4.5-HOUR WINDOW
• No age cutoff • Objective evidence of neurologic deficit on NIHSS (scale 0–42) • Symptom onset <3 hours (if unknown timing, last seen normal time used; if still unclear, exclude)	• Stroke or serious head trauma <3 months • Major surgery <14 days • Any current or history of ICH • SBP >185 or DBP >110 (see Question 28) • Rapidly improving or minor symptoms of stroke • Symptoms suggestive of SAH • GI or GU hemorrhage <21 days • Arterial puncture at noncompressible site <7 days • Seizure at onset of stroke • If on anticoagulation prior 48 hours, PT >15 seconds (or INR >1.7) • If on heparin previous 48 hours, PTT above normal range • Platelets <100,000 mm³ • Blood glucose <50 mg/dL and >400 mg/dL	• Age <18 or >80 years old • Severe stroke, defined as NIHSS >25 or imaging > of MCA territory • Combination of previous stroke and diabetes • Oral anticoagulation therapy (warfarin) • Major surgery or severe trauma <3 months • Other major disorders associated with an increased risk of bleeding *Note: must meet NINDS criteria as well*

DBP, Diastolic blood pressure; *ECASS,* European Cooperative Acute Stroke Study; *GI,* gastrointestinal; *GU,* genitourinary; *ICH,* intracranial hemorrhage; *INR,* international normalized ratio; *MCA,* middle cerebral artery; *NIHSS,* National Institutes of Health Stroke Scale; *NINDS,* National Institute of Neurological Disorders and Stroke; *PT,* prothrombin time; *PTT,* partial thromboplastin time; *SAH,* subarachnoid hemorrhage; *SBP,* systolic blood pressure.

concern surrounding conflict of interest, with many of the larger trials being sponsored by the drug manufacturer. However, proponents note that these studies do show significant improvement in patient functional mobility and ability to live alone, an important outcome given the burden of disability after stroke worldwide.

KEY POINTS: MORTALITY AND MORBIDITY OF tPA

1. tPA does not appear to confer a mortality benefit.
2. Patients appear to have improved functional outcomes.
3. There are serious risks associated with major bleeding complications.

29. **Is informed consent required before tPA administration?**
    Informed consent requirements will vary depending on institutional protocols. The practice of shared decision making, however, is critically important in all of these patients. If possible, the risks, benefits, and alternatives to tPA should be explained and confirmed to be understood by the patient or a surrogate decision maker. If the patient is able to refuse, it is important to explain the possible outcomes in that scenario as well. Patients will typically make some functional improvements even without receiving thrombolytics. In a patient whose current functional state impairs assessing his or her understanding and no surrogate decision maker is available, it is valid and supported by the AHA to administer tPA without a formal consent.

30. **What must I do after giving tPA?**
    Current guidelines recommend admission to the intensive care unit (ICU) for at least 24 hours with frequent neurologic checks to monitor for post tPA bleeding. Avoiding other antithrombotic agents (e.g., heparin, warfarin, aspirin, ticlopidine, and clopidogrel), maintaining BP below 180/105, and avoiding invasive procedures (e.g., venipuncture, catheter placement, and nasogastric tube) for this initial 24-hour period is also recommended.

KEY POINTS: SUCCESSFUL ADMINISTRATION OF tPA

1. Adhere to your institution's stroke alert protocol.
2. Be exact about the time of onset and document it.
3. Immediately consult with a neurologist.
4. Expedite the head CT and final radiology reading.
5. Send labs early (i.e., finger-stick glucose, complete blood count [CBC], prothrombin time [PT]/partial thrombo-plastin time [PTT], chemistry, and troponin).
6. Mix the tPA early; calculate your dosage (0.9 mg/kg actual body weight; max. 90 mg).
7. Double-check all inclusion and exclusion criteria.
8. Have shared decision making with the patient or proxies about the risks and benefits

31. What is a large vessel occlusion or LVO?

LVO is when a large intracranial vessel is block by clot proximally, leading to significant deficit due to the large area of infarct. The proximal location and large size of these lesions allow for the possibility of interventional radiology (IR)-guided mechanical thrombectomy which cannulates the vessel, breaks up the clot, and suctions it out to re-establish blood flow.

32. How should I approach a patient with a large vessel occlusion (LVO)?

Patients with LVO should be approached the same way as any other patient with stroke, including administration of tPA if indicated. The use of IV thrombolytics does not preclude a patient from receiving mechanical thrombec-tomy, and thus tPA administration should not be delayed. The identification of LVO does require vascular imaging, typically computed tomography angiography (CTA), which will show blood flow through the large vessels and can identify clot.

33. When should I evaluate a patient with stroke symptoms for an LVO?

There is no clear consensus as to when to get a CTA to evaluate for LVO. A meta-analysis from 2018 showed that the NIHSS performed the best when compared with other LVO prediction models. A score of >6 had a sensitivity of 87% and specificity of 52% for LVO on CTA, while a score >10 had a sensitivity of 73% and specificity of 74%. Neither of these thresholds has an acceptable sensitivity or specificity on their own, so it is important to follow your institutional guidelines and discuss with your consultants early in the patient's course.

34. Which patients are candidates for mechanical thrombectomy?

The initial studies on IR-guided mechanical thrombectomy included patients >18 years of age with a NIHSS >6, minimal functional deficits prior to stroke, and evidence of an LVO with salvageable tissue on CT scan who's last normal was less than 6 hours ago. The HERMES meta-analysis of the five largest randomized controlled trials (RCTs) showed significant patient functional benefit to receiving thrombectomy in this group (NNT=2.6) without increased risk of mortality or ICH at 90 days. Since then, the DEFUSE3 trial assessed thrombectomy between 6 and 16 hours, and the DAWN trial evaluated thrombectomy between 6 and 24 hours, showing improvement in functional outcomes when compared with standard of care. Embolectomy has been extremely promising over the last few years and will likely continue expanding its indications as more studies are published.

35. How should I manage ICH in the setting of tPA?

ICH should be considered if the patient has a sudden neurologic decline, new headache, nausea or vomiting, or sudden BP rise within 24 hours of receiving tPA. In this case, you should immediately stop the tPA, perform a noncontrast head CT, and send blood for laboratory testing (i.e., type and crossmatch, PT, PTT, platelets, fibrino-gen). There are no prospectively collected data on the therapy of ICH after administration of tPA; however, there are expert opinions provided in guidelines which recommend 10 units of cryoprecipitate, 6–8 units of platelets (or one single donor unit), and neurosurgical consultation for possible hematoma evacuation. Other reversal agents such as FFP, PCC, and TXA are options, but controversial.

36. How do I approach hypertension in the patient with acute ischemic stroke?

The benefits of lowering BP are reduced vascular damage, but, again, higher than normal BPs may be necessary to optimize cerebral perfusion. The AHA guidelines recommend lowering BP slowly by 15% if systolic BP (SBP) is ≥220 mmHg or diastolic BP (DBP) is ≥120 mmHg, or if the patient has another comorbid condition that would benefit from lower BP (e.g., heart failure, dissection, pre-eclampsia). However, if a patient has received tPA, the blood pressure should be maintained <180/105 for at least the first 24 hours.

37. How do I approach hypertension in the patient with acute hemorrhagic stroke?

Most patients will have an elevated blood pressure after ICH, and these high pressures have been shown to be associated with larger hematomas and increased morbidity and mortality. The INTERACT trial showed that target-ing a systolic BP goal of 110–140 mmHg did not change mortality rates, but did have modest improvements in patient's functional outcomes. The ATACH-II trial, which looked at similar BP goals, showed no difference in mor-tality or functional outcomes. Based on these two studies, the AHA guidelines state that lowering systolic BP to a goal of 140 mmHg in ICH is *safe* and may have functional outcome benefit.

38. **What is the treatment for patients who are not tPA or thrombectomy candidates?**
   All patients with acute ischemic stroke who are not candidates for tPA, have no evidence of associated ICH, and have no other contraindications for aspirin (e.g., allergy), should receive 324 mg of aspirin. In the International Stroke Trial, administration of aspirin within 48 hours reduced 14-day recurrent stroke from 3.9% to 2.8%. Other interventions include BP and glucose control to reduce risk of subsequent stroke and early rehabilitation with physical and occupational therapy.

39. **When should I consider extracranial arterial dissection as a cause of acute stroke?**
   Dissection of the extracranial carotid and vertebral arteries (also called *cervical arteries*) is an important etiology of acute ischemic stroke. Injury to these vessels can cause stroke from either thrombus embolization or vessel occlusion. Consider this source in those with neck trauma (including even minor trauma) or cervical spine fractures, young patients (<45 years old), and those with neck pain who present with neurologic deficits.

BIBLIOGRAPHY

American College of Emergency Physicians, American Academy of Neurology. Clinical policy: use of intravenous tPA for the management of acute ischemic stroke in the emergency department. *Ann Emerg Med.* 2013;61:225–243.

Anderson CS, Heeley E, Huang Y, et al. Rapid blood-pressure lowering in patients with acute intracerebral hemorrhage. The INTERACT-2 investigators. *N Engl J Med.* 2013;368:2355–2365.

Goyal M, Menon BK, van Zwam WH, et al. Endovascular thrombectomy after large-vessel ischaemic stroke: a meta-analysis of individual patient data from five randomised trials. The HERMES collaboration. *The Lancet.* 2016;387:1723–1731.

Khatri P, Kleindorfer DO, Devlin T, et al. Effect of alteplase vs aspirin on functional outcome for patients with acute ischemic stroke and minor nondisabling neurologic deficits: the PRISMS randomized clinical trial. *JAMA.* 2018;320(2):156–166. doi:10.1001/jama.2018.8496.

Perry JJ, Stiell IG, Sivilotti MLA, et al. Clinical decision rules to rule out subarachnoid hemorrhage for acute headache. *JAMA.* 2013;310(12):1248–1255. doi:10.1001/jama.2013.278018.

Powers WJ, Rabinstein AA, Ackerson T, et al. 2018 guidelines for the early management of patients with acute ischemic stroke: a guideline for healthcare professionals from the American Heart Association/American Stroke Association. *Stroke.* 2018;49:e46–e99.

Qureshi AI, Palesch YY, Barsan WG, et al. Intensive blood-pressure lowering in patients with acute cerebral hemorrhage. ATACH-2 trial investigators and the Neurological Emergency Treatment Trials Network. *N Engl J Med.* 2016;375:1033–1043.

Smith EE, Kent DM, Bulsara KR, et al. The American Heart Association Stroke Council: accuracy of prediction instruments for diagnosing large vessel occlusion in individuals with suspected stroke: a systematic review for the 2018 guidelines for the early management of patients with acute ischemic stroke. *Stroke.* 2018;49:e111–e122.

Thomalla G, Simonsen CZ, Boutitie F, et al. MRI-guided thrombolysis for stroke with unknown time of onset. The WAKE-UP investigators. *N Engl J Med.* 2018;379:611–622.

van der Hullo T, Kooiman J, den Exter PL, et al. Effectiveness and safety of novel oral anticoagulants as compared with vitamin K antagonists in the treatment of acute symptomatic venous thromboembolism: a systematic review and meta-analysis. *J Thromb Haemost.* 2014;12:320–328.

CHAPTER 27

MENINGITIS

Forrest Andersen, MD and Maria E. Moreira, MD, FACEP

1. **What is meningitis, and why is it important?**
   Meningitis is an inflammatory disease of the tissues surrounding the brain and spinal cord. The mortality rate from bacterial and fungal meningitis is 10%–30%. Prompt recognition and treatment of bacterial meningitis can lessen morbidity and mortality.

2. **What are the causes of meningitis?**
   See Table 27.1.

3. **Which organisms are most commonly involved in each age group?**
   See Table 27.2.

4. **Who is at risk for meningitis?**
   Individuals aged >60 years old and <5 years old are at highest risk. Medical conditions that put patients at risk include:
   - diabetes
   - alcoholism
   - cirrhosis
   - sickle cell disease
   - immunosuppressed states
   - history of splenectomy
   - thalassemia major
   - bacterial endocarditis
   - malignancy
   - history of ventriculoperitoneal shunt
   - intravenous drug abuse
        Other risks include recent exposure to others with meningitis, crowding, contiguous infection (e.g., sinusitis), and dural defect (e.g., traumatic, surgical, congenital).

5. **List the common presenting symptoms of meningitis.**
   - Fever (most sensitive sign)
   - Change in mental status
   - Headache
   - Photophobia
   - Stiff neck
   - Lethargy
   - Irritability
   - Malaise
   - Confusion
   - Seizures

KEY POINTS: CLASSIC CLINICAL TRIAD FOR MENINGITIS

1. The classic clinical triad of fever, neck stiffness, and altered mental status is present in less than two thirds of patients with meningitis.
2. The absence of all three signs of the classic triad virtually eliminates a diagnosis of meningitis.

6. **What clinical signs are characteristic of meningeal irritation?**
   - Nuchal rigidity
   - Brudzinski sign: flexion of the neck results in flexion of the knees and hips
   - Kernig sign: pain or resistance of the hamstrings when the knees are extended with the hips flexed at a 90-degree angle
   - Jolt accentuation: baseline headache increases when the patient turns the head horizontally two to three rotations per second. (This physical finding is found more reliably in meningitis than the previously mentioned physical findings.)

Table 27.1 Causes of Meningitis

INFECTIOUS CAUSES	NONINFECTIOUS CAUSES
Bacteria	Neoplastic
Viruses	Collagen vascular
Fungi	Drugs (i.e., antibiotics and anti-inflammatory medications)
Parasites	
Tuberculosis	

Table 27.2 Organisms Most Commonly Involved by Patient Group

AGE OR CONDITION	MOST COMMONLY ENCOUNTERED ORGANISMS
Newborns	Group B or D streptococci, non–group B streptococci, *Escherichia coli, Listeria monocytogenes*
Infants and children	*Streptococcus pneumoniae, Neisseria meningitides, Haemophilus influenzae, Listeria monocytogenes* (especially <3 months of age)
Adults	*S. pneumoniae, H. influenzae, N. meningitides,* staphylococci, streptococci, *Listeria* species
Patients with impaired cellular immunity	*Listeria monocytogenes,* gram-negative bacilli, *S. pneumoniae, N. meningitides*
Head trauma, neurosurgery, or CSF shunt	Staphylococci, gram-negative bacilli, *S. pneumoniae*

CSF, Cerebrospinal fluid.

While presence of these signs should guide providers to further evaluate for meningitis, their absence should not falsely reassure providers and be used in isolation to exclude the diagnosis.

7. **List the presenting signs of meningitis in infants.**
   - Bulging fontanel (may not be present if patient is dehydrated)
   - Paradoxic irritability (quiet when stationary, cries when held)
   - High-pitched cry
   - Hypotonia
   - Skin over the spine may have dimples, sinuses, nevi, or tufts of hair, indicating a congenital anomaly communicating with the subarachnoid space.

8. **If the symptoms are not specific and physical findings are absent, what are the indications for lumbar puncture (LP)?**
   LP should be done whenever meningitis is suspected, because analyzing cerebrospinal fluid (CSF) is the only way to diagnose meningitis.

9. **What tests should be done before doing an LP?**
   - *Funduscopic examination.* Check for papilledema and presence or absence of spontaneous venous pulsations. Alternatively, ocular ultrasound can be used to measure optic nerve sheath diameter to determine the presence of increased intracranial pressure.
   - *Computed tomography (CT) scan.* Order only if risk factors for cerebral herniation are present:
     - papilledema
     - absence of spontaneous venous pulsations
     - altered mental status
     - focal neurologic deficit
     - new-onset seizure
     - clinical suspicion for recent trauma or subarachnoid bleed
   - *Coagulation studies and platelet count.* Order if there is suspicion for bleeding disorder.

10. **What is the most common error in emergency department management of meningitis?**
    The most common error is delaying administration of antibiotics until the LP is done. If there is a clinical suspicion of bacterial meningitis, antibiotics should be administered promptly. Intravenous antibiotics given <2 hours before the LP (and ideally after blood and urine cultures are obtained) will not affect the results of the CSF analysis.

11. **Discuss the risks of LP.**
    - Transient leg paresthesias during LP: caused by irritation of nerve roots by the needle
    - Headache: most common sequela, seen in 5%–30% of patients
    - Tonsillar herniation: from increased intracranial pressure (no risk with normal CT)
    - Cauda equina syndrome: from hematoma in patients with coagulopathy (rare)
        Note that paralysis is a common fear, but exceedingly rare (needle inserted below level of spinal cord at L2 or below). A few case reports have been noted in the literature, due to post-LP spinal subarachnoid hemorrhage or arteriovenous fistula.

12. **What are the contraindications to performing an LP?**
    - There are no absolute contraindications.
    - Use caution in patients with possible increased intracranial pressure, thrombocytopenia or other bleeding diathesis, or suspected spinal epidural abscess.
    - In patients with severe thrombocytopenia (platelet counts $<50,000/mm^3$) or with an elevated international normalized ratio (INR >1.4), consider correcting the abnormality before performing the LP.

13. **What is the secret to performing LP successfully?**
    Proper positioning of the patient is crucial. If the LP is done with the patient lying down, be sure the shoulders and hips are in a straight plane perpendicular to the floor. The patient should be in the tightest fetal position possible. If the LP is done with the patient sitting up, have the upper body rest on a bedside table and have the patient push his or her back toward you as if he or she is an angry cat.

14. **When is it essential to perform the LP with the patient lying down?**
    This is important when you want to obtain an opening pressure. If you are unable to perform the LP with the patient lying down, you can place the needle with the patient sitting up and then have him or her lay down to obtain the opening pressure.

15. **What can cause a falsely elevated intracranial pressure?**
    Intracranial pressure can be elevated by a tense patient, the head being elevated above the plane of the needle, marked obesity, or muscle contraction.

16. **Which laboratory studies should be ordered on the CSF?**
    Four tubes are usually collected, each containing 1–1.5 mL of CSF. More CSF is needed if special tests are required.
    - Tube 1: Cell count and differential
    - Tube 2: Gram stain, culture, and sensitivities (special tests that may be ordered include viral cultures, tuberculosis cultures and acid-fast stain, fungal antigen studies and India ink stain, and serologic tests for neurosyphilis. Countercurrent immunoelectrophoresis, coagglutination, comparative proteomics, and latex agglutination can be used to rapidly detect specific bacterial antigens in the CSF)
    - Tube 3: Glucose and protein
    - Tube 4: Cell count and differential
        CSF procalcitonin may be helpful in differentiating between bacterial and viral or aseptic meningitis after neurosurgical procedures when CSF studies are difficult to interpret.
        In pediatric patients, three tubes are collected:
    - Tube 1: Microbiology
    - Tube 2: Glucose and protein
    - Tube 3: Cell count and differential

17. **What findings on LP are consistent with bacterial meningitis?**
    See Table 27.3.

KEY POINTS: CORRECTIONS FOR TRAUMATIC TAPS

1. In normal subjects, CSF from a traumatic LP contains ~1 white blood cell (WBC) per 700 red blood cells (RBCs).
2. When a traumatic LP has occurred, correct the CSF protein result for the presence of blood by subtracting 1 mg/dL of protein for each 1000 RBCs.
3. A high CSF protein level with a benign clinical presentation suggests fungal disease.

---

18. **Which antibiotics should be prescribed when the causative organism is unknown?**
    See Table 27.4.

19. **What about steroids?**
    Steroids may decrease pathophysiologic consequences, such as cerebral edema, increased intracranial pressure, altered cerebral blood flow, and hearing loss. The Infectious Disease Society of America (IDSA) includes

Table 27.3 Findings Consistent With Bacterial Meningitis

PARAMETER	FINDING
Opening pressure	In range of 20–50 cmH$_2$0
Appearance	Cloudy
White blood cell count	1000–5000 cells/mm^3
Cells	Neutrophil predominance >80%
Glucose	Low <40 mg/dL
Ratio of CSF to serum glucose	<0.4
CSF protein	Elevated (often >100 mg/dL)
CSF lactate	>3.5 mmol/L (more useful in postoperative patients than in community-acquired meningitis)

CSF, Cerebrospinal fluid.

Table 27.4 Recommendations for Known Organisms and Generalized Recommendations

ORGANISM	ANTIBIOTIC TREATMENT
Neisseria meningitides	Penicillin G 2 million IU IV every 2 hours, or ampicillin 2 g IV every 4 hours, or third-generation cephalosporin
Streptococcus pneumoniae	Vancomycin plus a third-generation cephalosporin
Haemophilus influenzae	Cefotaxime 2 g IV every 6 hours, or ceftriaxone 2 g IV every 12 hours, or chloramphenicol 50–100 mg/kg/day in four divided doses
Staphylococcus aureus	Nafcillin 2 g IV every 4 hours
Escherichia coli and other gram-negative enter-ics except *Pseudomonas aeruginosa*	Cefotaxime 2 g IV every 4 hours
P. aeruginosa	Ceftazidime 2 g IV every 8 hours, plus gentamicin, 3–5 mg/kg/day IV in three divided doses
Listeria monocytogenes	Ampicillin 2 g IV every 4 hours, plus gentamicin (as for *P. aeruginosa*)
Group B streptococci	Penicillin G 4 million units IV every 4 hours, or ampicillin 2 g IV every 4 hours
Generalized (Empiric Rx) Recommendations	
Age or condition	Antibiotic treatment
Age <3 months	Ampicillin + broad-spectrum cephalosporin
Age 3 months to 50 years	Vancomycin + broad-spectrum cephalosporin
Age >50 years	Ampicillin + broad-spectrum cephalosporin + vancomycin
Impaired cellular immunity	Ampicillin + ceftazidime + vancomycin
Head trauma, neurosurgery, CSF shunt	Vancomycin + ceftazidime
Patients with severe β-lactam allergies	Vancomycin + moxifloxacin + trimethoprim-sulfamethoxazole (if need *Listeria* coverage)

CSF, Cerebrospinal fluid; *IV,* intravenously; *Rx,* recipe or prescription.

dexamethasone in its treatment algorithm for children and adults. Dexamethasone should be given 10–20 minutes prior to antimicrobials or at least concomitant with them. Steroids should not be given after administration of antibiotics. Recommendations by age group:

- *Neonates.* The evidence is lacking.
- *Infants and children.* Use dexamethasone (0.15 mg/kg) in children with suspected or proven *Hemophilus influenzae* meningitis.

- *Adults.* Mortality benefit has been shown. Use dexamethasone (0.15 mg/kg) in adults with suspected or proven pneumococcal meningitis. Then only continue if CSF Gram stain shows gram-positive diplococci.

20. **Do people exposed to a patient with meningitis need antibiotics?**
Individuals who have had close contact with someone who has, or is suspected to have, meningococcal meningitis should take rifampin, 600 mg twice a day for 2 days (for children older than 1 month, 10 mg/kg every 12 hours; younger than 1 month, 5 mg/kg every 12 hours). Other accepted prophylaxis regimens for *Neisseria meningitides* include the following: ciprofloxacin 500 mg single dose (not recommended for pregnant or lactating women or patients <18 years of age); ceftriaxone 250 mg intramuscular (IM) dose for adults or 125 mg IM for children (used in pregnancy); or a single oral dose of azithromycin 500 mg for adults (pediatric dose 10 mg/kg). Note that azithromycin can be used if ciprofloxacin resistance has been detected but is not a first line agent. A 4-day course of rifampin is recommended for most individuals who have been in close contact with someone with *H. influenzae* type B meningitis. Rifampin dose recommended for *H. influenzae* prophylaxis is 20 mg/kg (maximum 600 mg) once daily for 4 days (10 mg/kg for children younger than 1 month). Individuals exposed to someone with other types of meningitis, especially viral, do not need prophylactic antibiotics.

Website
Infectious Diseases Society of America: www.idsociety.org; accessed January 22, 2019.

BIBLIOGRAPHY

Afhami S, Dehghan Manshadi SA, Rezahosseini O. Jolt accentuation of headache: can this maneuver rule out acute meningitis? *BMC Res Notes.* 2017;10(1):540. doi:10.1186/s13104-017-2877-1.

Alons IM, Verheul RJ, Kuipers I, et al. Procalcitonin in cerebrospinal fluid in meningitis: a prospective diagnostic study. *Brain Behav.* 2016;6(11):e00545.

Brouwer MC, McIntyre P, Prasad K, et al. Corticosteroids for acute bacterial meningitis. *Cochrane Database Syst Rev.* 2015;(9):CD004405.

Charalambous LT, Premji A, Tybout C, et al. Prevalence, healthcare resource utilization and overall burden of fungal meningitis in the United States. *J Med Microbiol.* 2018;67(2):215–227.

Heckenberg SG, Brouwer MC, Van de Beek D. Bacterial meningitis. *Handb Clin Neurol.* 2014;121:1361–1375.

Lundbo LF, Benfield T. Risk factors for community-acquired bacterial meningitis. *Infect Dis (Lond).* 2017;49(6):433–444.

Mount HR, Boyle SD. Aseptic and bacterial meningitis: evaluation, treatment, and prevention. *Am Fam Physician.* 2017;96(5):314–322.

Patterson DF, Ho ML, Leavitt JA, et al. Comparison of ocular ultrasonography and magnetic resonance imaging for detection of increased intracranial pressure. *Front Neurol.* 2018;9:278.

Sadoun T, Singh A. Adult acute bacterial meningitis in the United States: 2009 update. *Emerg Med Pract.* 2009;11:1–25.

BREATHING AND VENTILATION

Jeffrey Sankoff, MD and David B. Richards, MD, FACEP

CHAPTER 28

1. **How useful is the respiratory rate in the evaluation of a patient?**
   The respiratory rate is invaluable. Normal respiratory rate in children varies with age, whereas adults typically breathe 12–16 times per minute. As a testament to its usefulness, the respiratory rate can be helpful in the diagnosis of many conditions other than those with primary pulmonary pathology. For example, the respiratory rate can be elevated in patients with anemia, metabolic acidosis, pregnancy, febrile illness, anxiety, central nervous system pathology, arteriovenous fistula, cyanotic heart disease, and those at high altitude. It is important that the respiratory rate be counted carefully for at least 30 seconds to be accurate.

2. **Which breathing patterns are associated with pathologic conditions?**
   - Kussmaul respirations are deep, rapid breaths that are associated with metabolic acidosis.
   - Cheyne-Stokes breathing comprises respirations that wax and wane cyclically so that periods of deep breathing alternate with periods of apnea. Causes include congestive heart failure (CHF), hypertensive crisis, hyponatremia, high-altitude illness, and head injury.
   - Ataxic breathing is characterized by unpredictable irregularity. Breaths may be shallow or deep, and stop for short periods. Causes include respiratory depression and brain stem injury at the level of the medulla.

3. **Which pulmonary function tests are commonly used in the emergency department (ED)?**
   The most useful pulmonary function test for ED patients is the peak expiratory flow rate. It is measured by having a patient exhale forcefully at a maximum rate through a peak flowmeter. Normal values range from 350 to 600 L/min in adults. Lower levels are characteristic of increased airway resistance, as commonly seen in asthma and chronic obstructive pulmonary disease (COPD) exacerbations. Patients with values of less than 100 L/min have severe airflow obstruction. Comparing a patient's current peak expiratory flow rate to his or her personal best provides insight into the severity of respiratory distress and necessary treatment. Serial measurements are helpful for objectively quantifying response to treatment. A less commonly used test is the forced end-expiratory volume at 1 second, which helps quantify the severity of obstructive and restrictive lung disease.

   Peak inspiratory pressures can also be used to assess patients' ability to adequately ventilate when suffering from rib fractures, muscle weakness, or neurologic conditions.

4. **How does pulse oximetry work?**
   Pulse oximetry is based on a combination of spectrophotometry and plethysmography.
   - Spectrophotometry is based on the Beer-Lambert law, which holds that optical absorbance is proportional to the concentration of a substance and the thickness of the medium. Using this principle, the absorbance of light within a pulsatile vascular bed is used to distinguish between oxyhemoglobin (O_2Hb) and reduced hemoglobin (Hb).
   - Plethysmography measures the tissue displacement caused by an arterial pulse. This allows for assessment of the increase in light absorption caused by local arterial flow, compared with the background of composite tissues and venous blood. Plethysmography also allows determination of the pulse.

   Pulse oximeters function by placing a pulsatile vascular bed between a light-emitting diode (LED) and a detector. Light is transmitted through the tissue at two wavelengths, 660 nm (primarily absorbed by O_2Hb) and 940 nm (primarily absorbed by Hb), allowing differentiation of O_2Hb from Hb. The detector compares the concentration of O_2Hb and Hb and displays the result as a percent of saturation.

5. **When might the pulse recorded from the pulse oximeter be different than the heart rate shown on the cardiac monitor?**
   This occurs in situations where electrically conducted beats do not result in a subsequent pulse (i.e., electromechanical dissociation) and can provide valuable clinical information.

6. **How can pulse oximetry be useful?**
   Pulse oximetry is useful for monitoring O_2Hb saturation in:
   - cardiopulmonary disorders
   - procedural sedation or airway management
   - patients with a decreased level of consciousness
   - response to therapeutic interventions

7. **In which situations can pulse oximetry yield false readings?**
Situations in which the usefulness of pulse oximetry is limited include poor peripheral perfusion, excessive movement, low O_2Hb saturations (<83%), exposure of the measuring sensor to ambient light sources, and in the presence of certain types of nail polish. Oxygen saturation measurements may be falsely elevated in the presence of carboxyhemoglobin and falsely decreased in the presence of methemoglobin or sulfhemoglobin.

8. **Why can a good pulse oximetry reading be falsely reassuring?**
Clinicians often rely on the pulse oximeter as part of monitoring a patient's respiratory status, particularly when using procedural sedation. The pulse oximeter only measures oxygenation and provides no information regarding carbon dioxide (CO_2) exchange, and thus does not assess for adequate ventilation. A preoxygenated patient can be apneic for several minutes without an appreciable decrease in oxygen saturation, while significant hypercarbia is developing. Although the pulse oximeter has become indispensable, it only assesses one part of a patient's respiratory status.

KEY POINTS: PULSE OXIMETRY

1. Pulse oximetry measures oxygenation, not ventilation.
2. Poor peripheral perfusion is a common reason pulse oximeters provide unreliable readings.

9. **What is end-tidal CO_2 (EtCO_2) monitoring?**
An EtCO_2 monitor is used to evaluate ventilation and, when combined with the pulse oximeter, it provides a more complete evaluation of the patient's respiratory status. EtCO_2 monitors may be either qualitative or quantitative. Qualitative detectors (generally colorimetric) are often used immediately after intubation to detect the presence of CO_2 in exhaled gas, and are used only to determine the proper placement of the endotracheal tube. Quantitative EtCO_2 detectors continuously monitor exhaled CO_2, displaying its concentration in both numeric and graphic form. With a normal tidal volume, the CO_2 concentration in the breath correlates with the concentration of CO_2 in the alveoli. The CO_2 in the alveoli is dependent on the ventilation/perfusion (V/Q) relationship, which is influenced by a number of physiologic and pathologic states. Normal end-tidal CO_2 is in the range of 35–45 mmHg. A CO_2 increase or decrease may represent the earliest change in a patient's ventilation and perfusion status. Both the CO_2 level *and* the waveform must be used to interpret quantitative EtCO_2 detectors. For example, a low CO_2 level could be a result of shallow breathing (short flat waveforms) or hyperventilation (large rapid waveforms).

10. **When is EtCO_2 monitoring useful?**
EtCO_2 is used in a number of ways:
- during procedural sedation;
- in patients with sepsis or shock to monitor perfusion status;
- during cardiopulmonary resuscitation (CPR) to monitor effectiveness of resuscitation;
- for monitoring response to treatment in patients with COPD and asthma;
- to monitor for tube placement or dislodgement by emergency medical services (EMS) during intubation and transport;
- to monitor respiratory status in acutely intoxicated or overdose patients.

11. **What percentage of fraction of inspired oxygen (FiO_2) corresponds with the various types of oxygen delivery systems?**
The three primary means of oxygen delivery are nasal cannula, simple face mask, and face mask with an oxygen reservoir. A nasal cannula can be used to deliver oxygen at rates of 1–6 L/min. With a nasal cannula, every 1 L/min of flow increase causes the FiO_2 to rise by 4% over and above the atmospheric concentration (21% at sea level). As a result, a nasal cannula can deliver an FiO_2 between 25% and 45%. A simple face mask relies on an oxygen flow of 5–10 L/min, with a resulting FiO_2 ranging from 35% to 50%. A face mask with an oxygen reservoir has a constant flow of oxygen so that higher concentrations of oxygen can be achieved. A properly fitted face mask with an oxygen reservoir with a 15 L/min flow rate can deliver up to 85% FiO_2.

12. **What is noninvasive ventilation?**
It is a means of delivering positive-pressure ventilation without placement of a nasotracheal or endotracheal tube. As such, ventilatory assistance is possible without the risks of intubation and mechanical ventilation. Noninvasive ventilation can be a useful tool in carefully selected patients and may avoid the need for intubation.

13. **What forms of noninvasive ventilation are available to emergency physicians?**
The two most useful forms of noninvasive ventilation are continuous positive airway pressure (CPAP) and bilevel positive airway pressure (BiPAP). With each method, a tight-fitting mask is placed over the patient's face and high-flow air with or without supplemental oxygen is delivered through the circuit in order to augment the patient's breathing by positive pressure.
- CPAP delivers a continuous amount of positive airway pressure during and after inspiration and expiration.

- BiPAP not only provides a set positive pressure during exhalation but also delivers additional set inspiratory pressure when the patient initiates a breath. The inspiratory pressure is always set higher than the expiratory pressure, can be sustained for various periods, and stops when the patient ceases to inhale or begins to exhale, thus easing the work of breathing.

14. **In what circumstances would noninvasive ventilation be preferred over standard invasive ventilation?**
    Noninvasive ventilation has been shown to be useful in many conditions, including cardiogenic pulmonary edema, COPD, and nocturnal hypoventilation. There is some evidence to suggest that it may confer some benefit in patients with asthma and pneumonia with hypoxia. Noninvasive ventilation is most beneficial when the anticipated time needed for its use is short (e.g., in patients with acute exacerbations of CHF or COPD). In properly selected patients, CPAP is particularly useful in the treatment of pulmonary edema, and BiPAP can be useful in a patient with respiratory distress caused by COPD. With the use of noninvasive ventilation, patients with CHF exacerbation have been shown to improve more rapidly and are less likely to require intubation. Although overall mortality is not improved, this is likely the result of the underlying cardiac disease and not a failure of this modality. Patients with COPD are notoriously difficult to wean from mechanical ventilators, and noninvasive ventilation can often be used to reverse the course of patients with COPD in moderate respiratory distress who would otherwise have required standard invasive ventilation. The use of noninvasive ventilation has been shown to improve outcomes in this patient population. Lastly, some patients with advance directives forbidding intubation and mechanical ventilation may benefit from the respiratory support provided by noninvasive ventilation.

15. **When is noninvasive ventilation contraindicated?**
    Noninvasive ventilation cannot be used in patients with altered mental status or in the absence of spontaneous breaths. Other contraindications include:
    - risk for or active vomiting
    - inability to tolerate a tight-fitting mask
    - anticipated prolonged need for ventilation

16. **How do I determine the initial ventilator settings in someone who has just been intubated?**
    Ventilator settings should reflect the reason for intubation, and the patient's oxygenation, ventilation, and acid-base status. The primary method for affecting the oxygenation of a patient is to alter the FiO_2 and positive end-expiratory pressure (PEEP). Respiratory rate may also have an impact on oxygenation, but to a lesser degree. Initially, intubated patients should be given 100% oxygen or an FiO_2 of 1.00. Subsequently, if arterial blood gas analysis reveals that the partial pressure of oxygen (PaO_2) is high, the FiO_2 and PEEP should be lowered incrementally to maintain an adequate oxygen saturation. It is desirable to reduce FiO_2 to less than 0.6 as soon as possible, because sustained levels higher than this may lead to tissue damage via free radical formation.
    The main factors determining a patient's ventilatory status are tidal volume and respiratory rate. Changes in each are reflected by the partial pressure of carbon dioxide ($PaCO_2$) from arterial blood gas analysis. High respiratory rates and large tidal volumes decrease the CO_2 level, whereas the inverse elevates the CO_2 level. Initially, the tidal volume can be estimated to be 6–8 mL/kg; for a 70-kg patient, that is 420–560 mL. The initial respiratory rate varies depending on the clinical situation. On average, it should be set between 10 and 16 breaths per minute.

17. **Are ventilator settings always the same?**
    No. The ventilator is a means of treatment for a patient with respiratory failure. Since there are many reasons for respiratory failure necessitating intubation and mechanical ventilation, there are also many ways to use the ventilator. Ventilator settings will vary according to why the patient needed to be intubated and what is being treated. For example, a patient with an obstructive condition, such as asthma, does best with small tidal volumes, low respiratory rates, and low levels of PEEP. In contrast, a patient with pneumonia may need higher PEEP and airway pressures, but lower tidal volumes. Monitoring $EtCO_2$ and pulse oximetry can provide real-time feedback of the adequacy of the chosen settings. Other common ventilator settings for patients with closed head injury, CHF, metabolic acidosis, and sepsis are shown in Table 28.1. The most important thing to remember about ventilator settings is that they should not be static. As the patient's status changes over time, so too should the ventilator settings, reflecting the patient's need for more, or hopefully less, support as time goes on.

18. **Are there different methods of delivering ventilation?**
    Ventilation can be provided in two ways: (1) by providing a set tidal volume (volume control), or (2) by providing a set inspiratory pressure (pressure control). With volume control modes, the provider sets a tidal volume, and the pressures that arise within the patient are a result of the interaction between the volume and the patient's characteristics (e.g., a large tidal volume in a small patient will generate high pressures). With pressure control modes, the provider sets an inspiratory pressure, and the resulting tidal volume will be determined by the interaction between the pressure and the patient (e.g., high pressure and small patient results in a high tidal volume).

19. **What are the most commonly used methods?**
    The most commonly used volume control modes are assist control (AC) and synchronized intermittent mandatory ventilation (SIMV). With AC, all breaths administered by the ventilator are of the same tidal volume. The

Table 28.1 Initial Ventilator Settings According to Condition

CONDITION	TIDAL VOLUME (mL/kg)	RESPIRATORY RATE (BREATHS/MIN)	FiO₂	PEEP (cmH₂O)	COMMENTS
Asthma	5–8	6–10	100	5–10	Low RR will allow for lung deflation. Paralysis will be needed and hypercapnea WILL result. This may be tolerated until goals of treatment reached.
COPD	6–10	10–14	≤40	5	Lowest FiO₂ necessary to maintain SaO₂ of 90% or greater. Titrate down RR as soon as possible to allow patient to assume work of breathing.
Head injury	8	14	40	0	Normocapnea is goal. Low PEEP improves venous drainage from head and may improve cerebral perfusion pressure. Avoid hyperoxia if possible.
CHF	8	14	100	5	
Metabolic acidosis	8–10	18–22	50	5	If lungs are healthy, lower FiO₂ is all that is needed. If not, use higher concentration. High minute ventilation will offset metabolic acidosis.
Sepsis	6	12–16	100	5	Use higher PEEP to improve oxygenation. Avoid higher lung volumes.

CHF, Congestive heart failure; *COPD,* chronic obstructive pulmonary disease; *FiO₂,* fraction of inspired oxygen; *PEEP,* positive end-expiratory pressure; *RR,* respiratory rate.

machine will give a minimum number of breaths per minute. The patient may initiate additional breaths on top of that minimum set rate, although all additional breaths will be of the same tidal volume. With SIMV, the ventilator administers a set minimum number of breaths of a preset tidal volume, and additional breaths initiated by the patient have varying tidal volumes dependent on patient effort.

The most commonly used pressure control mode is pressure support ventilation (PSV). With PSV the patient must initiate all breaths because there is no minimum rate administered by the machine, and so spontaneous ventilation is a requirement for this mode. With each breath, the machine augments pressure to the predetermined rate, and tidal volume is determined by patient effort.

20. **What is PEEP?**

PEEP is positive end-expiratory pressure, or pressure that is applied during expiration. PEEP prevents collapse of alveoli at the end of expiration, leading to an increase in functional residual capacity and a recruitment of alveoli to participate in gas exchange. The end result is improved V/Q matching in the pulmonary circulation, thus improving oxygenation. On the flip side, higher PEEP can induce barotrauma, diminish venous return to the heart, and elevate intracranial pressure. PEEP is usually set at 2.5 or 5 cmH₂O. However, in certain clinical settings, especially those in which there is increased stiffness of the alveolar walls such as in acute respiratory distress syndrome (ARDS), much higher levels may be appropriate.

21. **What is auto-PEEP?**

Auto-PEEP occurs when gas is trapped in the lungs by small airways collapse prior to end expiration. This results in a positive pressure within the lungs at end expiration. Auto-PEEP is a significant problem for patients with advanced COPD and can contribute to respiratory failure by significantly impacting their work of breathing. Auto-PEEP can also be seen in patients with severe asthma. When on a mechanical ventilator, patients with significant auto-PEEP can have breath stacking and hyperinflation that leads to other potential complications, such as hypotension and barotrauma. The best solution to this is increasing expiratory time by decreasing the respiratory rate, thus allowing for more complete exhalation.

22. **What are the most common complications of mechanical ventilation?**
The most common direct complication seen in the ED is barotrauma. High pressure can cause rupture of the alveolar wall, which in turn can lead to pneumomediastinum, pneumothorax, tension pneumothorax, and subcutaneous emphysema. Pneumonia tops the list of ventilator complications overall, followed by sinusitis, tracheal necrosis, and local trauma to the nares and mouth.

23. **How do I approach a patient on a ventilator with acutely worsening oxygenation or ventilation?**
First, remove the patient from the ventilator and provide manual ventilation to the patient by using a bag ventilatory device. Many problems involving a $30,000 ventilator can be solved with a $15 resuscitation bag. The DOPE mnemonic taught in pediatric life support can be helpful in remembering the remainder of the approach.
Displacement: Confirm that the endotracheal tube is in the proper place by using some combination of auscultation, measurement of CO_2 exchange, radiography, and direct visualization.
Obstruction: Confirm that the endotracheal tube is patent by passing a suction catheter down the lumen. Sometimes an endotracheal tube can become kinked simply as a result of patient positioning.
Patient: Consider various causes within the patient. First and foremost is the possibility of secretions obstructing large bronchi. Vigorous suctioning may remedy this situation. Next, consider pneumothorax. Confirm that there is no evidence of barotrauma, usually by a combination of physical examination and a chest radiograph.
Equipment: Confirm that the ventilator circuit and ventilator itself are functioning properly.

KEY POINTS: VENTILATOR MANAGEMENT

1. Each clinical situation calls for a different approach to ventilator management.
2. Tidal volume and respiratory rate affect the patient's ventilation and $PaCO_2$.
3. FiO_2 and PEEP affect the patient's oxygenation and pO_2.
4. Oxygenation and ventilation problems in patients using mechanical ventilators can be managed by removing them from the ventilator and following the DOPE mnemonic.

ACKNOWLEDGMENT

The editors and authors of this chapter would like to acknowledge and thank Drs. John L. Kendall and Ryan D. Patterson for their previous contributions to this chapter.

BIBLIOGRAPHY

Kondo Y, Kumasawa J, Kawaguchi A, et al. Effects of non-invasive ventilation in patients with acute respiratory failure excluding post-extubation respiratory failure, cardiogenic pulmonary edema and exacerbation of COPD: a systematic review and meta-analysis. *J Anesth.* 2017;31(5):714–725.
Masip J, Peacock WF, Price S, et al. Indications and practical approach to non-invasive ventilation in acute heart failure. *Eur Heart J.* 2018;39(1):17–25.
Osadnik CR, Tee VS, Carson-Chahhoud KV, et al. Non-invasive ventilation for the management of acute hypercapnic respiratory failure due to exacerbation of chronic obstructive pulmonary disease. *Cochrane Database Syst Rev.* 2017;7:CD004104.
Paus-Jenssen ES, Reid JK, Cockcroft DW, et al. The use of noninvasive ventilation in acute respiratory failure at a tertiary care center. *Chest.* 2004;126:165–172.
Sankoff J, Tebb Z. Mechanical ventilation. *Crit Dec Emerg Med.* 2010;25:10–19.

CHAPTER 29

ASTHMA, CHRONIC OBSTRUCTIVE PULMONARY DISEASE, AND PNEUMONIA

Jeff Druck, MD, FACEP and Tom Califf, MD

ASTHMA

1. **What is asthma, and what are the presenting symptoms of asthma exacerbation?**
   Asthma is a heterogeneous chronic inflammatory disorder of the airways, resulting in recurrent episodes of wheezing, breathlessness, chest tightness, and coughing. Airway inflammation contributes to bronchial hyperreactivity, airflow obstruction, and chronic disease. This creates variable and reversible airflow limitation. The severity of disease is classified into four categories based on quality of life impact, frequency of short-acting bronchodilator use, pulmonary function tests (PFTs), and frequency of oral steroid use: intermittent (not requiring controller medication) versus mild, moderate, or severe persistent disease.

2. **In addition to asthma, what should be included in the differential diagnosis of wheezing?**
   - Chronic obstructive pulmonary disease (COPD)
   - Congestive heart failure (CHF)
   - Foreign body aspiration
   - Anaphylaxis
   - Tracheobronchitis
   - Epiglottitis
   - Viral respiratory infections and pneumonitis
   - Bronchiectasis (including cystic fibrosis)
   - Interstitial lung disease
   - Vocal cord dysfunction

3. **Which aspects of the asthmatic patient's history are important to the current exacerbation?**
   Primary considerations include exposure to common precipitants, such as:
   - environmental allergens
   - occupational exposure
   - viral upper respiratory tract infections
   - cold
   - exercise
   - aspirin or nonsteroidal anti-inflammatory drug use

   Also important are:
   - duration and severity of symptoms
   - past history and frequency of exacerbations
   - prior hospitalizations and intubations
   - number of recent emergency department (ED) visits
   - current medications
   - comorbidities

   Non-Caucasian race and lower socioeconomic standing are risk factors for increased severity requiring hospitalization.

4. **Are there any helpful ancillary diagnostic tests?**
   Bedside spirometry, which is dependent on the cooperation and effort of the patient, provides a rapid, objective assessment of airflow obstruction and serves as a guide to the effectiveness of therapy. The forced expiratory volume in 1 second (**FEV_1**) and the peak expiratory flow rate (**PEFR**) directly measure the degree of large airway obstruction.
   - Mild obstruction: FEV_1 or PEFR $\geq$70% of predicted or personal best
   - Moderate obstruction: FEV_1 or PEFR $\geq$40% and <70% of predicted or personal best
   - Severe obstruction: FEV_1 or PEFR <40% of predicted or personal best

   Pulse oximetry is a useful and convenient method for assessing oxygenation and monitoring oxygen saturation during treatment. Most other tests, including blood gases, complete blood counts, and electrocardiograms are not useful in the management of asthma except in cases of active or impending respiratory failure or diagnostic uncertainty. Asthmatic patients with PEFR >25% of predicted have been shown to be unlikely to have a notable respiratory acidosis on blood gas testing. Chest radiography is not typically indicated but may be helpful if the patient does not respond to initial treatment or if a pulmonary complication, such as foreign body obstruction, pneumonia, pneumomediastinum, pneumothorax, or CHF, is suspected.

5. **What are the key objectives when treating an asthma exacerbation? How are they achieved?**

The key objectives are to (1) **correct hypoxemia**, (2) **rapidly reverse airflow obstruction**, and (3) **reduce the likelihood of recurrence of severe airflow obstruction**.

First-line treatment includes inhaled β_2-agonists, systemic corticosteroids in moderate exacerbations, and supplemental oxygen if needed (Table 29.1). Hypoxemia is usually corrected by administration of supplemental oxygen with a goal oxygen saturation of >90%. Relief of bronchoconstriction is usually accomplished by administration of either intermittent or continuous doses of **aerosolized β_2-agonists**. Studies contain mixed conclusions as to whether there is any added clinical benefit to levalbuterol, an R-enantiomer form of albuterol that is thought to have a decreased effect on heart rate. Available evidence does not suggest an improved benefit from intravenous (IV) β_2-agonists compared with aerosol. **Early administration of systemic corticosteroids** addresses the inflammatory component of acute asthma and has been demonstrated to reduce hospitalizations, although beneficial effects of corticosteroids are often not noted until several hours after administration. There is no added benefit to IV corticosteroids compared with oral administration. Current research has failed to identify a difference in relapse of symptoms between patients receiving oral or intramuscular (IM) steroids; thus, patients who may have difficulty with postdischarge compliance may reasonably be given longer-acting IM steroids in the ED. High-dose inhaled corticosteroids may have some benefit in the acute setting and can be continued safely by patients already using inhaled steroids. Ipratropium, an anticholinergic agent, should be added when treating severe exacerbations to decrease the need for hospitalization, and is most effective in children and smokers. Epinephrine or terbutaline may be administered subcutaneously to patients unable to manage aerosolized treatments in severe exacerbations only. Theophylline is not recommended in the acute setting.

6. **How can I determine whether my patients are improving?**

Patients should be reassessed based upon (1) **subjective symptoms**, (2) **respiratory effort and lung sounds**, (3) **adequacy of oxygenation**, and (4) **objective measures of pulmonary function**. Either FEV_1 or PEFR

Table 29.1 Medications Used to Treat Asthma and COPD Exacerbations

MEDICATIONS	DOSAGE AND ROUTE
Inhaled Short-Acting β_2-Agonists	
Albuterol nebulizer solution (5 mg/mL)	2.5–5 mg inhaled every 20 min for three doses, then 2.5–10 mg every 1–4 h as needed; or 10–20 mg/h inhaled continuously; or 7.5 mg inhaled once
Albuterol MDI (90 μg/puff): *Must be used with spacer device*	4–8 puffs every 20 min up to 4 h, then every 1–4 h as needed
Systemic (Injected) β_2-Agonists[a]	
Epinephrine 1:1000 (1 mg/mL)	0.3–0.5 mg IM every 20 min for three doses
Terbutaline (1 mg/mL)	0.25 mg SQ every 20 min for three doses
Inhaled Anticholinergics	
Ipratropium nebulizer solution (0.25 mg/mL)	0.5 mg inhaled every 20 min for three doses, then every 2–4 h as needed
Ipratropium MDI (18 μg/puff): *Must be used with spacer device*	4–8 puffs as needed
Systemic Corticosteroids	
Prednisone or prednisolone	40–60 mg PO for 3–10 days (asthma); 40 mg PO for 5 days (COPD)
Methylprednisolone	125 mg IV or 160–240 mg IM (asthma only)
Dexamethasone	0.6 mg/kg, maximum 16 mg, PO or IM for 1–2 days
Triamcinolone	40–80 mg IM once (asthma only)

[a]Exercise extreme caution in patients with known coronary artery disease.
COPD, Chronic obstructive pulmonary disease; *MDI,* metered dose inhaler.

(the best of three attempts) should be obtained on presentation and after treatment and be compared with each patient's predicted or personal best FEV_1 or PEFR to determine the need for more aggressive therapy or hospitalization. Patients with incomplete response to initial medical therapies should be reassessed over 4–6 hours to determine the most appropriate disposition.

7. **What measures are available if my patient is not responding as expected?**
Magnesium, heliox, ketamine, and continuous positive-pressure ventilation may offer some benefits when conventional therapy has failed and patients remain in severe status asthmaticus. Intravenous magnesium sulfate, in conjunction with standard therapy, has been shown to reduce hospital admission in patients presenting with moderate to severe asthma exacerbation. Although widely discussed in the literature, the data for ketamine, heliox, and continuous positive-pressure ventilation are less compelling. Although it is often used with anecdotal success, data supporting use of noninvasive ventilation is lacking, particularly in reducing the need for intubation. Additionally, despite often being used for exacerbations of COPD, there is inconclusive evidence that antibiotics improve symptoms or objective measures of asthma exacerbation.

The only absolute indications for intubation during asthma exacerbations are apnea and coma. Relative indications for intubation include exhaustion, worsening respiratory distress, persistent or increasing hypercapnia, and depressed consciousness. Intubate semielectively, before the crisis of respiratory arrest, because intubation is often difficult in patients who have asthma. Patients should be sufficiently volume resuscitated to prevent periintubation hypotension. Once intubated, mechanical ventilation of patients with acute asthma presents special challenges, such as development of intrinsic positive end-expiratory pressure (auto-PEEP) and barotrauma (see Chapter 28). Patients should be ventilated with a strategy of permissive hypercapnia, targeting neutral to mildly acidotic pH and correction of hypoxemia over correction of hypercapnia.

8. **How should I decide whether a patient can be discharged or requires hospitalization?**
Disposition of patients is usually determined by their clinical response after up to three doses of aerosolized β_2-agonist therapy, ipratropium (if used), and corticosteroids. If patients have clear breath sounds, are no longer dyspneic or are back to baseline, and have an FEV_1 or PEFR that is at least 70% of predicted, they may be safely discharged home. Patients with an incomplete response to treatment (FEV_1 between 40% and 70% of predicted and mild dyspnea) can be considered for discharge after shared decision making. When feasible, observation for 4–6 hours after steroid administration can decrease the number of inpatient admissions and overall cost. Patients with a poor response to bronchodilators (FEV_1 less than 40% of predicted and continued moderate to severe symptoms after treatment) should be hospitalized.

9. **What should be considered at time of discharge?**
Patients who received corticosteroids acutely should continue oral steroid therapy at home for 3–10 days. For such brief courses of medication, no taper is required. Dosing parameters are controversial, so choose a moderate regimen – from 40 to 60 mg of prednisone per day. Alternatively, patients may similarly benefit from a single dose of IM corticosteroids in the ED if they are expected to have difficulty complying with outpatient oral therapy. All patients should be advised to use their short-acting β-agonists on a regularly scheduled basis for a few days and then as needed. Daily inhaled corticosteroids are now standard of care for asthma control, so patients with persistent asthma not previously on a regimen should be started on one. Patient education such as a "personalized asthma action plan" should be provided at discharge to reduce recidivism, as should instructions to make an appointment for a follow-up visit within several weeks for further long-term management of their disease.

10. **Does pregnancy change the management of acute asthma?**
No, pregnant women should receive standard therapy and dosages for asthma exacerbations. Patients should not be undertreated because of fear of teratogenicity, as the risks from respiratory failure and severe acute asthma are greater than from therapy with standard medications.

KEY POINTS: EMERGENCY TREATMENT OF ASTHMA

1. Relieve significant hypoxemia: Supplemental oxygen.
2. Reverse airflow obstruction: β-agonists and ipratropium.
3. Reduce the likelihood of recurrence: Early corticosteroids.
4. Provide objective measure of improvement: PEFR or FEV_1.
5. Provide adequate discharge planning: Education, medications, and follow-up care.

CHRONIC OBSTRUCTIVE PULMONARY DISEASE

11. **What is COPD, and what are the presenting symptoms of a COPD exacerbation?**
COPD is a disease characterized by **chronic airflow limitation** that is **progressive** and **not fully reversible**, associated with an abnormal inflammatory response to noxious particles or gases. Obstruction results from a combination of small airways disease and parenchymal destruction. COPD includes emphysema and chronic bronchitis, and it can overlap with asthma. The characteristic symptoms of COPD are **dyspnea**, **cough**, and

Box 29.1 COPD Differentiations per the Global Initiative for Chronic Obstructive Lung Disease (GOLD) Guidelines

GOLD I (mild)	$FEV_1 \geq 80\%$ of predicted
GOLD II (moderate)	$50\% \leq FEV_1 < 80\%$ of predicted
GOLD III (severe)	$30\% \leq FEV_1 < 50\%$ of predicted
GOLD IV (very severe)	$FEV_1 \leq 30\%$ of predicted

COPD, Chronic obstructive pulmonary disease; *FEV₁,* forced expiratory volume in 1 second.
From *2020 Global Strategy for Prevention, Diagnosis and Management of COPD.* Available at: https://goldcopd.org/gold-reports/. Accessed June 1, 2019.

sputum production. Tobacco smoking, exposure to occupational dusts and chemicals, genetic predisposition, and air pollution are the most common causes of COPD.

The formal diagnosis of COPD is made with spirometry, when the ratio of FEV_1 to forced vital capacity (FVC) following bronchodilator therapy is less than 70% of that predicted for a matched control. Differentiation of mild, moderate, and severe COPD relies on the FEV_1 and is staged per the Global Initiative for Chronic Obstructive Lung Disease (GOLD) guidelines shown in Box 29.1.

Exacerbations are characterized by increased airway inflammation, mucus production, and gas trapping, and are most often triggered by lower respiratory tract infections. These episodes are associated with **increased dyspnea**, often accompanied by **wheezing** and **chest tightness**, **increased cough and sputum**, and **change in color or thickness of sputum**.

12. **In addition to COPD, what should be included in the differential diagnosis?**
    In patients with wheezing:
    - CHF with cardiogenic pulmonary edema
    - pneumonia
    - asthma
    - bronchitis
    - foreign body aspiration
    - anaphylaxis

    In those who have dyspnea:
    - pulmonary embolism
    - pneumothorax
    - pneumonia
    - acute coronary syndrome
    - CHF
    - pericardial effusion $\pm$ cardiac tamponade
    - asthma
    - acute respiratory distress syndrome (ARDS)
    - pulmonary fibrosis
    - pleural effusion
    - metabolic disturbances such as severe acidosis
    - anemia
    - shock

13. **Which diagnostic tests are helpful in the management of COPD?**
    Diagnosing COPD as a chronic disease without formal PFTs is generally not possible in the ED. In contrast to asthma, spirometry measurements such as PEFR are less accurate diagnostic tools in the emergency setting. Pulse oximetry should be used in every patient with COPD, as titrated oxygen delivery improves mortality. Arterial blood gas measurements are useful to confirm hypercapnia and respiratory acidosis as a baseline for therapeutic endpoints, especially if compared with the patient's baseline values. Alternatively, venous blood gas measurements offer a good correlation to arterial pH, and venous partial pressure of carbon dioxide (pCO_2) ≤ 45 mmHg effectively rules out arterial hypercarbia. End tidal carbon dioxide ($ETCO_2$) measurements correlate well with the severity of carbon dioxide (CO_2) retention and cannot reliably be used in place of blood gas analysis.

    Chest radiographs are often appropriate in COPD exacerbations to help manage complications and concomitant disease, such as pneumothorax or pneumonia. Bedside ultrasound can also be used to differentiate alternative causes of dyspnea or to evaluate for complicating processes. In patients with *cor pulmonale*, continuous cardiac monitoring may identify any associated dysrhythmias. Although B-type natriuretic peptide (BNP) measurement does not reliably distinguish between CHF and COPD, elevated levels portend worse prognosis in patients admitted with respiratory failure. Testing to evaluate for pulmonary embolism is often warranted, particularly in patients with intermediate-to-high pretest probability or exacerbation requiring hospitalization.

Focused viral testing should be considered based on seasonal trends, as there is some evidence that patients with COPD benefit from neuraminidase inhibitors for influenza – except for zanamivir, which is associated with increased risk of bronchospasm. Sputum cultures rarely change management of true COPD exacerbations, and are, in general, not indicated.

14. **What are the key objectives when treating a COPD exacerbation, and how are they achieved?**
The key objectives are to (1) **ensure adequate oxygenation**, (2) **reverse airway obstruction**, (3) **treat infection if present**, and (4) **prevent invasive mechanical ventilation**. The cornerstone of initial management is treating hypoxia with supplemental oxygen, with a goal of oxygen saturation of 88%–92%. Excessive supplemental oxygen in patients with hypercapnic respiratory failure is theorized to reduce hypoxemia-induced ventilatory drive and is associated with worse outcomes. Despite adequate oxygen saturation, CO_2 retention owing to the obstructive nature of the disease can occur insidiously with little change in symptoms, necessitating close monitoring with repeated blood gas measurements in critically ill COPD patients. Administration of intermittent doses of aerosolized short-acting β_2-agonists, with or without anticholinergics such as ipratropium, are the main treatment regimen aimed to relieve airflow obstruction. Systemic corticosteroids should be given orally or parenterally, as they reduce the likelihood of treatment failure and hospital length of stay, but their use should be weighed against risk of steroid-related adverse events for patients with frequent exacerbations. Methylxanthines (theophylline, aminophylline) are generally not recommended due to their side-effect profiles; however, they may be considered when there is inadequate response to short-acting bronchodilators. Neither heliox nor magnesium (either IV or nebulized) have been shown to provide benefit in COPD exacerbations, in contrast to their use in acute asthma.

15. **How should the patient with respiratory failure be managed?**
Noninvasive positive-pressure ventilation (NIPPV) modalities such as continuous positive airway pressure (CPAP) and bilevel positive airway pressure (BiPAP) often can obviate the need for intubation by improving gas exchange, decreasing hypoxia, and reducing work of breathing. NIPPV is a well-studied means of decreasing hospital length of stay, intubation rates, and mortality in COPD exacerbations. High-flow nasal cannula (HFNC) is an emerging respiratory modality that may improve both hypoxemic and hypercapnic respiratory failure, but it has not been sufficiently studied in regard to patient-centered outcomes. Indications for invasive mechanical ventilation include inability to tolerate NIPPV or nonresponse to NIPPV, as evidenced by diminished consciousness, refractory hypoxemia, severe respiratory acidosis, shock, or respiratory arrest.

16. **What about antibiotics?**
Antibiotics have not been proven to deliver significant clinical benefits outside of patients admitted to the intensive care unit (ICU). However, the GOLD guidelines recommend antibiotic therapy for patients with **moderate to severe exacerbations** either (1) **requiring mechanical ventilation** or (2) with clinical signs of bacterial involvement, identified as **increased sputum purulence plus either increased sputum volume or worsened dyspnea**. The antibiotic choices should reflect local antibiotic sensitivity to common pulmonary pathogens such as *Streptococcus pneumoniae, Haemophilus influenzae,* and *Moraxella catarrhalis.* Guidelines for treatment of pneumonia, if present, should be considered, including exposure to methicillin-resistant *Staphylococcus aureus* (MRSA) and *Pseudomonas* species. Treatment should be continued for 5–7 days.

17. **How can I determine whether my patient is improving?**
Ask the patient how he or she feels, reexamine the patient's work of breathing and lung field aeration, and monitor his or her oxygen saturation. Measurements of respiratory acidosis and associated CO_2 retention on a blood gas demonstrate therapeutic response to bronchodilators and positive pressure ventilation. Subjective worsening should cue the need for further diagnostic studies, and periods of observation are indicated for patients who see little initial response to therapies. Failure of conservative measures may require intubation, although intubation remains a last resort intervention.

18. **How can I decide whether a patient can be discharged or requires hospitalization?**
Relapse rates remain high following COPD exacerbation, and hospitalization is associated with a 50% 5-year mortality. Unfortunately, no universally accepted discharge criteria exist for these patients. Failure of a patient's symptoms to improve in the ED, failed outpatient management, and complicating pulmonary processes are reasonable cause for hospitalization. However, patients who return to near baseline with improvement from ED treatment and have good social support systems in place may be discharged home with instructions for close follow-up monitoring.

19. **What should be considered at time of discharge?**
Patients who received corticosteroids acutely should continue oral steroid therapy at home for 5 days. There is significant heterogeneity of dosing regimens in clinical practice; however, studies to date generally support a moderate dose of corticosteroids without tapering. The GOLD guidelines suggest 40 mg of prednisone per day. Patients should continue to use their short-acting rescue medications. Adding inhaled anticholinergics plus long-acting β-agonists may improve lung function and help improve effectiveness of pulmonary rehabilitation. The

chronic use of inhaled corticosteroids is most beneficial for patients with moderate to severe COPD when used in conjunction with a long-acting β-agonist. Antibiotics should be considered as described above. Patients with resting hypoxemia should be evaluated for home oxygen therapy. Patients should be referred for pneumococcal and influenza vaccination, if not already received, to reduce mortality. Additionally, there is a demonstrated quality-of-life benefit from patients who enroll in pulmonary rehabilitation. Patient education should be provided at discharge, as should instructions to make an appointment for a follow-up visit within several days.

KEY POINTS: EMERGENCY TREATMENT OF COPD

1. Relieve significant hypoxemia: supplemental oxygen.
2. Reverse airflow obstruction: β-agonists with or without ipratropium.
3. Consider antibiotics in moderate to severe exacerbations.
4. Patients with COPD have less respiratory reserve and require admission more often than patients with asthma.
5. NIPPV may obviate the need for endotracheal intubation.
6. Adequate discharge planning includes education, medications, and careful follow-up observation, including consideration of pulmonary rehabilitation if available.

PNEUMONIA

20. **What is pneumonia, and what are the presenting symptoms of pneumonia?**
    Pneumonia is defined as an infection of the alveolar spaces of the lung. It commonly develops via inhalation or microaspiration of infectious particles or macroaspiration of oropharyngeal or gastric contents; less commonly, it occurs through hematogenous spread of infection, direct invasion from contiguous structures, direct inoculation, or reactivation of prior disease. Predisposing factors to developing pneumonia include:
    - impaired swallowing/airway protection
    - extremes of age
    - underlying lung parenchymal disease
    - chest wall disorders, including recent thoracic trauma
    - neuromuscular respiratory weakness
    - immunocompromise
    - recent hospitalization

      Overall, it is the seventh leading cause of death and the leading cause of death from infectious disease in the United States. The ED serves as the point of entry for the majority of these admissions. When patients are properly identified and treated as outpatients, the mortality of community-acquired pneumonia (CAP) decreases significantly. The role of the emergency physician is to diagnose pneumonia accurately, initiate timely antibiotic therapy, and make an appropriate disposition.

      Signs consistent with pneumonia include the following:
    - fever
    - tachypnea
    - tachycardia
    - decreased oxygen saturation
    - altered mental status, in cases of severe illness

      The physical examination may show evidence of alveolar fluid (inspiratory rales), consolidation (bronchial breath sounds), pleural effusion (dullness and decreased breath sounds), or bronchial congestion (rhonchi and wheezing).

21. **In addition to pneumonia, what should be considered on the differential diagnosis?**
    - CHF
    - Asthma
    - Bronchitis
    - Foreign body aspiration
    - Anaphylaxis
    - Pulmonary embolism
    - Pneumothorax
    - Acute coronary syndrome
    - Pericardial effusion ± cardiac tamponade
    - ARDS
    - Pulmonary fibrosis
    - Pleural effusion
    - Complications of pneumonia such as empyema or lung abscess
    - Metabolic disturbances such as severe acidosis
    - Shock

22. **What diagnostic studies are useful?**

Although some providers will treat healthy, low-risk patients with suspected pneumonia empirically, others feel a chest radiograph is mandatory in every patient with a history and symptoms suggestive of pneumonia. It is difficult to identify a set of specific criteria for ordering a chest radiograph, but all patients who have a cough do not need chest radiography. Clinical judgment must be used along with the presence of clinical indicators. The American Thoracic Society (ATS) and the Infectious Diseases Society of America (IDSA) suggest that a radiographically evident pulmonary infiltrate is required for the diagnosis of pneumonia. When chest radiography shows multifocal infiltrates, concomitant effusion, or abscess, or when alternate differential diagnoses such as pulmonary embolism are of high concern, computed tomography (CT) of the chest with contrast may better delineate intrathoracic pathology.

Although no tests are required in the management of patients with presumed pneumonia, some are more valuable than others. For example, an arterial or venous blood gas may augment the information obtained through pulse oximetry to assess the need for respiratory support. A complete blood count is frequently ordered to assess for concomitant anemia, while the white blood cell count is often used to assess severity of infection, although without much scientific evidence. A chemistry panel is also frequently ordered to identify electrolyte abnormalities or multiorgan dysfunction. Notably, results from these three tests are used in mortality risk prediction scores.

23. **Are there any newer tests to reduce unnecessary antibiotic use?**

Procalcitonin, a relatively new biomarker, is hypothesized to estimate bacterial-related inflammation and shows promise in guiding antibiotic therapy. As elevated procalcitonin levels are seen in bacterial infections, lower levels are more commonly associated with viral sources of pneumonia. Coupled with expanded viral diagnostics, future trends may be towards lower procalcitonin levels being treated without antibiotics. Despite initial evidence of this algorithm being an effective strategy, no current guidelines have been approved for implementation. Additionally, the turnaround time of a procalcitonin test remains a limiting factor for use in many ED settings.

24. **What is the role of microbiologic testing in evaluation of pneumonia?**

The value of the Gram stain for expectorated sputum is controversial, because it is uncertain how accurately expectorated sputum reflects lower respiratory tract secretions and pathology. Gram stain is commonly negative for specific organisms, and the results rarely change therapy. Gram stain may be more useful in high-risk or hospitalized patients and should be considered in this group. The use of sputum with other stains (such as acid-fast stains for mycobacteria) and techniques such as direct fluorescent antibody staining have a continuing and developing role, but are probably not helpful in ED management.

The utility of blood cultures to determine causative agents in unselected patients with CAP is only 5%–14% and rarely alters therapy for patients coming to the ED with pneumonia. More discriminatory use may potentially reduce resource utilization. However, in patients with severe symptoms or significant risk factors, blood cultures may demonstrate uncommon causative organisms or unexpected antibiotic resistance. The therapeutic benefit in noncritical patients of both Gram stains and cultures are questionable, but for patients that are critically ill or who have nosocomial pneumonia, both are still recommended by the ATS/IDSA.

New diagnostic modalities such as urine antigen testing and viral respiratory polymerase chain reaction (PCR) show some promise, with mixed sensitivity and specificity in available studies, but the implications on clinical practice are still unclear. However, their use may guide appropriate antibiotic therapy earlier in a patient's course.

25. **What are the clinical differences between community-acquired and nosocomial (hospital-acquired) pneumonias?**

Nosocomial pneumonias are rising rapidly, and in some cases, may account for 17% of pneumonias when patients return to the ED. Patients who develop a hospital-acquired pneumonia (HAP) have an attributable mortality of 27%–50%. The most recent IDSA/ATS guidelines strictly differentiate HAP and ventilator-acquired pneumonia (VAP) from CAP. HAP is defined as a pneumonia (1) not incubating at the time of hospital admission and (2) occurring 48 hours or more after admission. VAP is defined as a pneumonia occurring >48 hours after endotracheal intubation. CAP, by default, is all other pneumonias. Of note, the prior distinction of health care–acquired pneumonia (HCAP) is no longer specifically delineated, as in recent studies, the other patient characteristics, settings, and exposures align more with CAP-associated pathogens rather than drug-resistant organisms as previously supposed.

The causative organism is unknown in 30%–50% of patients with CAP. In those patients for whom the causative organism is known, *Streptococcus pneumoniae* is by far the most common agent. During hospitalization, exposure to more virulent organisms changes the pattern of infection. Gram-negative bacilli, particularly *Klebsiella* spp., *Pseudomonas aeruginosa*, and *Escherichia coli*, are responsible for more than 50% of these cases. *Staphylococcus aureus* accounts for another 10%–20% of HAPs and tends to be associated with more severe cases. The remainder of HAP cases are usually caused by anaerobic oral flora, *Streptococcus pneumoniae*, *Legionella* spp., and *Moraxella catarrhalis* (each accounting for <10% of cases).

26. **What treatments are indicated for pneumonia?**

Supportive care, including supplemental oxygen, NIPPV, or endotracheal intubation, should be provided as required. Rehydration, antipyretics, and pain control should also be started as needed. Antibiotic therapy, based on the most likely pathogens, should be initiated as soon as the diagnosis of pneumonia is made or strongly suspected. Studies have shown a decreased mortality and length of stay in a group of patients admitted for CAP when antibiotics were administered within 4–8 hours of arrival. All patients being admitted for pneumonia from the ED should receive their first dose of antibiotics before transfer to a hospital floor or ICU.

The choice of antibiotic is based on the site of treatment, suspected pathogens, and ability to tolerate oral medications. The antimicrobial suggestions in Table 29.2 should be used in consideration with the clinical picture, recent literature, local preference, and resistance patterns. Increasing evidence has strengthened the recommendation for combination empiric therapy for severe CAP. Presence of comorbidities, such as chronic heart, lung, liver, or renal disease; diabetes mellitus; alcoholism; malignancies; asplenia; and immunosuppressing conditions all influence the empiric choice of antimicrobials. Bronchodilator treatment has not been shown to benefit patients in the absence of reactive airways disease, but steroids have shown promise as an adjunctive treatment in pneumonia, decreasing mortality in severe CAP and decreasing duration of stay in CAP. Despite this evidence, steroids are still not a guideline-recommended therapy for pneumonia.

Table 29.2 Empiric Antimicrobial Therapy for Community-Acquired Pneumonia in Immunocompetent Adults

PATIENT/SETTING	COMMON PATHOGENS	IDSA/ATS CONSENSUS 2007 EMPIRIC THERAPY
Outpatient Previously healthy 　AND No comorbid diseases	*Streptococcus pneumoniae* *Mycoplasma pneumoniae* *Chlamydia pneumoniae* *Haemophilus influenzae* Viruses	Macrolide OR Doxycycline
Outpatient Presence of comorbid disease 　OR Antibiotic therapy within past 　3 months	*S. pneumoniae* (drug resistant) *M. pneumoniae* *C. pneumoniae* *H. influenzae* Viruses Gram-negative bacilli[b]	β-Lactam plus macrolide OR Respiratory fluoroquinolone[a]
Inpatient Not severely ill	*Staphylococcus aureus*[b] *S. pneumoniae* *H. influenzae* Polymicrobial Anaerobes *S. aureus* *C. pneumoniae* Viruses	Antipneumococcal β-lactam plus 　macrolide OR Respiratory fluoroquinolone
Inpatient Severely ill	*S. pneumoniae* *Legionella* spp. Gram-negative bacilli *M. pneumoniae* Viruses *S. aureus*	Antipneumococcal β-lactam plus 　azithromycin OR Antipneumococcal β-lactam plus 　respiratory fluoroquinolone
	Pseudomonas suspected	Antipneumococcal, antipseudomonal 　β-lactam plus ciprofloxacin/ 　levofloxacin OR Antipneumococcal, antipseudomonal 　β-lactam plus aminoglycoside plus 　azithromycin OR Antipneumococcal, antipseudomonal 　β-lactam plus aminoglycoside plus 　respiratory fluoroquinolone
	MRSA suspected[b]	Add vancomycin OR linezolid

[a]In the outpatient setting, many authorities prefer to reserve fluoroquinolones for patients with comorbid diseases/risk factors.
[b]In most cases, patients with pneumonias caused by these organisms should be hospitalized.
ATS, American Thoracic Society; *IDSA,* Infectious Diseases Society of America; *MRSA,* methicillin-resistant *Staphylococcus aureus.*

27. Where should patients be treated for pneumonia?

Once a diagnosis of pneumonia is strongly suspected and treatment initiated, the next decision is whether the patient is appropriate for discharge or requires hospital admission. Risk stratification scores, such as the CURB-65 criteria (Box 29.2; Table 29.3), or prognostic models, such as the Pneumonia Severity of Illness (PSI) score, are useful disposition aids. The PSI uses a combination of 20 parameters to evaluate patients, assign disease severity and mortality risk, and guide disposition (Tables 29.4 and 29.5; Box 29.3). Because of its prognostic accuracy,

---

Box 29.2 CURB-65 Score

Characteristic (+1 for Each)
- Confusion
- Blood urea nitrogen (BUN) >19 mg/dL
- Respiratory rate >30 per minute
- Systolic blood pressure (BP) <90 mmHg or diastolic BP ≤60 mmHg
- Age ≥65 years

Table 29.3 Using CURB-65 to Guide Disposition

SCORE	MORTALITY (%)	RECOMMENDED DISPOSITION
≤1	1.5	Outpatient
2	9.2	Inpatient versus observation
≥3	22	Inpatient

Table 29.4 Pneumonia Severity of Index (PSI) Score

PSI CHARACTERISTIC	POINTS GIVEN FOR PRESENCE OF CHARACTERISTIC
Age	Age in Years
Demographics	
Female sex	−10
Nursing home resident	+10
Coexisting Illnesses	
Neoplastic disease	+30
Liver disease	+20
CHF	+10
Cerebrovascular disease (TIA or CVA)	+10
Renal disease	+10
Physical Examination Findings	
Acute disorientation, stupor, or coma	+20
Respiratory rate ≥30 per minute	+20
Systolic blood pressure <90 mmHg	+20
Temperature <35°C or ≥40°C	+15
Heart rate ≥125 beats per minute	+10
Laboratory and Radiographic Findings (If Study Performed)	
Arterial pH <7.35	+30
Blood urea nitrogen ≥30 mg/dL	+20
Sodium <130 mmol/L	+20
Glucose ≥250 mg/dL	+10
Hematocrit <30%	+10
PaO_2 <60 mmHg or SpO_2 <90%	+10
Pleural effusion on chest x-ray	+10

CHF, Congestive heart failure; *CVA,* cerebrovascular accident; *TIA,* transient ischemic attack.

Table 29.5 Pneumonia Severity of Index (PSI) Class and Mortality[a]

PSI SCORE	CLASS	MORTALITY (%)	DISPOSITION
<51	I	0.1	Outpatient
51–70	II	0.6	Outpatient
71–90	III	0.9	Outpatient or observation
91–130	IV	9.5	Inpatient
>130	V	26.7	Inpatient

[a]Patients younger than 50 years and without any comorbid illnesses or vital sign abnormalities fall into class I. Patients not falling into risk class I require additional laboratory testing so that they may be assigned to risk classes II–V.

Box 29.3 Other Factors That Impact Disposition Decision

- Patient's clinical appearance
- Patient's ability to tolerate oral intake
- Patient's reliability
- Social factors, such as home support and ability to obtain antibiotics
- Clinical judgment of the physician (most important)

---

effectiveness, and safety as a decision aid, the PSI has become the reference standard for risk stratification. However, the CURB-65 criteria are still used in many hospitals due to simplicity of calculation. Although there are no clear guidelines for admission to an ICU, several rules have been published. In total, evidence to date suggests that less-restrictive ICU admission criteria for pneumonia may be associated with improved outcomes.

28. **What should be considered at time of discharge?**
    Antibiotics remain the mainstay of discharge treatment from the ED. Aside from appropriate duration and coverage for presumed pathogens, patient compliance and ability to obtain antibiotics need to be factored into the discussion. Symptomatic therapy, such as antitussives, decongestants, and mucolytics, have not shown any proven benefit, although there is also no evidence of harm. As such, the prescription of these adjuncts is left to provider discretion. All patients with pneumonia require follow-up to assure improvement. Patients with persistent or worsening symptoms need reevaluation for inadequate antibiotic coverage versus an alternate diagnosis.

KEY POINTS: EMERGENCY TREATMENT OF PNEUMONIA

1. Begin empiric treatment early based on suspected pathogens.
2. Support oxygenation, ventilation, and circulation as indicated by the patient's condition.
3. Consider classification of pneumonia to predict associated pathogens and guide antibiotic therapy.
4. Calculation of the PSI or CURB-65 scores reliably predicts mortality and assists with disposition decisions.

BIBLIOGRAPHY

Asthma

Kew KM, Kirtchuk L, Michell CI. Intravenous magnesium sulfate for treating adults with acute asthma in the emergency department. *Cochrane Database Syst Rev.* 2014;(5):CD010909.

McCracken JL, Veeranki SP, Ameredes BT, et al. Diagnosis and management of asthma in adults: a review. *JAMA.* 2017;318(3): 279–290.

Stefan MS, Shieh MS, Spitzer KA, et al. Association of antibiotic treatment with outcomes in patients hospitalized for an asthma exacerbation treated with systemic corticosteroids. *JAMA Intern Med.* 2019;179(3):333–339.

COPD

Global Initiative for Chronic Obstructed Lung Disease. *2020 Global Strategy for Prevention, Diagnosis and Management of COPD.* Available at: https://goldcopd.org/gold-reports/. Accessed June 1, 2019.

Osadnik CR, Tee VS, Carson-Chahhoud KV, et al. Non-invasive ventilation for the management of acute hypercapnic respiratory failure due to exacerbation of chronic obstructive pulmonary disease. *Cochrane Database Syst Rev.* 2017;7(8860):CD004104.

Vollenweider DJ, Frei A, Steurer-Stey CA, et al. Antibiotics for exacerbations of chronic obstructive pulmonary disease. Cochrane Airways Group, ed. *Cochrane Database Syst Rev.* 2018;10(3):CD010257.

Pneumonia

Guillon A, Aymeric S, Gaudy-Graffin C, et al. Impact on the medical decision-making process of multiplex PCR assay for respiratory pathogens. *Epidemiol Infect.* 2017;145(13):2766–2769.

Kalil AC, Metersky ML, Klompas M, et al. Management of adults with hospital-acquired and ventilator-associated pneumonia: 2016 clinical practice guidelines by the Infectious Diseases Society of America and the American Thoracic Society. *Clin Infect Dis.* 2016;63(5):e61–e111.

Mandell LA, Niederman MS. Aspiration pneumonia. *N Engl J Med.* 2019;380(7):651–663.

Stern A, Skalsky K, Avni T, et al. Corticosteroids for pneumonia. Cochrane Acute Respiratory Infections Group, ed. *Cochrane Database Syst Rev.* 2017;12(9977):CD007720.

Wunderink RG. Guidelines to manage community-acquired pneumonia. *Clin Chest Med.* 2018;39(4):726–761.

CHAPTER 30

VENOUS THROMBOEMBOLISM

Stephen J. Wolf, MD and Mario Andres Camacho, MD

1. **What is the Virchow triad of thromboembolism?**
   Venous stasis, vascular trauma, and hypercoagulable state

2. **What two diseases represent the continuum of venous thromboembolism (VTE)?**
   Deep venous thrombosis (DVT) and pulmonary embolism (PE)

3. **What percentage of patients diagnosed with DVT have concomitant PE when studied?**
   Fifty percent. Additionally, a similar percentage of patients with a diagnosed PE will have a concomitant DVT when studied.

4. **What are major risk factors for VTE?**
   - History of VTE
   - Immobilization (equivalent to bed rest ≥3 days)
   - Malignancy (treatment active, within 6 months, or palliative)
   - Postpartum (for up to 42 days)
   - Pregnancy (third > second > first trimester)
   - Recent surgery (≤4 weeks)
   - Major trauma

5. **List other minor risk factors for VTE.**
   - Advanced age
   - Cardiovascular disease (e.g., heart failure or congenital heart disease)
   - Circulating antiphospholipid antibodies (associated with systemic lupus erythematosus)
   - Estrogen use (e.g., hormone replacement or oral contraceptives)
   - Indwelling vascular access
   - Inflammatory bowel disease (i.e., Crohn disease, ulcerative colitis)
   - Inherited thrombophilia (i.e., antithrombin III deficiency, factor V Leyden thrombophilia, protein C or S deficiency, and prothrombin gene mutation)
   - HIV
   - Obesity
   - Neurologic disease (e.g., cerebrovascular event, paralysis)
   - Renal disease (e.g., chronic kidney disease, end-stage renal disease, dialysis, nephrotic syndrome, or renal transplant)

6. **Are there any signs or symptoms of PE that are diagnostic?**
   No, although the common clinical signs and symptoms of shortness of breath, chest pain, tachypnea, and tachycardia occur in upward of 97% of patients diagnosed with PE, they are nonspecific. Patient symptoms can range from mild shortness of breath to cardiovascular collapse.

7. **Why is a clinician's pretest probability for VTE so important?**
   Because no diagnostic test available for the evaluation of VTE is absolute (with a perfect sensitivity and specificity), the results of any given test must be considered in combination with the clinician's pretest probability to yield a posttest likelihood of disease. Thus, the pretest probability should be used to determine when to initiate a patient workup and how to interpret the results of any test. See Fig. 30.1 for a sample algorithm.

8. **When determining pretest probability for DVT, what are the Wells criteria?**
   - Malignancy (+1 point)
   - Paralysis/paresis/casted lower extremity (+1 point)
   - Recent immobilization or surgery (+1 point)
   - Tenderness along deep veins (+1 point)
   - Swelling of entire leg (+1 point)
   - 3-cm difference in calf circumference (+1 point)
   - Pitting edema (+1 point)
   - Collateral superficial veins (+1 point)
   - Alternative diagnosis more likely than DVT (−2 points)

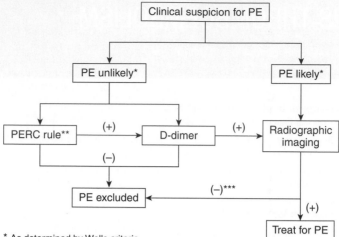

Fig. 30.1 Sample algorithm for the clinical suspicion for PE. *PE,* Pulmonary embolism; *PERC,* pulmonary embolism rule-out criteria.

9. **Once I have calculated a patient's Wells score for DVT, how do I interpret it?**
Using the Wells criteria for suspected DVT, patients are considered to have low (<2 points), moderate (2–6 points), or high (>6 points) pretest probability for a DVT. This correlates to an incidence of DVT of 3%, 17%, and 75%, respectively. Patients with a Wells score for DVT of less than 2 points are *DVT unlikely* and good candidates for a screening D-dimer.

10. **What is the pulmonary embolism rule-out criteria (PERC) rule for PE?**
PERC is a clinical decision rule that can be used to identify low pretest probability patients who do not require a laboratory or radiograph workup to exclude the diagnosis of PE. The criteria include:
- age younger than 50 years
- heart rate less than 100 beats per minute
- initial room air oxygen saturation level (SaO$_2$) greater than 94% at sea level
- no unilateral leg swelling
- no hemoptysis
- no recent surgery or trauma
- no history of VTE
- no exogenous estrogen use

11. **How do I use the PERC rule?**
In patients with a low gestalt clinical suspicion for PE, if all criteria are met, the patient has a less than 2% risk of PE, and further workup is not indicated. Patients with clinical suspicion who do not meet all criteria may require further evaluation. In patients with moderate or high clinical suspicion for PE, the PERC rule does not rule out PE.

12. **When determining pretest probability for PE, what are the Wells criteria?**
- Signs/symptoms of DVT (+3 points)
- No alterative diagnosis more likely than PE (+3 points)
- Heart rate greater than 100 beats per minute (+1.5 points)
- Recent immobilization or surgery (+1.5 points)
- History of previous VTE (+1.5 points)
- Hemoptysis (+1.0 point)
- Malignancy (+1.0 point)

13. **Once I have calculated the total Wells score for PE, how do I interpret it?**
Using the Wells criteria for suspected PE, patients can be considered to have low (<2 points), moderate (2–6 points), or high (>6 points) pretest probability for a PE. This correlates to an incidence of PE of 4%, 21%, and 67%, respectively.

Using a dichotomous approach, patients with a Wells score for PE of ≤4 points are considered *PE unlikely* and good candidates for a screening D-dimer test. Patients with a Wells score >4 are *PE likely,* requiring further study.

14. **What other clinical decision rules or PE management pathways have been validated to stratify patients with suspected VTE for risk?**
The Geneva score, Revised Geneva score, Charlotte criteria, Pisa model, and YEARS algorithm are other risk-stratification scoring systems that can be used to determine pretest probability in patients with suspected PE.

15. **What is a D-dimer test? How is it used?**
D-dimer, a degradation product of cross-linked fibrin, is found in increased levels of the circulation of patients with acute VTE. There are different assays available for measuring D-dimer with different sensitivities and specificities, including enzyme-linked immunosorbent assay (ELISA), rapid ELISA, turbidimetric assay, and whole-blood agglutination D-dimer assay. Different tests can report results as either fibrin equivalent units or D-dimer units. Older latex agglutination tests cannot be used in these algorithms because of poor negative predictive values. Although useful in ruling out VTE disease in select populations, owing to a lack of specificity, D-dimer has not proven useful at ruling in the diagnosis.

16. **Which patients can have VTE excluded, based on a negative D-dimer?**
Only patients considered to be DVT or PE unlikely (i.e., those with low to low-moderate pretest probability for disease) can have VTE excluded based on a D-dimer result. You would miss the diagnosis anywhere from 5% to 20% (depending on the type of assay) of the time if you used a negative D-dimer to rule out VTE in a patient with a higher pretest probability.

17. **Can the D-dimer cutoff value be adjusted for age?**
In patients older than 50 years, with low to low-moderate pretest probability for VTE, PE can be ruled out with an age-adjusted D-dimer. For D-dimer assays using fibrin equivalent units, use a cutoff of age $\times$ 10 $\mu g/L$. For assays using D-dimer units, use age $\times$ 5 $\mu g/L$.

18. **What are some clinical situations that cause a false-positive D-dimer test, lending to a decreased specificity?**
Advanced age, sepsis, disseminated intravascular coagulation (DIC), aortic dissection, pregnancy, recent surgery, and severe trauma

19. **What are two clinical situations that might cause a false-negative D-dimer result?**
Subacute thrombosis (>7 days) and recent anticoagulation

20. **What noninvasive imaging methods are available for the diagnosis of DVT?**
- Duplex ultrasound: Although often the test of choice, the sensitivity and specificity are operator dependent and related to patient symptomatology. Ultrasound can detect more than 95% of acute symptomatic proximal DVTs. However, its specificity for acute thrombosis decreases in the settings of chronic or recurrent VTE. Additionally, three-point compression Point of Care Ultrasound (POCUS) performed by emergency department (ED) clinicians looking for DVT have reported sensitivities >90%.
- Spiral multirow detector computed tomography venography (CTV): Although not often used in isolation, this modality has a sensitivity and specificity comparable to ultrasound. Venography is most often used in combination with a CT angiogram of the chest to increase the sensitivity of an evaluation for PE.
- Other less-used tests include magnetic resonance imaging (MRI) venography (useful in patients with contraindication to radiation or contrast dye), radio-fibrinogen leg scanning, and impedance plethysmography.

21. **Can a single duplex ultrasound exclude DVT in isolation?**
No. In patients with a moderate to high pretest probability for DVT, a negative D-dimer test or a repeat duplex ultrasound in 5–7 days is indicated to definitively exclude the diagnosis.

22. **Are there classic chest radiography findings in patients with PE?**
No. The chest radiograph may be normal in up to 30% of patients. Subtle abnormalities, such as focal atelectasis, slight elevation of a hemidiaphragm, or focal hyperlucency of the lung parenchyma, may be present. Local oligemia of vascular markings (Westermark sign) or a plural-based wedge-shaped infiltrate suggestive of pulmonary infarct (Hampton hump) are relatively uncommon.

23. **Are there classic electrocardiogram (ECG) findings in patients with PE?**
No, normal or near-normal ECGs with sinus tachycardia or nonspecific ST-T wave changes may be seen in up to 30% of patients. The findings classically associated with PE (i.e., S1, Q3, T3 pattern or a new right bundle-branch block) occur in less than 15% of patients and are nonspecific. Of note, precordial T-wave inversions should raise significant concern for right heart strain, and in the setting of PE, indicate worse prognosis.

24. **What imaging studies can be used to evaluate PE?**
- CT angiography (CTA) is the rapid test of choice. It is highly sensitive and specific in diagnosing central or segmental emboli and other intrathoracic pathology. However, it is not as sensitive in ruling out subsegmental clots. Outcomes data using newer-generation spiral multirow detector CTAs show higher sensitivities. In patients likely to have PE (i.e., those with moderate to high pretest probability), the sensitivity of a negative CTA can be improved with the finding of a negative CT venogram, lower extremity duplex ultrasound, or a D-dimer assay.

- Traditionally, a normal ventilation/perfusion (V/Q) scan has been used to rule out a diagnosis of PE with a post-test probability of disease <4%. Likewise, a high-probability scan is considered to rule in the diagnosis. Unfortunately, upward of 60% of V/Q scans are read as nondiagnostic (low or intermediate probability), particularly if the chest radiograph is abnormal, or if the patient has underlying cardiopulmonary disease. A nondiagnostic scan should be followed up with further diagnostic workup. Limitations of the V/Q scan include underlying lung pathology, technical support, availability, and interpretation variability.
- Other less frequently used studies include pulmonary angiogram and magnetic resonance angiogram (MRA).

25. What are the relative contraindications to CTA for PE?
- Contrast dye allergy
- Renal insufficiency
- Inability to lie flat
- Severe claustrophobia
- Morbid obesity exceeding the CT scanner's weight limit
- Clinical instability

26. What are the diagnostic test options for PE with the pregnant patient?
Although less specific in pregnancy and somewhat controversial, a D-dimer test can still be sensitive for excluding the diagnosis in patients with low pretest probability. For patients requiring diagnostic imaging, it is important to recognize that both CTA and the V/Q scan carry a radiation risk to the fetus that should be discussed with the patient. CTA (without concomitant CTV) has been shown to confer lower fetal radiation doses than the V/Q scan. CTV should be avoided because of the high pelvic radiation doses. When available, MRA is a diagnostic option that carries minimal radiation risk; however, it requires cardiac and respiratory gating in addition to significantly more time. Finally, the ultrasonographic identification of DVT in pregnant patients with respiratory complaint can obviate the need for thoracic testing.

27. What happens if the diagnosis of PE is missed?
PE is listed as one of the most common causes of death in the United States, and yet only about 25% of cases are diagnosed. Of the undiagnosed 75%, a small number die within 1 hour of presentation, so it is unlikely that diagnosis and intervention could improve outcome in that group. In the rest, however, the mortality from untreated PE is approximately 30%.

28. What is a massive PE?
A massive PE can be either anatomically described as the occlusion of greater than 50% of the pulmonary vasculature, or physiologically described as an embolus that is complicated by severe cardiopulmonary distress. These two definitions are not synonymous, because a young, healthy individual can lose 50% of pulmonary circulation without significant hemodynamic compromise, whereas a patient with significant underlying cardiopulmonary disease could suffer major hemodynamic compromise with a much smaller clot.

29. What is a submassive PE?
A submassive PE is generally felt to be one that is significant enough to cause right heart strain or impaired right heart function as evidenced by abnormal brain natriuretic peptide (BNP), troponin, ECG, or right ventricular strain on echocardiogram or CT, but without systemic hypotension. Although controversy exists on how to optimally treat patients with a submassive PE, options include catheter directed thrombolysis.

30. What is the treatment for DVT?
- Anticoagulation should be started in the ED. Traditionally, patients with proximal DVTs and temporary risk factors can receive heparin as an anticoagulation agent (80 mg/kg loading dose followed by 18 mg/kg/h infusion), followed by warfarin for 3 months. Patients with calf DVTs need to be treated for only 6 weeks. Patients with permanent risk factors potentially need lifelong treatment but should take anticoagulant medication for at least 3 months.
- Low-molecular-weight heparin (LMWH) is as effective as heparin for the treatment of DVT and probably should be considered the treatment of choice based on efficacy, low side-effect profile, and cost effectiveness. Outpatient management of DVT with LMWH is commonplace and has proved safe and effective.
- In select patients with DVT, recent studies recommend non–vitamin K antagonist oral anticoagulants (novel oral anticoagulants [NOACs]) as a safe and effective alternative.

31. What is the treatment for PE?
Initial treatment of acute PE is dependent on the patient's hemodynamic stability.
- Persistently unstable patients (e.g., massive PE) should be considered for systemic thrombolytic therapy with or without embolectomy.
- The treatment of hemodynamically stable patients who have evidence of significant right heart strain (i.e., submassive PE) with systemic or catheter-directed thrombolytic therapy is more controversial and should be considered on a case-by-case basis, weighing the risks and benefits to the patient.
- Patients with poor reserve or at high risk for embolization should be considered for inpatient management.

- In hemodynamically stable patients with acute PE who are not receiving thrombolytics, early anticoagulant therapy is the primary treatment for PE and should be started in the ED. Treatment regimens have evolved, and now include NOACS and LMWH, in addition to heparin and warfarin. In select patients with PE at low risk for adverse outcomes, outpatient treatment can be considered.
- In cases with isolated subsegmental PE, no anticoagulation can be considered using shared decision making with the patient.

32. **Which patients with PE are best suited for outpatient treatment?**
The pulmonary embolism severity index (PESI) or HESTIA criteria considers age; gender; history of cancer, heart failure, or chronic lung disease; vital signs (heart rate, systolic blood pressure, respiratory rate, oxygen saturation, and temperature); and mental status. Patients scored as low risk for adverse outcomes can be considered for close outpatient management.

33. **When can an inferior vena cava filter be considered in the treatment of VTE?**
    - Contraindication to anticoagulation
    - Recurrent VTE despite adequate anticoagulation

KEY POINTS

1. Use a clinical decision rule (e.g., Wells criteria) to help stratify a patient's pretest probability of disease when interpreting diagnostic test results as evaluation for VTE in the ED.
2. Use the D-dimer assay only in patients who are classified as PE unlikely, as determined by Wells criteria, to rule out PE.
3. In low-risk patients, use the PERC rule to determine which patients can forego radiographic and laboratory evaluation to exclude PE.
4. Consider additional diagnostic testing (e.g., CTV, lower extremity duplex ultrasound, or a D-dimer) to exclude PE in high-probability patients with a negative CT angiogram of the chest for PE.
5. Consider appropriate outpatient therapy for VTE when supported by the patient's clinical condition and risk-to-benefit ratio.

BIBLIOGRAPHY

Bibas M, Biava G, Antinori A. HIV-associated venous thromboembolism. *Mediterr J Hematol Infect Dis.* 2011;3(1):e2011030.
Fesmire FM, Brown MD, Espinosa JA, et al. ACEP: clinical policy: critical issues in the evaluation and management of adult patients presenting to the emergency department with suspected pulmonary embolism. *Ann Emerg Med.* 2011;57:628–652.
Pedraza Garcia J, Valle Alonso J, Ceballos Garcia P, et al. Comparison of the accuracy of emergency department-performed point-of-care-ultrasound (POCUS) in the diagnosis of lower-extremity deep vein thrombosis. *J Emerg Med.* 2018;54(5):656–664.
Reardon PM, Patrick S, Taljaard M, et al. Diagnostic accuracy and financial implications of age-adjusted D-dimer strategies for the diagnosis of deep venous thrombosis in the emergency department. *J Emerg Med.* 2019;56(5):469–477.
Righini M, Van Es J, Den Exter PL, et al. Age-adjusted D-dimer cutoff levels to rule out pulmonary embolism: the ADJUST-PE study. *JAMA.* 2014;311(11):1117–1124.

CHAPTER 31

CONGESTIVE HEART FAILURE AND ACUTE PULMONARY EDEMA

Jeffrey Sankoff, MD

1. **What is congestive heart failure (CHF)?**
   CHF is cardiac dysfunction that leads to an inability of the heart to work as a pump to meet the circulatory demands of the patient, resulting in edema. This edema can manifest as peripheral edema, hepatic congestion, and pulmonary edema.

2. **What causes CHF?**
   CHF results from any of the following four types of processes:
   1. Restrictive (e.g., hemochromatosis and pericardial disease)
   2. Ischemic (e.g., myocardial infarction)
   3. Congestive (e.g., volume overload of the ventricle from valvular insufficiencies)
   4. Hypertrophic (e.g., long-standing hypertension or valve stenosis)

3. **Describe the symptoms of CHF.**
   Common symptoms are dyspnea (the subjective feeling of difficulty breathing) and fatigue. Early in the course of CHF, the patient reports exertional dyspnea; the heart is able to supply enough cardiac output (CO) for sedentary activities but does not have the reserve to increase CO during exercise. As heart failure worsens, even minimal activity may be difficult. Patients also report orthopnea (dyspnea relieved by assuming an erect posture), paroxysmal nocturnal dyspnea (PND) (sudden onset of dyspnea at night), and nocturia. PND has the highest positive likelihood ratio (LR+ = 2.6) for diagnosing pulmonary edema in the emergency department (ED).

KEY POINTS: CARDINAL SYMPTOMS OF CHF

1. Exertional dyspnea
2. Fatigue
3. Paroxysmal nocturnal dyspnea
4. Orthopnea

4. **What causes these symptoms?**
   When the patient with CHF assumes a supine posture, venous return from the abdomen and lower extremities is improved, increasing right ventricular CO to the pulmonary vasculature. Because of limitations in left ventricle output, pulmonary hydrostatic pressure increases. The patient has difficulty lying flat and sleeps with several pillows or sits in a chair to relieve these symptoms. Redistribution of fluid may also lead to increased urine output and nocturia. In severe CHF, this volume redistribution may be sufficient to lead to acute pulmonary edema.

5. **Name the main determinants of cardiac function in CHF.**

   $$CO = \text{Stroke volume (SV)} \times \text{Heart rate (HR)}$$

   SV is determined by:
   - preload
   - afterload
   - myocardial contractility

6. **What is preload?**
   Within limits, the amount of work cardiac muscle can do is related to the length of the muscle at the beginning of its contraction. This relationship is shown graphically by the Frank-Starling curve, in which ventricular end-diastolic volume (VEDV) represents muscle length and SV represents cardiac work (Fig. 31.1). (It is easier to measure pressure than volume, so ventricular end-diastolic pressure [VEDP] is graphed versus SV.) Thus preload is measured as VEDP. As VEDP increases, SV increases. At higher VEDPs, the increase in SV is less for a given increase in VEDP.

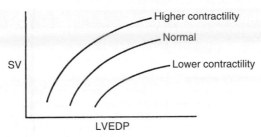

Fig. 31.1 Frank-Starling curves. *LVEDP,* Left ventricular end-diastolic pressure; *SV,* stroke volume.

7. **What are the effects of decreased contractility?**
   From Fig. 31.1, it can be seen that the heart can function on different Frank-Starling curves, depending on the contractility. A heart with better contractility will produce more CO than a heart with poorer contractility for the same preload. CHF results when the right and left ventricles begin to respond differently to similar preloads (i.e., operate on different Frank-Starling curves). If the right ventricular output for a given preload is better than the left for the same preload, the left ventricle cannot keep pace with the right. The difference in volume pumped re mains in the pulmonary vasculature, increasing hydrostatic forces and eventually leading to pulmonary edema.

8. **What about afterload?**
   Afterload refers to the pressure that the ventricle must overcome to eject blood from the heart (pressure work). The important components here are ventricular wall tension and systemic vascular resistance (SVR). As SVR increases (hypertension), the left ventricle must generate more force to push blood forward against this resistance. The result is an increase in ventricular wall tension that may compromise blood flow to myocytes. The response of the myocardium to chronic hypertension is to increase in size. This hypertrophy eventually compromises the ability of the heart to produce an adequate CO.

9. **What about HR?**
   Low HR may cause low CO even in normal hearts, because CO = SV × HR. But at excessively high HRs, there may be insufficient time to adequately fill the ventricle during diastole (diastolic filling time), leading to decreased left VEDP (LVEDP) and SV, so CO may become compromised despite the tachycardia.

10. **How does this physiology relate to treatment?**
    The goal of treatment of CHF is to improve CO. This can be accomplished by modifying each of these parameters. Diuretics, dietary salt, and water restriction decrease preload and improve volume work. Inotropic agents, such as digoxin or dobutamine, improve contractility. Vasodilators are helpful in reducing afterload and the pressure work required of the heart.

11. **Describe the role of B-type natriuretic peptides (BNPs) in CHF.**
    Natriuretic peptides are hormones produced by the heart in response to increased wall stress, and are secreted into the circulation. Pro-BNP is cleaved into BNP and amino-terminal pro-brain natriuretic peptide (NTproBNP). Both of these markers have been evaluated for their ability to predict the presence of CHF, and while each have unique properties and seem to have more favorable characteristics in specific clinical scenarios, the tests can on the whole be used interchangeably in clinical practice. BNP is an independent predictor of increased LVEDP, and levels correlate with symptoms and severity of disease. It has been suggested as a screening tool for the diagnosis of CHF in the ED, and for aiding the emergency physician in assessing the severity of CHF upon presentation. The single best instance when a BNP can be of value is in distinguishing the cause of dyspnea in a patient in whom both chronic obstructive pulmonary disease (COPD) and CHF are possibilities.

12. **How do I interpret BNP levels?**
    - Less than 100 pg/mL is unlikely to be CHF.
    - 100–500 pg/mL may be CHF.
    - 500 pg/mL is most consistent with CHF. (There is difficulty interpreting elevated BNP when a patient has known severe CHF, so their BNP should be evaluated in the context of previous BNP measurements.)

13. **How do patients with CHF appear upon arrival in the ED?**
    Patients with CHF come to the ED in one of two ways:
    1. With subacute gradual worsening, with slow progression of symptoms and signs;
    2. With an acute, dramatic change from baseline, with acute pulmonary edema.
       With respect to the first presentation, these patients tend to have evidence of worsening fluid overload, with elevated jugular venous distention and peripheral edema. They may have associated pulmonary edema as well, but it is usually mild to moderate with no respiratory distress. The second presentation is seen in patients who are generally euvolemic but have profound pulmonary edema as their main symptom.

1. Subacute, fluid overloaded
2. Acute flash pulmonary edema, euvolemic

14. **Discuss acute pulmonary edema.**
    The most dramatic presentation of CHF is acute pulmonary edema. To understand pulmonary edema, we must return to the physiologist Starling, who described the interaction of forces at the capillary membrane that lead to flow of fluid from capillaries to the interstitium. Simply put, there is a balance between hydrostatic pressure and osmotic pressure. Under normal circumstances, this leads to a small net movement of fluid from the capillaries into the lung interstitium. This fluid is carried away by lymphatics. In CHF, the left ventricular CO changes suddenly, whereas the right ventricle remains unchanged. As a result, there is a sudden increase in pulmonary vascular volume, and the capillary hydrostatic pressure increases to the point that the lymphatics no longer can handle the fluid. This then leads to interstitial edema and, subsequently, to alveolar edema.

15. **How do patients with acute pulmonary edema usually experience symptoms?**
    Patients develop acute shortness of breath and generally are fighting for air. These patients usually sit upright to decrease venous return (preload) and to redistribute edema to the dependent parts of the lungs. They may cough up frothy, red-tinged sputum. Auscultation of the lungs reveals wet rales throughout, and sometimes wheezes (resulting from bronchospasm or cardiogenic asthma). This presentation is a true emergency. Because of the stress response that this causes, patients have a large catecholamine release and are almost always very hypertensive. In these patients, hypertension is the response to, and usually not the cause of, the acute CHF. However, left unchecked, uncontrolled hypertension will result in an overall worsening.

16. **What is the treatment of acute pulmonary edema?**
    First, follow the ABCs (airway, breathing, and circulation). In severe hypoxia, airway and breathing may be compromised, requiring intubation. The use of noninvasive mask continuous or bilevel positive airway pressure (CPAP/BiPAP) has decreased the need for intubation in patients with pulmonary edema; however, this has not significantly affected in-hospital mortality. Intubation may also be avoided with prompt medical treatment. Patient symptoms can be dynamic, requiring frequent reevaluations for further medical management. Administer oxygen to maintain sufficient oxygen saturation (>90%), either by nasal cannula or nonrebreather mask, CPAP, or BiPAP. Continuously monitor oxygen saturation with pulse oximetry.

17. **What about drug therapy?**
    Drug therapy is aimed at decreasing preload. Nitrates are first-line drugs and are useful in the form of sublingual nitroglycerin (NTG) or intravenous (IV) NTG drip. NTG is predominantly a venodilator, reducing preload. However, NTG also dilates coronary arteries, and may be especially helpful in the setting of coronary artery disease. Diuretics should only be administered to patients with signs of obvious fluid overload (i.e., peripheral edema, elevated jugular venous distention). When indicated, furosemide is given as a 40-mg IV bolus (larger amounts if the patient is already taking diuretic medication, although high-dose diuretics are associated with worse outcomes). Initially, within 5–15 minutes of the injection, venodilation occurs, although this is of limited clinical benefit in the setting of nitrates. This action is followed within 30 minutes by diuresis.

1. Noninvasive mask ventilation may prevent the need for intubation.
2. Frequent reevaluation of the patient with an eye toward increasingly aggressive measures is important.
3. Nitrates are first-line pharmacotherapy.
4. Diuretic drugs should be reserved for patients with fluid overload.

18. **Are there other drugs that are useful in the treatment of acute pulmonary edema?**
    Yes, for the patient who is hypertensive, it is often helpful to lower the blood pressure (afterload). Hypertension and tachycardia generally result from reflex mechanisms because of the acute decompensation, and often correct spontaneously with the initial treatment outlined previously. With severe hypertension, nitroprusside is the treatment of choice. It is a venodilator and arterial dilator, reducing preload and afterload. Start the infusion at 10 µg/min and titrate upward every 5 minutes. It is important to monitor the blood pressure closely. If the patient becomes hypotensive, stopping the infusion causes a prompt increase in blood pressure because nitroprusside has such a short half-life. Generally, doses of 0.5–2 µg/kg/min are sufficient.

19. **What about giving positive inotropic drugs?**
    Digoxin has traditionally been used in the treatment of chronic CHF but has little role in the treatment of acute pulmonary edema. Increasingly, the effectiveness of digoxin has been questioned, even in outpatient settings. Inotropic agents that are helpful include dobutamine, dopamine, and milrinone. Dobutamine and dopamine are

positive inotropic agents. Dopamine has more alpha effect, especially at higher doses, and should be reserved for hypotensive patients. In cardiogenic shock that is refractory to these agents, milrinone infusion may be given. All of these agents may increase myocardial oxygen demand, potentially harmful in the setting of cardiac ischemia. These agents also increase myocardial irritability, thereby predisposing patients to dysrhythmias.

20. **When the initial treatment has begun, what else needs to be done?**
    After the patient's condition is stabilized, the most important next tests are a chest radiograph and electrocardiogram (ECG). Cardiac monitoring is begun; pulse oximetry is monitored continuously, and vital signs are recorded frequently. Closely monitor urine output. Attempt to discover the underlying reason for acute decompensation.

21. **Do all patients with CHF need to be admitted to the hospital?**
    Patients with a new diagnosis of CHF need an inpatient workup that includes serial cardiac enzymes and an echocardiogram. Patients with known CHF who have mild symptoms or signs may be managed on an outpatient basis, assuming that they are compliant with medications, have an appropriate home support, and attend follow-up appointments with their primary care physicians. Patients with acute pulmonary edema generally require admission.

22. **What are the usual precipitating causes of CHF exacerbations?**
    The most common cause of the subacute CHF exacerbation is undermedication, either as a result of patients not taking their medication or as a result of a change in medication under a physician's supervision. Dietary salt intake can also worsen symptoms; the patient gradually retains more and more fluid, resulting in eventual overload and a trip to the ED. Causes of acute pulmonary edema are principally cardiac and include acute myocardial infarction, dysrhythmias, and, rarely, severe hypertension. (As previously noted, hypertension is usually the result and not the cause of the acute exacerbation.) Noncardiac causes include infection and anemia. When precipitating factors are identified, specific therapy should be initiated.

23. **What is the outpatient treatment of CHF?**
    Angiotensin-converting enzyme (ACE) inhibitors are the mainstay of long-term treatment of CHF, leading to a decrease in mortality and an increase in functional capacity. Other drugs that act on the renin–angiotensin system (angiotensin receptor antagonists and spironolactone) also are effective. β-Blockers, particularly carvedilol, are useful in that they block the cardiac effects of long-term adrenergic stimulation, but they must be used cautiously because of their potential effects on cardiac contractility. Diuretics also are beneficial, especially in patients with volume overload. Digoxin has long been used as a means of improving the symptoms of chronic CHF, although it has been historically acknowledged that it does not have any impact on overall mortality. Recently though, the role of this medication has been increasingly questioned, with conflicting evidence. Consequently, the popularity of digoxin is waning. Combined therapy with hydralazine and isosorbide dinitrate has shown a decrease in mortality and is particularly useful in patients who have contraindications to other classes of drugs.

24. **How do ACE inhibitors work in CHF?**
    In response to cardiac decompensation, the renin–angiotensin system is activated. Angiotensin is a potent vasoconstrictor and leads to increased afterload. Stimulation of aldosterone causes sodium retention, extracellular fluid volume expansion, and increased preload. ACE inhibitors help to decrease afterload by decreasing angiotensin II–mediated vasoconstriction, and decrease preload by blocking sodium retention and volume expansion. Long term, they also improve outcomes through their effects on cardiac remodeling.

25. **What is the long-term prognosis for patients with CHF?**
    Prognosis depends on the cause and severity of the heart failure. The prognosis is good when the underlying cause can be corrected, such as in valvular heart disease. Patients with mild disease who can be controlled with ACE inhibitors with or without low doses of diuretics generally do well. Overall, however, patients with CHF have a 10%–20% yearly mortality, and fewer than half survive 5 years.

BIBLIOGRAPHY

Freeman JV, Yang J, Sung SH, et al. Effectiveness and safety of digoxin among contemporary adults with incident systolic heart failure. *Circ Cardiovasc Qual Outcomes.* 2013;6:525–533.

Long B, Koyfman A, Gottlieb M. Management of heart failure in the emergency department setting: an evidence-based review of the literature. *J Emerg Med.* 2018;55(5):635–646.

Maisel A, Hollander J, Guss D, et al. Primary results of the Rapid Emergency Department Heart Failure Outpatient Trial (REDHOT). A multi-center study of B-type natriuretic peptide levels, emergency department decision making, and outcome in patients presenting with shortness of breath. *JACC.* 2004;44(6):1328–1333.

Masip J, Roque M, Sánchez B, et al. Noninvasive ventilation in acute cardiogenic pulmonary edema: systematic review and meta-analysis. *JAMA.* 2005;294:3124–3130.

Matsue Y, Damman K, Voors AA, et al. Time-to-furosemide treatment and mortality in patients hospitalized with acute heart failure. *J Am Coll Cardiol.* 2017;69:3042–3051.

Weintraub NL, Collins SP, Pang PS, et al. Acute heart failure syndromes: emergency department presentation, treatment, and disposition: current approaches and future aims: a scientific statement from the American Heart Association. *Circulation.* 2010;122(19): 1975–1996.

CHAPTER 32

ISCHEMIC HEART DISEASE

Danya Khoujah, MBBS, MEHP and Amal Mattu, MD

1. **How is ischemic heart disease classified?**
   Chronic stable ischemic heart disease:
   - asymptomatic
   - with stable angina
   - after myocardial infarction (MI), with or without angina

   Acute coronary syndrome (ACS):
   - ST-segment elevation MI (STEMI)
   - non–ST-segment elevation acute coronary syndrome (NSTE-ACS), which includes:
       - unstable angina (UA)
       - non–ST-segment elevation MI (NSTEMI)

   These two entities are differentiated by the presence of elevated cardiac biomarkers in NSTEMI, and are otherwise similar in pathophysiology and treatment.

2. **What are the types of MI? Why is this distinction important?**
   MI is classified into five types based on pathologic, clinical, and prognostic differences, with subsequent differences in treatment strategies. Types 1 and 2 are the most clinically relevant in the emergency department (ED).
   - Type 1: spontaneous acute atherothrombosis in the artery supplying the infarcted myocardium that is usually precipitated by plaque disruption (rupture or erosion). The treatment revolves around revascularization and is the focus of discussion in this chapter.
   - Type 2: due to a mismatch between the myocardial oxygen supply and demand, but not due to atherothrombosis, this type can be caused by many conditions (Table 32.1) and usually occurs in the presence of underlying chronic coronary atherosclerosis. Treatment revolves around treating the imbalance between supply and demand and may include volume adjustment, blood pressure management, heart rate control, etc. Coronary evaluation may be indicated in select cases.
   - Type 3: sudden unexplained cardiac death.
   - Type 4: associated with percutaneous coronary intervention or stent thrombosis.
   - Type 5: associated with cardiac surgery.

3. **How do patients with acute ischemic heart disease experience symptoms?**
   The most common presenting symptom is chest pain. Typically, ischemic pain is described as heaviness, pressure, tightness, or squeezing. It is less commonly described as sharp or aching. Usually the pain lasts minutes, as opposed to seconds or hours. Patients may describe their pain as indigestion, which can lead to the misdiagnosis of reflux esophagitis. Although precordial discomfort is most common, it may be felt anywhere on the chest, the right or left shoulder or arm, the throat or jaw, or the upper abdomen. The pain often radiates to one of these locations as well. Less commonly, patients may simply have pain in other more unusual locations (e.g., left ear or upper back). Associated symptoms include dyspnea, nausea, vomiting, diaphoresis, lightheadedness or syncope, palpitations, or malaise. Diaphoresis and vomiting, in particular, increase the likelihood of ACS. One third of patients may not experience pain and just present with associated symptoms – in this case termed an *anginal equivalent* or *atypical angina*. The most common symptom is shortness of breath. This is more common in the elderly, women, and patients with diabetes.

4. **Which descriptors have the highest predictive value for true ACS?**
   Chest pain that radiates to one or both arms, chest pain accompanied by sweating or vomiting, and chest pain associated with exertion all have high predictive values for ACS.

5. **To understand the discomfort better, what information should be obtained?**
   Use the *OLDCAAAR* mnemonic when obtaining the history of present illness:
   Onset – when did the pain begin? Was it abrupt or gradual?
   Location of the pain
   Duration – if intermittent, how long do the episodes last?
   Character – is the pain sharp, dull, aching, pressure, or squeezing?
   Alleviating and aggravating factors – what makes the pain better or worse?
   Associated symptoms – dyspnea, nausea, vomiting, lightheadedness, diaphoresis
   Activity at onset
   Radiation – does the pain radiate to any other part of the body?

Table 32.1 Causes of Acute Myocardial Ischemia Secondary to Imbalance Between Oxygen Supply and Demand

DECREASED OXYGEN SUPPLY	INCREASED OXYGEN DEMAND
• Coronary artery spasm	• Sustained tachydysrhythmia
• Coronary artery dissection	• Severe hypertension
• Sustained bradydysrhythmia	
• Hypotension or shock	
• Systemic hypoxia	
• Severe anemia	

6. **Describe the typical features of chest discomfort in stable angina.**
   Typically, patients with stable angina have discomfort during exertion that is relieved within minutes by rest or nitroglycerin (NTG). The degree of exertion bringing on the discomfort (and rest/NTG required for relief) is predictable and constant (or stable) over time. The electrocardiogram (ECG) is unchanged and cardiac markers are normal.

7. **How do patients with unstable angina experience symptoms?**
   Patients with unstable angina usually have similar pain to those with stable angina, but it occurs with progressively less exertion or at rest, or is new in onset. Patients with unstable angina who have pain at rest also typically have pain with exertion. The ECG may show some ischemic changes. Cardiac markers do not meet the criteria for being positive, but frequently are in the indeterminate range and occasionally normal.

8. **What is Prinzmetal angina?**
   Prinzmetal angina is caused by coronary artery spasm, or "vasospasm." Patients with Prinzmetal angina typically have pain at rest, usually in the early morning hours, and often do not have exertional discomfort. Most patients with Prinzmetal angina have some underlying nonocclusive coronary artery disease. True vasospastic angina is uncommon.

9. **How does the pain of MI differ from that of angina?**
   Patients with acute MI typically have pain that is more severe than any preceding angina. It may be described as crushing, or it may be atypical (see Question 3). It is caused by myocardial necrosis. The ECG may show ST elevation (STEMI), or the cardiac markers may be elevated (NSTEMI).

10. **What other symptoms are associated with the chest discomfort of ischemic heart disease?**
    Shortness of breath commonly accompanies angina. Many conditions other than angina that cause chest discomfort, such as pulmonary disease and anxiety disorder, also are accompanied by shortness of breath. Diaphoresis occurs often with unstable angina or acute MI and should raise concern, because it does not typically occur with other disorders that cause chest pain. Nausea and vomiting are common with acute MI as well. The presence of diaphoresis or vomiting significantly increases the likelihood of true MI or unstable angina. Other symptoms that may occur include lightheadedness, syncope, and generalized weakness.

11. **Is there anything different about evaluating elderly patients?**
    The older the patient, the less likely it is that they will present with chest pain. Over the age of 70 years, only half of all patients will feel chest pain when they experience cardiac ischemia or acute MI. On the other hand, dyspnea is very common. Other presentations that become more common with advancing age include weakness, vomiting, abdominal pain, and syncope.

12. **Which patients are at high risk for unusual presentation?**
    • Patients with diabetes
    • The elderly
    • Women
    These groups tend to experience "anginal equivalents," such as dyspnea, vomiting, extreme fatigue, or lightheadedness rather than classic ischemic chest pain.

13. **What are the risk factors associated with ischemic heart disease?**
    Risk factors for ischemic heart disease are listed in Table 32.2.

14. **Should demographic features and the presence or absence of coronary risk factors change my mind about the diagnosis?**
    Yes and no. The presence or absence of these factors should raise or lower your suspicion for ischemic heart disease, but they are less important than the history of presenting illness or ECG findings. Most importantly, the absence of coronary risk factors should not obviate your concern for ischemic heart disease in a patient with a concerning history. For example, a young woman with no risk factors, but with pressure-like chest pain, shortness of breath, and ECG changes should still be suspected of having ischemic disease.

Table 32.2 Risk Factors for Ischemic Heart Disease

TRADITIONAL RISK FACTORS	NONTRADITIONAL RISK FACTORS
• Male gender • Age >55 years • Smoking • Hypertension • Hyperlipidemia • Diabetes mellitus • Family history	• Antiphospholipid syndrome • Rheumatoid arthritis • Systemic lupus erythematosus • Human immunodeficiency virus (HIV) • Chronic kidney disease • Cocaine abuse • Long-term steroid use • Obesity

15. **List the key elements of the initial evaluation of a patient with a suspected ACS.**
    - The patient should be placed on a cardiac monitor and have reliable intravenous (IV) access.
    - Supplemental oxygen should be applied if the patient is hypoxic (arterial oxygen saturation [SpO$_2$] <90%) or has signs of respiratory distress. Unnecessary oxygen may be harmful.
    - The patient should have an ECG performed and read by a qualified provider as soon as possible, ideally within 10 minutes of arrival to the ED.
    - The presence of abnormal vital signs, especially hypotension, should be addressed early.
    - A history of present illness directed at characterizing the pain and associated symptoms and a cardiovascular examination come next. The examination is useful for ruling out other diagnoses, such as pericarditis and aortic dissection, and also for assessing the presence of any complications of acute ischemia/infarction, such as acute heart failure or valvular dysfunction.
    - Administer chewable aspirin (162–324 mg) unless contraindicated (see Question 36).

16. **What is the significance of abnormal ST-segment changes on an ECG?**
    In a patient presenting with symptoms consistent with ischemic heart disease, ST elevation suggests acute myocardial injury (ongoing infarction). The current of injury that accompanies STEMI is typically a convex-upward elevation of the ST segment (resembling a tombstone). However, the elevation may be horizontal or concave upward instead. Causes of ST elevation are listed in Table 32.3.

    ST segment depression is typically caused by cardiac ischemia. However, ST depression in V1 and V2 can implicate a posterior STEMI. A particularly high-risk condition is when a patient demonstrates ST depression in multiple leads in conjunction with ST elevation in lead aVR. This combination of ST findings is predictive of left main coronary artery occlusion or, less commonly, triple vessel disease or proximal left anterior descending artery disease. In a patient with typical symptoms and any signs of instability, this pattern should be treated identically to a STEMI. In addition to cardiac ischemia, ST depression may be caused by such factors as ventricular hypertrophy, drugs (e.g., digoxin), and electrolyte abnormalities.

17. **How do I differentiate ST elevation caused by injury from other causes of ST elevation?**
    ST elevation caused by infarction may display one or more of the following:
    - *Morphology.* Convex upward ST elevation ("tombstone" morphology) is highly predictive of injury. However, the morphology may also be concave upward or horizontal.
    - *Reciprocal changes.* The presence of ST depression in another area of the ECG is highly predictive of injury, but is not always present.
    - ST elevation caused by injury is dynamic; serial ECGs usually show changes over time.

Table 32.3 Differential Diagnosis of ST Elevation on the Electrocardiogram

- Myocardial infarction
- Left ventricular hypertrophy
- Left bundle branch block
- Benign early repolarization
- Acute pericarditis
- Hyperkalemia
- Hypercalcemia
- Hypothermia
- Left ventricular aneurysm
- Ventricular rhythm
- Brugada syndrome
- Acute cerebral hemorrhage

ECG, Electrocardiogram.

18. **What is the typical course of ECG change in ischemic cardiac injury?**
    The first ECG abnormality is often the development of "hyperacute T waves" (Fig. 32.1). This consists of straightening of the initial portion (upward slope) of the T wave, as well as broadening of the base and an increase in the amplitude of the T wave. These T-wave changes may occur within the first minutes of ischemia. Next, the ST segment displays elevation (injury pattern, Fig. 32.2) or depression (ischemic pattern). ST-segment changes tend to occur in the first hour of ischemia, but they may be delayed by 1 or more hours. Therefore, serial ECGs are recommended during the first few hours of symptoms if the initial ECGs are nondiagnostic. Q waves may start to develop within 2–3 hours of transmural infarction. Significant Q waves should be at least 40 milliseconds in width and at least one third of the height of the R wave. As the ST segment returns to baseline, symmetrically inverted T waves evolve. This classic evolution is documented in approximately 65% of patients with acute MI.

19. **Can the ECG be normal while a patient is having cardiac ischemia or an acute MI?**
    Yes. Although serial ECGs showing evolving changes are found in acute MI in more than 90% of patients, 20%–50% of *initial* ECGs show nonspecific abnormalities, and up to 6% of initial ECGs may be completely normal (Fig. 32.3). The initial ECG is diagnostic for acute MI in only half of all patients. Therefore serial ECGs at 15- to 30-minute intervals in these patients are often helpful.

20. **Are cardiac markers useful in the ED?**
    Maybe. The most commonly used cardiac marker is troponin (TN), although creatine kinase-MB (CK-MB) is still used in some EDs. TN is used in preference to CK-MB because the elevation correlates with the magnitude of infarction and prognosis better than CK-MB. Commonly available TN assays demonstrate rising levels within 2–4 hours after the onset of myocardial necrosis with a sensitivity of 95%, and can remain elevated for up to 7–10 days. A newer generation of high-sensitivity TN T (hs-cTnT) is available in many other countries, and is

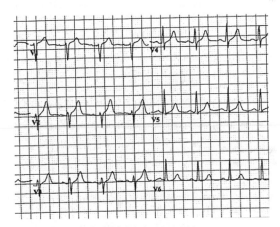

Fig. 32.1 Hyperacute T waves.

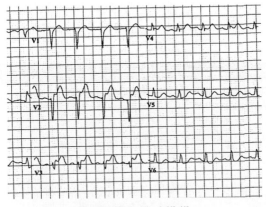

Fig. 32.2 ST elevation in V2–V3.

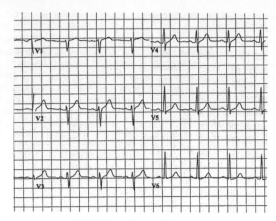

Fig. 32.3 Normalization of ST elevation.

becoming more widely available in the United States as well; hs-cTnT demonstrates elevations within 1–2 hours of infarction with a sensitivity of ≥99% and, as with all tests, the increased sensitivity comes at the cost of decreased specificity. In addition, it is critically important to remember that TNs are reliable markers only for infarction and are not reliable at detecting cardiac ischemia. Providers should not wait until TN level rise to make a decision to treat for ACS. The initial decision to treat a patient for ACS should be based on clinical suspicion, which is based on the history of present illness and the ECG.

21. **Can troponin be elevated in conditions other than myocardial ischemia?**
    TN elevations are noted in numerous cardiac and noncardiac conditions in which there is myocardial dysfunction or injury (Table 32.4).

22. **How is myocardial ischemia differentiated from other causes of myocardial injury?**
    Because of the lack of specificity of TN testing, the World Health Organization recommends that TNs should not be used alone to diagnose acute MI. Myocardial ischemia should be diagnosed with detection of a rise or fall of TN levels by ≥20% on serial TN testing over the course of 3–6 hours, with at least one value above the 99th percentile, and at least one of the following:
    • symptoms of myocardial ischemia;
    • new ischemic ECG changes;
    • development of pathological Q waves;
    • imaging evidence of new loss of viable myocardium or new regional wall motion abnormality in a pattern consistent with an ischemic etiology.

23. **How can echocardiography be useful in ED patients with suspected ACS?**
    The sensitivity of echocardiography in the acute setting is limited. The presence of cardiac wall motion abnormality is evidence that supports the diagnosis of ischemia, although it may be the result of an old rather than acute infarction. It may also provide information about complications, such as acute valvular dysfunction or acute heart failure with low ejection fraction. Echocardiography may also be helpful at distinguishing acute MI from pericarditis (looking for pericardial effusion) or large pulmonary embolus (looking for a right ventricle strain).

Table 32.4 Nonischemic Causes of Myocardial Injury/Dysfunction

CARDIAC CONDITIONS	SYSTEMIC CONDITIONS
• Heart failure (acute or chronic)	• Sepsis
• Myocarditis	• Burns
• Cardiomyopathy	• Critical illness
• Takotsubo syndrome	• Chronic kidney disease
• Catheter ablation	• Stroke
• Defibrillator shock	• Subarachnoid hemorrhage
• Cardiac contusion	• Pulmonary embolism
	• Infiltrative cardiac disease (e.g., amyloidosis, sarcoidosis)
	• Chemotherapeutic agents

A normal echocardiogram in the setting of a typical history and ECG does not rule out the diagnosis of an ACS. Waiting for the results of an echocardiogram may unnecessarily delay treatment.

24. **What is Takotsubo syndrome?**
Takotsubo syndrome, also known as stress or broken heart syndrome, is a type of nonischemic cardiomyopathy that presents acutely in the setting of severe emotional stress, most commonly in postmenopausal women. Patients typically present with similar symptoms to those with traditional ACS, and may develop cardiogenic shock, but their presentation is not caused by an acute coronary occlusion. Nevertheless, the ECG typically shows pronounced ischemic changes. Takotsubo cardiomyopathy is found in 1%–2% of patients presenting with a STEMI pattern on the ECG. In addition to ischemic ECG patterns, these patients also typically demonstrate elevations in serum TN. The differentiation from true thrombosis-related ACS is very difficult at the bedside. The diagnosis is typically made on formal echocardiography or coronary angiography, with the finding that the heart appears to have taken on an unusual but diagnostic elongated shape with apical ballooning. With aggressive supportive care, often including the use of vasopressors for shock, these patients usually have a good prognosis.

25. **What are the indications for reperfusion therapy in acute MI?**
Reperfusion therapy includes either percutaneous coronary intervention (PCI) or thrombolytics and is indicated in patients presenting with symptoms concerning for acute MI plus any of the ECG patterns listed in Table 32.5 that persist despite use of sublingual NTG. Of note, a new left bundle branch block alone is *no longer* an indication for acute reperfusion.

26. **What if ST elevation is not persistent and resolves on a repeat ECG?**
Management of ST elevation that self-resolves is controversial. The majority of these patients have significant underlying coronary disease. Therefore, many interventional cardiologists still take these patients for emergent catheterization. Others prefer to wait, closely observe these patients, and treat with anti-ischemic therapies with a plan for nonemergent catheterization. A decision on emergent catheterization should be made in conjunction with cardiology consultation. On the other hand, thrombolytics are generally withheld in patients who no longer have ST elevation on the ECG.

27. **What is the preferred method of reperfusion therapy in acute MI with STEMI – thrombolytic therapy or PCI?**
PCI is preferred over thrombolytic medication if done within 90 minutes of arrival. PCI shows a greater reduction in mortality, lower rates of reocclusion over the subsequent few days, and lower risks of intracranial bleeding. If PCI cannot be accomplished in such a timely manner, thrombolytic drugs should be used. There are notable exceptions to this rule, however. Thrombolytics are less effective for patients with cardiogenic shock (see Question 30), and also for patients whose symptoms have been ongoing for more than 6 hours. For these patients, the time window of benefit for PCI over thrombolytics can be extended. Management decisions for these patients should be made in conjunction with the interventional cardiologist.

28. **What if cardiac intervention is not available on site?**
If transfer from one hospital to a facility capable of intervention is needed for treatment of STEMI, the permissible time window for transfer and intervention is 120 minutes. Note that in this scenario, balloon inflation and not just the transfer should occur within 120 minutes. If intervention cannot be accomplished within this estimated window, thrombolytics should be promptly administered.

Table 32.5 ECG Findings Necessitating Reperfusion Therapy		
ECG CHANGE	**LOCATION**	**DESCRIPTION**
ST elevation	Leads V2–V3	≥2 mm for men ≥40 years of age
		≥2.5 mm in men <40 years of age
		≥1.5 mm in women
	In any other two anatomically contiguous leads	≥1 mm
Acute posterior MI	Leads V1–V3	ST-segment depression with tall R waves and upright T waves
	Posterior leads	ST-segment elevation ≥0.5 mm
Left bundle branch block with concordant Sgarbossa criteria	Any lead	Concordant ST elevation ≥1 mm
	Any of leads V1, V2, or V3	Concordant ST depression ≥1 mm

ECG, Electrocardiogram; *MI,* myocardial infarction.

29. **How do you choose which thrombolytic agent to use?**

    The choice of which thrombolytic to administer is of little importance. Alteplase, reteplase, and tenecteplase are all used and have similar efficacy. Typically, hospitals will stock one form of thrombolytic based on cost, and physicians will simply choose the drug that is on their formulary. Reteplase and tenecteplase have become more popular than alteplase, because they are administered as a bolus rather than an infusion. Regardless of which agent is chosen, it should be given within 30 minutes of arrival, and a dose reduction should be considered in patients aged 75 years or older.

30. **What is the preferred therapy for cardiogenic shock?**

    The only therapy shown to decrease the historically high mortality associated with this syndrome is invasive therapy (PCI or, in some cases, bypass surgery). PCI should be performed without delay. The added benefit of immediate transfer to a catheterization laboratory is that this facilitates insertion of an intraaortic balloon pump (IABP). An IABP has traditionally been considered to be superior to pharmacologic therapy for supporting blood pressure, decreasing afterload, and augmenting cardiac output; however, recent studies have demonstrated that the insertion of an IABP does not change mortality. Management decisions for patients with cardiogenic shock should be made in conjunction with a cardiology consultant. Vasopressors (such as norepinephrine) should be used to support the blood pressure in the meantime.

    Of note, hypotension caused by right ventricular infarction should be considered in patients with an acute MI and hypotension. This is not a true form of cardiogenic shock, but clinicians often confuse the two conditions. Right ventricular infarction should be suspected whenever hypotension accompanies an acute inferior MI. The presence of jugular venous distention and clear lungs are important clues to this diagnosis. These patients do not need vasopressors and their cases can often be managed successfully with volume replacement with IV fluids.

31. **List the contraindications to thrombolytic therapy in STEMI.**

    Contraindications to thrombolytic therapy are listed in Table 32.6.

32. **What other diagnoses should be considered before giving thrombolytic therapy?**

    Aortic dissection and acute pericarditis can mimic acute MI. Both may have fatal outcomes if thrombolytics are given. Dissection can be evaluated with a careful history, examination of peripheral pulses, and chest radiography. If significant concern for aortic dissection still exists, a chest computed tomography (CT) scan with IV contrast should be obtained to exclude the diagnosis before thrombolytics are given. Pericarditis can be excluded by carefully listening for a rub, examining the ECG for widespread, concave upward ST elevation, PR depression, and using point-of-care ultrasound to look for a pericardial effusion.

33. **What is the risk for fatal complications of thrombolytic therapy for acute MI?**

    Intracranial hemorrhage occurs in 2% of patients and is fatal in 0.5% of treated patients. Angioedema is rare, but can be fatal.

34. **What is the role of NTG in patients with ACS?**

    NTG is commonly used in patients with ongoing ischemic chest pain. NTG produces a reduction in preload, coronary vasodilatation, and might also improve coronary perfusion. NTG produces effective improvement in ischemic chest pain in most patients. In addition, NTG can be used to help control severe blood pressure in these patients. NTG can be administered sublingually at a dose of 0.3–0.4 mg every 3–5 minutes or can be given as an IV infusion. NTG should be used cautiously, if at all, in patients with borderline or low blood pressure, and it should be withheld in patients with right ventricular infarction, as it can produce or worsen hypotension. In addition, NTG can produce precipitous decreases in blood pressure when given to patients that have recently taken sildenafil or other phosphodiesterase inhibitors within the past 24–48 hours.

Table 32.6 Contraindications for Thrombolytic Therapy in STEMI	
ABSOLUTE CONTRAINDICATIONS	**RELATIVE CONTRAINDICATIONS**
• PCI immediately available • Active bleeding or bleeding diatheses • Suspected aortic dissection • Ischemic stroke within the past 3 months • History of hemorrhagic stroke • Intracranial or intraspinal surgery or trauma in the past 8 weeks • Intracranial or intraspinal neoplasm, aneurysm, or arteriovenous malformation	• Active peptic ulcer • Surgical or invasive procedure within the past 4 weeks • Significant trauma within the past 4 weeks • Pregnancy or 10 or fewer days postpartum • Prolonged (>10 min) or traumatic cardiopulmonary resuscitation • Hemorrhagic ophthalmic condition, especially diabetic retinopathy • Poorly controlled hypertension

PCI, Percutaneous coronary intervention; *STEMI,* ST-segment elevation myocardial infarction.

35. Is there any use for morphine in patients with acute MI?

Morphine has been used for decades to decrease pain in patients with acute MI. Pain produces a release of cate-cholamines, which can be detrimental to patients who are ischemic. Debate exists regarding the safety of morphine in patients with ACS because of a large nonrandomized study which demonstrated an association between the use of morphine and worse outcome in patients with acute MI. Additionally, morphine reduces the efficacy of thienopyridines (see below). Whether morphine itself causes harm is unclear but, ideally, ischemic pain should be treated with NTG. If the ischemic pain is intractable, IV morphine sulfate can be added in increments of 2–4 mg to alleviate these symptoms, and PCI should be planned for intractable ischemia.

36. What other medications are useful adjuvants to reperfusion therapy?

- *Aspirin.* Unless the patient has had a life-threatening allergic reaction to aspirin, it should be given immediately, because it reduces mortality independent of other therapies via its irreversible antiplatelet effects. The dosage is 162–324 mg of chewable aspirin; enteric-coated forms should be avoided because they have slow absorption rates.
- *Other antiplatelet agents.* The two major groups of additional antiplatelet agents are the thienopyridines (clopidogrel, ticagrelor, and prasugrel) and the glycoprotein IIb/IIIa (GP IIb/IIIa) receptor inhibitors (eptifibatide, tirofiban, and abciximab), referred to as GP IIb/IIIa inhibitors. Thienopyridines are most commonly used, because they have lower bleeding complications and are easier to administer than the GP IIb/IIIa inhibitors, and they are recommended for all patients who undergo reperfusion therapy. Ticagrelor is usually preferred to clopidogrel. Either of these medications can be given before or at the time of reperfusion therapy. Prasugrel is best reserved for use in the cardiac catheterization laboratory, and should not be given to patients with a history of stroke or transient ischemic attack. The GP IIb/IIIa inhibitors should be administered in consultation with cardiology, as combining them with thienopyridines may produce an increase in coronary artery patency at the expense of increased bleeding complications. The GP IIb/IIIa inhibitors are generally only indicated in patients who will be having PCI.
- *Heparin and other anticoagulants.* Anticoagulant medications are used in patients whether they undergo PCI or receive thrombolytics. When using alteplase, heparin should be initiated at least 1 hour before the completion of the thrombolytic infusion. Anticoagulants should be continued in the hospital for at least 48 hours after a patient has had thrombolytics or PCI. Options for anticoagulants include: unfractionated heparin, enoxaparin, and fondaparinux. Fondaparinux should not be used alone in patients receiving PCI due to the risk of catheter thrombosis. Bivalirudin is another option for anticoagulation only in patients receiving PCI, but is less commonly used.
- β-Blockers (see Question 38 below).
- High-dose statin such as atorvastatin in patients with no contraindication.

37. Which is better: low–molecular-weight heparin or unfractionated heparin?

Unfractionated heparin and low–molecular-weight heparin (enoxaparin) are equally effective and have a similar class rating. The real difference is in the practical considerations and the consulting cardiologist's preference. The advantage of low–molecular-weight heparin is that it can be given in the ED as a single bolus and does not require an infusion pump. The major disadvantage is that it is difficult to reverse if there is a bleeding complication or an invasive strategy is planned. Therefore, some cardiologists prefer unfractionated heparin because it enables them to measure levels of anticoagulation (activated partial thromboplastin time [aPTT]) and titrate with flexibility.

38. When should β-blockers be given?

β-Blockers should be given orally to patients with ACS within the first 24 hours of presentation to decrease heart rate and myocardial oxygen demand. Contraindications include heart failure, bradycardia (heart rate <55 beats per minute), advanced atrioventricular blocks, and bronchospasm. The most common β-blockers used in the setting of acute MI are metoprolol and atenolol. IV β-blockers are associated with an increased risk of the development of cardiogenic shock, and should be reserved for patients with severe hypertension refractory to NTG or tachydysrhythmias, such as rapid atrial fibrillation.

39. Which dysrhythmias occur with acute MI? How should they be treated?

Several dysrhythmias can occur with acute MI and are listed in Table 32.7. It is important to look for secondary causes such as drugs, electrolyte imbalance, and hypoxia.

40. What is the management of NSTE-ACS?

The management is similar to that for STEMI, except for reperfusion therapy (see below) and GP IIb/IIIa inhibitors. All patients with NSTE-ACS get aspirin, clopidogrel or ticagrelor, NTG for pain or severe hypertension, and anticoagulation if there is no contraindication. β-Blockers and high-dose statins should be administered within 24 hours in patients without contraindications.

41. Are there indications for emergent PCI in NSTE-ACS?

Yes. Immediate PCI (within 2 hours) is indicated in patients with any of the following features:

- Refractory angina (despite maximum medical therapy)
- Hemodynamic instability
- Electrical instability (sustained ventricular tachycardia or fibrillation)

Table 32.7 Dysrhythmias Commonly Occurring With Acute Myocardial Infarction

CATEGORY	ARRHYTHMIA		TREATMENT
Ventricular irritability	Isolated PVCs		Look for and treat the underlying cause
	Ventricular tachycardia	Nonsustained	Look for and treat the underlying cause
		Sustained (>30 sec)	If stable: lidocaine or amiodarone If unstable: synchronized cardioversion
	Accelerated idioventricular rhythm (heart rate 60–120 beats per minute)		Observation (treatment with antiarrhythmic results in asystole)
	Ventricular fibrillation		Defibrillation
Bradydysrhythmia	Second/third degree HB		With inferior MI: transient, no treatment usually necessary if stable, but use atropine if unstable
	Bifascicular block or LBBB plus first degree HB		With anterior MI: temporary pacemaker will likely be needed if the block is new

HB, Heart block; *LBBB,* left bundle branch block; *MI,* mycardial infarction; *PVC,* premature ventricular contraction.

- Early invasive reperfusion (within 24 hours) should be strongly considered in patients who have one of the following features (despite maximum medical therapy):
  - GRACE mortality risk score >140
  - temporal change in TN (increase or decrease by ≥20%)
  - new ST depression

KEY POINTS

1. Most predictive features of cardiac ischemia
   - Pain that radiates to arms
   - Pain associated with vomiting
   - Pain associated with diaphoresis
   - Pain that occurs or worsens with exertion
2. Key to the evaluation of patients with possible acute cardiac ischemia or MI
   - A good history of present illness is absolutely essential.
   - Chest pain is not universally present. Dyspnea is common in patients who do not have chest pain.
   - Three groups of patients are at high risk for atypical presentations of cardiac ischemia: elderly patients, patients with diabetes, and women.
3. ECG features most consistent with STEMI (versus a mimic)
   - ST elevation that is convex upwards (like a tombstone)
   - ST elevation that is associated with reciprocal ST-segment depression
   - Evolving changes of the ST segments and T waves, or development of new Q waves
4. PCI is preferable to thrombolytics for emergent management of STEMI unless there is an anticipated delay of more than 90–120 minutes to balloon inflation.
5. The most important medication for patients with suspected cardiac ischemia or MI is aspirin.

BIBLIOGRAPHY

Amsterdam EA, Wenger NK, Brindis RG, et al. 2014 AHA/ACC guideline for the management of patients with non–ST-elevation acute coronary syndromes: a report of the American College of Cardiology/American Heart Association task force on practice guidelines. *Circulation.* 2014;130:e344–e426.

Body R, Carley S, Wibberley C, et al. The value of symptoms and signs in the emergent diagnosis of acute coronary syndromes. *Resuscitation.* 2010;81:281–286.

Canto J, Rogers WJ, Goldbert RJ, et al. Association of age and sex with myocardial infarction symptom presentation and in-hospital mortality. *JAMA.* 2012;307:813–822.

Kontos MC, Diercks DB, Ho MP, et al. Treatment and outcomes in patients with myocardial infarction treated with acute beta-blocker therapy: results from the American College of Cardiology's NCDR. *Am Heart J.* 2011;161:864–870.

Kurz MC, Mattu A, Brady WJ. Acute coronary syndrome. In: Marx JA, Hockberger RS, Walls RM, et al., eds. *Rosen's Emergency Medicine: Concepts and Clinical Practice.* 8th ed. Philadelphia, PA: Saunders; 2014:997.

Newby LK, Jesse RL, Gersh BJ, et al. ACCF 2012 expert consensus document on practical clinical considerations in the interpretation of troponin elevations: a report of the American College of Cardiology Foundation task force on Clinical Expert Consensus Documents. *J Am Coll Cardiol.* 2012;60:2427–2463.

Thygesen K, Alpert JS, Jaffe AS, et al. Fourth universal definition of myocardial infarction. *J Am Coll Cardiol.* 2018;72:2231–2264.

CHAPTER 33

CARDIAC DYSRHYTHMIAS, PACEMAKERS, AND IMPLANTABLE DEFIBRILLATORS

Christopher B. Colwell, MD

1. **What is a sinus beat?**

   At the end of each heartbeat, all myocardial cells are depolarized and experience a refractory period. At this point, certain cardiac cells (sinoatrial and atrioventricular [AV] nodes and some ventricular cells) return toward threshold potential. It is like a race, and the sinoatrial node cells typically win this race, achieve threshold, fire, and assume the pacemaker function of the heart.

2. **What is the AV node?**

   The AV node is not simply a passive connection between the atria and ventricles. It is smart. Normally, all atrial impulses are conducted to the ventricles. When the ventricular rate becomes sufficiently rapid that cardiac output is compromised, conduction velocity begins to slow in the AV node. This progressive slowing filters the rapid atrial impulses so that serial atrial impulses are not conducted at all. This progressive AV nodal conduction block is a protective mechanism to prevent a dysfunctional rapid ventricular rate.

3. **Is it necessary to identify a dysrhythmia before treating it?**

   In general, if the patient is hemodynamically unstable, no. In the unstable patient, a general rule of thumb is to use electricity (perform electrical cardioversion) if the heart rate is fast, and if the heart rate is slow, pace the patient with a pacemaker.

4. **What is hemodynamic compromise?**

   In an adult, hemodynamic compromise is hypotension (a systolic blood pressure <90 mmHg) in combination with alteration in mental status, chest pain, or shortness of breath. In patients with underlying hypertension, hemodynamic compromise may occur at systolic blood pressures >90 mmHg.

5. **How do I know whether a patient's dysrhythmia is causing hemodynamic compromise?**

   Typically, if a patient's ventricular rate is between 60 and 100 beats per minute, hemodynamic instability is being caused by something else. It is unusual for a tachydysrhythmia at a rate <150 beats per minute to be the primary cause of hemodynamic instability.

6. **How do I treat bradydysrhythmias?**

   Do not treat bradycardia if the patient is hemodynamically stable and asymptomatic. Refer back to the rule of treating the patient, not a number. If the patient has a heart rate <60 beats per minute and is hemodynamically unstable:
   - Give 0.5 mg (0.01 mg/kg in a child; 0.02 mg/kg in a neonate; however, epinephrine is generally preferred in children) intravenous (IV) atropine (may be repeated).
   - Initiate pacemaker therapy, starting with external transcutaneous pacing. Placement of a transvenous pacemaker (especially without fluoroscopy) can take longer than you think.
   - Consider underlying causes such as cardiac ischemia, hyperkalemia, calcium channel toxicity, and β-blocker toxicity. Toxic and metabolic causes of bradycardia require specific therapy and often do not respond to pacing.

7. **How do I treat tachydysrhythmias?**

   Any unstable patient with a tachydysrhythmia that is believed to be the cause of the hemodynamic instability requires electric cardioversion, or in the case of unstable ventricular tachycardia, defibrillation. Supraventricular tachycardia (SVT) and atrial flutter often respond to low voltages (50 J), whereas most other tachydysrhythmias typically require at least 100 J to convert to a sinus rhythm. If the patient is hemodynamically stable, the next step is to identify whether they have a narrow- or wide-complex tachyarrhythmia.

8. **What is a narrow-complex tachycardia?**

   The AV node conducts impulses directly to the Purkinje system, which courses over the endocardial surface of the ventricles. An electrical impulse travels along the Purkinje fibers at 2–3 m/sec. If an impulse enters the ventricles from the AV node, it can rapidly activate the entire ventricular muscle mass in 0.12 seconds

(120 msec or three little boxes on electrocardiogram [ECG] paper). We see this as a narrow-complex QRS on the ECG, or a QRS complex with a width of less than 120 msec. A narrow-complex tachycardia must originate above the AV node. Sinus tachycardia, reentrant tachycardias, atrial fibrillation (AF) with rapid ventricular response, multifocal atrial tachycardia, and atrial flutter are examples of narrow-complex tachycardias.

9. **How do I make the diagnosis of AF when the ventricular rate is fast?**
AF is by definition an irregular rhythm, but very rapid AF may appear regular and be difficult to differentiate from SVT on a cardiac rhythm strip. The diagnosis of AF can be made by palpating a peripheral pulse and simultaneously auscultating the heart or visualizing the cardiac rhythm. AF is the only dysrhythmia that results in a pulse deficit (fewer beats palpable than observed or auscultated) and that has an irregular pulse with varying intensity of the pulse. Most irregularly irregular rhythms will be AF.

10. **How do I treat narrow-complex tachycardia in a hemodynamically stable patient?**
Because a narrow-complex tachycardia must originate above the AV node, to control the ventricular rate you will need to block the AV node. This is best done pharmacologically in the stable patient. If the patient has a rapid regular narrow-complex tachycardia that cannot be definitively identified, the best initial agent is adenosine, 6 mg IV rapid bolus followed by 12 mg, if needed (which also may be repeated). Because of the greater success of 12 mg over 6 mg, some have advocated for starting with 12 mg. For AV node reentrant tachycardia (AVNRT), a modified Valsalva maneuver (blowing on a syringe while lowering the head and raising the feet) has a conversion rate of 40%–50%. Adenosine has a response rate of 85%–90%, few serious side effects, and a very short half-life. Patients may experience chest tightness, nausea, and shortness of breath upon receiving adenosine and should be warned about these temporary unpleasant effects. Alternatively, verapamil 5–10 mg, or diltiazem 20 mg, intravenously over to 1–2 minutes, terminates or controls the ventricular response rate in 80%–90% of cases.

If the patient clearly has AF, rate control rather than conversion to a sinus rhythm has traditionally been the approach. Some authors are now advocating for rhythm control in patients that have been in AF for <48 hours or with therapeutic anticoagulation. For rate control, β-blockers (metoprolol 5–10 mg over 2 minutes) or calcium channel blockers (diltiazem 20 mg over 2 minutes) are effective AV nodal blocking agents in most patients with AF. 0.25 mg/kg for the diltiazem for those that like weight-based approaches.

Rarely, calcium channel blockers (especially verapamil) can cause hypotension, and there are case reports of life-threatening events after administration of adenosine, so it is important to have good IV access and an advanced cardiac life support (ACLS) cart nearby when giving any of these agents. Cardioversion for rhythm control can be electrical or pharmacologic. Success rates tend to be higher (80%–95%) with electrical conversion, which is generally done under sedation using 50–100 J with a biphasic defibrillator. A pharmacologic approach to AF can include procainamide, amiodarone, ibutilide, or flecainide.

11. **Is there a time when I should not use adenosine or a calcium channel blocker for a narrow-complex tachycardia?**
The one situation in which it would be potentially dangerous to use these agents is AF in the setting of Wolff-Parkinson-White (WPW) syndrome. In this disorder, there is an accessory pathway between the atria and the ventricles that bypasses the AV node. If an AV nodal blocking agent is given, conduction through the accessory pathway could speed up, making the tachycardia worse and potentially precipitating hemodynamic collapse. AF in WPW syndrome can present as narrow- or wide-complex tachycardia. It is difficult to determine on the ECG whether someone has WPW syndrome if the rhythm is very fast, but if the patient has a known history of the disorder, do not give adenosine or a calcium channel blocker. Procainamide or synchronized cardioversion should be used instead.

12. **Define premature ventricular contraction.**
A premature ventricular contraction occurs when a ventricular site wins the "race" among myocardial cells, and ventricular depolarization originates from an ectopic ventricular site.

13. **What is a wide-complex tachycardia?**
When an impulse originates from damaged or ischemic ventricular muscle instead of the sinoatrial or AV node, it does not use the Purkinje "superhighway" of conduction and therefore takes longer to activate the ventricular mass. Wide-complex tachycardia refers to any tachydysrhythmia accompanied by QRS duration of 0.12 seconds (120 msec or three small boxes on the ECG) or more.

14. **What is the most common cause of wide-complex tachycardia?**
Ventricular tachycardia (VT). Among awake patients coming to the emergency department (ED) with a wide-complex tachycardia, 70%–90% have VT, and only 10%–30% have SVT with aberrancy (see Question 16). VT is also more likely if the patient has a history of a prior myocardial infarction or congestive heart failure. For a new regular wide-complex tachycardia, assume VT until proven otherwise. Other causes of wide-complex tachycardia include ventricular fibrillation (VF), a wide-complex, irregular, non-perfusing rhythm that requires electrical defibrillation; and torsades de pointes, a wide-complex rhythm associated with prolonged QT interval.

Treatment of torsades de pointes is unsynchronized shock if the patient is unstable. If the patient is hemodynamically stable, treat with magnesium (1- to 2-g bolus over 5–10 minutes); if there is a prolonged QT interval, consider isoproterenol or ventricular pacing.

15. **Does VT always cause a patient to be hemodynamically unstable?**
No. Hemodynamic status should not be used to determine the nature of a wide QRS tachycardia. Do not assume that a wide-complex tachycardia cannot be VT just because the patient is hemodynamically stable.

16. **What is a supraventricular rhythm with aberrancy?**
Usually a supraventricular rhythm traverses the AV node and courses through the large endoventricular conduction fibers, activating the ventricles rapidly and resulting in a narrow QRS complex (<0.12 seconds). A wide-complex tachycardia typically represents a tachycardia of ventricular origin. Although less common, an impulse of supraventricular origin that travels through the ventricle in an aberrant fashion also can be wide and is called a *supraventricular rhythm with aberrancy*. One example is an SVT with an underlying bundle branch block. Another, as discussed in Question 11, is AF in the setting of WPW, a supraventricular dysrhythmia that can present as a narrow- or wide-complex tachycardia, depending on the direction of conduction through the accessory pathway.

17. **Differentiate VT from SVT with aberrancy based on findings on the 12-lead ECG.**
As stated earlier, always assume that the rhythm is VT and treat accordingly whenever there is any question.
Any of these findings on the 12-lead ECG strongly suggest VT:
- AV dissociation
- fusion or capture beats
- left- or right-axis deviation
- QRS width of >140 msec
- concordance of QRS complexes
- monophasic or biphasic QRS in lead V1
- RS or QS in lead V6
- history of coronary artery disease or congestive heart failure
- evidence of AV dissociation on physical examination (cannon A waves)

Heart rate is not an accurate way to differentiate VT from SVT with aberrancy. Again, if there is any doubt, assume VT. Treating SVT with aberrancy as if it were VT is less problematic than treating VT as if it were SVT with aberrancy.

18. **How do I treat wide-complex tachycardia?**
In the patient with a wide-complex tachycardia of unknown origin, assume VT and treat with cardioversion if unstable. Use procainamide or amiodarone if stable. Some authors have suggested procainamide has higher success and fewer adverse events. See Table 33.1.

Table 33.1 Treatment of Wide Complex Tachycardia

CLINICAL SITUATION	TREATMENT
Unstable patient	Cardioversion
Wide-complex tachycardia known to be SVT with aberrancy	Adenosine (6 mg IV push followed by 12-mg IV push if ineffective)
Wide-complex tachycardia of unknown type with preserved cardiac function (no clinical signs of congestive heart failure)	Amiodarone (150 mg IV given over 10–15 minutes) or procainamide (17 mg/kg IV at a rate of 20 mg/min, to be stopped if the dysrhythmia is suppressed, hypotension occurs, or the QRS complex widens by 50% of its original width)
Wide-complex tachycardia of unknown type in a patient with clinical evidence of congestive heart failure	Amiodarone
Rhythm known to be ventricular in origin	Amiodarone, procainamide, or lidocaine (1–1.5 mg/kg IV, repeated every 5 minutes to a maximum of 3 mg/kg); consider magnesium (2 g IV) if torsades de pointes suspected

IV, Intravenously; *SVT,* supraventricular tachycardia.
Modified from Shah CP, Thakur RK, Xie B, et al. Clinical approach to wide QRS complex tachycardias. *Emerg Med Clin North Am.* 1998;16:331–360.

19. **What does amiodarone do?**

Amiodarone is a class III antidysrhythmic drug that, among other effects, prolongs the action potential duration and refractory period, slows automaticity in pacemaker cells, and slows conduction in the AV node. It is approved for the treatment of ventricular and supraventricular arrhythmias, including AF, atrial flutter, and accessory pathway syndromes. Current ACLS guidelines suggest amiodarone be used as a first-line agent for stable VT, and it is also a good option to consider in a hemodynamically stable patient with a wide-complex tachycardia of unknown mechanism. Primary side effects are hypotension and bradycardia. The loading dose for adults is 150 mg intravenously given over 10–15 minutes. Amiodarone exhibits a slow onset of action and an even slower clearance.

20. **What drug is contraindicated in the treatment of any wide-complex tachycardia?**

Verapamil; because all wide-complex tachycardias must be considered to be of ventricular origin, verapamil carries a high risk of causing hypotension and may cause degeneration of the rhythm to VF or asystole.

21. **What is synchronized cardioversion?**

Synchronized cardioversion is synchronization of delivered energy to match the timing of the QRS complex. This reduces the chance that a shock will induce VF, which can occur when electrical energy impinges on the relative refractory portion of the cardiac electrical activity (downward slope of the T wave).

22. **How do I perform synchronized cardioversion?**

- Apply the defibrillation pads to the patient: one attaches to the anterior chest and the other is placed on the patient's back.
- Turn on the defibrillator.
- Select a lead on the monitor that clearly reveals an R wave of greater amplitude than the T wave.
- Engage the synchronization mode by pressing the synchronization control button, and look for markers on the R waves indicating the synchronization mode is functioning and capturing the QRS complex and not the T wave.
- You may need to adjust the R wave again until the synchronization markers occur with each QRS complex. Then select the appropriate energy level.
- Always remember to use adequate sedation in an awake patient.
  - If you are using defibrillation paddles, coat both paddles with conductive gel and apply 25 lbs. of downward pressure.

23. **Does it make sense to use cardioversion with asystole?**

Strictly speaking, no, it does not. Theoretically, electrical cardioversion synchronously depolarizes all myocardial cells simultaneously. All cells then should repolarize synchronously and spontaneously reinitiate sinus rhythm. With asystole, there is nothing to depolarize and no reason for cardioversion. Although the American Heart Association currently does not recommend routine shocking during asystole, there are two scenarios when cardioversion of apparent asystole may be helpful:

- Conceivably, if the major QRS vector is perpendicular to the axis of the ECG lead, VF may appear as asystole.
- It is also possible to have a fine (very low voltage) VF, which is difficult to distinguish from asystole on the monitor.

  If available, a point-of-care ultrasound of the heart is useful in these circumstances.

24. **When is it necessary to give anticoagulants to a patient with AF before cardioversion?**

Anticoagulation in patients who have AF for <48 hours is unnecessary. If the duration of AF has been >48 hours and the patient is stable, cardioversion may be delayed until the patient's blood is fully anticoagulated.

25. **Should I be using monophasic or biphasic waveform defibrillation in the ED?**

Theoretical advantages to biphasic waveforms include less energy required to achieve effective defibrillation and less postshock myocardial damage and dysfunction at equivalent energy levels. A study published in 2003 showed that biphasic waveforms were more likely to achieve a return to an organized rhythm with one shock than monophasic waveforms, but did not result in any statistically significant difference in overall survival. A 2006 study saw trends toward the requirement for fewer shocks, faster return of spontaneous circulation, and improved survival rates with biphasic waveforms. A 2016 Cochrane review concluded it is uncertain whether biphasic defibrillators have an important effect on defibrillation success in people with out-of-hospital cardiac arrest.

26. **What is a pacemaker?**

A pacemaker is an external source of energy used to stimulate the heart. It consists of a pulse generator (i.e., power source), an output circuit, a sensing circuit, a timing circuit, and pacing leads. In the ED, pacing is performed via a temporary external or transvenous pacemaker. Long-term therapy requires the placement of a surgically implanted device. It is usually possible to palpate these devices on physical examination; they are also visible as radiopaque foreign bodies on a chest radiograph.

27. **What are the indications for temporary pacemakers?**

Temporary emergency pacing is indicated for therapy of significant and hemodynamically unstable bradydys-rhythmias and prevention of bradycardia-dependent malignant dysrhythmias. In symptomatic or unstable patients who do not respond to atropine or other pharmacotherapies, emergency pacing should be initiated immediately for any of the following rhythms:

- Sinus node dysfunction
- Sinus bradycardia
- Sinus pauses greater than 3 seconds
- AV nodal block
- Second-degree AV block (Mobitz type I block)
- Complete heart block
- Infranodal block
- New bifascicular block associated with acute myocardial infarction (AMI)
- Alternating bundle-branch block with changing PR interval
- Complete heart block

  Pacemakers also can be used for overdrive pacing, to terminate VT by placing a ventricular extrasystole during the vulnerable period of the cardiac cycle. Prophylactic temporary pacing is indicated for insertion of a pulmonary artery catheter in a patient with an underlying left bundle-branch block or use of medications that may cause or exacerbate hemodynamically significant bradycardia.

28. **Where are external/transcutaneous pacemakers placed? How are they operated?**
Pacing pads and monitor leads are placed preferably in the midanterior chest and just below the left scapula. The desired heart rate is chosen, and the current is set to 0 mA. The external pacemaker is turned on, and the current is increased as tolerated until cardiac capture is achieved.

29. **What are the limiting factors in the use of external pacemakers.**
Skeletal muscle contraction can be quite uncomfortable for the patient, and often limits the use of external pacemakers. Placing electrodes over areas with the least skeletal muscle may minimize the discomfort. The physician should use the lowest effective current. Sedation should be strongly considered if these measures are inadequate.

30. **Can an external pacemaker be used if a permanent pacemaker malfunctions?**
Yes, but be careful to place the external pacer on a pace-only (fixed-rate) mode and not the sensing mode. Otherwise, it may sense the electrical spikes from the permanent pacemaker and not fire.

31. **What are the advantages of transvenous versus transcutaneous pacemakers?**
Transcutaneous leads are the easiest to use for rapid initiation of temporary pacing. Transvenous leads are more reliable and more comfortable, because external pacing requires 30–100 times the current needed for internal transvenous pacing.

32. **How are transvenous and transthoracic pacemakers placed?**
Semifloating or flexible balloon-tipped catheters can be placed with central venous access into the subclavian or internal jugular veins. In the ED, pacers can be placed blindly, using ECG, point-of-care ultrasound, or fluoroscopy. For blind placement, the pacer is set to pace at a fixed rate and maximal amplitude until capture is obtained. For ECG guidance, an alligator clip is connected to a precordial lead such as V1, with another clip attached to the pacing wire. When a current of injury (ST elevation) is seen on the monitor, indicating contact with the heart, the wire should be withdrawn slightly, leaving it in pacing position. For ultrasound, the probe is placed either parasternal or subxyphoid; when the balloon enters the ventricle, it can be visualized. If available, fluoroscopy is preferred to ensure proper placement.

33. **Can cardiopulmonary resuscitation (CPR) be performed with a pacemaker?**
CPR can be performed safely with the external pacing pads in place. Turning the external pacemaker off during CPR is advisable, in particular when performing defibrillation or cardioversion. If using separate defibrillator paddles, they should be placed at least 2–3 cm away from pacing pads to prevent arching of current.

34. **List the indications for a permanent pacemaker.**
Indications for permanent pacing are constantly evolving. As of 2019, permanent pacing is indicated for:

- sick sinus syndrome
- symptomatic sinus bradycardia
- tachycardia-bradycardia syndrome
- AF with a slow ventricular response
- complete heart block
- chronotropic incompetence (inability to increase the heart rate to match a level of exercise)
- long QT syndrome
  More controversial applications include:
- cardiomyopathies (hypertrophic or dilated)
- congestive heart failure (cardiac resynchronization therapy [CRT])
- severe refractory neurocardiogenic syncope
- paroxysmal AF (atrial pacing)

35. **Describe the complications of permanent pacemaker implantation.**

Routine placement of a pacemaker generator into a subcutaneous or submuscular pocket carries the risk of pocket hematoma, which if large enough to palpate may need surgical drainage. Pocket infection can also occur and manifests as local inflammation, fluctuance, and abscess formation or local cellulitis. Rarely, the pocket itself may erode with extrusion of the generator secondary to infection, trauma, or local tissue ischemia. Infection usually is caused by *Staphylococcus aureus* acutely and *Staphylococcus epidermidis* in chronic infections. Treatment is empiric antibiotics and, ultimately, removal of the device and reimplantation at a remote site.

Wound dehiscence may require admission for debridement and reapproximation of wound edges. Leadless pacemaker therapy is a new technology aimed at avoiding lead and pocket-related complications of conventional transvenous and epicardial pacing. Additional complications include upper extremity deep venous thrombosis (DVT) on the side of the pacer and ventricular perforation with a risk of pericardial effusion and tamponade.

36. **What does a pacer setting of DDD mean?**

The letters represent a pacing code. The code consists of five letters that describe the different types of pacer function; the first three letters are the most relevant to the emergency physician (Table 33.2). The first letter indicates the chamber paced; the second indicates the chamber in which electrical activity is sensed; and the third indicates the response to a sensed event. Fourth and fifth letters may be added to describe whether the pacemaker is programmable and whether special functions to protect against tachycardia are available. A DDD pacer is able to pace and sense atria and ventricles (**D**ual chambers) and has a **D**ual response to the sensed ventricular and atrial activity (i.e., it can pace either the atrium or the ventricle). Spontaneous atrial and ventricular activity inhibits atrial and ventricular pacing; atrial activity without ventricular activity triggers only ventricular pacing.

37. **How can the type of permanent pacemaker be identified in the ED?**

Patients will often carry a card with them providing information about their particular model. Most pacemaker generators have an x-ray code that can be seen on a standard chest radiograph. The markings, along with the shape of the generator, may assist with determining the manufacturer of the generator and pacemaker battery.

38. **What is the most common cause of permanent pacemaker malfunction?**

The most common cause of malfunction is lead dislodgement. Most pacemaker failures are the result of problems with the electrodes or the wires, and not the battery or the pulse generator. Because of greater technologic sophistication, patients with pacemaker problems come to the ED much less commonly now than in the past.

39. **What is the most reliable indicator of pacer malfunction?**

A good indication of malfunction is a rate that is inappropriate for the patient's paced heart. A nonpaced ventricular rate <60 beats per minute, or a paced rate >100 beats per minute, is probably secondary to pacemaker malfunction.

40. **What does a magnet do?**

Placing a pacemaker magnet over the pulse generator stops the pacemaker from sensing or responding to a sensed event. The pacemaker reverts to one of three fixed-rate modes:
1. AOO (atrium paced)
2. VOO (ventricle paced)
3. DOO (atrium and ventricle paced)

The purpose is to check the pacing rate, which should be done quickly because the pulse generator is no longer prevented from firing during the T wave or from inhibiting serious arrhythmias. Magnets can also be used to turn off some automatic implantable cardioverter defibrillators (AICDs; see Question 51).

41. **How do I assess a patient with potential pacemaker malfunction?**
- Take a focused history on symptoms related to pacemaker malfunction, including palpitations, weakness, fatigue, shortness of breath, hiccups, syncope, fever, or pain or erythema at the generator site.

Table 33.2 Modified Pacing Code		
FIRST LETTER: CHAMBER PACED TO A SENSED EVENT	**SECOND LETTER: CHAMBER SENSED**	**THIRD LETTER: RESPONSE TO SENSED EVENT**
A (atrium)	A (atrium)	I (inhibition)
V (ventricle)	V (ventricle)	T (triggering)
D (dual chamber)	D (dual chamber)	D (dual response)
O (none)	O (none)	O (no response)

- The physical examination should focus on vital signs, mental status, cardiovascular system, and inspection of the generator site.
- An ECG should be obtained to evaluate pacemaker function, and anteroposterior and lateral chest radiographs to check pacemaker lead placement and lead and connector integrity.
- Evaluate the ECG. Are there pacing spikes present? If pacing spikes are not present, apply a circular magnet over the pacemaker site. If the application of the magnet does not result in pacing spikes being produced, there is some mechanical failure present.
- If pacing spikes are present, look for capture (a P wave in response to an atrial spike or a QRS complex in response to a ventricle spike, or both, depending on the type of pacemaker). If there is failure to capture, it usually indicates mechanical failure, such as lead fracture or dislodgement, but ischemia, metabolic derangements, and certain drugs have also been implicated. If pacing is occurring at an inappropriately short interval between atrial or ventricular contractions, it may be because the pacer is oversensing. If a pacer spike is seen immediately after a native QRS complex, it may be because the pacer is undersensing. See Table 33.3 for a description of common pacemaker malfunctions.

42. What is pacemaker syndrome?
Pacemaker syndrome is a clinical spectrum of lightheadedness, fatigue, palpitations, syncope, dyspnea on exertion, and hypotension that usually is attributed to asynchronous AV contraction and loss of atrial functional support.

43. What is twiddler's syndrome?
Twiddler's syndrome is the most common cause of late lead dislodgement. It occurs when the patient twists (or twiddles) the pulse generator within its pouch, twisting leads around the generator box, shortening and dislodging them from their proper position. The pulse generator may erode through the skin.

44. What is pacemaker-mediated tachycardia?
A normally functioning pacemaker may initiate a tachydysrhythmia. Retrograde conduction of a ventricular beat may cause the atrium to trigger a second ventricular contraction that falls during the pacemaker's refractory period. Because this contraction is not sensed by the pacemaker, the pulse generator fires, initiating a reentrant tachycardia. Treatment consists of lengthening the AV time by any of the following methods:
- Programming an increase in the atrial refractory time
- Administering adenosine or verapamil
- Increasing atrial sensory threshold
- Applying a magnet to stop atrial sensing by the pacemaker

45. What is a runaway pacemaker?
Malfunction of the pacemaker that is manifested by tachycardia secondary to rapid ventricular pacing is known as a *runaway pacemaker*. The problem is recognized when rates are greater than the upper rate limit settings of the pacemaker, and may require drastic measures, such as cutting the pacer leads.

46. What happens as pacemakers lose battery power?
Pacemakers usually show a decline in the rate of magnet-mediated pacing, usually to a predetermined manufacturer's rate. Pacer response varies with manufacturer; some models may also change pacer mode (e.g., DDD to VVI).

Table 33.3 Malfunctions of Permanent PACEMAKERS	
COMPLICATION	**DESCRIPTION**
Oversensing	Occurs when a pacer incorrectly senses electrical activity and is inhibited from correctly pacing. This may be caused by muscular activity, electromagnetic interference, or lead insulation breakage.
Undersensing	Occurs when a pacer incorrectly misses intrinsic depolarization and paces despite intrinsic activity. This can be the result of poor lead positioning, lead dislodgement, magnet application, low battery states, or myocardial infarction.
Operative failures	This includes malfunction resulting from mechanical factors (such as a pneumothorax, pericarditis, infection, hematoma, lead dislodgement, or venous thrombosis).
Failure to capture	Occurs when a pacing spike is not followed by either an atrial or ventricular complex. This may be caused by lead fracture, lead dislodgement, a break in lead insulation, an elevated pacing threshold, myocardial infarction at the lead tip, drugs, metabolic abnormalities, cardiac perforation, poor lead connection, and improper amplitude or pulse width settings.

Table 33.4 Malfunctions Associated With an Automatic Implantable Cardioverter Defibrillator

COMPLICATION	DESCRIPTION
Operative failure	Similar to operative failures in pacemakers
Sensing failure	Oversensing and undersensing occur for reasons similar to pacemakers
Inappropriate cardioversion	May occur if a patient has atrial fibrillation or has received multiple shocks in rapid succession
Ineffective cardioversion	Can be seen because of T-wave oversensing, lead fracture, lead insulation breakage, electrocautery, MRI, or electromagnetic interference. Can also be caused by inadequate energy output, a rise in the defibrillation threshold because of antidysrhythmic medications, myocardial infarction at the lead site, lead fracture, insulation breakage, or dislodgement of the leads of the cardioversion patches
Failure to deliver cardioversion	Can be caused by failure to sense, lead fracture, electromagnetic interference, and inadvertent AICD deactivation

AICD, Automatic implantable cardioverter defibrillator; *MRI,* magnetic resonance imaging.
Modified from Higgins 3rd GL. The automatic implantable cardioverter-defibrillator: management issues relevant to the emergency care provider. *Am J Emerg Med.* 1990;8:342–347.

47. **Can a patient with a permanent pacemaker undergo defibrillation?**
Yes, but it is important to place the pads or paddles away from the pulse generator, preferably in the anteroposterior position. Defibrillation can damage the pulse generator. Temporary and even permanent loss of ventricular or atrial capture may occur secondary to elevation of the capture threshold of the pacer leads.

48. **What is an AICD?**
An AICD is a specialized device designed to treat a cardiac tachydysrhythmia. If the device senses a ventricular rate that exceeds the programmed cut-off rate of the implantable cardioverter defibrillator, the device performs cardioversion/defibrillation. Alternatively, the device may attempt to pace rapidly for a number of pulses, usually around 10, to attempt pace termination of the VT. Newer AICDs are a combination of implantable cardioverter defibrillator and pacemaker in one unit.

49. **Discuss malfunctions associated with an AICD.**
See Table 33.4.

50. **Name the most common type of AICD malfunction.**
Inappropriate cardioversion

51. **What will a magnet do when placed over an AICD?**
Use of a magnet over the AICD inhibits further shocks, but it does not inhibit bradycardic pacing should the patient require it. In older devices, application of a magnet produces a beep for each QRS complex. If the magnet is left on for 30 seconds, the AICD is disabled, and a continuous tone is produced. To reactivate the device, the magnet is removed and replaced. After 30 seconds, a beep returns for every QRS complex.

KEY POINTS: CARDIAC DYSRHYTHMIAS

1. An unstable patient with any tachydysrhythmia, regardless of the mechanism, requires electrical cardioversion.
2. If unable to determine if the rhythm your patient is in is VT or SVT with aberrancy, assume VT and treat accordingly.
3. The most common reason for early pacemaker malfunction is lead dislodgement.
4. Temporary transcutaneous or transvenous pacing should be used for hemodynamically unstable bradycardias, as well as for overdrive pacing to terminate VT.
5. Calcium channel blockers should not be used to treat wide-complex tachycardias.

BIBLIOGRAPHY

Ellison K, Sharma PS, Trohman R. Advances in cardiac pacing and defibrillation. *Expert Rev Cardiovasc Ther.* 2017;15(6):429–440.
Faddy FC, Jennings PA. Biphasic versus monophasic waveforms for transthoracic defibrillation in out-of-hospital cardiac arrest. *Cochrane Database Syst Rev.* 2016;2:CD006762. doi:10.1002/14651858.CD006762.pub2.

Foerster CR, Andrew E, Smith K, Bernard S. Amiodarone for sustained stable ventricular tachycardia in the prehospital setting. *Emerg Med Australas.* 2018;30(5):694–698.

Glikson M, Hayes DL. Cardiac pacing: a review. *Med Clin North Am.* 2001;85:369–421.

Greenspon AJ, Patel JD, Lau E, et al. Trends in permanent pacemaker implantation in the United States from 1993 to 2009. *Am J Coll Cardiol.* 2012;60(16):1540–1545.

Link MS. Evaluation and initial treatment of supraventricular tachycardia. *N Engl J Med.* 2012;367:1438–1448.

Martin A, Coll-Vinent B, Suero C, et al. Benefits of rhythm and rate control in recent-onset atrial fibrillation: the HERMES-AF study. *Acad Emerg Med.* 2019;26(6):1034–1043. doi:10.1111/acem.13703.

Mulpuru SK, Madhaven M, McLeod CJ, et al. Cardiac pacemakers: function, troubleshooting, and management: part 1 of a 2-part series. *J Am Coll Cardiol.* 2017;69(2):189–210.

Neumar RW, Otto CW, Link MS, et al. 2010 American Heart Association guidelines for cardiopulmonary resuscitation and emergency cardiovascular care. Part 8.2. Management of cardiac arrest. *Circulation.* 2010;122:S729–S767.

Ortiz M, Martin A, Arribas F, et al. Randomized comparison of intravenous procainamide vs. intravenous amiodarone for the acute treatment of tolerated wide QRS tachycardia: the PROCAMIO study. *Eur Heart J.* 2017;38:1329–1335.

Piela N, Kornweiss S, Sacchetti A, et al. Outcomes of the emergency department placement of transvenous pacemakers. *Am J Emerg Med.* 2016;34(8):1411–1414.

Squire B, Niemann JT. Implantable cardiac devices. In: Walls RM, Hockberger RS, Gaushe-Hill M, eds. *Rosen's Emergency Medicine: Concepts and Clinical Practice.* Philadelphia, PA: Elsevier; 2018:959–970.

Yealy DM, Kosowshy JM. Dysrhythmias. In: Walls RM, Hockberger RS, Gausche-Hill M, eds. *Rosen's Emergency Medicine: Concepts and Clinical Practice.* 9th ed. Philadelphia, PA: Elsevier; 2018:929–958.

CHAPTER 34

HYPERTENSION, HYPERTENSIVE EMERGENCY, AORTIC DISSECTION, AND AORTIC ANEURYSMS

Alexander S. Grohmann, MD and Madonna Fernández-Frackelton, MD, FACEP

HYPERTENSION AND HYPERTENSIVE EMERGENCY

KEY POINTS

1. Avoid precipitous or excessive drops in blood pressure (BP) with cerebrovascular emergencies.
2. Avoid the urge to treat "hypertensive urgency" in any other way than as if you were treating asymptotic hypertension (HTN); they are identical and should be treated with oral medication on an outpatient basis.
3. Avoid pure β-blockers for catecholamine-induced hypertensive emergencies. Treat with benzodiazepines first.
4. Understand that pain, anxiety, and just being in the emergency department (ED) might cause transient HTN.
5. Consider secondary causes of HTN in pediatric patients.

1. **What is the definition of HTN according to the Joint National Committee on Prevention, Detection, Evaluation, and Treatment of High Blood Pressure (JNC 7) report?**
   - Normal blood pressure (BP): lower than 120/80 mmHg
   - Prehypertension: systolic BP (SBP) 120–139 mmHg or diastolic BP (DBP) 80–89 mmHg
   - Stage 1 HTN: SBP 140–159 mmHg or DBP 90–99 mmHg
   - Stage 2 HTN: SBP >160 mmHg or DBP >100 mmHg

2. **How does the JNC 8 report differ from the JNC 7 report?**
   - JNC 8 does not address definitions, but rather thresholds for treatment.
   - There is strong evidence to treat patients >60 years of age. The goal BP should be less than 150/90 mmHg.
   - There is strong evidence to treat patients 30–59 years of age. The goal DBP should be less than 90 mmHg.
   - There is insufficient evidence for a goal SBP in patients <60 years of age, or for a goal DBP in patients <30 years of age. Expert recommendation in these age groups is <140/90 mmHg.

3. **What is the difference between primary and secondary HTN?**
   - Primary, or essential, HTN accounts for more than 90% of patients with HTN. Its cause is unknown, but likely related to a combination of genetics and environment.
   - Secondary HTN has an identifiable cause. It can result from:
     - Primary neurologic disorders that increase intracranial pressure (ICP), such as ischemic or hemorrhagic stroke, mass, or cerebral edema
     - Renal disorders (glomerulonephritis, polycystic kidney disease, chronic pyelonephritis, hemolytic uremic syndrome)
     - Vascular disorders (coarctation of the aorta, renal artery stenosis, fibromuscular dysplasia, Takayasu arteritis, polyarteritis nodosa)
     - Endocrine disorders (Cushing syndrome [increased cortisol], Conn syndrome [increased aldosterone], pheochromocytoma [increased catecholamines], thyroid disorders, renin-secreting tumor)
     - Pregnancy-induced HTN (preeclampsia and eclampsia)
     - Sleep apnea

4. **What might cause transient HTN in the ED?**
   - Anxiety or pain
   - Over-the-counter and prescription medications (estrogen containing medications, steroids, decongestants, diet pills, nonsteroidal anti-inflammatory drugs [NSAIDs], citrus aurantium)
   - Certain toxidromes (anticholinergic, sympathomimetic)
   - Serotonin syndrome and neuroleptic malignant syndrome

- Illicit drug use (e.g., cocaine, amphetamines, phencyclidine [PCP], or lysergic acid diethylamide [LSD])
- Alcoholism and alcohol withdrawal
- Lead intoxication
- Anti-HTN medication withdrawal

5. **How do I explain to patients the importance of treating HTN?**
Treatment results in a 35% reduction in stroke incidence, a 20% reduction in myocardial infarction (MI), and a 50% reduction in heart failure. It is estimated that achieving an SBP reduction of 12 mmHg for 10 years in patients with stage I HTN and modifying additional cardiovascular risk factors will prevent one death for every 11 patients treated. However, it is also important to convey that these treatment benefits are for long-term goals, and not necessarily short-term reductions in the ED. Short-term or drastic reductions can cause significant harm.

6. **Is diagnostic testing necessary in a patient with elevated BP and no symptoms in the ED?**
- Testing is generally not necessary. These patients should receive prompt follow-up with a primary care physician.
- In select patients, for whom follow-up care is uncertain, or if outpatient treatment is to be initiated by the emergency physician, a basic metabolic panel, including creatinine, is recommended (level C or expert consensus), as the results might affect disposition or medication selection.
- In a study of 109 patients with BP greater than 180/110 mmHg, 6% had laboratory abnormalities.
- An electrocardiogram (ECG) and chest radiography (CXR) may show abnormalities related to chronic HTN, but are unlikely to affect care.

7. **Should treatment be initiated in the ED in asymptomatic patients with elevated BP?**
- Generally, no. A significant number of patients, even with SBP >160 mmHg in the ED, will not have HTN on follow-up visits.
- If no follow-up visit can be arranged and the physician feels compelled to initiate treatment, it is recommended to start a thiazide diuretic (hydrochlorothiazide) or a calcium channel blocker (amlodipine) in the absence of renal or cardiac disease. For patients with SBP >180 mmHg or DBP >110 mmHg, consideration should be given to starting an antihypertensive agent. Patients with SBP >200 mmHg or DBP >120 mmHg should be started on an antihypertensive agent at discharge. Acute treatment to lower BP in the ED is not necessary.

8. **What is a hypertensive emergency, or crisis?**
- A hypertensive emergency is characterized by a severely elevated BP (typically 220/120 mmHg), with acute end-organ (brain, heart, kidneys) damage. The absolute BP is not a criterion. The terms *malignant HTN* and *accelerated HTN* are used in the *International Classification of Diseases (ICD)*, 10th edition.
- Examples include:
  - Hypertensive encephalopathy
  - Ischemic and hemorrhagic stroke
  - Subarachnoid hemorrhage (SAH)
  - Acute myocardial infarction (AMI)
  - Decompensated congestive heart failure (CHF) with pulmonary edema
  - Aortic dissection
  - Preeclampsia/eclampsia
  - Acute kidney injury (AKI): a controversial topic and requires special consideration as isolated elevations in creatinine may reflect chronic kidney disease and not an acute process.

9. **What is hypertensive urgency?**
- *Hypertensive urgency* is a term commonly used to describe severe asymptomatic HTN, where patients have very high BP (>220/120 mmHg) without evidence of acute end-organ damage. There may be a history of chronic HTN and chronic end-organ damage.
- BP should be controlled with oral medications over the next 48 hours, which can be done on an outpatient basis with appropriate follow-up care.
- There is no *ICD-10* code for hypertensive urgency, and the term refers more to the feeling the provider has about the HTN, rather than anything relevant to the treatment of the patient.

10. **What are the symptoms of hypertensive emergency?**
Signs and symptoms of hypertensive crisis are manifestations of the organ systems involved:
- Central nervous system involvement may cause headache, lethargy, dizziness, confusion, focal neurologic deficits, paresthesias, or vision changes. If left untreated, this can progress to seizures, blindness, and coma. (Headache alone is NOT a hypertensive emergency.)
- Chest pain, back pain, shortness of breath, and lower extremity swelling may be presenting signs and symptoms of CHF, AMI, or aortic dissection.
- Decreased urine output, nausea, and generalized malaise and weakness may suggest AKI.

11. **What physical examination findings support the diagnosis of hypertensive emergency?**
    - Central nervous system: confusion, altered level of consciousness, and focal neurologic findings.
    - Funduscopic examination: arteriovenous nicking, copper-wiring, flame hemorrhages, exudates, and papilledema.
    - Cardiopulmonary: rales, hepatomegaly, and lower extremity edema may be present, as well as a gallop, jugular venous distention, and a displaced point of maximal impulse.
    - Vascular: a pulsatile mass in the abdomen or unequal pulses may indicate an aortic aneurysm or dissection, respectively, but their absence does not rule out these diseases.

12. **What diagnostic studies should be considered in a patient with a hypertensive emergency?**
    - If neurologic symptoms or physical findings are present, a computed tomography (CT) of the head should be performed to evaluate for hemorrhagic or ischemic stroke, hypertensive encephalopathy, or subarachnoid bleed. If nondiagnostic, consider further investigation with magnetic resonance imaging (MRI) of the brain or a CT angiogram for aortic dissection.
    - An ECG should be performed in patients with chest pain or shortness of breath to evaluate for ischemia or infarction.
    - CXR should be performed in patients with chest pain or shortness of breath to evaluate for pulmonary edema or evidence of aortic dissection or aneurysm.
    - Point-of-care ultrasonography can be used to evaluate for B-lines in suspected pulmonary edema, abdominal aortic aneurysm (AAA) in patients with abdominal or back pain, or aortic root diameter in patients with suspected type A aortic dissection.
    - Troponin and hemoglobin tests should be ordered in patients with chest pain, back pain, shortness of breath, confusion, or altered level of consciousness.
    - If there is concern for aortic dissection or aneurysm, a CT angiogram should be obtained. These patients should also have a type and screen, as well as any other standard hospital protocol panels needed to prepare for surgical management, including a complete blood count (CBC), metabolic panel, coagulation profile, and ECG.
    - A chemistry panel should be considered to screen for renal insufficiency, and a urine sample can be obtained to check for protein, blood, and glucose. The results of the serum creatinine should not delay the CT angiogram in patients with a high suspicion for aortic dissection.

13. **How do I diagnose hypertensive encephalopathy?**
    - The classic triad is altered mental status (AMS), HTN, and papilledema.
    - Symptoms are reversible with appropriate BP reduction, but if left untreated, coma and death occur within hours.
    - Other causes of AMS should be evaluated, including cerebrovascular accident (CVA), intoxication, renal insufficiency, and microangiopathic hemolytic anemia.

14. **What is the pathophysiology of hypertensive encephalopathy?**
    Acute, severe elevations in BP cause cerebral autoregulation to fail, compromising the blood–brain barrier and increasing cerebral perfusion, resulting in overperfusion, vasospasm, and cerebral ischemia. This leads to cerebral edema and elevated ICP.

    Cerebral autoregulation works only within a certain range of mean arterial pressure (MAP), above or below which the cerebral blood flow (CBF) is significantly affected. CBF depends on cerebral perfusion pressure (CPP) and cerebrovascular resistance (CVR):

    $$CBF = CPP/CVR$$

    The CPP is defined as MAP minus venous pressure, in this case the ICP:

    $$CPP = MAP - ICP$$
    $$MAP = [(2 \times DBP) + SBP] \div 3$$

    To maintain CBF and CPP at relatively constant levels, cerebral arteries vasoconstrict when MAP increases, and vasodilate when MAP decreases. In normotensive individuals, cerebral autoregulation maintains constant CBF between a MAP of 60 and 120 mmHg. In hypertensive patients, the lower limit of autoregulation is raised. For both hypertensive and normotensive patients, the lower limit of autoregulation has been found to be approximately 25% below the resting MAP.

15. **How do I treat hypertensive encephalopathy?**
    - The goal of treatment is to carefully decrease the MAP by approximately 25% over the first hour, to a goal BP of 160/100 mmHg by 2–6 hours.
    - Medication selection should be based on patient parameters, physician experience, and hospital protocol.
    - Each medication works by different mechanisms, but should have three important properties in common:
      - Intravenous (IV) route for easy titration
      - Rapid onset
      - Short duration of action
    - IV nicardipine, labetalol, clevidipine, or esmolol are the currently recommended medications.

16. **What is the treatment threshold for HTN in ischemic stroke?**
    - There is an absence of conclusive data regarding treatment of HTN in the setting of ischemic stroke. The Stroke Council for the American Heart Association recommends cautiously lowering the BP in ischemic stroke only if the SBP is greater than 220 mmHg or DBP is greater than 120 mmHg. The BP should be lowered by 15% over the first 24 hours.
    - If the patient is eligible for thrombolysis, it is recommended to lower the BP to less than 185/110 mmHg. Decision making regarding BP management should be made in consultation with a neurologist or neurosurgeon, when possible.
    - It is important not to lower the BP too rapidly in these patients, because it may drop the CPP and lead to further ischemia.

17. **What are the recommendations regarding treatment of HTN in hemorrhagic stroke?**
    See Chapter 26.

18. **How do I treat HTN if it is associated with SAH?**
    - There are no definitive data on what BP is beneficial to these patients. The 2012 American Stroke Associate guidelines suggest that achieving an SBP of less than 160 mmHg is reasonable. Suggested medications are labetalol, esmolol, and nicardipine.
    - Nitroprusside and nitroglycerin should be avoided, because they can increase CBF and thus increase ICP.
    - Pain should be controlled with narcotic analgesics.

19. **How do I treat a patient with severe HTN and evidence of pulmonary edema?**
    Patients with pulmonary edema and severe HTN should be treated with a focus on afterload reduction, and other supportive care.
    - Sit the patient upright and provide oxygen and bilevel positive airway pressure (BiPAP) as needed.
    - Administer IV nitroglycerin with or without sodium nitroprusside for both preload and afterload reduction.
    - Provide angiotensin-converting enzyme (ACE) inhibitors, such as enalaprilat, for afterload reduction.
    - Loop diuretics, such as furosemide, may decrease the need for other antihypertensive agents.

20. **How do I treat a patient with severe HTN and chest pain caused by ischemia?**
    - Reduction of BP in the setting of angina or AMI is crucial to decrease myocardial workload and prevent ongoing ischemia. First-line treatment is IV nitroglycerin, in combination with an IV β-blocker if there is no evidence of CHF.
    - If this fails to control BP, nicardipine or fenoldopam can be added.
    - Sodium nitroprusside should be avoided, because it can cause a coronary steal phenomenon in patients with coronary artery disease, causing increased mortality in the presence of an AMI.
    - Hydralazine should be avoided because it can cause reflex tachycardia, thus increasing oxygen demand.

21. **What agents should I use to treat a patient with severe HTN and AKI?**
    - IV fenoldopam is a short-acting dopamine-1 receptor agonist that increases renal perfusion, creatinine clearance, sodium excretion, and diuresis. It is as effective as nitroprusside at lowering the BP without the risk of cyanide toxicity, but is more costly.
    - Other reasonable alternatives include nicardipine and labetalol.
    - ACE inhibitors should be avoided as they may worsen the glomerular filtration rate.

22. **What should I always think about in a pregnant or postpartum woman with HTN?**
    Preeclampsia; see Chapter 81.

23. **What antihypertensive medications, if stopped abruptly, can cause rebound HTN?**
    Short-acting sympathetic blockers, such as clonidine, and β-blockers.

24. **How do I treat a catecholamine-induced hypertensive emergency (i.e., stimulant ingestion and endogenous catecholamine overproduction)?**
    - Benzodiazepines are the first-line treatment of hyperadrenergic or catecholamine-induced HTN.
    - Antihypertensive agents that can be used for treatment of a catecholamine-induced hypertensive emergency include nicardipine, fenoldopam, phentolamine, and nitroprusside.
    - β-Blockers should be avoided, because they can cause unopposed α-adrenergic vasoconstriction and elevate BP further. In patients with cocaine ingestion, β-blockers fail to decrease heart rate, enhance coronary artery vasoconstriction, increase BP, decrease the seizure threshold, and increase mortality.
    - Labetalol, an α- and β-blocker, theoretically avoids the problem of unopposed α-adrenergic vasoconstriction, but still carries the risk of β > α blockade in patients with cocaine ingestion or pheochromocytoma.

25. **What are the common parenteral antihypertensive medications and their indications and contraindications?**
    See Table 34.1.

Table 34.1 Parenteral Antihypertensive Medications

DRUG	DOSAGE	ONSET	DURATION	INDICATIONS	CONTRAINDICATIONS
Nitroprusside	0.3–10 µg/kg/min IV	1–2 min	1–2 min	CHF, aortic dissection, catecholamine excess, hypertensive encephalopathy	Pregnancy, AMI, hepatic or renal insufficiency; caution with increased ICP and AKI
Nitroglycerin	10–200 µg/min IV	2–5 min	3–5 min	AMI, CHF	CVA
Nicardipine	5–15 mg/h IV	15 min	6 h	AMI, AKI, eclampsia, hypertensive encephalopathy, catecholamine excess	CHF, second- or third-degree AVB
Fenoldopam	0.1–1.6 µg/kg/min IV	5–15 min	1–4 h	AMI, CHF, AKI, aortic dissection, hypertensive encephalopathy, catecholamine excess	Glaucoma (can cause increased IOP)
Hydralazine	10–20 mg IV bolus; repeat every 2–4 h prn (max 40 mg)	10–20 min	3–8 h	Eclampsia	AMI, CVA, aortic dissection
Esmolol	500 µg/kg IV bolus over 1 min, then 50–300 µg/kg/min	1–2 min	10–20 min	CAD, aortic dissection	CHF, second- or third-degree AVB
Labetalol	20 mg IV bolus, then 40–80 mg every 10 min up to 300 mg or 2 mg/min IV	2–10 min	2–4 h	CAD, aortic dissection, hypertensive encephalopathy, eclampsia	CHF, second- or third-degree AVB, asthma
Phentolamine	5 mg IV, repeat every 10 min prn (max 20 mg)	1–2 min	10–30 min	Catecholamine excess	AMI

AKI, Acute kidney injury; *AMI*, acute myocardial infarction; *AVB*, atrioventricular block; *CAD*, coronary artery disease; *CHF*, congestive heart failure; *CVA*, cerebrovascular accident; *ICP*, intracranial pressure; *IOP*, intraocular pressure; *IV*, intravenously; *prn*, as needed.

26. **Can I use oral agents to treat hypertensive emergencies?**
There is no place for the use of oral or transdermal agents in a true hypertensive emergency. The therapeutic response is unpredictable and cannot be titrated.

27. **What disease processes should be considered in the hypertensive pediatric patient?**
Hypertension in the pediatric patient is described as a SBP or DBP greater than 90% of the upper limit of normal of the age adjusted measurements.
Neonates (0–30 days):
- Renal disorders: polycystic kidney disease, obstructive uropathy, renal dysplasia, renal venous thrombosis, renal artery thrombosis/stenosis
- Neoplasia: neuroblastoma, mesoblastic nephroma
- Cardiovascular: coarctation of the aorta
- Endocrinopathies: hyperthyroidism, adrenogenital syndrome
- Medications: steroids, phenylephrine eye drops, theophylline, caffeine, maternal cocaine use
6–10 Year olds:
- Essential hypertension
- Renal disorders: renal artery stenosis, glomerulonephritis, reflux nephropathy, pyelonephritis, vasculitis
- Endocrine disorders: corticosteroids, hyperaldosteronism, pheochromocytoma
10 Years to adolescence:
- Essential hypertension
- Renal disorders: glomerulonephritis, pyelonephritis, end-stage renal disease, vasculitis
- Pregnancy-related hypertensive disorders
- Drugs: amphetamines, sympathomimetics, and steroids

AORTIC DISSECTION AND ANEURYSMS

KEY POINTS

1. The triad of an AAA is abdominal pain, pulsatile mass, and hypotension.
2. Do not wait for a definitive study before calling a surgeon.
3. Point-of-care ultrasound is an excellent screening tool for AAA.
4. Contrast-enhanced CT is the gold standard for making the diagnosis of a ruptured AAA.

28. **How do aneurysms, pseudoaneurysm, and dissection differ?**
- An aneurysm involves dilation of all three layers of the arterial wall: the intima, media, and adventitia.
- A pseudoaneurysm, or false aneurysm, is typically caused by arterial injury, resulting in a tear in the arterial wall and consequent blood leak. The hematoma is contained within the outer tissue layer, but still communicates with the arterial lumen.
- Dissection is a distinctly different disease from an aneurysm, and involves a tear in the intima, resulting in a false lumen within the media. Blood can dissect in the wall either proximally or distally.
- The term *dissecting aneurysm* is not an accurate use of either term. Although it is possible for an aneurysm to dissect, dissection typically exists without an aneurysm present.

29. **Other than cardiac ischemia and aortic dissection, what causes chest pain in the hypertensive patient?**
Other life-threatening causes of chest pain include pulmonary embolism, tension pneumothorax, pericardial tamponade, and esophageal rupture.

30. **What are risk factors associated with aortic aneurysms?**
- Tobacco use, hypercholesterolemia, HTN, male gender, family history, and advanced age.
- Other rare causes include infection, such as tertiary syphilis (which leads to aneurysmal dilation in the aortic root/ascending aorta), blunt chest trauma (usually resulting in pseudoaneurysms), connective tissue diseases (such as Marfan syndrome and Ehlers-Danlos syndrome), and arteritis.
- Although true aneurysms can develop anywhere along the aorta, 75% are abdominal.

31. **What are the risk factors for aortic dissection?**
- HTN is present in 70% of patients (most common)
- Men are at higher risk than women
- Age older than 60 years
- The peak age for proximal dissection is 50–55 years, and for distal dissection is 60–70 years
- Bicuspid aortic valves
- History of aortic valve replacement or cardiac catheterization
- Cocaine or amphetamine use
- Genetic conditions (Marfan, Ehlers-Danlos, Loeys-Dietz, Noonan, and Turner syndromes)

- A family or personal history of dissection
- Known thoracic aortic aneurysm
- Pregnancy
- Weight lifting

32. **What symptoms may be present in a patient with thoracic aortic dissection?**
   - The patient experiences a sudden onset (85%) of severe chest pain with radiation to the jaw, neck, or back in the intrascapular region.
   - Pain is most severe at onset and is often described as sharp, ripping, or tearing in quality.
   - Pain starts in one region and moves to another (abdomen to chest or chest to abdomen).
   - The patient may have nausea, vomiting, diaphoresis, lightheadedness, and apprehension or a sense of impending doom.
   - Syncope can also be the presenting complaint, and in some cases may be the only symptom.
   - Proximal dissections may cause aortic regurgitation and pericardial effusion with tamponade (16%).
   - Occlusion of aortic branches may cause AMI (coronary artery involvement); stroke (carotid or vertebral artery involvement); or paresthesias and arm pain (subclavian artery involvement), which may be suggested by unequal BPs or pulses.
   - Spinal artery occlusion can cause neurologic compromise.
   - Hoarseness may result from recurrent laryngeal nerve compression.
   - Chest pain unrelieved by large doses of narcotic analgesics should raise the concern for this diagnosis.

33. **What physical examination findings may be present in a patient with thoracic aortic dissection?**
   - The patient often has high BP on arrival, but hypotension may be present if the patient develops tamponade, aortic regurgitation, MI, or rupture.
   - A new diastolic murmur of aortic regurgitation suggests dissection into the aortic root.
   - Unequal upper extremity BPs occur less than one third of the time; but, if present, are highly suggestive of proximal aortic dissection.
   - Pulses should be checked in all four extremities, because dissection can extend the entire length of the aorta and into the iliac arteries.
   - New focal neurologic deficit in the setting of chest pain.

34. **What diagnostic imaging should be performed when thoracic aortic dissection is suspected?**
   - CXR is abnormal in about 80% of cases, but the abnormalities are nonspecific. It may rule out other causes of chest pain, such as pneumothorax, but further imaging is usually required if dissection is suspected.
   - CT angiogram is the study of choice in the ED, because it is quick, accurate, and readily available in most practice settings.
   - MRI is sensitive and specific, but scan times are long and place the patient in a position inadequate for resuscitation if needed.
   - Transesophageal echocardiogram (TEE) is excellent for determining involvement of the aortic valve and coronary arteries and can detect the presence of pericardial effusion or tamponade, but the study requires sedation and an experienced cardiologist or technician.
   - If the patient is hypotensive, a bedside echocardiogram can rule out pericardial effusion with tamponade.
   - An ECG should be done to evaluate for MI.

35. **What might I see on the chest radiograph of a patient with a thoracic aortic dissection?**
   - Widened mediastinum
   - Loss of the aortic knob
   - Left pleural effusion
   - Tracheal (or nasogastric tube) deviation to the right
   - Apical pleural capping
   - Calcium sign (displacement of the intimal calcium layer >10 mm in the aorta)

36. **What other tests should I perform?**
   - Basic laboratory testing with CBC, metabolic panel, troponin, and lactate in addition to preoperative laboratory testing with type and screen, and coagulation panel.
   - D-dimer is elevated in 97% of aortic dissections. A D-dimer level <500 ng/mL has a negative predictive value of 95% for aortic dissection. A D-dimer level <500 ng/mL in a patient with a low pretest probability for aortic dissection has been prospectively shown to accurately and efficiently rule out aortic dissection.

37. **What is the Stanford classification for aortic dissection?**
   The Stanford classification describes the location of the dissection related to the recommended treatment modalities:
   - Type A dissections (67%) involve the ascending aorta proximal to the ligamentum arteriosum (with or without descending aorta involvement) and require emergent surgical repair. If the patient survives surgery, the in-hospital mortality is 30%.

- Type B dissections (33%) affect the descending aorta distal to the ligamentum arteriosum and are usually managed medically, but about one third will eventually require surgical or endovascular repair. Overall, in-hospital mortality is 10%, but it is only 8% if dissections are managed medically and 19% if vascular intervention is required.

38. How do I treat a patient with aortic dissection?

- Treatment should be initiated before imaging in patients with a high suspicion of aortic dissection.
- Opiate analgesics are appropriate to provide adequate pain control.
- IV antihypertensive medication should be initiated if the patient is hypertensive.
  - Rate control should start first with an IV β-blocker, such as esmolol, before the initiation of an antihypertensive to prevent reflex tachycardia and increased shear forces.
  - An antihypertensive agent such as nicardipine, fenoldopam, or nitroprusside should follow the administration IV β-blockers.
  - An alternative treatment regimen is IV labetalol used as a single agent.
  - Rapid reduction of SBP to a range of 100–110 mmHg and a heart rate of ~60 beats per minute is indicated.
- A cardiothoracic surgeon should be consulted emergently.
- If the patient is hypotensive, a bedside ultrasound should be performed to evaluate for pericardial tamponade.

ABDOMINAL AORTIC ANEURYSM

39. What are common presenting signs and symptoms of an AAA?

- Most patients with AAAs are asymptomatic, and the aneurysm is found incidentally.
- Patients with symptoms of acutely expanding AAA may have gradually increasing abdominal pain, low back pain, or flank pain radiating to the groin. It is often described as dull, throbbing, or colicky.
- 3% of men older than 50 years have an occult AAA.
- 75% of aneurysms >5 cm can be palpated.
- 5%–10% of patients with an AAA have an abdominal bruit.

40. What common diseases may mimic ruptured AAA?

- Renal colic, pancreatitis, perforated peptic ulcer, AMI, gallbladder pathology, diverticulitis, appendicitis, perforated viscus, bowel obstruction, musculoskeletal back pain, and intestinal ischemia.
- The diagnosis should be considered in patients >50 years of age with any one of the symptoms in the classic triad: pain, hypotension, and pulsatile mass.

41. What are the risks of rupture in AAA?

- The risk of rupture is minimal for an AAA measuring less than 4 cm.
- The risk increases dramatically at diameters >6 cm (Table 34.2).
- Rapid expansion is the greatest predictor of impending rupture, and routine screening of patients with known AAAs is important. All patients with an AAA ≥5 cm in diameter should have a follow-up consultation with a vascular surgeon.
- Expansion of >0.5 cm over 6 months, or >1 cm per 1 year is a risk factor for rupture, regardless of aneurysm size.

42. What is the presentation of a ruptured AAA?

- The classic triad of ruptured AAA is pain, hypotension, and a pulsatile abdominal mass. Oftentimes, patients only have one or two of these symptoms, and sometimes, none.
- Hypotension, syncope, or low hematocrit may signify significant blood loss.
- Rarely, AAAs can rupture into the intestines and present as a massive gastrointestinal (GI) bleed (aortoenteric fistula). GI bleeding in a patient with previous aortic repair may suggest fistula formation between the wall of the aorta and the small or large bowel.
- Radicular pain may occur if the bleeding is retroperitoneal. Leg ischemia may occur because of peripheral embolization of mural plaques.

Table 34.2 Risk of Rupture in Abdominal Aortic Aneurysm (AAA)	
AAA DIAMETER	**RISK OF RUPTURE**
6–7 cm	10%–20%
7–8 cm	20%–40%
>8 cm	30%–50%

43. How do I treat a patient with a suspected ruptured AAA?

- Place two large-bore IVs; type and cross-match for at least six units of packed red blood cells.
- Call a vascular surgeon to get the patient to the operating room as soon as possible. Transport should not be delayed for definitive studies or to attempt full resuscitation in the ED.
- A bedside ultrasound can be done quickly to screen for an AAA. The ultrasound can confirm AAA, but rarely detects rupture because most AAAs rupture into the retroperitoneum.
- CT scans are appropriate in hemodynamically stable patients, and have a 100% sensitivity for detecting AAA, and 77%–100% sensitivity for picking up retroperitoneal bleeding. The CT can be performed without contrast if there is concern for the patient's kidney function. The mortality for elective repair of an unruptured AAA is approximately 5%, compared with greater than 50% mortality associated with acute repair of an already ruptured AAA.

44. What are the dilemmas of aggressive fluid resuscitation in a hypotensive patient with ruptured AAA?

There are no prospective studies to guide optimal fluid resuscitation in ruptured AAA. The goal is to achieve intravascular volume replacement adequate to maintain end-organ perfusion. Allowing some degree of hypotension may slow bleeding and allow for clot formation. Excessive fluid can have the opposite effect, and may cause an increased BP and dilutional coagulopathy, increasing bleeding. We recommend that crystalloid and blood products be used to maintain a MAP of 60–65 mmHg.

45. When should a symptomatic unruptured AAA be repaired?

- Aneurysms ≥5.5 cm should be repaired.
- There is debate over when to operate on patients with aneurysms 4–5.4 cm in diameter.
- A threshold of 5 cm has been suggested for women, as they have a higher rupture rate.
- Current guidelines do not address expansion rate and need for surgery. However, expansion of >0.5 cm over 6 months, or >1 cm per 1 year are generally considered for repair.

46. How are AAAs surgically repaired?

AAAs can be repaired with open surgery or endovascular stenting. The acute risks of open surgery are higher and the hospital stay is longer, but it corrects the problem. Stenting involves the insertion of a graft through a small incision in the groin and positioning of the stent with a balloon. The acute risks are lower, and the recovery period is shortened.

47. What are the complications of endovascular aortic repair (EVAR)?

The long-term mortality rates of patients who have undergone EVAR seem to be equal to the open approach. And while the short-term outcomes of EVAR also seem equal or favorable to open repair, EVAR has shown higher reintervention rates and AAA rupture rates. Many of the complications of EVAR are similar to the complications of open surgical repair. Certain complications have decreased in incidence with the evolution of the technique and advances in materials used.

Complications of EVAR include:

- Endoleak is the most common complication and occurs in up to one fourth of all patients who have undergone EVAR. Some types of endoleaks place the patient at a higher risk of AAA rupture.
- Graft infection, which can lead to aortoenteric fistula formation, commonly presenting as upper GI bleed
- Limb ischemia caused by arterial occlusion
- Stent migration
- Continued aneurysmal sac expansion (endotension)

BIBLIOGRAPHY

Chaikof EL, Dalman RL, Eskandari MK, et al. The Society for Vascular Surgery practice guidelines on the care of patients with an abdominal aortic aneurysm. *J Vasc Surg.* 2018;67(1):2–77.e2.

Claude J, Greenberg SM, Anderson CS, et al. Guidelines for the management of spontaneous intracerebral hemorrhage. *Stroke.* 2015;46(7):2032–2060.

James PA, Oparil S, Carter BL, et al. 2014 evidence-based guidelines for the management of high blood pressure in adults. Report from the panel members appointed to the Eighth Joint National Committee (JNC 8). *JAMA.* 2014;311:507–520.

Morgenstern LB, Hemphill JC, Becker K, et al. Guidelines for the management of spontaneous intracerebral hemorrhage: a guideline for health care professionals from the American Heart Association/American Stroke Association. *Stroke.* 2010;41:2108–2129.

Moulakakis KG, Mylonas SN, Dalainias I, et al. Management of complicated and uncomplicated acute type B dissection: a systemic review and meta-analysis. *Ann Cardiothorac Surg.* 2014;3:234–246.

Nazerian P, Morello F, Vanni S, et al. Combined use of aortic dissection detection risk score and D-dimer in the diagnostic workup of suspected acute aortic dissection. *Int J Cardiol.* 2014;175(1):78–82.

Powers WJ, Rabinstein AA, Ackerson T, et al. 2018 Guidelines for the early management of patients with acute ischemic stroke: a guideline for healthcare professionals from the American Heart Association/American Stroke Association. *Stroke.* 2018;49(3):e46–e110.

Wolf SJ, Lo B, Shih RD, et al. Clinical policy: critical issues in the evaluation and management of adult patients in the emergency department with asymptomatic elevated blood pressure. *Ann Emerg Med.* 2013;62:59–68.

Wylie T, Khan N. Hypertensive emergencies. In: Baren JM, Rothrock SG, Brennan JA, Brown L, eds. *Pediatric Emergency Medicine.* Philadelphia, PA: Saunders/Elsevier; 2008:506–513.

CHAPTER 35

PERICARDITIS AND MYOCARDITIS

Christopher B. Colwell, MD

PERICARDITIS

1. **Describe a normal pericardium.**
   The pericardium is 1–2 mm thick, is relatively inelastic, and envelops the heart. It has two layers. Between the two layers is the pericardial space, which normally contains 25–50 mL of fluid.

2. **What is pericarditis?**
   Inflammation of the pericardium.

3. **What causes pericarditis?**
   - Idiopathic pericarditis accounts for the vast majority of cases, and is thought to be caused by the antibody-mediated autoimmune reaction that occurs 2–4 weeks after a viral illness (Table 35.1).
   - Infectious agents, such as viruses and bacteria, can cause pericarditis as a result of spread of infection to the pericardium.
   - An autoimmune reaction to cardiac antigens may occur after cardiac instrumentation or acute myocardial infarction (MI).
   - The likelihood of postinfarction pericarditis is reduced by half (from approximately 12%–6%) when a thrombolytic agent is used.

4. **Who is most susceptible to infectious pericarditis?**
   Viral and idiopathic pericarditis occur most commonly in healthy people between 20 and 40 years old. Bacterial pericarditis can occur in patients with a bacterial infection of the lungs, endocardium, or blood. Patients with immunosuppression are susceptible to pericarditis caused by opportunistic infections.

5. **Describe the clinical presentation of pericarditis.**
   The most common symptom is chest pain, often described as midline and sharp. The pain is generally worse with movement and breathing, and relief is obtained from sitting up and leaning forward. The discomfort may radiate to the neck, back, or shoulders (more commonly the left shoulder along the ridge of the trapezius). Dyspnea, malaise, and fever may occur. The pathognomonic clinical finding is a friction rub, which is a scratchy noise, similar to creaking leather. The optimal patient position for a rub is to be auscultated is sitting up, leaning forward, and in full expiration. The diaphragm of the stethoscope should be pressed firmly to the chest at the lower left sternal border. A little luck may be needed to detect a rub, because it occurs intermittently and can be difficult to hear in a loud environment like the ED.

6. **What are the electrocardiograph (ECG) findings in pericarditis?**
   The ECG typically evolves through the following four stages:
   1. In stage 1, the first hours to days of illness may show ST-segment elevation and PR-segment depression in all leads except aVR and V1, in which reciprocal changes occur. The ST-segment displacement is attributed to the associated subepicardial myocarditis, whereas the PR segment depression is attributed to subepicardial atrial inflammation.
   2. In stage 2, the ST and PR segments normalize, and the T waves flatten.
   3. In stage 3, deep T-wave inversion occurs.
   4. In stage 4, the ECG reverts to normal. Occasionally, stage 4 does not occur, which results in permanent generalized or focal T-wave inversions and flattenings.

7. **How can acute pericarditis be distinguished from acute MI?**
   ST-segment elevations in stage 1 of acute pericarditis tend to be upwardly concave rather than convex, and simultaneous T-wave inversions are not typically seen. The progression to T-wave inversions in stage 2 tends to occur after the ST segments have returned to baseline, whereas in acute MI, the T-wave inversion is more likely to accompany ST-segment elevation. The ST-segment elevations in acute pericarditis typically are diffuse, as opposed to an anatomic distribution, which is more likely to be seen in the setting of an acute MI. There are no reciprocal ST depressions in pericarditis.
   Patients with acute pericarditis are more likely to be younger, to be otherwise healthy, and to have a history of a preceding viral illness and pleuritic-type chest pain. Patients with acute MI are more likely to be older with risk factors for coronary artery disease. Ventricular arrhythmias are not associated with isolated pericardial disease and suggest the presence of underlying cardiac disease.

Table 35.1 Causes of Pericarditis

INFECTIOUS	IMMUNOLOGIC MEDIATED DISEASES	TRAUMA	DRUGS	OTHER
Viral: Coxsackie B Herpesvirus Mumps virus HIV	Autoimmune disorders	Blunt	Procainamide	Sarcoidosis
Bacterial: *Staphylococcus*	Acute rheumatic fever	Penetrating	Hydralazine	Amyloidosis
Tuberculosis (most common cause in the developing world)	Rheumatoid arthritis	Post-cardiac injury syndrome	Cromolyn sodium	Uremia
Fungal	Connective tissue diseases	Post-pericardiotomy		Radiation
Parasitic	Lupus erythematosus			Neoplasm
Rickettsia	Postinfarction			Aortic dissection

8. **How can acute pericarditis be distinguished from musculoskeletal chest pain?**
Musculoskeletal chest pain generally is not relieved by sitting up, and the characteristic friction rub and ECG abnormalities of pericarditis are not present. In general, pericarditis does not cause reproducible chest pain on examination.

9. **Is pericardial effusion a concern in patients with pericarditis?**
Pericardial effusion can lead to cardiac tamponade, a life-threatening increase in pericardial fluid that can reduce cardiac output by impairing right ventricular filling. The most common cause of nontraumatic tamponade is secondary to cancer. In general, pericardial effusion occurs most commonly in patients with acute viral or idiopathic, neoplastic, postradiation, or posttraumatic pericarditis.

10. **Besides pericardial effusion, can acute pericarditis cause an MI?**
No, acute MI is not a known complication of acute pericarditis.

11. **How much pericardial effusion is significant?**
The answer depends entirely on the clinical situation. A patient with a stab wound to the heart may be able to accommodate only 80–200 mL of pericardial fluid before tamponade develops. Patients with long-standing pericardial fluid collections can gradually stretch their pericardium, and may tolerate 2000 mL or more without hemodynamic compromise.

12. **How can a pericardial effusion be diagnosed?**
The physical examination is unreliable in detecting or excluding a pericardial effusion. Similarly, the cardiac silhouette is not enlarged on chest radiograph until at least 250 mL of fluid has accumulated. Echocardiography has excellent sensitivity and specificity; it can detect as little as 15 mL of pericardial fluid.

13. **What is cardiac tamponade?**
Cardiac tamponade exists when accumulating pericardial fluid leads to increased pericardial pressure to the point that it prevents the atria and ventricles from filling adequately during diastole, decreasing the volume of blood available to be pumped during systole and causing hemodynamic compromise. Although any form of pericarditis may lead to cardiac tamponade, acute tamponade usually is caused by trauma. Subacute tamponade occurs most commonly in neoplastic pericarditis.

14. **How is cardiac tamponade diagnosed?**
The first step is to confirm the presence of a pericardial effusion by echocardiography at the bedside (point-of-care ultrasound [POCUS]). Absence of a pericardial effusion rules out cardiac tamponade. If an effusion is present, a combination of physical examination and echocardiographic findings can confirm the diagnosis of tamponade. Physical examination findings suggestive of tamponade include the following:
- tachycardia
- hypotension
- cyanosis
- dyspnea
- jugular venous distention
- pulsus paradoxus
- elevated central venous pressure (>15 mmHg)

Echocardiographic findings are more specific and develop sequentially as pericardial pressure increases: systolic right atrial collapse, diastolic right ventricular collapse, and bowing of the interventricular septum. Another helpful finding is to perform the sniff test. Instruct the patient to inhale quickly through the nose while the ultrasonographer visualizes the inferior vena cava. Incomplete collapse of the inferior vena cava correlates well with elevated central venous pressure measurements.

15. **What is pulsus paradoxus?**
Pulsus paradoxus is an abnormally large (>10 mmHg) drop in the systolic blood pressure with inspiration. Kussmaul termed this phenomenon *paradoxical* because of the disappearance of the pulse during inspiration when the heart was obviously beating. Pulsus paradoxus is a pulse – not pressure – change and is an exaggeration of the normal inspiratory fall in arterial flow and systolic pressure. Inspiration favors right-sided heart filling by decreasing pericardial pressure, whereas expiration favors left-sided heart filling. Pulsus paradoxus usually signals large reductions in ventricular volumes and equilibration of mean pericardial and all cardiac diastolic pressures. The detection of pulsus paradoxus on physical examination suggests (and may be one of the earliest clues to) the existence of cardiac tamponade.

16. **What is the appropriate ED management of pericarditis?**
Anti-inflammatory agents, such as ibuprofen 600 mg four times a day for 1 week or indomethacin (Indocin) 25 mg three times a day for 1 week, should be administered. As shown in several randomized controlled trials, the addition of colchicine to nonsteroidal anti-inflammatory drugs (NSAIDs) reduces recurrence of pericarditis. The use of corticosteroids is controversial. Although corticosteroids are effective anti-inflammatory agents, 10%–20% of patients develop recurrent pericarditis with tapering. Echocardiography is indicated to rule out pericardial effusion. If cardiac tamponade is present, the first intervention is to infuse intravenous fluids to increase rapidly to increase preload and right-sided filling pressures. If this fails, or the patient is in extremis, percutaneous pericardiocentesis should be performed to relieve pericardial pressure.

17. **What is the prognosis for patients with pericarditis?**
Most patients recover fully, although up to 20% have a recurrence, probably because of an autoimmune mechanism. NSAIDS are used for recurrences. If these agents are ineffective, corticosteroid therapy is initiated. Colchicine holds promise as an adjunctive therapy in recurrent pericarditis. If medical interventions fail, pericardiectomy may be indicated.

18. **Do pediatric patients get pericarditis?**
Yes, in fact, pericarditis accounts for about 5% of all children who come to the pediatric ED with chest pain. Children with pericarditis usually have sharp, stabbing, retrosternal chest pain, fever, and shortness of breath. Like in adults, the chest pain is typically worse with inspiration and relieved by sitting up and leaning forward. Referral to a cardiologist is recommended. The reported recurrence rate for children is as high as 36%.

MYOCARDITIS

19. **What is myocarditis?**
An inflammation of the myocardium in the absence of ischemia

20. **What causes myocarditis?**
In the United States, myocarditis is caused most commonly by viruses. Enteroviruses, especially the Coxsackie B virus, predominate as causative agents. Infectious agents cause myocardial damage by three basic mechanisms:
1. Direct invasion of the myocardium.
2. Production of a myocardial toxin (e.g., diphtheria).
3. Immunologically mediated myocardial damage. The immunologically mediated destruction of cardiac tissue from infiltration of host cellular immune components is probably the more common mechanism in adults, whereas in neonates, damage from direct viral invasion is more likely.

Worldwide, Chagas disease is the leading cause of myocarditis. Other organisms that are known to infiltrate the myocardium include:
- Influenza A and B
- Adenovirus
- Hepatitis A and B
- Tuberculosis
- *Chlamydia pneumoniae*
- *Borrelia burgdorferi* (Lyme disease)
- *Legionella pneumophila*
- Cytomegalovirus
- *Toxoplasma gondii*
- *Trichinella spiralis*
- *Corynebacterium diphtheriae*
- *coronavirus*

21. **When should a diagnosis of myocarditis be considered in the emergency department?**
Diagnosing myocarditis in the emergency department (ED) can be a challenge. Because the presenting symptoms and signs are typically nonspecific, this is often a diagnosis of exclusion. Nonspecific symptoms include fatigue, myalgias, nausea, vomiting, fever, dyspnea, palpitations, and precordial discomfort. Chest pain may reflect associated pericarditis. Patients may have dilated cardiomyopathy without evidence of ischemia or valvular disease. Myocarditis should be considered in any previously healthy person who develops dyspnea, orthopnea, decreased exercise tolerance, palpitations, or syncope when no other obvious cause is found. Patients should be asked about concomitant or recent upper respiratory or gastrointestinal illness.

22. **What clinical findings may be present in myocarditis?**
Tachycardia is common and can be disproportionate to the temperature or apparent toxicity. This may be the only clue that something more serious than a simple viral illness exists. Clinical evidence of congestive heart failure occurs only in more severe cases. A pericardial friction rub may be auscultated if pericarditis is also present. Complications of myocarditis include ventricular dysrhythmias and left ventricular aneurysms.

23. **Are there any chest radiograph or ECG abnormalities in myocarditis?**
- The chest radiograph may be normal or abnormal, depending on the extent of disease. The cardiac silhouette may be enlarged, which can be the result of dilated cardiomyopathy or a pericardial effusion.
- The ECG commonly shows a sinus tachycardia and may show low voltages. Nonspecific ST-segment and T-wave abnormalities, a prolonged corrected QT interval, atrioventricular block, or an acute MI pattern may also occur. Atrial dysrhythmias have been described.

24. **How is myocarditis diagnosed?**
Making the diagnosis clinically can be difficult. Endocardial biopsy is considered the gold standard, although it has highly variable sensitivity and specificity. Cardiac enzyme like troponin may be elevated in only 50% of patients. The white blood cell count and erythrocyte sedimentation rate may be elevated, but are nonspecific. Echocardiography often shows global dysfunction that does not correspond to a specific coronary artery distribution. Cardiac gated magnetic resonance imaging (MRI) can demonstrate myocarditis.

25. **How can acute myocarditis be distinguished from acute MI?**
Myocarditis occurs primarily in young, healthy patients without significant cardiac history or risk factors for coronary artery disease. Chest pain, dyspnea, ECG abnormalities, and cardiac enzyme elevation may occur in both conditions. In the ED, it may be impossible to distinguish between these two entities, in which case treatment for acute MI should be initiated.

26. **Is myocarditis a concern in AIDS?**
Yes, the incidence of myocarditis found at autopsy of AIDS patients has been reported as high as 52%, compared with less than 10% in the population as a whole. The increased risk of myocarditis in patients with AIDS may be the result of an abnormal autoimmune reaction, opportunistic infections, or HIV itself.

27. **In what other clinical situations should myocarditis be considered?**
Myocarditis and dilated cardiomyopathy have been associated with cocaine use. Myocarditis is a common autopsy finding in patients who have died from cocaine abuse.

28. **Describe the appropriate ED management of a patient with myocarditis.**
In general, myocarditis is treated like other types of cardiomyopathies and congestive heart disease (CHF). Exercise increases mortality, and competitive sports should be avoided for a minimum of 4–6 weeks. All patients with suspected myocarditis should be admitted to a monitored bed in the hospital. Antibiotics are appropriate when a bacterial cause is suspected. In severe cases, temporary pacing and external circulatory support may be needed. Patients with a fulminant clinical course may require cardiac transplantation.

29. **What is the prognosis for patients with acute myocarditis?**
Mortality for patients with myocarditis has been reported to be 20% at 1 year and 56% at 4 years, although many patients do recover completely.

30. **Does myocarditis present differently in children?**
Pediatric myocarditis rarely presents with specific cardiac symptoms and should be considered in children with nonspecific clinical presentations, particularly those with symptoms and signs of hypoperfusion, especially syncope or seizure.

KEY POINTS: PERICARDITIS AND MYOCARDITIS

1. The physical examination or chest radiography is neither sensitive nor specific for pericardial effusion; echocardiography is the gold standard.
2. Myocarditis should be considered in patients with significant tachycardia that cannot otherwise be explained or in any patient with the combination of viral symptoms and evidence of cardiac disease.
3. Viruses are the most common causes of pericarditis and myocarditis, and a history of preceding or concurrent viral illness is quite common.
4. Myocarditis is very common in patients with AIDS, with rates at autopsy as high as 52%.

BIBLIOGRAPHY

Alerhand S, Carter JM. What echocardiographic findings suggest a pericardial effusion is causing tamponade? *Am J Emerg Med.* 2019;3(2):321–326.

Bergmann KR, Kharbanda A, Haveman L. Myocarditis and pericarditis in the pediatric population: validated management strategies. *Pediatr Emerg Med Pract.* 2015;12(7):1–22.

Hooper AJ, Celenza A. A descriptive analysis of patients with an emergency department diagnosis of acute pericarditis. *Emerg Med J.* 2013;30:1003–1008.

Imazio M, Gaita F. Acute and recurrent pericarditis. *Cardiol Clin.* 2017;35(4):505–513.

Lilly LS. Treatment of acute and recurrent idiopathic pericarditis. *Circulation.* 2013;127:1723–1726.

Sagar S, Liu PP, Cooper LT. Myocarditis. *Lancet.* 2012;379:738–747.

Shu-Ling C, Bautista D, Kit CC, et al. Diagnostic evaluation of pediatric myocarditis in the emergency department. *Pediatr Emerg Care.* 2013;29:346–351.

CHAPTER 36

ESOPHAGUS AND STOMACH DISORDERS

Rakesh Talati, MD, MBA and Kent McCann, MD

1. **How are gastrointestinal (GI) problems differentiated from acute myocardial infarction?**
Esophageal or gastric pain can present with visceral chest pain (e.g., ache, pressure), or upper abdominal pain and nausea that are difficult to differentiate from pain and nausea related to myocardial ischemia or infarction. For patients with descriptions of pain concerning for cardiac etiology or significant risk factors for cardiac disease, regular use of an electrocardiogram (ECG) will minimize clinical errors. Response to therapeutic interventions cannot be relied on to differentiate the two. Patients with esophageal spasm may respond to nitroglycerin and antacids, and GI cocktails may provide a placebo-like benefit to patients with cardiac ischemia.

2. **What is a GI cocktail?**
The most commonly used GI cocktails contain:
   - Antacid (e.g., 30 mL of aluminum hydroxide/magnesium hydroxide liquid) with or without a combination of the following:
     - Viscous lidocaine (10 mL)
     - Atropine, hyoscyamine, phenobarbital, and scopolamine (Donnatal; 10 mL)
     - Dicyclomine (Bentyl; 20 mg)
     These cocktails may provide temporary symptomatic relief of minor esophageal and gastric irritation.
     Note: It has been concluded that the addition of Donnatal or lidocaine does not provide more relief than an antacid alone.

3. **What is heartburn?**
Heartburn is a retrosternal burning discomfort that may radiate to the sides of the chest, neck, or jaw. The description of the pain may be similar to the pain of cardiac ischemia. Heartburn is characteristic of reflux esophagitis and often is made worse by bending forward or lying recumbent after meals. It may be relieved by upright posture, liquids (including saliva or water), or, more reliably, antacids. Heartburn is probably caused by heightened mucosal sensitivity to acid. Painful swallowing (odynophagia) is not typical of heartburn and may indicate a more severe disease process.

4. **How is reflux esophagitis treated?**
Medications
   - Antacids (e.g., Maalox, tums)
   - H_2-blockers (e.g., cimetidine)
   - Proton pump inhibitors (PPIs; e.g., omeprazole)
Other general measures
   - Elevation of the head of the bed
   - Weight reduction
   - Elimination of factors that increase abdominal pressure (e.g., tight fitting clothes)
   - Avoiding alcohol, chocolate, coffee, fatty foods, mint, orange juice, smoking, ingestion of large quantities of food and drink, and certain medications (e.g., anticholinergics or calcium channel blockers)
     Treatment is usually for 1–2 months, and the disease may recur.

5. **What are the esophageal causes of odynophagia?**
Odynophagia, or painful swallowing, is a characteristic of nonreflux esophagitis. Infectious esophagitis is a common cause and usually occurs in immunocompromised patients. It can be traced to fungal (e.g., monilial), viral (e.g., herpes, cytomegalovirus), bacterial (e.g., *Lactobacillus,* β-hemolytic streptococci), or parasitic organisms. Other types of nonreflux esophagitis include radiation, corrosive, and pill-induced esophagitis (e.g., certain antibiotics, nonsteroidal anti-inflammatory drugs [NSAIDs], bisphosphonates), as well as esophagitis related to certain systemic diseases (e.g., Behçet's syndrome, Crohn's disease, pemphigus vulgaris, Stevens-Johnson syndrome). Odynophagia is unusual in reflux esophagitis but may occur with a peptic ulcer of the esophagus (Barrett ulcer).

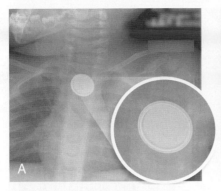
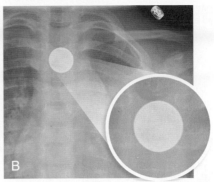

Fig. 36.1 Anterior-posterior radiographs. (A) Double ring, or halo sign, of a button battery in the esophagus of a child. (B) Homogeneous appearance of a coin in the esophagus of a child. (From Jatana KR. Button battery injuries in children: a growing risk. *Everything Matters in Patient Care.* 2013;26:9–10. Columbus, OH: Nationwide Children's Hospital.)

6. **How does esophageal obstruction present?**

   Except in infants, esophageal obstruction usually presents with a history of eating or swallowing something that is followed by the onset of chest pain, odynophagia, inability to swallow, hypersalivation, or regurgitation of undigested food. Foreign bodies usually lodge at one of four locations: cervical esophagus, upper esophageal sphincter, aortic arch, and lower esophageal sphincter. Obstruction by food may occur wherever there is narrowing of the lumen because of stricture, carcinoma, or a lower esophageal ring. The most dangerous esophageal foreign body is a disc (button) battery, which can cause a chemically induced perforation in as few as 4 hours and has a characteristic appearance on plain radiographs (Fig. 36.1).

7. **How is esophageal obstruction treated?**

   All foreign bodies stuck in the esophagus should be removed within 24 hours. Meat tenderizer should not be used to facilitate passage of obstructed meat. Intravenous (IV) glucagon (0.5–2 mg) has historically been given to allow foreign bodies to pass by relaxing smooth muscle of the lower esophagus. However, no studies have shown that it decreases the need for endoscopy for ED patients. In addition, it often causes vomiting, which may increase risk of aspiration or esophageal perforation.

8. **What is Mallory-Weiss syndrome?**

   Mallory-Weiss syndrome is a mucosal tear that usually involves the gastric mucosa near the squamocolumnar mucosal junction between the stomach and esophagus; it also may involve the esophageal mucosa. It usually is caused by vomiting and retching, and it often is seen in patients with heavy alcohol use. Patients with a Mallory-Weiss tear may experience upper GI bleeding and may require resuscitation. Endoscopy is recommended for any patient with signs of active bleeding. Tears usually heal within days without further complications, but some patients require repeat endoscopy, or, in rare cases, surgery.

9. **What causes esophageal perforation, and how is it diagnosed and treated?**

   Esophageal perforation, a true emergency, can be caused by iatrogenic damage during instrumentation, trauma (most often penetrating, but sometimes blunt), increased intraesophageal pressure associated with forceful vomiting (Boerhaave syndrome), or diseases of the esophagus (e.g., corrosive esophagitis, ulceration, neoplasm). It often presents with mild, nonspecific symptoms. More than half of all patients are initially misdiagnosed. Symptoms can quickly progress to chest pain that becomes severe and may be worsened by swallowing or breathing. Chest radiography may reveal pleural effusion or air within the mediastinum, pericardium, pleural space (pneumothorax), or subcutaneous tissue. Esophageal perforation may lead to leakage of gastric contents into the mediastinum and secondary infection (i.e., mediastinitis), rapidly progressing to sepsis. Esophageal perforation is confirmed radiographically with imaging enhanced by the enteral contrast diatrizoic acid (Gastrografin). Treatment includes broad-spectrum antibiotics, gastric suction, and surgical repair and esophageal fluid drainage as soon as possible.

10. **What are causes of abdominal pain that are gastric or duodenal in origin?**

    An estimated 10% of cases of abdominal pain seen in the emergency department (ED) are caused by gastric or duodenal disease. Gastritis and peptic ulcer disease (PUD; ulcer of the stomach or duodenum resulting from gastric acid) account for most patients with abdominal pain secondary to gastric or duodenal disease (Fig. 36.2). Perforated PUD and gastric volvulus are the two most serious conditions of esophageal or duodenal etiology that present with abdominal pain requiring immediate diagnosis and treatment.

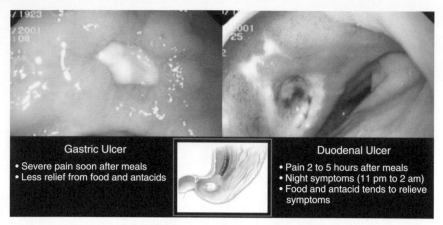

Fig. 36.2 Clinical comparison of gastric ulcer and duodenal ulcer. (Reproduced with permission from RoshReview.)

11. What are the common causes of gastritis and PUD?

Gastritis is associated with alcohol, salicylates, NSAIDs, and hiatal hernia. Almost all non–NSAID-related ulcers are caused by *Helicobacter pylori*. It is the only bacterium to be classified as a class I carcinogen by the World Health Organization (WHO), because it is a precursor to gastric carcinoma. First-line treatment for patients with *H. pylori* is the combination of a PPI, clarithromycin, and amoxicillin. NSAIDs are the second most common cause of PUD. They suppress protective prostaglandins in the stomach. Up to 25% of chronic NSAID users develop ulcer disease.

12. How do perforated PUDs present and how are they managed?

Sudden onset of abdominal pain that is not often related to eating is a common presentation for both gastric volvulus and perforated PUD. Patients with perforated PUDs typically have a history of dyspeptic symptoms, but some patients have "silent" ulcers without significant heralding symptoms. Perforated PUD pain typically radiates to the back, but also may radiate to the chest or upper abdomen. The pain is usually steady and refractory to antacids. Free air may cause referred pain to either or both shoulders. Vomiting is present in approximately 50% of cases. On physical examination, patients appear to be in acute distress and often have tachycardia. Blood pressure may be elevated secondary to pain, or decreased secondary to extensive fluid loss from generalized peritonitis. Patients usually lie still and avoid movement. Involuntary guarding, rebound tenderness, and abdominal rigidity are common. Free air is present on an upper right chest radiograph or the abdominal left lateral decubitus view in more than 70% of patients. Prompt surgical consultation should be obtained. Broad-spectrum antibiotics should be given, and the patient should be prepared for emergent laparotomy.

13. What differentiates upper from lower GI hemorrhage?

Upper GI hemorrhage is bleeding proximal to the ligament of Treitz, and lower GI bleeding is distal. Bloody or coffee-ground vomit, known as *hematemesis,* or dark, tarry stools, known as *melena,* most often represents upper GI bleeding. Lower GI bleeding most often produces bright red or maroon blood, known as *hematochezia.* Note, brisk upper GI bleeds can present with bright red or maroon blood per rectum as well. Although generally reliable, false-negative and false-positive results may occur when using Hemoccult and Gastroccult cards.

14. Do all patients with only lower GI bleeding require nasogastric (NG) tube placement?

The routine use of NG aspiration was once advocated to rule out occult upper GI bleeding. However, NG aspiration, with or without lavage, has a low sensitivity and poor negative likelihood ratio, limiting its role in ruling out an upper GI source of bleeding in patients with melena or hematochezia without hematemesis. NG tube placement is a painful procedure with potential complications, including aspiration and perforation.

15. How is a patient with an upper GI bleed classified as low risk?

The Glasgow-Blatchford score (GBS) is a risk stratification tool applied to patients with acute nonvariceal upper GI bleeding. The GBS is calculated by totaling points assigned for laboratory and clinical risk markers (Table 36.1). A score >0 is 99.6% sensitive in predicting high-risk patients who will require clinical interventions, including blood transfusion, endoscopy, or surgery. Low-risk patients with a score of 0 are candidates for outpatient management.

Table 36.1 Glasgow-Blatchford Score

ADMISSION RISK MARKER	SCORE
Blood Urea Nitrogen (mg/dL)	
6.5–7.9	2
8–9.9	3
10–25.0	4
≥25	6
Hemoglobin (g/dL) for Men	
12–13	1
10–11.9	3
<10	6
Hemoglobin (g/dL) for Women	
10–11.9	1
<10	6
Systolic Blood Pressure (mmHg)	
100–109	1
90–99	2
<90	3
Other Markers	
Pulse ≥100 (beats per minute)	1
Presentation with melena	1
Presentation with syncope	2
Hepatic disease	2
Cardiac failure	2

16. **What are the causes of upper GI bleeding?**
    - PUD (45%)
    - Gastric erosions (23%)
    - Varices (10%)
    - Mallory-Weiss tear (7%)
    - Esophagitis (6%)
    - Duodenitis (6%)

17. **Discuss the initial management and assessment of upper GI bleeding.**
    Begin by rapidly assessing and managing the patient's airway, breathing, and cardiovascular status. Patients should be undressed, connected to cardiac and arterial oxygen saturation (SaO_2) monitors, and given supplemental oxygen if SaO_2 is less than 93%. A large-bore, peripheral IV catheter with infusion of normal saline should be started. A focused physical examination should be done, checking for signs of shock (e.g., altered mental status, tachycardia, hypotension, cool extremities, and delayed capillary fill). Patients who have abnormal vital signs or signs of shock should have two or more IV lines placed and are given rapid infusion of crystalloid. Blood should be drawn for type and cross-matching; hemoglobin and hematocrit tests; platelet count; prothrombin time; and obtaining electrolyte, blood urea nitrogen (BUN), and creatinine levels. Stool should be tested for occult or gross blood. Elderly patients, patients with a history of cardiovascular disease or chest pain, and patients who are severely anemic should have an ECG to evaluate for signs of cardiac ischemia. An upright chest radiograph should be obtained to rule out pneumoperitoneum or pulmonary aspiration.

18. **What medications improve GI bleeding outcomes?**
    Infusion of high-dose PPIs (e.g., 80 mg IV pantoprazole) before endoscopy has been shown to accelerate the resolution of signs of bleeding in ulcers and reduce the need for endoscopic therapy. Patients with upper GI bleeding from suspected esophageal varices (severe liver disease, previous variceal bleed, history of alcoholism, or highly abnormal liver function tests) should receive an infusion of octreotide (50-μg IV bolus, followed by 50-μg/h infusion). Antibiotics should be considered in these patients as well.

19. **How should a patient with continued GI bleeding be managed?**
    Surgery and gastroenterology consultation should be initiated emergently. Patients who do not respond promptly (i.e., remain hypotensive) to a 30 mL/kg infusion of crystalloid should be given O-negative blood if type-specific blood is not yet available. Cross-matched blood usually takes approximately 45–60 minutes to become available. Upper GI bleeding can often be stopped with endoscopy, but emergent operative repair may be required in patients with persistent GI bleeding.

20. **Is placement of an NG or orogastric tube contraindicated in someone with esophageal varices?**
    There is no evidence that a properly placed NG or orogastric tube results in a significantly increased risk of tearing varices or increased size of a Mallory-Weiss tear; however, diagnostic NG or orogastric tubes are unnecessary if the patient vomits gastric contents in the ED, because this may be inspected for the presence of blood.

21. **Should most patients with upper GI bleeding undergo endoscopy?**
    Yes, because endoscopy is the most accurate diagnostic tool available for the evaluation of patients with upper GI bleeding. Endoscopy will identify a lesion in 78%–95% of patients if it is done within 12–24 hours of hemorrhage. Accurate identification of the bleeding site allows risk stratification with respect to predicting rebleeding and mortality. Risk stratification facilitates a proper disposition decision.

22. **What is the disposition for patients with GI bleeding?**
    GI bleeding usually stops spontaneously, and no further ED management is necessary. Low-risk patients with upper GI bleeding can often be discharged home with clear instructions, including signs and symptoms of worsening GI bleeding, and a plan for urgent outpatient follow-up care. Lower GI bleeding with definitive source from hemorrhoids, fissure, or proctitis can also be managed on an outpatient basis. All other patients with upper and lower GI bleeding are admitted for further evaluation and intervention.

23. **When can a patient with low-risk upper GI bleeding be sent home?**
    - No comorbid diseases
    - Normal vital signs
    - Normal or trace positive stool guaiac
    - Normal or near-normal hemoglobin and hematocrit levels
    - Proper understanding of signs and symptoms of significant bleeding
    - Good home support
    - Follow-up consultation arranged within 24 hours
    - Immediate access to emergent care, if needed

KEY POINTS: ESOPHAGUS AND STOMACH DISORDERS

1. Epigastric pain may be caused by myocardial ischemia, so an ECG should be obtained in adult patients with epigastric discomfort, visceral-type pain, or cardiac risk factors.
2. Antacids often provide symptomatic relief of abdominal discomfort related to gastroesophageal disease.
3. *H. pylori* is the most common cause of PUD, and the only bacteria classified as a class I carcinogen by the WHO.
4. Esophageal perforation can present with vague nonspecific symptoms and rapidly progress to sepsis and death.
5. Patients with upper GI bleeding who are hemodynamically unstable should receive rapid IV crystalloid infusion, urgent surgery, and gastroenterology consultation.

BIBLIOGRAPHY

Ali Khan M, Howden CW. The role of proton pump inhibitors in the management of upper gastrointestinal disorders. *Gastroenterol Hepatol (NY)*. 2018;14(3):169–175.

Arora S, Galich P. Myth: glucagon is an effective first-line therapy for esophageal foreign body impaction. *CJEM*. 2009;11:169–171.

Banister T, Spiking J, Ayaru L. Discharge of patients with an acute upper gastrointestinal bleed from the emergency department using an extended Glasgow-Blatchford Score. *BMJ Open Gastroenterol*. 2018;5(1):e000225.

Jatana KR. Button battery injuries in children: a growing risk. *Everything Matters in Patient Care*. 2013;26:9–10.

Moises G. Mallory-Weiss syndrome. In: Saltzman JR, ed. *UpToDate*. Waltham, MA: UpToDate Inc. Available at: http://www.uptodate.com. Accessed on January 10, 2019.

Palamidessi N, Sinert R, Falzon L, et al. Nasogastric aspiration and lavage in emergency department patients with hematochezia or melena without hematemesis. *Acad Emerg Med*. 2010;17:126–132.

Ware-McGee DM, Wheaton N. Diseases of the stomach. In: Adams JG, ed. *Emergency Medicine Clinical Essentials*. 2nd ed. Philadelphia, PA: Elsevier Saunders; 2013:279–285.

CHAPTER 37

BOWEL DISORDERS

Morgan P. Eutermoser, MD, DTMH and Patricia Klingenbjerg, MD

1. **When do I consider evaluating a patient for appendicitis?**
   Appendicitis can occur at any age, but is most prevalent in the teens and 20s. With the high incidence of appendicitis in the population, atypical presentations are common. Appendicitis is one of the most commonly missed diagnoses in emergency medicine, and it is the most common nonobstetric emergency during pregnancy.

2. **What is the pathogenesis of acute appendicitis?**
   The appendiceal lumen becomes obstructed, most commonly by a fecalith, leading to bacterial overgrowth and dilation of the appendix. Early on, the distended lumen causes dull, diffuse abdominal pain. Inflammation progresses to a localized peritonitis, producing the classic right lower quadrant (RLQ) pain with rebound on physical examination.

3. **How does appendicitis present clinically?**
   The classic presentation of appendicitis is nonspecific, umbilical abdominal pain that migrates over several hours to the RLQ of the abdomen. Associated symptoms include nausea, anorexia, and fever. However, variation of the appendix location leads to varied clinical presentations. For example, a retrocecal appendix may cause back or flank pain, and can be mistakenly diagnosed as pyelonephritis or nephrolithiasis. An abnormally long appendix with an inflamed tip may produce left lower quadrant pain. In pregnancy, the appendix is displaced into the right upper quadrant and, when inflamed, may be mistaken for symptomatic cholelithiasis or cholecystitis. Other diagnoses of RLQ pain should also be considered (Table 37.1). Prediction rules for pediatric appendicitis such as the Pediatric Appendicitis Score and the Alvarado Score are available, but have not been proven to be superior over clinical judgment.

4. **Is the physical examination reliable in appendicitis?**
   Unfortunately, the classic physical examination findings of appendicitis – RLQ guarding and rebound, and positive psoas, obturator, or Rovsing signs – are neither specific nor sensitive enough to accurately diagnose appendicitis. Standard laboratory test results may raise or lower clinical suspicion, but only an abdominal computed tomography (CT) scan or direct visualization with surgery can reliably diagnose an inflamed appendix. Commonly, nonspecific RLQ pain and tenderness are the only clinical findings of appendicitis.

5. **What laboratory tests are helpful in evaluating RLQ pain?**
   Although no laboratory test is diagnostic of appendicitis, tests can aid in the evaluation of the patient and exclude other diagnoses:
   - White blood cell count: more than 10,000/mm^3 in approximately 90% of cases.
   - Urinalysis: to exclude nephrolithiasis or urinary tract infection; however, mild hematuria or pyuria may be present when an inflamed appendix lies near the bladder or ureter.
   - β-Human chorionic gonadotropin: to exclude ectopic pregnancy.

6. **What radiologic study is best at imaging the appendix?**
   Abdominal and pelvic CT is the imaging modality of choice for appendicitis. The scan is routinely done with intravenous (IV) contrast alone, but oral or rectal contrast enhancement can be added. It has a reported accuracy of 93%–98% in ruling in or out the diagnosis of appendicitis, and is more sensitive and specific than any combination of physical examination and laboratory findings. CT without contrast has a sensitivity of 88%–96%, but is dependent on body habitus, as intraperitoneal fat improves sensitivity.
   Consider ultrasound imaging in children, pregnant patients, and thin patients. The sensitivity is 88%–94%, dependent on the patient's body habitus and the sonographer's and radiologist's experience. Ultrasound is useful to confirm a suspicion of appendicitis, but it is not as useful to exclude it. An appendiceal diameter greater than 6 mm is considered abnormal. Obtain abdominal and pelvic CT imaging with IV contrast if the ultrasound is indeterminate, or if it is normal despite a high clinical suspicion for appendicitis. Magnetic resonance imaging (MRI) may also be used but it can be difficult to obtain after hours and takes longer to perform.

7. **What is the treatment for appendicitis?**
   Appendectomy is the definitive treatment. However, some data suggest that antibiotics for up to 10 days and 1–3 days of in-hospital observation may be used in patients who have uncomplicated appendicitis and are poor surgical candidates or have a strong desire to avoid surgery. Patients should be advised that there is up to a 10% failure rate for antibiotic therapy during the initial hospitalization, resulting in the need for rescue surgery.

Table 37.1 Differential Diagnosis for Right Lower Quadrant Abdominal Pain

Acute ileitis	Inflammatory bowel disease
Diverticulitis	Acute cholecystitis
Perforated gastric or duodenal ulcer	Volvulus
Intussusception	Small bowel obstruction
Inflammation of Meckel's diverticulum	Uterine or tuboovarian pathologic abnormality (e.g., tuboovarian abscess, ovarian torsion, ovarian cysts)
Incarcerated inguinal hernia	Ectopic pregnancy
Testicular torsion or epididymitis	Mittelschmerz
Mesenteric adenitis	Pyelonephritis, symptomatic nephrolithiasis

There is also up to a 40% chance of recurrence of appendicitis within 5 years if nonoperative management is chosen; nonoperative management may miss appendiceal neoplasm. Once appendicitis has been diagnosed, or is highly suspected, a surgical consultation should be obtained. In these cases, start IV fluid resuscitation, advise the patient not to eat or drink, provide pain control, and start broad-spectrum antibiotics while waiting for surgery. A delay in diagnosis and treatment increases perforation risk.

8. **What is mesenteric ischemia?**
Mesenteric ischemia is caused by insufficient blood supply to the intestines, leading to tissue ischemia and infarction. The common causes are arterial emboli (most common) or thrombus, venous thrombosis, or nonocclusive hypoperfusion states. Patients should be assessed for risk factors of mesenteric ischemia (Table 37.2).

9. **How do patients with mesenteric ischemia experience symptoms?**
Patients complain of a diffusely painful abdomen. In the early stage, patients complain of severe pain but have minimal physical findings (i.e., the classic *pain out of proportion to the examination*). As infarction of bowel develops, peritoneal signs occur. Vomiting, hematochezia, hematemesis, abdominal distention, fever, and shock are late signs that indicate infarcted bowel.

10. **How do I diagnose mesenteric ischemia?**
The combination of clinical suspicion, radiographic imaging, and laboratory findings can help make the diagnosis. Direct surgical visualization of the bowel is the gold standard. Abdominal CT angiography with IV contrast or MR angiography can show the location of the vascular occlusion and secondary findings consistent with ischemia such as air within the bowel wall, intestinal wall thickening, and local inflammation. The CT should be performed without oral contrast as this can obscure the mesenteric vessels and bowel wall enhancement.
Laboratory findings may include leukocytosis, hemoconcentration, metabolic acidosis, and an elevated lactate level. These laboratory findings may indicate ischemic bowel; however, they have poor sensitivity and specificity.

11. **How is mesenteric ischemia treated?**
Initial treatment includes vigorous resuscitation, parenteral antibiotics, correction of predisposing factors, and early surgical consultation. Definitive management involves selective vasodilator infusion, anticoagulation in venous occlusion, or embolectomy. Laparotomy is necessary for resection of necrotic bowel.

12. **What is intussusception?**
Intussusception occurs when an intestinal segment invaginates and telescopes into an adjacent segment. This is a disease predominantly seen in children (see Chapter 65), but it can occur in adults. Typical pathologic lesions include tumors, Meckel's diverticulum, and inflammatory lesions. The high incidence of mass lesions in adults usually mandates surgical exploration.

Table 37.2 Risk Factors for Mesenteric Ischemia

Age older than 50 years	Recent myocardial infarction
Valvular or atherosclerotic heart disease	Dysrhythmias (e.g., atrial fibrillation)
Peripheral vascular disease	Critical illness with hypotension or sepsis
Congestive heart failure	Diuretics or vasoconstrictive drugs

13. **What is inflammatory bowel disease (IBD)?**
    IBD is an idiopathic, chronic inflammatory disease of the intestine. IBD includes two main groups:
    1. Crohn disease (CD), also known as regional enteritis or granulomatous ileocolitis
    2. Ulcerative colitis (UC)
    CD and UC are rising in incidence. Common clinical features are summarized in Table 37.3.

14. **How do CD and UC present?**
    Although they are pathologically distinct diseases, CD and UC can appear similar and affect all age groups (see Table 37.3). Both diseases may present with diarrhea, abdominal pain, fever, anorexia, weight loss, and bloody diarrhea; however, UC is more likely to present with bloody diarrhea. The diagnosis can be confirmed by endoscopy or barium enema.

15. **What is the ED management for IBD?**
    Patients with mild disease and no signs of life-threatening complications can be treated as outpatients. Treatment usually consists of sulfasalazine, steroids (oral or rectal), steroid-sparing agents such as 6-mercaptopurine, antidiarrheal agents (e.g., loperamide, Lomotil, and cholestyramine), and analgesia. Antidiarrheal agents should be used with caution, because they can predispose a patient to toxic megacolon. Metronidazole may help treat the chronic perirectal complications of CD. Patients should be admitted if they have severe pain, heavy bleeding, signs of hemorrhagic shock, peritonitis, or any life-threatening complications. Extraintestinal manifestations of IBD can also occur (Table 37.4).

16. **Describe what happens during intestinal obstruction.**
    When the large and small bowels become obstructed, loss of the normal forward flow of digested food and secretions occurs. Proximal to the obstruction, a buildup of bowel gas, gastric secretions, and food develops. The bowel then becomes distended, causing pain, vomiting, and decreased oral intake. The cause of the obstruction can be mechanical or adynamic. Mechanical obstruction from adhesions or tumors commonly requires surgical intervention, whereas an adynamic ileus usually resolves spontaneously within a few days.

Table 37.3 Common Features for Inflammatory Bowel Disease

CLINICAL FEATURE	CROHN DISEASE	ULCERATIVE COLITIS
Weight loss	Common	Fairly common
Fever	Common	Fairly common
Diarrhea	Fairly common	Very common
Rectal bleeding	Fairly common	Very common
Perianal disease	Common	None
Site		
Colon	Two-thirds of patients	Exclusively
Ileum	Two-thirds of patients	None
Jejunum, stomach, or esophagus	Uncommon	None
Intestinal Complications		
Stricture	Common	Unknown
Fistulas	Fairly common	None
Toxic megacolon	None	Unknown
Perforation	Uncommon	Unknown
Cancer	Common	Fairly common
Endoscopic Findings		
Friability	Fairly common	Very common
Aphthous and linear ulcers	Common	None
Cobblestone appearance	Common	None
Rectal involvement	Fairly common	Very common
Radiologic Findings		
Distribution	Discontinuous, segmental	Continuous
Ulceration	Deep	Superficial
Fissures	Common	None
Strictures for fistulas	Common	Rare
Ileal involvement	Narrowed, nodular	Dilated

Modified from Podolsky DK. Inflammatory bowel disease. *N Engl J Med.* 2002;347:417–429.

Table 37.4 Common Extraintestinal Manifestations of Inflammatory Bowel Disease

CLINICAL CATEGORY	DISORDER
Ocular	Uveitis, episcleritis
Dermatologic	Erythema nodosum, pyoderma gangrenosum
Musculoskeletal	Ankylosing spondylitis, peripheral arthritis, sacroiliitis
Hepatobiliary	Cholelithiasis, pericholangitis, hepatitis, fatty liver, primary sclerosing cholangitis, cholangiocarcinoma, pancreatitis
Hematologic	Thromboembolic disease, chronic anemia
Renal	Nephrolithiasis, amyloidosis leading to renal failure

17. **What are the common causes of mechanical small bowel obstruction (SBO)?**
    Overall, adhesions, hernias, and cancer account for more than 90% of mechanical SBO cases. Postoperative adhesions are the most common cause of an SBO (56%), followed by incarcerated hernia (25%) and cancer (10%). Other less common causes include:
    - IBD
    - gallstones
    - volvulus
    - intussusception
    - radiation enteritis
    - abscesses
    - congenital lesions
    - bezoars

18. **What are the clinical features of SBO?**
    Patients have diffuse abdominal pain, distention, and, occasionally, vomiting. Early on, the pain is mild, crampy, and colicky. An early SBO can be difficult to diagnose. The patient has pain but continues to have flatus and passage of some stool. As the obstruction progresses, the intestinal contents build up proximally, leading to nausea and vomiting. The intestine distal to the obstruction empties of stool and has decreased peristaltic motion, leading to obstipation (inability to pass feces or flatus). Auscultation may reveal high-pitched, hyperactive tinkling sounds compared with absent sounds found in paralytic ileus.

19. **Describe the radiographic findings in SBO.**
    The classic finding on abdominal plain films is multiple air-fluid levels and distended loops of small bowel. When the obstructed intestine contains more fluid than gas, small round pockets of air may line up to form the string of pearls sign. A paucity of stool and gas is noted distal to the obstruction. Plain films have a sensitivity of 41%–86% and a specificity of 25%–88%. An abdominal CT scan has a higher sensitivity (100%) and specificity (83%). Additionally, a CT scan can reveal the location of the obstruction and help identify the cause (e.g., mass or infection such as appendicitis or diverticulitis); however, waiting for a CT should not delay surgical consultation when the suspicion is high and the plain film supports the diagnosis.

20. **What is the treatment for SBO?**
    The initial emergency management includes electrolyte replacement, decompression with a nasogastric tube, and IV fluid resuscitation. Patients lose a large amount of fluid into the obstructed bowel and can be significantly intravascularly depleted. SBOs can often be managed nonoperatively with observation, IV fluid resuscitation, and bowel rest. However, some complete SBOs or mechanical obstructions require surgery.

21. **What are the characteristics of an ileus?**
    The terms *ileus* and *adynamic ileus* are synonymous for a paralyzed intestine. The bowel is unable to perform peristalsis. Causes of an ileus include infection (e.g., pancreatitis, peritonitis), drugs (e.g., narcotics, anticholinergics), electrolyte imbalance (e.g., hypokalemia), spinal cord injuries, and recent bowel surgery. Patients have symptoms of abdominal distention, nausea and vomiting, and obstipation. Abdominal examination reveals hypoactive bowel sounds, mild tenderness, and absence of peritoneal signs. Radiographs usually show minimally distended bowel throughout the entire gastrointestinal (GI) tract, with diffuse air-fluid levels in the small bowel.

22. **How is an ileus treated?**
    Management is similar to SBO. Limit oral intake, resuscitate with IV fluids, and correct electrolyte abnormalities, particularly hypokalemia. If abdominal distention is present, place a nasogastric tube to decompress the stomach. Limit administration of medications, such as opioids, that slow intestinal motility. If the ileus is prolonged (>3–5 days), obtain additional imaging to search for an underlying cause.

23. **What are the causes of large bowel obstruction (LBO)?**

LBO is caused most commonly by colon cancer (60%), volvulus (20%), and diverticular disease (10%). Primary adenocarcinoma accounts for most cancerous lesions. Other less likely causes include metastatic carcinoma, gynecologic tumors, IBD, intussusception, and fecal impaction. In infants, consider congenital disorders, such as Hirschsprung disease or an imperforate anus. Hernias and adhesions are uncommon causes of LBO.

24. **What are diverticula and what are common complications?**

Diverticula are saclike outpouchings of the colon that occur through weakened areas of the muscularis of the colon wall. They commonly occur in persons of industrialized nations and increase in incidence with age. It is estimated that one-third of the US population will develop diverticula by age 50, and two-thirds by 85 years. Complications from diverticula include bleeding and diverticulitis, a localized infection. Diverticulitis is caused by obstruction of the opening of diverticula, usually by stool, leading to infection from the proliferation of colonic bacteria and buildup of bowel secretions within the diverticula.

25. **How does diverticulitis clinically present?**

The most common symptom of diverticulitis is abdominal pain. The pain usually evolves over 1–2 days from dull, diffuse abdominal pain to more intense, typically left lower quadrant pain. Patients may complain of fever, nausea, vomiting, and decreased appetite. Diverticulitis occurs most commonly in the descending and sigmoid regions of the colon but can occur throughout the colon. The abdominal CT scan with IV contrast is the diagnostic procedure of choice and can show evidence for abscesses, bowel perforation, and severity of disease.

26. **How do I manage diverticulitis?**

Diverticulitis management depends on whether it is uncomplicated or complicated. In 2015, the American Gastroenterology Association Institute released updated guidelines for diverticulitis. The guideline now suggests that "antibiotics should be used selectively, rather than routinely, in patients with AUD (adult uncomplicated disease)." The committee cited an earlier randomized controlled trial (RCT) showing that there was no significant difference in complication rates between patients treated with antibiotics and those not treated with antibiotics. Patients with comorbidities, abscess, fistula, bleeding, or bowel perforation require hospitalization, IV antibiotics, and serial examinations. Surgery may be required for repeat episodes or for bowel perforation. Abscess requires surgical or interventional radiology evaluation.

27. **What are common causes of lower GI bleeding?**

Patients often arrive in the emergency department (ED) with complaints of rectal bleeding. Lower GI bleeds occur from many causes, and a thorough history and examination are vital to diagnose the bleeding source. Investigating anatomically from the rectum proximally, evaluate for hemorrhoids and rectal fissures, then, based on history and examination, consider diverticulosis, polyps, cancer, arteriovenous (AV) malformation, IBD, ischemic colitis, infectious diarrhea, and finally an upper GI source.

28. **How do I perform anoscopy?**

Anoscopy can provide a direct view of the anus and distal rectum. A lubricated anoscope with the obturator in place is advanced gently through the anal orifice. The obturator is removed to view the distal rectal mucosa; a light source is shined into the barrel of the anoscope, and the anoscope is withdrawn slowly while searching for internal hemorrhoids, fissures, abscess, masses, or bleeding proximal to the rectum.

29. **What are hemorrhoids?**

Hemorrhoids are engorged vascular cushions composed of internal or external hemorrhoidal veins and present most often with bleeding, pain, or rectal itching. They are associated with prolonged increase in resting pressure in the anal canal, most often from constipation but also seen in pregnancy, excessive straining, and in certain occupations (e.g., truck driver).

30. **How do internal and external hemorrhoids differ?**

- Internal hemorrhoids arise above the dentate line, are covered by mucosa, and are not usually palpable or painful. They are seen during anoscopy and typically present as bright red blood in the toilet bowl or on toilet paper.
- External hemorrhoids are covered by skin and are easily visible and palpable at the anal orifice. They are commonly enlarged and tender. A common complication of external hemorrhoids is thrombosis, which is painful and requires excision of the thrombus.

31. **How are hemorrhoids treated?**

Treat mildly symptomatic hemorrhoids with the following:
- irrigation during the shower or bath
- stool softeners
- high-fiber diet
- bulk laxatives (e.g., psyllium or methylcellulose)
- increased fluid consumption
- proper anal hygiene
- analgesics if necessary

Nonthrombosed prolapsed hemorrhoids should be gently reduced. Thrombosed hemorrhoids should be excised. Patients with intractable symptoms need surgical referral.

32. What is an anal fissure?

An anal fissure is a linear crack or ulcer in the epithelium in the distal anal canal. Anal fissures are the most common cause of rectal pain. Most are idiopathic, but any anal canal trauma can cause a fissure. Most benign anal fissures occur in the posterior midline, followed by the anterior midline. Fissures in other locations are associated with CD, infection, malignancy, or immunodeficiency.

33. How do I treat an anal fissure?

Most anal fissures can be managed conservatively with sitz baths, stool softeners, high-fiber diet, bulk laxatives (e.g., psyllium or methylcellulose), additional fluid consumption, proper anal hygiene, and analgesics. Recent studies have shown good success with the use of topical 0.2% nitroglycerin ointment applied twice daily for 6 weeks or a single botulinum injection. Fissures that do not improve with conservative therapies should be referred to a surgeon for consideration of a lateral internal sphincterotomy.

34. Can I drain anorectal abscesses in the ED?

Small, isolated *perianal* abscesses can be drained successfully in the ED. These abscesses can be painful, requiring both local anesthetic and oral or parenteral sedation. For complicated or deep rectal abscesses, consult surgery for operative drainage.

KEY POINTS: BOWEL DISORDERS

1. Appendicitis is common, and unusual presentations occur often; therefore always consider appendicitis in a patient with abdominal pain. Nonoperative management can be an option with antibiotics, observation, and discussion regarding risks and complications.
2. A patient with atrial fibrillation and abdominal pain has mesenteric ischemia until proven otherwise.
3. Surgical adhesions are the most common cause of SBO.
4. Patients with SBO should be aggressively resuscitated with IV fluids in the ED because of the extensive depletion of intravascular fluid.
5. Acute uncomplicated diverticulitis should be treated with antibiotics only in selected patients. There is no significant difference in complication rates in patients treated with antibiotics compared with those not treated with antibiotics.
6. IBD can cause complicated rectal abscesses or fissures that require surgical consultation.

BIBLIOGRAPHY

Brisinda G, Maria G, Bentivoglio AR, et al. A comparison of injections of botulinum toxin and topical nitroglycerin ointment for the treatment of chronic anal fissure. *N Engl J Med.* 1999;341:65–69.
Podolsky DK. Inflammatory bowel disease. *N Engl J Med.* 2002;347:417–429.
Salminen P, Tuominen R, Paajanen H, et al. Five-year follow-up of antibiotic therapy for uncomplicated acute appendicitis in the APPAC randomized clinical trial. *JAMA.* 2018;320(12):1259–1265.
Sceats LA, Trickey AW, Morris AM, et al. Nonoperative management of uncomplicated appendicitis among privately insured patients. *JAMA Surg.* 2019;154(2):141–149. doi:10.1001/jamasurg.2018.4282.
Segatto E, Mortelé KJ, Ji H, et al. Acute small bowel ischemia: CT imaging findings. *Semin Ultrasound CT MR.* 2003;24:364–376.
Stollman N, Smalley W, Hirano I, et al. American Gastroenterology Association Institute guideline on the management of acute diverticulitis. *Gastroenterology.* 2015;149:1944–1949.

LIVER AND BILIARY TRACT DISEASE

CHAPTER 38

Barbara K. Blok, MD

1. **What are the common manifestations of biliary disease?**

   Cholelithiasis is the presence of gallstones in the gallbladder without evidence of infection. Among adults, 8% of men and 17% of women have gallstones, and the incidence increases with age, with an incidence as high as 27% in the elderly.

   - Biliary colic is right upper quadrant or epigastric pain sometimes radiating to the right shoulder or scapula. It usually lasts less than 6 hours, is persistent (i.e., not colicky), often occurs after a fatty meal, and is thought to be the result of transient obstruction of the cystic duct by a gallstone.
   - Of patients with biliary colic, 30% progress to cholecystitis, inflammation of the gallbladder resulting from obstruction of the cystic duct by a stone. Pain with cholecystitis is similar to biliary colic but persists beyond 6 hours, is accompanied by a Murphy sign, and can be present with or without fever or leukocytosis.
   - Choledocholithiasis occurs when a gallstone lodges in the common bile duct (CBD), and can cause cholecystitis, pancreatitis (if the ampulla of Vater is obstructed), or both.
   - Ascending cholangitis is a severe infection of the biliary tract from complete biliary obstruction (most commonly in the CBD) in the presence of a bacterial infection. It presents as right upper quadrant pain, fever and chills, and jaundice (Charcot triad), although only 25% of patients have all three. It may include shock and mental status changes (Reynold pentad), more commonly seen with gangrenous or emphysematous cholecystitis.
   - Emphysematous cholecystitis is caused by complete cystic duct obstruction with subsequent abscess formation in the gallbladder wall by gas-forming bacteria. It is seen with vascular insufficiency, severe burns, and trauma. It is more common in men and diabetic patients and often is accompanied by sepsis.

2. **Do all gallstones produce pain? Does a lack of stones preclude cholecystitis?**

   Of patients with gallstones, 80% are asymptomatic. Of asymptomatic patients, 15%–30% develop symptoms within 15 years. Although 90%–95% of cholecystitis cases are in the setting of gallstones, 5%–10% are not secondary to cholelithiasis and are termed *acalculous cholecystitis*, a difficult diagnosis, because it is often a complication of another process such as diabetes, burns, multisystem trauma, AIDS, or sepsis.

3. **What is the Murphy sign?**

   The patient is asked to take a deep breath while the examiner applies pressure over the area of the gallbladder. If the gallbladder is inflamed, the descending diaphragm forces it against the examiner's fingertips, causing pain and often a sudden halt to inspiration. A sonographic Murphy sign uses the ultrasound probe instead of the examiner's fingers and is positive when the site of maximal tenderness localizes to the gallbladder. The finding is 97% sensitive for acute cholecystitis.

4. **Can a plain radiograph of the abdomen aid diagnosis?**

   Maybe; however, ultrasound is the preferred first-line diagnostic test. Only 10%–20% of gallstones contain sufficient calcium to be radiopaque. Air can be seen in the biliary tree or the gallbladder wall when infection is caused by gas-forming bacteria or there is a biliary-intestinal fistula.

5. **What is the gold standard for diagnosing cholecystitis?**

   Although ultrasound is the test of choice in the emergency department (ED), a hepatobiliary iminodiacetic acid (HIDA) scan is the gold standard, with 95% accuracy if the gallbladder does not fill with radioisotope within 4 hours after injection.

6. **Describe the ultrasound findings in cholecystitis.**

   Gallstones as small as 2 mm can be detected directly, or sometimes their presence can be inferred by interference with transmission of ultrasound waves (acoustic shadowing; Fig. 38.1). Other helpful findings include a thickened gallbladder wall (>3 mm), fluid collections around the gallbladder (pericholecystic fluid), and CBD dilation (>6 mm). As noted, the sonographic Murphy sign is very sensitive for cholecystitis. In fact, it has been found to be even more sensitive in the hands of emergency physicians than ultrasound technicians or radiologists. Ultrasound overall is 94% sensitive and 78% specific for identifying cholecystitis.

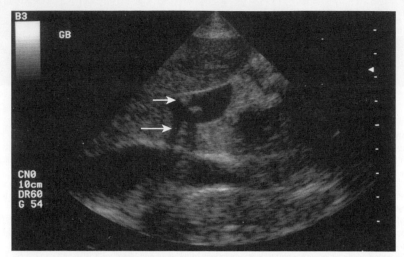

Fig. 38.1 Ultrasound image reveals an anechoic gallbladder containing two echogenic stones, which are creating acoustic shadowing inferiorly. The *short arrow* is pointed to the gallstones within the gallbladder, and the *long arrow* points to the shadowing effect of the stones.

KEY POINTS: ULTRASOUND FINDINGS OF CHOLECYSTITIS

1. Presence of gallstones
2. Gallbladder wall thickening greater than 3 mm
3. Pericholecystic fluid
4. CBD dilation greater than 6 mm

7. **When should elective surgery be considered in patients with asymptomatic cholelithiasis?**
   Cholecystectomy for asymptomatic cholelithiasis should be considered for Native Americans due to increased risk of gallbladder cancer and in patients with chronic hemolytic disease where prophylactic cholecystectomy has shown improved outcomes. *It is no longer recommended for patients with porcelain gallbladder or in the setting of bariatric surgery.*

8. **What are Courvoisier law, Klatskin tumor, and Fitz-Hugh–Curtis syndrome?**
   - The Courvoisier law states that a palpable gallbladder in the setting of painless jaundice is unlikely to be due to gallstones.
   - A Klatskin tumor is a cholangiocarcinoma occurring where the hepatic ducts form the CBD.
   - Fitz-Hugh–Curtis syndrome is caused by pelvic inflammatory disease extending up the right paracolic gutter, causing inflammation of the capsule of the liver (perihepatitis); it can lead to adhesions between the liver and abdominal wall.

9. **What is porcelain gallbladder?**
   Porcelain gallbladder is a gallbladder with calcified walls leading to a characteristic bluish discoloration and brittle walls. It is often an incidental finding on abdominal imaging and is associated with a small increased risk of gallbladder cancer.

10. **Are all gallstones created equal?**
    No, the most common are cholesterol stones that are usually found in the stereotypic female patient who is overweight, age ≥40 years, and is not yet menopausal. Patients of Asian descent, those with parasitic infections (*Ascaris lumbricoides*), chronic liver/biliary disease, or chronic hemolysis states (i.e., sickle cell disease, spherocytosis) are more likely to have pigmented stones.

11. **What are the common causes of biliary obstruction in patients with acute cholangitis? What are the typical organisms?**
    Choledocholithiasis is by far the most common cause of biliary obstruction in patients presenting with acute cholangitis. Other common causes include benign or malignant biliary strictures and obstructed biliary stents. The typical organisms are those from the gastrointestinal tract with *Escherichia coli* being most common, followed by *Klebsiella* and *Enterobacter* species.

12. **What is Mirizzi syndrome?**
Acute cholangitis-like symptoms resulting from compression and obstruction of the common hepatic duct by a large stone in the adjacent cystic duct or Hartman's pouch of the gallbladder.

13. **What is endoscopic retrograde cholangiopancreatography (ERCP)? What is the most common complication seen in the ED after an ERCP procedure?**
ERCP is a procedure that examines the pancreatic and bile ducts for disease or irregularities with the ability of removing lodged stones and opening narrowed ducts with stents. The most common serious complication is pancreatitis, which occurs in 5%–10% of cases.

14. **What are liver function tests?**
Aspartate aminotransferase (AST) and alanine aminotransferase (ALT) are markers of acute liver injury, but they have no correlation with liver function. Liver function is analyzed best by measuring factors affected by hepatic protein synthesis. Acute liver failure results in a decrease in vitamin K–dependent coagulation factors (except factor VIII), leading to a prolonged prothrombin time (PT). The liver also synthesizes albumin, although its longer half-life makes it a better marker of subacute or chronic liver disease.

15. **What is the difference between conjugated and unconjugated bilirubinemia?**
Bilirubin is a breakdown product of hemoglobin and heme-related proteins. In its unconjugated, hydrophobic form, it is unable to be excreted into bile, although it can traverse the blood–brain barrier and placenta. Bilirubin is conjugated in the liver with glucuronic acid, making it more water soluble for excretion into the bile. A predominance of unconjugated bilirubin occurs when there is overproduction (hemolysis) or decreased conjugation (decreased intrinsic metabolic activity of the liver by acute or chronic injury). A primarily conjugated bilirubinemia results from reflux into the plasma from impaired excretion and is secondary to biliary obstruction from cholestasis, gallstones, tumors, or strictures.

16. **How can you use the AST, ALT, and alkaline phosphatase to differentiate the cause of hyperbilirubinemia and jaundice?**
A predominately elevated AST and ALT suggest hepatocellular damage, as in viral hepatitis or toxin exposure, while a predominately elevated alkaline phosphatase suggests cholestasis either from biliary obstruction or intrahepatic cholestasis. If both are normal, then the hyperbilirubinemia is likely due to hemolysis or impaired bilirubin uptake in the liver.

17. **State the major causes of acute hepatitis.**
Hepatitis is caused by viruses such as hepatitis A through E, Epstein-Barr virus, herpes simplex virus (HSV), Coxsackie virus, and cytomegalovirus. It also can result from exposure to toxins such as ethanol, *Amanita phalloides* mushrooms, carbon tetrachloride, acetaminophen, halothane, and chlorpromazine.

18. **What are the risk factors for viral hepatitis? Which can result in a carrier state?**
Hepatitis B and C are transmitted via blood and body fluid exposures as occur through sexual intercourse, injection drug use, blood transfusions, tattoos or body piercings, hemodialysis, and needle sticks. Hepatitis A and E are transmitted via fecal/oral exposure (i.e., foreign travel, raw seafood ingestion, poor hygiene or sewage management, and close contact with a person infected with hepatitis). Hepatitis A and E are often self-limited, whereas hepatitis B and C can result in a carrier state from chronic infection and progress to chronic hepatitis. Hepatitis D requires coinfection with hepatitis B to replicate, but when present imparts higher risk of a more severe course and progression to fulminant hepatitis.

19. **What is the recommended treatment for hepatitis C?**
Several new direct-active antiviral medications are available to treat hepatitis. These medications are typically given for chronic infection and have a 90% cure rate. Initially cost prohibitive, there are now few barriers to treatment.

20. **What is the most common form of liver disease in the United States?**
Alcoholic hepatitis is the most common form of liver disease and is most often diagnosed by history, but highly suggestive associated findings include spider angiomas, gynecomastia, palmar erythema, ascites, and elevated AST and ALT in a ratio of greater than 2:1.

21. **What are discriminant function, the Model for End-Stage Liver Disease (MELD) score, and the Glasgow Alcoholic Hepatitis score?**
These are scores that provide the clinician with an indication of the severity of alcoholic hepatitis.
- Maddrey discriminant function is calculated as

$$[4.6 \times (\text{Patient's PT} - \text{Control PT})] \times \text{serum bilirubin level}$$

- PT is reported in seconds, and serum bilirubin level is reported in milligrams per deciliter. Higher values, especially greater than 32, imply more severe hepatitis and should prompt the physician to consider initiating specific corticosteroid treatment to decrease mortality.

- The MELD score incorporates bilirubin, international normalized ratio (INR), and creatinine to create a score that gives an indication of disease severity and risk of death at 3 months while a patient is awaiting liver transplant for alcoholic hepatitis. Multiple calculators online are available. A higher score indicates a worse prognosis.
- The Glasgow Alcoholic Hepatitis score incorporates bilirubin, PT, creatinine, age, and serum albumin to create a score that gives an indication of 28- and 84-day survival. Multiple calculators are available online. Higher values, especially if greater than 9, indicate a worse prognosis and more severe hepatitis, and should prompt the physician to consider initiating specific corticosteroid treatment to decrease mortality.

KEY POINTS: CRITERIA FOR ADMISSION IN A PATIENT WITH HEPATITIS

1. Coagulopathy, INR greater than 3
2. Active bleeding
3. Encephalopathy
4. Unable to tolerate intake by mouth
5. Social barriers making follow-up care and compliance problematic

22. **What is the initial treatment of hepatic encephalopathy? What is asterixis?**
Hepatic encephalopathy is the accumulation of nitrogenous waste products normally metabolized by the liver. Ammonia is produced in the intestines and liver as a by-product of protein metabolism and intestinal flora. When portal hypertension occurs, portal systemic shunting causes the ammonia to bypass the liver, where it would normally be metabolized. These increased levels of systemic ammonia cause it to cross the blood–brain barrier, resulting in impaired neurotransmission and neuronal dysfunction. Hepatic encephalopathy, a clinical diagnosis, comprises a spectrum of clinical presentations ranging from lethargy to coma. Precipitating cause should be considered and include gastrointestinal (GI) bleeding, infection (including spontaneous bacterial peritonitis), and renal failure. Serum ammonia levels should not be used to make or exclude the diagnosis. In addition to supportive care, lactulose and rifaximin are the mainstays of treatment. Lactulose reduces ammonia absorption by increasing GI motility and by trapping ammonia as ammonium in the stool via fecal acidification in the form of lactic acid; rifaximin is a minimally absorbed antibiotic that reduces gut bacteria that produce ammonia.
Asterixis is a clinical manifestation of moderate hepatic encephalopathy in which the hands flap (low-amplitude alternating flexion and extension) when the arms are held straight and the wrists are held in extension.

KEY POINTS: TREATMENT OF HEPATIC ENCEPHALOPATHY

1. Supportive care
2. Lactulose 30–45 mL orally (PO every 6–8 hours)
3. Rifaximin 550 mg PO twice daily

23. **What are complications of chronic liver disease to watch for in the ED?**
The most common complication of cirrhotic ascites is spontaneous bacterial peritonitis (SBP), which can present with fever, abdominal pain, or mental status changes. A benign abdominal examination does not exclude the diagnosis of SBP, so have a low threshold for diagnostic paracentesis. Ascites fluid neutrophil count >250 cells/mm^3 or positive Gram stain supports a diagnosis of SBP, which is confirmed by positive fluid culture, most commonly *E. coli*. Portal hypertension causes the development of esophageal varices, which can lead to massive GI bleeding. Management should focus on resuscitation, local control (balloon tamponade or endoscopic ligation/sclerotherapy), reduction of portal pressure with octreotide, and initiation of prophylactic antibiotics (IV 1 g ceftriaxone). If necessary, emergent transjugular intrahepatic portosystemic shunt may be indicated to further reduce portal pressure. Patients with chronic liver disease are at greatly increased risk of bleeding because of deficits of the coagulation cascade proteins, platelet abnormalities, and increased fibrinolysis. Renal failure in cirrhotic patients with structurally normal kidneys represents hepatorenal syndrome (HRS). One study showed a 38% 1-year survival rate in patients with HRS. Of note, rapidly progressive renal failure in HRS developing over 2 weeks indicates a more fulminant course, has an extremely high mortality, and is an indication for referral for liver transplantation which can be curative. Patients with cirrhosis and chronic hepatitis B or C are at risk of developing hepatocellular carcinoma, and should be suspected with deterioration of a previously stable patient.

KEY POINTS: PERITONEAL FLUID CRITERIA FOR SBP

1. Neutrophil count >250 cells/mm^3
2. Positive Gram stain
3. Positive culture result (gold standard)

24. **Are there any special issues to watch for in the patient who has had a liver transplant?**
    Transplant rejection is common and manifests as fever, pain, and elevated transaminases and bilirubin. This can be treated with high-dosage steroids or increased immunosuppressive medications. Other causes of transplant dysfunction include biliary strictures, recurrence of viral hepatitis, and vascular thrombosis. Immunosuppressive therapy can cause nephrotoxicity, neurotoxicity, and hypertension. As with other immunosuppressed patients, opportunistic infections, such as cytomegalovirus, Epstein-Barr virus, mycobacteria, *Pneumocystis,* and fungal infection should be considered.

ACKNOWLEDGMENTS

The editors and author of this chapter would like to acknowledge and thank Drs. Elan S. Levy, Kaushal H. Shah, and Molly E.W. Thiessen for their previous contributions to this chapter.

BIBLIOGRAPHY

Bass NM, Mullen KD, Sanyal A, et al. Rifaximin treatment in hepatic encephalopathy. *N Engl J Med.* 2010;362:1071–1081.
Ely R, Long B, Koyfman A. The emergency medicine-focused review of cholangitis. *J Emerg Med.* 2018;54:64–72.
Herrera JL. Management of acute variceal bleeding. *Clin Liver Dis.* 2014;18:347–357.
Horsley-Silva JL, Vargas HE. New therapies for hepatitis C virus infection. *Gastrointerol Hepatol (N Y).* 2017;13:22–31.
Ibrahim M, Sarvepalli S, Morris-Stiff G, et al. Gallstones: watch and wait, or intervene? *Cleve Clin J Med.* 2018;323–331.
Kochar B, Akshintala VS, Afghani E, et al. Incidence, severity, and mortality of post-ERCP pancreatitis: a systematic review by using randomized, controlled trials. *Gostrointest Endosc.* 2015;81:143–149.e9.
Kowdley K, Gordon SC, Reddy KR, et al. Ledipasvir and sofosbuvir for 8 or 12 weeks for chronic HCV without cirrhosis. *N Engl J Med.* 2014;370:1879–1888.
Lucey MR, Mathurin P, Morgan TR. Alcoholic hepatitis. *N Engl J Med.* 2009;360:2758–2769.
Privette TW Jr, Carlisle MC, Palma JK. Emergencies of the liver, gallbladder and pancreas. *Emerg Med Clin North Am* 29:293–317, 2011.
Yokoe M, Hata J, Takada T, et al. Tokyo guidelines 2018: diagnostic criteria and severity grading of acute cholecystitis (with videos). *J Hepatobiliary Pancreat Sci.* 2018;24:41–54.

CHAPTER 39

RENAL COLIC AND SCROTAL PAIN

Christopher M.B. Fernandes, MD

1. What are the most common forms of renal stones?
Calcium stones account for 80% of all renal stones: two-thirds are calcium oxalate, and the remainder are calcium phosphate. Struvite (magnesium ammonium phosphate), uric acid, and cystine account for 20% of renal stones.

2. List factors that predispose to stone formation.
Calcium stones
• Chronic dehydration
• Antacid use
• Hypercalciuria
• Hyperoxaluria
• Acidic urine
• Ingestion of vitamins A, C, and D
Struvite stones
• Chronic infection by urea-splitting organisms
Cystine stones
• Cystinuria

3. What lethal conditions are sometimes misdiagnosed as renal colic?
Aortic and iliac aneurysms are sometimes misdiagnosed. A careful search for bruits and pulsatile masses are mandatory when renal colic is suspected. Imaging should include this consideration when the diagnosis of an aneurysm cannot be excluded.

4. What clinical features help distinguish renal colic from other causes of abdominal pain?
Renal colic usually begins abruptly, causing terrible flank, costovertebral angle, lateral abdominal, and genital pain. Patients often are profoundly distressed, more so than patients with other abdominal pathologies. Pallor, diaphoresis, restlessness, and nausea are prominent. Renal colic causes flank tenderness, but in contrast to other causes of lateralized abdominal pain (e.g., appendicitis, diverticulitis, cholelithiasis, and ectopic pregnancy), it produces minimal or no abdominal tenderness.

5. In which patients would imaging be absolutely indicated to confirm the diagnosis of renal colic? What factors predict a high probability of ureteral stones?
• Patients with first episode of renal colic
• Patients in whom diagnosis is unclear
• Patients in whom a proximal urinary tract infection, in addition to a calculus, is suspected
• Elderly patients
Five factors most predictive of ureteral stones include:
• male sex
• short duration of pain
• nausea or vomiting
• microscopic hematuria

6. What is the role of the abdominal flat plate in diagnosing renal colic?
The abdominal flat plate, or *kidneys-ureter-bladder (KUB),* is less sensitive and less specific than the clinical examination and, by itself, has no role in the workup of suspected renal colic. If a stone is diagnosed on ultrasound, it may be appropriate to view the stone on a plain film. Subsequent radiographs may be helpful to document stone progression.

7. Has helical computed tomography (CT) now supplanted the intravenous pyelogram (IVP) as the diagnostic test of choice for suspected ureteral calculi? Why or why not?
Helical noncontrast CT has replaced IVP as the preferred diagnostic test. The IVP pinpoints stone size and location, clarifies the degree of obstruction, and shows ongoing renal function. Helical CT has been shown to be 97% sensitive and 96% specific in diagnosing renal stones. Used for this purpose, helical CT does not require intravenous (IV) contrast material and is faster than IVP – requiring only 1–2 minutes of scanner time to complete a

study. Even though helical CT provides no information about renal function, this can be ascertained by a urinalysis and serum creatinine. The marginal cost is less, and it can identify other important causes of flank pain.

8. **Is pregnancy a contraindication to CT KUB/IVP?**
   Ultrasound is the study of choice in pregnant patients, but if ultrasound is nondiagnostic, a limited IVP (scout film and 20-minutes' post-injection film, preferably coned to the area of concern) may be appropriate to reduce radiation from CT KUB.

KEY POINTS: MOST COMMON FORMS OF RENAL STONES

1. Calcium stones (80%)
   (a) Calcium oxalate (50%)
   (b) Calcium phosphate (5%)
   (c) Mixture of both (45%)
2. Struvite, uric acid, and cystine (20%)

9. **Name the most common sites of ureteral stone impaction.**
   The ureteropelvic junction, the pelvic brim (where the ureter crosses the iliac vessels), and the ureterovesical junction (the most narrow point in the ureter).

10. **Can the likelihood of spontaneous passage be predicted based on the size and location of the stone?**
    Stones reaching the distal ureter are more likely to pass than those impacting proximally. Stones 2–4 mm pass 95% of the time; stones 4–6 mm pass 50% of the time; and stones >6 mm pass 10% of the time. When estimating stone size, remember that the x-ray image is magnified; the actual size is 80% of what is measured on the films.

11. **What if the imaging study is normal, but the patient still appears to have renal colic?**
    Re-examine the patient carefully to ensure that you have not missed another cause of pain and that the patient is not developing a condition requiring surgery. If the physical examination is still compatible with renal colic, treat the patient, not the test result. Occasional false-negative results occur with all tests, and imaging modalities may miss small stones, but this may not be clinically relevant because small stones are unlikely to require specific therapy. Persistent severe flank pain can be caused by a leaking abdominal aortic aneurysm (AAA).

12. **Isn't an ultrasound just as accurate as helical CT or an IVP?**
    Ultrasound is safe and noninvasive but is more prone to false-negative results than the other studies. Ultrasound is sensitive for stones in the bladder and renal pelvis but often fails to visualize those in the mid and distal ureter – the most common sites for stone impaction. When ultrasound fails to identify a stone, however, it may show dilation of the renal collecting system, providing evidence of ureteral obstruction.

13. **List secondary signs of ureteral obstruction shown on helical CT.**
    - Unilateral obstruction
    - Stranding of perinephric fat
    - Hydronephrosis
    - Nephromegaly

14. **What is the soft-tissue rim sign on helical CT? How is it useful?**
    This sign shows soft-tissue attenuation around a ureteral calculus and helps differentiate a calculus from a phlebolith.

15. **What other tests are useful in the emergency department (ED) in patients with renal calculi?**
    Urine dipsticks are sensitive for microscopic hematuria, which is present in 80% of patients with renal colic. Urinalysis is recommended to rule out pyuria and bacteriuria. Urine culture is indicated if symptoms, signs, or urinalysis findings suggest infection. Determination of blood urea nitrogen (BUN), creatinine, and electrolyte levels is helpful if the patient has been vomiting or if presence of an underlying renal disease is suspected. There is usually no need for a more extensive metabolic workup in the ED.

16. **Why is coexistent infection a major problem?**
    Bacteria in an obstructed collecting system can cause abscess formation, renal destruction, bacteremia, and sepsis. The presence of infection in an obstructed ureter mandates immediate consultation with a urologist and IV antibiotics.

17. **Has lithotripsy supplanted percutaneous and open surgical methods of stone removal?**
    Not always. Optimal therapy depends on the size, type, and location of the stone. Ureteroscopic techniques probably are still preferable for lower ureteral stones. Extracorporeal shock wave lithotripsy (ESWL) is optimal for

stones 2 cm in size, particularly those in the renal pelvis. Percutaneous stone removal techniques are indicated for larger stones, when there is obstructive uropathy, and when less-invasive techniques have failed. For some stones, a combination of ESWL followed by percutaneous instrumentation is optimal. Some large stones still require open surgery. The method of removal is best determined by a urologist. Of note, newer technologies for treatment have led to an increased frequency of procedural interventions.

18. **What are the basics of ED treatment of renal colic?**
Hydration, analgesia, and antiemetics are the mainstay of treatment. Patients who have clinical dehydration secondary to vomiting and decreased oral intake, and if a radiocontrast media study is planned, should receive IV fluid hydration. However, on their own, neither fluids nor diuretics have been shown to be useful. Various analgesics and antiemetics are available for rapid control of symptoms (Table 39.1). IV pain control is the mainstay of ED treatment. Analgesic treatment should not be delayed waiting for test results. Rectal or IV nonsteroidal anti-inflammatory drugs (NSAIDs), which inhibit renal prostaglandin synthesis and interrupt ureteral spasm, are effective. A systematic review suggested that NSAIDs achieve slightly better pain relief, reduce the need for rescue analgesia, and produce much less vomiting than do opioids. Optimal ED pain control often involves the combined administration of NSAIDs and opioids. There is some emerging data supporting the use of IV preservative-free cardiac lidocaine (1.5 mg/kg in 100 mL normal saline (NS) over 10 minutes) as an approach to sparing opioid use to treat renal colic in patients without renal, liver, or cardiac disease.

Table 39.1 Analgesics and Antiemetics for Renal Colic

Opioid Analgesics			
Anileridine (Leritine)	PO 50 mg	q 4 h	prn
Hydromorphone (Dilaudid)	IV 1–2 mg	q 2–4 h	
	IM 1–2 mg/kg	q 2 h	prn[a]
Meperidine (Demerol)	IV 25–50 mg	q 5–10 min	prn
Morphine sulphate	IV 3–5 mg	q 5–10 min	prn
	IM 0.1–0.2 mg/kg	q 3 h	prn[a]
Oxycodone and acetaminophen (Percocet)	PO 2 tabs	q 4 h	prn
Oxycodone and acetylsalicylic acid (Percodan)	PO 2 tabs	q 4 h	prn
Antiemetics			
Metoclopramide (Reglan)	IV 10–20 mg	q 15 min	prn
Perphenazine (Trilafon)	IM 5 mg	q 6 h	prn[a]
	PO 4 mg	q 6 h	prn
Prochlorperazine (Compazine)	IV 5–10 mg	q 4 h	prn
	IM 5–10 mg	q 6 h	prn[a]
	PO 5–10 mg	q 4 h	prn
Ondansetron (Zofran)	IV 4 mg		
Nonsteroidal Analgesics			
Diclofenac (Voltaren)	50- or 100-mg suppositories, 150 mg/day		
Indomethacin	50- or 100-mg suppositories, 200 mg/day		
Ketorolac (Toradol)	IV 30 mg	q 6 h	
	IM 30 mg	q 6 h	
Other Lidocaine (preservative free)	IV 1.5 mg/kg		

[a]Intramuscular route not recommended for ED management of acute, severe pain.
IM, intramuscularly; *IV*, intravenously; *PO*, per os (by mouth); *prn*, as needed; *q*, every.

19. **Who requires hospitalization and /or urology consultation?**
Consider patients with high-grade obstruction, intractable pain or vomiting, associated urinary tract infection, a solitary or transplanted kidney, and in whom the diagnosis is uncertain. Obtain urologic consultation for patients with stones larger than 5 mm in diameter, urinary extravasation, a urinary tract infection with obstruction, and renal insufficiency regardless of symptoms.

20. **What advice should I give to patients being discharged from the ED?**
Patients should be advised to drink plenty of fluids, strain their urine (e.g., through a coffee filter), and return to the ED if they develop symptoms of infection or recurrent severe pain. Follow-up with a urologist within 1 week should be recommended.

21. **Which analgesics are recommended for outpatient pain control?**
Gastrointestinal irritation limits the usefulness of oral NSAIDs in patients with renal colic; however, rectal NSAIDs (diclofenac, indomethacin) may provide adequate analgesia. If necessary, oral opioids can be combined with NSAIDs in patients with documented ureteral calculi.

KEY POINTS: INDICATIONS FOR UROLOGY CONSULTATION FOR POSSIBLE HOSPITALIZATION

1. High-grade obstruction
2. Intractable pain or vomiting
3. Associated urinary tract infection
4. Solitary or transplanted kidney
5. Urinary extravasation
6. Renal insufficiency regardless of symptoms
7. Stones >5 mm requiring urology procedure to pass

---

22. **Why should patients be given a urine strainer on discharge?**
If the stone can be analyzed, the patient can then receive follow-up counseling on dietary modification or medications that may reduce the risk of recurrence.

23. **When should patients return to the ED?**
Patients should be instructed to seek medical care immediately if they have continued or increasing pain, nausea and vomiting, fever or chills, or any other new symptoms.

24. **What medical alternatives to active stone removal are available?**
In patients with ureteral stones <10 mm and whose symptoms are controlled with medications, observation with periodic evaluation is an option. In such patients, α-blocker therapy can be used, with some data suggesting faster passage with tamsulosin. One study suggested that 5–10 mm stones dislodge faster with tamsulosin, though other studies showed no improvement with either tamsulosin or nifedipine.

25. **What is the differential diagnosis in a patient presenting with an acutely painful scrotum?**
The differential diagnosis of acute scrotal pain includes testicular torsion, torsion of the testicular or epididymal appendages, epididymitis, orchitis, scrotal hernia, testicular tumor, renal colic, Henoch–Schönlein purpura, and Fournier's gangrene. Although not life threatening, testicular torsion may be a significant cause of morbidity and sterility in males. Thus any case of an acute scrotum should be considered testicular torsion until proven otherwise.

26. **What is testicular torsion?**
Testicular torsion results from maldevelopment of the normal fixation that occurs between the enveloping tunica vaginalis and the posterior scrotal wall. This maldevelopment then allows the testis and the epididymis to hang freely in the scrotum (the so-called bell-clapper deformity), allowing the testis to rotate on the spermatic cord. The degree of testicular ischemia is dependent on the number of rotations of the cord.

27. **When is testicular torsion most likely to occur?**
The annual incidence of testicular torsion is estimated to be 1 in 400 for males younger than 25 years of age. Testicular torsion has a bimodal distribution, with peak incidence in the neonate within the first few days of life, and in preadolescence.

KEY POINTS: SIX DIFFERENTIAL DIAGNOSES OF ACUTE SCROTUM

1. Testicular torsion
2. Torsion of the testicular or epididymal appendages
3. Epididymo-orchitis

4. Scrotal hernia
5. Testicular tumor
6. Fournier's gangrene

28. **What history is suggestive of testicular torsion?**
Usually, there is a history of trauma or strenuous event before the onset of scrotal pain in testicular torsion. One study reported sudden onset of scrotal pain to be present in 90% of patients with testicular torsion, compared with 58% of patients with epididymitis and 78% of patients with normal scrotum. Fever was present in 10% of patients with testicular torsion compared with 32% of patients with epididymitis.

29. **What clinical features are suggestive of testicular torsion?**
In testicular torsion, the affected testis usually is firm, tender, and aligned in a horizontal rather than a vertical axis. The presence of the cremasteric reflex appears to be one of the most helpful signs in ruling out testicular torsion, with 96% negative predictive value. It is elicited by gently stroking the inner aspect of the involved thigh and observing >0.5 cm of elevation in the affected testis.

30. **What is the proper management of testicular torsion?**
The proper management of a suspected testicular torsion is immediate urologic consultation and surgical exploration. If surgical consultation is not immediately available, manual detorsion should be attempted.

KEY POINTS: PROPER MANAGEMENT OF TESTICULAR TORSION

1. Emergent urologic consultation
2. Attempt at manual detorsion

31. **How is manual detorsion performed?**
This procedure is best done by standing at the foot or right side of the patient's bed. The torsed testis is detorsed in a fashion similar to opening a book. The patient's right testis is rotated counterclockwise, and the left testis is rotated clockwise. A testis viability rate is directly related to time of symptoms: 100% viability for <6 hours; 70% for 6–12 hours; and 20% for 12–24 hours.

32. **Is imaging testing helpful to confirm the diagnosis of testicular torsion?**
Testicular torsion is mainly a clinical diagnosis. Urology should be consulted at the time testicular torsion is suspected, and should precede testing due to the time-dependent nature of outcomes. However, imaging tests can be helpful to confirm the diagnosis or when other testicular conditions are on the differential diagnoses.

33. **What are the diagnostic imaging tests that can be used to evaluate the acute scrotum?**
Doppler ultrasound has supplanted radionuclide scintigraphy as the diagnostic imaging study of choice in evaluation of the acute scrotum. Both measure the blood flow to the testis; Doppler ultrasound carries a sensitivity of 86% and 97% accuracy, whereas radionuclide scintigraphy has 80% sensitivity and 97% specificity. Most urologists prefer confirmation of testicular torsion on a Doppler ultrasound study prior to surgical intervention.

34. **How is testicular torsion treated surgically?**
The involved testis must be detorsed and then checked for viability. If it is viable, it is fixed (orchiopexy). Since approximately 40% of patients have a bell-clapper deformity of the contralateral testis, the unaffected testis should be fixed to prevent recurrence.

35. **What are testis and epididymal appendix?**
The appendix testis is a müllerian duct remnant that is attached to the superior pole of the testicle and rests in the groove between the testis and epididymis. The appendix epididymis is a wolffian duct remnant, which is attached to the head of the epididymis.

36. **What are clinical features of torsion of testis and epididymal appendix?**
Both torsion of testis and epididymal appendix result in unilateral pain. The pain of epididymal appendix torsion typically is more gradual in onset and is usually not quite as severe as that associated with true testicular torsion. The most important aspect of the physical examination is pain and tenderness localized to the involved appendix. However, late in its course, generalized scrotal swelling and tenderness may be encountered, making it difficult to differentiate from testicular torsion. The classic blue dot sign (visualization of the ischemic or necrotic appendix testis through the scrotal wall on the superior aspect of the testicle) is pathognomonic for appendix testis torsion, but is also relatively uncommon.

37. **How is torsion of testis or epididymal appendix treated?**

   Torsion of epididymal and testicular appendix are self-resolving, benign processes. Rest, scrotal elevation, and analgesia are the mainstays of treatment. Resolution of the swelling and pain should be expected within 1 week.

38. **What is epididymitis?**

   Epididymitis arises from swelling and pain of the epididymis. It usually occurs secondary to infection or inflammation from the urethra or bladder. Patients with epididymitis present with increasing, dull, unilateral scrotal pain during a period of hours to days. Possible associated symptoms include fever, urethral discharge, hydrocele, erythema of the scrotum, and palpable swelling of the epididymis. Involvement of the ipsilateral testis is common, producing epididymitis-orchitis.

39. **List the most common causes of epididymitis.**

   The most common causes of epididymitis in males >35 years are gram-negative organisms such as *Escherichia coli, Klebsiella,* and *Pseudomonas* species. Among sexually active men <35 years, epididymitis is often caused by *Chlamydia trachomatis* or *Neisseria gonorrhoeae. E. coli* infection also may occur in men who are insertive partners during anal intercourse.

40. **What is the treatment for epididymitis?**

   Admission should be considered for any febrile, toxic-appearing patient with epididymitis or with testicular or epididymal abscess. In-patient therapy includes bed rest, analgesia, scrotal elevation (performed by taping a towel under the scrotum and over the proximal anterior thighs in the supine position), NSAIDs, and parenteral antibiotics. When sexually transmitted disease is suspected to be the cause of epididymitis, or in males <35 years old, urethral culture should be taken for *Chlamydia* and gonorrhea, followed by empirical treatment with ceftriaxone 250 mg intramuscularly once, plus doxycycline 100 mg orally twice a day for 10 days *or* ofloxacin 300 mg orally twice a day for 10 days. When gram-negative bacilli are suspected to be the cause for epididymitis, or in males >35 years old, treatment includes ciprofloxacin 500 mg orally twice a day or levofloxacin 500 mg once a day for 10 days. If patients are at risk for both, treat with ceftriaxone 250 mg intramuscularly once and levofloxacin or ciprofloxacin for 10 days. Treatment in all patients should include bed rest, analgesia, and scrotal elevation. Follow-up with a urologist within 5–7 days is recommended.

41. **What is Fournier's gangrene?**

   Fournier's gangrene, a surgical emergency, is a life-threatening disease characterized by necrotizing fasciitis of the perineal and genital region. It is generally the result of a polymicrobial infection from bacteria that are normally present in the perianal area. The diagnosis and treatment of Fournier's gangrene are similar to those of necrotizing fasciitis. Diabetes mellitus, alcohol abuse, and local trauma are known risk factors. Empirical broad-spectrum antibiotics with early surgical debridement are the mainstays of therapy. Re-exploration is commonly needed, and some patients require diverting colostomies or orchiectomies.

42. **What organisms are commonly seen with Fournier's gangrene?**

   This is typically a polymicrobial infection, with an average of four isolates/case. *E. coli* is the predominant aerobe, and *Bacteroides* the predominant anaerobe.

BIBLIOGRAPHY

Alelign T, Petros B. Kidney stone disease: an update of current concepts. *Adv Urol.* 2018;2018:3068365.

DaJusta DG, Granberg CF, Villanueva C, et al. Contemporary review of testicular torsion: new concepts, emerging technologies and potential therapeutics. *J Pediatr Urol.* 2013;9(6 Pt A):723–730.

Furyk JS, Chu K, Banks C, et al. Distal ureteric stones and tamsulosin: a double-blind, placebo-controlled, randomized, multicenter trial. *Ann Emerg Med.* 2016;67:86–95.

Holdgate A, Pollock T. Systematic review of the relative efficacy of non-steroidal anti-inflammatory drugs and opioids in the treatment of acute renal colic. *BMJ.* 2004;328:1401–1406.

Pickard R, Starr K, MacLennan G, et al. Medical expulsive therapy in adults with ureteric colic: a multicentre, randomised, placebo-controlled trial. *Lancet.* 2015;386:341–349.

Preminger GM, Tiselius HG, Assimos DG, et al. 2007 Guideline for the management of ureteral calculi. *J Urol.* 2007;178:2418.

Salim Rezaie. IV lidocaine for renal colic: another opioid sparing option? REBEL EM blog, December 6, 2016. https://rebelem.com/iv-lidocaine-for-renal-colic-another-opioid-sparing-option/.

Smith-Bindman R, Aubin C, Bailitz et al. Ultrasonography versus computed tomography for suspected nephrolithiasis. *N Engl J Med.* 2014;371:1100–1110.

Worster AS, Supapol WB. Fluids and diuretics for acute ureteric colic. *Cochrane Database Syst Rev.* 2012;12. https://www.cochranelibrary.com/cdsr/doi/10.1002/14651858.CD004926.pub3/full. Accessed December 19, 2018.

CHAPTER 40

ACUTE URINARY RETENTION

Benjamin Li, MD and Bonnie Kaplan, MD

1. **What is acute urinary retention (AUR)?**
   AUR is characterized by painful inability to urinate. It is most commonly the result of bladder outlet obstruction, but it also may result from neurogenic, pharmacologic, or other causes of detrusor muscle dysfunction. Urine is produced normally but is retained in the bladder, which manifests as distention and discomfort.

2. **Is there chronic urinary retention?**
   Yes, it generally represents prolonged retention. The hallmarks of chronic urinary retention are the absence of pain and overflow incontinence. It most commonly occurs in neurologically compromised patients.

3. **What is the most common cause of AUR? Who gets it?**
   Obstruction of the lower urinary tract (bladder and urethra) is the most common cause encountered in the emergency department (ED). In general, AUR is a disease of older men, although it is occasionally encountered in women. The usual site of obstruction is the prostate gland, but lesions of the urethra or penis also may cause retention. Patients with indwelling catheters (urethral or suprapubic) are at risk for episodes of retention because of obstruction or dysfunction of non-native drainage systems.

4. **How does benign prostatic hypertrophy (BPH) cause AUR?**
   BPH with bladder neck obstruction is the most common cause of AUR. By 50 years old, at least half of men are affected by BPH with lower urinary tract symptoms. As the prostate hypertrophies, urine outflow is obstructed by enlargement of the median lobe of the gland impinging on the internal urethral lumen. The typical patient with BPH gives a progressive history suggestive of urinary outlet obstruction. Symptoms such as urgency, frequency, hesitancy, straining, dribbling, nocturia, and the sensation of incomplete bladder emptying may precede an episode of AUR. New medications or increased fluid load may also precipitate an acute episode of retention in patients.

5. **List the other causes of AUR.**
   Obstructive:
   - BPH
   - Prostate carcinoma
   - Prostatitis
   - Urethral stricture
   - Posterior urethral valves
   - Phimosis
   - Paraphimosis
   - Balanitis
   - Meatal stenosis
   - Calculi
   - Blood clots
   - Circumcision
   - Urethral foreign body
   - Constricting penile ring
   - Clogged or crimped catheter

   Neurogenic
   - Spinal cord injuries
   - Herniated lumbosacral disks (cauda equina syndrome)
   - Central nervous system (CNS) tumors
   - Stroke
   - Diabetes
   - Multiple sclerosis
   - Encephalitis
   - Tabes dorsalis
   - Syringomyelia
   - Herpes simplex
   - Herpes zoster

Pharmacologic
- Anticholinergics
- Antihistamines
- Antidepressants
- Antispasmodics
- Narcotics
- Sympathomimetics
- Antipsychotics
- Antiparkinsonian agents

Psychogenic
- Diagnosis of exclusion

6. **What are the important features in the history and physical examination?**
Any history of prostate or urethral conditions should be elicited. Patients often have a history of chronic voiding hesitancy, slow urinary stream, a feeling of incomplete bladder emptying, or nocturia. Information about neurologic symptoms, trauma, previous instrumentation, back pain, and current medication is essential. On physical examination, the distended bladder is often palpable above the pubic rim and indicates at least 150 mL of urine in the bladder. The penis or vulva, and particularly the urethra, should be examined carefully for any signs of stricture evident on palpation. A rectal examination is essential and often provides clues to the diagnosis of BPH, prostate carcinoma, or prostatitis. A careful neurologic examination, including rectal tone and perineal sensation, is essential in any patient suspected of having a neurologic lesion.

7. **Are there any red flags in the history and physical examination that might indicate a more serious (e.g., surgical) cause?**
Yes, new urinary symptoms, particularly retention, in patients with a history of trauma or back pain should alert the examiner to the possibility of spinal cord compression resulting from disk herniation, fracture, epidural hematoma, epidural abscess, or tumor. Be especially suspicious if there is no prior history of bladder, prostate, or urethral disorders.

8. **How do I treat AUR?**
Treat AUR with catheterization and bladder decompression using a Foley catheter.

9. **What if I cannot pass a Foley catheter?**
Occasionally, simple passage of a 16- or 18-French Foley catheter cannot be accomplished. One trick which often helps is to fill a 30-mL syringe with lidocaine jelly and inject it into the urethral meatus. If one is still unable to pass the catheter, consider an 18- or 20-French coudé catheter. The coudé (elbow, in French) tip catheter has a slight bend in the distal 3 cm that, when pointed upward, can maneuver over the enlarged prostate. Never force a catheter through an area of significant resistance, because this can cause urethral perforation, a false lumen, and subsequent stricture formation.

10. **Is a bigger catheter better?**
If you are unable to pass a 16-French (standard adult) catheter, it is generally recommended to move up in size to an 18- or 20-French Foley catheter. Usually, the stiffness and larger bulk of the bigger catheter are more successful in passing through the bladder neck than a smaller, more flexible catheter. Remember, never force a catheter through significant resistance.

11. **What if nothing is working?**
If you still cannot pass a catheter, the obstruction may be more severe than anticipated, or a stricture may be present. One clue to the presence of a stricture in adult males is the obstruction occurs less than 16 cm from the external urethral meatus. If this is the case, an attempt may be made using a pediatric-sized urinary catheter. If this fails, more sophisticated instrumentation may be required, such as filiformes and followers or catheter guides. These techniques should be done only by a urologist or practitioner with extensive training. If AUR cannot be relieved by transurethral bladder catheterization, placement of a suprapubic catheter may be necessary.

12. **What is suprapubic catheterization? How is it performed?**
Suprapubic catheterization is a procedure used to pass a urinary catheter percutaneously into the bladder through the lower anterior abdominal wall (Fig. 40.1). It is indicated when bladder drainage is necessary and other methods have failed, or when urethral damage from trauma is suspected. The procedure is done under sterile conditions with local anesthesia or procedural sedation. The location and presence of a distended bladder is preferentially confirmed by ultrasound (which can also identify overlying bowel), or percussion. A small midline incision is made 2 cm above the symphysis pubis. The bladder is then penetrated through the incision using either a needle and Seldinger technique, or directly using a trocar. Contraindications to suprapubic catheterization without simultaneous cystoscopy are a history of lower abdominal surgery, nonvisualizable distended bladder by ultrasound, and pelvic cancer.

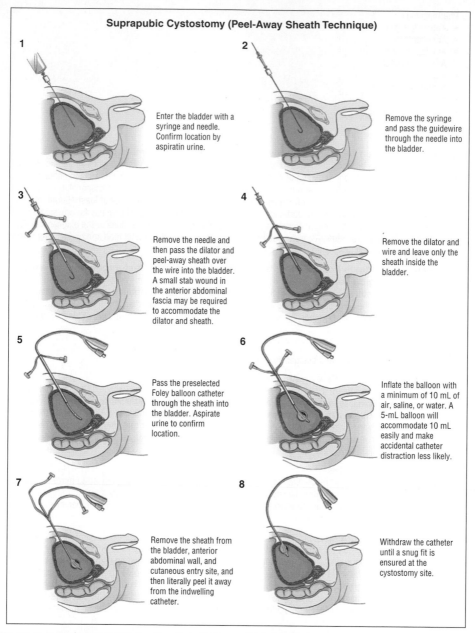

Suprapubic Cystostomy (Peel-Away Sheath Technique)

1 Enter the bladder with a syringe and needle. Confirm location by aspiratin urine.

2 Remove the syringe and pass the guidewire through the needle into the bladder.

3 Remove the needle and then pass the dilator and peel-away sheath over the wire into the bladder. A small stab wound in the anterior abdominal fascia may be required to accommodate the dilator and sheath.

4 Remove the dilator and wire and leave only the sheath inside the bladder.

5 Pass the preselected Foley balloon catheter through the sheath into the bladder. Aspirate urine to confirm location.

6 Inflate the balloon with a minimum of 10 mL of air, saline, or water. A 5-mL balloon will accommodate 10 mL easily and make accidental catheter distraction less likely.

7 Remove the sheath from the bladder, anterior abdominal wall, and cutaneous entry site, and then literally peel it away from the indwelling catheter.

8 Withdraw the catheter until a snug fit is ensured at the cystostomy site.

Fig. 40.1 (A–D) Suprapubic catheterization. (From Davis JE, Silverman MA. Urological procedures. In: Roberts JR, ed. *Roberts and Hedges' Clinical Procedures in Emergency Medicine*. 6th ed. Elsevier; 2019, Fig. 55.29.)

KEY POINTS: TREATMENT OPTIONS FOR AUR

1. Foley catheter placement
2. Coudé catheter placement
3. Filiformes and followers
4. Suprapubic catheterization

13. **What diagnostic studies are useful in the evaluation of AUR?**
   Bedside ultrasonography can be helpful during the initial evaluation, and, if needed, may facilitate suprapubic as-piration. Always check a urinalysis with microscopic examination and urine culture. It is generally recommended to check blood urea nitrogen and creatinine levels to evaluate renal function, especially in cases of suspected chronic retention.

14. **Which medications may cause AUR?**
   Table 40.1 presents the broad categories, as well as specific medications, that can cause AUR.

Table 40.1 Medications That Can Cause Acute Urinary Retention
Sympathomimetics (α-Adrenergic)
Ephedrine
Pseudoephedrine (Sudafed, Actifed)
Phenylephrine hydrochloride (Neo-Synephrine, Dimetapp)
Phenylpropanolamine hydrochloride (Contac)
Amphetamine
Cocaine
Sympathomimetics (β-Adrenergic)
Isoproterenol
Terbutaline
Antidepressants
Tricyclic
Fluoxetine (Prozac)
Antidysrhythmics
Quinidine
Disopyramide (Norpace)
Procainamide
Anticholinergics
Atropine
Dicyclomine (Bentyl)
Antihistamines
Chlorpheniramine (Chlor-Trimeton)
Diphenhydramine (Benadryl, Unisom)
Hydroxyzine (Atarax, Vistaril)
Antiparkinsonian Agents
Benztropine (Cogentin)
Amantadine (Symmetrel)
Levodopa (Sinemet)
Trihexyphenidyl (Artane)
Hormonal Agents
Progesterone
Estrogen
Testosterone

Continued on following page

Table 40.1 Medications That Can Cause Acute Urinary Retention *(Continued)*

Antipsychotics

Haloperidol

Chlorpromazine (Thorazine)

Prochlorperazine (Compazine)

Risperidone (Risperdal)

Clozapine (Clozaril)

Quetiapine (Seroquel)

Antihypertensives

Nifedipine (Procardia)

Hydralazine

Nicardipine

Muscle Relaxants

Diazepam (Valium)

Cyclobenzaprine (Flexeril)

Narcotics

Morphine sulfate

Codeine

Meperidine (Demerol)

Hydromorphone hydrochloride (Dilaudid)

Miscellaneous

Indomethacin

Metoclopramide (Reglan)

Carbamazepine (Tegretol)

Mercurial diuretics

Dopamine

Vincristine

MDMA (3,4-methylenedioxymethamphetamine; ecstasy)

Cannabis

15. **Summarize the different neurogenic causes of AUR.**
    - *Upper motor neuron lesions.* Lesions located in the spinal cord above the sacral micturition center (L2 vertebral level, S2–S4 spinal segments) result in a spastic or reflex bladder. Common causes are spinal cord trauma, tumor, and multiple sclerosis. Lesions of the cerebral cortex (e.g., stroke, bleed) usually cause chronic loss of bladder control and incontinence, except in the acute phase, when the lesions typically produce AUR.
    - *Lower motor neuron lesions.* Lesions at the micturition center in the cauda equina interrupt the sacral reflex arc and produce vesical dysfunction. There is loss of sensation of bladder fullness, leading to overstretch, muscle atony, and poor contraction. Large residuals are common. The most common causes include spinal trauma, tumor, herniated intervertebral disks, and multiple sclerosis.
    - *Bladder afferent and efferent nerve dysfunction.* Dysfunction in this pathway disrupts the micturition reflex arc that is necessary for proper urination, causing AUR. Common causes include diabetes, herpes simplex infection, and postoperative states.

16. **Name the most common complications of AUR.**
    Complications include infection, hemorrhage, and postobstruction diuresis. All three are more common in patients with chronic urinary retention.

17. **What is autonomic dysreflexia/hyperreflexia, and what does it have to do with AUR?**
    Autonomic dysreflexia/hyperreflexia is an abnormality of the autonomic nervous system seen in patients with long-standing cervical or high thoracic spinal cord lesions (e.g., patients with quadriplegia and high paraplegia). It is caused primarily by unchecked reflex sympathetic discharge secondary to visceral or somatic stimuli below the level of the spinal injury. This potentially life-threatening syndrome includes severe paroxysmal hypertension, diaphoresis, tachycardia or bradycardia, anxiety, headache, and flushing. Uncontrolled, it may result in seizures and coma. Morbidity has resulted from cerebrovascular events, subarachnoid hemorrhage, and respiratory arrest. One of the most common precipitating stimuli is overdistention of the bladder (AUR) from a plugged or kinked catheter; therefore, it is always important to evaluate catheter patency in this population.

18. **What is postobstruction diuresis? How is it managed?**
    The inappropriate excretion of salt and water after relief of urinary obstruction is called *postobstruction diuresis.* Patients with abnormal renal function or chronic urinary retention are most susceptible. A physiologic diuresis is normal, because the kidneys excrete the overload of solute and volume retained while the urinary system is obstructed. If urine output persists at high levels, significant fluid and electrolyte abnormalities may develop. Any patient who exhibits a continuous diuresis after clinical euvolemia is reached requires hospitalization for hemodynamic monitoring and fluid and electrolyte repletion.

19. **Who can I send home? Who needs admission? Can I remove that catheter?**
    Most patients with AUR caused by an obstruction require urethral catheterization with continuous drainage. Reliable patients in good health and without signs of serious systemic infection are candidates for careful outpatient management with a leg bag and timely urologic follow-up (within 2 weeks). The use of prophylactic antibiotics in these patients is controversial. Patients with new neurogenic causes, severe infection, systemic toxicity, or any lesion that may need surgical intervention require hospital admission. Some younger patients with pharmacologic urinary retention may have the catheter removed after decompression. The causative medication should be discontinued, and the patient should be discharged with instructions to return if symptoms recur. If the catheter is removed, it is prudent to confirm patients can spontaneously void before discharge from the ED.

20. **Do medications play any role in the treatment of AUR?**
    Although the mainstay of treatment is bladder decompression, medications play an important adjunctive role in the treatment of this condition. Urinary tract infections in the setting of AUR should be treated with antibiotics, guided by your local antibiogram. Patients with a suspected prostatic or bladder cause may benefit from an α_1-adrenergic blocking agent such as doxazosin, prazosin, or tamsulosin. These agents work at the prostate and bladder neck to decrease resistance and ease micturition, and are generally recommended for men without another obvious precipitating cause.

ACKNOWLEDGMENTS

The authors would like to thank John P. Marshall, MD, for his prior contributions.

BIBLIOGRAPHY

Egan KB. The epidemiology of benign prostatic hyperplasia associated with lower urinary tract symptoms: prevalence and incidence rates. *Urol Clin North Am.* 2016;43:289–297.

Georgopoulos P, Apostolidis A. Neurogenic voiding dysfunction. *Curr Opin Urol.* 2017;27:300–306.

Granieri MA, Wang HS, Routh JC, et al. A nationwide assessment of emergency department management of acute urinary retention due to urethral stricture. *Urology.* 2017;100:79–83.

Manjunath AS, Hofer MD. Urologic emergencies. *Med Clin North Am.* 2018;102:373–385.

Marshall JR, Haber J, Josephson EB. An evidence-based approach to emergency department management of acute urinary retention. *Emerg Med Pract.* 2014;16:1–24.

Sliwinski A, D'Arcy FT, Sultana R, et al. Acute urinary retention and the difficult catheterization: current emergency management. *Eur J Emerg Med.* 2016;23:80–88.

Yoon PD, Chalasani V, Woo HH. Systematic review and meta-analysis on management of acute urinary retention. *Prostate Cancer Prostatic Dis.* 2015;18:297–302.

CHAPTER 41

URINARY TRACT INFECTION: CYSTITIS, PYELONEPHRITIS, AND PROSTATITIS

Monica Noori, MD and Renee A. King, MD, MPH

1. **Define terminology pertinent to the range of urinary tract infections (UTIs).**
   - Bacteriuria: the occurrence of bacteria within the urinary tract. Significant bacteriuria is defined as 10^5 colony-forming units (CFU)/mL.
   - Cystitis: inflammation of the bladder caused by significant bacteriuria with bladder mucosal (urothelium) invasion. Clinicians commonly use the term *UTI* to mean *cystitis*.
   - Pyelonephritis: infection of the parenchyma and collecting system of the kidney. Usually seen with flank pain, fever, and significant bacteriuria.
   - Urethritis and acute urethral syndrome: dysuria, frequency, and urgency in the absence of significant bacteriuria.
   - Prostatitis: inflammation of the prostate. It is classified as asymptomatic, acute, or chronic bacterial prostatitis, or chronic nonbacterial inflammatory or noninflammatory prostatitis.

KEY POINTS: CHARACTERISTICS OF CYSTITIS

1. Dysuria
2. Frequency
3. Urgency
4. Suprapubic pain
5. Significant bacteriuria

2. **What are the most common causes of UTI?**
   Most UTIs are caused by one pathogen. The most common etiology is *Escherichia coli*, accounting for up to 95% of acute UTIs. *Staphylococcus saprophyticus* is the second most common cause of acute cystitis. Complicated UTIs may have a broader range of microbes, including *Enterococcus, Providencia, Pseudomonas, Serratia*, and *Staphylococcus*, and occasionally fungi.

3. **What is asymptomatic bacteriuria?**
   The presence of 10^5 CFU/mL in a clean-catch midstream urine sample from a patient without symptoms is consistent with asymptomatic bacteriuria. If two successive specimens result in the same microbe at the same concentration, the likelihood of true bacteriuria is 80%–95%.

4. **Should asymptomatic bacteriuria be treated?**
   Healthy females who are not pregnant do not need treatment for asymptomatic bacteriuria.

   A pregnant female with asymptomatic bacteriuria does need treatment with antibiotics, since 20%–40% of these patients go on to develop UTI or pyelonephritis, which is associated with prematurity and low birth weight.

   Preoperative patients should be treated with antibiotics, because this has been shown to decrease the potential for postoperative infections.

   Evidence indicates that antibiotic treatment is not needed for patients with indwelling catheters who have asymptomatic bacteriuria as this only leads to resistance.

5. **List the differential diagnoses of dysuria.**
   - Infectious causes: cystitis, epididymitis, prostatitis, pyelonephritis, urethritis (gonococcal vs. nongonococcal), vulvovaginitis
   - Structural causes: calculi, neoplastic lesions
   - Traumatic causes: blunt trauma, chemical irritants, sexual intercourse or assault

6. **When should a pelvic examination be performed in a female patient with dysuria?**
   If the history and physical examination raise concern for a cause other than classic UTI, then a pelvic examination should be performed. Clinical symptoms such as external inflammation indicative of vulvovaginitis, low abdominal

or bilateral flank discomfort, and any person with risk factors for sexually transmitted infection (STI) or sexual assault should receive a pelvic examination to rule out conditions, such as pelvic inflammatory disease and trauma. Furthermore, patients who are unresponsive to empiric antibiotic treatment for cystitis or who have negative urine studies should undergo a pelvic examination.

7. **What tests can be done to evaluate for UTI?**
Urinalysis with dipstick or microscopy is the first step in evaluating for presence of a UTI. Urine culture with a Gram stain is not the first choice of testing because of the lengthier process and expense. However, culture is useful for the selection of appropriate antibiotic therapy, especially in patients with risks for complicated UTI. Common forms of urinalysis include the following:
- Dipstick test: includes blood, glucose, leukocyte esterase ($\geq +1$), nitrite, and protein. A positive dipstick is a good screening test (about 75%–90% sensitive, with 75%–85% specificity), but if the history obtained is strongly suggestive of a UTI, a negative dipstick does not reliably rule out infection.
- Microscopy
  - Bacteriuria: a finding of 10^5 CFU/mL is used to define significant bacteriuria in an asymptomatic patient. However, as few as 10^2 CFU/mL with symptoms and pyuria are suggestive of a UTI.
  - Epithelial cells: the presence of epithelial cells is used mainly to estimate perineal contamination of midstream specimens. Although epithelial cells are present throughout the urinary tract, their occurrence on urinalysis is typically of vaginal epithelial cell origin, but is not necessarily predictive of urine contamination.
  - Leukocyte esterase: this enzyme is present in neutrophils, and is able to convert indoxyl carboxylic acid to an indoxyl moiety in leukocytes. A positive test is indicative, but not confirmatory, of pyuria.
  - Nitrite: present in acute cystitis, it is produced from nitrate by nitrate reductase, an enzyme that is found in gram-negative microbes. A first morning specimen is ideal given the longer incubation time. This test is specific, but not sensitive for acute cystitis.
  - Pyuria: ≥ 10 leukocytes/mL observed by direct microscopy correlates significantly with acute cystitis.

8. **When should a urine culture be ordered?**
For uncomplicated cystitis in healthy patients, urine culture is unnecessary. A culture with sensitivities is useful in cases of complicated UTI or pyelonephritis.

9. **What comprises a complicated UTI?**
A complicated UTI is any underlying condition that predisposes the patient to infection and reduces the effectiveness of standard treatments.

KEY POINTS: RISK FACTORS FOR COMPLICATED UTI

1. Anatomic abnormality of the urinary tract
2. Male sex
3. Diabetes
4. Foreign body (urethral catheter, nephrostomy tube)
5. Kidney failure
6. Multidrug resistant organism
7. Obstruction of urinary tract (prostate hypertrophy, stone, stenosis)
8. Pregnancy
9. Renal failure/renal transplant
10. Immunosuppression

---

10. **What is the treatment for uncomplicated UTI?**
Without treatment, approximately 25%–42% of uncomplicated cystitis resolves spontaneously, but standard therapy involves antibiotics. Choosing the appropriate antibiotic depends on efficacy, including local resistance patterns and geographic variation of pathogen resistance, cost, risk of adverse effects, and antibiotic availability.
First-line treatment for uncomplicated UTI in women includes nitrofurantoin 100 mg twice daily for 5–7 days, trimethoprim-sulfamethoxazole (TMP-SMX) 160/800 mg twice daily for 3 days, or fosfomycin 3 g one-time dose. Local recommendations for therapy may vary in different geographic regions.

11. **Is there a role for nonantibiotic treatment?**
In some cases of cystitis, phenazopyridine (Pyridium), a urinary analgesic, may be useful. A 48-hour course of 200 mg three times daily after meals is the usual regimen. This medication can cause false-positive nitrite dipstick results. Patients should be warned that body fluids may turn orange. Pyridium should not be used longer than 2 days, as it may mask symptoms that would prompt reevaluation. Supratherapeutic doses can also lead to methemoglobinemia.

12. **What is the treatment for pyelonephritis?**

In healthy, nonpregnant patients, extended antibiotic regimens based upon local resistance patterns are recommended. Fluoroquinolones such as ciprofloxacin, levofloxacin, and ofloxacin are considered therapies for uncomplicated pyelonephritis. Other options include cefdinir, cefixime or cefpodoxime. A one-time dose of gentamicin or ceftriaxone can be used parenterally if needed. Nitrofurantoin is not recommended for treatment of pyelonephritis as it does not attain therapeutic levels in the renal parenchyma.

KEY POINTS: SIGNS AND SYMPTOMS OF PYELONEPHRITIS

1. Fever
2. Flank pain
3. Significant bacteriuria
4. Costovertebral angle tenderness

13. **Which patients with pyelonephritis require admission?**

Admission for pyelonephritis should be considered for patients who have a ureteral obstruction, are unable to tolerate oral medications or fluids, immunocompromised, severely ill or in extreme pain, and patients with little or no support or resources. Admission should also be considered for women who are pregnant. Although some in the early first trimester may be discharged with oral antibiotics, discussion with an obstetrician is advised.

14. **When should imaging be obtained for pyelonephritis?**

If fevers or positive blood cultures persist for longer than 48 hours, there is concern for obstruction (e.g., by a urethral stone), sudden clinical deterioration, symptoms persist despite antibiotic therapy, the patient is immunocompromised, severely diabetic or an organ transplant recipient, then obtaining an ultrasound or computed tomography may be warranted to evaluate for an abscess or obstruction.

KEY POINTS: POSSIBLE ADMISSION CRITERIA FOR PYELONEPHRITIS

1. Complicated cystitis
2. Inability to tolerate oral medication or hydration
3. Lack of support/resources
4. Pregnancy
5. Ureteral obstruction
6. Sepsis/extreme illness

15. **What are the differences when treating complicated cystitis?**

The length of treatment in complicated UTIs is longer. Treatment should be extended to 7–10 days. If the patient is pregnant, antibiotics should be compatible with pregnancy. Common medications based upon local resistance patterns may include amoxicillin, cephalexin, cefdinir, and nitrofurantoin. Intravenous (IV) antibiotics, such as ceftriaxone, may also be needed, especially if the patient cannot tolerate oral medications.

16. **What is the presentation of acute bacterial prostatitis?**

Most patients (80%) experience dysuria, frequency, and urgency. About 60% of these patients are febrile. Myalgias, perineal pain, and rigors can also be seen with bacterial prostatitis.

17. **What is the treatment for acute prostatitis?**

A urinalysis should be obtained to evaluate for bacterial infection. Catheterization and prostate massage should not be performed because of pain and the risk of bacteremia. Antibiotics are the mainstay of treatment. Common medications utilized, pending upon resistance patterns, include aminoglycosides, fluoroquinolones, and cephalosporins. TMP-SMX may also be used, although it has decreased sensitivity. Duration of treatment should be 4–6 weeks to resolve symptoms and prevent chronic prostatitis. Consider STI in all patients.

18. **What are signs and symptoms of chronic bacterial prostatitis?**

Chronic bacterial prostatitis is a recurrent subacute infection which is the primary cause of recurrent UTI in males. Examination is variable, but common symptoms include pain with urination, frequency, and urgency. Other complaints include back pain, pain in the scrotum and perineum, painful ejaculation, and hematospermia. Fevers and chills are not usually seen. Symptoms may be present for 3 or more months.

19. **What is the treatment for chronic bacterial prostatitis?**

Treatment can be difficult because of the relapsing nature of the illness. Generally, long-term treatment with a 12-week course of therapy is needed. Referral to a urologist is recommended.

ACKNOWLEDGMENTS

The editors and authors of this chapter would like to acknowledge and thank Dr. Sara M. Krzyzniak for her previous contributions to this chapter.

BIBLIOGRAPHY

Bent S, Nallamothu BK, Simel DL, et al. Does this woman have an acute uncomplicated urinary tract infection? *JAMA*. 2002;287: 2701–2710.

Grabe M, Bjerklund-Johansen TE, et al. *Guidelines on urological infections*. Arnhem, Netherlands: European Association of Urology; 2013.

Gupta K, Trautner B. In the clinic. Urinary tract infection. *Ann Intern Med*. 2012;156:ITC3-1–ITC3-15.

Lutters M, Vogt-Ferrier NB. Antibiotic duration for treating uncomplicated, symptomatic lower urinary tract infections in elderly women. *Cochrane Database Syst Rev*. (3):CD001535; 2008.

Wang A, Nizran P, Malone MA, et al. Urinary tract infections. *Prim Care*. 2013;40:687–706.

CHAPTER 42

RENAL FAILURE

Andrew Brookens, MD and Lily Cervantes, MD

1. **How should you manage fluids in patients with renal failure?**
   Volume overload plagues patients with end-stage renal disease (ESRD), whether from patient nonadherence to dietary restrictions or from iatrogenic over-administration of fluids. Whether acute kidney injury (AKI), chronic kidney disease (CKD), or ESRD, patients in shock should be treated with the resuscitative standard of care. Fluid restraint may be beneficial in patients with clear volume overload. If your patients are alert, ask if they still make urine and how much. Knowing their ability to later excrete volume helps you juggle concerns of organ hypoperfusion and the risk of progressive volume overload.

2. **How should you manage medications in patients with renal failure?**
   The effects of renal failure on drug metabolism and disposition are complex; therefore, it is advisable to check recommended dosage adjustments for patients with renal failure before administering or prescribing medications. Medications and drug interactions are a frequent reason for emergency department (ED) visits and complicate the management strategy.

KEY POINTS: HIGH-YIELD PEARLS FOR MANAGING MEDICATIONS IN RENAL FAILURE

1. *Hold* angiotensin-converting enzyme (ACE) inhibitors and ARBs (angiotensin-receptor blockers) in renal failure in the ED.
2. Consider holding all blood pressure (BP) medicines with hypotension.
3. *Hold* nonsteroidal anti-inflammatory drugs (NSAIDs) when renal failure is diagnosed, as they cause different renal injury patterns including hemodynamic, allergic, and electrolyte imbalance.
4. Diuretics *should be held* in suspected renal failure. *However*, in fluid overload (e.g., pulmonary edema), *use* diuretics as a primary treatment.
5. *Hold* metformin in severe acidosis and renal failure where the glomerular filtration rate (GFR) is <30 mL/min. Its principal risk in the kidney is of lactic acidosis and not AKI.
6. *Hold* SGLT2 (sodium-glucose co-transporter 2-inhibitors, e.g., empagliflozin, dapagliflozin, and canagliflozin) in hypotension and renal failure, as they act like diuretics in the kidney.
7. Calcineurin inhibitors (cyclosporine and tacrolimus) to prevent transplant rejection *should be held in AKI*. If you hold them, *communicate this* to admitting and outpatient providers. Documenting their levels should only be done 12 hours after a patient's last scheduled dose.

3. **What is dialysis and its forms?**
   Most patients with renal failure and ESRD requiring renal replacement therapy are on hemodialysis (HD). The HD treatment involves exposing the patient's blood to a chemically balanced aqueous solution inside a dialyzer filter. Both convection (pressure) and diffusion (down a concentration gradient) move waste products out of the patient's blood. Chronic dialysis patients undergo this treatment over approximately 4 hours, three times per week. Hemodialysis access to the patient's blood occurs through either a high-flow dialysis catheter or a surgically created vascular access (e.g., a fistula or artificial graft).

   As an alternative to HD, an increasing proportion of patients are on peritoneal dialysis (PD) where the patient's peritoneal membrane serves as the semipermeable barrier between the blood and a sterile dextrose dialysate solution. Access occurs through a surgically placed catheter in the low peritoneum, avoiding direct vascular exposure.

KEY POINTS: DIALYSIS TRIAGE FOR RENAL FAILURE

1. Intermittent HD is the preferred treatment for a dialysis emergency in the hospital where rapid treatment is needed over several hours and the patient can be hemodynamically stabilized.
2. Continuous renal replacement therapy (CRRT) is offered to patients less hemodynamically stable or who need gentler treatment, including steady, large-volume removal continuously over several days.
3. Urgent-start PD is increasingly an option for patients with renal failure who prefer to do dialysis at home, are too busy for hemodialysis clinics, or have an aversion to hemodialysis.

Table 42.1 A Mnemonic for Emergency Dialysis

"AEIOU" is Useful But Imperfect	
A	Acidosis
E	Electrolyte disorder
I	Ingestion or intoxication
O	Overload (fluid)
U	Uremia

4. **When is dialysis emergent?**
   Emergency dialysis is a potentially life-saving intervention that is not without risks. Indications include acute pulmonary edema, life-threatening electrolyte abnormalities such as hyperkalemia, severe metabolic acidosis, and life-threatening intoxication or overdose secondary to dialyzable toxins ordinarily are excreted by the kidneys.

KEY POINTS: INDICATIONS FOR EMERGENCY DIALYSIS

1. Life-threatening hyperkalemia
2. Severe metabolic acidosis
3. Acute pulmonary edema
4. Life-threatening intoxication or overdose with agents normally excreted by the kidneys
5. Severe uremic symptoms in advanced renal failure

(Table 4.1)

5. **What is the most common problem relating to hemodialysis vascular access in the ED?**
   Arteriovenous (AV) fistula, using a patient's own anatomy, is the optimal dialysis vascular access. Other options including a vascular graft, a tunneled central venous catheter (nontunneled for urgent in-hospital treatment). The AV fistula projects a palpable thrill and audible bruit by auscultation to the skin, and patients on dialysis are taught to monitor this regularly. Suspect thrombosis when patients report loss of a bruit or thrill in the fistula. More often, they come to the ED when there has been a problem establishing adequate flow during a hemodialysis session, something frequently caused by thrombosis or intravascular stenosis. Consult interventional radiology, or, if unavailable, nephrology or a vascular surgeon to establish an action plan. A special angiogram called a fistulagram defines the nature and extent of the obstruction.

KEY POINTS: MOST COMMON PROBLEMS WITH VASCULAR ACCESS

1. Thrombosis
2. Stenosis
3. Infection
4. Hemorrhage

6. **How do I diagnose and treat a vascular access infection?**
   Infection is obvious when the patient has signs of inflammation localized to the access site. The difficulty is that many dialysis patients have few or atypical signs such as fever, lethargy, or hypotension, and they may not have specific localizing signs. Obtain blood cultures early when suspected. Stable patients, with AV fistulae and a clear infectious nidus, may be discharged from the ED if close outpatient dialysis follow-up can be confirmed. Many dialysis units stock limited intravenous (IV) antibiotics such as vancomycin and cefazolin and see these patients frequently enough to be the sole provider of such antibiotics.

KEY POINTS: DIALYSIS VASCULAR ACCESS INFECTIONS

1. Fever, lethargy, hypotension, or mental status changes in a dialysis patient are nonspecific but may be the only sign of an access infection.
2. Dialysis access points with a foreign body (catheters, grafts) are more likely to require admission and more involved intervention.
3. Vancomycin IV 15–20 mg/kg once is the first-line treatment for access infections because most infections are staphylococcal and it may not be possible to determine MRSA (methicillin-resistant *Staphylococcus aureus*) status. The drug's duration of action in a dialysis ESRD patient is up to 5 days.

4. Obtain nares swab to help narrow to cefazolin (Ancef). Cefazolin 2–3 g IV can be dosed with dialysis treatments.
5. A third- or fourth-generation cephalosporin is the first-line treatment if gram-negative infection is suspected or if source is not clearly skin. An aminoglycoside is an acceptable alternative, and careful follow-up observation must be arranged with the dialysis center.

7. **How to approach vascular access in the ED?**
Hemodialysis patients are instructed to never permit a blood draw or IV infusion through their dialysis access site outside a dialysis setting. This is to protect the access device, which is truly the patient's *lifeline*. Even in emergency situations, obtaining intraosseous (IO) lines or peripheral lines far away from, or *distal* to, AV access is preferable to using the dialysis access site. For both HD and PD, allow only dialysis-trained staff to use the dialysis access site.

KEY POINTS: HOW TO APPROACH A DIALYSIS VASCULAR ACCESS IN THE ED

1. Do not access if possible.
2. Prioritize IO, peripheral access on a different limb, or, if not possible, *distal* to AV access.
3. Dialysis access should be performed *only* by a trained person in relatively stable patients.

8. **How is PD-associated peritonitis diagnosed?**
Peritonitis associated with PD occurs about once every 1–2 years in the average patient. The diagnosis is often suspected by the patient based on new cloudiness in the dialysis effluent or abdominal discomfort; a minority of cases present with SIRS (systemic inflammatory response syndrome) criteria. It is confirmed by an elevated neutrophil count in an effluent sample. PD fluid samples should be obtained either by a dialysis-trained nurse, under their direct supervision, or even by the patient or her trained dialysis partner. In contrast to other types of peritonitis, PD-associated peritonitis tends to be milder clinically, and most cases can be managed without hospital admission and instead with close coordination with the dialysis unit. PD-associated peritonitis is caused most commonly by gram-positive organisms, which are thought to be introduced during the home dialysate exchange procedure through improper technique.

KEY POINTS: DIAGNOSING PD-ASSOCIATED PERITONITIS

1. Suspect PD-associated peritonitis in the presence of cloudy abdominal effluent.
2. A sample of PD fluid should be obtained by a dialysis-trained registered nurse or with a trained person directly supervising.
3. Send fluid samples for culture, cell count, and differential after a minimum dwell time of 2 hours.
4. The diagnosis is confirmed by an elevated white blood cell (WBC) count $>100/\mu L$ with $>50\%$ polymorphonuclear neutrophils (PMN).
5. A small amount of abdominal free air with otherwise benign findings may result from the normal procedure of PD and does not constitute an acute surgical emergency. However, consider diagnosing an acute surgical abdomen rather than PD-associated peritonitis in a patient with localized peritoneal findings.
6. Vancomycin (15–30 mg/kg) plus a third- or fourth-generation cephalosporin or an intraperitoneal (IP) aminoglycoside is initial therapy; administer IV if safe and IP access is not guaranteed.
7. Consult nephrology or the dialysis unit, as each center has its own protocols.
8. Admit for severe pain, nausea/vomiting, a toxic appearance, or difficulty establishing a safe outpatient follow-up plan.

9. **What should I pay attention to in the urinalysis?**
The urinalysis is critical to working up and treating renal disease. The results offer varying clues to diagnosing conditions. Its highest yield in the ED is in detecting urinary tract infection (UTI; look for leukocyte esterase [LE], nitrites or WBCs). It has significant utility in managing electrolyte disorders (e.g., specific gravity, for hyponatremia), severe acidosis (pH and ketones), edema and anasarca (protein), and general renal failure (hemoglobin, red blood cells [RBCs], WBCs, specific gravity [SG], casts). A dipstick is useful even if full urinalysis with cellular reporting is not available.

Table 42.2 A Rough Association Between Urinalysis Specific Gravity and Osmolality

1.005	<≈	200 mOsm/L	(dilute)
1.01	≈	300 mOsm/L	
1.02	≈	600 mOsm/L	
1.03	≈	900 mOsm/L	(concentrated)

KEY POINTS: PEARLS FOR THINKING ABOUT URINALYSIS

1. Send urine *with reflex to microscopic analysis and culture* on any patient with suspected renal failure.
2. Consider sending urinalysis on patients with altered mental status – particularly in the elderly and immunocompromised.
3. For more accurate laboratory results in patients with a chronic urinary catheter, send a urinalysis with culture *after* replacing the catheter. If the catheter is suprapubic, or if the patient has a history of difficult catheterization, consult urology.
4. In assessing hematuria, the "hemoglobin" sensor can be triggered by myoglobin, hemoglobin, and full blood cells. Only "RBC" consistently denotes true hematuria.
5. Protein on the urinalysis sensor reflects albumin in the urine and may miss a nonalbumin protein such as immunoglobulin or light chain (e.g., in myeloma kidney disorders).
6. Diagnose UTI with clinical picture plus urinalysis result, noting that a negative urinalysis may miss UTI, more often in children. Positive LE suggests UTI but is a product of WBC breakdown and can be falsely positive in sterile pyuria (think interstitial nephritis and/or autoimmune conditions). Positive nitrites suggest UTI with fewer false positives but has low sensitivity (negative does not rule it out).
7. Specific gravity can be higher in new renal failure, particularly where renal hypoperfusion is at issue (volume depletion, cirrhosis, and or heart failure).
8. In hyponatremia, order urinalysis, urine sodium, and urine osmolality. In SIADH (syndrome of inappropriate antidiuretic hormone secretion), isotonic IV fluids may worsen the condition, dropping serum sodium further. You can use urinalysis SG to roughly assess urine osmolality (varying by pH and contaminating secretions), which can inform your fluid administration strategy (e.g., to limit isotonic fluids when SG < 1.02).

(Table 42.2)

10. **What is unique about a dialysis patient with cardiac arrest?**
    Two potentially reversible entities always should be considered in a patient with renal failure and cardiac arrest:
    1. Severe hyperkalemia may cause severe rhythm disturbances and ultimately cardiac arrest without any other warning or clinical signs. When a patient suffers an arrest from whatever cause, respiratory and metabolic acidosis and the efflux of potassium from cells can be expected to produce hyperkalemia secondarily. In the patient who already may have a tendency toward hyperkalemia, this further increase could cause the patient to be refractory to standard advanced cardiac life support (ACLS) interventions. Patients with CKD who are in cardiac arrest should receive IV calcium if they do not respond immediately to the first round of ACLS measures.
    2. Acute pericardial tamponade may result from the accumulation of pericardial fluid or spontaneous bleeding into the pericardial sac, and patients with uremia are more susceptible. Patients with tamponade tend to display refractory hypotension, pulseless electrical activity, or both. Consider pericardial tamponade in patients for whom other measures have failed. Bedside ultrasound may be diagnostic, and emergency pericardiocentesis may be life saving.

11. **How should I treat hyperkalemia in a patient with renal failure?**
    The approach is similar to that taken with patients who do not receive dialysis. In all cases of acute hyperkalemia, recheck serum potassium levels often, and repeat electrocardiograms (ECGs) or obtain continuous ECG monitoring. Ask if the patient makes urine to guide your approach to therapy (to assess utility of diuretics).
    Stabilize the cardiac membrane. To stabilize the cardiac membrane, use calcium IV infusion (10 mL of a 10% solution; calcium chloride or calcium gluconate), which mitigates the cardiotoxic effects of hyperkalemia by stabilizing the myocyte membrane. It does not lower serum potassium. Its effect occurs within minutes but is transient. Redose within 10 minutes if the desired improvement in cardiac rhythm is not achieved. This should be used only as a temporizing measure in patients with cardiovascular compromise or a widened QRS complex on the ECG. Calcium chloride has more elemental calcium and enhanced effect over typical gluconate formulations but is more irritating to tissue on infusion.

Shift potassium. To shift potassium out of the plasma space, use insulin, β-agonists, and bicarbonate solution. Insulin (typically 5–10 U regular-dosed once) and dextrose (50 g as a slow IV infusion, to maintain normoglycemia) move potassium into cells but require close serial monitoring of blood glucose levels. Insulin's actions are more powerful in renal failure due to decreased urinary elimination. Albuterol (10–20 mg inhaled nebulizer solution) acts within minutes to shift potassium into cells. It is easy to administer, generally has minimal side effects, and is effective for a few hours. Sodium bicarbonate (50 mEq ampule over 5 minutes) similarly shifts potassium intracellularly but is less effective, can exacerbate volume overload, and can acutely decrease serum ionized calcium.

Eliminate potassium. To eliminate potassium from the body, use diuretics patients who make urine. High-dose IV loop diuretics such as furosemide work within 1–2 hours in a patient able to make urine, and are more effective than Kayexalate (sodium polystyrene sulfonate, a sodium-potassium exchange resin; see later). For this reason, ask patients if and how much urine they produce daily. Failing their effectiveness or, in addition, promptly arrange hemodialysis in particular in existing dialysis patients. Kayexalate is typically given orally to enhance passage through the gut. It acts less quickly (hours to days) and therefore has limited efficacy in emergencies; it can exacerbate cases of intestinal ischemia. Hold medications that elevate serum potassium levels, such as ACE inhibitors, ARBs, potassium-sparing diuretics, and possibly β-blockers.

KEY POINTS: THERAPIES FOR ACUTE HYPERKALEMIA WITH CARDIAC FINDINGS

1. Calcium, chloride or gluconate, IV infusion
2. Insulin + dextrose
3. Albuterol nebulizer
4. Bicarbonate ampule or infusion
5. Diuretics, such as furosemide 40–80 mg IV once
6. Hemodialysis
7. Sodium polystyrene sulfonate (SPS, or Kayexalate)

12. **What is the differential diagnosis of hypotension in a patient with CKD?**
The principal mediator of BP in a dialysis patient is volume. The most common etiologies for hypotension are hypovolemia after dialysis, sepsis, hemorrhage, and acute pericardial tamponade. Have a very low threshold to send blood cultures in the dialysis patient, as sepsis frequently presents more subtly in this population.

13. **What are unique causes of altered mental status in patients with renal failure?**
In the patient on dialysis, consider disequilibrium syndrome, which is caused by rapid solute shifts during hemodialysis. Consider also side effects of drugs with sedating properties, as these are ineffectively eliminated in renal failure. The differential also includes spontaneous intracranial hemorrhage to which patients with renal failure have increased susceptibility related to uremic platelet dysfunction.

BIBLIOGRAPHY

Agency for Healthcare Research and Quality. *Statistical Brief #238. Healthcare Cost and Utilization Project (HCUP).* Rockville, MD: Agency for Healthcare Research and Quality; 2018. Available at: https://www.hcup-us.ahrq.gov/reports/statbriefs/sb238-Emergency-Department-Age-Payer-2006-2015.jsp. Accessed February 7, 2019.

Chawla LS, Eggers PW, Star RA, et al. Acute kidney injury and chronic kidney disease as interconnected syndromes. *N Engl J Med.* 2014;371:58–66.

Imran S, Eva G, Christopher S, et al. Is specific gravity a good estimate of urine osmolality? *J Clin Lab Anal.* 2010;24(6):426–430.

Koyner JL, Davison DL, Brasha-Mitchell E, et al. Furosemide stress test and biomarkers for the prediction of AKI severity. *J Am Soc Nephrol.* 2015;26(8):2023–2031.

Lazarus B, Wu A, Shin JI, et al. Association of metformin use with risk of lactic acidosis across the range of kidney function: a community-based cohort study. *JAMA Intern Med.* 2018;178(7):903–910.

Li PK, Szeto CC, Piraino B, et al. ISPD peritonitis recommendations: 2016 update on prevention and treatment. Available at: http://www.pdiconnect.com/content/36/5/481.full. Accessed February 13, 2019.

Li PK, Szeto CC, Piraino B, et al. Peritoneal dialysis-related infections recommendations: 2010 update. *Perit Dial Int.* 2010;30:393–423.

Oliveira LG, Luengo J, Caramori JC, et al. Peritonitis in recent years: clinical findings and predictors of treatment response of 170 episodes at a single Brazilian center. *Int Urol Nephrol.* 2012;44(5):1529–1537.

United States Renal Data System. Chapter 4: Hospitalizations, readmissions, emergency department visits, and observation stays, 2018. Available at: https://www.usrds.org/2018/view/v2_04.aspx?zoom_highlight=emergency. Accessed February 7, 2019.

Wolfson AB. Chronic kidney disease and dialysis-related emergencies. In: Wolfson AB, Cloutier RL, Hendey GW, et al, eds. *Harwood-Nuss' Clinical Practice of Emergency Medicine.* 6th ed, Philadelphia: Wolters Kluwer; 2015:615–621.

HEMOSTASIS AND COAGULOPATHIES

Mitchell Jay Cohen, MD, FACS

CHAPTER 43

1. What is meant by hemostasis?

Hemostasis is a balance between excessive bleeding and thrombosis. It is an active milieu of protease and cellular activity resulting in clot formation and degradation in response to injury of a blood vessel or a local inflammatory state. This response normally occurs through the coordinated efforts of the endothelium, red blood cells, the plasma (including proteins comprising the clotting factor cascade), immune cells, platelets, and a complex system of fibrinolysis.

KEY POINTS: PHASES OF HEMOSTASIS

1. Initiation of coagulation from endothelial injury or contact pathway activation.
2. Initial thrombin production, platelet aggregation, and fibrin clot formation.
3. Fibrinolysis.

---

2. What are the main causes of coagulopathies encountered in the emergency department?

Most hemostatic abnormalities result from drugs (e.g., new oral anticoagulants [NOACs], heparin, warfarin, aspirin) or associated diseases (i.e., liver or kidney failure). Acute traumatic coagulopathy is a significant cause of coagulation disturbances after trauma and shock. The hemophilias remain important but are less common issues for the emergency physician.

3. Do I really need to know the whole clotting cascade to manage patients?

A working knowledge of the basics of the three phases of hemostasis, understanding of coagulation disturbances, knowledge of anticoagulant medications, and familiarity with basic testing and therapeutics improves patient management.

- *Initiation of hemostasis.* After injury, subendothelial tissue factor results in a small amount of thrombin production. Additionally, platelets and von Willebrand factor (vWF) from the endothelium interact to form a plug (platelet adhesion). Platelet activation and aggregation occur, along with vessel constriction. Disorders include problems with platelet quantity and function, vWF problems, and vascular abnormalities (i.e., hereditary telangiectasia). Platelet count and bleeding time are used to assess this phase of hemostasis.
- *Coagulation cascade.* The platelet plug is reinforced with cross-linked fibrin from the coagulation cascade (factor XIII causes covalent cross-links, resulting in final strength). Effective functioning of the cascade may be impaired by deficiencies of coagulation factor activity (hemophilia A and B), endogenous inhibitors to specific coagulation factors, anticoagulant inhibition (protein C, antithrombin [AT]), and exogenous therapeutics (warfarin, heparin, NOACs, etc.) that interrupt coagulation at specific steps in the cascade or impair production of proteases.
- *Fibrinolysis.* The fibrin clot is enzymatically broken down by plasmin. Endothelial cells release plasminogen activator, which converts plasminogen to plasmin. The plasmin breaks down fibrin and fibrinogen into fibrin split products and D-dimers. Excessive fibrinolytic activity or deficiencies of fibrinolytic inhibitors can increase bleeding. Conversely, impaired fibrinolysis, termed "fibrinolytic shutdown," results in thrombosis and thromboinflammation.

4. What are the contact and tissue factor coagulation pathways? How can I tell the difference?

The tissue factor pathway (formerly known as the extrinsic pathway) is activated by tissue damage, exposing subendothelial tissue factor at the site of injury. The contact pathway (formerly known as the intrinsic pathway) is initiated by blood exposure to a negatively charged surface. While defects in the tissue factor pathway affect the prothrombin time (PT), defects in the contact pathway affect partial thromboplastin time (PTT). Both pathways converge to activate factor X, which activates prothrombin to thrombin (common pathway). In the setting of a prolonged PTT and a normal PT, the defect is in the contact pathway. If the PT is prolonged and the PTT is normal, the defect is in the tissue factor coagulation pathway. Prolongation of both PT and PTT implies the defect is in the common pathway.

5. What parts of the history and physical examination can help me assess a suspected bleeding abnormality?

Ask about medications, medical history (especially liver, kidney, and malignant disease), previous problems with bleeding (i.e., with surgeries and dental work), and family history of bleeding disorders. In patients with known bleeding disorders, ask about the nature of their disease and previous therapies. They are commonly knowledge-able about their individual diseases. On examination, platelet disorders commonly result in petechia, purpura, epistaxis, and gum and other mucosal bleeding. These disorders are common in women and usually acquired. In contrast, problems with coagulation factors are more commonly congenital, found more often in men, and are likely to present as deep muscle or joint bleeding.

6. **How do I interpret PT, PTT, and international normalized ratio (INR)?**
PT tests the factors of the tissue factor and common pathways. It is prolonged by deficiencies of prothrombin, fibrinogen, and factors V, VII, and X. A PT 2 seconds more than the control is significant. PTT tests the contact and common pathways, including all factors except VII and XIII. INR reduces interlaboratory variation by indexing thromboplastin test lot activity to an international standard and hence is commonly utilized instead of the PT. Liver disease, warfarin use, and other abnormalities of the vitamin K–sensitive factors (i.e., II, VII, IX, X) affect the PT and INR. An INR of 1 is normal. An INR between 2 and 3 indicates a therapeutic level of warfarin.

7. **What are the causes of thrombocytopenia?**
- Decreased production: marrow disease, chemotherapy, alcohol, thiazide effect
- Immune destruction: idiopathic thrombocytopenic purpura (ITP), systemic lupus erythematosus (SLE), lymphoma, quinine, quinidine, postinfectious disease
- Toxic destruction: disseminated intravascular coagulation (DIC), thrombotic thrombocytopenic purpura (TTP), hemolytic uremic syndrome (HUS), hemolysis with elevated liver enzymes and low platelets (HELLP) syndrome
- Splenic sequestration (hypersplenism, rare): hematologic malignancy, portal hypertension, autoimmune hemolytic anemia, hereditary spherocytosis
- Dilution: massive transfusion
- Laboratory error

8. **What are the differences between idiopathic and chronic thrombocytopenic purpura?**
ITP is a diagnosis of exclusion after considering SLE, antiphospholipid syndrome, human immunodeficiency virus (HIV), and lymphoproliferative disorders. It is associated with antiplatelet antibody immunoglobulin G (IgG). The acute form is seen in children 4–6 years old several weeks after a viral prodrome. It is self-limited, with a 90% rate of spontaneous remission. Morbidity and mortality rates are low, and steroid therapy does not seem to alter the course.

Chronic ITP is found in adults. It is three times more common in women than in men. Severity waxes and wanes, with only 1% mortality, but spontaneous remissions are rare. It may respond to therapy with glucocorticoids or intravenous (IV) immunoglobulin. Splenectomy, monoclonal antibody therapy, and immunosuppressive agents can be considered in patients refractory to this treatment. Platelet transfusion is reserved for life-threatening bleeds because it may increase antiplatelet antibodies.

9. **What are the five clinical signs of TTP?**
- Fluctuating change in mental status
- Thrombocytopenia
- Fever (in 90% of patients)
- Microangiopathic hemolytic anemia
- Renal impairment

Only 40% of patients have all five.

10. **What causes TTP? Is it worse than ITP?**
TTP results from subendothelial and intraluminal deposits of fibrin, and platelet aggregation in capillaries and arterioles. Prostacyclin and abnormal platelet aggregation are thought to contribute to its origins. It may affect patients of any age or gender, although most are between 10 and 40 years of age and 60% are female. When untreated, there is 80% mortality at 3 months as a result of microthrombi in the heart, brain, and kidneys. Plasmapheresis has reduced this rate to 17%. Other therapies include steroids, splenectomy, α-globulin, vincristine, and antiplatelet agents such as aspirin and dipyridamole (Persantine). Platelet transfusions may cause additional microcirculatory thrombi and should be avoided unless bleeding is life threatening.

11. **What is HUS?**
HUS is similar to TTP. They both present with hemolytic anemia, fever, neurologic abnormality, and renal dysfunction. However, HUS causes less change in mental status and more renal dysfunction. Patients with HUS tend to be younger (children are more common than adults), and onset is often associated with a bacterial gastroenteritis such as *Escherichia coli O157:H7* and *Shigella* species.

12. **What is unique during large-volume blood product resuscitation?**
Stored banked blood is platelet poor, as platelets only have a 5-day life span. Platelet counts should be monitored, and transfusion of platelets should be based on the clinical situation and viscoelastic (thromboelastography [TEG] or rotational thromboelastometry [ROTEM]) measures of coagulation. Massive transfusion is defined as the replacement of the patient's total body volume of blood, or the transfusion of 10 units or more of packed red blood cells

(PRBCs) over 24 hours. In a patient who has sustained major trauma and is likely to require massive transfusion, a ratio of 1:1:1 of PRBCs to platelets to fresh frozen plasma (FFP) is recommended.

13. What do I need to know about trauma induced coagulopathy (TIC) and trauma resuscitation?

Trauma induced coagulopathy (TIC; acute traumatic coagulopathy) occurs in approximately 30% of trauma patients when severe tissue injury is combined with shock. TIC manifests with hypocoagulability measured by conventional coagulation tests (PT and PTT) or viscoelastic tests (TEG or ROTEM). While clearly a mix of overlapping phenotypes, TIC results in impaired coagulation that results in more bleeding, increased need for resuscitation, a 4 $\times$ mortality rate, and increased inflammatory and organ failure morbidity. Phenotypically, TIC is a mix of impaired coagulation through dysfunction of the coagulation cascade, anticoagulant pathways including protein C, dysregulated fibrinolysis, and platelet dysfunction. Trauma resuscitation is based on the principle that in order to resuscitate a severely injured patient the biochemical mechanisms of clotting must be restored or maintained in order to first allow sufficient coagulation to restore hemostasis and stop bleeding and secondly to repair or fix the dysregulation of the inflammatory, immune and endothelial systems.

14. How does aspirin increase bleeding?

Aspirin blocks cyclooxygenase, which decreases thromboxane formation, leading to decreased platelet aggregation and less vasoconstriction. Aspirin poisons this reaction for the life of the platelet. Nonsteroidal anti-inflammatory drugs (NSAIDs), such as indomethacin, have this effect only while in the circulation. Uremia has a similar reversible effect.

15. What are the indications for platelet transfusions?

Platelet transfusion should be delayed in ITP and TTP to avoid disease-specific complications and alloimmunization. It is more commonly indicated for primary bone marrow problems.
- Platelet count >50,000/mL → hemorrhage unlikely.
- Platelet count of 10,000–50,000/mL → variable risk of bleeding with trauma, ulcer, and invasive procedures. Choosing when to transfuse at these levels is not an exact science.
- Counts <10,000 → platelet transfusion is indicated because there is a significant risk of spontaneous hemorrhage.

Each bag of random donor platelets may be expected to raise the platelet count 5000/mL. They are usually ordered six at a time.

16. What is the most common inherited bleeding disorder?

It is von Willebrand disease (5–10 cases per million). It is usually autosomal dominant. There is a deficiency or dysfunction of vWF and a mild factor VIII defect. Treatment is with desmopressin (DDAVP [desamino-D-arginine vasopressin]) in the mild, most common, type I form of the disease. In more severe types, therapy is with factor VIII concentrate, with dosing based on the patient's factor VIII level.

17. Do people with hemophilia A have low levels of factor VIII?

It is the activity of factor VIII that is impaired, not its level. Seventy percent of cases are transmitted by sex-linked recessive (X chromosome) inheritance and 30% by spontaneous mutation. Severe disease has less than 1% activity, and spontaneous bleeding (joints, deep muscles, urinary tract, and central nervous system [CNS]) is a problem. Between 1% and 5% activity is considered moderate disease, with problems occurring mostly after trauma and surgery. Above 5% is considered mild disease, but some trauma and surgical risks persist. PTT is only prolonged with less than 35% activity.

Note: One unit of factor VIII per kilogram increases the activity level by 2% (unless adversely affected by antifactor VIII antibodies [IgG], which develops in up to 20% of patients). Recombinant DNA factor VIII is the replacement of choice and lacks the hepatitis B, C, and HIV risks of FFP and cryoprecipitate.

18. How is factor VIII dosed in hemophilia A?

Use 25 U/kg for moderate bleeding, and 50 U/kg for severe hemorrhage or life-threatening bleeding sites (gastrointestinal [GI], neck, sublingual, retroperitoneal, intraabdominal, head injury, CNS bleed, and necessary surgical procedures). Because the half-life is 8–12 hours, redose with half the loading dose after 8–12 hours. Recombinant factor VIII unit concentration is noted on the label. Cryoprecipitate (from FFP) is assumed to be 80–100 U of factor VIII per bag.

19. What is Christmas disease?

Christmas disease is hemophilia B, which involves decreased factor IX activity. The clinical presentation is the same as that for hemophilia A. The genetic pattern is the same, although it is less prevalent in the population, with only one fifth of the number of cases. Treatment is with factor IX 50 U/kg, or FFP.

Pearl: There is no factor IX in cryoprecipitate.

20. What does DDAVP do?

DDAVP is a synthetic analog of antidiuretic hormone. It causes release of vWF from endothelial storage sites, thus increasing levels of factor VIII in hemophilia A and some cases of von Willebrand disease. The dosage is 0.3 µg/kg IV; it lasts 4–6 hours and is most effective in mild to moderately deficient patients. Administration of DDAVP can also be helpful in obtaining hemostasis in patients with bleeding caused by uremia (i.e., patients with end-stage renal disease or those receiving dialysis).

21. **What factors are affected by vitamin K deficiency, warfarin, liver disease, and banked blood?**
    - Vitamin K deficiency affects factors II, VII, IX, and X, the same ones affected by warfarin.
    - Hepatic insufficiency affects all factors except factor VIII.
    - Stored blood is low in factors V and VIII, and platelets.

KEY POINTS: HEMOSTATIC DEFICIENCIES

1. Hemophilia A and B: bleeding time is normal (as is the PT and the PTT in mild and moderate cases).
2. von Willebrand disease: bleeding time is increased.
3. PT reflects a tissue factor pathway abnormality through factor VII-deficient activity.
4. Factor VII has the shortest half-life of the factors (3–5 hours) and causes the first manifestations of production deficiency.
5. An INR of 2–3 is recommended with most warfarin therapy.
6. Deficiency of factors VIII, IX, and XI accounts for 99% of inherited bleeding disorders. If a congenital bleeding disorder is suspected, FFP at 15 mL/kg will support hemostasis while a definitive diagnosis is being made.

22 **What happens in DIC?**
Platelets and clotting factors (especially factors V, VIII, and XIII) are consumed. Thrombin formation overwhelms fibrinolysis and activates fibrinogen. Fibrin is deposited in small vessels of multiple organ systems. Fibrin degradation products are released; platelet function, as well as fibrin polymerization, is decreased. Definitive treatment is to treat the underlying cause (e.g., sepsis), but the coagulopathy is temporized with transfusion of platelets and FFP. Heparin may be used if fibrin deposition and thrombosis dominate the clinical picture.

23. **What are heparin-induced thrombocytopenia (HIT) and HIT with thrombosis (HITT)?**
HIT type I is a nonimmune-mediated thrombocytopenia that usually resolves without treatment or complication. The more serious HIT type II (the form usually referred to when discussing HIT) is caused by antibodies to heparin/platelet factor IV complex. It results in platelet activation and clot formation. It usually occurs 5–10 days after exposure to heparin, but may occur after as few as 10 hours. It occurs in 2% of patients receiving unfractionated heparin anticoagulation therapy and 0.2% of patients receiving low-molecular-weight heparin (LMWH). Platelet counts drop to 50,000–100,000/mL. HITT develops in 50% of the patients with HIT. HIT and HITT require discontinuation of heparin (including heparin flushes). Prophylactic platelet transfusions should be avoided. A direct thrombin inhibitor is indicated in patients with thrombosis (i.e., lepirudin or argatroban). Doppler ultrasound of the legs is indicated as studies have found subclinical deep venous thrombosis (DVT) in up to 50% of patients with HIT.

24. **Need help with HELLP?**
HELLP criteria:
    - Microangiopathic hemolytic anemia
    - Serum aspartate transaminase levels greater than 70 U/L
    - Platelets less than 100,000/mL

    The HELLP syndrome is a form of preeclampsia. Gestational thrombocytopenia (100,000–150,000/mL) is found in 5%–10% of third trimester pregnancies. It is even more common in pregnancies complicated by preeclampsia (15%–20%) and eclampsia (40%–50%). Fetal and maternal mortality are increased. Treatment is primarily supportive, although platelet transfusion may be required before cesarean section. DIC may develop.

25. **How do heparin and LMWH work?**
Heparin catalyzes the inactivation of thrombin and factor X by AT. It also has some effect on factors II, IX, and XI. Factor VII is not affected. At usual dosages, it will prolong the PTT (and thrombin time [TT]) but not the PT. Occult GI bleeding is a relative contraindication to its use, and clearance is prolonged in hepatic and renal dysfunction.

    LMWH is derived from smaller pieces of the heparin molecule. Weight-based subcutaneous dosing of LMWH without anticoagulation monitoring has proven safe and effective in clinical trials. Because LMWH inactivates factor X more than it does thrombin, PTT is not significantly affected and is not used to monitor clinical effect and therapeutic plasma concentrations. Weight-based pharmacokinetic predictions for LMWH are not reliable in patients weighing more than 100 kg, pregnant patients, and those with decreased creatinine clearance. If LMWH is used in these patients, anti-X activity must be monitored. Unfractionated heparin often becomes the drug of choice in these patients.

26. **How do I treat hemorrhage secondary to heparin therapy?**
With major bleeding episodes, heparin can be 100% reversed with protamine sulfate at a dosage of 1 mg/100 U of circulating heparin to a maximum dosage of 50 mg. It is given intravenously over 10 minutes. Rapid infusion

increases the risk of anaphylaxis. Protamine is only 60% effective in reversing LMWH, so unfractionated heparin is usually preferred in cases when surgery or invasive procedures are likely.

KEY POINTS: DIAGNOSIS AND TREATMENT OF COAGULOPATHIES

1. Thrombocytopenia: increased bleeding time, epistaxis, purpura, petechia, mucosal bleeding, six bags random donor platelets yields 30,000/mL increase
2. PT and INR: tissue factor and common paths (i.e., factors II, VII, IX, and X), warfarin
3. PTT: contact and common paths (all factors except VII and XIII), heparin
4. Severe bleeding with hemophilia A: 50 U/kg factor VIII
5. To support hemostasis until definitive diagnosis: FFP 15 mL/kg

27. **How does warfarin work? How do I deal with elevated INR?**
Warfarin (an oral anticoagulation therapy [OAT]) inhibits the reduction of vitamin K to its active form, causing depletion of factors II, VII, IX, and X. The starting dosage is 5 mg/day, with 4–5 days required for the full anticoagulant effect. Heparin or LMWH is continued in the interim, owing to the early inactivation of proteins C and S, which causes a temporary procoagulant effect. The target is usually an INR of 2–3. Significant bleeding occurs in 3% of patients receiving chronic OAT. Drug interactions are common, and INR must be monitored.
   Approach to elevated INR:
   - Asymptomatic with elevated INR → stop warfarin.
     - INR >10 or high risk of bleeding: give oral vitamin K.
   - Minor bleeding + elevated INR → withhold doses of warfarin ± oral vitamin K.
     - Consider the underlying need for anticoagulation.
   - Serious bleeding + elevated INR → treat with FFP (10–15 mL/kg) or prothrombin complex concentrate (PCC) + 10 mg IV vitamin K (given slowly).
     - FFP provides immediate effect; vitamin K's effect takes hours.
   - Head computed tomography (CT) evaluation should be performed even in minor head trauma with therapeutic dosing.

28. **What about PCCs?**
PCC is a concentrate powder not requiring thawing that can be used to reverse warfarin. PCCs have been shown to reverse elevated INR much faster than FFP. It is usually given via slow IV push and leads to lower volume infusion than with FFP. All PCCs contain factors II, IX, and X. Factor VII is also present in some PCC variants. PCCs with normal amounts of factor VII are known as *4-factor PCCs* and also contain proteins C and S; those without factor VII are called *3-factor PCCs*.

29. **What are all these new oral anticoagulants I keep hearing about?**
NOACs have shown stable metabolism across patients and fewer food or drug interactions. Because of this, they do not require monitoring of the INR. Some examples are rivaroxaban and apixaban (factor Xa inhibitors) and dabigatran (a direct thrombin inhibitor). These agents have been found to be as effective as warfarin with less risk of bleeding.

30. **That sounds great! So what's the catch?**
Cost is an issue, and caution is needed with the factor Xa inhibitors in patients with renal disease. However, the biggest concern in the ED is the availability of reversal agents as their mechanism of action makes vitamin K and FFP ineffective. Currently, three reversal agents are in different stages of development.

31. **So what do I do if someone taking a factor Xa or thrombin inhibitor comes in with severe bleeding?**
Start with large-bore IV access for fluid administration and prepare cross-matched blood. PT/PTT and INR are not reliable measurements of the degree of anticoagulation from Xa or thrombin inhibitors, so they cannot be used to guide management. Although normal PT and PTT essentially rule out any significant amount of active medication in the blood stream, elevated values do not correlate with degree of toxicity or anticoagulation. There may be a role for PCC, activated PCC (aPCC; also known as *antiinhibitor coagulant complex [Feiba]*), and recombinant factor VIIa. In aPCC, factor VII is in its activated form. Although animal studies have shown decreased bleeding with these agents, human in vivo studies are lacking.

32. **Can anything be done to control massive hemorrhage from trauma?**
Although not approved by the US Food and Drug Administration (FDA) for this indication, tranexamic acid (TXA) is an antifibrinolytic agent with some mixed evidence showing a potential mortality benefit for use in patients with significant hemorrhage from trauma. As a plasmin and plasminogen activation inhibitor, TXA works by inhibiting clot breakdown rather than promoting clot formation. A large trial with controversial data taking place primarily in the developing world showed maximum mortality benefit when given less than 3 hours after initial injury, and most effective when given within 1 hour after injury. Administration more than 3 hours after onset of bleeding

was associated with increased mortality. Newer data suggested that TXA may be deleterious, especially in patients with impaired fibrinolysis (fibrinolysis shutdown) after injury. Taken together, TXA should be given in a bleeding patient with documented hyperfibrinolysis. Additional data from current ongoing studies are needed before more empiric recommendations can be made and its use should be garnered with caution.

Clotting agents used by the military to stabilize traumatic bleeding in the combat field include:

- QuickClot (Z-Medica, Wallingford, CT) – kaolin-impregnated gauze shown to be the most effective in controlling hemorrhage in areas not amenable to tourniquet placement. Kaolin is a nonbotanical, nonhuman, nonanimal mineral compound that promotes the activation of factor XII and platelet-associated factor XI.
- HemCon (HemCon Medical Technologies, Portland, OR) bandage – made of chitosan, a substance with muco-adhesive properties. It becomes extremely sticky when in contact with blood and seals the wound to control bleeding.
- Dry fibrin-sealant dressing – contains human fibrinogen, human thrombin, and calcium chloride; does not transmit human viruses as older fibrin sealants. Human studies ongoing.

BIBLIOGRAPHY

Arepally GM. Heparin-induced thrombocytopenia. *Blood.* 2017;129(21):2864–2871.

Baumann Kreuziger LM, Keenen JC, Morton CT, et al. Management of the bleeding patient receiving new oral anticoagulants: a role for prothrombin complex concentrates. *Biomed Res Int.* 2014;2014:583794.

Cohen MJ, Kutcher M, Redick B, et al. Clinical and mechanistic drivers of acute traumatic coagulopathy. *J Trauma Acute Care Surg.* 2013;75(1 suppl 1):S40–S47.

Janz TG, Hamilton GC, et al. Disorders of hemostasis. In Marx JA, Hockberger RS, Walls RM, editors: *Rosen's emergency medicine: concepts and clinical practice.* 8th ed. Philadelphia: Elsevier; 2014:1606–1616.

Kunitake RC, Howard BM, Kornblith LZ, et al. Individual clotting factor contributions to mortality following trauma. *J Trauma Acute Care Surg.* 2017;82(2):302–308.

Levy JH, Douketis J, Weitz JI. Reversal agents for non-vitamin K antagonist oral anticoagulants. *Nat Rev Cardiol.* 2018;15(5):273–281.

The CRASH-2 Collaborators. Effects of tranexamic acid on death, vascular occlusive events, and blood transfusion in trauma patients with significant haemorrhage (CRASH-2): a randomised, placebo-controlled trial. *Lancet.* 2010;376:23–32.

CHAPTER 44

SICKLE CELL DISEASE

Daniel Willner, MD

1. What is sickle cell disease (SCD)?

SCD is an inherited disorder of hemoglobin (Hb) that causes repeated vasoocclusive episodes and anemia. SCD is caused by a single nucleic acid substitution of valine for glutamic acid within the β-globin gene, which codes for the β-globin component of the Hb tetramer ($\alpha_2\beta_2$). This Hb molecule (HbS) is poorly soluble in deoxygenated conditions and polymerizes with other Hb molecules in the circulating erythrocyte, creating linear Hb polymers, the cause of the erythrocyte's sickled shape.

2. What are the variants of SCD?

In SCD, both copies of the β-globin gene produce the abnormal Hb (HbSS). Patients with sickle cell trait have one normal copy of the β-globin gene and one mutant copy (HbAS); they are asymptomatic carriers and don't suffer from the same complications as individuals with SCD.

Several other variants of SCD exist, including HbC, which is the substitution of lysine for glutamic acid, and β-thalassemia, which causes decreased β-globin production. In β-thalassemia there is clinical heterogeneity based upon the degree of inhibition of β-globin synthesis. Patients with HbSβ$^+$-thalassemia have a milder clinical course than individuals with HbSS. Patients with HbSβ^0-thalassemia produce only HbS and are at risk for the same set of clinical complications as patients with SCD.

3. What is the epidemiology of SCD?

SCD affects approximately 1 in 500 African Americans, with 1 in 12 African Americans carrying the sickle cell trait. Between 70,000 and 100,000 Americans have SCD. More than half of patients with SCD now survive into the fifth decade of life, and more than 90% of children in the United States survive into adulthood. Median life expectancy varies significantly depending on the sickle cell genotype. Overall, life expectancy is increasing as therapies to manage complications improve.

4. What is the pathophysiology of SCD?

The clinical manifestations of SCD are the result of the conformational change induced in HbS while in the deoxygenated state. Oxygen is unloaded from hemoglobin as the erythrocyte travels through the microvasculature; in patients with SCD, this deoxygenated state promotes polymerization of HbS. This process occurs repeatedly as the erythrocyte passes through the capillary system, and this stress causes changes to the red blood cell (RBC). These changes include decreased deformability of the RBC (making capillary transit more difficult), changes to the erythrocyte cell membrane, and increased expression of cell surface markers, which promote adherence to the vascular endothelium. The increased cellular stress decreases the life span of a circulating erythrocyte from 120 days to between 16 and 20 days.

5. What are the typical laboratory findings?

Patients with SCD have mild to moderate anemia (hematocrit 20%–30%), reticulocytosis (3%–15%), baseline leukocytosis and thrombocytosis, elevated L-lactate dehydrogenase (LDH) and unconjugated bilirubin, and decreased haptoglobin. Creatinine rises over time because of progressive renal dysfunction from microvascular infarcts. A peripheral blood smear demonstrates sickled cells, polychromasia from reticulocytes, and Howell-Jolly bodies from functional asplenia. Erythrocytes are normochromic and normocytic. Patients with SCD may show elevations in acute-phase reactants, including C-reactive protein (CRP), fibrinogen, LDH, interleukin (IL)-2, and tumor necrosis factor (TNF).

6. What are the causes of acute anemia in SCD?

Acute anemia is described as a drop in Hb of at least 2 g/dL. Splenic sequestration, aplastic anemia, and increased hemolysis are the three principal causes of acute anemia in SCD.

1. Splenic sequestration is an emergency. It occurs more commonly in infants and children who have not yet undergone splenic infarctions and fibrosis. It is characterized by splenomegaly with or without tenderness, acute anemia, thrombocytopenia, and reticulocytosis. Patients may develop hemodynamic instability because of the shift of blood volume into the spleen and require aggressive supportive care. Transfusion is indicated for severe anemia; care must be taken to not overtransfuse because the sequestered erythrocytes can cause a hyperviscosity syndrome and increase the risk of vasoocclusion when the blood reenters the circulation.
2. Aplastic anemia is the arrest of erythropoiesis and is most often caused by infection. Clinical manifestations include lethargy, fatigue, and possibly syncope or fever. Laboratory assessment demonstrates a decrease in the reticulocyte count (<1%). The most common cause is parvovirus B19, which directly invades erythrocyte progenitor cells. Many other infections, including *Streptococcus pneumoniae, Salmonella,* and Epstein-Barr virus (EBV), may also trigger an aplastic crisis.

3. Increased hemolysis may play a role in a small subset of patients with SCD. Hemolysis should be a diagnosis of exclusion after other causes have been ruled out.

7. What is an acute pain episode?

An acute pain episode (previously known as *sickle cell* or *vasoocclusive crisis*) is a paroxysmal event caused by vasoocclusion at the capillary level and it is the most common reason a patient with SCD will seek medical care. It is most often the result of vasoocclusion and ischemia within bone or bone marrow; pain occurs most commonly in the back, chest, and extremities. Acute pain episodes in infants and children may present as pain in the hands or feet, a condition termed *dactylitis*. The frequency of acute pain episodes in adults correlates with higher mortality.

8. What are the triggers of acute pain episodes?

A variety of triggers, including infection, stress, dehydration, changes in weather, cigarette smoke, and hypoxia, can cause acute pain episodes. An acute pain episode is a clinical diagnosis; there is no laboratory test or vital sign that can accurately diagnose an acute pain episode.

9. How is an acute pain episode treated?

Patients experiencing an acute pain episode should receive intravenous (IV) hydration until they are clinically euvolemic. Supplemental oxygen should be provided if the oxygen saturation (SpO_2) is below 95%. Treat expediently with IV opioid pain medicine; however, meperidine should be avoided due to accumulation of the metabolite normeperidine, which can lead to central nervous system toxicity and seizures. Pain should be reassessed promptly, and, if not adequately controlled, a second dose of opioid pain medicine should be administered. If pain persists, consider the use of patient-controlled analgesia (PCA) using a PCA pump. Adjuvant therapies with nonsteroidal anti-inflammatory drugs (NSAIDs), such as ketorolac, as well as pain-dose ketamine may also be considered. Nonpharmacologic adjuvant therapies, such as heat, may be employed. Patients needing ongoing pain control should be admitted.

10. Are patients with SCD at increased risk of infection?

Yes, patients with SCD are functionally asplenic as a result of repeated splenic infarctions. In addition to the scheduled childhood vaccinations, these patients should receive vaccinations against the encapsulated organisms (*S. pneumoniae*, *Haemophilus influenzae*, and *Neisseria meningitidis*) and a yearly inactivated influenza vaccination. Pediatric patients should be asked about the use of prophylactic penicillin.

11. How should I manage fever in a patient with SCD?

Fever in a patient with SCD should always prompt a thorough evaluation for a source of infection. Any patient with a temperature above 38.5°C (101.3°F) should have a complete blood count (CBC) with differential, reticulocyte count, blood cultures, urinalysis, and urine culture. Any respiratory symptoms necessitate a chest radiograph to evaluate for acute chest syndrome (ACS). Bone tenderness with or without swelling and erythema necessitates an evaluation for osteomyelitis. Focal neurologic findings require computed tomography (CT) of the head and lumbar puncture to evaluate for infection. First-line antibiotic therapy is with a third-generation cephalosporin (and a macrolide if there are respiratory symptoms). Admit patients with temperatures above 39.5°C (103.1°F).

12. What is ACS?

ACS is distinguished by a new infiltrate visible on the chest radiograph and at least one of the following: chest pain, cough, wheezing, tachypnea, fever, or hypoxia. ACS is the second leading cause of hospitalization and the most common cause of death in SCD. Causes of ACS include viral or bacterial infection, fat or bone marrow embolism, bone (rib, sternum, or vertebrae) infarction causing splinting and hypoventilation, atelectasis, and asthma exacerbation. Localized vasoocclusion leads to ischemia, infarction, and inflammatory changes. The most common infectious causes of ACS include *Mycoplasma pneumoniae*, *Chlamydia pneumoniae*, and respiratory viruses. ACS is often preceded by an acute pain episode. There are no specific laboratory values or vital signs that confirm or exclude ACS. Physical examination findings may include rales; however, a normal physical examination is common.

13. What is the treatment of ACS?

Patients with ACS require pain control, antibiotics (a third-generation cephalosporin *and* macrolide), IV fluids, supplemental oxygen to maintain SpO_2 above 95%, incentive spirometry, and possibly transfusion. Simple transfusion is indicated in symptomatic anemia and Hb that has fallen more than 1 g/dL below baseline. Exchange transfusion is indicated in refractory hypoxemia ($SpO_2 < 90\%$ despite supplemental oxygen), rapidly progressive disease (increasing respiratory distress or worsening infiltrate seen on the chest radiograph), or worsening anemia despite simple transfusion. Patients with ACS always require admission.

14. Are patients with SCD at increased risk of cardiac complications?

Yes, chronic anemia leads to a high-output cardiac state, which over time can lead to dilated cardiac chambers and heart failure. Patients with SCD are prone to arrhythmias, which can be secondary to abnormal chamber size and prolonged QT intervals. Patients may also develop cardiac ischemic secondary to vasoocclusion or anemia.

15. **What are the neurologic effects of SCD?**

Children and adults with SCD are at increased risk of stroke; nearly 25% of patients will have a stroke by age 45. Many children will experience silent ischemic events leading to neurologic and functional impairment. Children with SCD are screened with transcranial Doppler ultrasound to detect abnormal blood flow in the brain, a marker of increased stroke risk. Early identification and treatment with preventive exchange transfusions have significantly decreased stroke incidence. In children or adults that present with focal neurologic findings, emergent neuroimaging and prompt consultation with hematology and neurology is indicated. Therapies for acute ischemic stroke include transfusion – both simple and exchange – and thrombolysis with tissue plasminogen activator (tPA). The decision on specific therapy should be made in consultation with hematology and neurology. Other neurologic sequelae of SCD include intracranial hemorrhage, seizure, spinal cord infarction, hearing loss, posterior reversible encephalopathy (PRES), and cerebral venous sinus thrombosis (CVST).

16. **How does SCD affect pregnancy?**

SCD increases the risk of both fetal and maternal complications during pregnancy. Fetal risks, including fetal demise, growth restriction, and preterm labor, are usually related to abnormal blood flow to the placenta or placental abruption. Maternal risks include preeclampsia/eclampsia, infections, thromboembolic events, and higher rates of cesarean section. Pregnant women are more susceptible to acute pain episodes and have increased rates of hospitalization.

17. **What is the role and indication for blood transfusion in SCD?**

Transfusion of RBCs dilutes the amount of HbSS in the circulation and suppresses the production of abnormal Hb. This offsets the direct effects of sickled cells in the circulation as well as the effects on the vascular endothelium, inflammatory cells, and clotting. Risks of transfusion include infection, allergic reaction, increased blood viscosity, and alloimmunization, which may limit the ability to receive future transfusions. Patients with SCD have compensated chronic anemia; transfusion should only be considered for specific indications, such as aplastic crisis, splenic sequestration, preparation for surgery, ACS, and stroke.

18. **What are the types of transfusions that are available?**

Blood can be given via simple transfusion or exchange transfusion. Simple transfusion involves giving packed RBCs and only requires a peripheral IV line. A simple transfusion increases the hematocrit level and blood viscosity, which increases risk of vasoocclusive events. Exchange transfusion involves removing a patient's sickled RBCs and replacing them with normal donor RBCs. In addition to exposing the patient to more donor blood, exchange transfusion usually requires a central line and specialized equipment. The benefit is that the amount of sickled hemoglobin is significantly reduced without increasing viscosity or causing iron overload.

19. **What are the interventions for priapism in SCD?**

Priapism is a common occurrence in male patients with SCD and is described as a sustained erection lasting longer than 4 hours. Stuttering priapism is also common. Recurrent episodes can lead to impotence over time. First-line treatment for priapism includes aggressive hydration and pain control. Therapy with α-agonists including oral pseudoephedrine and injection of phenylephrine into the corpus cavernosum is also indicated. Local aspiration and irrigation of the corpus cavernosum may be performed. Exchange transfusion may be used if these measures are unsuccessful. Urology should be consulted and surgical management may be indicated if other interventions are unsuccessful.

20. **What are the ocular complications of SCD?**

SCD patients with trauma to the eye are at risk of traumatic hyphema. Sickled blood cells are unable to drain from the chamber, leading to ischemia and increased intraocular pressure. Hyphema is considered an ocular emergency in patients with both SCD and sickle cell trait. Failure to quickly treat hyphema can result in glaucoma, central retinal artery occlusion, and optic nerve ischemia. An ophthalmologist should be emergently consulted and most patients should be admitted for serial examinations and ocular pressure measurements. Patients with SCD are at an increased risk of central retinal artery occlusion, retinopathy, retinal detachment, and orbital infarction.

21. **What are the orthopedic complications of SCD?**

Patients with SCD are at increased risk of avascular necrosis caused by repeated sickling events in the bone marrow, with the hip being the most common site. Infarcted bone is at higher risk of infection, leading to an increased incidence of osteomyelitis. *Salmonella* is the most common infectious agent identified. Historical features, such as fever and location of pain, can help in differentiating between osteomyelitis and vasoocclusive crisis.

KEY POINTS: TREATMENT OF ACS

1. Antibiotics
2. Fluids
3. Supplemental oxygen to maintain SpO_2 greater than 95%
4. Incentive spirometer
5. Consider transfusion
6. Admission

KEY POINTS: FEVER WORKUP IN PATIENTS WITH SCD AND NO CLEAR SOURCE

1. CBC with differential
2. Blood, urine, and throat cultures
3. Chest radiograph
4. Urinalysis
5. Lumbar puncture
6. Joint aspiration if isolated joint pain present

KEY POINTS: CLINICAL PEARLS

1. Acute pain episodes are the most common reason that patients with SCD come to the emergency department (ED). Most patients with SCD have chronic anemia and should not receive transfusions unless there is an additional indication.
2. ACS, a leading cause of death in patients with SCD, should be suspected in any patient with chest pain and any respiratory or infectious symptoms. All patients with ACS should be treated with antibiotics, admitted to the hospital, and transfusion should be considered.
3. Children with SCD may have uncommon diseases for the pediatric population, such as stroke and thromboembolic events.

ACKNOWLEDGMENT

The editors and authors of this chapter would like to acknowledge and thank Drs. Brad Talley and Louisa Canham for their contributions to previous editions of this chapter.

BIBLIOGRAPHY

Buchanan GR, Yawn BP. *Evidence-based management of sickle cell disease: expert panel report, 2014.* National Institutes of Health; National Heart, Lung, and Blood Institute; 2014. https://www.nhlbi.nih.gov/health-topics/evidence-based-management-sickle-cell-disease. Accessed February 1, 2019.

Debaun MR, Vichinsky EP. Vaso-occlusive pain management in sickle cell disease. *UpToDate* October 2018. https://www.uptodate.com/contents/vaso-occlusive-pain-management-in-sickle-cell-disease. Accessed February 2, 2019.

Elmariah H, Garrett ME, De Castro LM, et al. Factors associated with survival in a contemporary adult sickle cell disease cohort. *Am J Hematol.* 2014;89(5):530–535.

Field JJ, Vichinsky EP, DeBaun MR. Overview of the management and prognosis of sickle cell disease. *UpToDate* September 2018. https://www.uptodate.com/contents/overview-of-the-management-and-prognosis-of-sickle-cell-disease. Accessed January 30, 2019.

Glassberg J. Evidence-based management of sickle cell disease in the emergency department. *Emerg Med Pract.* 2011;13:1–20.

Kassim AA, Galadanci NA, Pruthi S, et al. How I treat and manage strokes in sickle cell disease. *Blood* 125(22):3401–3410, 2015.

Miller AC, Gladwin MT. Pulmonary complications of sickle cell disease. *Am J Respir Crit Care Med.* 2012;185:1154–1165.

Roseff SD. Sickle cell disease: a review. *Immunohematology.* 2009;25:67–74.

CHAPTER 45

ONCOLOGIC EMERGENCIES

Nicholas J. Jouriles, MD and Donald Norris, MD

1. What is an oncologic emergency?

An oncologic emergency is a life- or limb-threatening problem in a patient with a diagnosed or undiagnosed neoplasm. These problems may be caused by the cancer, its systemic effects, the therapeutic interventions against the cancer, or the resulting psychosocial issues.

2. Is this important in the emergency department (ED)?

Yes. Cancer is the second leading cause of death in the United States. As treatments improve and patients with cancer live longer, there will be an ever-increasing number of ED patients with complications and oncologic emergencies.

3. Can cancer be cured?

Modern therapies offer excellent success with medical (e.g., testicular cancer, lymphoma, leukemia), surgical (e.g., lung, colon, and breast cancer), and combination treatments (e.g., radiotherapy and chemotherapy, head and neck, anal cancers). Many patients today survive for a long time, giving them ample opportunity to develop complications and morbidities that in later years need emergency care.

4. Name several oncologic emergencies.

See Table 45.1.

5. How is an oncologic emergency diagnosed?

In any patient with cancer, a complication should be suspected. This includes patients who have been previously cured of their cancer, as well as those with risk factors but no diagnosis. We often make the initial cancer diagnosis in the ED.

6. Which of the entities listed in Table 45.1 is life threatening?

Life-threatening emergencies can be divided into the standard categories of shock: volume loss (bleeding) or impaired vascular return (superior vena cava syndrome [SVCS]), pump impairment (cardiac tamponade), and derangement of systemic vascular resistance (sepsis). There are also serious metabolic derangements (hypercalcemia, hyperkalemia) and disabling neurologic impairment (spinal cord compression [SCC]).

7. Describe these.

- *SVCS* is caused by narrowing of the superior vena cava. Most cases are caused by a neoplastic process. Lung cancer is the most common cause, usually the small cell or squamous types. Breast cancer and lymphoma are also common. Metastatic lesions from distant primary sites may also cause SVCS. The diagnosis is made clinically and verified by imaging. Treatment usually involves a combination of radiation therapy, chemotherapy, or endovascular stenting.

- *Cardiac tamponade* of oncologic etiology usually occurs secondary to metastatic disease involving the pericardium. Patients with cardiac tamponade usually have a large tumor burden and an unlikely 6-month survival. Malignant cardiac tamponade occurs most commonly in lymphoma, lung cancer, and breast cancer. An enlarged cardiac silhouette on chest radiography is suspicious for cardiac tamponade as are muffled heart sounds and jugular venous distention on examination. Pericardial effusion with wall motion abnormalities on bedside ultrasound confirms the diagnosis. Treatment involves pericardial drainage either in the ED with ultrasound guidance or by operative window.

- *Febrile neutropenia* ($T > 38.0°C$ and absolute neutrophil count < 500 cells/mm^3) puts patients at risk for myriad infections; place the patient in protective isolation and obtain cultures from all potential infection sources. Administer broad-spectrum antibiotics quickly. Most patients with febrile neutropenia require admission. A stable patient may be assessed using the Multinational Association for Supportive Care in Cancer (MASCC) risk score (Table 45.2). If patients are low risk, have the ability and desire to follow up, and you have coordinated care with their oncologist, they may be discharged home on ciprofloxacin and amoxicillin/clavulanate (clindamycin if penicillin allergic), thus avoiding complications of hospitalization and broad-spectrum antibiotic use.

- *Hypercalcemia* occurs in up to 30% of patients with cancer. It is the most common life-threatening oncologic emergency. Common presenting signs are anorexia, lethargy, constipation, and altered mental status. The mnemonic "stones, groans, bones, thrones (GI symptoms), and psychiatric overtones" is helpful to remember the symptoms. Lymphoma, breast cancer, and multiple myeloma are often responsible. Treatment involves

Table 45.1 Emergencies in Patients With Underlying Neoplastic Diseases (Partial List)

Mechanical/Structural Airway compromise Intestinal obstruction Intestinal perforation Obstructive jaundice Obstructive uropathy Spinal cord compression Superior vena cava syndrome Pain	**Psychosocial** Emotional stress related to death and dying DNR orders Family issues
	Cardiac Pericardial effusion Cardiac tamponade Cardiac toxicity
Endocrine Adrenal crisis SIADH	**Immunologic** Graft versus host disease
Metabolic Tumor lysis syndrome (TLS) Hypercalcemia (unrelated to TLS)	**Genitourinary** Hemorrhagic cystitis (chemotherapy or radiotherapy induced)
Hematological Bleeding from primary mass Low platelet count or abnormal clotting factors due to liver mass	**Pulmonary** Pulmonary toxicity
Infection Infection associated with neutropenia Postobstructive pneumonia	

DNR, Do not resuscitate; *SIADH,* syndrome of inappropriate secretion of antidiuretic hormone.

Table 45.2 MASCC Score[a]

CATEGORY	POINTS
Burden of current illness: no or mild symptoms	5
Systolic BP > 90 mmHg	5
No COPD	4
Solid tumor or no previous fungal infection	4
Outpatient – applies to all ED patients	3
Burden of tumor: moderate symptoms	3
No dehydration	3
Age < 60 years old	2

[a]A score equal to or greater than 21 is low risk.
BP, Blood pressure; *COPD,* chronic obstructive pulmonary disease; *ED,* emergency department; *MASCC,* Multinational Association for
  Supportive Care in Cancer.
From Multinational Association for Supportive Care in Cancer. https://www.mascc.org/mascc-fn-risk-index-score.

hydration with normal saline and bisphosphates such as pamidronate or zoledronic acid. Calcitonin or the
monoclonal antibody denosumab may be needed in refractory cases.
- *SCC* occurs in up to 5% of all patients with metastatic disease. The spinal cord or nerve root is directly
  compressed by an extradural mass, resulting in neurologic dysfunction. The most common cancers
  causing SCC are lung, breast, prostate, and multiple myeloma. The most common presenting symptom is
  back pain. Any patient with an underlying malignancy who presents with back pain, motor loss, paresthesias, or incontinence should be evaluated for SCC. Prompt diagnosis with emergent magnetic resonance imaging (MRI) can save neurologic function. Up to 40% of patients with SCC may have normal
  plain radiographs. Steroids should be given in the ED. Treatment includes emergent radiation therapy or
  surgical decompression. The strongest predictor of neurologic outcome is the neurologic deficit at the
  time of initial ED diagnosis.

KEY POINTS: PATIENT WHO IS NEUTROPENIC AND FEBRILE

1. Early antibiotics improve outcome.
2. ED antibiotics should be broad spectrum and reflect local infection and resistance patterns.
3. Protective isolation should be used while neutropenia is being confirmed.
4. If truly low risk, the patient may meet criteria for discharge with close follow-up.

KEY POINTS: SPINAL CORD COMPRESSION

1. Negative plain films do not rule out SCC; up to 40% of patients with SCC have normal plain radiographs.
2. Suspicion of SCC is an indication for emergent MRI.
3. Steroids and analgesics are the initial ED management while arranging for appropriate definitive treatment.

8. **Are these life-threatening complications common?**
Of the life-threatening emergencies, SCC, febrile neutropenia, and hypercalcemia are relatively common.

9. **What symptoms can be related to an underlying oncologic emergency?**
Common ED complaints such as chest pain (SVCS or cardiac tamponade), abdominal pain (colon cancer), headache (metastatic disease), or back pain (SCC) can be the initial presentation of an oncologic process. Unfortunately, any ED presenting symptom can be caused by a neoplasm. A neoplastic process should be considered in any patient who complains of chronic pain, unexplained weight loss, weakness, dizziness, altered mental status, bowel obstruction, or new-onset seizures.

10. **What other problems are common in patients with an underlying malignancy?**
After pain, the most common problems are complications of cancer treatment. Each chemotherapeutic agent has side effects. Nausea, vomiting, and diarrhea are common. Renal involvement and pulmonary and cardiac toxicity occur frequently enough to be seen often in the ED.

KEY POINTS: TUMOR LYSIS SYNDROME (TLS)

1. Metabolic abnormalities include hyperkalemia, hyperphosphatemia, hypocalcemia, and hyperuricemia.
2. Patients with dehydration or underlying renal abnormalities are at increased risk for developing TLS.
3. TLS is most commonly seen in the week following treatment.

11. **What is tumor lysis syndrome (TLS)?**
TLS is characterized by hyperkalemia, hyperphosphatemia, hypocalcemia, and hyperuricemia. TLS is commonly seen in cancer patients with a large tumor burden such as leukemia or lymphoma. Additional risk factors include baseline kidney injury and dehydration. Although it can occur spontaneously, it is more common in the week following treatment. Symptoms can be nonspecific but include symptoms specific for the metabolic derangements listed above. Treatment is targeted at reversing metabolic abnormalities. Those with significant kidney injury may require dialysis.

12. **What about immune therapy for cancer?**
Some newer cancer treatments involve immunotherapy. Adverse effects of these treatments include inflammation, most notably colitis, diarrhea, skin changes (rash and itching), although any organ can be involved. Treatment is supportive when symptoms are mild. For advanced symptoms, steroids may be needed. Since steroids occasionally interfere with cancer treatment, the emergency physician should contact the patient's oncologist to coordinate care.

13. **When should the patient be admitted?**
Patients in whom the diagnosis of an oncologic process is first made in the ED are usually admitted. Patients with acute end-organ damage usually require admission. A special group of patients who need to be admitted are those who lack resources at home. It is not uncommon for families to give so much of themselves that they need a break, and respite care is indicated.

14. **Anything special about care plans?**
It is best to discuss treatment plans, including admission, with the patient, family, and primary physician. Most patients with cancer have a primary oncologist who knows the patient's situation best. The emergency physician should balance the current medical problem with the patient's preferences. Many patients have already spent much time at the hospital and would like to be home with their loved ones as much as possible. Care plans evolve over time. Talk with the patient and provide them the help they need. Sometimes it is not medical treatment.

15. **How is a patient with a terminal neoplastic disease treated?**

Often the best treatment for a patient with a terminal malignancy is a kind word, adequate analgesia, comfort measures, and supportive care. The emergency physician can also be challenged by issues related to "do not resuscitate" orders, especially in the out-of-hospital arena. It is vital to communicate well with the patient so as to arrive at the very best individualized treatment plan. Beginning palliative care in the ED is often the best treatment option (see Chapter 7).

BIBLIOGRAPHY

Baugh CW, Wang TJ, Caterino JM, et al. Emergency department management of patients with febrile neutropenia: guidelines concordant or overly aggressive? *Acad Emerg Med.* 2017;24:83–91.

Coyne C, Le V, Brennan J, et al. Application of the MASCC and CISNE risk-stratification scores to identify low-risk febrile neutropenic patients in the emergency department. *Ann Emerg Med.* 2017;69:755–764.

Gupta A, Moore JA. Tumor lysis syndrome. *JAMA Oncol.* 4:895, 2018.

Halfdanarson TR, Hogan WJ, Madsen BE. Emergencies in hematology and oncology. *Mayo Clin Proc.* 2017;92:609–641.

Minisola S, Pepe J, Piemonte S, et al. The diagnosis and management of hypercalcemia. *BMJ.* 2015;350:h2723.

Ristić AD, Imazio M, Adler Y, et al. Triage strategy for urgent management of cardiac tamponade: a position statement of the European Society of Cardiology Working Group on myocardial and pericardial diseases. *Eur Heart J.* 2014;35:229–2284.

Ropper AE, Ropper AH. Spinal cord compression. *N Engl J Med.* 2017;376:1358–1369.

Talapatra K, Panda S, Goyle S, et al. Superior vena cava syndrome: a radiation oncologist's perspective. *J Can Res Ther.* 2016;12:515–519.

CHAPTER 46

FLUIDS AND ELECTROLYTES

Corey M. Slovis, MD and H. Evan Dingle, MD

1. **What is the anion gap?**
   The anion gap (AG) measures the amount of negatively charged ions in the serum (unmeasured anions) that are not bicarbonate (HCO_3^-) or chloride (Cl^-). The AG is calculated by subtracting the sum of HCO_3^- and Cl^- values from the sodium (Na^+) value, the major positive charge in the serum. Potassium (K^+) values are not generally used in the calculation, because of the huge amount of intracellular K^+ (155 mEq/L) and the relatively low amount of K^+ in the serum (only about 4 mEq/L). The formula for determining AG is as follows:

   $$AG = Na^+ - (Cl^- + HCO_3^-)$$

   The normal AG is generally accepted as ranging from 8 to 12 ± 2.

2. **Why is it important to always calculate the AG?**
   An elevated AG means there is some unmeasured anion, toxin, or organic acid in the blood. If you do not calculate the gap, you could miss one of the only clues to a potentially life-ending disease or overdose. The AG also allows acidosis to be divided into two types: wide gap (AG >12–14) and normal gap.

3. **What is hyperchloremic metabolic acidosis?**
   Hyperchloremic acidosis is just another name for normal gap metabolic acidosis. Since the formula for AG is $Na^+ - (Cl^- + HCO_3^-)$, and assuming no unmeasured anions, Cl^- has to rise when HCO_3^- goes down – hence the name *hyperchloremic metabolic acidosis*.

4. **Is there an easy way to remember the differential diagnosis for wide gap metabolic acidosis?**
   The authors' favorite mnemonic is called *MUKPILES.*
   Methanol
   Uremia
   Diabetic **k**etoacidosis (DKA), alcoholic **k**etoacidosis (AKA), and starvation **k**etoacidosis
   Phenformin/metformin and **p**aracetamol overdose *(the English version of acetaminophen)*; **P**ropylene glycol
   Isoniazid (INH) and **i**ron
   Lactic acidosis
   Ethylene glycol
   Salicylates and **s**olvents

5. **What are the clues to each of the entities in MUKPILES?**
   See Table 46.1.

6. **What are the causes of narrow gap acidosis?**
   Memorize the mnemonic *HARDUPS.*
   Hyperventilation (chronic)
   Acetazolamide, **a**cids (e.g., hydrochloric), **A**ddison's disease
   Renal tubular acidosis
   Diarrhea
   Ureterosigmoidostomy
   Pancreatic fistulas and drainage
   Saline (in large amounts)
   If you do not want to memorize anything, it is important to know that diarrhea, especially in children, and renal tubular acidosis, especially in adults, are the two most common causes of a narrow gap acidosis.

7. **Intravenous (IV) fluid goes into which three compartments?**
   1. Inside blood vessels (intravascular)
   2. Into cells (intracellular)
   3. In between the two (interstitial)
   Normal saline (NS) and lactated Ringer (LR) solution are the preferred fluids for IV fluid resuscitation, as 25%–33% of the solutions stay in the intravascular compartment. In contrast, for each liter of half (0.45) NS provided, only 125–175 mL stay in blood vessels; each liter of D_5W adds only about 80 mL into the vasculature.

Table 46.1 Clues to the Differential Diagnosis of Wide Gap Metabolic Acidosis

DISEASE OR TOXIN	CLUES
Methanol	Alcoholism, blindness or papilledema, profound acidosis
Uremia	Chronically ill-appearing, history of chronic renal failure, BUN >100 mg/dL, and creatinine >5 mg/dL
DKA	History of diabetes, polyuria, and polydipsia, glucose >500 mg/dL
AKA	Alcoholism, glucose <250 mg/dL, nausea and vomiting
Starvation ketoacidosis	Poor PO intake, eating disorders, prolonged fasting
Phenformin/metformin	Diabetes, medication history, recent contrast study
Paracetamol	Acetaminophen use, hepatotoxicity, fulminant hepatic failure
Propylene glycol	Large amounts of IV diazepam or lorazepam (propylene glycol used as diluent)
INH	Tuberculosis, suicide risk, refractory status seizures
Iron	Pregnant or postpartum, hematemesis, radiopaque tablets on abdominal film (unreliable finding)
Lactic acidosis	Hypoxia, hypotension, sepsis
Ethylene glycol	Alcoholism, oxalate crystals in urine with or without renal failure, fluorescent mouth or urine (from drinking antifreeze; unreliable finding)
Salicylates	History of chronic disease requiring aspirin use (e.g., rheumatoid arthritis), mixed acid-base disturbance (primary metabolic acidosis plus primary respiratory alkalosis), aspirin level >20–40 mg/dL
Solvents	History of exposure or huffing; spray paint on face

AKA, Alcoholic ketoacidosis; *BUN,* blood urea nitrogen; *DKA,* diabetic ketoacidosis; *INH,* isoniazid; *IV,* intravenous; *PO,* per os (by mouth, orally).

8. **What are "balanced" crystalloids?**
   Balanced crystalloids are fluids with electrolyte compositions, osmolality, and pH similar to plasma. Two of the most common balanced crystalloids are LR and Plasmalyte. These solutions have much lower sodium and chloride content than NS. For example, LR has a Na^+ of 130 mEq/L and a Cl^- of 109 mEq/L, versus 155 mEq/L of each in NS. The solution is called *lactated,* because it has 28 mEq/L of bicarbonate in the form of lactate, which is converted to HCO_3^- by the liver. Unlike NS, LR solution also has 4 mEq/L of K^+ and 3 mEq/L of calcium.

9. **Which solution is better – NS or balanced crystalloids?**
   Because balanced crystalloids are "more physiologic" and have less chloride in them, patients do not develop a hyperchloremic metabolic acidosis that occurs when large volumes of sodium chloride are administered. Critically ill patients who receive balanced crystalloids, as opposed to NS, have been shown to have lower overall mortality and lower incidence of kidney injury. In most situations, Plasmalyte or LR is preferred when giving large volumes. However, NS can be given for standard fluid resuscitation, particularly in patients with protracted vomiting who have a hypochloremic metabolic alkalosis from vomiting stomach contents (rich in hydrogen and Cl^-).

10. **What is the most dangerous electrolyte abnormality? What are its most common causes?**
    Hyperkalemia is the most dangerous electrolyte abnormality. It may result in sudden arrhythmogenic death because of its effect on the cells' resting membrane potentials. The most common explanation for hyperkalemia is often referred to as *laboratory error.* Actually, the laboratory does the right analysis, but the serum sample has hemolyzed after (or while) being drawn.
    Other common causes of hyperkalemia are:
    - Chronic renal failure (No. 1 true case).
    - Acidosis (K^+ moves out of the cell as the pH falls).
    - Drugs or medications (including nonsteroidal anti-inflammatory drugs, K^+-sparing diuretics, digoxin, angiotensin-converting enzyme inhibitors, and administration of IV potassium chloride).
    - Cell death (when K^+ comes out of injured muscle or red cells), including burns, crush injuries, rhabdomyolysis, tumor lysis syndrome, and intravascular hemolysis.
       Much less common causes include adrenal insufficiency, hyperkalemic periodic paralysis, and hematologic malignancies.

11. **What is the most important study to order in patients with suspected hyperkalemia?**
    An electrocardiogram (ECG) is the most important study to obtain in the setting of suspected hyperkalemia
    (e.g., a patient with chronic renal failure or an unexplained bradycardic rhythm). The first ECG changes in hyper-
    kalemia are tall peaked *T waves* which occur as K$^+$ values rise to 5.5–6.5 mEq/L. Loss of the *p wave* may follow
    as K$^+$ levels rise to 6.5–7.5 mEq/L. The most dangerous ECG finding (typically at levels >8 mEq/L) is widening of
    the *QRS complex*, which may merge with the abnormal *T wave* and create what appears to be a sine wave of
    ventricular tachycardia.

12. **Summarize the best treatment for hyperkalemia.**
    Treatment is based on the presence or absence of ECG changes, serum levels, and the patient's underlying renal
    function. If the patient has life-threatening ECG changes of hyperkalemia (widening QRS complex, a sine wave–like
    rhythm or bradycardia/heart block), 10% calcium chloride should be given (10 mL, preferably through a central
    line) to temporarily stabilize the myocardial cell membranes. Although calcium is relatively fast-acting, its effect
    lasts only 30–60 minutes, requiring additional measures to lower K$^+$ levels. However, most patients with hyperka-
    lemia will not have QRS widening, and only require K$^+$ moved intracellularly, and then removed from the body.

13. **How can K$^+$ be moved intracellularly?**
    The most effective way is by giving glucose and insulin. Glucose and insulin work by activating the glucose
    transport system to move glucose into the cell. As glucose is carried intracellularly, K$^+$ is carried along. The usual
    dosage of glucose is two ampules of dextrose 50% in water (D$_{50}$W; 100 mL) and 10 U of regular insulin; however,
    emerging evidence supports the use of lower doses of insulin (given risk for hypoglycemia with higher doses)
    while still producing similar decreases in K$^+$ levels. Another excellent first-line method of driving K$^+$ into the cell
    is use of inhaled β-agonist bronchodilators. β-Agonists may be especially helpful in a patient who has renal fail-
    ure with fluid overload, additionally treating bronchospasm from pulmonary edema. HCO$_3^-$ may also be used to
    drive K$^+$ into the cell, but it is effective only in acidotic patients. Usually one to two ampules of HCO$_3^-$ (50 mEq of
    HCO$_3^-$ per ampule) are given over 1–10 minutes, depending on patient acuity.

14. **What is BRASH syndrome?**
    BRASH stands for **b**radycardia, **r**enal failure, **A**V-nodal blockers, **s**hock, and **h**yperkalemia. These patients present
    with bradycardia and hyperkalemia in the setting of renal failure, acidosis, and, typically, the use of an AV-nodal
    blocking agent such as a β-blocker or calcium channel blocker. In BRASH, renal failure causes hyperkalemia
    and accumulation of the patient's nodal blocking agent, both of which worsen bradycardia. In a dangerous cycle,
    bradycardia then leads to shock, further worsening renal perfusion, and so on.

KEY POINTS: HYPERKALEMIA

1. Hyperkalemia itself is often asymptomatic; check the ECG.
2. The ECG changes seen as K$^+$ rises are tall, peaked *T waves*, followed by loss of P waves, and, finally, widening
   of the QRS complex.
3. Administering glucose and insulin, supplemented by an inhaled β-agonist, is the most effective method to drive
   K$^+$ into the cell and acutely lower serum K$^+$.
4. HCO$_3^-$ only works to lower serum K$^+$ in acidotic patients.
5. Only give calcium for hyperkalemia if there is a wide QRS complex or life-threatening bradycardia.

15. **After K$^+$'s electrical effects have been counteracted (if indicated) and K$^+$ has been driven
    intracellularly, how do I remove it from the body?**
    K$^+$ can be removed from the body by diuresis, K$^+$-binding resins, and hemodialysis. Renal diuresis with saline,
    supplemented by furosemide, is an excellent way to lower total body K$^+$. Most hyperkalemic patients, however,
    have renal failure and do not produce urine, which is how they became hyperkalemic in the first place. Sodium
    polystyrene sulfonate (Kayexalate) is an Na$^+$-containing resin that exchanges its Na$^+$ content for the patient's K$^+$
    in the gastrointestinal (GI) tract. Each 1 g of Kayexalate can remove about 1 mEq of K$^+$ from the patient's body.
    We do not recommend mixing it with sorbitol, a practice associated with colonic necrosis and perforation.
    Kayexalate takes many hours, with variable efficacy, and so is not a useful tool for rapid potassium lowering in
    the emergency department. The best method of lowering K$^+$ is by hemodialysis, the method of choice for any
    severely ill, acidotic, or profoundly hyperkalemic patient.

16. **Discuss the most common causes of hyponatremia.**
    Hyponatremia is a serum Na$^+$ <135 mEq/L. Most patients with mild hyponatremia (125–130 mEq/L) have
    hyponatremia from a diuretic medication, or from some degree of fluid overload as a result of heart failure, re-
    nal failure, or liver disease. Diuretic-induced hyponatremia is the most common cause of hyponatremia in the
    elderly. Patients with heart failure, liver failure, or renal failure develop hyponatremia as a result of secondary
    hyperaldosteronism. Renal hypoperfusion causes the release of aldosterone, resulting in fluid retention, volume

overload, and a dilutional hyponatremia (even in the face of total body Na^+ excess). Moderate to severe hyponatremia (levels <125 mEq/L) is most commonly caused by the syndrome of inappropriate secretion of antidiuretic hormone (SIADH), psychogenic polydipsia (compulsive water drinking), or excessive free water ingestion (marathon runners and ecstasy users).

17. What is SIADH?
SIADH results from abnormally high levels of antidiuretic hormone (ADH) from the posterior pituitary gland. Normally, when Na^+ levels fall, levels of ADH, which blocks free water excretion, also decrease, resulting in urinary loss of water (diuresis). In SIADH, ADH release is unregulated, causing serum Na^+ levels to fall as more excess free water is retained (antidiuresis). The hallmark of this syndrome is relatively concentrated urine, rather than the maximally diluted expected. Patients cannot be given this diagnosis if they are taking diuretics or have a reason to be fluid overloaded (e.g., congestive heart failure, chronic renal failure, and liver failure).

18. What are neurologic signs of hyponatremia?
Na^+ affects the brain through its effects on osmolality, influencing neuron shrinkage and expansion. Symptoms of hyponatremia include dizziness, confusion, coma, and seizures.

19. How fast should hyponatremia be corrected?
There has been much debate over how rapidly Na^+ should be corrected, ranging from 0.5 to 2.0 mEq/L/h. In most patients, if serum Na^+ is <120 mEq/L, serum Na^+ should be corrected slowly, rising by no more than 0.5 mEq/h. This approach avoids the possible development of central pontine myelinolysis (which is also called *osmotic demyelinating syndrome* by some purists), a catastrophic neurologic illness seen with too-rapid Na^+ correction: coma, flaccid paralysis, and usually death.

20. Should Na^+ levels ever be increased quickly?
There are some specific indications for raising a patient's Na^+ rapidly, by infusing 3% saline. In general, patients who have serum Na^+ levels of <120 mEq/L *and* acute alterations in mental status, seizures, or new focal neurologic findings should have their levels raised about 4–6 mEq/L over a few hours. Hypertonic saline should be given carefully to these acutely ill patients (100 mL over 10 minutes, with a possible second 100 mL bolus over the next 50 minutes). Other than these rare patients with severe, symptomatic hyponatremia, gradual correction by water restriction, often with a slow infusion of saline, is all that is required.

21. What is the osmolality gap?
Osmolality is calculated by multiplying the serum Na^+ by 2 and adding the amount of glucose (GLU) divided by 18, plus the blood urea nitrogen (BUN) level divided by 2.8. Normal is approximately 280–290 mOsm. If ethanol (EtOH) is present, its added value is divided by 4.6:

$$\text{Calculated serum osmolality} = 2 \times Na + (GLU/18) + (BUN/2.8) + (EtOH/4.6)$$

The osmolal gap is the difference in the laboratory's measured osmolality and the calculated osmolality, and should be only about 10. If the osmolal gap is >10, other osmols are in the serum (e.g., an alcohol, IV contrast media, toxic alcohol, mannitol, etc.).

22. How do I use the osmolal gap to figure out whether someone has ingested methanol or ethylene glycol?
If the osmolal gap is elevated, you should measure the patient's serum ethanol level in percent of milligrams and divide it by 4 for a rapid estimation of ethanol's osmolar contribution. If the alcohol level is 100 mg/dL, alcohol will contribute ~25 additional osmols.

   If there is a higher gap, these unaccounted osmols may represent methanol, ethylene glycol, or isopropyl alcohol. Clues to a wide anion gap metabolic acidosis are delineated in Table 45.1.

23. What are the most common causes of hypercalcemia? How do they present?
Mild hypercalcemia is usually caused by dehydration, thiazide diuretics, or hyperparathyroidism. It is often asymptomatic, but mild fatigue, renal stones, or nonspecific GI symptoms may be present. Severe hypercalcemia, often secondary to a malignancy, with levels greater than 2–3 mg/dL above normal, usually presents as depressed mental status along with signs and symptoms of profound dehydration. ECG changes in hypercalcemia include shortened *QT intervals*, flattened *T waves*, and rarely, *QRS* widening.

24. Describe the emergency treatment of hypercalcemia.
Symptomatic hypercalcemia is treated by rapid volume resuscitation with NS, supplemented by furosemide after intravascular volume has been normalized. Once the volume status is normalized, patients should receive approximately 150–200 mL of NS per hour, plus enough furosemide to keep urine output at 1 mL/kg/h or higher. Saline blocks the proximal tubules from absorbing calcium; furosemide, once thought to block distal tubular absorption, assists in maintaining diuresis. Older patients and patients with impaired cardiac function must be closely monitored during saline infusion to avoid iatrogenic congestive heart failure.

KEY POINTS: FLUIDS AND ELECTROLYTES

1. An elevated AG should alert you to a potentially serious disease or overdose.
2. Large quantities of NS can cause a normal gap hyperchloremic metabolic acidosis.
3. Raise serum Na^+ by no more than 0.5 mEq/L/h, *or* by more than 12 mEq/L/day in patients with Na^+ concentrations <120 mEq/L.
4. Seizures, coma, and acute neurologic findings in a previously normal patient are the only indications to give hypertonic saline in patients with severe hyponatremia.
5. The therapy of hypercalcemia centers on a saline-induced diuresis, carefully supplemented by furosemide.

BIBLIOGRAPHY

Hoffman RS, Charney AN. Fluid electrolyte and acid-base principles. In: *Goldfrank's Toxicologic Emergencies.* 10th ed. New York: McGraw-Hill; 2015: 248–261.
Pfennig C, Slovis CM. Electrolyte disorders. In: Walls RM, Hockberger RS, Gausche-Hill M, eds. *Rosen's Emergency Medicine: Concepts and Clinical Practice.* Vol 2, 9th ed. Philadelphia: Elsevier; 2018: 1516–1532.
Semler MW, Self WH, Wanderer JP, et al. Balanced crystalloids versus saline in critically ill adults. *N Engl J Med.* 2018;378(9):829–839.
Sterns RH. Disorders of plasma sodium – causes, consequences, and correction. *N Engl J Med.* 2015;372:55–65.
Sterns RH, Rojas M, Bernstein P, et al. Ion-exchange resins for the treatment of hyperkalemia: are they safe and effective? *J Am Soc Nephrol.* 2010;21:733–735.

CHAPTER 47

ACID-BASE DISORDERS

John Rague, MD and Jenelle H. Badulak MD

1. **Which laboratory values do I need to determine a patient's acid-base status?**
   You need a basic metabolic panel (BMP) and either a venous or arterial blood gas. The BMP is used to measure the bicarbonate, calculate the anion gap (AG), and gather additional information about the etiology of the acid-base disorder (e.g., glucose, sodium, and renal disorders). The blood gas is used to measure the pH and the venous or arterial partial pressure of carbon dioxide (PCO_2). In general, the venous blood gas (VBG) will provide all the information required to determine a patient's acid-base status using the pH and venous partial pressure of carbon dioxide ($PvCO_2$). The pH from a VBG is usually slightly lower, and the $PvCO_2$ slightly higher, than the arterial pH, and the arterial partial pressure of carbon dioxide ($PaCO_2$), respectively. If the patient is suffering from circulatory shock, or has significant hypercarbia, the VBG becomes more unreliable. A VBG from a central vein is more accurate and gives additional information about oxygenation. An arterial blood gas (ABG) is the most accurate and gives additional information about oxygenation.

2. **Which six questions do I need answered to determine a patient's acid-base status?**
   1. Is the pH acidemic (pH < 7.35), alkalemic (pH > 7.45), or normal?
   2. Is the primary acid-base disturbance respiratory or metabolic?
   3. If a primary respiratory disturbance is present, is it acute or chronic?
   4. Is there an increased AG?
   5. Is there adequate compensation?
   6. Is there more than one primary disorder (mixed disorder)?

3. **How do I determine if the primary acid-base disturbance is respiratory or metabolic?**
   Increases or decreases in the PCO_2 and bicarbonate (HCO_3^-) are evaluated to determine the cause of the alkalemia or acidemia. If an increase/decrease in the PCO_2 corresponds with the acidemia/alkalemia, the primary disorder is respiratory. If an increase/decrease in the HCO_3^- corresponds with the alkalemia/acidemia, the primary disorder is metabolic (Table 47.1).

4. **How do I determine whether a primary respiratory disturbance is acute or chronic?**
   The rate at which the pH changes is determined by the acute or chronic nature of the change in ventilation. Acute changes lead to larger changes in pH, and chronic changes lead to smaller changes in pH (Table 47.2).

5. **How do I determine whether compensation is adequate, and what is the physiologic limit of compensation?**
   Proportional changes in the PCO_2 (lungs) and HCO_3^- (kidneys) are made to correct the pH. Note that compensation will never completely return the pH to normal (Table 47.3).

6. **What are the three ways I can identify more than one primary acid-base disturbance (a mixed disorder)?**
   1. If the compensation is higher or lower than anticipated:
      - If the PCO_2 is too low or high, there is an additional respiratory alkalosis or acidosis, respectively.
      - If the HCO_3^- is too low or high, there is additional metabolic acidosis or alkalosis, respectively.
   2. If the pH is normal, but the PCO_2, HCO_3^-, or AG is abnormal (Table 47.4):
      - If the PCO_2 and HCO_3^- are high, there is respiratory acidosis and metabolic alkalosis.
      - If they are both low, there is respiratory alkalosis and metabolic acidosis.
      - If the PCO_2 and HCO_3^- are normal but the AG is elevated, there is AG metabolic acidosis (AGMA) and metabolic alkalosis.
      - If the PCO_2, HCO_3^-, and AG are normal, there is either no acid-base disturbance or there is non-AGMA and metabolic alkalosis.
   3. If the AG is increased
      - The delta-delta ($\Delta AG/\Delta HCO_3^-$) should be calculated to determine whether there is additional non-AGMA or metabolic alkalosis (see later).

7. **How do I calculate the AG and how do I calculate the delta-delta ($\Delta AG/\Delta HCO_3^-$)?**
   The AG can be calculated using values from the BMP:

$$AG = Na^+ - (Cl^- + HCO_3^-)$$

Table 47.1 Primary Acid-Base Disorders

ACID-BASE DISORDER	pH	HCO_3^-	PCO_2	EXAMPLE
Metabolic acidosis	↓	↓↓	↓	Lactic acidosis in sepsis
Metabolic alkalosis	↑	↑↑	↑	Protracted vomiting
Respiratory acidosis	↓	↑	↑↑	Chronic obstructive pulmonary disease with CO_2 retention
Respiratory alkalosis	↑	↓	↓↓	Hypoxemic drive leading to hyperventilation

HCO_3^-, Bicarbonate; PCO_2, arterial or venous partial pressure of carbon dioxide.

Table 47.2 Chronicity of Respiratory Acid-Base Disorder

Acute respiratory acidosis	↓0.08 pH = ↑10 PCO_2
Chronic respiratory acidosis (3–5 days)	↓0.03 pH = ↑10 PCO_2
Acute respiratory alkalosis	↑0.08 pH = ↓10 PCO_2
Chronic respiratory alkalosis (2–3 days)	↑0.03 pH = ↓10 PCO_2

PCO_2, Arterial or venous partial pressure of carbon dioxide.

Table 47.3 Renal/Pulmonary Compensation

PRIMARY DISORDER	ANTICIPATED COMPENSATION	LIMIT OF COMPENSATION
Metabolic acidosis	$PCO_2 = (1.5 \times HCO_3^-) + 8 \pm 2$	
	PCO_2 = last 2 digits of pH	PCO_2 down to 10
Metabolic alkalosis	↑$PCO_2 = 0.75 \times \Delta HCO_3^-$	PCO_2 up to 60 (limited by hypoxemia)
Acute respiratory acidosis	↑1 HCO_3^- = ↑10 PCO_2	
Chronic respiratory acidosis	↑4 HCO_3^- = ↑10 PCO_2	
Acute respiratory alkalosis	↓2 HCO_3^- = ↓10 PCO_2	HCO_3^- down to 18
Chronic respiratory alkalosis	↓5 HCO_3^- = ↓10 PCO_2	HCO_3^- down to 12–15

HCO_3^-, Bicarbonate; PCO_2, arterial or venous partial pressure of carbon dioxide.

Table 47.4 Mixed Acid-Base Disorders With a Normal pH

MIXED ACID-BASE DISORDER	pH	HCO_3^-	PCO_2	AG
Respiratory acidosis and metabolic alkalosis	Normal	↑	↑	Normal
Respiratory alkalosis and AGMA (or non-AGMA)	Normal	↓	↓	↑ (or normal)
Metabolic alkalosis and AGMA	Normal	Normal	Normal	↑
Metabolic alkalosis and non-AGMA or Normal acid-base status	Normal	Normal	Normal	Normal

AG, Anion gap; AGMA, anion gap metabolic acidosis; HCO_3^-, bicarbonate; PCO_2, arterial or venous partial pressure of carbon dioxide.

If an AGMA is detected, the $\Delta AG/\Delta HCO_3^-$ should be calculated to find additional acid-base disorders:

$$\Delta AG = \text{calculated AG} - \text{normal AG}, \Delta HCO_3^- = \text{normal HCO}_3^- - \text{measured HCO}_3^-$$

- $\Delta AG/\Delta HCO_3^- < 1$ indicates there is an AGMA and simultaneous non-AGMA
- $\Delta AG/\Delta HCO_3^- = 1\text{--}2$ indicates this is a pure AGMA
- $\Delta AG/\Delta HCO_3^- > 2$ indicates there is an AGMA and (simultaneous metabolic alkalosis *or* compensated respiratory acidosis)

8. **What are four major etiologies of an AGMA, and which laboratory tests differentiate them?**
   1. Lactic acidosis: lactate level
   2. Ketoacidosis: urine dipstick acetoacetate (AcAc) or serum β-hydroxybutyrate (βHB) level
   3. Renal failure and uremia: blood urea nitrogen (BUN) and creatinine levels
   4. Toxic ingestion: aspirin level, acetaminophen level, toxic alcohol levels (ethanol (EtOH), methanol, ethylene glycol, propylene glycol), cyanide level, carbon monoxide level, iron level, elevated osmolal gap

   CAT MUDPILES is also a common mnemonic.
   Cyanide
   Alcoholic ketoacidosis
   Toluene
   Methanol, metformin
   Uremia
   Diabetic ketoacidosis (DKA)
   Propylene glycol, paraldehyde
   Isoniazid, iron
   Lactate, linezolid
   Ethylene glycol
   Salicylates

9. **Name three types of lactic acidosis, their causes, and examples of each.**
   See Table 47.5.

10. **List disorders that can cause a hyperketonemic state.**
    - DKA
    - Alcoholic ketoacidosis (AKA)
    - Starvation
    - Isopropyl alcohol intoxication
    - Hyperemesis gravidarum
    - Salicylate toxicity
    - Paraldehyde intoxication
    - Stress hormone excess

11. **In a patient with DKA who is clinically improving with appropriate therapy, why might the urine ketones increase?**
    There are three ketone bodies: βHB, AcAc, and acetone. βHB and AcAc are acids; acetone is not. The proportion of βHB to AcAc depends on the oxidation-reduction status of the patient. Patients experiencing DKA are often severely dehydrated, and the preponderance of ketone bodies may be in the form of βHB. The urine test by which ketones are detected is the nitroprusside reaction test (Acetest, Ketostix), which measures AcAc and acetone but is not

Table 47.5 The Three Types of Lactic Acidosis

LACTIC ACIDOSIS	CAUSE	EXAMPLE
Type A	Impaired tissue oxygenation and lactate overproduction through anaerobic metabolism	Shock, respiratory failure, sepsis, ischemic bowel, carbon monoxide, cyanide, severe anemia
Type B	Compromised lactate metabolism without tissue hypoxia, usually toxicologic ingestion often causing uncoupling of oxidative phosphorylation, or increased glycolytic flux	Biguanides (metformin), antiretrovirals, isoniazid, salicylates, valproic acid, iron, liver disease, thiamine deficiency, catecholamine excess, malignancies, inherited metabolic deficit in lactate clearance
D-lactic acidosis	Metabolism by-product of bacteria in the gut	Accumulates in patients with short gut syndrome or gastric bypass. Note that this type of lactate is not detected by traditional laboratory assays

sensitive to βHB. As fluids and insulin therapy are instituted, the amount of βHB converted to AcAc increases. The nitroprusside reaction, which initially may have been weakly positive or even negative, becomes increasingly positive. In a case where DKA is suspected but the urine nitroprusside test is negative, a serum βHB level can be tested.

12. **How can glucose and albumin affect calculation of the AG?**
A high glucose can cause a hypertonic hyponatremia, and a correction factor must be used to determine the calculated concentration of sodium (Na^+) (for each 100 mg/dL increase in glucose greater than 100 mg/dL, increase the Na^+ by 1.6 mEq/L); however, when calculating the AG, use the measured, not the calculated, Na^+.

A patient's expected AG is dependent upon the concentration of albumin.

$$Expected\ AG = (Albumin) \times 2.5$$

Therefore if the patient is hypoalbuminemic, he or she could have AGMA at a lower calculated AG (e.g., expected AG = 10 if albumin is 4 g/dL; expected AG = 5 if albumin is 2 g/dL).

13. **How can a patient have a metabolic acidosis without evidence of an elevated AG?**
A patient with a hyperchloremic metabolic acidosis (non-AGMA) may have no evidence of an elevated AG. This condition is caused by adding hydrogen chloride to the serum. The fall in serum HCO_3^- is offset by the addition of Cl^-; consequently, there is no increased AG. Non-AGMAs are disorders caused by inappropriate hydrogen ion (H^+) retention or HCO_3^- excretion, usually caused by either the kidneys (positive urine AG) or the gastrointestinal (GI) tract (negative urine AG).

14. **How can I remember some of the causes of non-AGMA?**
Use the mnemonic *USED CARP.*
Ureteroenterostomy
Small bowel fistula
Extra chloride (normal saline intravenous [IV] fluid)
Diarrhea
Carbonic anhydrase inhibitors
Adrenal insufficiency
Renal tubular acidosis
Pancreatic fistula

15. **Which electrolyte is most commonly affected by a change in acid-base status?**
Serum potassium (K^+) is affected. Because of H^+/K^+ cell membrane exchange pumps, a change in pH of 0.1 will cause an inverse change in serum K^+ of about 0.5 mEq/L (range, 0.3–0.8 mEq/L). If the pH is elevated by 0.1, the serum K^+ falls by about 0.5 mEq/L; if the pH is diminished by 0.1, the serum K^+ increases by about 0.5 mEq/L. For example, in DKA, although the patient's total body K^+ may be severely depleted, serum K^+ levels may be elevated because of acidemia. As the patient is treated and acidosis resolves, K^+ supplementation is indicated, because serum levels may fall precipitously as K^+ moves intracellularly.

16. **What are potential causes of a metabolic acidosis in a patient with chronic alcohol use?**
AKA is a common metabolic disturbance in patients with chronic alcohol-use disorder. The patient is often undernourished, resulting in depletion of glycogen stores. This increases the mobilization and delivery of fatty acids to the liver, where they are converted to ketone bodies. Alcohol metabolism results in an increased ratio of nicotinamide adenine dinucleotide + H (NADH) to nicotinamide adenine dinucleotide (NAD^+), which favors the formation of βHB. This NAD^+/NADH redox ratio also causes inhibition of gluconeogenesis, leading to hypoglycemia. Administering dextrose-containing fluids treats AKA. Chronic alcohol users are also at risk for thiamine deficiency, which can lead to a type B lactic acidosis. Liver insufficiency, AKA, alcohol withdrawal seizures, and acute alcohol intoxication can all lead to lactic acidosis. Ingestion or co-ingestion of other toxic alcohols should be considered as well.

17. **What are the etiologies of a metabolic alkalosis?**
- Patients with saline responsive states have a low urine chloride (<10 mEq/L) and are usually hypovolemic. Causes include GI losses (vomiting, nasogastric tube drainage, high-volume ileostomy, villous adenomas) and renal losses (prior diuretic use).
- Patients with saline resistant states have a high urine chloride (>20 mEq/L). Patients are either hypertensive, which is caused by hyperaldosteronism, or are hypotensive or normotensive, which is caused by current diuretic use, severe hypokalemia, exogenous alkali ingestion, licorice or Bartter or Gitelman syndromes.

18. **How does a patient with metformin-associated lactic acidosis (MALA) present, and what is the treatment?**
These patients have a very high lactate and a low pH, out of proportion to clinical presentation. Chronic toxicity usually arises from the patient who develops renal failure for some reason and continues to take therapeutic doses of his or her metformin. Because metformin is cleared by the kidneys, it starts to accumulate, resulting in a significantly elevated lactate and acidemia. The mechanism for the elevated lactate and acidemia is due to inhibition of complex I in the electron transport chain by metformin. The treatment is emergent dialysis for patients with renal failure and a severe acidosis.

19. **How can the osmolal gap and the AG be used to differentiate toxic alcohol ingestions?**
All toxic alcohols cause an elevated osmolal gap. Osmolal gap = measured osmoles − calculated osmoles.

$$\text{Calculated osmoles} = (2 \times Na) + (Glucose/18) + (BUN/2.8) + (EtOH/4.6)$$

An osmolal gap is considered elevated when it is greater than 10. Isopropyl alcohol is the only toxic alcohol that does not produce an elevated AG, because it is metabolized to acetone (which is not an anion). All the other toxic alcohols (EtOH, methanol, ethylene glycol, propylene glycol) lead to an elevated AG.

20. **Infusion of what medications can cause an AGMA?**
Both lorazepam and diazepam infusions can cause an AGMA. These medications are suspended in propylene glycol. The accumulation of propylene glycol during prolonged infusions of these medications can cause an elevated AG.

21. **What etiologies should be considered when evaluating a patient with respiratory acidosis? How are they treated?**
- Central causes: sedatives, intracranial trauma, obesity hypoventilation syndrome
- Upper airway causes: obstructive sleep apnea, laryngospasm, acute airway obstruction
- Lower airway causes: chronic obstructive pulmonary disease (COPD), asthma, lung protective permissive hypercapnia for acute respiratory distress syndrome (ARDS)
- Muscular causes: Guillain-Barré syndrome, myasthenia gravis, amyotrophic lateral sclerosis, muscular dystrophy, severe hypophosphatemia, botulism
- Thoracic cage causes: chest wall trauma, severe scoliosis, pectus carinatum or excavatum
  Respiratory acidosis is treated by increasing alveolar ventilation. This is accomplished by increasing respiratory rate, increasing tidal volume, and decreasing dead space.

22. **Why do patients suffer carpopedal spasms during hyperventilation?**
Hyperventilation leads to a respiratory alkalosis that increases the pH of the blood. As albumin is alkalinized, its affinity for calcium increases, thus decreasing the amount of available ionized (not bound to albumin) calcium for use by the muscles, leading to tetany.

KEY POINTS: ACID-BASE DISORDERS

1. Fully evaluating a patient's acid-base status requires a blood gas and chemistry panel.
2. Physiologic compensatory mechanisms to achieve a normal pH include the HCO_3^- buffering system in the blood, alveolar ventilation in the lungs, and renal excretion or retention of HCO_3^-.
3. AG metabolic acidosis is common and life threatening; the four major causes are lactic acid, ketones, renal failure, and toxic ingestions.

ACKNOWLEDGMENT

The editors and authors of this chapter would like to acknowledge and thank Drs. Stephen L. Adams, Morris S. Khrasch, and Jason A. Hoppe for their previous contributions to this chapter.

BIBLIOGRAPHY

Andersen LW, Mackenhauer J, Roberts JC, et al. Etiology and therapeutic approach to elevated lactate levels. *Mayo Clin Proc.* 2013;88:1127–1140.
Bruno CM, Valenti M. Acid-base disorders in patients with chronic obstructive pulmonary disease: a pathophysiological review. *J Biomed Biotechnol.* 2012;2012:915150.
Byrne AL, Bennett M, Chatterji R, et al. Peripheral venous and arterial blood gas analysis in adults: are they comparable? A systematic review and meta-analysis. *Respirology.* 2014;19(2):168–175.
Dzierba AL, Abraham P. A practical approach to understanding acid-base abnormalities in critical illness. *J Pharm Pract.* 2011;24: 17–26.
Gomez H, Kellum JA. Understanding acid base disorders. *Crit Care Clin.* 2015;31(4):849–860.
Kelly AM. Review article: can venous blood gas analysis replace arterial in emergency medical care. *Emerg Med Australas.* 2010;22:493–498.
Kraut JA, Mullins ME. Toxic alcohols. *N Engl J Med.* 2018;378(3):270–280.
Lalau JD. Lactic acidosis induced by metformin: incidence, management and prevention. *Drug Saf.* 2010;33:727–740.
Lee Hamm L, Hering-Smith KS, Nakhoul NL. Acid-base and potassium homeostasis. *Semin Nephrol.* 2013;33:257–264.
Palmer BF, Clegg DJ. Electrolyte disturbances in patients with chronic alcohol-use disorder. *N Engl J Med.* 2017;377(14):1368–1377.
Rice M, Ismail B, Pillow MT. Approach to metabolic acidosis in the emergency department. *Emerg Med Clin North Am.* 2014;32: 403–420.
Treger R, Pirouz S, Kamangar N, et al. Agreement between central venous and arterial blood gas measurements in the intensive care unit. *Clin J Am Soc Nephrol.* 2010;5:390–394.

CHAPTER 48

DIABETES MELLITUS

C. Ryan Keay, MD, FACEP

1. **Describe the classifications of diabetes.**
   - Type I disease is characterized by autoimmune pancreatic β-cell destruction, which causes an absolute insulin deficiency. Patients with type I disease have little or no endogenous production of insulin and develop diabetic ketoacidosis (DKA) without exogenous supplementation of insulin. This makes insulin essential to the treatment of type I diabetes.
   - Type II disease is characterized by peripheral insulin resistance, with progressive defective insulin production by pancreatic β-cells. Glucose levels often respond to oral dietary modification, weight loss, exercise, and oral hypoglycemic agents; however, insulin is sometimes necessary to control glucose levels.
   - Type 1.5 diabetes, also known as latent autoimmune diabetes in adults (LADA), shares characteristics with type I and type II diabetes. It has a gradual onset, like type II, and is often mis-diagnosed as such, but is characterized by loss of beta cell functioning in the pancreas. It cannot be reversed with diet and exercise.
   - Diabetes from other causes is a subset of diabetes caused by other hereditary or organ system dysfunctions leading to pancreatic disruption. These include etiologies such as cystic fibrosis, disrupting the exocrine function of the pancreas; toxicologic causes; mutations in insulin function; and drug/chemical causes, such as treatment for HIV/AIDS or transplantation medications.
   - Gestational diabetes mellitus (GDM) is diagnosed in the second or third trimester and is a state of insulin resistance and impaired insulin production diagnosed in pregnancy that is not overt diabetes and often resolves postpartum.

2. **What are the diagnostic criteria for diabetes mellitus?**
   The 2019 diagnostic criteria for diabetes – as agreed upon by the American Diabetes Association (ADA), International Diabetes Federation (IDF), and the European Association for the Study of Diabetes (EASD) – are outlined below and in Box 48.1. Patients are diagnosed with diabetes based on:
   - 8-Hour fasting plasma glucose (FPG) ≥126 mg/dL (7 mmol/L), **OR**
   - Hemoglobin A1c (HbA1c) level ≥6.5% (48 mmol/mol), **OR**
   - 2-Hour oral glucose tolerance test (OGTT) ≥200 mg/dL (11.1 mmol/L), **OR**
   - Classic symptoms of hyperglycemia or hyperglycemic crisis and random glucose levels of ≥200 mg/dL (11.1 mmol/L). Two separate measurements are recommended to increase sensitivity of testing.

3. **List the physiologic complications of hyperglycemia.**
   - Osmotic diuresis (polyuria)
   - Dehydration
   - Electrolyte abnormalities
   - Coronary artery disease
   - Cerebral vascular disease
   - Peripheral vascular disease
   - Nephropathy
   - Retinopathy
   - Neuropathy
   - Infection secondary to impaired leukocyte function
   - Cutaneous manifestations
   - Ketoacidosis (in type I and some type II patients)

4. **Describe the pertinent clinical and laboratory findings of DKA.**
   A patient with DKA has polyuria and polydipsia because of osmotic diuresis. This results in dehydration, drowsiness, and potentially altered mentation. Nausea, vomiting, and abdominal pain are symptoms secondary to gastric distention or stretching of the liver capsule. Other clinical signs include weight loss, tachypnea or Kussmaul respirations, and fruity breath odor from ketosis. Laboratory findings include hyperglycemia, metabolic acidosis, elevated serum potassium (intracellular potassium migration to the extracellular space), hyponatremia (and pseudohyponatremia from hyperglycemia), hypochloremia, hypocalcemia, hypomagnesemia, and hypophosphatemia.

5. **What causes DKA?**
   DKA is a state of insulin deficiency and infection is the single most common cause. Other precipitants include medication errors or noncompliance (15%), new-onset diabetes (10%), other physiologic stressors (5%), and no identified cause (40%). Insulin is the primary anabolic hormone produced by the pancreas. Without insulin, cells cannot take up glucose, resulting in an increase in the body's catabolic hormones: glucagon, catecholamines, cortisol, and growth hormone. Catabolism stimulates lipolysis, breaking down fatty acids, which are then oxidized

---

Box 48.1 Diagnostic Criteria for Diabetes

HbA1c ≥6.5%
or
FPG ≥126 mg/dL (7 mmol/L)
or
OGTT with 2-hour glucose ≥200 mg/dL (11.1 mmol/L)
or
Classic symptoms of hyperglycemia and random glucose levels ≥200 mg/dL (11.1 mmol/L)

FPG, Fasting plasma glucose; *HbA1c,* hemoglobin A1c; *OGTT,* oral glucose tolerance test.

---

to acetoacetate and β-hydroxybutyrate, resulting in a metabolic acidosis. These breakdown products are the ketones measured in DKA. The overall shift in metabolism during DKA is from a state of carbohydrate metabolism to fat metabolism.

6. **How do I make the diagnosis of DKA?**
   DKA can be mild, moderate, or severe, based on laboratory values. (Table 48.1) Often in early DKA, an anion gap can be present with a normal or only mildly low serum bicarbonate.
   - Blood glucose >250 mg/dL (>13.9 mmol/L)
   - Low bicarbonate (<15 mEq/L)
   - Low pH (<7.3) with ketonemia and ketonuria

7. **How should DKA be treated in the emergency department (ED)?**
   - *Fluid resuscitation in adults.* Patients often have a fluid deficit of 5–10 L. Normal saline (NS) should be administered by giving 15–20 mL/kg/h in the first hour. After this, titrate fluid resuscitation to urine output, blood pressure, heart rate, mental status, and serum electrolytes. If patients are eunatremic or hypernatremic, give 0.45% saline at 250–500 mL/h. In patients with hyponatremia, continue 0.9% sodium chloride (NaCl) at 250–500 mL/h. The goal is to replace all fluid deficits in the first 24 hours.
   - *Fluid resuscitation in pediatrics.* In normotensive children, give 10 mL/kg/h of fluid for the first hour. Over the next 4 hours, most patients should receive two more 10-mL/kg/h boluses with electrolyte repletion (potassium acetate/potassium phosphate). Overaggressive fluid resuscitation in children has been associated with (although not proven directly causative of) cerebral edema.
   - *Insulin.* Initial dosage is 0.1 U/kg intravenous (IV) bolus, followed by an infusion of 0.1 U/kg/h. Alternatively, start a 0.14-U/kg/h infusion without a bolus, with no difference in clinical outcome between the two methods. Blood sugar level should be checked frequently, with a goal of dropping the glucose level by 50–75 mg/dL/h. Do not start insulin before checking a potassium level, and replete potassium to greater than 3.5 mEq/L before starting insulin. In children, do not give bolus insulin. After initial fluids, start an insulin infusion at 0.1 U/kg/h.
   - *Potassium replacement.* Although serum potassium is often elevated, the serum potassium will drop as it moves intracellularly with correction of the metabolic acidosis. Once the serum potassium is <5.5 mEq/L, adding 20–40 mEq in each 1 L bag of crystalloid will help correct the deficit slowly. Goal levels are between 4 and 5 mEq/L.

Table 48.1 Diagnostic Criteria for Diabetic Ketoacidosis and Hyperosmolar Hyperglycemic State

	DKA			HHS
	Mild	Moderate	Severe	
Plasma glucose (mg/dL)	>250	>250	>600	>600
Arterial pH	7.25–7.30	7–7.24	<7.00	>7.30
Serum bicarbonate (mEq/L)	15–18	10 to <15	<10	>15
Serum ketones	Positive	Positive	Positive	Small
Urine ketones	Positive	Positive	Positive	Small
Serum Osms (mOsm/kg)	Variable	Variable	Variable	>320
Anion gap	>10	>12	>12	Variable
Mental status	Alert	Alert/drowsy	Stupor/coma	Stupor/coma

DKA, Diabetic ketoacidosis; *HHS,* hyperosmolar hyperglycemic state; *Osms,* osmolality.

- *Phosphate.* Randomized studies showed no benefit in phosphate repletion in DKA. In addition, it may cause hypocalcemia in some patients.
- *Bicarbonate.* Patients with a pH of 6.9 or greater do not require bicarbonate therapy. There are no prospective randomized trials studying bicarbonate in patients with pH less than 6.9. Given the adverse effects of severe acidosis, critically ill patients with expected deterioration may get 100 mmol of sodium bicarbonate ($NaHCO_3$) in 400 mL of sterile water with 20 mEq of potassium chloride (KCl) at a rate of 200 mL/h for 2 hours until the pH is greater than 7.
- *Glucose.* When the serum levels drop <200 mg/dL, IV fluids should be switched to half NS with the addition of 5% dextrose, and decrease the insulin infusion to 0.02–0.05 U/kg/h. Insulin infusion is still required until serum ketones are eliminated, at which point the patient can be transitioned to subcutaneous insulin. The goal for glucose in DKA is 150–200 mg/dL.
- *Magnesium and calcium.* Levels should be monitored and replaced accordingly.

8. **List the potential complications of therapy for DKA in the ED.**
   - Hypoglycemia
   - Hypokalemia (risk of dysrhythmias)
   - Hypophosphatemia
   - Adult respiratory distress syndrome
   - Cerebral edema

9. **What is the hyperosmolar hyperglycemic state (HHS)?**
   HHS (formerly termed *hyperosmolar hyperglycemic nonketotic coma*) is a life-threatening emergency, defined as severe hyperglycemia (usually >600 mg/dL), elevated plasma osmolality (>320 mOsm/kg), serum bicarbonate greater than 15 mEq/L, arterial pH greater than 7.3, negative serum ketones (can be mildly positive), and altered mental status (see Table 48.1).

10. **How is plasma osmolality determined?**

$$\text{Osmolality (mOsm/kg water)} = 2(\text{Serum sodium}) + (\text{Serum glucose}/18 + \text{BUN}/2.8)$$

   where *BUN* is *blood urea nitrogen.*

11. **What occurs pathophysiologically to cause HHS?**
    HHS is a rare presentation that usually occurs in older patients with type II diabetes and significant comorbidities. The pathophysiology is similar to DKA, without the marked generation of ketones. As in DKA, elevated glucose levels result in glucosuria and osmotic diuresis, leading to profound dehydration. Why these patients are not ketotic remains controversial. There may be some available insulin in HHS, inhibiting lipolysis. Additionally, there are lower levels of catabolic hormones found in HHS patients compared with their DKA counterparts, which is poorly understood.

12. **What are the precipitants of HHS?**
    Patients with type II diabetes and comorbid conditions, such as chronic renal disease and heart failure, are at risk of developing HHS, especially when combined with an event leading to dehydration. Causes include infections, such as pneumonia and urinary tract infections (UTIs); stroke; intracranial hemorrhage; myocardial infarction; and pulmonary embolism. Drugs are commonly implicated, including thiazide diuretics, β-blockers, histamine-2 blockers, antipsychotics, alcohol, cocaine, and total parenteral nutrition (TPN).

13. **What are the four key points in ED management of patients with HHS?**
    - *Fluid administration.* Administer 15–20 mL/kg of NS in the first hour. Fluid deficits may be as high as 10 L; however, judicious rehydration should be observed in cardiac and renal patients. Be aware of correcting hypernatremia too quickly; rehydration can usually be achieved slowly with administration of 0.45% saline at 250–500 mL/h.
    - *Potassium.* Replace at 10–20 mEq/h in patients with normal renal function.
    - *Insulin.* Low-dose insulin infusion protocols used in DKA are appropriate for HHS. Do not give an insulin bolus in HHS, and consider starting a lower dose infusion of 0.05–0.1 U/kg/h.
    - *Glucose.* Add 5% dextrose to IV fluids when levels are 300 mg/dL or less, and decrease the insulin infusion to 0.02–0.05 U/kg/h.

14. **Describe hypoglycemia.**
    Outside of the neonatal period, hypoglycemia is a serum glucose level <70 mg/dL (3.9 mmol/L), although symptoms usually occur at <50 mg/dL (2.8 mmol/L).

15. **Who develops hypoglycemia?**
    Patients who are taking hypoglycemic medications are at greatest risk for hypoglycemia. Sulfonylurea drugs (e.g., glipizide and glimepiride) and meglitinides (e.g., repaglinide and nateglinide) stimulate release of insulin from pancreatic β cells and may inhibit both gluconeogenesis in the liver and lipolysis. These drugs have long-acting metabolites, and their pharmacokinetics are affected by other medications, including antibiotics. Overdoses can

result in prolonged hypoglycemia, and usually require admission for monitoring of repeat hypoglycemic episodes. Other causes include accidental or intentional overdose (e.g., insulin, pentamidine, aspirin, haloperidol), insulinomas, renal failure, sepsis, adrenal insufficiency, alcoholism, and heart failure.

16. **Which overdoses of oral hypoglycemic agents do not cause hypoglycemia?**
    The medications listed below are often referred to as "antihyperglycemics," as they do not directly lower blood sugar.
    - Metformin overdose does not cause hypoglycemia, because it decreases hepatic production of glucose and increases insulin sensitivity. Instead, symptoms of overdose include nausea, vomiting, and abdominal pain. Lactic acidosis is a known complication of therapeutic and supratherapeutic doses of metformin. Lactic acidosis may be treated with $NaHCO_3$ or hemodialysis.
    - Thiazolidinediones (glitazones) increase peripheral tissue glucose use and do not cause hypoglycemia. Hepatotoxicity has been reported with these drugs.
    - α-Glucosidase inhibitors decrease gastrointestinal glucose absorption and do not cause hypoglycemia. Symptoms of overdose include bloating, abdominal pain, and diarrhea.
    - DPP-4 inhibitors (e.g., sitagliptin) lower blood glucose through the release of glucagon-like peptide-1 (GLP-1). It is metabolized in the liver and overdose is associated with mild to no clinical effects. Only rarely has hypoglycemia been reported in overdose.

17. **What are the presenting signs of hypoglycemia?**
    As blood glucose falls, the counter-regulatory hormones (adrenalin, glucagon) cause shakiness, diaphoresis, tachycardia, pallor, mydriasis, hunger, nausea, and vomiting. As glucose levels drop in the brain, there are neurologic manifestations that include a wide range of symptoms, such as decreased level of consciousness, slurred speech, pins-and-needles sensation, emotional lability, lethargy, coma, seizures, bizarre and sometimes violent behavior, and focal neurologic deficits. Symptoms should reverse with administration of glucose. If symptoms do not resolve, seek an alternative diagnosis.

18. **Which patients with hypoglycemia require admission to the hospital?**
    Admit patients who:
    - have a persistent altered mental status or hypoglycemia after glucose administration;
    - have taken excessive amounts of oral hypoglycemic agents or long-acting insulin;
    - are unable to tolerate oral intake.

19. **Can patients who have been treated for hypoglycemia by paramedics refuse transport?**
    Yes, this is a common scenario. Patients most commonly have taken their normal or recently adjusted dose of insulin and have skipped a meal. If these patients can eat and have decision-making capacity by all other measures (e.g., not intoxicated, not suicidal, no head injury), they may refuse transport. Patients who may have taken an intentional overdose of insulin or oral hypoglycemic agents should be transported. In addition, patients taking therapeutic dosages of oral hypoglycemics with repeat hypoglycemic episodes should be transported.

20. **Describe gestational diabetes mellitus (GDM).**
    GDM is any degree of glucose intolerance that develops in the second or third trimester of pregnancy, with clear evidence of no pre-existing type I or II diabetes, and occurs when a woman's pancreatic function cannot overcome the insulin resistance created by placental anti-insulin hormones. International consensus guidelines (2010) define GDM as a:
    - FPG level >92 mg/dL (5.1 mmol/L), OR
    - 1-hour glucose level >180 mg/dL (10 mmol/L), OR
    - 2-hour glucose level >153 mg/dL (8.5 mmol/L).
    GDM affects approximately 4% of women in the United States but varies according to ethnicity. These women are at increased risk of developing type II diabetes later in life. Untreated GDM can have serious health effects for the fetus, including fetal macrosomia, hypoglycemia, hypocalcemia, and hyperbilirubinemia.

21. **What types of infections are seen more commonly in patients with diabetes than in other patients?**
    Diabetic patients are more susceptible to UTIs, candidal vaginitis, cystitis, balanitis, pneumonia, influenza, tuberculosis, lower-extremity skin and soft-tissue infections, and bacteremia.
    - Rhinocerebral mucormycosis is a rare, rapidly progressive invasive saprophytic fungal infection of the nasal and paranasal sinuses. A computed tomography (CT) scan should be obtained to define extent of disease. Early surgical debridement is essential for good outcomes, with a mortality rate as high as 50% despite optimal management. The IV antifungal of choice is amphotericin B.
    - Malignant otitis externa is usually caused by *Pseudomonas aeruginosa*. Patients have unilateral otalgia, swelling, and discharge. The external auditory canal is initially affected; it can then cause adjacent cellulitis, osteomyelitis, and temporoparietal abscess. A CT scan should be used to image affected regions. IV antipseudomonal antibiotics, debridement, and hyperbaric oxygen are required for extensive disease.

- Emphysematous pyelonephritis and cholecystitis are more common in diabetic patients. Findings include gas on plain film, although CT may be required for diagnosis. IV antibiotics and surgical treatment are indicated. Even with prompt treatment, mortality rates can be as high as 40%.

22. **What are the common manifestations of diabetic neuropathy?**
    Patients typically exhibit a peripheral symmetric neuropathy, which often follows a stocking-glove pattern. Symptoms include bilateral pain, hyperesthesia, and anesthesia. Neuropathic pain is opioid resistant and is better treated with duloxetine (60 mg daily), gabapentin, and amitriptyline. Mononeuropathy multiplex affects motor and sensory nerves, often resulting in wrist or foot drop and affecting cranial nerves III, IV, and VI.

KEY POINTS: DIABETES MELLITUS

1. Infections in diabetic patients must be aggressively treated, because they may spread rapidly and can precipitate DKA/HHS.
2. Always measure the serum glucose in patients who are agitated, violent, diaphoretic, or comatose to rule out hypoglycemia as an easily treatable cause of these findings.
3. Because of the risk of cerebral edema, crystalloid volume replacement for DKA in children should not exceed 10 mL/kg in the first hour.

BIBLIOGRAPHY

American Diabetes Association. Classification and diagnosis of diabetes: standards of medical care in diabetes 2019. *Diabetes Care.* 2019;42(suppl 1):S13–S28.

Goyal N, Miller JB, Sankey SS, et al. Utility of initial bolus insulin in the treatment of diabetic ketoacidosis. *J Emerg Med.* 2010;38: 422–427.

IADPSG Consensus Panel. International association of diabetes and pregnancy study groups recommendations on the diagnosis and classification of hyperglycemia in pregnancy. *Diabetes Care.* 2008;33:676–682.

Kitabchi AE, Umpierrez GE, Miles JM, et al. Hyperglycemic crises in adult patients with diabetes. *Diabetes Care.* 2009;32:1335–1343.

Nattrass M. Diabetic ketoacidosis. *Medicine.* 2010;38:667–670.

Nyenwe EA, Kitabchi AE. Evidence-based management of hyperglycemic emergencies in diabetes mellitus. *Diabetes Res Clin Pract.* 2011;94:340–351.

Van Ness-Otunnu R, Hack JB. Hyperglycemic crisis. *J Emerg Med.* 2013;45(5):797–805.

CHAPTER 49

THYROID AND ADRENAL DISORDERS

Rob Klemisch, MD

1. **What thyroid-related conditions are considered true emergencies?**
   The two true emergencies are thyroid storm (severe hyperthyroidism) and myxedema coma (severe hypothyroidism). Rarely, eye complications from Graves' disease may also require emergent treatment.

2. **What are the common clinical signs and symptoms of thyrotoxicosis?**
   - Constitutional: fatigue, heat intolerance, diaphoresis, weight loss, and uncommonly fever
   - Neuropsychiatric: tremor, hyperreflexia, apathy, anxiety, irritability, emotional lability, and uncommonly psychosis
   - Ophthalmologic: exophthalmos (only seen with Graves' disease), lid lag, injection, and uncommonly diplopia and reduced visual acuity
   - Cardiovascular: tachycardia, palpitations, and, uncommonly, atrial fibrillation, chest pain, and congestive heart failure
   - Gastrointestinal: increased frequency of bowel movements or frank diarrhea, nausea, and uncommonly vomiting
   - Reproductive: amenorrhea, infertility in women, and, uncommonly gynecomastia in males
   - Dermatologic: hair loss, onycholysis

3. **What are the most common causes of hyperthyroidism and how do they present?**
   Conditions with excessive thyroid hormone production:
   - Graves' disease (85% of all cases): diffuse homogenous enlargement of the thyroid gland, often present with proptosis
   - Toxic multinodular goiter: multiple thyroid nodules and more common with advanced age
   - Hyperfunctioning nodule: large thyroid nodule, with the rest of the gland reduced in size or suppressed
   Conditions with excessive release of thyroid hormone:
   - Subacute thyroiditis: usually presents with pain and tenderness over the thyroid gland, and thought to be caused by viral infection
   - Painless thyroiditis: same as subacute thyroiditis, but without thyroid pain/tenderness
   - Postpartum thyroiditis: painless thyroiditis that occurs 1–6 months after childbirth
   - Drug-induced thyroiditis: induced by amiodarone, lithium, cytokines (e.g., interferon-α), and tyrosine kinase inhibitors that typically resolves when the drug is discontinued
   - Radiation-induced inflammation: exacerbation of Graves' disease that occurs 7–10 days after the administration of radioactive iodine therapy
   Exogenous thyroid hormone administration
   - Thyrotoxicosis factitia: thyroid hormone is taken to cause illness
   - Thyroid hormone overdose: may occur because the patient takes too much hormone (often for weight loss) or the physician prescribes too much

4. **What laboratory tests should be ordered in a patient with suspected hyperthyroidism?**
   While thyroid-stimulating hormone (TSH) level is a reasonable screening test, if thyrotoxicosis is strongly suspected, also obtain serum triiodothyronine (T_3) and a free thyroxine (T_4) level. When hyperthyroidism is caused by overproduction of thyroid hormone, TSH should be completely suppressed (<0.01 mIU/L). A patient with suppressed TSH and a normal T_3 and T_4 level has subclinical hyperthyroidism.

5. **What is apathetic thyrotoxicosis?**
   Apathetic thyrotoxicosis is a commonly missed presentation of hyperthyroidism seen most often in the elderly, but which may present at any age, even in children. Classic findings such as tremor and heat intolerance are often absent. The typical apathetic thyrotoxic patient is 70–80 years of age without goiter but with unexplained weight loss, muscle weakness, and depressed or "apathetic" affect.

6. **What is thyroid storm?**
   Thyroid storm is simply severe hyperthyroidism with serious morbidity and mortality. Clinical features characteristic of thyroid storm are temperature greater than 38°C (100.4°F), cardiovascular decompensation, and altered mental status. The challenge is that these symptoms mimic far more commonly seen emergency disorders, such as drug intoxication, alcohol withdrawal, sepsis, or cardiac disease.

7. **What is the Burch-Wartofsky score?**
   The Burch-Wartofsky score is a point scale that helps assess the degree of thyrotoxicosis independent of thyroid hormone levels. The criteria included are temperature, central nervous system effects, gastrointestinal–hepatic dysfunction, cardiovascular dysfunction, and the presence of a precipitating event. A score greater than 45 is highly suggestive of thyroid storm (Table 49.1).

8. **Which patients with hyperthyroidism should be admitted to the hospital?**
   Patients with suspected thyroid storm should be admitted. Because severe hyperthyroidism is a hypercoagulable state, those with atrial fibrillation should be admitted and anticoagulated to prevent atrial thrombus. Patients with

Table 49.1 Burch-Wartofsky Thyroid Storm Diagnostic Criteria

PARAMETERS	SCORE[a]
Thermoregulatory Dysfunction	
Oral Temperature (°F)	
99–99.9	5
100–100.9	10
101–101.9	15
102–102.9	20
103–103.9	25
≥104	30
Cardiovascular Dysfunction	
Tachycardia (beats/min)	
90–109	5
110–119	10
120–129	15
130–139	20
≥140	25
Congestive Heart Failure	
Absent	0
Mild (pedal edema)	5
Moderate (bilateral rales)	10
Severe (pulmonary edema)	15
Atrial Fibrillation	
Absent	0
Present	10
Central Nervous System Symptoms	
Absent	0
Mild agitation	10
Moderate (delirium, psychosis, extreme lethargy)	20
Severe (seizure, coma)	30
Gastrointestinal/Hepatic Dysfunction	
Absent	0
Moderate (diarrhea, nausea, vomiting, abdominal pain)	10
Severe (unexplained jaundice)	20
Precipitating Event	
Absent	0
Present	10

[a]Scores >45 are highly suggestive of thyroid storm; 25–44 are suggestive of thyroid storm; and a score <25 indicates that thyroid storm is improbable.

Modified from Burch HB, Wartofsky L. Life-threatening thyrotoxicosis. Thyroid storm. *Endocrinol Metab Clin North Am*. 1993;22:263–277.

heart failure should be admitted to determine the appropriate dosage of β-blockers in the outpatient setting. Tachycardia alone is not an indication for admission in otherwise healthy patients; β-blockade can safely be instituted as an outpatient.

9. **What conditions are included in the differential diagnosis of thyroid storm?**
A history of goiter, thyroid disease, or previous treatment with an antithyroid medication is helpful in distinguishing thyroid storm from the following other conditions:
- sympathomimetic (i.e., cocaine, amphetamine) and anticholinergic ingestion.
- alcohol, benzodiazepine, γ-hydroxybutyrate, or baclofen withdrawal
- infections such as encephalitis, meningitis, and sepsis

10. **What conditions precipitate thyroid storm?**
Thyroid storm can be precipitated by the following:
- infection
- surgery
- trauma
- childbirth
- myocardial infarction, stroke, or pulmonary embolus
- withdrawal of antithyroid therapy
- recent ^{131}I thyroid ablation therapy

11. **How is hyperthyroidism treated in the emergency department (ED)?**
For most patients, treatment with a β-blocker can be initiated if there is no evidence of overt heart failure or other contraindications to β-blockers. Although propranolol blocks the conversion of T_4 to T_3, it needs to be taken at least three times a day in the patient with hyperthyroidism because of more rapid metabolism. Metoprolol or atenolol are alternatives which are taken once to twice daily, with potentially better compliance. Methimazole or propylthiouracil can be initiated, though their use interferes with thyroid scanning. Typically, start with a β-blocker and refer the patient for follow-up. ED management of thyroid storm is outlined in Table 49.2. Recent literature suggests that patients with intolerance or allergy to medications, or refractory thyroid storm, can also be treated with therapeutic plasmapheresis.

KEY POINTS: THYROID DISORDERS

1. Thyroid disease is common but thyroid storm and myxedema coma are rare.
2. Thyroid storm is a life-threatening emergency.
3. Thyroid storm presents similarly to infection, stimulant ingestion, and alcohol withdrawal. The diagnosis is easily missed; keep it on your differential.

Table 49.2 Stepwise Therapy for Thyroid Storm

1. Supportive Measures
- General: oxygen, cardiac monitor, intravenous fluids
- Fever: external cooling, acetaminophen (aspirin is contraindicated as it may increase free T_4)
- Nutrition: glucose, multivitamins including folate (deficient secondary to hypermetabolism)
- Cardiac decompensation: β-blockers
  - Propranolol 60–80 mg every 4 hours (preferred in thyroid storm as it blocks T_4 to T_3 conversion)
  or
  - Esmolol 50–100 μg/kg/min (preferred with significant heart failure)
- Treat precipitating event as indicated

2. Inhibition of Hormone Biosynthesis: Thionamides
- PTU 500–1000 mg load followed by 250 mg every 4 hours (preferred over methimazole as it also blocks conversion of T_4 to T_3)
  or
- Methimazole 60–80 mg/day

3. Blockade of Hormone Release: Iodides (at least 1 hour after step 2)
- SSKI 5 drops every 6 hours (alternative: Lugol's solution)

4. Blockade of the Peripheral Conversion of T_4 to T_3
- Hydrocortisone 300 mg IV load, then 100 mg every 8 hours (alternative: dexamethasone)

IV, Intravenous; *PTU,* propylthiouracil; *SSKI,* supersaturated potassium iodide; T_3, triiodothyronine; T_4, thyroxine.
From Ross DS, Burch HB, Cooper DS, et al. 2016 American Thyroid Association guidelines for diagnosis and management of hyperthyroidism and other causes of thyrotoxicosis. *Thyroid.* 2016;26:1343–1421.

12. **What is Graves' ophthalmopathy (orbitopathy)?**

Graves' ophthalmopathy is an autoimmune disorder of the eye and surrounding structures closely related to Graves' disease. Clinical features include periorbital edema, proptosis, eyelid retraction, chemosis, diplopia, reduced eye movement, and exposure keratopathy. A loss in visual acuity is a particularly concerning finding.

13. **When is treatment of Graves' ophthalmopathy an emergent condition?**

Patients with compression of the optic nerve or corneal ulceration require immediate ophthalmologic evaluation. Visual and diminished color brightness suggests compression of the optic nerve. High-dose steroids remain first line, but newer immune suppressing agents are being used more frequently, and surgical decompression of the orbit or external orbital radiation may also be required. Intravenous (IV) steroids have been shown to be superior to oral doses, but often a prolonged course is required, so discussing with an ophthalmologist is beneficial. Severe proptosis can cause keratitis or corneal ulceration, and may present as eye pain, photophobia, conjunctival infection, visual loss, and cell and flare in the anterior chamber. Corneal ulcers, with or without keratitis, require topical antibiotics.

14. **What is thyrotoxic periodic paralysis?**

Thyrotoxic periodic paralysis is a rare condition typically seen in Asian men who have episodic muscle weakness and hypokalemia in the setting of hyperthyroidism (most commonly Graves' disease). This disorder is distinct from hypokalemic periodic paralysis, but has been linked to genetic mutations in genes which code for specific ion channels, and is also associated with hypokalemia. Appropriate treatment includes potassium replacement, followed by treatment of the hyperthyroidism.

15. **What are the common clinical manifestations of hypothyroidism?**
- Constitutional: fatigue, cold intolerance, weight gain, lethargy, hoarse or deep voice, slow speech, facial puffiness, and drowsiness
- Neuropsychiatric: delayed relaxation of deep tendon reflexes, depression, moodiness, and, rarely, dementia or psychosis
- Cardiovascular: bradycardia and, less commonly, congestive heart failure, and, rarely, pericardial effusion
- Respiratory: dyspnea, obstructive sleep apnea, hypoventilation, and, rarely, pleural effusions
- Gastrointestinal: constipation, anorexia
- Musculoskeletal: joint swelling, myalgias, muscle weakness, carpal tunnel syndrome
- Dermatologic: cool, dry skin and hair loss
- Gynecologic: menometrorrhagia

16. **What are the most common causes of hypothyroidism?**

The two main categories of hypothyroidism are primary and secondary. Primary hypothyroidism is caused by thyroid gland dysfunction (TSH is increased and T_4 is decreased). A patient with an increased TSH but a normal T_4 has subclinical hypothyroidism.
- *Autoimmune thyroid destruction.* Hashimoto thyroiditis (most common cause), thyroid gland may be firm or small.
- *Thyroiditis.* After a period of hyperthyroidism, the gland may be hypofunctioning permanently (or transiently over 1–2 years).
- *Hypothyroidism* after thyroidectomy or radioactive iodine treatment.

    Secondary hypothyroidism is caused by pituitary or hypothalamic insufficiency, resulting in inadequate TSH secretion. TSH is typically normal (or low), and T_4 is also low. These patients typically show signs and symptoms of follicle-stimulating hormone (FSH)/luteinizing hormone (LH) deficiency (amenorrhea in women, hypogonadism in men) and may have signs of adrenocorticotropic hormone (ACTH) deficiency.
- Pituitary tumor
- Pituitary infarction: Sheehan syndrome (after childbirth) or pituitary apoplexy (hemorrhage into a preexisting pituitary tumor)
- Meningioma or craniopharyngioma near the hypothalamus

17. **What additional features are present in severe hypothyroidism (or myxedema coma)?**

The hallmark clinical features of myxedema are hypothermia and altered mental status (ranging from lethargy to coma) but patients will often have bradycardia, hypoventilation, and hypotension. Laboratory evaluation may reveal anemia, hyponatremia, hypoglycemia, hypercarbia with associated respiratory acidosis, or respiratory failure. An electrocardiogram (ECG) may show bradycardia with low voltages that may be caused by a pericardial effusion. The chest radiograph may show cardiomegaly, pleural effusions, or pulmonary edema.

18. **What precipitates myxedema coma in the patient with hypothyroidism?**

As with thyroid storm, myxedema coma is typically precipitated by concurrent illness, sedatives and anesthetic agents, trauma, myocardial infarction, cerebrovascular accident, or gastrointestinal hemorrhage. Prolonged cold exposure may also be a trigger. Even moderate hypothyroidism may be life threatening in patients with underlying hypoxia, hypercapnia, or congestive heart failure.

Table 49.3 Treatment for Myxedema Coma
• Supportive care
• Airway control, oxygen, IV access, and cardiac monitor (ABCs)
• Hypotension: crystalloids and vasopressors as indicated (often ineffective without thyroid hormone replacement)
• Hypothermia: passive rewarming (e.g., Bair Hugger warming system)
• Identification and treatment of precipitating factors and measure baseline thyroid studies
• Measure cortisol and treat empirically with stress dose glucocorticoids (such as IV hydrocortisone 100 mg every 8 hours). This can avoid precipitating adrenal insufficiency when thyroid hormone is replaced
• Thyroid replacement therapy
• Give IV T_4 (200–400 µg load followed by IV 1.2 µg/kg/day until oral medication is tolerated)
• Treatment of concomitant metabolic abnormalities, including hyponatremia, hypoglycemia, and hypercalcemia

ABCs, Airway, breathing, circulation; *IV,* intravenous; T_4, thyroxine.
Adapted from Jonklaas J, Bianco AC, Bauer AJ, et al. Guidelines for the treatment of hypothyroidism. *Thyroid.* 2014;24:1670–1751.

19. **What is the treatment for myxedema coma?**
    See Table 49.3.

20. **What advice should be given to the patient when a thyroid nodule is palpated on examination or incidentally found on a radiologic study?**
    Thyroid nodules are very common (4%–7% of the population has a palpable node), and though typically benign, approximately 5% are cancerous. All patients with a newly discovered thyroid nodule should have serum TSH measured and a thyroid sonography with cervical lymph nodes performed. These can be done as an outpatient in clinically stable patients. Depending on the results of the ultrasound and TSH levels, more testing is often indicated as an outpatient.

21. **What are the adrenal emergencies that I need to worry about?**
    The two most serious adrenal emergencies, acute adrenal insufficiency (adrenal crisis) and pheochromocytoma crisis, are discussed in more detail below.
    Hypercortisolism can be caused by a pituitary tumor secreting ACTH, ectopic ACTH secretion from a nonpituitary tumor, or an adrenal tumor secreting cortisol. It may present with weight gain, hypertension, amenorrhea, insulin resistance, or frank diabetes. The specific physical findings in this condition include wide (>1 cm) purple striae, easy bruising, and proximal muscle weakness.
    Hyperaldosteronism is an underrecognized cause of hypertension that may present with hypokalemia, which may be particularly severe when the patient is also taking a thiazide diuretic.

22. **What is the difference between primary and secondary adrenal insufficiency?**
    • Primary adrenal insufficiency, also referred to as Addison disease, is caused by failure of the adrenal gland.
    • Secondary adrenal insufficiency is the result of inadequate production of ACTH by the hypothalamic–pituitary axis.

23. **List the signs and symptoms of primary adrenal insufficiency.**
    Thomas Addison described primary adrenal insufficiency in 1855 as including weakness, fatigue, anorexia, salt craving, abdominal pain, hyperpigmentation, and orthostatic hypotension.
    • *Hyperpigmentation.* Marked "tanning" in palmar creases, as well as mucosal membranes, is seen in primary adrenal insufficiency due to increased melanocyte-stimulating hormone (MSH), which is oversecreted, along with ACTH.
    • *Gastrointestinal symptoms.* Nausea, vomiting, abdominal pain, and diarrhea occur, and abdominal pain may be severe and mimic an acute abdomen.
    • *Neurologic symptoms.* Clouded sensorium to coma may occur depending on severity.
    • *Hypotension.* This typically presents with orthostatic changes but can be more severe. Think of adrenal insufficiency when hypotension does not respond to vasopressors.
    • *Fever.* Temperatures as high as 40°C (104°F) may be seen in acute adrenal insufficiency.

24. **List the causes of adrenal insufficiency.**
    See Table 49.4.

25. **What are the most common causes of primary adrenal insufficiency?**
    Up to 90% of cases are the caused by autoimmune disorders in Western countries, but infectious diseases make up a larger proportion worldwide, with tuberculosis being among the most common. Other etiologies include granulomatous diseases, uncontrolled HIV infection, metastatic cancer, and adrenal hemorrhage.

Table 49.4 Causes of Adrenal Insufficiency

PRIMARY ADRENAL INSUFFICIENCY	SECONDARY ADRENAL INSUFFICIENCY
Idiopathic (autoimmune)	Exogenous glucocorticoid administration
Tuberculosis	Pituitary or suprasellar tumor
Bilateral adrenal hemorrhage or infarction	Pituitary irradiation or surgery
AIDS	Head trauma
Drugs	Infiltrative disorders of the pituitary or hypothalamus
Aminoglutethimide	Sarcoidosis
Etomidate	Hemochromatosis
Ketoconazole	Histiocytosis X
Infections	Metastatic cancer
Fungal or bacterial sepsis	Lymphoma
Infiltrative disorders	Infectious diseases
Sarcoidosis	Tuberculosis
Hemochromatosis	Meningitis
Myeloidosis	Fungus
Lymphoma	Isolated ACTH deficiency
Metastatic cancer	
Bilateral surgical adrenalectomy	
Hereditary	
Adrenal hypoplasia	
Congenital adrenal hyperplasia	
Adrenoleukodystrophy	
Familial glucocorticoid deficiency	

ACTH, Adrenocorticotropic hormone.

26. What is the most common cause of secondary adrenal insufficiency?
Long-term glucocorticoid therapy is the most common cause of secondary adrenal insufficiency and is the result of suppression of the hypothalamic–pituitary–adrenal (HPA) axis.

27. How long must a patient be treated with steroids to cause suppression of the HPA axis, and how long does it take them to recover normal function?
Patients receiving maximal stress doses of steroids (e.g., $\geq$60 mg/day of prednisone) for over 1 week may have a blunted response to ACTH, though these short courses do not often cause clinically significant adrenal deficiency. The time it takes to suppress the hypothalamic–pituitary axis to a significant degree depends on the dose of steroids, length of use, and the individual patient. If a person has been taking maximal stress doses of steroids for many months or years and then the medications are gradually tapered, they may be able to make enough cortisol for normal daily functioning. However, when ill or injured, they may exhibit signs and symptoms of adrenal insufficiency even 1–2 years later.

28. What are the characteristic laboratory findings of primary adrenal insufficiency?
Hyperkalemia may be present from lack of aldosterone as well as cortisol deficiency. Hyponatremia may be present and is caused by lack of aldosterone and the syndrome of inappropriate secretion of antidiuretic hormone (SIADH). Cortisol is one of the counter-regulatory hormones that increase liver glucose production with fasting. In the setting of adrenal insufficiency, hypoglycemia may develop if the patient has not eaten. Anemia and an increase in eosinophils may be seen. Rarely, adrenal insufficiency causes hypercalcemia.

29. How is the presentation of secondary adrenal insufficiency different from that of primary adrenal insufficiency?
In secondary adrenal insufficiency, there is no deficiency of aldosterone secretion. As a result, these patients do not have hyperkalemia. Hypotension, hypoglycemia, and hyponatremia can be seen in both primary and secondary adrenal insufficiency. Patients who have adrenal insufficiency from a suppressed HPA axis (i.e., chronic steroid use) may have a cushingoid appearance. If the patient has a pituitary or hypothalamic cause for the adrenal insufficiency, findings may include symptoms of other pituitary hormone deficiencies, such as hypothyroidism, amenorrhea in women, or hypogonadism in men.

30. What is adrenal crisis?
Adrenal crisis is an acute and more severe form of adrenal insufficiency. It typically presents in patients with chronic adrenal insufficiency and an acute stressor (e.g., an acute myocardial infarction, systemic infection, surgery, or trauma) who are unable to increase their circulating cortisol levels. No current well-accepted scoring system or definition exists, but major clinical features are hypotension and hypovolemia.

31. **What is the most common iatrogenic cause of acute adrenal crisis?**
The most common iatrogenic cause of acute adrenal crisis is rapid withdrawal of steroids in patients who have been taking long-term steroids.

32. **How is adrenal crisis diagnosed?**
Although many of the signs and symptoms are nonspecific (e.g., fever, abdominal pain, hypotension, fatigue, anorexia), they should raise your suspicion if the patient has a history of being treated with steroids, has a history of a pituitary tumor, has AIDS, or has known metastatic cancer or other predisposing conditions. A rapid ACTH stimulation test can confirm the diagnosis. Presumptively treating without testing precludes a definitive diagnosis and also makes future testing difficult so avoid this in clinically stable patients. A random cortisol level is often indeterminate.

33. **How is the rapid ACTH stimulation test performed?**
A baseline cortisol level is determined at time 0 and is followed by an IV 0.25-mg dose of cosyntropin (synthetic ACTH). Cortisol levels are then checked 30 and 60 minutes later.

34. **What if the patient needs emergent treatment with steroids? Should I withhold treatment until the rapid ACTH stimulation test has been done?**
No. If your patient is unstable, begin treatment using a glucocorticoid that will not cross react with the cortisol assay. A test for cortisol levels can be done and then followed by IV dexamethasone (4–10 mg). Cosyntropin 0.25 mg is then given, and serum cortisol levels are checked 30 and 60 minutes later.

35. **How is acute adrenal insufficiency/adrenal crisis treated?**
Stress-dose steroids should be promptly administered once the diagnosis of acute adrenal insufficiency is considered and the ACTH stimulation test has been initiated. Initial treatment includes 100 mg of IV hydrocortisone and a bolus of 1000 mL of crystalloid containing 5% dextrose. After the initial boluses, give further IV fluids as needed and begin an IV hydrocortisone infusion of 200 mg/day. Decrease the infusion to 100 mg/day the following day. Perform a detailed history and examination to identify any precipitant of the adrenal insufficiency. In unstable patients, begin empiric broad-spectrum antibiotics while waiting for culture results. Mineralocorticoid replacement is usually unnecessary with hydrocortisone.

KEY POINTS: ADRENAL CRISIS

1. Consider adrenal crisis in all hypotensive patients, especially if they are unresponsive to vasopressors.
2. All patients in adrenal crisis require rapid administration of IV steroids.
3. Dexamethasone may be initiated in adrenal crisis without affecting the cosyntropin (ACTH) stimulation test.
4. Prolonged high-dose steroid use can cause adrenal suppression, making a patient more prone to adrenal crisis.

36. **What should be done for the patient with chronic adrenal insufficiency who has an illness or injury?**
Administer a dose of hydrocortisone that is between the daily replacement dosage and the maximal stress dosage, depending on the degree of illness. Simple home management of a febrile illness may warrant doubling the home dose of steroid until recovery for fever >38°C or tripling it for fever >39°C. More severe stresses such as a major surgery may require the same dosing as for adrenal crisis. All patients should be counseled to have a medical identification bracelet for future episodes, should they be critically ill and not able to communicate.

37. **What are the signs and symptoms of pheochromocytoma?**
Pheochromocytoma is a tumor of the adrenal medulla or sympathetic ganglia that makes excessive catecholamines (e.g., epinephrine, norepinephrine, or dopamine). The classic symptoms of a pheochromocytoma include severe headache, palpitations, and sweating. These symptoms, occurring in the setting of severe hypertension, especially if symptoms are episodic, should raise suspicion for pheochromocytoma. Other symptoms include nervousness, tremor, weight loss, and hyperglycemia.

38. **Which patients with hypertension should be evaluated for pheochromocytoma?**
Only around 0.2%–0.6% of outpatients with hypertension will have pheochromocytoma. Though rare, patients with episodic hypertension, hypertension that requires four or more medications to control, or hypertension that began before age 35 years or after age 60 should raise suspicion for pheochromocytoma. Also, patients that have symptoms provoked by medications, such as β-blockers, sympathomimetics, or dopamine antagonists, should also raise suspicion and prompt testing. Patients who are hypertensive and have a family history of severe episodic hypertension, or components of multiple endocrine neoplasia type 2 (medullary thyroid cancer, hyperparathyroidism, and pheochromocytoma) are also at higher risk.

39. **What is unique about the treatment of hypertension in a patient with pheochromocytoma?**
   The most important thing to remember is to not to use β-blockers as the first-line treatment. β-Blockade will result in unopposed α-receptor activation, which will increase vasoconstriction and worsen hypertension. Institute α-blockade early, with medications like phenoxybenzamine or prazosin. Labetalol or carvedilol, having both α- and β-blocking activities, may also be used.

BIBLIOGRAPHY

Allolio B. Extensive expertise in endocrinology: adrenal crisis. *Eur J Endocrinol* . 2015;172:R115–R124.

Chiha M, Samarasinghe S, Kabaker AS. Thyroid storm: an updated review. *J Intensive Care Med.* 2015;30:131–140.

Galindo RJ, Hurtado CR, Pasquel FJ, et al. National trends in incidence, mortality, and clinical outcomes of patients hospitalized for thyrotoxicosis with and without thyroid storm in the United States, 2004-2013. *Thyroid.* 2019;29:36–43.

Garber JR, Cobin RH, Gharib H, et al. Clinical practice guidelines for hypothyroidism in adults: cosponsored by the American Association of Clinical Endocrinologists and the American Thyroid Association. *Endocr Pract.* 2012;18:988–1028.

Hampton J. Thyroid gland disorder emergencies: thyroid storm and myxedema coma. *AACN Adv Crit Care.* 2013;34:325–332.

Haugen BR, Alexander EK, Bible KC, et al. 2015 American Thyroid Association management guidelines for adult patients with thyroid nodules and differentiated thyroid cancer. *Thyroid.* 2016;26:1–133.

Jonklaas J, Bianco AC, Bauer AJ, et al. Guidelines for the treatment of hypothyroidism: prepared by the American Thyroid Association task force on thyroid hormone replacement. *Thyroid.* 2014;24:1670–1751.

Lenders JW, Duh QY, Eisenhofer G, et al. Pheochromocytoma and paraganglioma: an Endocrine Society clinical practice guideline. *J Clin Endocrinol Metab.* 2014;99:1915–1942.

Meseeha M, Parsamehr B, Kissell K, Attiac M. Thyrotoxic periodic paralysis: a case study and review of the literature. *J Community Hosp Intern Med Perspect.* 2017;7:103–106.

Ross DS, Burch HB, Cooper DS, et al. 2016 American Thyroid Association guidelines for diagnosis and management of hyperthyroidism and other causes of thyrotoxicosis. *Thyroid.* 2016;26:1343–1421.

Simsir IY, Ozdemir M, Duman S, et al. Therapeutic plasmapheresis in thyrotoxic patients. *Endocrine.* 2018;62:144–148.

Tu X, Dong Y, Zhang H, et al. Corticosteroids for Graves' ophthalmopathy: systematic review and meta-analysis. *Biomed Res Int.* 2018;2018:4845894.

CHAPTER 50

SEPSIS SYNDROMES AND TOXIC SHOCK

Stephen J. Wolf, MD and Paul A. Leccese, MD

1. How is sepsis defined?
Sepsis is now defined as life-threatening organ dysfunction caused by a dysregulated host response to infection. There are two working definitions for the diagnosis of sepsis in clinical use. The first, and older definition, is the combination of SIRS (systemic inflammatory response syndrome) criteria with suspicion for an infectious source. The second, recommended by the Surviving Sepsis Campaign published in 2016, is two out of the three qSOFA (quick sequential organ failure assessment) criteria.

2. What SIRS?
As its name implies, it is a syndrome of inflammation, not necessarily infection.

3. What are the SIRS criteria?
A patient must meet two of the following four criteria to be diagnosed with SIRS:
1. Temperature $>100.4°F$ ($38°C$) or $<95°F$ ($35°C$)
2. Heart rate >90 beats per minute
3. Respiratory rate >20 breaths per minute or arterial partial pressure of carbon dioxide ($PaCO_2$) <32 mmHg
4. Serum white blood cell count $> 12,000$ mm^3 or < 4000 mm^3, or 10% band forms

4. What are the qSOFA criteria?
A patient must fulfill two out of the following three criteria to be diagnosed with sepsis:
1. Tachypnea with respiratory rate at least 22/minute
2. Hypotension with systolic blood pressure <100 mmHg
3. Altered mental status, defined as Glasgow Coma Scale (GCS) <15

5. What is the diagnostic performance of SIRS compared with qSOFA for predicting patients at risk of decompensating due to sepsis?
The qSOFA criteria were 60.8% sensitive and 72% specific for mortality in a recent meta-analysis; SIRS criteria were 88.1% sensitive and 25.8% specific for mortality. Research is ongoing to determine the best criteria to use, but neither will be perfect.

6. What distinguishes sepsis from septic shock?
Septic shock is now defined as a subset of sepsis with circulatory and cellular/metabolic dysfunction associated with a higher risk of mortality. Clinically, septic shock can be defined as patients meeting the above criteria for sepsis with hypotension refractory to fluid resuscitation. The older definition of severe sepsis (sepsis complicated by organ dysfunction), while no longer endorsed by the Surviving Sepsis Campaign, is still in widespread clinical use.

7. What is the significance of an elevated lactate level in sepsis?
An elevated serum lactate concentration identifies tissue hypoperfusion. Although lactate measurements may be useful and correlate with mortality, they lack precision as a measure of tissue metabolic status. As an example, multiple studies have correlated a serum lactate >4 mmol/L with increased mortality (30%–40% in some studies).

8. What organ systems can become dysfunctional, suggesting severe sepsis?
- Cardiovascular: vasodilation, poor myocardial contractility and increased cardiac oxygen demand, systemic hypotension, or cardiac ischemia
- Central nervous system: altered mental status
- Global tissue hypoperfusion: elevated lactate of 4 mmol/L or greater
- Hematologic: increasing prothrombin time (PT), international normalized ratio (INR), partial thromboplastin time (PTT), hemolysis and thrombocytopenia, or disseminated intravascular coagulation (DIC)
- Liver: coagulopathy, jaundice, or elevated transaminases
- Renal: acute renal failure determined by increase in blood urea nitrogen (BUN) and creatinine, or decreased urine output to less than 0.5 mL/kg/h
- Pulmonary: acute respiratory distress syndrome, respiratory failure, or unexplained hypoxia

9. What is the mortality rate of sepsis versus septic shock?
The mortality rate of sepsis is as high as 20%, whereas septic shock has an up to 40% mortality rate.

10. **What is the primary goal of resuscitation in a septic patient?**
Resuscitation aims to ensure that oxygen delivery meets oxygen demand of tissues affected by the septic state. Essential components of resuscitation include fluids to restore tissue perfusion and ensuring adequate source control.

11. **Describe early goal-directed therapy (EGDT). What benefits was it shown to have?**
Historically, EGDT was shown to decrease mortality by 16% in severe sepsis and septic shock compared with what was, at the time, usual care. It was a protocol for resuscitation, including fluids and vasopressors to optimize central venous pressure (CVP) and mean arterial pressure (MAP), ensure adequate urine output, transfuse packed red blood cells to a hematocrit of at least 30%, and maintain a central venous oxygen saturation ($ScvO_2$) of at least 70% using inotropes.

12. **What is the current role of EGDT in the management of septic shock?**
Many large, multicenter randomized controlled trials have shown that protocolized management of sepsis to specific goals to be no better than liberal fluids, early vasopressors, and source control. Most notably, the routine use of inotropes, CVP monitoring, $ScvO_2$ monitoring, and transfusion strategies to hematocrit of 30% are no longer favored, because they have been shown to have no influence on mortality.

13. **What are the benefits to early, protocol-guided resuscitation of septic patients?**
While EGDT as a protocol-driven strategy is no longer recommended by the Surviving Sepsis Campaign guidelines, the general principles still apply. For example, multiple studies have shown an association between early antibiotics and improved outcomes. However, it is essential to note that source control often requires more than just appropriate antimicrobial coverage, and may require procedural intervention in some cases. Other studies have shown an association between adherence to the 3-hour sepsis "bundle" with improved outcomes.

14. **What are the components to the sepsis "bundle?"**
The Centers for Medicare and Medicaid Services (CMS) has provided a panel of interventions that it recommends are completed within 3 hours of patients with suspected sepsis arriving to the emergency department (ED). The components include administration of a 30 mL/kg fluid bolus, blood cultures collected prior to administration of antibiotics, early antibiotics to cover the suspected source, and checking a lactate level. Notably, antibiotics should not be delayed if blood cultures cannot be quickly obtained.

15. **Which fluid type should be used for resuscitation of the septic patient?**
Historically, colloids such as albumin were administered in order to prolong the amount of time the fluid would stay in the vascular space. However, studies showed no benefit to colloid as compared with crystalloids such as normal saline (NS) or lactated Ringer's (LR) solution. There have been many studies examining the difference in outcomes between balanced crystalloid, such as LR, or unbalanced fluids, such NS, with conflicting outcomes. However, a recent large randomized controlled trial did show a benefit (reduced rates of kidney injury and renal replacement therapy) to the use of balanced fluids compared with NS.

16. **When should vasopressors be administered?**
Vasopressors should be considered any time the patient's shock (tissue hypoperfusion) is felt to be unresponsive to further fluid resuscitation. There is currently no accepted standard for exactly what volume of fluids should be given. There is at least one study that has shown that earlier administration of vasopressors improved outcomes in patient with sepsis and hypotension. Multiple markers of end-organ perfusion should be followed, such as mental status, urine output, and lactate clearance, to determine whether a septic patient is continuing to display shock physiology and might benefit from vasopressors. The goal MAP in septic patients is typically 65 mmHg.

17. **Which vasopressor should be used in septic shock?**
Norepinephrine is typically used as the first-line vasopressor in septic shock. There is some weak, and conflicting, evidence in the literature for the use of vasopressin as a second-line vasopressor for shock refractory to norepinephrine. Inotropes such as dobutamine no longer have a role in septic shock. Dopamine, while historically favored in septic shock, has now been shown to be inferior to norepinephrine. Epinephrine can be considered as a second-line agent for shock refractory to other agents.

18. **What other pharmacologic therapies can be used as adjuncts?**
The mainstays of treatment include adequate fluid resuscitation, early source control, and vasopressors. However, some studies have shown a benefit to steroids (usually glucocorticoids, though mineralocorticoids have also been used in some cases) while others have not. This is a source of controversy in the literature. Vitamin C and thiamine are new, and still controversial, therapies that have shown some benefit in small retrospective studies.
A large randomized controlled trial is currently underway to study this further.

19. **What is the role of glycemic control in sepsis syndromes?**
There are data to demonstrate that, in critically ill patients, there is a reduction in intensive care unit (ICU) mortality with appropriately controlled glucose (level between 110 and 180 mg/dL). Protocols aiming for tighter glycemic control (<110 mg/mL) have been shown to be associated with higher rates of severe hypoglycemia and mortality. It is recommended that an appropriate insulin-controlled glucose protocol be started in critically ill patients in the ED.

20. **What is toxic shock syndrome (TSS)?**
    TSS is a clinical syndrome characterized by shock and multiorgan failure. It is characterized by a rapidly progressing constellation of symptoms, caused by one of several different bacterial exotoxins that act as a superantigen to stimulate an excessive immune response. Symptoms include high fever, headache, confusion, conjunctival hyperemia, and gastrointestinal symptoms, which are accompanied by a characteristic scarlatiniform rash and severe shock.

21. **Which bacteria are associated with TSS?**
    Although originally linked to *Staphylococcus aureus,* the same toxin-mediated syndrome has been described with other bacterial infections, including community-acquired methicillin-resistant *S. aureus* (MRSA), group A streptococcus, and certain clostridial infections, each of which cause TSS-like symptoms through the production of different endotoxins.

22. **Who gets TSS?**
    Menses was associated with 91% of cases reported by 1980, which quickly pointed to the use of new high-absorbency tampons as a risk factor. Such tampons, made with cross-linked carboxymethylcellulose and polyester foam, were thought to provide an ideal environment for the expression of TSS toxin and subsequently were removed from the market. Current risk factors include air-containing foreign bodies (e.g., tampons, nasal packing), recent surgery, postpartum state, burns, local trauma (bruising or open skin wounds), and focal infections (e.g., cutaneous and subcutaneous lesions, mastitis, sinusitis, and wound infections).

23. **Describe the pathophysiology of TSS.**
    Three stages have been identified:
    1. Local proliferation of the toxin-producing strain of bacteria
    2. Toxin production
    3. Immune response to the toxin, which sets off the inflammatory cascade and leads to multisystem organ involvement
       Although many different bacteria from a wide variety of sources have been reported to cause TSS, the common link between infection and TSS is the production of a superantigen, which stimulates massive cytokine release and a systemic inflammatory response leading to shock.

24. **List the criteria for defining a case of TSS caused by *S. aureus.***
    - Temperature >102°F (38.9°C)
    - Hypotension
    - Diffuse macular erythematous rash with desquamation, usually of the palms or soles, after 1–2 weeks after symptom onset
    - Involvement of three or more of the following organ systems:
      - Gastrointestinal: vomiting or diarrhea
      - Muscular: myalgias or elevated creatine phosphokinase (twice normal)
      - Mucous membrane: vaginal, oropharyngeal, or conjunctival hyperemia
      - Renal: elevated BUN or creatinine (twice normal), or pyuria in the absence of urinary tract infection
      - Hepatic: total bilirubin, alanine aminotransferase, aspartate aminotransferase levels at least twice the upper limit of normal
      - Hematologic: platelet count less than 100,000/mm^3
      - Central nervous system: disorientation or alteration in consciousness without focal neurologic signs (when fever and hypotension are absent)
    - Negative results for the following, if obtained:
      - Blood, throat, or cerebrospinal fluid cultures (blood cultures may be positive for *S. aureus*)
      - Rise in titer to Rocky Mountain spotted fever, leptospirosis, or rubeola

25. **How is the diagnosis of streptococcal TSS made?**
    Diagnosis requires the isolation of streptococci from a sterile or nonsterile site, hypotension, and multisystem organ involvement (at least two or more of the following):
    - Renal impairment
    - Coagulopathy causing DIC or thrombocytopenia
    - Hepatitis
    - Adult respiratory distress syndrome
    - Necrotizing soft-tissue infections
    - Skin changes similar to those seen in *S. aureus* TSS

26. **Describe the rash associated with TSS.**
    The rash is a macular erythroderma that blanches and is not pruritic. It may be diffuse or localized and often is described as being like a sunburn. It appears early in the illness and fades in about 3 days. It may be subtle and can be missed in dark-skinned patients.

27. When is desquamation likely to occur?

Loss of skin, usually of the distal extremities, invariably occurs in survivors 5–12 days after the illness starts. Delayed alopecia and fingernail loss may occur later, and seem to depend on the level of hypotension during the acute illness.

28. Given the previously mentioned criteria for TSS, list the differential diagnoses.

- Colorado tick fever
- Drug reactions
- Erythema multiforme
- Kawasaki disease
- Leptospirosis
- Measles
- Meningococcemia
- Rocky Mountain spotted fever
- Sepsis
- Staphylococcal scalded skin syndrome
- Stevens-Johnson syndrome
- Streptococcal scarlet fever
- Toxic epidermal necrolysis

29. Summarize the treatment for TSS.

- Supportive care with EGDT
- Identification and removal of the source of infection (e.g., tampon, abscess, nasal packing)
- Appropriate antibiotics
- Intravenous immunoglobulin (IVIG) can be considered for streptococcal, but not staphylococcal, toxic shock syndrome

30. What antibiotics should I use?

Vancomycin should be used to cover MRSA infections, which are becoming increasingly prevalent. Clindamycin is a mainstay of therapy for the added advantage of a direct antitoxin effect. In addition, administer broad-spectrum antibiotics, such as a penicillin/β-lactamase inhibitor combination (e.g., piperacillin-tazobactam). If not tolerated, such as due to allergy, a carbapenem (e.g., meropenem) can be substituted.

31. Are there other therapies that can help control the immune response to the toxin?

A recent meta-analysis provided some clarity regarding the use of IVIG for streptococcal TSS, showing an absolute mortality benefit of 18%. However, data regarding IVIG in staphylococcal TSS are limited, and most authorities currently do not recommend routine use of IVIG in these patients. While corticosteroids would theoretically help attenuate the systemic response to the toxin, there are no prospective studies to show efficacy in TSS. Furthermore, steroid use in sepsis is still a matter of controversy in the literature.

32. Do all patients with TSS need admission?

Patients in whom TSS is suspected should be admitted, because this toxin-mediated disease can progress rapidly. In most patients, the systemic signs of illness (e.g., hypotension, fever, and multisystem organ involvement) are present in the ED, clearly indicating the need for inpatient supportive care.

33. What about the asplenic patient?

Any asplenic patient who meets SIRS criteria should be presumed to have pneumococcal sepsis and should immediately be treated with the appropriate antibiotics.

KEY POINTS: SEPSIS SYNDROMES AND TOXIC SHOCK

1. Use protocol-driven resuscitation to manage sepsis in all patients who come to the ED with SIRS and a presumed infectious source.
2. In patients with severe sepsis, initiate early fluid resuscitation and antibiotic or other therapy to achieve source control to reduce mortality.
3. Consider norepinephrine as the first-line vasopressor for treatment of sepsis with hypotension refractory to the initial fluid bolus.
4. Consider TSS in any patient with a rapidly progressive shock syndrome and diffuse erythematous rash, and ensure there is no removable infected source of endotoxin production.

BIBLIOGRAPHY

Annane D, Renault A, Brun-Buisson C, et al. Hydrocortisone plus fludrocortisone for adults with septic shock. *N Engl J Med.* 2018;378:809–818.

ARISE Investigators and the ANZICS Clinical Trials Group. Goal-directed resuscitation for patients with early septic shock. *N Engl J Med.* 2014;371:1496–1506.

Fernando SM, Tran A, Taljaard M, et al. Prognostic accuracy of the quick sequential organ failure assessment for mortality in patients with suspected infection: a systematic review and meta-analysis. *Ann Intern Med.* 2018;168(4):266–275.

Lappin E, Ferguson AJ. Gram-positive toxic shock syndromes. *Lancet.* 2009;9:281–290.

Levy MM, Rhodes A, Phillips GS, et al. Surviving Sepsis Campaign: association between performance metrics and outcomes in a 7.5-year study. *Intensive Care Med.* 2014;40:1623–1633.

Mouncey PR, Osborn TM, Power GS, et al. Trial of early, goal-directed resuscitation for septic shock. *N Engl J Med.* 2015;372: 1301–1311.

Parks T, Wilson C, Curtis N, et al. Polyspecific intravenous immunoglobulin in clindamycin-treated patients with streptococcal toxic shock syndrome: a systematic review and meta-analysis. *Clin Infect Dis.* 2018;67(9):1434–1436.

ProCESS investigators. A randomized trial of protocol-based care for early septic shock. *N Engl J Med.* 2014;370:1683–1693.

Rhodes A, Evans LE, Alhazzani W, et al. Surviving Sepsis Campaign: international guidelines for management of sepsis and septic shock. *Crit Care Med.* 2016;45(3):486–552.

Semler MW, Self WH, Wanderer JP, et al. Balanced crystalloids versus saline in critically ill adults. *N Engl J Med.* 2018;378:829–839.

Seymour CW, Liu VX, Iwashyna TJ, et al. Assessment of clinical criteria for sepsis: for the Third International Consensus Definitions for sepsis and septic shock (Sepsis-3). *JAMA.* 2016;315(8):762–774.

Vasu TS, Cavallazzi R, Hairani A, et al. Norepinephrine or dopamine for septic shock: systematic review of randomized clinical trials. *J Intensive Care Med.* 2012;27:172–178.

Venkatesh B, Finfer S, Cohen J, et al. Adjunctive glucocorticoid therapy in patients with septic shock. *N Engl J Med.* 2018;378:797–808.

Young P, Bailey M, Beasley R, et al. Effect of a buffered crystalloid solution vs saline on acute kidney injury among patients in the intensive care unit: the SPLIT randomized clinical trial. *JAMA.* 2015;314(16):1701–1710.

CHAPTER 51

SOFT-TISSUE INFECTIONS

Jason J. Lewis, MD and Joshua S. Kolikof, MD

1. **How is cellulitis different from an abscess?**
   Cellulitis is an acute skin and subcutaneous tissue infection characterized by pain, warmth, swelling, and erythema. An abscess is a localized collection of purulent material (pus) that usually presents as a red, painful, indurated, and fluctuant mass.

2. **How does cellulitis occur and progress?**
   Cellulitis is most often caused by group A *Streptococcus* (i.e., *Streptococcus pyogenes*) and *Staphylococcus aureus*. Usually the first sign is local skin discomfort, which is followed by tenderness, erythema, and swelling. Over the course of 24 hours, the area noticeably expands. Lymphangitic "streaking" can occur from the primary area and is a very specific diagnostic sign for cellulitis. The most common areas are the lower extremities, upper extremities, and face, respectively.

3. **How do cutaneous abscesses occur and progress?**
   Abscesses can occur in any part of the body through localized breaks in the skin. *S. aureus* is the most common infecting organism, but *Streptococcus*, gram-negative rods, and *Pseudomonas* also must be considered.
   Abscesses are most commonly seen on the extremities, axilla, and perirectal regions. Untreated follicular infection can evolve into a cutaneous abscess. Blockage of the apocrine glands can lead to abscess formation in the axilla and groin, whereas blockage of Bartholin gland ducts can lead to vaginal abscesses. Obstruction of a sebaceous gland can lead to abscess formation on the head and neck. Superficial abscesses may rupture spontaneously, but often they continue to enlarge until they are incised and drained.

4. **Who is at increased risk for abscesses?**
   People with diabetes, inflammatory bowel disease, and other immune disorders are at greater risk. Intravenous (IV) drug users are at increased risk for cutaneous abscesses caused by community-acquired methicillin-resistant *S. aureus* (CA-MRSA).

5. **What is pus and what does its presence signify?**
   Pus is a mixture of cellular debris and bacteria in various stages of digestion by polymorphonuclear leukocytes. The presence of pus signifies abscess formation.

6. **How do I know if pus is present?**
   Physical examination can indicate the presence of purulent material, or pus. A painful area of localized fluctuance and induration is indicative of an abscess. There may also be a small focus of purulent drainage from the abscess. A computed tomography (CT) scan and ultrasound are not often needed to identify obvious cutaneous abscesses; however, they may be required in suspected deep-tissue abscesses.

7. **How can I easily distinguish abscesses from cellulitis at the bedside?**
   Point-of-care ultrasound is useful in situations where clinical suspicion for an abscess is high, but the physical examination is indeterminate or does not demonstrate a fluctuant mass. In fact, ultrasound has a higher sensitivity and specificity for diagnosing an abscess than physical examination alone. In one study, the incidence of unnecessary incision and drainage decreased by 20% with the utilization of ultrasound. Abscesses will appear as an anechoic fluid collection. Furthermore, ultrasound can be useful in guiding incision and drainage.

8. **State the differential diagnoses for cellulitis.**
   - Thrombophlebitis: a superficial clot of the vein leading to inflammation and irritation must be considered, particularly on the lower extremities
   - Viral exanthems and drug-induced rashes
   - Dermatitis: often associated with pruritus and scaling
   - Insect stings: associated with less pain, pruritus edema
   - Fungal infections: particularly *Candida*, which are characteristically located in the intertriginous areas and have a moist, red appearance with satellite locations

9. **State the differential diagnoses for abscesses.**
   - Acne vulgaris
   - Fungal infections
   - Insect bites
   - Noninfectious nodular lesions, including cutaneous cysts, tumors or other growths, and granulomas

- Recurrent or multiple abscesses may signify disease processes that are more complicated (e.g., hidradenitis suppurativa) or systemic (e.g., endocarditis)

10. What is folliculitis?
Folliculitis is irritation and inflammation of the hair follicles, typically caused by infection, chemical irritation, or injury to the skin. It most commonly involves the apocrine areas, but can occur in any hair-bearing region. Infecting organisms include *S. aureus* (most common), streptococci, and gram-negative rods (including *Pseudomonas*).

11. What is erysipelas?
Erysipelas is a distinctive form of cellulitis caused primarily by group A streptococci. It is characterized by a shiny red, sharply demarcated, and palpable lesion that can rapidly expand. It is typically associated with fever and an elevated white blood cell (WBC) count.

12. What is the role of wound culturing for cellulitis or abscesses?
Although abscesses are commonly caused by CA-MRSA, they are treated with incision and drainage and do not require culturing. Typically, cellulitis is caused by group A *Streptococcus* or *S. aureus*. However, culturing can be useful for patients who are immunocompromised or in those whose initial treatment fails.

13. What is the role of blood cultures in the management of cellulitis?
Blood cultures are typically not warranted in immunocompetent patients with uncomplicated cellulitis. In immunocompromised hosts or those suspected cases of *Haemophilus influenzae* type B, blood cultures may be collected, because bacteremia has been reported in up to 90% of these cases. However, a retrospective study of blood culturing of complicated cellulitis in immunocompromised patients found that results changed empiric management only 2% of the time, with most alterations narrowing antibiotic coverage.

14. What is CA-MRSA?
CA-MRSA has become increasingly prevalent since its first recognition as a community-associated pathogen in skin and soft-tissue infections. Today, CA-MRSA causes 21%–80% of skin infections and abscesses. It is important to note that CA-MRSA is genetically and phenotypically distinct from hospital-associated MRSA infections and has different antibiotic sensitivities and susceptibilities.

15. Who is at risk for CA-MRSA?
Patients at risk for CA-MRSA include those who are incarcerated, men who have sex with men, those with multiple abscesses, and patients who use IV drugs. Others at higher risk include those with chronic medical conditions, such as end-stage renal disease with dialysis, diabetes, peripheral vascular disease, or immunosuppression. Athletes who share equipment or play on artificial turf are also at risk.

16. Should I order routine laboratory tests?
No. Consider laboratory tests (e.g., WBC count, lactate) and blood cultures for immunocompromised patients or those who appear systemically ill.

17. What is the appropriate emergency department (ED) treatment for cellulitis?
Uncomplicated cellulitis can be treated as on an outpatient basis with a 7- to 14-day course of oral antibiotics with strict return precautions (e.g., spreading infection, persistent fevers, or increasing pain).

18. What is the appropriate ED treatment of an abscess?
1. After appropriate analgesia with or without sedation, prepare the area with betadine or chlorhexidine.
2. Using a scalpel, incise approximately two-thirds the diameter of the abscess cavity to allow for instrument-assisted breaking of loculations and full drainage.
3. Instruct patients to attend a follow-up appointment in 48–72 hours for a wound check.
   Although it used to be recommended to routinely pack abscesses after incision and drainage, there is recent literature that demonstrates no difference in outcomes. Additionally, there has been recent literature that indicates no difference with routine irrigation.

19. What is the treatment for suspected CA-MRSA?
While most simple abscesses with suspected CA-MRSA are adequately treated with incision and drainage, there have been several studies showing administration of oral antibiotics reduces treatment failure. Trimethoprim-sulfamethoxazole, clindamycin, and doxycycline are optional oral agents. For more serious infections, start IV vancomycin, daptomycin, or linezolid.

20. What are the concerning anatomic areas that may be affected by cellulitis and/or abscess formation?
- *Midface.* The orbital spaces are very concerning and should be treated with early surgical consultation and IV antibiotics, as abscesses can cause blindness, extend into the intracranial space, form brain abscess, or cause other intracranial infections with significant morbidity and mortality. These infections can also result in cavernous sinus thrombosis.
- *Perirectal or perianal space.* Perianal abscesses originate from anal crypts and can dissect proximally into the ischiorectal space, becoming perirectal abscesses, which require surgical management.

- *Bartholin gland.* Abscesses arise from duct obstruction and infection from vaginal flora, causing pain in the vaginal vestibule and labia minora.
- *Retropharyngeal space or sublingual tissues (e.g., Ludwig angina).* An abscess here can lead to airway compromise and may require surgical intervention. These can lead to descending mediastinitis.
- *Deep space abscess (e.g., in the neck and groin).* These commonly require surgical intervention, given the proximity to neurovascular structures.

21. **Describe the physical examination findings that help differentiate orbital cellulitis from preseptal cellulitis.**
Pain with extraocular movements is one of the most sensitive findings of orbital cellulitis. Patients may also present with proptosis, ophthalmoplegia, fever, systemic symptoms, and toxicity; however, up to 30% of patients with orbital soft-tissue infections are afebrile.

22. **How do I appropriately treat a Bartholin abscess?**
The two most commonly used treatments are incision and drainage or needle aspiration. There is literature that suggests that the outcomes may be similar. The traditional treatment is placement of a small balloon-tipped catheter into the abscess cavity after incision of the medial portion of the abscess cutting parallel to the labia minora, closer to the vaginal introitus. The catheter typically stays in place for 4–6 weeks, with the patient having twice-daily sitz baths.

23. **Who requires hospital admission or ED observation?**
Along with IV antibiotics, any patient who appears systemically ill or septic needs admission or ED observation, as well as those whose treatment has failed or who have progressing disease. Any concern for necrotizing soft-tissue infection (necrotizing fasciitis) or perineal soft-tissue infection (Fournier gangrene) requires immediate surgical consultation, resuscitation, and broad-spectrum antimicrobial therapy. Patients with infections of the hand may need observation to monitor for neurovascular compromise, or in more severe cases, evaluation by a hand specialist. Those with retropharyngeal/sublingual space infections should be monitored until ongoing airway patency is assured and receive an oral maxillofacial surgical or ENT (ear, nose, and throat) evaluation.

24. **What is necrotizing fasciitis?**
Necrotizing fasciitis or necrotizing soft-tissue infection is a rapidly progressive, polymicrobial infection of the skin and soft tissues that is limb and life threatening, rapidly progressing to vascular occlusion and tissue necrosis. Mortality rates range from 25% to 75%. The most common etiology is a mixed bacterial picture of gram-negative enteric bacilli, gram-positive *Streptococcus*, and other anaerobes. However, it can be caused by a single organism, such as group A *Streptococcus* with toxic superantigens. Although bacteria can be introduced from skin trauma, abdominal surgery, perirectal infections, cutaneous ulcers, or IV drug use, the entry point often goes unidentified.

25. **How does necrotizing fasciitis progress?**
Bacterial exotoxins cause an acute onset of severe systemic toxicity. Early in the presentation, the skin appears erythematous and is minimally painful. As the disease progresses, there is separation of the dermal connective tissues, inflammation, and necrosis, and painful rapidly expanding edema. Gas can form under the skin, manifesting as crepitus on physical examination. If not treated aggressively with early broad-spectrum IV antibiotics and surgical debridement, limb ischemia, septicemia, and death can occur.

26. **How do I diagnose necrotizing fasciitis?**
You should suspect necrotizing fasciitis in patients with severe pain and tenderness that is out of proportion to the degree of visible cellulitis. Feel for crepitus, which is sometimes also appreciated on plain radiographs. Outline the area of visible infection to monitor for rapidly expanding signs of infection. CT or magnetic resonance imaging (MRI) can help evaluate the extent of the disease. Patients may appear septic, but this can occur later in the course of the disease.

27. **What is the laboratory risk indicator for necrotizing fasciitis (LRINEC) score?**
The LRINEC score is an objective scoring system that was retrospectively developed to help distinguish necrotizing fasciitis from other soft-tissue infections. It is calculated from six predictive factors, as seen in Table 51.1. While a score greater than or equal to 6 may predict the presence of necrotizing fasciitis and the likelihood of increased mortality and amputation rates, sensitivity is only ~50%, which highlights the importance of clinical suspicion rather than reliance on this scoring system.

28. **Who should be consulted for patients with suspected necrotizing fasciitis?**
A surgeon should be consulted upon suspicion of necrotizing fasciitis, a surgical emergency that must be treated early with extensive operative debridement.

29. **What antibiotics should I order if I suspect necrotizing fasciitis?**
Broad-spectrum IV antibiotics need to be initiated immediately. Use vancomycin or daptomycin *plus* clindamycin *plus* piperacillin/tazobactam *or* a carbapenem (imipenem, meropenem or ertapenem).

Table 51.1 The LRINEC Score	
VARIABLE	**SCORE**
C-Reactive Protein Level (mg/L)	
<150	0
≥150	4
Total White Blood Cell Count (per mm³)	
<15	0
15–25	1
>25	2
Hemoglobin Level (g/dL)	
>13.5	0
11–13.5	1
<11	2
Sodium Level (mmol/L)	
≥135	0
<135	2
Creatine Level (μmol/L)[a]	
≤141	0
>141	2
Glucose Level (mmol/L)[a]	
≤10	0
>10	1

[a]To convert the values of creatinine to milligrams per deciliter (mg/dL), multiply by 0.01131. To convert the values of glucose to mg/dL, multiply by 18.015.
LRINEC, Laboratory risk indicator for necrotizing fasciitis.

30. **What other treatment is beneficial?**
Hyperbaric oxygen (HBO) produces a tissue oxygenation level of 300 mmHg, which can result in bacteriostasis, halting the release of tissue toxins. HBO treatment (in combination with early surgical intervention and IV antibiotics) may help arrest the spread of infection.

31. **What is Fournier gangrene?**
Fournier gangrene is a fulminant, necrotizing soft-tissue infection involving the perineal, genital, or perianal regions; the mortality rate reaches 30%. Men are most commonly affected. It is typically caused by mixed flora, and is usually localized in the genitourinary tract, lower gastrointestinal tract, or groin skin. Patients exhibit a rapidly spreading necrotizing fasciitis with significant scrotal and perineal swelling and induration, which can progress to scrotal wall necrosis and sepsis with multiorgan failure.

32. **Who is at increased risk for Fournier gangrene?**
Patients at risk include those with diabetes mellitus, chronic alcoholism, and immunosuppression.

33. **What is the treatment for Fournier gangrene?**
Like other necrotizing soft-tissue infections, Fournier gangrene is a surgical emergency that requires early and extensive surgical debridement. ED management includes early consultation with a general surgeon or urologist, IV fluid resuscitation, and broad-spectrum antibiotics.

34. **Is any other needed treatment for patients with cellulitis or abscess?**
Tetanus prophylaxis is needed for patients who are not up to date on their immunizations.

35. **What about bites?**
See Chapter 73.

KEY POINTS: SOFT-TISSUE INFECTIONS

1. Cellulitis is an infection of the soft tissues and should be treated with antibiotics.
2. Simple abscesses are treated with incision and drainage, and do not require antibiotics.
3. If you are unsure if there is an abscess, a bedside ultrasound can confirm the presence or absence of a fluid collection.
4. Necrotizing infections are a surgical emergency that requires emergent operative debridement, IV fluid resuscitation, and broad-spectrum IV antibiotics.

ACKNOWLEDGMENT

The editors and authors of this chapter would like to acknowledge and thank Drs. Harvey W. Meislin and Megan A. Meislin for their previous contributions to this chapter.

BIBLIOGRAPHY

Blaivas M, Adhikari S. Unexpected findings on point of care superficial ultrasound imaging before incision and drainage. *J Ultrasound Med*. 2011;30(10):1425–1430.

Hloch O, Mokra D, Masopust J, et al. Antibiotic treatment following a dog bite in an immunocompromised patient in order to prevent *Capnocytophaga canimorsus* infection: a case report. BMC Res Notes. 2014;7:432.

Pallin DJ, Camargo CA, Schuur JD. Skin infections and antibiotic stewardship: analysis of emergency department prescribing practices, 2007-2010. *West J Emerg Med*. 2014;15:282–289.

Peterson D, McLeod S, Woolfrey K, et al. Predictors of failure of empiric outpatient antibiotic therapy in emergency department patients with uncomplicated cellulitis. *Acad Emerg Med*. 2014;21:526–531.

Rudloe TF, Harper MB, Prabhu SP, et al. Acute periorbital infections: who needs emergent imaging? *Pediatrics*. 2010;125:e719–e726.

Stevens DL, Bisno AL, Chambers HF, et al. Practice guidelines for the diagnosis and management of skin and soft tissue infections: 2014 update by the Infectious Diseases Society of America. *CID*. 2014;59(2):e10–e52.

CHAPTER 52

SEXUALLY TRANSMITTED INFECTIONS AND HUMAN IMMUNODEFICIENCY VIRUS

Sarah Rowan, MD and Jason Haukoos, MD, MSc

1. **What are the most common sexually transmitted infections (STIs)?**
   The true incidence of most STIs is unknown, because not all cases are reported. The Centers for Disease Control and Prevention (CDC) report that 2.3 million cases of chlamydia, gonorrhea, and syphilis were diagnosed in the United States in 2017, an increase of 200,000 cases from 2016. Half of reported STIs occur in persons aged 15–24 years.
   - Chlamydia is the most common *reportable* STI in the United States. In 2017, 1.7 million cases were reported in the United States, marking a 7% increase from 2016. Chlamydia can be a significant health problem for young women if it leads to pelvic inflammatory disease (PID) and the possible sequelae of infertility, ectopic pregnancy, and chronic pelvic pain.
   - Gonorrhea is the second most prevalent reportable STI in the United States. Incidence increased 75% from 2009 to 2017 with 550,000 cases reported to the CDC in 2017. Gonorrhea is also a major cause of PID and its sequelae. Gonorrheal resistance to antibiotics has been increasing in recent years, posing a major public health threat.
   - In 2017, 30,644 cases of primary and secondary syphilis were reported. The incidence of syphilis has been increasing since 2000, largely driven by an increase in cases among men who have sex with men (MSM). Syphilis rates are highest among Blacks, occurring at 4.5 times the rate of syphilis among Whites.
   - Trichomoniasis is the most common curable STI in young, sexually active women. The CDC estimates that 3.7 million people have trichomoniasis, 70% of whom are asymptomatic.
   - Genital human papillomavirus (HPV) is the most common (nonreportable) STI in the United States, with a prevalence of genital infection of 43% among individuals aged 18–59 years. HPV types 16 and 18 cause about 66% of cervical cancers in the United States. These viruses are also responsible for vulvar, vaginal, anal, penile, and oropharyngeal cancers. Types 6 and 11 cause 90% of genital warts.
   - Herpes simplex virus type 2 (HSV-2) infection is present in approximately 12% of adolescents and adults aged 14–49 years in the United States, with many unaware. Annually, 776,000 people in the United States are estimated to contract genital herpes. The age-adjusted prevalence of HSV-2 in the United States decreased from 18% in 2000 to 12% in 2016. HSV-2 infection is much more prevalent among non-Hispanic Blacks (35%) than non-Hispanic Whites (8%).
   - Worldwide, approximately 38 million people are living with human immunodeficiency virus (HIV), and in 2019, 690,000 people died of acquired immunodeficiency syndrome (AIDS)-related complications. Approximately 1.1 million people in the United States are living with HIV, and 15% of those individuals are estimated to be undiagnosed. In 2017, nearly 39,000 people in the United States were diagnosed with HIV. The number of annual new diagnoses in the United States has not changed significantly since 2012.
   - Hepatitis B (HBV) can be transmitted through sexual contact or blood-to-blood exposure. Approximately 21,000 individuals are estimated to acquire HBV annually in the United States. While 80% of adults who acquire HBV will clear the infection without medications, the other 20% will go on to have chronic HBV infection. Chronic HBV can be controlled with medications, but at this time, it is not curable. Hepatitis C (HCV) is more closely associated with blood-to-blood transmission, but cases of sexual transmission have been reported. HIV-positive MSM are the group most at risk for sexual transmission of HCV. The incidence of HCV is increasing, with an estimated 41,000 new infections occurring in 2016, mostly acquired through injection drug use. Approximately 30% of individuals who acquire HCV will clear without treatment, while 70% will have chronic infection. HCV can be cured with short courses (8–12 weeks) of well-tolerated and highly effective direct acting antiviral medications.

2. **How should I evaluate symptomatic vaginal discharge?**
   - Take a complete sexual history. The CDC recommends "the 5 P's" for sexual history taking. These include number and gender of sex **p**artners over the past 12 months, sexual **p**ractices (vaginal, anal, or oral sex), **p**rotection from STIs (condoms), **p**ast history of STIs, and **p**revention of pregnancy.
   - Obtain a pregnancy test to guide treatment.
   - Perform a pelvic examination and note any discharge, and take a sample for wet preparation and gonorrhea/chlamydia testing.

- Vulvovaginal candidiasis (not an STI) causes a white, curd-like discharge that clings to vaginal walls. Hyphae are present on potassium hydroxide preparation. Recent antibiotic use is a risk factor, as are diabetes and HIV. Treatment is single-dose oral fluconazole or any of the topical imidazoles.
- Bacterial vaginosis (not an STI) is an alteration of the microbial ecosystem, with overgrowth of *Gardnerella vaginalis* and other species. Diagnosis is made by noting clue cells on the wet preparation, and treatment is with metronidazole (preferred) or clindamycin.
- *Trichomonas vaginitis* infection is a true STI and causes a green, frothy discharge, with an erythematous and friable "strawberry" cervix. Diagnosis is usually based on finding the motile trichomonads on wet preparation or in urine. Treatment is with metronidazole. Individuals who are allergic to metronidazole should meet with an allergist for desensitization.
- Chlamydia and gonorrhea can also cause abnormal vaginal discharge. The best tests are nucleic acid amplification tests (NAATs). If detected, treatment is ceftriaxone 500 mg IM (intramuscular) once for gonorrhea (dose increased to 1g IM for individuals weighing > or = to 150 kg) and doxycycline 100 mg PO BID for 7 days for chlamydia. If a person is pregnant, azithromycin 1g PO once may be given for chlamydia. However, the infections are often treated presumptively while awaiting results of the polymerase chain reaction (PCR).

3. **How do I evaluate a sexually active young man with dysuria?**
Dysuria in young men is usually the result of urethritis from an STI. Likely pathogens include *Neisseria gonorrhoeae, Chlamydia trachomatis, Mycoplasma genitalium, Trichomonas vaginalis,* and HSV. A purulent discharge is often caused by *N. gonorrhoeae,* whereas a mucoid discharge or dysuria without discharge is more likely to be caused by chlamydia. Gram stain from a urethral swab may show gram-negative intracellular diplococci, which is diagnostic for gonorrhea, or white blood cells. Urinalysis often reveals positive leukocyte esterase or white blood cells. Urine NAAT for gonorrhea and chlamydia should be ordered any time gonococcal or nongonococcal urethritis is suspected.

4. **Should patients be tested for extragenital gonococcal or chlamydial infection?**
Yes. Gonorrhea and chlamydia can cause many types of extragenital infections, but the most common are rectal and oropharyngeal disease. Many cases are asymptomatic, though they may present with signs or symptoms of proctitis – tenesmus, pain, bleeding, or discharge – or pharyngitis – sore throat, exudates, or cervical lymphadenitis. Rectal or pharyngeal NAATs may be ordered, depending on symptoms and sites of exposure.

5. **Are there any single-dose treatment regimens for uncomplicated chlamydial infections?**
Single-dose treatment for chlamydia is no longer preferred due to decreased efficacy of azithromycin compared to doxycycline. However, azithromycin 1 g PO once is considered an acceptable alternative for patients who cannot take doxycycline including those who are pregnant or in whom pregnancy has not been excluded.

6. **What is the treatment for gonorrhea?**
Uncomplicated urethral, endocervical, or rectal gonorrheal infections should be treated with 500 mg of ceftriaxone IM once for individuals weighing less than 150 kg and 1 g of IM ceftrixone once for individuals weighing ≥150 kg. Dual therapy with azithromycin is no longer recommended. If injectable cephalosporins are not available, cefixime 800 mg PO once is an alternative, though this is not preferred due to risk of treatment failure. In cases of severe cephalosporin allergy, gentamicin 240 mg IM plus high-dose azithromycin (2 g PO) is the preferred alternative. In these cases, test of cure with a repeat NAAT is recommended 14 days after treatment.

7. **What is the significance of finding mucopurulent cervicitis (MPC) in a woman with lower abdominal pain?**
The normal endometrial secretion should be transparent. The presence of mucopurulent secretions from the os, which may appear yellow when viewed on a white cotton-tipped swab, or friability suggest MPC. MPC, most commonly caused by *N. gonorrhoeae* or *C. trachomatis,* is a precursor to upper genital tract infection: PID or tubo-ovarian abscess.

8. **What are the most common causes of genital ulcers?**
Genital ulcers can represent infection with HSV, syphilis, lymphogranuloma venereum (LGV), or chancroid. Patient history and key physical examination findings can suggest the diagnosis.
- *HSV.* Genital herpes resulting from HSV-1 or HSV-2 is the most common cause of genital ulcers in the United States, presenting as itching, pain, and burning with ulcerating vesicles or pustules. Patients with primary HSV infection may have myalgias, headache, and fever with associated tender inguinal adenopathy. Lesions heal in 2–3 weeks. Diagnosis is made by viral culture, PCR, or direct fluorescent antibody testing. Most patients with primary HSV will experience a recurrent episode in the first year, and ongoing recurrences are common. Patients may shed the virus while they are asymptomatic. HSV cannot be cured, but treatment with antiviral agents can shorten the duration of symptoms. Long-term suppressive therapy can prevent outbreaks of ulcers.
- *Syphilis.* Primary syphilis presents 2–4 weeks after exposure with a painless, indurated ulcer called a *chancre.* Secondary syphilis represents systemic disease and may present with a wide variety of manifestations, including rash, fever, malaise, mucous patches, hepatitis, alopecia, or condyloma lata. Syphilis infection may also be asymptomatic (latent syphilis). Direct testing for syphilis through darkfield microscopy is not widely available. Therefore, serologic testing with nontreponemal and treponemal-specific antibody tests are

recommended. Nontreponemal tests – rapid plasma reagin (RPR) and Venereal Disease Research Laboratories (VDRL) – are traditionally done first, followed by treponemal-specific testing (fluorescent treponemal antibody absorption [FTA-ABS], enzyme immunoassay [EIA], chemiluminescence immunoassay [CIA], or *Treponema pallidum* particle agglutination assay [TPPA]) for confirmation. The "reverse algorithm," employing treponemal-specific testing followed by nontreponemal testing, is being employed more frequently as syphilis EIAs have become more widely available. Nontreponemal tests are typically a marker of disease activity, while more specific treponemal-specific tests are required for a definitive diagnosis but will be positive for life. Primary, secondary, or early latent syphilis can be treated with a single IM injection of 2.4 million units of benzathine penicillin. Doxycycline 100 mg PO for 2 weeks is the recommended alternative for penicillin-allergic individuals. Neurosyphilis should be considered in any patient with suspected syphilis and neurologic, otic, or ophthalmologic symptoms. Neurosyphilis is treated with 2 weeks of intravenous (IV) penicillin.

- *LGV* is caused by *C. trachomatis* strains L1, L2, and L3. LGV was once rare in the United States, but over the past decade several outbreaks have been reported, most often among MSM. The lesion of primary LGV is usually a painless, small papule, or herpetiform erosion. Secondary LGV is marked by painful inguinal lymphadenopathy (bubo), which may drain, or anorectal syndrome that presents with ulcerative anal lesions or proctocolitis. Diagnosis of LGV is challenging. NAAT will be positive for *C. trachomatis,* but distinguishing LGV serotypes requires specialized testing that is not widely available. If the diagnosis is suspected by history and examination, treatment may be initiated with doxycycline 100 mg PO twice daily for 21 days while awaiting results of testing.
- *Chancroid.* Also called *soft sore,* this disease is caused by *Haemophilus ducreyi,* a bacterium that is difficult to culture. Clinically, this syndrome causes an ulcer that is painful and not indurated, distinguishing it from a syphilitic chancre. Painful inguinal adenopathy is found in more than 50% of cases. Treatment options include single-dose azithromycin (1 g) or ceftriaxone (250 mg).

9. **What is the Jarisch-Herxheimer reaction?**
After initiation of treatment for syphilis (most commonly with penicillin), the patient may experience onset of fever, chills, myalgias, headache, tachycardia, increased respirations, increased neutrophil count, and mild hypotension. Though not well understood, this is believed to occur though an immune response to killed spirochetes. It occurs approximately 2–5 hours after initiation of treatment, with peak temperatures at approximately 7 hours, and defervescence at 12–24 hours. This reaction occurs in 10%–35% of patients. In patients with secondary syphilis, lesions may become more edematous and erythematous.

10. **What is proctitis and how is it managed?**
Any individual, male or female, with the onset of acute proctitis symptoms (e.g., rectal pain, discharge, tenesmus) who has recently had condomless receptive anal intercourse is at risk for proctitis. These patients should be examined by anoscopy and tested for gonorrhea, *Chlamydia*, and HSV. All patients should have testing for syphilis and empiric treatment for gonorrhea and chlamydial infection. If ulcers are apparent on anoscopy, consider empirical antiviral therapy with acyclovir or empiric treatment for LGV (as described earlier).

11. **How do I evaluate a sexually active young person who has an acutely swollen, warm, painful right ankle?**
This patient, with acute monoarticular arthritis, should be presumed to have disseminated gonococcal infection (DGI). There are two syndromes: (1) a triad of dermatitis, tenosynovitis, and septic arthritis; and (2) a purulent arthritis without skin lesions, with knees, ankles, and wrists most commonly involved. Patients with DGI do not usually have concurrent genital symptoms. To evaluate suspected DGI, two sets of blood cultures should be ordered, and arthrocentesis should be performed on the involved joint. The fluid should be sent for Gram stain, cell count, and bacterial culture, with specific request for gonococcal culture. Gonorrhea is cultured from less than 50% of joints. NAAT testing for gonorrhea should be sent using specimens from all potential sites of exposure. Patients with the polyarthritis triad form may yield a better result from blood cultures. A patient suspected of having DGI should be admitted and treated with parenteral antibiotics, starting with ceftriaxone 1 g IM/IV daily plus a single dose of azithromycin 1 g orally.

12. **Do I need to report STI cases to the health department?**
Yes, accurate reporting of STIs is essential to national and local STI control efforts. HIV, gonorrhea, chlamydia, and syphilis are reportable infections in every state. It is the responsibility of each clinician to know his or her local reporting requirements. If you are unsure of what to report about a specific patient, contact your local health department.

13. **What are the important points for the aftercare instructions for patients with STIs?**
- Education about STIs is the responsibility of every emergency physician, because you may be the only contact the patient has with the medical system.
- Instruct patients to refer all of their sexual partners for evaluation and treatment. Expedited partner therapy (EPT) is the practice of providing prescriptions or medications for sex partners of patients diagnosed with gonorrhea or chlamydia without examining the partner. This approach is endorsed by CDC for male partners of women diagnosed with gonorrhea or chlamydia, but the legal status of EPT varies by state so should be

reviewed at the state and institutional level prior to prescribing EPT. A resource guide for legal status of EPT by jurisdiction can be accessed on the CDC's website.
- Patients should be instructed to avoid sexual contact for 7 days after a single-dose treatment or until a full 7-day course of treatment has been completed, and until all their sex partners are treated.

14. **What is the significance of HIV in patients seen in the emergency department (ED)?**
Patients with all stages of HIV, ranging from undiagnosed to an advanced immunocompromised state (AIDS), are encountered commonly in the ED. Seroprevalence among ED patients varies greatly, depending on the location and type of hospital. Among ED patients in an inner city, seroprevalence ranges from approximately 1% to 5%. Knowledge of HIV infection and its related diseases is essential to diagnose and treat patients appropriately.

15. **How is the diagnosis of HIV made?**
To make the diagnosis of HIV infection, the CDC recommends a multitest algorithm consisting of a positive initial HIV-1/2 antibody (third generation) or combination antigen/antibody test (fourth generation) and a subsequent positive result from an HIV-1/HIV-2 antibody differentiation immunoassay. If the screening test or follow-up test is negative or indeterminate but acute HIV is suspected, an HIV-1 RNA test is used to make the diagnosis. AIDS is diagnosed by laboratory evidence of HIV infection plus the presence of an AIDS-defining illness or CD4 lymphocyte level <200 cells/micro.

16. **When should HIV infection be suspected?**
HIV should be suspected in all patients with known behavioral risk factors or with presenting symptoms suggestive of an opportunistic infection, including thrush. Additionally, HIV infection should be suspected in any patient thought to be immunocompetent but with an infectious disease (e.g., community-acquired pneumonia or cellulitis in an otherwise healthy adult), those with unexplained leukopenia or lymphopenia, and those who have chronic nonspecific symptoms (e.g., weight loss, fever, or diarrhea). Questioning the patient directly about risk factors may be crucial to diagnosing HIV-related disease. High-risk behaviors commonly associated with HIV infection include condomless sexual intercourse with multiple partners or a partner living with untreated HIV, and injection drug use.

17. **What is acute HIV infection and how do I differentiate it from other viral syndromes?**
Acute HIV infection, also referred to as acute HIV or retroviral syndrome, occurs in the weeks following HIV transmission and resembles many more general systemic viral illnesses. The clinical syndrome is marked by fever, fatigue, and rash, and commonly also includes headache, lymphadenopathy, pharyngitis, myalgias, nausea, and diarrhea. Although this syndrome is not common, the ED serves as an important clinical site to identify patients with acute HIV infection. These patients often have very high viral loads and, therefore, are more likely to transmit HIV to others. Approximately 15% of patients diagnosed with HIV in the ED have acute infections, although the overall prevalence of acute HIV is 0.05% of those screened for HIV. Making the diagnosis requires astute clinical suspicion, and differentiating it clinically from other viral syndromes may be challenging. These patients are more likely to have a prolonged duration, rash, and diarrhea, which may help differentiate it from other viral illnesses.

18. **Should EDs test for HIV infection?**
Yes, in 2014 the CDC released new recommendations for diagnostic HIV testing, including use of fourth-generation assays and confirmation with an HIV-1/HIV-2 antibody differentiation assay. The most common HIV testing approach is diagnostic testing (i.e., where physicians are able to test patients based on clinical signs or symptoms). However, some agencies, including the CDC, have advocated for performing routine opt-out rapid HIV screening, which means that unless patients refuse testing they would be tested. In addition to the CDC, the US Preventive Services Task Force also endorses routine screening. An increasing number of EDs are now performing HIV screening, recognizing that integrating a more routine form of HIV testing into ED operations is possible and with minimal impact on patient flow. Regardless of whether or not HIV testing is performed in the ED, outpatient referral for high-risk patients is appropriate.

19. **Which diagnoses are unique to patients with HIV?**
Patients with HIV are susceptible to all common illnesses. In cases of advanced immunosuppression, opportunistic infections must also be considered. Patients may have involvement of virtually any organ system. Because of the wide spectrum of diseases related to HIV infection, many specific diagnoses cannot be made definitively in the ED; treatment focuses on recognition of disease, institution of initial therapy, and admission to the hospital or close outpatient follow-up.
- **Neurologic complications.** Patients with CD4 cell counts <200 cells/micro are at higher risk for meningitis and central nervous system lesions caused by opportunistic infections or HIV-associated tumors. HIV-associated neurocognitive disorders (HAND) may occur at any level of immunosuppression but are more common with greater immunosuppression. Evaluation for patients presenting with altered mental status, seizures, headache, or focal neurologic deficits should include a complete neurologic examination, computed tomography (CT) with and without IV contrast or magnetic resonance imaging (MRI), and lumbar puncture. Specific cerebrospinal fluid studies may include cell count and glucose and protein levels, Gram stain, bacterial culture, viral culture, fungal

culture, cryptococcal antigen tests, coccidioidomycosis titers, VDRL, and select PCR studies such as JC virus or HSV. The most common causes of meningitis among patients with HIV and advanced immunosuppression include *Cryptococcus neoformans, Mycobacterium tuberculosis,* syphilis, and progressive multifocal leukoencephalopathy (PML). If imaging reveals CNS lesions, toxoplasma encephalitis and lymphoma should be considered. HAND range in severity from asymptomatic neurocognitive impairment to HIV-associated dementia (HAD). Although HAD is increasingly uncommon with more widespread use of antiretroviral therapy (ART), less severe forms of HAND continue to be prevalent.

- **Gastrointestinal complications.** Diarrhea is common among people living with HIV, though it is less common now in the era of widespread ART use. The causes of infectious diarrhea vary with the immune status of the patient. With higher CD4 cell counts, pathogens are similar to those of the HIV-uninfected patient, though duration of illness may be longer. Bacterial infections *(Clostridia, Salmonella, Shigella, Campylobacter)* and *Giardia* are common causes and are associated with prolonged watery or bloody diarrhea. At lower CD4 cell counts, infections caused by *Cryptosporidium, Isospora, Cyclospora, Histoplasma,* cytomegalovirus (CMV), and *Mycobacterium avium* complex should be suspected. Noninfectious causes of diarrhea include lymphoma or Kaposi's sarcoma. Stool multiplex PCR, culture, examination for ova and parasites, and *Clostridium difficile* toxin assay can all be helpful diagnostic studies. In some cases, such as CMV colitis, endoscopy with biopsy is required to confirm the diagnosis. Esophageal complaints are common and may be most commonly caused by *Candida* esophagitis, CMV, or herpes simplex esophagitis. Patients with esophagitis should receive a 2-week empiric course of oral antifungal agents, followed by endoscopy if the condition is not successfully treated.
- **Pulmonary complications.** Common presenting pulmonary complaints are cough, hemoptysis, shortness of breath, and chest pain. After history and lung examination, arterial blood gases, chest radiography, sputum culture, Gram stain, acid-fast stain, and blood cultures should be obtained if clinically indicated. Compared with the general population, patients with HIV have a 10- to 25-times increased risk of developing bacterial pneumonia (usually *Streptococcus* caused by *Streptococcus pneumoniae*); recurrent bacterial pneumonia is an AIDS-defining illness. Pneumococcal septicemia is 100 times more common in patients living with HIV. *Pneumocystis jiroveci* pneumonia (PJP; previously known as *Pneumocystis carinii* pneumonia or *PCP*) is less common with ART and PJP prophylaxis but still occurs in untreated patients. It typically presents with subacute onset of dyspnea, dyspnea with exertion, nonproductive cough, fever, and hypoxemia. Rapid institution of therapy with trimethoprim-sulfamethoxazole (TMP-SMX) and oral steroids (for patients with arterial partial pressure of oxygen [PaO$_2$] breathing room air $\leq$70 mmHg or alveolar-arterial oxygen gradient $\geq$35 mmHg) may prevent excessive morbidity and mortality. Other causes of pulmonary disease in patients with HIV include *Mycobacterium tuberculosis* pneumonia, *Histoplasma capsulatum,* other traditional community-acquired pneumonia organisms, and neoplasm.
- **Cutaneous manifestations.** Kaposi's sarcoma is the most common unique cutaneous manifestation of HIV. Usually it involves the lower extremities, mucous membranes, or genitals, though it can occur anywhere in the body. The primary treatment is ART. Exacerbation of underlying dermatologic conditions is also common in patients living with HIV. Complaints such as xerosis (dry skin) and pruritus are common, particularly in the setting of low CD4 cell counts. Xerosis may be treated with emollients and, if necessary, with mild topical steroids. Pruritus may respond to oatmeal baths and, if necessary, antihistamines. Other dermatologic conditions that occur with increased incidence in patients with HIV include drug reactions to ART (especially TMP-SMX), seborrheic dermatitis, psoriasis, atopic dermatitis, and alopecia. Consult an infectious disease specialist and a dermatologist, and admit patients with any disseminated cutaneous infection requiring IV antibiotics or antiviral agents.
- **Ocular complications.** Eye complaints such as change in visual acuity, floaters, photopsia (flashing lights), photophobia, redness, and pain are common and may represent retinitis or invasion of eye or periorbital tissues with a malignant or infectious process. CMV retinitis occurs in up to 25% of patients with AIDS who are not on ART. It has a characteristic appearance of fluffy white retinal lesions, often perivascular (sometimes referred to as *tomato and cheese pizza* appearance). Ophthalmology consultation is indicated, followed by treatment with foscarnet or ganciclovir for 2 weeks and long-term maintenance therapy.

20. **Should patients with HIV receive tetanus and other immunizations?**
    According to the US Public Health Service Immunizations Practices Advisory Committee, routine immunization recommendations apply to individuals with HIV who have CD4 cell counts >200 cells/micro. Additionally, it is recommended that individuals with HIV receive immunizations for pneumococcal infection, HPV up through age 26 years, HBV, hepatitis A (HAV), and meningococcal infection. For individuals with CD4 cell counts <200 cells/micro, vaccines may be less effective, and live vaccines including MMR, varicella, zoster, and yellow fevers should be avoided.

21. **What's new with HIV treatment?**
    ART is recommended for all patients living with HIV, regardless of CD4 count. In addition to opportunistic infections, HIV viremia is a risk factor for coronary artery disease (CAD), renal disease, neurocognitive deficits, liver disease, and non–HIV-associated malignancy, all of which are largely mitigated by ART. ART is also recommended for the prevention of HIV transmission. Multiple large studies have now demonstrated that among persons with suppressed viral loads, there is effectively no risk for sexual transmission of HIV. For the most part, ART regimens are dosed

once daily, and many single-tablet regimen options exist. In addition to being highly effective at suppressing HIV, the medications are now much easier to take, with very few short- or long-term side effects. Life expectancy for people with HIV who are diagnosed before significant immune damage has occurred is nearly the same as that of individuals who do not have HIV.

22. **How can health care providers protect themselves from acquiring HIV?**
With the use of universal precautions, the risk of acquiring HIV infection by occupational exposure is extremely low. However, because HIV infection is often undiagnosed, the use of universal precautions is imperative and should be performed in all patients, including the appropriate use of gown, gloves, mask, and goggles for procedures. The *Needlestick Safety and Prevention Act* of 2000 mandates that safety-engineered devices be used whenever possible, and that institutions maintain exposure control plans.

23. **What constitutes high-risk exposure to HIV?**
    - **Nonoccupational exposures.** Exposure through the vagina, rectum, eye, mouth, or other mucous membrane, or non-intact skin to blood, semen, vaginal, or rectal secretions, or breast milk from a source that is known to be HIV positive is considered high risk. When the HIV status of the source patient is unknown, the risk is considered intermediate.
    - **Occupational exposures.** Higher-risk percutaneous exposures associated with an increased likelihood of transmission include deep injuries, visible blood on a device, and injuries sustained when placing a catheter in a vein or artery. Percutaneous exposures that are superficial or involve solid needles are considered lower-risk exposures. High-risk sources are patients with symptomatic HIV, AIDS, acute seroconversion, or high viral load. Patients with asymptomatic HIV or viral load <15,000 copies/mL are considered lower risk.

24. **Should post-exposure prophylaxis (PEP) be administered after exposure to blood and body fluids?**
PEP should be considered after all occupational and nonoccupational exposures. Decisions to treat should be based on the type of exposure, the risk of HIV in the source patient, and careful consideration of the risks and benefits of therapy. PEP must be started within 72 hours of exposure to be effective and usually consists of two nucleoside reverse transcription inhibitors, such as combination tenofovir-emtricitabine, plus an integrase inhibitor such as dolutegravir or raltegravir. Ideally, each health care institution should have written protocols that are formulated in consultation with occupational medicine and infectious disease specialists for occupational exposures in health care workers and patients with nonoccupational exposures.

25. **What is PrEP?**
Pre-exposure prophylaxis (PrEP) to HIV involves taking a daily medication to prevent HIV acquisition. The only two currently Food and Drug Administration (FDA)-approved options for PrEP are Truvada and Descovy, both of which are combinations of two antiretroviral agents, tenofovir and emtricitabine. When taken as prescribed, PrEP is over 92% effective at preventing HIV acquisition. PrEP is indicated for all individuals who are at higher risk for HIV acquisition, such as MSM who have condomless sex with multiple partners, or individuals with history of certain STIs. Monitoring for patients on PrEP involves HIV and STI testing every 3 months and monitoring for renal toxicity every 6 months. The CDC estimates up to 1.1 million people in the United States have indications for PrEP.

KEY POINTS: STIs

1. STIs affect 20 million people per year in the United States, 50% of whom are aged 15–24 years.
2. Annual targeted screening is recommended for all STIs.
3. Chlamydial infection is the most prevalent reportable STI in the United States, and it is often asymptomatic.
4. Every patient with HIV should be treated with ART to prevent comorbidities and transmission.

BIBLIOGRAPHY

CDC and Association of Public Health Laboratories. Laboratory testing for the diagnosis of HIV infection: updated recommendations. https://stacks.cdc.gov/view/cdc/50872. Published June 2014; updated January 2018.

Centers for Disease Control and Prevention. Occupational exposure to blood. https://www.cdc.gov/oralhealth/infectioncontrol/faqs/occupational-exposure.html. Accessed February 17, 2019.

Centers for Disease Control and Prevention. Preexposure prophylaxis for the prevention of HIV infection in the United States; 2017 Update. https://www.cdc.gov/hiv/pdf/risk/prep/cdc-hiv-prep-guidelines-2017.pdf. Accessed February 22, 2019.

Centers for Disease Control and Prevention. Sexually transmitted disease surveillance; 2017. https://www.cdc.gov/std/default.htm. Accessed February 17, 2019.

Centers for Disease Control and Prevention. Sexually transmitted diseases treatment guidelines; June 5, 2015. https://www.cdc.gov/std/tg2015/. Accessed February 22, 2019.

Department of Health and Human Services. Guidelines for the prevention and treatment of opportunistic infections in HIV-infected adults and adolescents; January 10, 2020. https://aidsinfo.nih.gov/contentfiles/lvguidelines/adult_oi.pdf . Accessed July 21, 2020.

Department of Health and Human Services. Guidelines for the use of antiretroviral agents in adults and adolescents living with HIV. https://aidsinfo.nih.gov/contentfiles/lvguidelines/adultandadolescentgl.pdf. Accessed February 22, 2019.

Dombrowski JC, Wierzbicki MR, Newman L, et al. A randomized trial of azithromycin vs. doxycycline for the treatment of rectal chlamydia in men who have sex with men. Presented at the National STD Prevention Conference, Atlanta, GA, September 14–24, 2020.

Grant RM, Lama JR, Anderson PL, et al. Preexposure chemoprophylaxis for HIV prevention in men who have sex with men. *N Engl J Med.* 2010;363(27):2587–2599.

Kong FY, Tabrizi SN, Law M, et al. Azithromycin versus doxycycline for the treatment of genital chlamydia infection: a meta-analysis of randomized controlled trials. *Clin Infect Dis.* 2014;59:193–205.

Kuhar DT, Henderson DK, Struble KA, et al. Updated US Public Health Service guidelines for the management of occupational exposures to human immunodeficiency virus and recommendations for postexposure prophylaxis. *Infect Control Hosp Epidemiol.* 2013;34: 875–892.

McCormack S, Dunn DT, Desai M, et al. Pre-exposure prophylaxis to prevent acquisition of HIV-1 infection (PROUD): effectiveness results from the pilot phase of a pragmatic open-label randomised trial. *Lancet.* 2016;387(10013):53–60.

MMWR; December 2020. https://www.cdc.gov/mmwr/volumes/69/wr/mm6950a6.htm.

Papp JR, Schachter J, Gaydos CA, et al. Recommendations for the laboratory-based detection of *Chlamydia trachomatis* and *Neisseria gonorrhoeae*: 2014. *MMWR Recomm Rep.* 2014;63(RR-02):1–9.

Patton ME, Su JR, Nelson R, et al. Primary and secondary syphilis: United States; 2005–2013. *MMWR Morb Mortal Wkly Rep.* 2014; 63:402–406. www.cdc.gov/mmwr/preview/mmwrhtml/mm6318a4.htm?s_cid=mm6318a4_w. Accessed February 17, 2019.

Stanley K, Lora M, Merjavy S, et al. HIV prevention and treatment: the evolving role of the emergency department. *Ann Emerg Med.* 2017;70:562–572.

White DAE, Giordano TP, Pasalar S, et al. Acute HIV discovered during routine HIV screening with HIV antigen-antibody combination tests in 9 U.S. emergency departments. *Ann Emerg Med.* 2018;72:29–40.e2.

World Health Organization. Sexually transmitted infections (STIs); 2019. https://www.who.int/news-room/fact-sheets/detail/sexually-transmitted-infections-(stis). Accessed February 17, 2019.

CHAPTER 53

TETANUS, BOTULISM, AND FOODBORNE ILLNESSES

James Dazhe Cao, MD, FACEP, FACMT

TETANUS

1. **What is the causative agent of tetanus, and what is its mechanism of action?**
   Clostridium tetani is an obligate anaerobic bacterium that produces tetanospasmin. Tetanospasmin travels in a retrograde fashion into the central nervous system (CNS), where it irreversibly cleaves synaptic vesicle–docking proteins, and disables inhibitory neurotransmitter (γ-aminobutyric acid [GABA] and glycine) release in both the autonomic and somatic nervous systems. Decreased inhibition causes dysautonomia and increased muscle spasticity seen in clinical tetanus. Although *C. tetani* is heat- and oxygen-sensitive, spores are extremely resilient and able to survive household disinfectants, extremes in temperatures and humidity, and being autoclaved for up to 15 minutes.

2. **What are the forms of tetanus?**
   - Generalized tetanus (>80% of cases in the United States) involves rigidity and spasm of all muscles in the body, usually starting cranially and proceeding caudally.
   - Localized tetanus is seen with lower toxin loads in peripheral injuries. Spasm, rigidity, and pain are usually limited to the injured area.
   - Cephalic tetanus occurs after a head wound, presents as cranial nerve paralysis (most commonly lower motor neuron weakness of cranial nerve VII), and often proceeds to generalized tetanus.
   - Neonatal tetanus, although rare in developed countries, is the most common form of tetanus worldwide because of lack of immunizations and poor umbilical hygiene.
   - Since 2001, annual incidence of tetanus in the United States is around 29 cases, with a fatality rate of about 13%.

3. **How is tetanus contracted?**
   Tetanus generally originates from a deep, usually grossly contaminated wound (soil, manure, or metal), that facilitates anaerobic bacterial growth. Other sources include burns, ulcers, snakebites, middle ear infections, tattooing, piercings, septic abortions, childbirth, surgery, and intramuscular injections. A prior episode of tetanus does not confer lifelong immunity.

4. **What are the presentation and prognosis of neonatal tetanus?**
   Neonatal tetanus presents commonly during the first week of life in infants of nonimmunized mothers. The bacteria enter through the umbilical cord stump, especially after the application of mud or feces, a practice in some developing countries. Irritability and poor feeding progress to generalized spasms, pneumonia, and pulmonary or CNS hemorrhage. Toxin load is high, and the mortality rate ranges from 40% to 95%. In 2017, an estimated 61,000 neonates died from neonatal tetanus.

5. **What is the presentation of generalized tetanus?**
   Initial symptoms proceed head to toe, including trismus (from masseter and parapharyngeal spasm – "lock jaw"), dysphagia, neck muscle spasm/pain, *risus sardonicus* (the sardonic smile of tetanus from facial muscle spasm), and opisthotonos (painful arching of neck and back from paraspinous and abdominal wall muscle spasm). Minor stimuli (e.g., light touch, drafts, or noises), pain, and anxiety may trigger severe spasms. Death can result from glottic spasm, respiratory failure, and autonomic instability (e.g., labile hypertension, dysrhythmias, hyperpyrexia, tachycardia, or myocardial infarction). Autonomic instability is the most common cause of death from tetanus in developed countries.

6. **What is the differential diagnosis for generalized tetanus?**
   - Strychnine poisoning
   - Dystonic reactions
   - Dental infections leading to trismus
   - Seizure

7. **What is the time course of tetanus?**
   The incubation period after exposure averages from 8 to 11 days (range, 3–21 days). In neonatal tetanus, the incubation period is 4–14 days from birth, averaging about 7 days. The first week of illness is characterized by

muscle rigidity and spasm, followed by autonomic disturbances that last for 1–2 weeks. Muscle spasms generally subside after 2–3 weeks, but patients may experience persistent stiffness.

8. **How do I treat generalized tetanus in the emergency department (ED)?**
Initial management requires close attention to the patient's airway, including potential endotracheal intubation, and liberally administered benzodiazepine for sedation. Administer tetanus immunoglobulin (500 units) intramuscularly to bind free tetanotoxin at the site of the wound and before any wound cleaning/debridement. Administer metronidazole 7.5 mg/kg intravenous, max of 4 g/day every 6 hours; doxycycline, macrolides, clindamycin, and cephalosporins are alternatives.

9. **Where should I admit patients with tetanus?**
Patients with tetanus should be admitted to an intensive care unit (ICU) setting in a dark and quiet environment to minimize external stimuli.

10. **How do I prophylactically vaccinate someone against tetanus?**
  - First, determine if the patient has received a three-dose primary series of tetanus immunization. If not, administer Tdap (tetanus, diphtheria, and acellular pertussis), followed by second dose (Td – tetanus and diphtheria booster) 4 weeks later, and a third booster 6–12 months later. If the wound is tetanus prone, including but not limited to devitalized tissue, gross contamination, or wounds from crush injuries, administer the tetanus immunoglobulin (Table 53.1).
  - If the patient is fully immunized, determine when their last dose of tetanus toxoid (TT) was administered. For clean wounds, administer TT if last dose was over 10 years ago. If the wound is tetanus prone, administer TT if last dose was over 5 years ago.
  - TT choice: children <7 years old should receive higher diphtheria toxoid dose in either DT or DTaP. Between ages 7 and 64 years old, Tdap should be administered at least once; the remainder of boosters can be the Td formulation. For patients >65 years old, Tdap is preferred.

11. **What are the side effects of tetanus vaccine?**
Side effects are generally limited to local reactions, such as erythema, induration, tenderness, nodule, or sterile abscess at the site of infection. Mild systemic reactions can occur and include fever, drowsiness, fretfulness, and anorexia, but all are self-limited.

12. **Is the tetanus vaccine safe for pregnant and immunocompromised patients?**
The tetanus vaccine is a toxoid (inactivated toxin) that is safe and effective in pregnancy and can help prevent neonatal tetanus. All pregnant women should receive Tdap immunization during each pregnancy, irrespective of prior vaccination status. The tetanus vaccine is also safe for administration in immunocompromised patients.

KEY POINTS: TETANUS

1. Initial management of generalized tetanus is to monitor the airway and to provide adequate sedation to control spasms and pain.
2. Human tetanus immunoglobulin, surgical debridement, and metronidazole are initial treatments of choice.
3. In developed countries with ICU capabilities, autonomic instability is the most common cause of mortality.

Table 53.1 Postexposure Tetanus Prophylaxis

	Clean, Minor Wounds		All Other Wounds[a]	
VACCINATION HISTORY	**TT**	**TIG**	**TT**	**TIG**
Unknown primary series or <3 doses	Yes	No	Yes	Yes
Primary series ≥3 doses				
≥10 years since most recent dose	Yes	No	Yes	No
5–9 years since most recent dose	No	No	Yes	No
<5 years since most recent dose	No	No	No	No

[a]Wounds greater than 1 cm in depth, incurred more than 6 hours earlier, or with stellate or avulsion configuration; crush injuries or burn injuries; devitalized tissue; and wounds contaminated with dirt, feces, or saliva.
TT, Tetanus toxoid; *TIG*, tetanus-specific immune globulin.
From Hodowanec A, Bleck TP. Tetanus (*Clostridium tetani*). In: Bennett JE, Dolin R, Blaser MJ, eds. *Mandell, Douglas, and Bennett's Principles and Practice of Infectious Diseases.* 8th ed. Philadelphia: Churchill Livingstone; 2015:2757–2762.

BOTULISM

13. What is the causative agent of botulism, and what is its mechanism of action?

Botulism is caused by toxins produced by an obligate anaerobic bacterium, *Clostridium botulinum*. Botulinum toxins are taken up preferentially by skeletal and autonomic peripheral cholinergic nerve terminals, where the toxins irreversibly cleave synaptic vesicle docking and prevent the release of acetylcholine, producing a life-threatening paralytic illness. By weight, botulinum toxin is the most potent toxin known. Annually, 100–200 cases of botulism are reported in the United States.

14. How does the mechanism of botulism differ than that of tetanus?

Both botulinum toxin and tetanospasmin irreversibly cleave proteins in the synaptic vesicle docking mechanism to prevent neurotransmitter release. Botulism remains in the nerve terminals of acetylcholine-releasing neurons. However, tetanus is conveyed by retrograde transport to inhibitory GABA- and glycine-releasing neurons in the peripheral and central nervous system. Botulism inhibits activating neurons, leading to paralysis, whereas tetanus inhibits inhibitory neurons, leading to unopposed muscle contraction.

15. What are the six types of botulism?

- Infant botulism (70%–80% of US cases) is caused by the ingestion of spores, which proliferate in the gastrointestinal (GI) tract in the absence of competitive flora. Age of patients ranges from 6 days to 1 year, with a median age of 10 weeks. The source is unknown in most cases, but may be related to contaminated soil; contaminated raw honey ingestion accounts for 20% of cases
- Foodborne botulism (10%–20% of US cases) results from the foodborne ingestion of preformed toxin. Undercooked home-canned foods, fermented foods, and pruno (prison wine) are common sources.
- Wound botulism (5%–20% of US cases) is caused by the contamination of cutaneous wounds with spores. US cases are almost exclusively in "'black-tar" heroin users who "skin-pop" (injection into subcutaneous tissue).
- Iatrogenic botulism results from complications of cosmetic or therapeutic injections; it may be focal or generalized.
- Inhalational botulism is rare. Cases have been reported from insufflation of contaminated cocaine. Bioterrorism use of aerosolized botulinum toxin has been theorized.
- Botulism of undetermined etiology describes cases in which the patient's stool contains *C. botulinum* with signs and symptoms of clinical botulism, yet no contaminated food or wound can be identified.

16. What are the differential diagnoses of botulism?

- Electrolyte disorders: hypomagnesemia, hypokalemia, hypophosphatemia
- Guillain-Barré syndrome (especially Miller Fisher variant)
- Lambert-Eaton myasthenic syndrome
- Myasthenia gravis
- Neuromuscular blocker poisoning
- Organophosphate poisoning
- Paralytic shellfish poisoning
- Stroke syndromes
- Tetrodotoxin poisoning
- Tick paralysis

17. What is the presentation of infant botulism?

Constipation is often the first presenting symptom, followed by a weak cry, prolonged or poor feeding, hypotonia, and decreased gag or suck reflex. In severe cases, infants can have upper airway obstruction and respiratory failure. As in adults, infants can develop descending motor weakness, flaccid paralysis, and autonomic dysfunction.

18. How does an adult patient with foodborne botulism present?

- Early symptoms are nonspecific, usually begin 12–36 hours after ingestion (range, 6 hours to 8 days), and include nausea, vomiting, weakness, malaise, and dizziness.
- Next, prominent anticholinergic symptoms ensue, including extreme dry mouth, decreased lacrimation, constipation, or urinary retention.
- Then, symmetric cranial nerve palsies follow (up to 3 days after anticholinergic symptoms), including ptosis, diplopia, blurred vision, photophobia, dysphonia, or dysphagia.
- Finally, a descending symmetric flaccid paralysis of the voluntary muscles may follow and lead to respiratory failure.

19. How is botulism diagnosed?

The clinical diagnosis is based on history and examination with *treatment initiated based on clinical suspicion*. The most sensitive means of confirmatory diagnosis is toxin detection or anaerobic cultures of serum, stool, or implicated food products. Testing should be performed with coordination of your state health department or the Centers for Disease Control and Prevention (CDC).

20. **What is the treatment of foodborne botulism?**
Treatment is mostly supportive, including early elective intubation of patients at risk for respiratory failure. Heptavalent equine-derived antitoxin is also recommended within 24 hours to arrest progression, and shorten duration, of paralysis.

21. **What is treatment for infant botulism?**
Treatment of infant botulism includes supportive care with close monitoring of respiratory function. Human botulinum immune globulin (BabyBIG) reduces duration of hospitalization, mechanical ventilation, and tube feedings. The California Department of Health Services Infant Botulism Treatment and Prevention Program should be contacted for assistance in management and delivery of BabyBIG (510-231-7600, www.infantbotulism.org). Equine-derived antitoxin is not recommended for infant botulism.

22. **Are systemic antibiotics indicated for infant botulism?**
No, and aminoglycosides are absolutely contraindicated because they may potentiate neuromuscular blockade and increase duration of symptoms. Antibiotic administration may cause bacterial lysis in the gut and theoretically increase the free toxin load.

23. **Are antibiotics indicated in wound botulism?**
In addition to surgical debridement, antibiotics (penicillin G or metronidazole) may be of use in wound botulism, but benefit is unproven.

KEY POINTS: BOTULISM

1. Adult botulism presents as nonspecific anticholinergic symptoms followed by symmetric cranial nerve palsies and descending paralysis.
2. Infant botulism usually presents as constipation, followed by weak cry, prolonged or poor feeding, hypotonia, and decreased gag or suck reflex.
3. Human botulinum immune globulin (BabyBIG) is available for infant botulism.

FOODBORNE ILLNESSES

24. **Name the causes of foodborne illnesses.**
    * Viruses (e.g., *Enterovirus*, hepatitis, *Norovirus*, *Rotavirus*, or *Sapovirus*)
    * Direct bacterial invasion or endotoxins (e.g., *Campylobacter*, *Escherichia coli*, *Listeria monocytogenes*, *Salmonella*, *Shigella*, *Vibrio*, or *Yersinia enterocolitica*)
    * Parasites (e.g., *Entamoeba histolytica*, *Cryptosporidium*, or *Giardia lamblia*)
    * Mushrooms (e.g., *Amanita phalloides*, *Chlorophyllum*)
    * Secreted/preformed exotoxins (e.g., *Bacillus cereus*, *Clostridium perfringens*, *Shigella*, shellfish-associated algal toxins, *Staphylococcus aureus*, or tetrodotoxin)

25. **What is the time course of traveler's diarrhea?**
    * Onset: (1) Secreted/preformed exotoxins – hours. (2) Bacterial/viral pathogens – 6–72 hours. (3) Protozoal pathogens – 1–2 weeks.
    * Duration: although about 10% of patients have more than 1 week of symptoms, traveler's diarrhea usually lasts 3–7 days; 2% of patients have more than 1 month of symptoms.

26. **What is the geographic incidence of traveler's diarrhea?**
    * High-risk destinations (20%–90% incidence for a 2-week stay): most of Africa, most of Asia, Central America, Mexico, the Middle East, and South America.
    * Intermediate-risk destinations (8%–20% incidence): some Caribbean islands, Eastern Europe, and South Africa.
    * Low-risk destinations (<8% incidence): Australia, Canada, Northern/Western Europe, Japan, New Zealand, and the United States.
    * Overall, approximately 30%–70% of travelers will be affected, and of those, 3%–30% of individuals will have symptoms of dysentery (e.g., bloody stool, fever).

27. **What are some of the more serious complications of traveler's diarrhea? What are the causative agents?**
    * Amebic hepatitis and amebic abscesses: *Entamoeba*
    * Bacteremia leading to endocarditis, aortitis, septic arthritis, osteomyelitis: *Salmonella, Yersinia*
    * Ekiri syndrome (lethal toxic encephalopathy): *Shigella*
    * Erythema nodosum: *Campylobacter, Salmonella, Shigella, Yersinia*
    * Glomerulonephritis: *Campylobacter, Shigella, Yersinia*
    * Guillain-Barré syndrome: *Campylobacter*
    * Hemolytic anemia: *Campylobacter, Yersinia*

- Hemolytic uremic syndrome (HUS): *Shigella dysenteriae* and Shiga toxin–producing *Escherichia coli (STEC, O157:H7)*
- Intestinal perforation: *Campylobacter, Entamoeba, Salmonella, Shigella, Yersinia*
- Meningitis: *Listeria, Salmonella* (in infants ≤3 months)
- Postinfectious irritable bowel syndrome: *Campylobacter, Giardia, Salmonella, Shigella, STEC*
- Reactive arthritis [formerly Reiter syndrome]: *Campylobacter, Salmonella, Shigella, Yersinia*

28. **What is the ED management of infectious diarrhea?**
The primary goal of resuscitation is rehydration. Mild to moderate symptoms should be managed by reduced-osmolarity oral rehydration solution. Intravenous fluids may be necessary for severe dehydration. Antimotility drugs (e.g., loperamide) and antiemetic drugs (e.g., ondansetron) are adjunctive and should not replace fluid resuscitation. Avoid antimotility drugs in cases suspecting toxic megacolon or diarrhea with fever/bloody stools (Fig. 53.1).

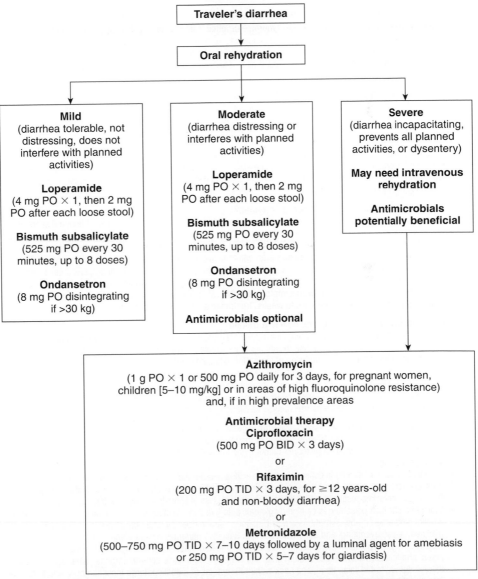

Fig. 53.1 Approach to traveler's diarrhea. *BID,* Twice daily; *PO,* orally *(per os)*; *TID,* three times daily.

29. **Should antibiotics be used for infectious diarrhea?**
Empiric antibiotics should *not* be used in well-appearing immunocompetent patients with infectious diarrhea. The treatment of certain bacterial pathogens with antibiotics may decrease duration of symptoms by 1 day. However, the benefits are typically outweighed by risk of increasing antibiotic resistance and risk of HUS with antibiotic-induced lysis of STEC-releasing endotoxins. Empiric antibiotics may be considered in the following patient populations:
   - Infants <3 months old with suspected bacterial source.
   - Ill-appearing patients with dysentery.
   - Patients who have traveled internationally with fever or sepsis.

   Antimicrobial choice: First-line – single oral dose of ciprofloxacin 3-day regimen of ciprofloxacin 500 mg twice daily. Alternative regimen (for children and pregnant women) is azithromycin 1 g (5–10 mg/kg) PO (orally), as a single dose or 500 mg PO daily for 3 days. In areas where amebiasis and giardiasis are endemic, consider metronidazole 500–750 mg PO three times daily for 7–10 days followed by a luminal agent (iodoquinol 650 mg PO three times daily for 20 days or paromomycin 25–35 mg/kg/day PO in 3 divided doses for 7 days) for amebiasis or 250 mg PO three times daily for 5–7 days for giardiasis (see Fig. 53.1).

30. **Which diarrhea-producing agent is associated with febrile seizures in children?**
Shigella in young children can cause Ekiri syndrome or lethal toxic encephalopathy. Symptoms include high fevers, generalized toxic appearance, abdominal cramps, bloody mucoid stool, and seizures with or without encephalopathy. Other complications include dehydration, hyponatremia, hypoglycemia, and surgical emergencies (e.g., toxic megacolon, rectal prolapse, or intestinal perforation). Endemic *Shigella* is responsible for 75% of diarrhea-related deaths in developing countries.

31. **What is scombroid poisoning, and how is it treated?**
Scombroid fish poisoning is caused by ingestion of improperly refrigerated fish, with bacterial conversion of naturally occurring histidine to histamine. Fish with high histidine content including the Scombridae family (e.g., tuna, albacore, bonito, mackerel, skipjack), mahi-mahi, and bluefish have been implicated. Affected fish typically retain normal appearance and odor but may taste peppery. Not a true fish allergy, poisoning causes histaminergic symptoms minutes to hours after ingestion, typically an urticarial rash of the face, neck, and upper chest. Other symptoms include flushing, vomiting, diarrhea, headache, palpitations, and a metallic taste in the mouth. Rarely, severe cases may cause hypotension resembling anaphylactic shock and require pressor support. Treatment with H_1- and H_2-antagonists is generally effective.

32. **What is ciguatera poisoning, and how is it treated?**
Ciguatera poisoning occurs after the ingestion of coral reef fish (barracuda, sea bass, parrot fish, red snapper, grouper, amber jack, kingfish, and sturgeon) that contain ciguatoxin, a heat-stable toxin from *Gambierdiscus toxicus* that opens sodium channels. Contaminated fish have no distinctive appearance, odor, or taste. A constellation of gastrointestinal and neurologic symptoms start within hours of ingestion, including vomiting, watery diarrhea, abdominal pain, diaphoresis, headache, reversal of temperature perception, facial/perioral paresthesias, sensation of loose/painful teeth, ataxia, and coma. Other findings include bradycardia, hypotension, arthralgias, myalgias, itching, dysuria, and dyspareunia. Most symptoms resolve within a few days; however, severe neurologic and cardiac symptoms may persist for days to weeks. Treatment is largely supportive care.

33. **What is tetrodotoxin poisoning, and how is it treated?**
Tetrodotoxin is found in puffer fish (fugu), blue-ringed octopus, horse shoe crabs, and rough-skinned newt. The toxin blocks sodium channels, inhibiting axonal nerve transmission. Tetrodotoxin is resistant to cooking and is most concentrated in the viscera and skin of the puffer fish. Safe consumption is predicated on expert chefs removing these areas. Symptoms begin with perioral paresthesias, which can spread to the entire body, as well as vomiting and dizziness; most patients develop a rapid ascending paralysis. Respiratory failure ensues if unmanaged and is followed by cardiovascular collapse, coma, and death within 6 hours on average. Treatment should be focused on airway management, mechanical ventilation, and supportive care.

34. **Describe the toxic syndromes associated with ingestion of shellfish.**
Algal toxins are produced by numerous species of marine algae that contaminate shellfish, crustaceans, and some fish. Diagnosis is based on history of recent ingestion and clinical picture; treatment is supportive. Syndromes include:
   - Amnesic shellfish poisoning is caused by domoic acid, a neuroexcitatory toxin, found primarily in squid, scallops, mussels, and razor clams. Symptoms start within 24 hours of ingestion and can include vomiting, dizziness, headache, confusion, respiratory difficulty, and coma, with loss of short-term memory that may be permanent.
   - Diarrhetic shellfish poisoning is caused by okadaic acid found in affected mussels, cockles, scallops, oysters, whelks, and green crabs. Symptoms are self-limited, characterized by acute onset within 30 minutes of severe diarrhea, nausea/vomiting, and abdominal cramps. Recovery generally occurs within 3–4 days.
   - Paralytic shellfish poisoning is caused by saxitoxin in affected mussels, clams, oysters, scallops, abalone, crabs, and lobster, which blocks sodium channels of nerve and muscle cell membranes. Initial perioral paresthesias spread to the face, head, and neck within 30 minutes of ingestion; large ingestion may lead to respiratory arrest and death within 2 hours.

- Neurotoxic shellfish poisoning is caused by the brevotoxin family of toxins, commonly found in cockles, mussels, and whelks off the coast of Florida and the Gulf of Mexico. Symptoms begin 15 minutes to 18 hours after ingestion, last up to 48 hours, and can include perioral paresthesias, abdominal pain, dizziness, diplopia, gait deficits, chills, reversed temperature perception, headache, musculoskeletal pain, bradycardia, and respiratory difficulty. Mechanism and symptoms are similar to ciguatoxin poisoning but without long-term sequelae.

35. **Which population of patients is at risk of invasive *Vibrio* disease from eating raw oysters?**
Patients with preexisting liver diseases (cirrhosis and hemochromatosis), immunodeficiency, or hematologic disorders with elevated iron levels have an 80 times higher risk of invasive *Vibrio* disease. Consumption of raw oysters, especially from warmer waters between April and November, has a high incidence of *Vibrio vulnificus* and *Vibrio parahaemolyticus*.

36. **Describe the four stages of *Amanita phalloides* mushroom toxicity.**
    - *Stage 1.* Patient remains asymptomatic for 6–24 hours postingestion, an important distinction from most GI-irritant mushrooms. After the initial latent period, patients experience violent onset of nausea, vomiting, diarrhea (often bloody), and severe abdominal pain lasting 1–2 days, which is often misdiagnosed as viral gastroenteritis. This stage may include acid-base disturbances, electrolyte abnormalities, hypoglycemia, dehydration, and hypotension. Physical examination may be significant for epigastric tenderness and hepatomegaly with normal liver function tests.
    - *Stage 2.* The quiescent stage begins 24–48 hours after ingestion and is characterized by transient clinical improvement despite continued hepatic deterioration.
    - *Stage 3.* Beginning suddenly 2–4 days postingestion, the patient develops multisystem organ failure with marked rise in liver function tests, acute kidney injury, cardiomyopathy, hepatic encephalopathy, convulsions, coma, and death.
    - *Stage 4.* Recovery stage for survivors.

KEY POINTS: FOODBORNE ILLNESSES

1. Antibiotics are not recommended in children with bloody diarrhea with concern for toxin release and development of HUS.
2. Patients with liver disease are at highest risk for invasive *Vibrio* disease from eating raw oysters.
3. Patients with *A. phalloides* toxic poisoning may appear to be improving before experiencing rapid deterioration.

ACKNOWLEDGMENT
The editors gratefully acknowledge the contributions of John E. Houghland, MD, Kevin Dean, MD, and Scott Rudkin, MD, MBA, authors of this chapter in the previous edition.

BIBLIOGRAPHY
Connor BA. The pretravel consultation. In: Brunette GW, ed. *Centers for Disease Control and Prevention. CDC Yellow Book 2018: Health Information for International Travel.* New York: Oxford University Press; 2017.
Diaz JH. Amatoxin-containing mushroom poisonings: species, toxidromes, treatments, and outcomes. *Wilderness Environ Med.* 2018;29:111–118.
Isbister G, Kiernan M. Neurotoxic marine poisoning. *Lancet Neurol.* 2005;4:219–228.
Hodowanec A, Bleck TP. Botulism (*Clostridium botulinum*). In: Bennett JE, Dolin R, Blaser MJ, eds. *Mandell, Douglas, and Bennett's Principles and Practice of Infectious Diseases.* 8th ed. Philadelphia: Churchill Livingstone; 2015:2763–2767.
Hodowanec A, Bleck TP. Tetanus (*Clostridium tetani*). In: Bennett JE, Dolin R, Blaser MJ, eds. *Mandell, Douglas, and Bennett's Principles and Practice of Infectious Diseases.* 8th ed. Philadelphia: Churchill Livingstone; 2015:2757–2762.
Neil MA, Carpenter CCJ. Other pathogenic vibrios. In: Bennett JE, Dolin R, Blaser MJ, eds. *Mandell, Douglas, and Bennett's Principles and Practice of Infectious Diseases.* 8th ed. Philadelphia: Churchill Livingstone; 2015:2480–2483.
Shane AL, Mody RK, Crump JA, et al. 2017 Infectious Diseases Society of America clinical practice guidelines for the diagnosis and management of infectious diarrhea. *Clin Infect Dis.* 2017;65:1963–1973.
Suguitan MA, Rao RB. Scombroid. In: Brent J, ed. *Critical Care Toxicology: Diagnosis and Management of the Critically Poisoned Patient.* 2nd ed. New York: Springer; 2017:2075–2083.
Tetanus. In: Hamborsky J, Kroger A, Wolfe S, eds. *Centers for Disease Control and Prevention. Epidemiology and Prevention of Vaccine-Preventable Diseases.* 13th ed. Washington, DC: Public Health Foundation; 2015:341–352.

CHAPTER 54

TRAVEL MEDICINE AND VECTOR-BORNE DISEASES

Evangelina Murray, MD and Jennifer J Whitfield, MD, MPH

1. What is travel medicine?
Travel medicine refers to the prevention and management of health problems in travelers.

2. Why is travel medicine important?
International tourism and business travel are growing industries; more than 1 billion international arrivals occurred worldwide, and nearly 55 million international trips were taken by Americans in 2018. Approximately 8% of travelers from high-income to developing countries become ill enough to seek medical care. Health care providers and medical students are increasingly traveling internationally to provide charitable health care and to participate in clinical rotations. Greater than 25% of graduating medical students in 2018 took part in an international medical elective before graduation, compared with 6% in 1984.

3. Should I visit a travel clinic before my trip?
Fewer than half of patients treated after travel report a pretravel clinic visit. Travelers, especially those going to developing countries, should visit a travel medicine clinic 4–8 weeks before departure to obtain required vaccinations and antimalarial prophylaxis, if necessary. Dental, gynecologic, and primary health care visits are also recommended, particularly before prolonged travel to areas with few health care resources. The traveler should assemble a medical kit with the basics: first-aid supplies, antidiarrheal medicines, contraceptives, water disinfectant, sunscreen, insect repellent, prescribed medications, and antihistamines.

4. What other pretravel preparation should take place?
Travelers should have a basic understanding of health risks particular to their journey, activities, and destination, and take relevant precautions before, during, and after travel. The Centers for Disease Control and Prevention (CDC) *Yellow Book* provides information regarding country and region-specific health risks, and is an invaluable resource for both travelers and health professionals. Travelers should register with the Smart Traveler Enrollment Program of the US Department of State to receive up-to-date information on travel warnings and to facilitate seeking medical care or repatriation if needed. The US Department of State also provides health-related information, including detailed country-specific safety concerns, instructions for finding hospitals and arranging medical evacuation while abroad, and links to travel insurance plans. Travel insurance is highly recommended and should cover hospitalizations and acute care in the destination country, as well as medical evacuation if necessary.

5. How should I prepare before embarking on volunteer clinical work overseas?
Physicians should volunteer with organizations that have a long-standing and integrated role within the local health care system. Volunteers should have expertise treating diseases common in the region, speak the local language, and understand the cultural and social influences on health care provision. Participation in a tropical or wilderness medicine course is advised.

6. What clinical history should I obtain from the ill traveler?
Find out about the location of travel, including layovers, type of transportation, dates of travel, accommodations, activities, and exposures. Ask specifically about use of insect repellents, bed nets, food and water safety, exposure to fresh water, insect and animal bites, body fluid exposures, and pretravel preparation, including vaccines and use of malarial prophylaxis. Careful investigation of the timing of symptom onset and associated symptoms is crucial as well. The CDC's website is an excellent resource for researching common health conditions by geographic region, presenting signs and symptoms, and season, as well as updates on recent outbreaks.

7. What are the most common illnesses affecting returned travelers?
- Diarrhea and other gastrointestinal illness (34%)
- Febrile illnesses (23%)
- Skin conditions (20%)

    From 1997 to 2011, 19% of returned febrile travelers tracked by the GeoSentinel Global Surveillance System were diagnosed with *Plasmodium falciparum* malaria.

8. What causes traveler's diarrhea (TD)?
Acute diarrheal illness, or TD, is the most common illness in persons traveling from high-income to low-income regions. Travelers to developing countries who consume inadequately prepared food, and fruits and vegetables

that are not peeled or washed in treated water are at highest risk. Most TD is caused by an unspecified pathogen; a recent surveillance study found that about 23% bacterial, most commonly enterotoxigenic *Escherichia coli*, followed by *Campylobacter jejuni*, *Shigella* spp., and *Salmonella* spp. *Giardia* (13%) and amebiasis (4%) are less common causes. An overview of foodborne illness is available in Chapter 53.

9. **What are the most common skin conditions seen in returned travelers?**
Most skin conditions seen in travelers are similar to those seen domestically and caused by the same organisms, including insect bites, cellulitis, nonspecific dermatitis, and fungal infections. A few notable exceptions include cutaneous leishmaniases, cutaneous larva migrans, and rashes associated with systemic illnesses such as dengue, rickettsial infections, and chikungunya fever. Diagnosis relies heavily on knowing the location and timing of travel; if there is a history of animal, insect, or arthropod bites, stings and scratches, and sexual activity.

10. **What is leishmaniasis?**
A vector-borne disease transmitted by sand flies, leishmaniasis can present in myriad ways, but most commonly with cutaneous ulcers on exposed skin called *localized cutaneous leishmaniasis (LCL)*. It begins as a pink papule that eventually enlarges into a painless ulceration with an indurated border. Symptoms can start weeks or months after initial exposure, and it is most common among travelers to the Middle East, North Africa, and Central and South America. Diagnosis is made via identification of the protozoa from a suspicious ulcer though culture or polymerase chain reaction (PCR).

11. **How is LCL treated?**
It can be reasonable to manage localized, noncomplicated LCL with observation. Treatment of LCL can decrease risk of scarring and disfigurement, as well as the risk of extension to one of the many other manifestations of the disease, such as mucosal and diffuse cutaneous leishmaniasis. Topical agents are first-line treatment; thermotherapy or cryotherapy can be performed by an experienced dermatologist. Therapies like pentavalent antimonials and topical paromomycins are not available in the United States commercially.

12. **What are the most important tools in diagnosing these vector-borne diseases?**
A detailed history and a skin examination are critical. Many of these illnesses initially present with a nonspecific syndrome of fever, headache, and myalgias. A history of travel, exposure to the vector, or a characteristic rash can provide the key to a difficult diagnosis.

13. **What causes malaria?**
Malaria is caused by one of four species of the protozoan *Plasmodium*: *P. falciparum*, *P. vivax*, *P. ovale*, and *P. malariae*. Malaria is usually acquired by the bite of a protozoan-infected *Anopheles* mosquito, but it also may be transmitted by transfusion of infected blood or from mother to child in utero. *P. falciparum*, the most common and most life-threatening type, causes virtually all of the 1 million annual malaria deaths worldwide.

14. **Can malaria be prevented?**
Although no one method of protection is 100% effective, proper use of prophylactic drugs, bed nets, and insect repellent, as well as proper patient education, can prevent most cases of traveler's malaria seen in the United States.

15. **What is the presentation of malaria in emergency department (ED) patients?**
Symptoms develop 10–14 days after *P. falciparum* infection, but may be latent for 1 year with *P. vivax*. Patients complain of flulike symptoms, with fever, chills, headache, nausea, vomiting, abdominal pain, cough, and myalgias. Physical examination may reveal jaundice, hepatomegaly, or splenomegaly, but is often normal. The presence of a rash or significant lymphadenopathy suggests another diagnosis or coinfection. Anemia, thrombocytopenia, and hemoglobinuria are common laboratory findings. Patients may develop renal failure, pulmonary edema, shock, disseminated intravascular coagulation, profound anemia, acidosis, and hypoglycemia. Cerebral malaria, the most common fatal manifestation of malaria in adults, presents with altered mental status, seizures, and coma.

16. **How is malaria diagnosed?**
A high index of suspicion is the key to an early clinical diagnosis and survival, because early initiation of treatment is a time-critical action. Definitive diagnosis is made by visualization of protozoa on blood smears using microscopy. Thick blood smears are more sensitive, but thin blood smears are necessary for speciation and calculation of parasitemia percentage. Despite recommended repeat blood smears at least three times at 12-hour intervals, false-negative results will still occur. Rapid antigen detection kits are useful in case of limited access to an experienced laboratory technician.

17. **How is malaria treated?**
Unless *P. falciparum* infection can be ruled out, prompt treatment should be initiated empirically and the patient admitted. Severe malaria is treated with intravenous artesunate, or with quinine plus doxycycline or clindamycin (to avoid resistance), if artesunate is not available. There are several oral options for treating uncomplicated malaria. In chloroquine-resistant areas, the World Health Organization (WHO) recommends artemisinin-based combination therapies (ACTs) as first-line treatment, including artesunate-mefloquine, artesunate-amodiaquine, and artemether-lumefantrine (Coartem). Central America and most of the Middle East are chloroquine-sensitive areas, and infections in travelers visiting these regions can be treated as such. Treatment should be initiated

according to the CDC, which has a 24-hour hotline for clinicians, as well as comprehensive online resources. Those receiving intravenous medications should receive telemetry monitoring, as quinine and quinidine cause dysrhythmogenic QT prolongation.

KEY POINTS: MALARIA

1. Malaria is a common and lethal disease of the returning traveler or recent immigrant.
2. Normal blood smears do not rule out the disease.
3. Begin early empiric treatment in a sick patient with the right travel history.
4. More people die from malaria than from any other bite- or sting-induced disease.

18. What is dengue, and where does it occur?

Dengue is a mosquito-borne flavivirus endemic to tropical regions transmitted by *Aedes aegypti*. The WHO estimates 50–100 million infections occur yearly. The CDC reported a fourfold increase in reported cases from 1989 to 2007 in Central America, South America, Mexico, and the Caribbean. There have been outbreaks in the United States in Texas and Florida.

19. How does dengue fever present?

Many infections, especially in children, are asymptomatic or go unnoticed as a mild febrile illness. Classic dengue fever occurs 5–6 days after incubation and lasts about 1 week, with most patients fully recovering. Presenting symptoms include fever, retroorbital headache, nausea, vomiting, arthralgias, and severe myalgias, earning it the nickname of *breakbone fever*. The characteristic confluent, blanching, macular rash occurs in 50% of cases. A small proportion of patients go on to develop severe dengue, which is characterized by vascular permeability with consequent pulmonary effusions, ascites, hemorrhage, and multiorgan failure. Severe, untreated dengue carries a mortality rate of greater than 40%.

20. How do I diagnose and treat dengue fever?

Dengue fever should be suspected in patients returning from endemic areas with suspicious symptoms and laboratory markers. The diagnosis can be made with enzyme-linked immunosorbent assay (ELISA) serology, but it is often negative during acute illness and may cross react with antibodies to other arboviruses, such as West Nile virus. Laboratory abnormalities include thrombocytopenia, leukopenia, and nonspecific elevation of liver enzymes. Progression to severe dengue is marked by hemoconcentration, hypoproteinemia, and rapid decrease in platelet count. Treatment is supportive: oral rehydration and analgesics in the outpatient setting for mild disease all the way to intensive care for severe disease with shock. Nonsteroidal anti-inflammatory drugs (NSAIDs) and aspirin must be avoided because of their platelet inhibition. A vaccine is available as of 2019 in the United States and was already available in Europe; however, it is not recommended for travelers and only for children 9–16 years old with documented serologic evidence of previous infection in endemic areas.

21. What is chikungunya virus and where does it occur?

Chikungunya virus is an alphavirus transmitted by *Aedes aegypti* and *Aedes albopictus* mosquitoes. It is endemic in West Africa, but outbreaks have occurred elsewhere, including the Caribbean, Puerto Rico, and Florida.

22. What are the symptoms of chikungunya?

Onset occurs after an incubation period of 3–7 days with mild fever, significant arthralgias that are typically bilateral and distal. It can also present with a maculopapular rash.

23. How do I diagnose and treat chikungunya virus?

It is diagnosed using reverse transcription polymerase chain reaction (RT-PCR) of viral RNA in serum. Treatment is supportive.

24. What is Zika virus and where is it prevalent?

Zika virus is a flavivirus transmitted by *Aedes* mosquitos. From 2014 to 2017 there was an epidemic of Zika virus infections in Central and South America. In 2016 the WHO declared the Zika epidemic in the Americas a Public Health Emergency of International Concern (PHEIC). Outbreaks have also occurred in Africa, Southeast Asia, and the Pacific Islands. From 2015 to 2019, 231 cases of presumed local transmission were reported in Florida and Texas.

25. What are the clinical manifestations of Zika virus infection?

Onset is 2–14 days after insect bite, with fever, pruritic maculopapular rash, arthralgias in hands and feet, and conjunctivitis. However, some infected individuals are asymptomatic. Postviral Guillain-Barré syndrome has been described and associated regionally with outbreaks of Zika in multiple countries.

26. How do I diagnose and treat Zika virus infections?

RT-PCR for viral RNA in serum, urine, or whole blood. Treatment is supportive. Prevention is primarily through prevention of insect bites and avoiding unprotected sex with infected individuals. There is currently no vaccine available. Treatment is supportive care.

27. **What are the risks of Zika infection in pregnant women?**
Congenital microcephaly and fetal loss are the primary concerning complications of Zika virus infection in pregnancy. These risks are much higher in the first trimester of pregnancy. Current recommendations for couples trying to become pregnant are to abstain from unprotected sex for at least 3 months if the male partner was infected, and at least 8 weeks if the female partner was.

KEY POINTS: DENGUE, ZIKA, AND CHIKUNGUNYA

1. Coinfections are increasingly common.
2. Definitive diagnosis requires expensive laboratory tests.
3. Treatment is supportive.
4. Pregnant women should avoid travel in areas endemic with Zika.

---

28. **What is West Nile virus?**
The West Nile virus is a flavivirus acquired through the bite of *Culex* mosquitoes. It is endemic in Africa, the Middle East, southern Europe, Southwest Asia, and Australia. Peak incidence in the United States was ~10,000 in 2003, with a decrease since.

29. **What are the symptoms of West Nile infections?**
Only one-fifth of infections leads to symptoms; only one in approximately 200 present with central nervous system (CNS) involvement. Symptomatic infection with the West Nile virus occurs 2–14 days after exposure, and 94% of patients in the United States report symptom onset between July and September. Initial symptoms include fever, headache, weakness, nausea, vomiting, and a maculopapular rash predominantly on the torso and extremities, sparing the palms and soles. Those with CNS involvement most commonly have an encephalitic syndrome that includes altered mental status or seizures. Isolated aseptic meningitis also occurs. More rarely, patients suffer polio-type paralysis or parkinsonian movement disorders. The elderly are at much higher risk for severe disease and death. Neuropsychiatric sequelae occur in more than 50% of those with severe disease.

30. **How is West Nile encephalitis diagnosed and treated?**
Diagnosis is made with ELISA antibody assays on serum or cerebrospinal fluid (CSF). Treatment is supportive.

31. **Are ticks a significant vector of disease?**
Yes, they are responsible for the greatest variety and steadily increasing numbers of vector-borne human illness in North America. There are two major families of ticks: the hard ticks and the soft ticks. Hard ticks transmit all tick-borne diseases, with the exception of relapsing fever. Ticks typically spread disease in the summer months, when ticks are actively seeking blood meals, and when most potential human hosts are engaged in outdoor activities.

32. **List the principal vectors and distribution of tick-borne diseases.**
See Table 54.1.

Table 54.1 Principal Vectors and Distribution of the Tick-Borne Diseases

DISEASE	VECTOR	PATHOGEN	US DISTRIBUTION	FIRST-LINE TREATMENT
Babesiosis	*Ixodes scapularis*	*Babesia microti*	Northeast, upper Midwest	Azithromycin and atovaquone
Colorado tick fever	*Dermacentor andersoni*	*Coltivirus*	Western mountains	Supportive
Ehrlichiosis	*Amblyomma americanum*	*Ehrlichia chaffeensis*	Southeast, South Central	Doxycycline
Anaplasmosis	*Ixodes* species	*Anaplasma phagocytophila*	Same as Lyme disease	Doxycycline
Lyme disease	*Ixodes* species	*Borrelia burgdorferi*	Northeast, Midwest, West	Doxycycline
Tick-borne relapsing fever	*Ornithodoros* species	*Borrelia* species	Western mountains	Tetracycline

Continued on following page

Table 54.1 Principal Vectors and Distribution of the Tick-Borne Diseases *(Continued)*

DISEASE	VECTOR	PATHOGEN	US DISTRIBUTION	FIRST-LINE TREATMENT
RMSF	*Dermacentor* species	*Rickettsia rickettsii*	Nationwide, mostly Southeast	Doxycycline
STARI	*A. americanum*	*Borrelia lonestari*	South	Doxycycline
Tick paralysis	Multiple	Toxins	Nationwide	Tick removal
Tularemia	*A. americanum* and *Dermacentor* species	*F. tularensis*	West, South Central	Streptomycin

RMSF, Rocky Mountain spotted fever; *STARI,* southern tick-associated rash illness.

33. **How is Lyme disease transmitted?**
    Ixodes scapularis ticks transmit Lyme disease in eastern and central North America, whereas *Ixodes pacificus* is the vector on the Pacific Coast. Tick nymphs pick up the *Borrelia* spirochetes from mice and transmit the Lyme infections to people. Transmission of Lyme disease rarely occurs before 48 hours of attachment. Acute Lyme diseases peak between April and September.

34. **Describe the three clinical stages of lyme disease.**
    1. *Early acute or localized infection.* In 80% of infections, the classic skin lesion, erythema migrans (EM), develops at the bite site within 3–30 days. Up to 75% of patients with EM will not recall a tick bite. EM expands slowly as an erythematous macule with central clearing that is usually painless but at times pruritic. Many individuals will develop systemic flulike symptoms with fever, suggesting some degree of early dissemination. Untreated, EM will typically resolve spontaneously over 3–4 weeks.
    2. *Early disseminated disease.* Untreated, this may occur days to weeks after the tick bite. Most will have fever and adenopathy, and many will have multiple secondary skin lesions that are smaller than the initial EM. Neurologic manifestations include cranial neuritis, such as unilateral or bilateral lower facial nerve palsy, and aseptic meningitis. Other neurologic manifestations include radiculoneuritis, similar to postherpetic neuralgia, with burning and paresthesias. Carditis, most commonly presenting with atrioventricular blocks, occurs in <10% of cases.
    3. *Late or chronic disease.* Late manifestations occur months to years after infection. Lyme arthritis is most common, presenting in 10% of those untreated and affecting one or several large joints, usually the knee. There is typically no joint destruction, and symptoms may spontaneously resolve after several years. Chronic neurologic disease may include polyneuritis, multiple sclerosis–like encephalomyelitis (0.1%), and subtle encephalopathy. Chronic dermatitis (acrodermatitis chronicum atrophicans) and keratitis are relatively rare in the United States.

35. **How is Lyme disease diagnosed?**
    The typical EM rash in an endemic area is sufficient for diagnosis. ELISA serology is used to detect Lyme antibodies; however, clinical findings are essential to make the diagnosis, as positive serology does not prove active infection in an endemic area. A positive test in an asymptomatic individual is not an indication for treatment. Blood cultures have low sensitivity, and thus are of little diagnostic value.

36. **How is Lyme disease treated?**
    Oral therapy with doxycycline (first line) or amoxicillin is effective for early disease and for mild early disseminated disease. Neurologic and cardiac manifestations (with the exception of an isolated Bell palsy) typically require parenteral therapy with ceftriaxone over 2–3 weeks, with a good prognosis. Given the risk of progression, Lyme carditis usually necessitates admission to telemetry, even for a first-degree atrioventricular block if the PR interval is greater than 300 milliseconds. Temporary pacing may be needed for third-degree blocks, with late disease not always responsive to treatment.

37. **Can Lyme disease be prevented?**
    The mainstays of prevention remain avoiding tick exposure, preventing attachment with protective clothing, and removing ticks promptly if they attach (twice-daily tick checks). The only vaccine was removed from the market in 2002.

38. **An ED patient has a tick bite; should you treat prophylactically for Lyme disease?**
    Yes and no; if you practice in an endemic area, if you can identify the tick as *I. scapularis*, and it was likely attached for more than 48 hours (suggested by engorgement, or known exposure time), treatment with a single 200-mg dose of doxycycline is effective in preventing Lyme disease (pediatric dosage is 4 mg/kg up to

maximum dose of 200 mg). If you cannot meet these three conditions, simply give your patient appropriate return precautions.

KEY POINTS: LYME DISEASE

1. It is the most common vector-borne disease in the United States.
2. A classic EM rash develops at site of tick bite.
3. Heart block, lower motor facial nerve palsy, and arthritis develop in advanced disease.
4. Positive serology test is not diagnostic of infection.
5. Treatment is doxycycline (first line), amoxicillin, or ceftriaxone.

39. **What on earth is STARI and what can be done about it?**
STARI stands for *southern tick-associated rash illness* and causes EM just like Lyme disease. It is caused by a spirochete, *Borrelia lonestari*, transmitted by the lone star tick, *Amblyomma americanum*. If a patient comes to the ED in the southern United States, an area nonendemic for Lyme disease, the diagnosis is likely to be STARI. Treat it just as you would early localized Lyme disease.

40. **What is tick-borne relapsing fever?**
Tick-borne relapsing fever (TBRF) is caused by several *Borrelia* species transmitted by soft ticks. Most cases are linked to stays in rural, rodent-infested cabins in the mountains of the western United States. Abrupt onset of flulike symptoms (i.e., fever, myalgias, headache, and vomiting) occurs 2–18 days after exposure. After 3 days of fever, symptoms resolve and then relapse on a weekly basis up to 10 times, with declining severity. Diagnosis is made by detection of spirochetes on stained thick and thin blood smears or by special culture. The disease responds well to doxycycline and erythromycin, but a Jarisch-Herxheimer reaction may occur (malaise and hypotension).

41. **What is Rocky Mountain spotted fever (RMSF)?**
RMSF is a life-threatening infection caused by *Rickettsia rickettsii* and transmitted by *Dermacentor*, or dog ticks. Currently, most cases are reported from the southeastern and south-central United States in spite of the name. Abrupt-onset fever, severe headache, and myalgias 5–7 days after the tick bite are the most common presenting symptoms. The rash is petechial, occurring initially on the wrists and ankles, spreading to the palms and soles, and then the trunk, and often progressing into purpuric lesions. Although the rash is rarely present during the first 3 days of illness, ~90% will develop a rash, and ~60% of infections will develop with the classic triad of rash, fever, and tick exposure.

42. **How dangerous is RMSF? What can be done about it?**
Untreated, RMSF mortality rates range from 20% to 80%. The rickettsial pathogen induces a vasculitis that leads to end-organ dysfunction, including confusion, respiratory failure, and renal failure. Death is most typically a result of disseminated intravascular coagulation. Appropriate and timely antibiotics can reduce the mortality rate to less than 5%. Doxycycline remains the drug of choice. Consider early empiric treatment in the spring and summer in endemic regions.

43. **What are ehrlichiosis and anaplasmosis?**
Ehrlichiosis and anaplasmosis are tick-borne diseases caused by the rickettsia-like bacteria, *Ehrlichia chaffeensis* and *Anaplasma phagocytophilia*. Ehrlichiosis is transmitted by *A. americanum* in the southeastern and south-central United States, whereas anaplasmosis is transmitted by *Ixodes* ticks in a similar distribution to Lyme disease. Both diseases present with fever and flulike symptoms and progress to coma, with respiratory and renal failure in severe cases. Rash may occur in ehrlichiosis, but not in anaplasmosis.

44. **How are ehrlichiosis and anaplasmosis diagnosed and treated?**
High clinical suspicion is needed in endemic areas during the summer months. Thrombocytopenia, leukopenia, and mildly elevated liver enzymes, in the context of possible tick exposure or bites, are highly suggestive and should prompt treatment. Microscopic examination of buffy coat or peripheral blood may reveal characteristic inclusion bodies in monocytes or neutrophils. Doxycycline is first-line therapy.

45. **What is Colorado tick fever?**
Colorado tick fever is caused by an RNA *Coltivirus* that is transmitted by *Dermacentor* ticks in the western United States. Patients generally seek treatment 3–6 days after a bite, with sudden fever, headache, myalgias, and photophobia. A transient petechial rash may occur. In about 50% of cases, symptoms resolve and then recur in 3 days. Prognosis is excellent, although complications such as encephalitis, meningitis, and pericarditis have been reported. Diagnosis is by serology, and treatment is supportive.

46. **What is babesiosis?**
Babesiosis is a malaria-like illness, caused by the *Babesia microti* protozoan. It is transmitted by *Ixodes* ticks in the northeastern and upper midwestern United States. Patients have fever, drenching sweats, myalgias, and

headache. Although most disease is mild, life-threatening disease occurs in elderly and asplenic patients. Concurrent infection with Lyme disease occurs in 30%, causing a more severe illness. Diagnosis is made by serology, or by detecting ring forms on stained thin or thick blood smears. Treatment typically consists of azithromycin plus atovaquone for mild infection, and quinine plus clindamycin for more severe cases.

47. What is tularemia?

Tularemia is a rare disease caused by *Francisella tularensis*, a virulent gram-negative coccobacillus. Transmission occurs through tick bites or contact with infected tissue of rabbits or rodents; cases have been reported in all US states except Hawaii. The more common ulceroglandular form manifests with an ulcer at the tick bite, painful regional adenopathy, fever, headache, and myalgia. The severe typhoidal form presents with abdominal pain, fever, and prostration without skin and lymphatic manifestations. Untreated, the mortality rate is 30%–60% from septic shock. Streptomycin remains the drug of choice to treat both forms of the disease.

48. What is tick paralysis?

Tick paralysis is a syndrome caused by neurotoxins in the saliva of gravid female ticks. The syndrome usually presents as an ascending paralysis similar to that of Guillain-Barré disease, with sparing of sensorium and sensory function. Young girls in western North America are at highest risk, especially after prolonged tick attachment. Mortality can occur as a result of respiratory failure. Tick removal usually brings about prompt and complete recovery; treatment is otherwise supportive.

49. What is the proper method for tick removal?

Use direct traction with a gloved hand and forceps as close as possible to the tick mouthparts, avoiding twisting. It is not necessary to dig after embedded mouthparts. Cleanse the area well after removal.

Websites

American Society for Tropical Medicine and Hygiene: www.astmh.org; accessed February 11, 2019.

Centers for Disease Control, Travelers Health: Yellow Book: https://wwwnc.cdc.gov/travel/yellowbook/2020/table-of-contents; accessed February 11, 2019.

US Department of State: US Passports and International Travel: https://travel.state.gov/content/travel/en/international-travel.html.

World Health Organization: www.who.int; accessed February 11, 2019.

ACKNOWLEDGMENT

The editors and authors of this chapter would like to acknowledge and thank Dr. Andrew M. Kestler for his previous contributions to this chapter.

BIBLIOGRAPHY

Baud D, Gubler DJ, Schaub B, et al. An update on Zika virus infection. *Lancet.* 2017;390:2099–2109.

Centers for Disease Control and Prevention. Summary of notifiable diseases: United States, 2017. *MMWR Morb Mortal Wkly Rep.* 2017;64:1–143.

Centers for Disease Control and Prevention. *Yellow book*, chapter 5: post-travel evaluation, 2018 [online]. Available at https://wwwnc.cdc.gov/travel/yellowbook/2018/post-travel-evaluation/general-approach-to-the-returned-traveler. Accessed September 2, 2019.

Guzman MG, Harris E. Dengue. *Lancet.* 2015;385:453–465.

Harvey K, Esposito DH, Han P, et al. Surveillance for travel-related disease: GeoSentinel Surveillance System, United States, 1997–2011. *MMWR Surveill Summ.* 2013;62:1–23.

Leder K, Torresi J, Libman MD, et al. GeoSentinel surveillance of illness in returned travelers, 2007–2011. *Ann Intern Med.* 2013;158(6):456–468.

Lindsey NP, Lehman JA, Staples JE, et al. West Nile virus and other arboviral diseases: United States, 2013. *MMWR Morb Mortal Wkly Rep.* 2014;63:521–526.

Lindsey NP, Staples JE, Fischer M. Chikungunya virus disease among travelers—United States, 2014–2016. *Am J Trop Med Hyg.* 2017;98(1):192–197.

Peterson LR, Brault AC, Nasci RD. West Nile virus: review of the literature. *JAMA.* 2013;310:308–315.

Petersen LR, Jamieson DJ, Powers AM, et al. Zika virus. *N Engl J Med.* 2016;374(16):1552–1563.

Simmons CP, Farrar JJ, Nguyen VV, et al. Dengue. *N Engl J Med.* 2012;366:1423–1432.

Stanek G, Wormser GP, Gray J, et al. Lyme borreliosis. *Lancet.* 2012;379(9814):451–473.

Weaver SC, Lecuit M. Chikungunya virus and the global spread of a mosquito-borne disease. *N Engl J Med.* 2015;372(13):1231–1239.

CHAPTER 55

ARTHRITIS

James D. Whitledge, MD and Nicole M. Dubosh, MD

1. What are the signs and symptoms of arthritis?

Arthritis refers to the inflammation of a joint. The process may be monoarticular (involving a single joint) or polyarticular (involving multiple joints). Common presenting symptoms include pain, swelling, redness, and limitation of motion about the involved joint. With an infectious or autoimmune etiology, systemic symptoms such as fevers, chills, and fatigue may be present as well. On examination, there may be tenderness, swelling, effusion, erythema, and decreased range of motion. Preverbal children may have a limp or avoid using the extremity. There are many different etiologies of arthritis, some of which are more serious than others and can result in permanent joint damage and increased mortality.

2. What are the common causes of acute arthritis?

Arthritis has many causes, including:
- Infection (bacterial, fungal, or viral)
- Trauma (fracture, overuse)
- Hemorrhage (traumatic hemarthrosis, inherited coagulopathy, or anticoagulant induced)
- Crystal deposition disease (gout or pseudogout)
- Neoplasm (metastasis)
- Inflammatory conditions (rheumatoid arthritis, rheumatic fever, systemic lupus erythematosus [SLE], Reiter syndrome)
- Degenerative conditions (osteoarthritis [OA])

3. What is the difference between an intraarticular and a periarticular process?

An intraarticular process involves inflammation of the synovium. This results in diffuse, generalized joint pain, warmth, effusion, and an increase in pain with range of motion about the joint and with axial loading. Arthritis is an intraarticular process. A periarticular process has a more localized area of tenderness, lack of joint effusion, and pain with stretching muscles and tendons over the affected surfaces, as opposed to with moving the joint throughout its entire range. Bursitis and tendinitis are examples of periarticular processes.

4. What are some examples of diseases that are monoarticular, polyarticular, and periarticular?

See Table 55.1 for a list of diseases by the number of joints involved.

5. What other physical findings may be helpful in diagnosing a patient with arthritis?

A careful physical examination may provide additional clues to certain diseases. Examples include genital ulcerations, purulent urethral discharge, and conjunctivitis in Reiter syndrome; urethral or cervical discharge in gonococcal arthritis; tophi or concomitant renal stones in gout; malar rash in SLE; swan-neck deformity in rheumatoid arthritis; erythema chronicum migrans rash in Lyme disease; and evidence of joint surgery or cellulitis overlying a prosthetic joint in septic arthritis.

6. What does the location and distribution of the joint pain reveal about the diagnosis?

Some diseases have a predilection for certain joints. Gout most commonly affects the first metatarsophalangeal (MTP) joint, whereas pseudogout frequently affects the knee. Rheumatoid arthritis commonly affects the metacarpophalangeal (MCP) and proximal interphalangeal (PIP) joints. OA often affects the distal interphalangeal (DIP) and the first MCP joints. Septic joints most commonly involve the knee (>50%) and the hip.

7. Is radiography helpful in the diagnosis of arthritis?

Oftentimes, the only radiographic evidence of inflammation is soft-tissue swelling. Plain radiographs may reveal foreign bodies, fractures, effusions, osteoporosis, or osteomyelitis. The radiographic changes of degenerative arthritis include asymmetric joint-space narrowing, marginal osteophytes, ligamentous calcifications, and subchondral sclerosis. In advanced gout, there may be "punched out" subchondral and marginal erosions, joint-space narrowing, and periarticular calcified tophi. Pseudogout radiographs may show chondrocalcinosis. Rheumatoid arthritis radiographic findings can include periarticular osteopenia progressing to bony erosion, as well as narrowing of the joint space. There is an emerging role for ultrasound in emergency department evaluation of arthritis, including identification of effusions difficult to appreciate on physical examination and differentiation of cellulitis overlying a joint from true effusion.

8. Are the erythrocyte sedimentation rate (ESR) and peripheral white blood cell (WBC) count useful for the evaluation of acute arthritis?

No. Peripheral WBC, ESR, and C-reactive protein (CRP) are nonspecific markers of inflammation and are not useful in acute arthritis. A 2011 meta-analysis found no reduction in posttest probability of a septic joint based on these

Table 55.1 Joints Involved in Disease

MONOARTICULAR	POLYARTICULAR	PERIARTICULAR
Septic arthritis	Systemic lupus erythematosus	Cellulitis
Gout and pseudogout	Rheumatoid arthritis	Bursitis
Osteoarthritis	Rheumatic fever	Tendinitis
Hemarthrosis	Osteoarthritis	
Trauma	Reiter syndrome	
	Lyme disease	
	Serum sickness	

findings. The ESR and WBC represent the body's acute-phase reaction to inflammation and infection, and are neither sensitive nor specific enough to confirm or exclude any particular disease. False-negative ESRs in septic arthritis can be as high as 30%. Likewise, the peripheral WBC count does not contribute meaningfully to the diagnosis of an inflamed joint.

9. **What is the most important diagnostic test for determining the etiology of acute arthritis?**
Arthrocentesis is the most important diagnostic procedure for evaluation of an acutely inflamed joint. Synovial fluid analysis provides rapid, critical diagnostic information and should be performed on all patients with an acute joint effusion who have no contraindications. An arthrocentesis can drain a tense hemarthrosis and enable a caregiver to inject an analgesic or anti-inflammatory medication into the joint. The procedure is simple and safe, and complications are rare when performed under sterile conditions with proper technique. If a prosthetic joint infection is suspected, an orthopedic consultation should be obtained before joint aspiration.

10. **What are the general steps of an arthrocentesis?**
    1. Place the patient in a comfortable position with the joint exposed.
    2. Palpate the bony landmarks. Ultrasound can be used to identify landmarks or an effusion.
    3. Cleanse and prep the skin, and drape the patient with sterile drapes.
    4. Provide anesthesia by local infiltration with an anesthetic, such as 1% or 2% lidocaine.
    5. Using an 18-gauge needle (or smaller, depending on joint size) attached to a syringe, aspirate gently while carefully advancing the needle into the joint. Avoid puncture of the articular cartilage.
    6. Withdraw as much synovial fluid as possible.
    7. If necessary, inject anesthetic solution into the joint for pain relief.
       Send the synovial fluid for WBC count with differential, crystals, Gram stain, culture, and, if possible, synovial lactate tests. If you only retrieve one drop of fluid, it should be sent for culture.

11. **What are some causes of arthritis with fever?**
Diseases causing arthritis with fever include septic arthritis, Lyme disease, rheumatic fever, Reiter syndrome, and toxic synovitis.

12. **How do I interpret the results of the arthrocentesis?**
See Table 55.2 for interpretation of synovial fluid analysis.

13. **Does a synovial fluid WBC counts <50,000 cells/mm³ completely rule out the diagnosis of a septic joint?**
No. Typical synovial fluid counts in septic arthritis are >50,000 WBC/mm³, with predominantly polymorphonuclear neutrophilic (PMN) WBCs, and a gram-positive stain for bacteria. However, some patients with septic arthritis have synovial fluid counts of less than <50,000 cells/mm³, particularly those with prosthetic joints. For this reason, the threshold for starting antibiotics should be low if the clinical examination suggests bacterial arthritis.

14. **Are there any other synovial fluid tests for arthritis?**
There is evidence to suggest that synovial fluid lactate level >10 mmol/L is highly suggestive of septic arthritis, whereas levels <4.3 mmol/L make septic arthritis very unlikely.

15. **What is the most serious cause of arthritis?**
Nongonococcal bacterial arthritis is by far the most serious cause of acute monoarticular arthritis, as it can cause rapid cartilage destruction and in-hospital mortality. The most important risk factor for septic arthritis is preexisting joint disease, including prosthetic joints and rheumatoid arthritis. Almost half of patients with septic arthritis have previous joint problems. Permanent joint damage may occur in as little as 7 days if untreated, and this can result in chronic disability and pain. In children, septic arthritis can cause epiphyseal damage, resulting in growth impairment and limb length discrepancy.

16. **What organisms cause bacterial arthritis?**
Septic arthritis is grouped into gonococcal and nongonococcal, as the disease process and management differs. *Neisseria gonorrhoeae* is the most common cause of septic arthritis in young, healthy, sexually active adults.

Table 55.2 Synovial Fluid Analysis

DIAGNOSIS	APPEARANCE	TOTAL WBC COUNT (per mm³)	PMN (%)	MUCIN CLOT TEST	FLUID/BLOOD GLUCOSE (diff.) (mm/dL)	MISCELLANEOUS (CRYSTALS/ORGANISMS)
Normal	Clear, pale	0–200 (200)	<10	Good	NS	—
Group I (Noninflammatory; Degenerative Joint Disease, Traumatic Arthritis)						
	Clear to slightly turbid	50–4000 (600)	<30	Good	NS	—
Group II (Noninfectious, Mildly Inflammatory; SLE Scleroderma)						
	Clear to slightly turbid	0–9000 (3000)	<20	Good (occasionally fair)	NS	Occasionally LE cell, decreased complement
Group III (Noninfectious, Severely Inflammatory)						
Gout	Turbid	100–160,000 (21,000)	70	Poor	10	Uric acid crystals
Pseudogout	Turbid	50–75,000	70 (14,000)	Fair-poor	Insufficient data	Calcium pyrophosphate
Rheumatoid arthritis	Turbid	250–80,000	70	Poor	30	Decreased
Group IV (Infectious, Inflammatory)						
Acute bacterial	Very turbid	150–250,000 (80,000)	90	Poor	90	Positive culture for bacteria
Tuberculosis	Turbid	2,500–100,000 (20,000)	60	Poor	70	Positive culture for *Mycobacterium tuberculosis*

LE, Lupus erythematosus; *NS,* not significant; *PMN,* polymorphonuclear cells; *SLE,* systemic lupus erythematosus; *WBC,* white blood cell.
From Wyngaarden JB, Smith LH, eds. *Cecil Textbook of Medicine.* 18th ed. Philadelphia: Saunders; 1988:1994, with permission.

The most common cause of nongonococcal septic arthritis is *Staphylococcus aureus,* followed by *Streptococcus* species. Methicillin-resistant *S. aureus* (MRSA) causes up to half of septic arthritis cases, with risk factors including advanced age, comorbid medical conditions, and recent hospitalization. Other causative organisms include *Escherichia coli, Pseudomonas aeruginosa, Kingella kingae,* and *Haemophilus influenzae.* In children, the incidence of septic arthritis due to *H. influenzae* has decreased by 95% since widespread vaccination.

17. **How is bacterial arthritis treated?**
Patients with bacterial arthritis require admission to the hospital and immediate orthopedic consultation for arthroscopic joint drainage, open joint drainage, or daily joint aspirations. Intravenous (IV) antibiotics should be administered based on the Gram stain and culture of the synovial aspirate if available, and are generally continued for about 3–4 weeks or 6 weeks if there is accompanying osteomyelitis. Culture results should not delay initiation of IV antibiotics. Vancomycin and a third-generation cephalosporin is the recommended empiric coverage. If the patient is allergic to penicillins or cephalosporins, aztreonam or a fluoroquinolone can be substituted. See Table 55.3 for a list of antibiotic recommendations for each organism. If the Gram stain is negative, then empiric antibiotics can be administered according to the patient's epidemiology. MRSA and antpseudomonal coverage should be administered if the patient has risk factors such as being elderly, a recent hospitalization, comorbid medical conditions, IV drug use, or living in a location with a high prevalence of community-acquired MRSA.

18. **What causes crystal-induced arthritis?**
Crystal-induced arthropathies include gout and pseudogout. They are more common than septic arthritis and often mimic a septic joint. Gout is caused by monosodium urate crystal precipitation into a joint, whereas pseudogout develops when calcium pyrophosphate crystals precipitate into the joint. Both are released from the cells lining the synovium and initiate an inflammatory reaction. Under polarized light microscopy, gout crystals are needle shaped and negatively birefringent, whereas pseudogout crystals are rhomboid in shape and positively birefringent.

19. **What are the risk factors for gout, and which joints are most commonly affected?**
Risk factors for gout include obesity, hypertension, diabetes, dietary excess, alcohol consumption, proximal loop diuretics, increased uric acid levels, and stress (illness or surgery). Middle-aged men and postmenopausal women are at an increased risk for gout. The MTP joint of the great toe is the most commonly affected joint (up to 75%). In this joint, gout is known as *podagra.* Other commonly involved joints are the tarsal joints, the ankle, and the knee. Gout is polyarticular in many cases.

20. **What medications can be used to treat gout in the acute setting?**
Nonsteroidal anti-inflammatory drugs (NSAIDs) are the primary agents used to treat gout. For example, indomethacin is given at a dosage of 50 mg orally three times daily with discontinuation 2–3 days after resolution of symptoms. Colchicine is also effective in treating acute attacks and works by inhibiting microtubule formation, resulting in a decreased inflammatory response. It may be administered orally at an initial dose of 1.2 mg at

Table 55.3 Antibiotic Treatment for Septic Arthritis

ORGANISM	GRAM STAIN	ANTIBIOTICS	DOSAGE
Methicillin-sensitive *Staphylococcus aureus*	Gram-positive cocci clusters	Cefazolin, nafcillin, or oxacillin	Cefazolin 2 g IV q8h Nafcillin 2 g IV q4h Oxacillin 2 g IV q4h
Methicillin-resistant *S. aureus*	Gram-positive cocci clusters	Vancomycin	Vancomycin 15–20 mg/kg IV q12h
Streptococcus pneumoniae	Gram-positive cocci chains	Penicillin G or ampicillin	Penicillin G 12–24 mU IV q24h, divided
Penicillin sensitive			Ampicillin 2 g IV q4h
S. pneumoniae, penicillin resistant	Gram-positive cocci chains	Ceftriaxone or cefepime	Ceftriaxone 2 g IV q24h Cefepime 2 g IV q8h
Neisseria gonorrhoeae	Gram-negative cocci	Ceftriaxone or cefepime	Ceftriaxone 1 g IV q24h Cefepime 2 g IV q8h
Pseudomonas aeruginosa	Gram-negative rods	Ceftazidime or cefepime plus gentamicin	Ceftazidime 2 g IV q8h Cefepime 2 g IV q8h Gentamicin 5 mg/kg IV daily in 2–3 divided doses

IV, Intravenously; *mU,* million units; *q,* every.

the first sign of a flare, followed by 0.6 mg 1 hour later, followed by 0.6 mg twice daily until the flare subsides. Providers must be aware of the narrow therapeutic window and toxicity in overdose when prescribing colchicine. Once bacterial infection has been ruled out, oral corticosteroids may also be administered: for example, prednisone 0.5 mg/kg/day orally for 5–10 days. Drugs that alter serum uric acid levels, such as allopurinol and probenecid, should not be administered acutely because changing serum uric acid levels can exacerbate the condition.

21. Which tick-borne infection causes arthritis?

Lyme disease, caused by the bacteria *Borrelia burgdorferi,* can cause arthritis as a late manifestation of the disease. Synovial fluid polymerase chain reaction (PCR) testing should be ordered for *B. burgdorferi* if clinical suspicion is high. The Infectious Diseases Society of America recommends treatment with a 28-day course of oral antibiotics (doxycycline 200 mg daily divided into two doses, amoxicillin 1.5 g daily divided into three doses, or cefuroxime 1000 mg daily divided into two doses) for patients without neurologic manifestations of the disease.

22. What are the signs and symptoms of OA?

OA, or degenerative arthritis, is the most common joint disease and is more prevalent in the elderly. Symptoms include chronic, progressive joint pain; morning stiffness; crepitus; Heberden nodes at the distal phalangeal joints; and Bouchard nodes at the PIP joints. The joint pain is generally worse with weight bearing, improves with rest, and worsens over the course of the day.

23. What are the treatment options for OA?

Acetaminophen and NSAIDs are efficacious. Regimens include acetaminophen 1000 mg every 6 hours or ibuprofen 400–800 mg every 6 hours. Acetaminophen and NSAIDs can be combined with a synergistic effect. Topical NSAID creams such as diclofenac gel are another option that reduces the side-effect profile of systemic NSAIDs. Topical capsaicin cream can also be considered, though skin irritation is a common side effect. Intraarticular corticosteroid joint injections with methylprednisolone, triamcinolone, or betamethasone may provide relief.

KEY POINTS

1. Septic arthritis is a medical emergency, requiring prompt diagnosis by arthrocentesis, followed by management with IV antibiotics and orthopedic consultation for joint washout.
2. Normal serum inflammatory markers, including WBC count, ESR, and CRP, cannot be used to rule out a septic joint. A synovial fluid WBC count greater than 50,000/mm^3 and predominantly PMN WBCs are commonly seen in septic arthritis but are not absolute.
3. Gout and pseudogout are types of arthritis caused by crystal precipitation in the joint and can mimic septic arthritis.

ACKNOWLEDGMENT

The editors and authors of this chapter would like to acknowledge and thank Dr. Catherine B. Custalow for her previous contributions to this chapter.

BIBLIOGRAPHY

Carpenter CR, Schuur JD, Everett WW, et al. Evidence-based diagnostics: adult septic arthritis. *Acad Emerg Med.* 2011;18:781–796.

Couderc M, Pereira B, Mathieu S, et al. Predictive value of the usual clinical signs and laboratory tests in the diagnosis of septic arthritis. *CJEM.* 2015;17(4):403–410. doi:10.1017/cem.2014.56.

Ross JJ. Septic arthritis of native joints. *Infect Dis Clin North Am.* 2017;31(2):203–218. doi:10.1016/j.idc.2017.01.001.

Sanchez E, Vannier E, Wormser GP, et al. Diagnosis, treatment, and prevention of Lyme disease, human granulocytic anaplasmosis, and babesiosis: a review. *JAMA.* 2016;315(16):1767–1777. doi:10.1001/jama.2016.2884.

Shu E, Farshidpour L, Young M, et al. Utility of point-of-care synovial lactate to identify septic arthritis in the emergency department. *Am J Emerg Med.* 2019;37(3):502–505. doi:10.1016/j.ajem.2018.12.030.

Situ-LaCasse E, Grieger RW, Crabbe S, et al. Utility of point-of-care musculoskeletal ultrasound in the evaluation of emergency department musculoskeletal pathology. *World J Emerg Med.* 2018;9(4):262–266. doi:10.5847/wjem.j.1920-8642.2018.04.004.

Sivera F, Andres M, Carmona L, et al. Multinational evidence-based recommendations for the diagnosis and management of gout: integrating systematic literature review and expert opinion of a broad panel of rheumatologists in the 3e initiative. *Ann Rheum Dis.* 2014;73(2):328–335. doi:10.1136/annrheumdis-2013-203325.

Taylor N. Nonsurgical management of osteoarthritis knee pain in the older adult: an update. *Rheum Dis Clin North Am.* 2018;44(3):513–524. doi:10.1016/j.rdc.2018.03.009.

CHAPTER 56

SKIN DISEASES

Monica Noori, MD and Avery MacKenzie, MD

1. **What are the terms used to describe skin lesions?**
   Use characteristics such as color, contour, depth, distribution, location, and texture. Common terminology for skin lesions is listed in Table 56.1.

2. **How can skin disorders lead to life-threatening conditions?**
   Disruptions of the skin's barrier function can impair the body's ability to regulate fluid and electrolyte balance, cause heat dysregulation, and allow for introduction of pathogens that lead to infection. Mucosal lesions of the oral cavity may compromise life if they are severe enough to prevent food or fluid intake.

3. **What categories of skin conditions are life threatening or associated with life-threatening disease?**
   - Diseases resulting in extensive compromise to the cutaneous barrier (e.g., erythroderma, toxic epidermal necrolysis [TEN]/Stevens-Johnson syndrome [SJS], pemphigus vulgaris, toxic shock syndrome, staphylococcal scalded skin syndrome)
   - Skin infections (e.g., cellulitis, necrotizing fasciitis)
   - Cancers (e.g., melanoma, cutaneous T-cell lymphoma, Kaposi's sarcoma)
   - Skin signs of systemic infection (e.g., meningococcemia, disseminated intravascular coagulation [DIC], Rocky Mountain spotted fever [RMSF])
   - Angioedema with airway compromise or anaphylaxis
   - Skin signs of vascular compromise (including hemorrhage, emboli, thrombi, and vasculitis)
   - Skin findings of an introduced toxin (e.g., venomous spider or snake bite)
   - Skin signs of physical abuse/trauma

4. **Identify the skin lesions found in the potentially life-threatening diseases of meningococcemia, RMSF, toxic shock syndrome, and necrotizing fasciitis.**
   - Meningococcemia: petechiae or purpura with dusky centers, commonly found on the trunk and limbs. Lesions may also be found on palms and soles.
   - RMSF: on the fourth day after fever, lesions originate on distal extremities, may include the palms and soles, and spread centrally. After 1–2 days, skin findings evolve into petechiae or purpura. The rash can be difficult to differentiate from meningococcemia. Eliciting a history of hiking or tick exposure and considering geographic location can be helpful.
   - Toxic shock syndrome: lesions include a sunburn-like rash, edema of the face and limbs, conjunctival erythema, and mucosal redness within oral or genital areas. Desquamation of hands and feet 1–2 weeks after initial lesions may be seen.
   - Necrotizing fasciitis: briskly advancing tender erythema, progressing to duskiness and necrosis with or without blisters. Overlying skin findings may belie the necrosis occurring underneath, but findings may be subtle (e.g., pain out of proportion to examination).

5. **Distinguish pemphigus vulgaris from bullous pemphigoid.**
   - Pemphigus vulgaris: autoantibodies against desmogleins in the cell membrane result in loss of cell-to-cell adhesion in the epidermis and formation of flaccid, painful blisters that rupture easily. Blisters appear on the face, trunk, intertriginous and mucosal areas. Nikolsky sign is positive. Onset between 40 and 60 years of age. Frequently fatal unless treated with immunosuppression.
   - Bullous pemphigoid: autoantibodies against the basement membrane result in large, tense subepidermal blisters that may be intensely pruritic. Oral lesions are uncommon. Typical age of onset is 60–80 years.

6. **What is Nikolsky sign and in which diseases is this sign positive?**
   Firm sliding pressure with a finger separates normal-appearing epidermis, creating erosion. Nikolsky sign is observed in blistering diseases such as staphylococcal scalded skin syndrome, pemphigus vulgaris, and TEN.

7. **What are the characteristics of melanoma?**
   Recognition of melanoma and referral for surgical removal before metastasis can be life saving. Findings suggestive of melanoma are irregular pigment and borders, and presence of red, white, or blue-black color. A nevus is concerning if no other lesions appear similar, even if it appears evenly pigmented, small, and entirely round. A change in nevus appearance is a risk factor, as is a personal or family history of melanoma.

Table 56.1 Basic Dermatologic Terms

SKIN LESION	DESCRIPTION	EXAMPLE
Macule	Flat, nonpalpable, circumscribed discoloration <1 cm	Café-au-lait spot
Patch	Flat discoloration >1 cm	Vitiligo
Papule	Elevated, solid lesion <1 cm	Molluscum contagiosum
Plaque	Elevated, flat-topped lesion >1 cm	Psoriasis
Nodule	Elevated, solid lesion. Size and depth distinguishes from papule.	Erythema nodosum
Vesicle	Raised, fluid-filled lesion <1 cm	Varicella
Bulla	Raised, fluid-filled lesion >1 cm	Bullous pemphigoid
Pustule	Superficial cavity containing exudative fluid	Folliculitis
Petechiae	Non-blanching foci of capillary hemorrhage <0.3 cm	Rocky Mountain spotted fever
Purpura	Non-blanching foci of capillary hemorrhage 0.3–1 cm	Meningococcemia
Cyst	Cavity containing liquid or semisolid to solid material	Epidermoid cyst
Wheal	Evanescent, flat-topped or rounded edematous lesion	Urticaria

KEY POINTS: LOOK FOR ABCDE SIGNS OF MELANOMA

1. Asymmetry
2. Border: irregular or poorly defined
3. Color: irregular pigmentation
4. Diameter: generally >6 mm (size of a pencil eraser)
5. Evolving: different from patient's other pigmented lesions or changing in color, shape, or size

8. **What other skin findings can mimic melanoma?**
   - Seborrheic keratosis: common, benign, darkly pigmented or unevenly colored growths that typically occur in middle age. Growths commonly have scales, but they may not be easy to visualize with the naked eye.
   - Blue nevus: solitary blue-colored nevus that is generally benign.
   - Venous lakes: vascular growths that often appear on the helix of the ears and on the lips of older persons with sun damage. The purple color may mimic that of melanoma. Pressing firmly on the lesion drains much of the blood and reveals it as a vascular growth.

9. **Describe erythema multiforme (EM).**
   EM is an acute onset eruption that is characterized by multiple fixed red papules with a dusky center as a result of keratinocyte necrosis leading to a target-shaped appearance. Lesions are found on the dorsal hands and extensor extremities, with palms and soles commonly involved. Mucous membranes are usually spared or mildly affected. Significant involvement should raise suspicion for another diagnosis, such as SJS.

   Most EM is caused by infections (herpes simplex virus [HSV] and *Mycoplasma* pneumonia), although medications, malignancy, autoimmune diseases, and immunizations have been implicated. The eruption may last 2–3 weeks, but can recur. Symptomatic management consists of antihistamines. Topical or oral steroids are not indicated.

10. **Which illness can mimic EM?**
    Acute urticaria may mimic EM. Unlike urticaria, the lesions of EM have a dark center, often involve the mucosa, and do not move around the body. Unlike urticaria, the lesions of EM do not improve with diphenhydramine or epinephrine.

11. **Differentiate erythema multiforme, erythema migrans, erythema marginatum, and erythema nodosum.**
    - Erythema multiforme: morbilliform rash usually on the palms and soles, resulting from viral/bacterial infections or medications.
    - Erythema migrans: bull's-eye rash that usually expands (rather than migrates). Common manifestation of early Lyme disease.
    - Erythema marginatum: evanescent, nonpruritic rash that typically involves the trunk and extremities while sparing the face. Part of the Jones' criteria for diagnosis of rheumatic fever.
    - Erythema nodosum: acute inflammatory reaction leading to appearance of red, painful tender nodules on the lower legs. Diverse (and often idiopathic) etiologies.

12. **How do drug-induced rashes typically present?**
The vast majority of drug-induced rashes are mild, type IV hypersensitivity reactions that can be termed drug-induced exanthems. Most commonly morbilliform in appearance, they typically present several days to 2 weeks after exposure. Most are mild in severity without significant morbidity. Management involves discontinuing the causal medication. Use of antihistamines may relieve itching and discomfort.

13. **Which illness commonly mimics drug-induced exanthems?**
Viral exanthems have similar skin and histologic findings, relying on a thorough history to differentiate them. Eosinophilia supports the diagnosis of a drug eruption. Ten to twenty percent of exanthematous eruptions in children are medication related, versus 50%–70% in adults.

14. **Which medications are most commonly implicated in drug eruptions?**
   - Antibiotics: β-lactams, sulfonamides, penicillins, macrolides
   - Anticonvulsants: phenytoin, carbamazepine, lamotrigine
   - Nonsteroidal anti-inflammatory drugs (NSAIDs): ibuprofen
   - Antiretrovirals: abacavir, nevirapine

15. **What clinical signs should alert concern for a severe drug-induced hypersensitivity reaction?**
Signs of severe reactions include facial edema, hepatosplenomegaly, mucosal petechiae, significant eosinophilia, painful dark-colored papules or blisters, and skin sloughing. Clinical features that can help identify and differentiate SJS, TEN, and drug reaction with systemic symptoms (DRESS) can be found in Table 56.2.

KEY POINTS: SEVERE DRUG ERUPTIONS

1. An exanthematous drug eruption may be an early sign of a severe hypersensitivity reaction such as SJS, TEN, or DRESS. Warning signs include evolution of morbilliform rash to erythroderma, fever >38°C, facial edema, mucositis, skin tenderness, or blistering.
2. Consider transfer to a burn center as these patients require wound care and resuscitation similar to that of a burn patient.

16. **Describe findings seen in each childhood skin rash.**
See Table 56.3.

17. **How can you identify tinea versicolor?**
The rash consists of well-marginated oval or round macules that scale when gently abraded and appear hypo- or hyperpigmented, depending on skin color. Lesions are generally asymptomatic, although patients may report mild pruritus. Lesions are caused by an overgrowth of *Malassezia furfur,* which fluoresces blue-green under Wood's lamp. Treatments include selenium sulfide or ketoconazole shampoo and oral or topical azoles.

18. **Which papulosquamous rash is classically preceded by a herald patch?**
Pityriasis rosea presents as scaly, salmon-colored oval patches on the trunk and proximal extremities in a "Christmas tree–like" distribution along the Langer's lines. Classically, this diffuse rash is preceded by a herald patch 1 week prior. The disease is self-limiting and generally resolves within 6–8 weeks. The exact etiology is unknown, but human herpes virus 6 and 7 have been implicated. Consider ruling out syphilis. Treatment is focused on symptomatic control of pruritus with antihistamines and topical steroids.

19. **Distinguish folliculitis, furuncle, and carbuncle.**
   - Folliculitis: superficial pustule involving the hair follicle. Etiologies include bacteria, fungi, virus, and mites.
   - Furuncle: generally evolves from folliculitis extending into subcutaneous tissue.
   - Carbuncle: coalescence of furuncles.

20. **What is the treatment for hidradenitis suppurativa?**
Hidradenitis suppurativa is a chronic disease of the apocrine gland-bearing skin requiring a multimodal treatment approach. For acute painful nodules, consider intralesional triamcinolone followed by incision and drainage of the abscess. For chronic disease, oral antibiotics such as clindamycin with rifampin or tetracycline can be useful. Surgery with wide excision may be necessary. Other considerations include tobacco cessation, weight loss in obese patients, and laser hair removal.

21. **Which skin lesions mimic cellulitis?**
   - Stasis dermatitis: erythema, serous drainage, and superficial desquamation with edema of bilateral lower extremities.
   - Contact dermatitis: area of erythema generally confined to site of contact with allergen or irritant. Requires removal of the offending agent along with topical corticosteroids. Systemic corticosteroids for 2–3 weeks may be necessary for severe reactions.

Table 56.2 Characteristics of Severe Drug Eruptions

	TBSA INVOLVED	SIGNS/SYMPTOMS	MORTALITY	TREATMENT
SJS	<10% body surface area	Upper respiratory prodrome 1–14 days before onset of mucosal involvement. Morbilliform rash progresses to painful papules, vesicles, and bullae that blister and slough. Mucosal necrosis and sloughing of two membranes (commonly mouth and eyes).	1%–5%	Prompt withdrawal of offending agent. Symptomatic management is similar to burn treatment and should include tetanus prophylaxis. Oral lesions are managed with mouthwashes and topical anesthetics to tolerate oral rehydration. Areas of denuded skin must be cleansed and covered to prevent infection and dehydration.
TEN	>30% body surface area	Onset with fever 1–2 weeks before appearance of painful, red macules that progress, darken, and then coalesce. Areas of hypopigmentation may also be interspersed, then blisters and sloughing are seen.	25%–35% Poor prognostic factors: advanced age, delay in withdrawing offending agent, and greater extent of epidermal involvement.	Prompt withdrawal of offending agent. Symptomatic management is similar to ICU/burn treatment. Controversies exist in the management of TEN with the use of steroids and other immuno-modulators. Early administration of intravenous immunoglobulin may be beneficial.
DRESS	Typically > 50% body surface area involved	Long latency (2–8 weeks) between exposure and disease onset. Facial edema is a hallmark. Fever, morbilliform rash, lymphadenopathy, eosinophilia, and atypical lymphocytosis are common features. Involves at least one internal organ (liver/kidney/lung).	10%–20% Liver failure is the most common cause of death.	Prompt withdrawal of the offending agent is imperative. Systemic steroids are commonly used, although effectiveness is unverified in controlled clinical trials.

Note: 10%–30% involvement considered SJS/TEN overlap.

DRESS, Drug reaction with systemic symptoms; *ICU,* intensive care unit; *SJS,* Stevens-Johnson syndrome; *TBSA,* total body surface area; *TEN,* toxic epidermal necrolysis.

Table 56.3 Childhood Skin Rashes

DISEASE	ETIOLOGY	CLINICAL FINDINGS	COMPLICATIONS
Erythema infectiosum (fifth disease)	Parvovirus B19	"Slapped cheeks" followed by lacy, reticular-like pattern. Rash follows resolution of fever and clinical improvement. Rash can last for months, precipitated by changes in temperature, sun, exercise, and stress.	Aplastic anemia
Roseola (exanthema subitum)	Herpes virus 6	Illness begins with 2–3 days of persistent fever, followed by sudden defervescence and the development of a pink maculopapular rash.	Febrile seizures
Rubella (German measles)	Rubivirus	Morbilliform rash spreading from face down. Associated with mild illness, low-grade fever, and posterior cervical lymphadenopathy.	In utero infections can cause major birth defects and death
Rubeola (measles)	Paramyxovirus	Morbilliform rash spreading from face down. Associated with high fever, Koplik spots (white spots on the buccal mucosa), cough, coryza, and conjunctivitis (the 3 C's).	Diarrhea, pneumonia, and acute disseminated encephalomyelitis (ADEM)
Varicella (chickenpox)	Varicella zoster virus	Groups of faint macules evolve into papules and then vesicles over 1–2 days ("dew drop on a petal" appearance). Vesicles acquire a moist crusty appearance and eventually erode into shallow lesions. Begins on the trunk and extends peripherally. Hallmark is lesions in various phases of development.	Bacterial superinfection, encephalitis, transverse myelitis, and Reyes syndrome in those given aspirin
Hand-foot-mouth	Coxsackie virus	Sudden onset of scattered papules on palms, soles, buttocks, and mucosa that develop into vesicles with a red rim.	Dehydration in setting of painful oral lesions Meningitis (rare)
Kawasaki disease (KD)	Unknown; likely immune phenomenon	High fever for at least 5 days with four of the following: • Cervical lymphadenopathy • Edematous or desquamating extremities • Exanthema • Mucosal changes • Nonpurulent limbal-sparing conjunctivitis In patients with suspected KD without four of five criteria, incomplete KD is possible and labs can support diagnosis.	Coronary artery aneurysms develop in 1:5 patients, leading to myocardial infarction and arrhythmias. Treat with IVIG and aspirin.
Scarlet fever	Group A streptococcus	Red macules and papules beginning on the neck, extend to the trunk and extremities. Skin can have a distinct sandpaper texture. Pastia lines formed by confluent petechiae in major skin folds may be seen. "Strawberry tongue" with circumoral pallor may develop.	Otitis media, pneumonia, throat abscesses, rheumatic fever, and poststreptococcal glomerulonephritis
Staphylococcal scalded skin syndrome	Certain strains of *Staphylococcus*	Preferentially affects neonates and infants. Begins with upper respiratory infection, followed by erythema of the face, neck, and axilla, with crusting around eyes, mouth, and in skin folds. Mucous membranes are not affected. Nikolsky positive.	Significant desquamation can lead to electrolyte imbalances, and superinfection. With anti-staphylococcal antibiotics, wound care, and fluid replacement, mortality is low.

IVIG, Intravenous immunoglobulin.

Table 56.4 Topical Steroids

POTENCY/CLASS	AREAS OF USE	EXAMPLES
Superpotency: Class 1	Used to treat prolonged, refractory illnesses, especially on thick skin, including the palms and soles. Requires outpatient monitoring.	0.05% clobetasol 0.05% betamethasone dipropionate 0.05% halobetasol 0.05% diflorasone
High potency: Class 2 and 3	Best for thicker-skinned areas. Can cause adverse effects when used >2 weeks.	0.05% fluocinonide 0.1% halcinonide 0.25% desoximetasone
Moderate potency: Class 4 and 5	Neck and body; not on thin-skinned areas. Commonly used in the emergency department setting.	0.025% fluocinolone 0.1% triamcinolone 0.2% hydrocortisone valerate
Low potency: Class 6 and 7	All areas, including thin-skinned areas: face, breasts, axilla, and groin.	1% hydrocortisone 2.5% hydrocortisone 0.05% desonide

- Lymphedema: localized edema, induration, and erythema of an affected extremity. Absence of warmth, pain, and systemic symptoms.
- Papular urticaria: hypersensitivity reaction to arthropod bite associated with significant itching rather than pain.
- Deep vein thrombosis (DVT): skin overlying clot in leg may be red, warm and swollen.

KEY POINTS: CELLULITIS

1. Cellulitis is rarely bilateral.
2. Cellulitis is often associated with systemic symptoms of fever and elevation of inflammatory markers.

22. **Debridement is generally contraindicated in which lower extremity eruption?**
    Pyoderma gangrenosum.

23. **Should oral steroids be used to treat eczema?**
    Topical steroids are generally used to treat chronic dermatitis by targeting the primary problem of skin barrier defect. They also avoid systemic side effects and rebound of disease when oral steroids are tapered. Patients with acute dermatitis that is expected to be self-limited, such as poison ivy dermatitis, may be given systemic steroids based on disease severity and if there are no contraindications.

24. **Should steroids be used in psoriasis?**
    Patients with psoriasis have different treatment options. In mild disease, topical creams and other emollients should suffice. Moderate psoriasis may require the addition of phototherapy. Although systemic treatments may become necessary in severe psoriasis, steroids are not generally recommended because rebound pustular psoriasis may develop once steroid medication is withdrawn.

25. **What are the different classes of steroids, and on which part of the body can they be applied?**
    See Table 56.4.

26. **Which formulation of topical steroids is most potent?**
    Ointments, creams, and lotions contain different proportions of oil to water. An ointment is 80% oil and 20% water, while a cream is 50% oil and 50% water. Ointments have the greatest potency, followed by gels, creams, lotions, solutions, and sprays.

ACKNOWLEDGMENTS

The editors and authors of this chapter would like to acknowledge and thank Drs. Renee A. King, Lela A. Lee, and Joanna M. Burch for their previous contributions to this chapter.

BIBLIOGRAPHY

Mockenhaupt M. Epidemiology of cutaneous adverse drug reactions. *Chem Immunol Allergy.* 2012;97:1–17.
Mockenhaupt M. Stevens-Johnson syndrome and toxic epidermal necrolysis: clinical patterns, diagnostic considerations, etiology, and therapeutic management. *Semin Cutan Med Surg.* 2014;33:10–16.
Wolff K, Johnson RA, Saavedra AP. *Fitzpatrick's Color Atlas and Synopsis of Clinical Dermatology.* 7th ed. New York: McGraw-Hill Medical; 2013.

CHAPTER 57

LIGHTNING AND ELECTRICAL INJURIES

David S. Young, MD, MS, FAWM and Tracy Cushing, MD, MPH, FAWM

LIGHTNING INJURIES

1. **What causes lightning?**
   Lightning is a large discharge of electrical energy. When warm and cold air meet within the atmosphere, warm air rises and cold air descends, forming cumulonimbus clouds, more commonly known as *thunderheads.* The air within a cloud contains water molecules, some in liquid state and others in ice crystals, depending on the temperature within the cloud. The movement of these molecules within a convectively active cloud creates an electric charge and separation of polar (oppositely charged) ends of the cloud. Generally, the upper cloud portion retains a positive charge, and the lower portion is negatively charged. Air acts as an insulator between the opposite charges within clouds, as well as between the cloud and the ground. Once the charge exceeds the insulating capacity of the air, lightning is discharged, which equalizes the charged regions within the atmosphere. Lightning can discharge between opposite charges within a cloud, between clouds (cloud flashes), or between the opposite charges of the cloud and the ground (cloud-to-ground lightning). When a cloud-to-ground strike occurs, it is initiated by the formation of a stepped leader, a path of negatively charged electricity descending from the cloud in a series of short, zig-zagged spurts; simultaneously, a positively charged upward streamer is generated from the ground. When these currents meet at approximately 50–100 m above ground, the return stroke is initiated, commonly known as the *lightning bolt.* Usually there are four to five return strokes, which are high-voltage, high-current, and high-velocity electrical discharges that strike objects within 30–50 m from the point of the upward streamer.

2. **What is a "bolt from the blue?"**
   This phenomenon is a cloud-to-ground strike that travels a relatively long distance, sometimes through an apparently cloudless sky, to strike an object up to 25 miles away from the thunderstorm.

3. **What causes thunder?**
   Thunder is an acoustic wave caused by lightning. The energy created in the electrostatic discharge of a bolt of lightning heats the surrounding air to greater than 50,000°F (27,760°C) within a few milliseconds, creating a high-pressure region within the column of air. The pressurized air then expands outward, causing an acoustic sound wave heard as thunder.

4. **Is lightning direct current (DC) or alternating current (AC)?**
   Technically, it is neither, but it behaves most like DC. It has a very high voltage (100 million to 2 billion volts [V]), very large current (20,000–300,000 amperes [amps, A]), and very high energy (1 billion joules [J] to 280 kilowatt-hours [kWh]); however, it has a very short duration, lasting only 0.1–1 millisecond.

5. **Is it true that lightning never strikes twice in the same place?**
   No. Contrary to popular belief, lightning can and does strike the same place twice. The Empire State Building in New York is struck around 23 times per year. In contiguous United States, ~20,000,000 cloud-to-ground strikes have been detected annually since 1989.

6. **How does lightning cause injury?**
   A bolt of lightning is a massive discharge of electrical energy, with current ranging from 30,000 to 110,000 A. There are five types of lightning injuries.
   1. Direct strike: an uninterrupted connection between the victim and the bolt of lightning
   2. Contact injury: a transfer of electrical energy from touching an object that is struck directly
   3. Side splash: an injury from current "splashing" or jumping from nearby objects to a victim's body
   4. Ground current: when lightning strikes the ground or an object nearby and travels through the ground from the strike point to the victim
   5. Upward streamer: when positively charged current passes up from the ground through the victim that does not connect with the pilot strike or stepped leader
      In addition to electrical injury from a lightning strike, there may also be injuries from blunt or blast trauma. Common findings associated with blunt and blast trauma include tympanic membrane rupture, pulmonary contusions, loss of consciousness, fractures or dislocations, and clothing/shoes being blown off.

7. What types of injuries does lightning cause?

Lightning injuries vary from minor to catastrophic. Nearly all organ systems can be affected. The most significant morbidity is sudden cardiac death, usually from a direct strike. Cardiac arrest is caused by a fatal cardiac arrhythmia such as asystole or ventricular fibrillation, but may also result from coronary vasospasm or myocardial contusion. Return of spontaneous circulation can precede recovery of the respiratory system, because the medullary respiratory control center or the respiratory muscles themselves have been affected by the strike. This can cause a secondary cardiac arrest secondary to hypoxia. Lightning electricity travels the path of least resistance through body tissues. Nerves have lowest resistance, followed by blood, muscle, skin, fat, and then bone. While any tissue can sustain injury, those that conduct electricity with least resistance are more often affected by lightning. See Table 57.1 for common injuries by organ system.

8. Are there any long-term sequelae of being struck by lightning?

Most people survive lightning strikes (estimates range from 70% to 90%), but about 70% will have some sort of long-lasting morbidity from the strike. Permanent injuries include those sustained at the time of the strike, including hypoxic encephalopathy, disability from severe musculoskeletal injuries, scarring from burns, and hearing loss. However, many of the long-lasting sequelae are neurologic, including sleep disturbances, headaches, seizures, and neuropathies. In addition, psychiatrists are uncovering significant mental health issues following lightning strike, including posttraumatic stress disorder (PTSD), personality changes, depression, adjustment disorders, and cognitive

Table 57.1 Lightning Injuries by Organ System	
ORGAN SYSTEM	**INJURIES**
Cardiovascular	Injuries range from benign ECG changes to sudden cardiac death. Direct strikes are commonly associated with asystole and ventricular fibrillation, both of which have high mortality. ECG changes include ST elevation, T-wave inversion, QT prolongation, atrial fibrillation, ventricular tachycardia, and ventricular fibrillation. Severe cardiomyopathy and cardiogenic shock may occur, as well as labile blood pressures and autonomic instability.
Respiratory	Respiratory control centers in the midbrain or the diaphragm are commonly affected, causing respiratory depression. Also, pulmonary contusion, pulmonary hemorrhage, hemothorax, and pneumothorax may be caused directly by the strike or by the blast injury that may result.
Nervous	Injuries range from transient to permanent, and can have immediate or delayed onset. Transient symptoms include loss of consciousness, seizure, headache, paresthesias, weakness, confusion, disorientation, memory loss, and autonomic dysfunction (including pupillary dysfunction). Keraunoparalysis, transient paralysis caused by a lightning strike, is thought to be secondary to overstimulation of the autonomic nervous system and a hyperadrenergic state. Permanent symptoms include hypoxic encephalopathy, intracranial hemorrhage, and basal ganglia or brain stem injury. Delayed neurologic injuries include myelopathy and neuropathy.
Dermatologic	Lichtenberg figures ("feathering" or "ferning" pattern) are pathognomonic for lightning strike. Linear burns (partial-thickness burns from the vaporization of sweat into steam), or flashover, punctate burns (small, <1 cm, full-thickness circular burns from exit current), and thermal burns may be secondary to burning clothing, fabric, and the surrounding environment.
Musculoskeletal	Fractures, dislocations, muscle necrosis, and compartment syndrome
Renal	Myoglobinuria can be seen. Rhabdomyolysis is common after severe injuries.
Ophthalmologic	Lightning strike may affect both anterior and posterior chambers, and can occur from current injury, blunt and blast trauma, vasoconstriction, and heat. The lens is the most commonly injured portion of eye, with cataracts being the most common injury. There may also be mydriasis, loss of light reflex, anisocoria, and Horner's syndrome.
Otologic	Tympanic membrane rupture is a common occurrence secondary to blast trauma. Tinnitus and hearing loss may occur.
Psychiatric	Depression, posttraumatic stress disorder, memory impairment, personality changes, storm apprehension, and phobias are common even years after the strike.

ECG, Electrocardiogram.

deficits in verbal memory, executive functioning, and attention. Most cardiac manifestations are not permanent. Electrocardiogram (ECG) changes and cardiomyopathies tend to resolve over the course of weeks to days.

9. **Am I safe from a lightning strike in my car, because of the insulation of the rubber tires?**
No. It is true that being inside a metal-topped car (rather than a convertible) with the windows and doors closed is safer than no shelter at all; however, you are not entirely protected. The metal body, rather than the rubber tires, offers some protection, by acting as a Faraday cage, which allows the flow of electricity around the exterior of the car, rather than through it. This does not, however, protect occupants from splash current or induced electromagnetic currents through the interior.

10. **Am I safe from lightning if I am indoors?**
No. While being indoors is safer than no shelter at all, a significant number of lightning injuries actually occur in occupants of buildings. Strike can be from side flash through plumbing, telephone wires, and electrical appliances that are connected to the exterior of the building.

11. **Does lightning ever hit airplanes? What are the consequences?**
Yes. Fortunately, the consequences of lightning strikes to airplanes are minimal. On average, commercial airlines report that each aircraft is struck 1–2 times per year. Most strikes occur at an altitude of around 10,000–15,000 feet. Most aircraft skins are composed primarily of aluminum, which conducts electric current very well. The lightning flashes over the aircraft, leaving only minor, if any, damage. By ensuring that no gaps exist in the exterior, aircraft engineers are able to ensure that lightning flashes over the plane. The bright flash of lightning can temporarily blind pilots, and the electromagnetic effect can temporarily interrupt aircraft lighting and aviation controls. The last confirmed commercial plane crash in the United States directly attributable to lightning occurred in 1967, when lightning ignited the fuel tank and caused a catastrophic explosion.

12. **How common is lightning? How common are injuries or deaths?**
Lightning strikes occur around 100 times per second worldwide; about 20% of strikes result in cloud-to-ground strikes. Within the contiguous 48 states of the United States, there are an average of 20 million cloud-to-ground strikes annually. Within the United States, the incidence of lightning-related fatalities has been declining over the past 50 years, in part because of a decrease in rural populations, improved quality of dwellings, and improved medical care. In 2018, only 20 people were killed in the United States by lightning, the lowest annual incidence ever recorded. Unfortunately, rates of death internationally remain high in developing countries. This is attributed to tropical locations where thunderstorms are prevalent, there are many outside laborers, few cars, and poor quality of dwellings.

13. **Who tends to get struck by lightning? Where do most strikes occur?**
Males are >5 times more likely to be struck by lightning than women. Most victims are between the ages of 20 and 45 years, and >90% of deaths occur in the summer months. Within the United States, the lifetime risk of getting struck by lightning is around one in 12,000. Individuals in Florida, Colorado, and Texas have the highest risk. Globally, thunderstorms occur commonly in the tropics, where there is warm weather and heavy rainfall. Activities commonly associated with lightning strikes include hiking, boating, swimming, golfing, outdoor occupations, and land-line telephone use.

14. **I am treating a hiker who was found unconscious on the trail after a thunderstorm passed. How can I tell if he was struck by lightning?**
First, ensure the scene safety. If you can safely move the patient to a nearby safe environment, it is reasonable to do so. Assuming the thunderstorm has passed, initiate your assessment with a primary survey. Given the patient is unconscious, it is essential to establish a patent airway and adequate circulation.
Several physical examination findings can help you make the diagnosis. First, examine his skin, looking for "ferning" or "feathering" patterns, known as *Lichtenberg figures*. These skin findings are pathognomonic for a lightning strike. The skin findings will usually be present within 1 hour of the lightning strike and resolve over several hours. Unfortunately, Lichtenberg figures are only present in about 20% of confirmed lightning strikes. If possible, examine ears for evidence of tympanic membrane rupture, which occurs in approximately 50% of lightning strikes. Next, you should examine for evidence of other burns on his skin, as well as damage to his clothing, shoes, and equipment. See Table 57.1 for additional physical examination findings.

15. **The hiker has a palpable carotid pulse, but he does not appear to be breathing on his own. Why?**
The primary cause of death in lightning-strike victims is cardiac arrest, caused by a sudden depolarization of the entire myocardium. Often, the intrinsic cardiac automaticity will spontaneously restore organized cardiac activity along with a perfusing cardiac rhythm. However, there may be simultaneous respiratory arrest as a result of spasm of the thoracic muscles and stunning of the central nervous system (CNS) respiratory center. You should continue to give ventilatory support, in the form of rescue breathing, or a secondary hypoxic cardiac arrest can occur.

16. **The hiker is now breathing spontaneously. He is tachycardic, hypertensive, and has cool, pale skin with diminished peripheral pulses. He is awake, confused, and unable to move his extremities. Why?**
The victim is most likely experiencing *keraunoparalysis*, which is a transient paralysis after a lightning strike. It is secondary to overstimulation of the autonomic nervous system, which causes vasospasm and hypoperfusion. The

symptoms usually resolve within several hours. However, other injuries may have occurred, including traumatic spinal cord injuries that can also cause neurologic deficits. Regarding the victim's confusion, most direct-strike victims have no recollection of the event. Victims of indirect strikes may initially have some recollection of the events; however, they often develop anterograde amnesia.

17. **How should I approach rescuing multiple victims of a lightning strike?**
Lightning strikes are the one exception to the mass casualty triage principle. In the situation of a lightning strike, first priority should go to victims who are not breathing or moving. These patients are typically triaged "black" in traditional mass causality incidents. This is because for victims who are in cardiac arrest, the risk of death is the highest. However, in cardiac arrest due to lightning, there is a high likelihood of successful resuscitation. For victims without cardiopulmonary arrest, there is little chance of death, which means in this situation, the first priority is patients in cardiopulmonary arrest.

18. **Is prolonged cardiopulmonary resuscitation (CPR) beneficial in lightning-strike victims?**
No, there is little evidence to support prolonged CPR, or to suggest that it improves survival. If reversible causes of cardiopulmonary arrest have been ruled out, it would be reasonable to stop CPR after 30 minutes, just as you would do in a non–lightning-strike situation. However, fixed and dilated pupils cannot be used as an indicator of brain death or to gauge prognosis, as lightning strikes can cause autonomic dysfunction, including an abnormal pupillary response.

19. **Do victims of lightning strike typically suffer extensive burns?**
No. Contrary to popular folklore, victims do not burst into flames. In fact, of the victims who do suffer thermal burns, only 10% require skin grafting. Lightning usually flashes over a victim, with few, if any, deep-tissue burns. Victims with burns usually have linear, punctate, or partial-thickness thermal burns. Of note, victims with cranial burns have a threefold increase in mortality and are twice as likely to have cardiac arrest as victims with burns elsewhere. Those with metal near their body, such as necklaces, zippers, or belt buckles, are more likely to have full-thickness burns as a result of the metal becoming heated.

20. **What are the best ways to prevent lightning-related injury or death?**
   - *Behavioral strategies.* Avoid exposure to lightning by paying close attention to the weather in high-risk areas like beaches, open water, mountain tops, and golf courses. When there is a risk of lightning strike, seek shelter. *When thunder roars, go indoors* is the current recommendation from the National Weather Service.
   - *Shelter.* The center of the largest, most substantial building is the best shelter choice. Small open huts may increase the risk of side flashes. Avoid use of land-line telephones and electrical appliances. You can also seek shelter in a metal-topped vehicle – be sure to close the windows and doors. If you find yourself outdoors with no obvious shelter available, seek shelter deep in a cave (twice as deep as the opening), far into a dense forest, or deep ravine. Avoid shallow caves, open picnic shelters, or solitary trees because of the risk of ground current and side splash. According to the National Weather Service 30:30 rule, wait a minimum of 30 minutes after hearing the last thunder clap before returning outdoors.
   - *Lightning position.* Cracking sounds, hair standing on its end, or a visible glow (St. Elmo's fire) are signs of imminent strike. In these situations or very nearby lightning strikes with no shelter in sight, assume a lightning position by sitting or crouching on a ground pad.
   - *Avoid groups.* Separate members of a group by at least 20 feet to limit possibility of ground current and side splash affecting all members of the party.

21. **What are the differences between lightning and electrical injuries?**
See Table 57.2.

ELECTRICAL INJURIES

22. **What are the basic physics of electricity?**
Simply put, electricity is the flow of charged particles, known as *electrons*. The electric potential difference between two points is known as *voltage*. The number of electrons flowing past a specific point is known as *electric current*, and it is measured in amperes. The resistance to electron flow is a property of the material through which the electrons are flowing, and it is measured in ohms. These factors are related with Ohm's law, which states that current equals voltage divided by resistance.

23. **What is an easy and common way to classify electrical injuries? Does this help determine the nature and severity of electrical injuries?**
Electrical injuries can be divided into two categories: high voltage (>1000 V) and low voltage (<1000 V). Electrical injuries are related to the current, tissue resistance, and duration of contact. Current contributes most to tissue injury; however, in reality, voltage is often used as a surrogate for amperage (high voltages are usually associated with high amperages).

24. **How does the type of circuit relate to injury?**
Electrical current flows in two types of circuits: direct current (DC) and alternating current (AC). AC is the most common type of electricity in homes and is supplied in either 120 V or 240 V. High-voltage (>1000 V) DC can

Table 57.2 Comparison of Lightning With High-Voltage and Low-Voltage Electrical Injuries

	LIGHTNING	HIGH-VOLTAGE INJURY	LOW-VOLTAGE INJURY
Voltage (V)	$>30 \times 10^6$	>1000	<600 (<240)
Current (A)	>200,000	<1000	<240
Duration	Instantaneous	Brief	Prolonged
Type of current	DC	DC or AC	Mostly AC
Cardiac arrest (cause)	Asystole	Ventricular fibrillation	Ventricular fibrillation
Respiratory arrest (cause)	Direct CNS injury	Indirect trauma or tetanic contractions of respiratory muscles	Tetanic contractions of respiratory muscles
Muscle contraction	Single	DC, single; AC, tetanic	Tetanic
Burns	Rare, superficial	Common, deep	Usually superficial
Rhabdomyolysis	Uncommon	Very common	Common
Blunt injury (cause)	Blast effect; shock wave	Muscle contraction, fall	Fall (uncommon)
Mortality (acute)	Very high	Moderate	Low

AC, Alternating current; *CNS,* central nervous system; *DC,* direct current.

cause large single-muscle contractions, resulting in the victim being thrown away from source. This results in a short duration of contact. High-voltage AC is much more dangerous, because the cyclic flow of current causes muscle tetany and prolonged exposure to the source.

25. How common are electrical injuries?
There are approximately 500–1000 deaths per year in the United States from electrical injuries, more than 25 times the frequency of lightning strikes. High-tension electrical injuries account for ~7% of burn unit admissions (3%–5% for pediatric populations). Reported mortality rates of all electrical injuries are as high as 15%. Serious electrical burns have a mortality rate of up to 40%. In victims of low-voltage electrical injuries who do not suffer immediate cardiac death, mortality is low, but there may be significant morbidity, including oral trauma in children and hand trauma in adults.

In general, there is a bimodal age distribution for electrical injuries, with a peak in young children, and another around age 20. The peak in children is secondary to developmental stages in which children are exploring electrical outlets and cords. The peak around age 20 is because of occupational exposures and accidents, with electrical and construction workers accounting for a large percentage of these incidents. Electrical injury is the fourth leading cause of occupational deaths in the United States.

26. What should I do if I am a responder to the scene of an electrical injury?
The first priority is to not become a victim yourself – take time to ensure scene safety. Turn off all power sources that pose a threat to the rescuers or the victim. As with any trauma, airway, breathing, and circulation (ABCs) are the mainstay of initial resuscitation. Assume trauma has occurred and consider immobilizing the spine if there is a high suspicion for spinal injuries. Cardiac arrest from electrical injury is treated with CPR and general resuscitation principles. Additionally, given the propensity for large burns and extensive tissue damage, fluid resuscitation should begin early.

27. How does tissue resistance relate to electrical injury?
Within the body, different tissue types have different resistance, which affects how electric currents travel through them, resulting in different patterns of injury. Nerves have the least amount of resistance, meaning that electrical currents penetrate the deepest through nerves but cause them the least amount of heat injury. Blood and blood vessels have the next least resistance, followed by mucous membranes, muscle, skin, tendons, fat, and then bones. With the highest resistance in bone, it has the least penetration but the most thermal injury.

Of note, skin resistance is variable, depending on thickness, moisture content, and vascularity. Thick, dry, calloused skin, as on feet and hands, is much more resistant than thin, wet skin. Skin that is immersed in water has even lower resistance. When exposed to electrical energy, the thick skin of the hands and feet, with its high resistance, experiences thermal burns. As the skin is burned and charred in these areas, resistance drops, allowing for deeper penetration of electrical current and more extensive injury.

28. Which organ systems are affected by electrical injury? What types of injuries occur?
See Table 57.3.

Table 57.3 Common Presentations of Electrical Injuries by Organ System

ORGAN SYSTEM	INJURY
Skin	Skin may show a variety of burns, usually thermal. Typically, in AC burns, the entrance and exit burns are similar in size and shape. In DC burns, the exit is larger than the entrance wound. Flexor crease burns and mouth commissure burns, which may cause delayed bleeding from the labial artery when the eschar separates, may also be seen.
Cardiovascular	Patients often experience VF, and occasionally asystole. Usually VF is caused by low-voltage AC, whereas asystole is caused by high-voltage AC or DC. Can also see atrial and ventricular ectopy, atrial fibrillation, first-degree and second-degree heart block, QT prolongation, bundle-branch blocks, and acute myocardial infarction (rare). Long-term cardiac complications are rare.
Vascular	Hemorrhage, venous or arterial thrombosis, vasospasm and ischemia, necrosis (presumed to be from skip lesions where the current skips from the blood to the vessel wall)
Nervous	Electrical burns can cause central or peripheral injuries, including transient amnesia, confusion, or loss of consciousness; and seizure, apnea, respiratory depression, paralysis, and paresthesias. Peripheral nerve damage (motor nerves injured more commonly than sensory nerves) has a poor recovery rate.
Musculoskeletal	Compartment syndrome, fractures, dislocations, muscular pain, muscle necrosis (leading to rhabdomyolysis), tendon rupture, "electroporation" (formation of cell membrane pores in bone), aseptic necrosis, and periosteal burns.
Respiratory	Chest wall muscle spasm from tetanic contractions may cause respiratory arrest. Can also see respiratory arrest from inhibition of respiratory center within brain stem.
Gastrointestinal	Hollow organ and solid organ injury (rare); stress ulcers.
Renal	Acute tubular necrosis (from rhabdomyolysis and myoglobinuria), renal failure, hyperkalemia, hypocalcemia, acidosis.
ENT	Ruptured tympanic membranes, facial burns, cataracts (develop in approximately 6% of victims, usually 6–24 months after incident), corneal burns, intraocular hemorrhage, retinal edema, retinal detachment, uveitis, optic nerve atrophy.
Genitourinary	Can see spontaneous abortion in pregnant victims (fetal death rate is 73%), oligohydramnios, and IUGR. (Amniotic fluid and fetal tissues conduct 200 times better than dry, intact adult skin.)
Psychiatric	Depression, posttraumatic stress disorder, memory impairment, personality changes.

AC, Alternating current; *DC,* direct current; *ENT,* ear, nose, and throat; *IUGR,* intrauterine growth retardation; *VF,* ventricular fibrillation.

29. **What are the most common long-term complications of electrical injuries?**
Electrical injury can cause serious long-term sequelae, including neurologic symptoms such as numbness, weakness, paresthesias, memory problems, and chronic pain. Psychiatric symptoms include anxiety, poor concentration, depression, nightmares, insomnia, and PTSD. Victims of high-voltage injury have significantly more complications related to contact burns.

30. **Does the Parkland formula, which is applied to cutaneous burns, apply to those caused by electrical injury?**
Burn victims are usually resuscitated using a formula, such as the Parkland formula (4 mL × weight in kilograms × total body surface area affected) to determine fluids; however, these equations do not apply in situations of electrical burns. This is because the surface damage does not reflect the degree of deeper tissue damage. In this scenario, fluid replacement should be administered at a rate that produces 1–1.5 mL/kg/h of urine output. Fluids should be given early in the resuscitation of patients with electrical burn to prevent renal failure secondary to rhabdomyolysis.

31. **Should I obtain a computed tomography (CT) scan of the head or is close observation enough in the patient with electrical injury?**
You should consider a head CT scan in any victim of high-voltage electrical injury who has CNS symptoms on presentation or shortly after the event. Neural tissue has low resistance, and thus conducts electricity well. Traumatic subarachnoid hemorrhage can occur as a result of high-voltage shocks. Additionally, every patient with electrical injury should be evaluated as a trauma patient; therefore, CT of the head may be indicated to rule out other intracranial injuries as a result of blunt head trauma.

Table 57.4 Type of Exposure and Initial Presentation of Electrical Injuries

TYPE OF EXPOSURE	PRESENTATION
Low-voltage AC without LOC or cardiac arrest	<1000 V exposure; usually in home/office setting. Children typically are seen after biting cord; generally suffer oral burns. Adults come to emergency department with hand burns after working on home appliances. May have significant injuries if prolonged exposure with tetanic muscle contractions.
Low-voltage AC with LOC or arrest	Consider respiratory arrest secondary to thoracic muscle spasm or cardiac arrhythmias; consider whenever unwitnessed arrests occur.
High-voltage AC without LOC or arrest	Devastating thermal burns.
High-voltage AC with LOC or arrest	Rare; usually no LOC or arrest.
DC injury	Typically single-muscle contraction that throws victim from source. Rarely associated with LOC, unless secondary head trauma. Victims can usually remember what happened.
Conducted electrical devices/weapons (CEWs)	Example: Taser gun used in law enforcement. Delivers high-voltage current, is neither true AC nor DC, but is more like a series of low-amplitude DC shocks. No evidence of cardiac arrhythmias or death in healthy volunteers.

AC, Alternating current; *DC,* direct current; *LOC,* loss of consciousness.

32. Are presentations from high-voltage electrical injury similar to lightning-strikes?

No. Lightning strikes and high-voltage electricity cause different injury patterns and thus require a different approach. While many similarities do exist, there are important differences. High-voltage injuries often cause deep burns that may lead to rhabdomyolysis and renal failure, require focused fluid repletion, and may need further interventions, such as fasciotomies if compartment syndrome develops (Table 57.4). Victims of high-voltage electrical injury will often exhibit ventricular fibrillation. In contrast, victims of lightning rarely have deep or severe burns, rarely need aggressive fluid resuscitation, and generally do not require fasciotomies. They also are more likely to be asystolic from massive cardiac depolarization. Long-term neurologic and psychiatric consequences have been found to be similar.

33. Are there any medications to consider for electrical or lightning injury victims?

There is no pharmacotherapy indicated specifically for lightning or electrical injuries. In patients with electrical injury who have rhabdomyolysis, liberal fluid resuscitation with normal saline is beneficial. Sodium bicarbonate can also be used to alkalize the urine, which in turn increases myoglobin clearance. As with all burns, attention to appropriate pain control is important.

34. Who needs to be admitted for lightning-strike or electrical injuries?

Any patient with cardiac abnormalities (detected in the field or the emergency department [ED]), neurologic findings, or significant burns warrants hospital admission. See Table 57.5 for admission and cardiac monitoring indications. Patients who meet admission criteria and have suffered a high-voltage or lightning-strike injury should receive cardiac monitoring for 24 hours. Serial ECGs and echocardiography may be indicated. Patients who suffered low-voltage injuries and demonstrated ECG abnormalities should also receive cardiac monitoring. Patients with traumatic injuries or burns should be stabilized and then considered for transfer to a trauma center or burn unit. Asymptomatic patients who have sustained a low-voltage injury and no loss of consciousness may be discharged from the ED with appropriate follow-up instructions as needed. Patients should have repeat laboratory studies in several days to evaluate for rhabdomyolysis. Patients should also be referred for an ophthalmologic follow-up appointment within 3 months, as well as otolaryngologic, neurologic, and psychiatric follow-up care as needed.

35. What laboratory studies are helpful in assessment of severity for those suffering electrical injuries?

Elevated serum creatinine kinase can be used as a prognostic factor, and help determine the need for early fasciotomy to prevent limb loss in high-voltage burn victims. Serial creatine kinase (CK) levels should be followed if initially elevated to guide treatment for rhabdomyolysis, and electrolyte abnormalities corrected (see Chapter 46). Troponin may be useful in determining the level of cardiac damage, but an elevated level does not suggest ongoing ischemia. Patients with suspected abdominal involvement should receive liver function, lipase, and coagulation studies. A urinalysis should also be sent to evaluate for myoglobinuria. Patients with burns or trauma will typically exhibit leukocytosis, but this has no prognostic value.

Table 57.5 Criteria for Admission and Cardiac Monitoring Versus Discharge

ADMIT (CONSIDER TRANSFER TO BURN OR TRAUMA CENTER)	DISCHARGE
• Cardiac arrest/required CPR • Documented loss of consciousness • Abnormal ECG; dysrhythmia observed in prehospital or ED setting • Presence of significant risk factors for cardiac disease • Concomitant injury severe enough to warrant admission • Suspicion of conductive injury: High-voltage injury, especially with transthoracic current path • Hypoxia • Chest pain • Neurologic abnormalities • Major burns; circumferential burns, hand/face/groin burns • Myoglobinuria • OB/GYN consult for pregnant patients	• Asymptomatic low-voltage injury • No ECG findings • No significant burns • No other significant injuries [a]Ophthalmology follow-up examination in 3 months for lightning injury [a]ENT, neurology, psychiatry follow-up examinations as needed [a]Close ENT or plastic surgery follow-up monitoring and counseling about eschar formation in mouth commissure burns in pediatric patients

[a]If discharged, these referrals and follow-up arrangements should be made.
CPR, Cardiopulmonary resuscitation; *ECG,* electrocardiogram; *ENT,* ear, nose, and throat; *OB/GYN,* obstetric, gynecologic.

36. What about children who get injured by a household electrical cord or appliance? Should I admit them to the hospital for observation, or can I discharge them home from the ED?

Most often, children sustain electrical injuries in the home. These injuries are usually associated with electrical cords (60%–70%), with contact to an extremity or the mouth, or with wall outlets (15%–20%). Healthy children exposed to common household currents (120–240 V) without water contact can be discharged home, as long as they are asymptomatic at presentation with no evidence of ventricular arrhythmia or cardiac arrest in the field. Those with nonfatal arrhythmias or nonspecific ECG abnormalities typically resolve within 24 hours without intervention. Therefore healthy children exposed to common household electrical currents do not require initial screening ECG or admission for cardiac monitoring. For children with oral burns from chewing an electrical cord, consultation with plastic surgery is recommended, although most labial artery complications tend to happen when the eschar falls off in 5–7 days.

37. What about pregnant patients who sustain electrical injuries?

When a fetus is exposed to electrical current, just as in adults, it is at risk of cardiac arrest. The risk may be higher in a fetus, however, because fetal tissue offers less resistance than postnatal tissue. Fetal skin is 200 times less resistant than postnatal skin; exposure of the fetus to even low voltage can be lethal. When considering the risk to the fetus, the critical consideration is the current path, and whether the current passed through the uterus. This is most often seen in hand-to-foot passage. Pregnant patients should be monitored for 24 hours if there are any signs of fetal distress or decreased fetal movement on initial ultrasound. Care for the mother should be the same as with nonpregnant patients.

KEY POINTS: LIGHTNING AND ELECTRICAL INJURIES

1. Secure the scene; rescuers should not become victims.
2. Traditional triage rules do not apply to lightning victims; remember to reverse triage and concentrate on victims who appear to be in cardiopulmonary arrest. Assume occult trauma and remember that entrance/surface burns may be indicators of underlying tissue damage. It is not possible to predict the degree of underlying tissue damage based on the extent of cutaneous injury.
3. AC exposure is far more dangerous than DC exposure of the same voltage, secondary to the potential for tetanic muscle contractions and prolonged contact with AC current.

Websites
American Burn Association: http://ameriburn.org/; accessed January 15, 2019.
American Heart Association: http://circ.ahajournals.org/; accessed January 15, 2019.
Lightning Injury Research Program: https://chicago.medicine.uic.edu/departments/academic-departments/emergency-medicine/research/previously-funded/lightning-injury/; accessed January 15, 2019.
Lightning and Atmospheric Electricity Research at Global Hydrology and Climate Center: https://ghrc.nsstc.nasa.gov/lightning/; accessed January 19, 2019.
National Weather Service: US Lightning Deaths in 2018. https://www.weather.gov/safety/lightning-fatalities; accessed January 15, 2019.

ACKNOWLEDGMENT

The authors and editors gratefully acknowledge the contributions of Gabrielle A. Jacquet and Timothy R Hurtado, authors of this chapter in previous editions.

BIBLIOGRAPHY

Altalhi A, Al-Manea W, Alqweai N, et al. Cardiac rhythm recorded by implanted loop recorder during lightning strike. *Ann Saudi Med.* 2017;37(5):401–402.

Andrews CJ, Reisner AD, Cooper MA. Post-electrical or lightning injury syndrome: a proposal for an American Psychiatric Association's Diagnostic and Statistical Manual formulation with implications for treatment. *Neural Regen Res.* 2017;12(9):1405–1412.

Azzena B, Tocco-Tussardi I, Pontini A, et al. Late complications of high-voltage electrical injury might involve multiple systems and be related to current path. *Ann Burns Fire Disasters.* 2016;29(3):192–195.

Biswas A, Dalal K, Hossain J, et al. Lightning injury is a disaster in Bangladesh? – Exploring its magnitude and public health needs. *F1000Res.* 2016;5:2931.

Christophides T, Khan S, Ahmad M, et al. Cardiac effects of lightning strikes. *Arrhythm Electrophysiol Rev.* 2017;6(3):114–117.

Davis C, Engeln A, Johnson E, et al. Wilderness medical society practice guidelines for the prevention and treatment of lightning injuries. *Wilderness Environ Med.* 2012;23:260–269.

Gibran N. *Electrical Injuries. Burn Care for General Surgeons and General Practitioners.* Cham: Springer; 2016:193–200.

Hansen SM, Riahi S, Hjortshoj S, et al. Mortality and risk of cardiac complications among immediate survivors of accidental electric shock: a Danish nationwide cohort study. *BMJ Open.* 2017;7:e015967.

Luz DP, Millan LS, Alessi MS, et al. Electrical burns: a retrospective analysis across a 5-year period. *Burns.* 2009;35:1015–1019.

Mulder MB, Msalu L, Caro T, et al. Remarkable rates of lightning strike mortality in Malawi. *PLoS One.* 2012;7(1):e29281.

Reisner D. Delayed neural damage induced by lightning and electrical injury: neuronal death, vascular necrosis and demyelination? *Neural Regen Res.* 2014;9(9):907–908.

Teodoreanu R, Popescu SA, Lascar I. Electrical injuries: biological values measurements as a prediction factor of local evolution in electrocutions lesions. *J Med Life.* 2014;7(2):226–236.

Zijlmans M, Rinkel G. Electrical injury to the brain. *J Neurol Neurosurg Psychiatry.* 2012;83:933–934.

CHAPTER 58

DROWNING

Andrew Schmidt, DO, MPH and Jedd Roe, MD, MBA, FACEP

1. Define drowning.

In 2002, the World Congress on Drowning developed the following standard definition for drowning: *The process of experiencing respiratory impairment due to submersion or immersion in a liquid.* The following descriptive terms should **not** be used, as they cause confusion and do not have clinical value: *near, dry, wet, active, passive,* and *secondary drowning.*

2. How many people drown each year?

Each year in the United States, more than 3500 people die from drowning (an estimated 400,000 worldwide), and it is the second most common cause of injury-related death in pediatric patients 1–14 years old. Approximately 8 million nonfatal drownings occur worldwide each year, many of which may lead to severe morbidity.

3. Who drowns, and why?

Drowning is primarily a disease of youth, and the incidence peaks in two groups: toddlers and teenagers. The most vulnerable group is toddlers (ages 1–4 years); they are inherently inquisitive and often physically unable to extricate themselves from hazards such as pools, buckets, tubs, toilets, or washers. Inadequate supervision, even for brief moments, is the primary cause of drowning in toddlers. Providers should consider the possibility of abuse when evaluating a child drowning victim, because inflicted submersions account for up to 8% of child abuse cases in those <5 years of age. In people ages 15–24 years, ~80% of drowning victims are male. Young males are often victims because of risk-taking behavior during swimming, boating, diving, or other water-related activities. Alcohol is a contributing factor in more than 60% of all teenage and young adult drownings.

Other risk factors in all age groups are as follows:

- Inability to swim
- Seizure disorder
- Cardiac diseases
- Substance abuse
- Trauma (diving in shallow water, boating)
- Hypothermia
- Freediving training (hyperventilation)

4. What kills a drowning victim?

The primary cause of morbidity and mortality in drowning is hypoxia. Historically, a misguided focus has been placed on the type of water aspirated (salt versus fresh), the volume of water aspirated, and whether laryngospasm occurred. Additionally, the actual volumes of water commonly aspirated are much smaller than originally postulated. Therefore, a resuscitative strategy focused on expelling water from the lungs, instead of reversing hypoxia, will do more harm than good.

5. What happens in a drowning?

The first event is an unexpected or prolonged submersion. The victim begins to struggle and panic. Fatigue begins, and air hunger develops. Reflex inspiration ultimately overrides breath holding. The victim inhales water, and aspiration occurs, causing laryngospasm that may last for several minutes. Hypoxemia worsens, and unconsciousness ensues. If the victim is not rescued and resuscitated promptly, central nervous system (CNS) damage begins within minutes.

6. Describe the presenting symptoms of drowning victims.

The presenting symptoms are varied, from asymptomatic to cardiac arrest. The patient may have a mild cough, show mild dyspnea and tachypnea, or be in fulminant pulmonary edema. The spectrum of CNS findings may range from normal to confusion or lethargy to coma.

7. What is the pulmonary pathophysiology?

The central clinical feature of all submersion incidents is hypoxemia caused by airway obstruction by a liquid medium. The partial pressure of oxygen (PO_2) decreases, the partial pressure of carbon dioxide (PCO_2) increases, and there is a combined respiratory and metabolic acidosis. If the patient is successfully resuscitated, the recovery phase often is complicated by aspirated water or vomitus. Aspiration can cause airway obstruction by particulates, bronchospasm by direct irritation, acute respiratory distress syndrome (ARDS) caused by pulmonary edema from parenchymal damage, atelectasis from loss of surfactant, and pulmonary bacterial infections. Some patients may later develop pulmonary abscesses or empyema.

8. How is the cardiac system affected in drowning?

Cardiac decompensation and dysrhythmias (most commonly asystole or pulseless electric activity [PEA]) are caused by hypoxemia and complicated by the ensuing acidosis. The heart is relatively resistant to hypoxic injury, and with proper resuscitation resumption of cardiac activity is common, although severe CNS damage often occurs. Response of the heart to therapy, particularly antiarrhythmic medications and defibrillation, may be limited by hypoxia, acidosis, and hypothermia. Primary therapy is aimed at reversal of these three problems.

9. What is the prehospital treatment?

The most important part of treatment of a drowning victim is delivered in the prehospital phase with immediate resuscitation. Therapy must correct hypoxia as rapidly as possible. If a submersion victim has appropriate airway management and ventilation is rapidly established, anoxic brain injury can be avoided, and prompt and full recovery may be possible. Establish a patent airway and administer oxygen with positive pressure ventilation as indicated by the patient's condition. This may not necessarily include endotracheal intubation if interventions like bag-valve-mask or supraglottic devices are successful. Although cervical spine immobilization is important for suspected spinal injury, the incidence of this in drowning cases is very low. If there is high suspicion for cervical spine injury (witnessed diving or fall from height, known ethanol ingestion, facial trauma), appropriate precautions should be taken with in-line stabilization. However, cervical spine immobilization should never delay proper ventilation in the critical patient. If the patient is pulseless, cardiopulmonary resuscitation (CPR) (with ventilations) should be initiated using advanced cardiac life support (ACLS) protocols.

Note: There is no evidence supporting the use of abdominal thrusts or postural drainage maneuvers, and their use is not recommended.

10. When is endotracheal intubation indicated?

Any person with altered mentation or an inability to protect the airway should be considered for intubation. In the initial resuscitation, if noninvasive maneuvers are successful (bag-valve-mask, supraglottic device, noninvasive positive airway pressure), these may be used to ensure early reversal of hypoxia. Inability to maintain a $PO_2 > 90$ mmHg with high-flow oxygen by nonrebreather mask is suspicious for ARDS. Stable patients may be bridged with continuous positive airway pressure (CPAP), while those with hemodynamic instability, worsening respiratory failure despite CPAP, or altered mental status require intubation. Early airway management with positive pressure ventilation, and positive end-expiratory pressure, can help decrease intrapulmonary shunting.

11. If aspiration is suspected, what treatment is needed?

Treatment of aspiration is primarily supportive. Close observation and appropriate aftercare instruction for signs of a developing pulmonary infection or ARDS are needed. Rarely, cases with significant aspiration may require bronchoscopy to remove particulate matter and tenacious secretions. Bronchodilator therapy with β-agonists is appropriate if bronchospasm is evident.

12. Does a normal chest radiograph rule out pulmonary injury?

No. A normal initial chest radiograph does not predict extent of injury or clinical course. Findings on chest radiograph vary and may be delayed, but patients with severe injury often display a pattern similar to that seen in ARDS.

13. Is there a role for prophylactic antibiotics?

When highly contaminated water is involved (e.g., sewage), prophylactic antibiotics may be considered. In all other instances, prophylactic antibiotics are of no proven benefit. Their use is indicated if the presence of clinical evidence suggests pneumonia, which is rare and would only be expected in a delayed fashion after drowning.

14. Discuss the approach to patients with a decreased level of consciousness or coma.

Hypoxic injury leads to cerebral edema and a concomitant rise in intracranial pressure. Although there was initial enthusiasm for treatment of presumed elevated intracranial pressure with the usual modalities of muscle paralysis, hyperventilation, mannitol, barbiturate coma, hypothermia, and steroids, more recent studies have shown no improvement in outcome with these therapies. Supportive care is the mainstay of therapy. Be attentive to the possibility of cranial or spinal injuries in all boating or diving injuries in patients with altered level of consciousness. Do not forget the possibility of a suicide attempt or child abuse. If the history is in doubt, assume a cranial and a cervical injury, as long as the treatment of such does not delay airway support. Consider concomitant ingestions and substance use.

15. Are glucocorticoids, barbiturate coma, or induced hypothermia indicated?

In the case of glucocorticoids and barbiturate coma, no. These therapies are unproven and remain controversial. However, targeted temperature control (e.g., hypothermia) has been shown to be of benefit in cardiac arrest, and case reports have suggested similar outcomes for victims of submersion. This should be initiated only after proper resuscitation, with a focus on oxygenation and ventilation, and only in facilities with the proper policies, equipment, and training to initiate and maintain the hypothermia for 24–48 hours.

16. What is unique about cold-water submersion?

Cases in which victims of prolonged submersion in cold water have been resuscitated successfully without apparent neurologic sequelae are reported occasionally. The number remains small, however. The induced hypothermia causes a decrease in metabolic demand, reducing potential hypoxic injury from prolonged asphyxia. Cold water does have potentially deleterious effects. Most significant are the induced cardiac irritability from hypothermia, exhaustion, and altered mental status. Resuscitation of hypothermic drowning victims should be continued until patients are rewarmed or to the level required for therapeutic hypothermia (see Chapter 59). Extracorporeal membrane oxygenation (ECMO) has received increased attention in the literature for the treatment of drowning patients. If available, this may be considered for severe or refractory hypothermia or hypoxemia.

17. What is swimming-induced pulmonary edema (SIPE)?
Swimming-induced pulmonary edema or SIPE is a form of pulmonary edema in swimmers that is unrelated to aspiration of water. It happens more commonly in patients who are exposed to cold water and in patients who are wearing tight-fitting wetsuits. Additionally, female gender and older age predispose to this condition. The condition has four diagnostic criteria: (1) acute onset of dyspnea during or shortly after swimming; (2) hypoxia; (3) chest x-ray consistent with pulmonary edema; and (4) absence of preceding infection or aspiration. There is no consensus on treatment for the condition.

18. When should resuscitative efforts be withheld?
In general, all patients should receive initial resuscitative efforts. There are numerous reports of survival after prolonged submersion, especially in small children who have drowned in extremely cold water, although this is by no means the usual circumstance. In general, a submersion time longer than 10 minutes, or resuscitation time longer than 25 minutes, has been shown to correlate with a poor prognosis (death or survival with poor neurologic outcome). Historically, the philosophy has been to resuscitate the victim until the core temperature is greater than 32°C. However, it is important to acknowledge the often devastating neurologic outcomes patients (and families) endure after prolonged submersion and resuscitation.

19. What is the disposition of a submersion victim?
All submersion victims with cardiac arrest deserve effective prehospital and in-hospital resuscitation efforts, with a focus on reversing hypoxia. All other submersion victims require close observation. Some respiratory complications of drowning are delayed in presentation and usually appear within 4–6 hours. After initial resuscitation and stabilization, any patient with continued respiratory complaints or symptoms, altered mentation, chest radiograph abnormalities, or a demonstrated oxygen requirement should be monitored closely in a hospital for at least 24 hours. Patients without any symptoms and completely normal evaluation may be discharged after 4–6 hours of observation with instructions to return immediately for any new respiratory symptoms.

20. What are the most important factors in estimating prognosis?
The most consistent prognostic indicator found in the literature is duration of submersion, and this highlights the pivotal role that hypoxia plays in the injury process. Other factors that have been found to have some prognostic value are:

- Delay in initiation of CPR
- Delay in arrival of emergency medical services (EMS)
- Need for prolonged resuscitation
- A Glasgow Coma Scale score ≤5
- pH <7
- Asystole on arrival to the emergency department (ED)

  Dr. David Szpilman has proposed a clinical classification based on the analysis of 1831 cases of submersion seen in Brazil over 19 years. The classification is based on clinical findings in the field, and the mortality rates are shown in Table 58.1.

21. Can we prevent drowning?
Many of the factors contributing to death by drowning are preventable and can be directed at those groups at risk, particularly children. Efforts include:

- Participating in swim lessons
- Fencing of private and public swimming pools

Table 58.1 Szpilman Classification of Drowning

GRADE	CLINICAL FINDINGS	MORTALITY RATE (%)
1	Normal pulmonary auscultation ± cough	0
2	Rales or crackles in some lung fields	0.6
3	Crackles in all fields without hypotension	5.2
4	Crackles in all fields with hypotension	19.4
5	Respiratory arrest without cardiac arrest	44
6	Cardiopulmonary arrest	93

- Using personal flotation devices
- Improving supervision of infants and young children near water
- Increasing public knowledge of the risks of the day's water conditions
- Understanding the limitations of personal health conditions
- Stressing the separation of alcohol from water-related activities

KEY POINTS: SUBMERSION INCIDENTS

1. Toddlers and teenagers are most at risk for death from submersion.
2. Prehospital treatment is critical and directed at correcting underlying hypoxia.
3. A normal chest radiograph does not rule out pulmonary injury.
4. Asymptomatic drowning victims can often be safely discharged after 4–6 hours of observation.
5. Most drownings are preventable.

Websites
www.drowninglit.com; accessed June 6, 2019.

BIBLIOGRAPHY

Cantu RM, Pruitt CM, Samuy N, et al. Predictors of emergency department discharge following pediatric drowning. *Am J Emerg Med.* 2018;36(3):446–449.

Centers for Disease Control and Prevention. *Unintentional drowning: get the facts.* 2016 https://www.cdc.gov/homeandrecreationalsafety/water-safety/waterinjuries-factsheet.html. Accessed November 7, 2017.

Dyson K, Morgans A, Bray J, et al. Drowning related out-of-hospital cardiac arrests: characteristics and outcomes. *Resuscitation.* 2013;84:1114–1118.

Quan L, Mack CD, Schiff MA. Association of water temperature and submersion duration and drowning outcome. *Resuscitation.* 2014;85:790–794.

Schmidt A, Sempsrott J. Drowning in the adult population: emergency department resuscitation and treatment. *Emerg Med Pract.* 2015;17(5):1–22.

Sempsrott J, Schmidt A, Hawkins S, et al. Submersion injuries and drowning. In: Auerbach P, Cushing TA, Harris NS, eds. *Wilderness Medicine.* 7th ed. Philadelphia, PA: Elsevier; 2017:1530–1549.

Shenoi RP, Allahabadi S, Rubalcava DM, et al. The pediatric submersion score predicts children at low risk for injury following submersions. *Acad Emerg Med.* 2017;24(12):1491–1500.

Szpilman D. Near-drowning and drowning classification: a proposal to stratify mortality based on the analysis of 1,831 cases. *Chest.* 1997;112:660–665.

Szpilman D, Bierens JJ, Handley AJ, et al. Drowning. *N Engl J Med.* 2012;366:2102–2110.

CHAPTER 59

HYPOTHERMIA AND FROSTBITE

Martin R. Huecker, MD and Daniel F. Danzl, MD

HYPOTHERMIA

1. What is accidental hypothermia?

Accidental hypothermia is an unintentional decrease in core temperature to less than 35°C (95°F).

2. What factors are important in the epidemiology of hypothermia?

Primary accidental hypothermia results from direct exposure to the cold. Although outdoor exposure is common, many elderly victims are found indoors. Secondary hypothermia is a natural complication of many systemic disorders, including sepsis, cancer, and trauma. The mortality rate of secondary hypothermia is much higher.

3. How is body temperature normally regulated?

The normal physiology of temperature regulation is activated by cold exposure, producing reflex vasoconstriction and stimulating the hypothalamic nuclei, which normally maintains temperature within 1°C. Heat preservation mechanisms include shivering, autonomic and endocrine responses, and adaptive behavioral responses. Although acclimatization to heat stress is efficient, humans cannot acclimate to sudden, extreme, or prolonged exposure to cold.

KEY POINTS: COMMON MECHANISMS OF HEAT LOSS

1. Radiation
2. Conduction
3. Convection
4. Respiration
5. Evaporation

---

4. Describe the common findings in mild, moderate, and severe hypothermia.

- Mild hypothermia (32.2°C–35°C [90°F–95°F]) depresses the central nervous system (CNS) and increases the metabolic rate, pulse, and amount of shivering thermogenesis. Dysarthria, amnesia, ataxia, and apathy are common findings.
- Moderate hypothermia (27°C–32.2°C [80°F–90°F]) progressively depresses the level of consciousness and the vital signs. Shivering is extinguished. Patients are at significant risk of dysrhythmia. The QT interval is prolonged, and a J wave (Osborn wave) may appear at the junction of the QRS complex and ST segment. Patients cannot rewarm spontaneously. A cold diuresis results from an initial central hypervolemia, which is caused by the peripheral vasoconstriction.
  - As the body's temperature drops from moderate to severe hypothermia, patients may exhibit paradoxical undressing, as mentation is altered and peripheral vessels suddenly dilate, tricking the already-compromised brain into thinking the body is too warm.
- Severe hypothermia (< 27°C [80°F]) results in coma and areflexia with profoundly depressed vital signs. Carbon dioxide production decreases 50% for each 8°C fall in temperature; there is little respiratory stimulation.

5. What factors predispose a patient to hypothermia?

- Decreased heat production
- Increased heat loss
- Impaired thermoregulation

6. What decreases heat production?

Decreased heat production is common with the following conditions:

- Age extremes
- Inadequate stored fuel
- Endocrine or neuromuscular insufficiency

Neonates are poorly adapted for cold, even without being subjected to emergent deliveries and resuscitations. The elderly have progressively impaired thermal perception. Anything from hypoglycemia to more severe malnutrition impairs temperature regulation. Examples of endocrine failure include myxedema, hypopituitarism, and hypoadrenalism.

7. **What are common causes of increased heat loss?**
   Increased heat loss results mainly from exposure or dermatologic problems that interfere with the skin's integrity. Iatrogenic causes include emergency childbirth, cold infusions, trauma resuscitation, and heat stroke treatment.

8. **What are the ways in which thermoregulation can be impaired?**
   Impairment can occur via central, peripheral, metabolic, or pharmacologic mechanisms. A variety of CNS processes, including traumatic or neoplastic lesions and degenerative processes, affect hypothalamic function, inducing hypothermia. Acute spinal cord transection extinguishes peripheral vasoconstriction, preventing heat conservation. The abnormal plasma osmolality common with metabolic derangements, including diabetic ketoacidosis and uremia, can also impair thermoregulation. Finally, many medications and toxins can also impair central thermoregulation in either toxic or therapeutic doses.

9. **When should hypothermia be suspected?**
   The diagnosis is facilitated with a history of cold exposure. The history may not be available or helpful, however, and subtle presentations are far more common in urban areas. Ataxia and dysarthria may mimic a cerebrovascular event or intoxication. You can avoid missing the diagnosis by measuring the patient's core temperature.

10. **Are there keys in the physical examination that help distinguish primary from secondary hypothermia?**
    If there is tachycardia disproportionate to the temperature, suspect hypoglycemia, an overdose, or hypovolemia. Hyperventilation during moderate or severe hypothermia suggests a CNS lesion or systemic acidosis (e.g., diabetic ketoacidosis or lactic acidosis). A cold-induced rectus spasm and ileus may mask or mimic an acute abdomen. Suspect an overdose, alcohol intoxication, or CNS insult whenever the decreased level of consciousness is not consistent with the temperature.

11. **What options are available to measure the core temperature?**
    The gold standard is pulmonary artery temperature measurements; however, this is rarely performed. Rectal, esophageal, and bladder sites can be measured. The rectal temperature may lag or be falsely low if the probe is in cold feces. Esophageal temperature is falsely elevated during heated inhalation.

12. **How does temperature depression affect the hematologic evaluation of patients?**
    The hematocrit increases 2% per 1°C drop in temperature, which can mask anemia. Leukocytes often are sequestered, which may result in low white blood cell counts despite infection. There are no safe predictors of values – the increased viscosity seen with cold hemagglutination can result in either thrombosis or hemolysis, and a type of disseminated intravascular coagulation syndrome can occur. Coagulopathies of hypothermia are not reflected by the deceptively normal international normalized ratio (INR), because this test is done routinely on blood rewarmed to 37°C.

13. **Should arterial blood gases be corrected for temperature?**
    No. A pH of 7.4 and a partial pressure of carbon dioxide (PCO_2) of 40 mmHg confirm acid-base balance at all temperatures.

14. **What is the key decision regarding rewarming?**
    The primary initial decision is whether to rewarm the patient passively or actively. Passive rewarming is noninvasive and involves simply covering the patient in a warm environment. This technique is ideal for previously healthy patients with mild hypothermia.

15. **What conditions necessitate active rewarming?**
    - Cardiovascular instability
    - Temperature less than 35°C (90°F)
    - Age extremes
    - Neurologic or endocrine insufficiency

16. **What is core temperature afterdrop?**
    Core temperature afterdrop is the commonly observed continued drop in core temperature after initiation of external rewarming. There are two causes:
    1. Temperature equilibration between tissues
    2. The circulatory return of cold peripheral blood to the core

17. **Are there unique considerations with active external rewarming?**
    The external transfer of heat to a patient is accomplished most safely when the heat is applied directly to the trunk. In chronically hypothermic patients, rapidly rewarming the vasoconstricted extremities may overwhelm a depressed cardiovascular system and result in cardiovascular collapse. Forced heated-air rewarming blankets (such as Bair Hugger), circulating water blankets, and warming lights are commonly used. Monitoring in a heated tub can be difficult, and vasoconstricted skin is burned easily by electric blankets.

18. **What constitutes active core rewarming?**
    Active core rewarming involves techniques that deliver heat directly to the core. Options include: heated inhalation; heated infusion; heated central venous catheters; bladder lavage, gastric lavage, thoracic lavage, and peritoneal

lavage; and extracorporeal rewarming using extracorporeal membrane oxygenation (ECMO), dialysis, or cardiopulmonary bypass circuits.

19. When is airway rewarming indicated?
Heated, humidified oxygen can be administered via mask or endotracheal tube. Heat transfer is not as significant by mask, but respiratory heat loss is eliminated while the patient is rewarmed gradually.

20. What are the techniques for heated irrigation?
Irrigation (or lavage) should be considered only in severe cases and in combination with other techniques. Thoracostomy tube irrigation with two tubes is a more efficient method in severe cases. Intravenous (IV) fluids heated to 40°C–42°C are particularly helpful during major volume resuscitations. Double-catheter peritoneal lavage can efficiently rewarm seriously hypothermic patients. Infuse 2 L of isotonic dialysate at 40°C–45°C, and suction after 20 minutes dwell time. Heat transfer from irrigation of the gastrointestinal tract is minimal and risks aspiration. Bladder irrigation also has minimal effect.

21. When is extracorporeal rewarming indicated?
Cardiopulmonary bypass, ECMO, continuous arteriovenous and venovenous rewarming, and hemodialysis can be life saving in cardiac arrest situations; this can also allow for concomitant treatment of completely frozen extremities, severe rhabdomyolysis, and major electrolyte fluxes.

22. What are the contraindications to cardiopulmonary resuscitation (CPR) in accidental hypothermia?
CPR should be initiated unless do-not-resuscitate status is verified, lethal injuries are identified, no signs of life are present, or the chest wall is frozen and cannot be compressed. Because a profoundly hypothermic patient may appear dead, and because vital signs may be difficult to obtain, a cardiac monitor should be applied for 30–45 seconds to ensure that there are no signs of life.

23. Are there unique pharmacologic considerations during hypothermia?
Protein binding increases as body temperature drops, and most drugs become ineffective; pharmacologic manipulation of the pulse and blood pressure should generally be avoided.

24. What is the significance of atrial and ventricular dysrhythmias?
Atrial dysrhythmias normally have a slow ventricular response. They are innocent and should be left untreated. Preexistent ventricular ectopy may resurface during rewarming and confuse the picture. Ventricular dysrhythmia treatment is problematic, because the cold heart may be unresponsive to cardiovascular agents. If the patient is in ventricular fibrillation, only one defibrillation attempt (2 J/kg) is indicated until the core temperature exceeds 30°C–32°C. Patients who are moderately or severely hypothermic are at high risk of decompensation into ventricular dysrhythmia with movement, endotracheal intubation, and jugular or subclavian catheter placement.

FROSTBITE

25. What is frostbite?
Frostbite is the most common freezing injury of tissue. It occurs whenever the tissue temperature decreases to <0°C (<32°F). Ice crystal formation damages the cellular architecture, and stasis progresses to microvascular thrombosis.

26. Which factors predispose a patient to frostbite?
Tissue rapidly freezes when in contact with good thermal conductors, including metal, water, and volatiles. Direct exposure to cold wind (wind-chill index) quickly freezes acral areas (e.g., fingers, toes, ears, nose). A variety of conditions can impair the peripheral circulation and predispose a person to frostbite. Constrictive clothing and immobility reduce heat delivery to the distal tissues. Vasoconstrictive medications, including nicotine, can exacerbate cold damage, especially when coupled with underlying vascular conditions, such as atherosclerosis.

27. What peripheral circulatory changes precede frostbite?
Humans possess a life-versus-limb mechanism that helps prevent systemic hypothermia. Arteriovenous anastomoses in the skin shunt blood away from acral areas to limit radiative heat loss.

28. Before frostbite occurs, what other cutaneous events take place in the prefreeze phase?
As tissue temperatures decrease to <10°C, anesthesia develops. Endothelial cells leak plasma, and microvascular vasoconstriction occurs. Crystallization is not seen as long as the deeper tissues conduct and radiate heat.

29. What happens during the freeze phase of frostbite?
The type of exposure determines the rate and location of ice crystal formation. Usually, ice initially forms extracellularly, causing water to exit the cell, and inducing cellular dehydration, hyperosmolality, collapse, and death.

30. Immediately after thawing, what may occur?
In deep frostbite, progressive microvascular collapse develops. Sludging, stasis, and cessation of flow begin in the capillaries and progress to the venules and the arterioles. The tissues are deprived of oxygen and nutrients. Plasma leakage and arteriovenous shunting increase tissue pressures and result in thrombosis, ischemia, and necrosis.

31. What is progressive dermal ischemia?

This is an additional insult to potentially viable tissue that is partially mediated by thromboxane. Arachidonic acid breakdown products are released from underlying damaged tissue into the blister fluid. The prostaglandins and thromboxanes produce platelet aggregation and vasoconstriction.

32. What delayed physiologic events occur?

Edema progresses for 2–3 days. As the edema resolves, early necrosis becomes apparent if nonviable tissue is present. Final demarcation often is delayed for more than 60–90 days. Hence the aphorism, "Frostbite in January, amputate in July."

33. What are the symptoms of frostbite?

Sensory deficits are always present, affecting light touch, pain, and temperature perception. Frostnip produces only a transient numbness and tingling. This is not true frostbite, because there is no tissue destruction. In severe cases, patients report a "chunk of wood" sensation and clumsiness.

34. What imaging techniques might help assess frostbite severity?

Routine radiography at presentation and 4–10 weeks postinjury may demonstrate soft-tissue swelling or frank bony destructions. Standard or digital subtraction angiography and Fluorescence microangiography can be used to assess utility of thrombolytic therapy. Technetium (Tc)-99m scintigraphy and single-photon emission computed tomography (SPECT) may predict tissue loss and help monitor efficacy of treatment. Magnetic resonance imaging and magnetic resonance angiography can assess tissue viability and may predict tissue demarcation.

35. What is chilblain (pernio)?

Repetitive exposure to dry cold can induce chilblain (cold sores), especially in young women. Pruritus, erythema, and mild edema may evolve into plaques, blue nodules, and ulcerations. The face and dorsa of the hands and feet are commonly affected.

36. What is trench foot?

Prolonged exposure to wet cold above freezing results in trench foot (immersion foot). Initially, the feet appear edematous, cold, and cyanotic. The subsequent development of vesiculation may mimic frostbite. However, liquefaction gangrene is a more common sequela with trench foot than with frostbite.

37. How should frostbite be classified?

Classification by degrees, as is done with burns, is unnecessary and of poor prognostic value. Superficial or mild frostbite does not result in actual tissue loss; deep or severe frostbite does.

38. What do the various signs of frostbite indicate?

The initial presentation of frostbite can be deceptively benign. Frozen tissues appear yellow, waxy, mottled, or violaceous to white. Favorable signs include normal sensation, warmth, and color after thawing. Early clear bleb formation is more favorable than delayed hemorrhagic blebs. These result from damage to the subdermal vascular plexi. Lack of edema formation also suggests major tissue damage.

39. How should frozen tissues be thawed?

Rapid, complete thawing by immersion in circulating water at 40°C–41°C is ideal. Reestablishment of perfusion is intensely painful, and parenteral narcotics are needed in severe cases. Premature termination of thawing is a common mistake, because an incomplete thaw increases tissue loss. Never use dry heat or allow tissues to refreeze. Rubbing or friction massage may be harmful.

KEY POINTS: COMMON SEQUELAE OF FROSTBITE

1. Paresthesias
2. Hyperhidrosis
3. Thermal misperception
4. Epiphyseal damage
5. Nail deformities

40. What steps should immediately follow thawing?

- Handle tissues gently, and elevate the injured parts to minimize edema formation.
- If cyanosis is still present after thawing, monitor the tissue compartment pressures.
- Consider streptococcal and tetanus prophylaxis.
- Avoid compressive dressings, and use daily whirlpool hydrotherapy.
- Consider phenoxybenzamine (α-blocker that reduces vasoconstriction) in severe cases.
- Whenever possible, defer surgical decisions regarding amputation until clear demarcation is demonstrated.
- Magnetic resonance angiography may predict demarcation earlier than clinical demarcation.

41. How are blisters treated?

Clear blisters may temporarily be left intact or aspirated under sterile conditions. After debridement, apply antibiotic ointment or a specific thromboxane inhibitor, such as topical aloe vera. When coupled with systemic ibuprofen, this strategy can minimize accumulation of arachidonic acid breakdown products. In contrast, hemorrhagic blisters should be left intact to prevent tissue desiccation.

42. Are any ancillary treatment modalities beneficial?

A variety of vasodilatory treatment regimens, including medical and surgical sympathectomies, dextran, heparin, tissue plasminogen activator, and a variety of anti-inflammatory agents do not conclusively increase tissue salvage. In select cases, with <6 hours of warm ischemia time, thrombolytic therapy may decrease the need for amputation.

Website

www.uptodate.com; accessed July 8, 2020.

BIBLIOGRAPHY

Danzl DF, Huecker MR. Accidental hypothermia. In: Auerbach PS, Cushing TA, Harris NS, eds. *Auerbach's Wilderness Medicine: Concepts and Clinical Practice*. 7th ed. Philadelphia, PA: Mosby Elsevier; 2017:135–161.

Dow J, Giesbrecht GG, Danzl DF, et al. Wilderness Medical Society Clinical Practice Guidelines for the out-of-hospital evaluation and treatment of accidental hypothermia: 2019 update. *Wilderness Environ Med.* 2019;30(4S):S47–S69.

Zafren K, Danzl DF. Frostbite and nonfreezing cold injuries. In: Marx JA, Hockberger RS, Walls RM, eds. *Rosen's Emergency Medicine: Concepts and Clinical Practice.*, 9th ed. Philadelphia, PA: Mosby Elsevier; 2017:1735–1742.

CHAPTER 60

HEAT ILLNESS

Christopher B. Colwell, MD

1. **How does the body regulate temperature?**
   The hypothalamus controls thermoregulation. The posterior region functions to conserve heat, while the preoptic region is involved in heat dissipation. Information on body temperature is transmitted from cutaneous and core receptors to the hypothalamus, which then sends signals to regulate increase or decrease blood flow to the periphery (for cooling) or to the core (for warming). This is a critical function, because human body systems operate under a narrow range of temperatures (35°C–38.2°C [95°F–100.8°F]). In addition, the sympathetic system regulates sweat production, which helps to cool the body.

2. **What are the four mechanisms for heat dissipation?**
   1. Conduction: passive transfer of heat from one object (the body) to another through direct contact via a temperature gradient
   2. Convection: heat loss to air or water molecules circulating around the body
   3. Radiation: heat transfer by electromagnetic waves; accounts for 65% of heat loss in cool environments, and is a major source of heat gain in hot climates
   4. Evaporation: conversion from a liquid to a gaseous phase (e.g., sweat)

3. **Which mechanism is the most effective for cooling?**
   Although there is lack of high-quality evidence, there is general consensus that ice water submersion is preferred. However, this may not be feasible in the emergency department, especially in patients who may require other interventions.

4. **How does the relative humidity of the atmosphere affect the normal body mechanisms of cooling?**
   The moisture gradient has to be such that the air is dryer than the body for evaporation to occur. As humidity rises, evaporation becomes less effective. Heat is removed from the body at a slower rate, causing greater heat retention. At humidity levels exceeding 75%, sweat evaporation ceases.

5. **Is there any way to predict heat stress?**
   Wet bulb globe temperature (WBGT) accounts for absolute temperature, radiant heat absorption, and humidity. This and other measurements are used on a larger scale to predict hyperthermia occurrence in a given environment and can inform whether an activity should be attempted or not (e.g., whether a competitive event, such as a marathon, should be postponed). Tests such as the Heat Tolerance Test (HTT) have been used in the military, and have been shown to be valid in predicting likelihood of recurrence of heat illness events.

6. **How does heat harm the body?**
   Heat is directly toxic to cells, causing protein denaturation, as well as breakdown of cellular membranes and nuclei, leading to cell apoptosis and necrosis. Stress from heat causes the release of several inflammatory cytokines, which can precipitate a severe systemic inflammatory response syndrome (SIRS). In addition, heat directly injures the vascular endothelium, causing increased vascular permeability, activation of the coagulation cascade, and disseminated intravascular coagulation (DIC). Heat also may accelerate biochemical reactions, which in turn may cause metabolic abnormalities.

   Temperatures >41.6°C (106.9°F) are considered to be above the critical thermal maximum for humans and can cause cellular damage within hours of exposure. Temperatures >49°C (120°F) can cause immediate cell death and necrosis. Lower temperatures over longer periods can cause the same degree of damage as higher temperatures over shorter periods, and increases in humidity can both worsen the heat index and impair the body's ability to dissipate heat.

7. **Why is this epidemiologically important?**
   According to the Centers for Disease Control and Prevention (CDC), there are on average more than 600 US deaths annually attributed to excessive heat exposure. Heat-related illness is the leading cause of morbidity and mortality among US high school athletes. The rate of heat-related illness appears to be increasing.

8. **Why might someone be unable to dissipate heat appropriately?**
   - Increased energy production (e.g., exercise, delirium, seizures, fever, sympathomimetic drugs, thyroid storm)
   - Damaged conducting system (e.g., atherosclerosis, diabetes)
   - Thermostat malfunction (e.g., hypothalamic injury)

- Pump malfunction/decreased cardiac output (e.g., cardiac disease, β-blockers)
- Low coolant levels/dehydration (e.g., inadequate intake, diarrhea, vomiting, diuretics)
- Decreased ability to sweat (e.g., cystic fibrosis, scleroderma)
- Radiator malfunction (e.g., skin disease, anhidrosis, occlusive clothing, anticholinergic drugs)

9. **What risk factors can lower the threshold for heat stroke?**
   In addition to the previously mentioned factors, age (infants, young children, and the elderly), inability to care for oneself, alcohol abuse, obesity, and failure to acclimatize can limit the ability to respond to changes in temperature.

10. **Why are young children at higher risk for heat illness?**
    They have a higher surface to mass ratio, which increases their absorption of heat. In addition, they have a lower proportion of sweat glands to regulate heat loss.

11. **List the spectrum of heat illnesses and briefly describe them.**
    - Heat edema: transient swelling of hands, feet, and ankles because of dependent pooling of interstitial fluid via peripheral vasodilatation, commonly occurring in individuals who have not acclimatized. Usually resolves spontaneously, and may be amendable to compression stockings and elevation. Diuretics are not useful and should be avoided as they may worsen heat illness.
    - Prickly heat (also known as *heat rash, miliaria rubra,* or *lichen tropicus*): pruritic vesicular rash on an erythematous base caused by excessive sweating and blockage of sweat ducts, primarily occurring on parts of the body covered by tight clothing. Blocked ducts can become infected and can be treated with chlorhexidine cream and small amounts of salicylic acid 1% to localized areas. Routine use of talcum or baby powder should be avoided.
    - Heat cramps (exercise-associated muscle cramps): painful involuntary spasms of large muscle groups occurring after exertion or during exertion. Heat cramps should trigger additional evaluation for volume depletion and other heat-related illness. Treated with oral salt solutions (not salt tablets, which can delay gastric emptying) or intravenous fluids. Stretching the effected muscle, cooling the patient, and rest can help as well.
    - Heat syncope: loss of consciousness caused by a precipitous drop in blood pressure as a result of peripheral vasodilatation shunting blood from the core, characterized by rapid return to normal mental status and functional ability. Worsened by dehydration and prolonged standing.
    - Heat exhaustion: excessive dehydration and electrolyte depletion, leading to fatigue and other symptoms (e.g., nausea, headaches, muscle cramps). Patient may be hypotensive. Core temperatures are usually between 38.3°C and 40°C (100.9°F and 104°F).
    - Heat stroke: a medical emergency caused by neurologic dysfunction and hyperthermia at a temperature >40°C (104°F). Neurologic changes may range from confusion and delirium to seizures and coma.
      Some have advocated for describing heat illness in basically two categories: heat stroke, and everything else that can occur in a hot environment that may or may not be directly caused by heat exposure (e.g., electrolyte repletion and exercise leading to cramps, syncope, and exhaustion).

12. **How are heat-related illnesses treated?**
    Management includes removing the patient from the hot environment into a shady or air-conditioned area and replacing fluid loss with oral electrolyte and salt solutions when feasible. In more severe cases, intravenous fluids may be indicated.
    Immediate cooling should be initiated, especially in the case of heat stroke. Active cooling is most efficiently achieved by removing all of the patient's clothing, wetting the patient, and using a fan to circulate air over the patient (allows for both convective and evaporative heat loss). Cold packs to the groin and axillae may also be applied, but have limited effect. Immersion in ice water baths is a very effective way of cooling patients (takes advantage of water's 25 times greater conduction rate than air); however, this is not practical in some settings. Cooling blankets are of limited use and should not replace evaporative cooling methods. Invasive cooling techniques, such as iced gastric, peritoneal, or rectal lavage and cardiopulmonary bypass, do not have a clear advantage over evaporative cooling and can cause delays in initiating treatment.
    Core temperature should be monitored (rectal or Foley thermometry is considered the gold standard). Free water deficits should be replaced slowly as overcorrection of hypernatremia can lead to cerebral edema in rare instances.

13. **Tell me more about heat exhaustion.**
    Heat exhaustion is caused by either water or salt depletion, or both. With water depletion, there is progressive dehydration resulting from inadequate water consumption when working in a hot environment (termed *voluntary dehydration,* because individuals commonly only replace two-thirds of their water loss). This can progress to heat stroke. In the salt depletion form, excessive sweating is replaced by free water, which leads to hyponatremia and hypochloremia with near-normal body temperature.
    Regardless of the primary cause, symptoms can be variable, and include fatigue, weakness, headache, impaired judgment, vertigo, nausea/vomiting, and muscle cramps (if salt depletion). Orthostatic dizziness and syncope is possible, and sweating may be profuse. Heart rate may be increased, but can be normal as well.

Body temperature will be modestly elevated (<40°C [104°F]) or may be normal. Signs of major central nervous system (CNS) dysfunction such as sustained altered mental status or seizures indicate heat stroke.

14. Why is heat stroke so bad?

Heat stroke is a life-threatening medical emergency characterized by an elevated core body temperature (>40°C [104°F]), and CNS dysfunction with varying degrees of shock and multi-organ collapse. Skin is hot. The patient may or may not be sweating. Symptoms include muscle twitching, confusion, drowsiness, disorientation, ataxia, anxiety, psychosis, seizures, and coma. Ataxia and mild confusion are often earlier signs of heat stroke, in part because the cerebellum is more sensitive to heat. In addition, vasoconstriction of the renal and splanchnic circulation can lead to acute renal failure, hepatic damage, and intestinal ischemia. SIRS or DIC may develop, resulting from hepatic injury–mediated coagulopathy, activation of clotting factors, thrombocytopenia, fibrinolysis, and direct thermal injury of the vascular endothelium

15. Describe the two types of heat stroke.

Classic heat stroke (CHS) occurs during periods of sustained high ambient temperatures and humidity, and particularly affects individuals who are in poorly ventilated areas (no air-conditioning). People who are particularly vulnerable to this condition include those of low socioeconomic status, the elderly, infants, alcoholics, and patients with chronic medical conditions or taking medications that alter the ability to adapt to the hot environment. Anhidrosis is common, and laboratory abnormalities are generally mild.

Exertional heat stroke (EHS) is observed in active, young, healthy individuals (such as athletes and military recruits) whose normal adaptive responses to a hot climate are overwhelmed by endogenous heat production (strenuous activity). Sweating is often preserved. Lactic acidosis, rhabdomyolysis, and renal failure is common, as is hypoglycemia resulting from depleted glycogen stores and increased glucose metabolism.

16. How do I treat a patient with heat stroke?

After addressing the airway, breathing, and circulation (ABCs), immediate and rapid cooling should be initiated with a goal temperature <38.9°C (102°F) within 30 minutes of presentation to minimize organ damage. Cooling should not be delayed to determine exact temperature, although core temperature should be monitored during treatment. Unlike warming hypothermic patients, who can be harmed when warmed too rapidly, patients with heat stroke should be cooled as quickly as possible. Cold water immersion has been shown to be effective for patients with EHS. Evaporative cooling is effective for both CHS and EHS.

Resuscitation with intravenous fluids is necessary for concomitant dehydration, although cooling efforts can increase blood pressure via peripheral vasoconstriction. Electrolyte repletion should be appropriately tailored to specific laboratory derangements. Hemodynamics and urine output should help guide resuscitation efforts. Over-resuscitation should be avoided, because it may exacerbate pulmonary edema.

Rhabdomyolysis is typically treated with fluid resuscitation but may warrant urinary alkalinization. In oliguric patients, mannitol should be avoided, and hemodialysis should be considered in severe cases.

Tachyarrhythmias that may develop because of heat stroke commonly resolve with cooling, and electrical cardioversion should be avoided if possible because it may worsen myocardial damage.

17. Are any medications indicated in the treatment of heat stroke, and are there any that should be avoided?

As mentioned, evaporative cooling and supportive care is paramount. Antipyretic agents such as acetaminophen or salicylic acid has not been shown to be beneficial, and may cause harm by worsening hepatic damage (acetaminophen) or worsening hyperthermia and coagulopathy (salicylates). α-Adrenergic agents, such as norepinephrine, should be avoided, because they can worsen vasoconstriction and decrease cutaneous heat exchange (therefore compromising cooling treatment). Atropine and other anticholinergics that inhibit sweating should also be avoided.

18. What laboratory abnormalities are seen in patients with heat illness?

Patients with severe heat exhaustion and heat stroke may have evidence of acute renal failure (elevated creatinine), hemoconcentration (elevated hemoglobin/hematocrit), rhabdomyolysis (elevated creatinine kinase), hypernatremia or hyponatremia (depending on free water intake), hyperkalemia or hypokalemia, leukocytosis, and DIC (prolonged prothrombin time and partial thromboplastin time, elevated D-dimer). Liver transaminases may be in the tens of thousands with heat stroke, but may take more than 24 hours to rise.

19. What is the differential diagnosis of heat stroke?

- Infection
  - Generalized (e.g., sepsis, malaria, typhoid, tetanus)
  - CNS (e.g., encephalitis, meningitis, brain abscess)
- Drugs/toxins
  - Intoxication (e.g., phencyclidine, amphetamines, cocaine, anticholinergics, salicylate, diuretics, antipsychotics phenothiazines)
  - Withdrawal (e.g., ethanol)
  - Serotonin syndrome
  - Neuroleptic malignant syndrome

- Malignant hyperthermia
- Drug-induced fever
- Endocrine derangements
  - Thyroid storm, pheochromocytoma
- Neurologic conditions
  - Status epilepticus, cerebral hemorrhage
- Blood clots
  - Deep vein thrombosis, pulmonary embolism, deep-seated hematomas

20. **What is the mortality rate associated with heat stroke?**
The mortality rate varies because of a number of factors, such as age, underlying comorbidities, and, most important, the degree and duration of hyperthermia; it can range from 20% to 60%. Poor prognostic indicators include advanced age, persistent hypotension requiring vasopressor therapy, and respiratory failure requiring intubation.

21. **How do I prevent heat-related illness?**
Maximize heat loss with lightweight, loose-fitting clothing (which allows for enhanced convection and evaporation), and ensure adequate hydration and electrolyte repletion before and during any strenuous activity in a hot environment. Decrease heat stress by limiting exertion as much as possible in extreme heat. Identify vulnerable populations during heat waves in your community and advocate for developing plans to address their needs.

22. **What about acclimatization?**
Acclimatization is the physiologic adaptation a normal person develops that results from repeated exposure to heat stress, which allows for earlier onset of sweating (at a lower core temperature), increased sweat volume, and decreased electrolyte concentration of sweat. Additionally, heart rate generally lowers, and stroke volume becomes more robust as the cardiovascular system adapts to the hot environment. The process can take 1 week or more, and involves limiting exertional activity during that period.

KEY POINTS: HEAT ILLNESS

1. Heat stroke is life threatening and is defined by a temperature $>40°C$ ($104°F$) and altered mental status. Heat stroke victims may or may not be sweating.
2. Cooling should be initiated immediately upon suspicion of heat stroke. You cannot cool a patient too quickly.
3. Evaporative cooling is quick, safe, and effective.
4. Antipyretics are not effective for environmental hyperthermia.

BIBLIOGRAPHY

Atha WF. Heat-related illness. *Emerg Med Clin North Am.* 2013;31:1097–1108.
Gaudio FG, Grissom CK. Cooling methods in heat stroke. *J Emerg Med.* 2016;50(4):607–616.
Hajat S, O'Conner M, Kosatsky T. Health effects of hot weather: from awareness of risk factors to effective health protection. *Lancet.* 2010;375:856–863.
Joslin J, Mularella J, Worthing R. Heat-related illness: time to update our lexicon. *Wilderness Environ Med.* 2014;25:249–251.
Lipman GS, Eifling KP, Ellis MA, et al. Wilderness Medical Society practice guidelines for the prevention and treatment of heat-related illness. *Wilderness Environ Med.* 2013;24:351–361.
O'Brien KK, Leon LR, Kenefick RW, et al. Clinical management of heat-related illnesses. In: Auerbach PS, Cushing TA, Harris NS, eds. *Auerbach's Wilderness Medicine.* 7th ed. Philadelphia, PA: Mosby Elsevier; 2017:267–274.
Patz JA, Frumkin H, Holloway T, et al. Climate change – challenges and opportunities for global health. *JAMA.* 2014;312:1565–1580.
Schermann H, Heled Y, Fleischmann C, et al. The validity of the heat tolerance test in prediction of recurrent exertional heat illness events. *J Sci Med Sport.* 2018;21(6):549–552.

CHAPTER 61

ALTITUDE ILLNESS AND DYSBARISMS

Hillary E. Davis, MD, PhD and Chris Davis, MD

1. **What are three disease states that comprise high-altitude illness?**
   1. Acute mountain sickness (AMS)
   2. High-altitude pulmonary edema (HAPE)
   3. High-altitude cerebral edema (HACE)
      HACE and HAPE are much less common than AMS, but are potentially fatal.

2. **How is AMS defined?**
   AMS is most often described as feeling similar to a "hangover," but is formally defined as the presence of a headache in the setting of recent ascent to high altitude, along with additional symptoms described by the Lake Louise Acute Mountain Sickness Score. The 2018 updated Lake Louise criteria are:
   - Headache (which *must* be present)
   - Gastrointestinal symptoms
   - Fatigue or weakness
   - Dizziness/light-headedness

3. **How quickly do symptoms of AMS develop, and what is the minimum elevation at which AMS occurs?**
   Usually, symptoms begin within 6–12 hours of ascent. AMS most often occurs at elevations greater than 2500 meters (m) (8200 feet [ft]), but has been documented in susceptible individuals to as low as 1500 m (4900 ft).

4. **How do I prevent AMS?**
   Gradual ascent, pre-acclimatization, acetazolamide, dexamethasone, and ibuprofen have all demonstrated prophylactic benefits. In general, preventive strategies are based on ascent profile, previous susceptibility to high-altitude illness, patient preference, and availability of resources. Gradual ascent is defined as no more than 500 m/day (1600 ft/day) of sleeping altitude when above 2500 m (8200 ft), along with an additional rest day every 3–4 days. The recommended prophylactic adult dose for acetazolamide is 125 mg twice daily. Dexamethasone is effective for prophylaxis, but is not typically recommended due to the associated risks of this drug. These include adrenal insufficiency, steroid psychosis, and ulcers. The prophylactic dose is 2 mg every 6 hours or 4 mg every 12 hours. Larger doses (4 mg every 6 hours) can be considered in high-risk situations during which rapid rise to elevation is expected, such as in military excursions or rescue missions.

KEY POINTS: PREVENTION OF AMS OR HACE

1. Acclimatization
2. Slow ascent
3. Acetazolamide

5. **How do I treat AMS?**
   AMS is usually a self-limited disease that resolves with acclimatization over a period of 1–2 days as long as there is no further ascent. All high-altitude illnesses, including AMS, can be treated with oxygen and descent. However, oxygen is not always available, and descent is not always logistically feasible or always necessary. For mild AMS, avoiding further ascent and taking over-the-counter analgesics such as ibuprofen is a reasonable approach. Other treatment options include the use of acetazolamide, dexamethasone, or simulated descent with portable hyperbaric chambers. The adult treatment dose of acetazolamide is 125 mg twice daily. Dexamethasone is 8 mg followed by 4 mg every 6 hours (intramuscular [IM], intravenous [IV], or oral [PO]).

6. **What are risk factors for AMS?**
   Risk factors for the development of AMS are increased rate of ascent, altitude reached (especially the sleeping altitude), and an individual's genetic susceptibility. The strongest independent risk factor for developing AMS is a history of AMS during previous ascents. Alcohol should be avoided as it is a respiratory depressant. Contrary to popular belief, aggressive hydration does not prevent AMS, but it does prevent dehydration, which has a similar but confounding symptom profile.

7. What is HACE?

HACE is widely viewed as the end stage of a disease spectrum that starts with AMS. The defining symptoms of HACE are ataxia or altered mental status. HACE may progress to coma and death, typically through brain herniation. Magnetic resonance imaging (MRI) findings in patients with HACE include vasogenic edema and microhemorrhages in the corpus callosum, a thick band of nerve fibers that connects the right and left halves of the brain. The distribution of microhemorrhages in HACE differs from other diseases like vasculitis. However, HACE is a clinical diagnosis and MRI is rarely helpful in the acute management of HACE patients.

8. When does HACE occur?

The onset of HACE usually occurs 2–5 days after arrival at elevation.

9. What is the treatment for HACE?

HACE is a life-threatening medical emergency requiring immediate descent. HACE victims should be supervised during descent. Other treatments include supplemental oxygen and dexamethasone. If descent is not possible, a portable, hyperbaric chambers should be used as a stabilizing measure until descent is possible. Acetazolamide and diuretics are not indicated for the treatment of HACE.

KEY POINT: BEST TREATMENT FOR HACE

1. Immediate descent!

10. Is there anything that will prevent HACE?

Because HACE is thought to be the end point on the spectrum of altitude illness, prevention strategies for HACE are the same as those for AMS. Those that have experienced HACE during prior trips to elevation are more likely to develop it again and should carefully consider the risk of a repeat high-altitude exposure. Previous victims of HACE should seek the help of a qualified physician should a future ascent be necessary

11. What is HAPE?

HAPE is two of the following symptoms in the setting of a recent ascent, typically >2500 m (8200 ft):
- Dyspnea at rest
- Cough
- Weakness or decreased exercise tolerance
- Chest tightness or congestion *and* two of the following signs:
  - Crackles or wheezing in at least one lung field
  - Central cyanosis
  - Tachypnea
  - Tachycardia

HAPE is thought to be noncardiogenic pulmonary edema resulting from an exaggerated pulmonary hypertension leading to failure of the alveolar-capillary barrier. Cold stress and heavy exertion also increase pulmonary arterial pressure, which may further exacerbate the resulting pulmonary edema.

12. When does HAPE occur?

Classically, HAPE occurs on the second night after arrival to a new altitude above 2500 m (8200 ft). The development of HAPE *may or may not* be preceded by AMS.

13. How do I prevent HAPE?

The best prevention strategy to avoid HAPE is slow ascent. Pharmacologic strategies include nifedipine (30 mg extended release, administered twice daily), tadalafil (10 mg twice daily), and dexamethasone. Roles for salmeterol and acetazolamide in HAPE prevention remain unclear.

14. How do I treat HAPE?

Similar to HACE, the most important treatment for HAPE is immediate descent or oxygen. If descent is not possible, supplemental oxygen should be initiated immediately to maintain oxygen saturations above 90%. If oxygen is readily available, and the patient's work of breathing is minimal, descent may not be necessary. Other adjuncts include portable hyperbaric chambers and nifedipine. Tadalafil can be considered if nifedipine is not available. Positive pressure ventilation such as continuous positive airway pressure (CPAP) has demonstrated a limited benefit as well. The use of acetazolamide, salmeterol, and diuretics are not currently indicated for the management of HAPE.

15. What findings on imaging can be expected in HAPE?

Chest x-rays may demonstrate patchy alveolar infiltrates with a normal-sized mediastinum and heart. Lung ultrasounds have evidence of B-lines consistent with pulmonary edema.

16. **Will I ever see HAPE, HACE, or AMS at the same time?**
    HACE is thought to be end-stage AMS, so you will not see both at the same time. HACE often occurs in association with HAPE, but you can see HAPE without any signs of AMS or HACE.

17. **Which form of altitude illness is most common, and which is most deadly?**
    The incidence of altitude illnesses depends on the altitude achieved in the group studied.
    - AMS: incidence, 15%–70% (most common); mortality rate, 0%
    - HACE: incidence, 1%–2%; mortality rate unknown because of usually coexistent HAPE
    - HAPE: incidence, 1%–15%; mortality rate, as high as 50% when left untreated

18. **What is dysbarism?**
    Dysbarism refers to pressure-related diseases, but is classically limited to diseases resulting from SCUBA diving injuries. This category includes diseases specifically related to pressure changes and their physical effects (e.g., middle ear barotrauma [MEBT], pneumothorax, arterial gas embolism [AGE], pneumomediastinum, and barosinusitis), as well as disease related to bubble formation (e.g., pulmonary decompression sickness [DCS], spinal decompression sickness, and the bends).

19. **How much pressure does a diver experience at 10 m (33 ft) underwater?**
    Each 10 m (33 ft) is equivalent to 1 atm. Because sea level is equivalent to 1 atm, 10 m (33 ft) underwater is 2 atm, which is equal to 29.4 psi or 1520 mmHg. Pressure underwater is directly proportional to depth. Hence, 20 m (66 ft) is equivalent to 3 atm.

20. **What is DCS?**
    Decompression sickness is a disorder that occurs when there is supersaturation of inert gases in the blood and tissues that produces free gas formation upon ascent. There are two types: type 1 or "simple DCS" affects the skin, musculoskeletal system, or lymphatic systems, while type 2 or "serious DCS" typically involves the pulmonary or neurologic systems. Of note, AGE is generally considered a separate disorder, the result of injection of air into the circulation.

21. **What are the bends?**
    The bends, also known as *caisson disease* (named after caisson workers, who work in pressurized underwater chambers), is one of the more common forms of dysbarism and is classified as a type 1 DCS. It occurs when nitrogen comes out of solution (during ascent) and forms bubbles in tissues, causing muscle and joint pain. The most common location to experience pain is in the shoulder.

22. **When would I see someone with the bends?**
    People experience the bends when they ascend too rapidly from SCUBA diving. Although the bends can occur immediately after ascent, over half of cases will occur after 1 hour of dive completion.

23. **Why would nitrogen precipitate in tissues?**
    According to Boyle's law of gases, pressure is inversely proportional to volume. Furthermore, Henry's law states that the amount of gas in solution is directly proportional to the partial pressure of that gas. Thus with increased pressure underwater, the volume of gas decreases, and the amount of gas in solution (dissolved) increases. However, with rapid ascent, gas will expand and come out of solution, resulting in increased gas bubble size and possible precipitation in tissues. With a slow ascent, the gradual increase in bubble size and slow change in amount of gas in solution allow the gases to remain dissolved in circulating blood and be expelled through the respiratory system.

24. **Why should divers not immediately fly on aircraft?**
    Time is required to achieve equilibrium between inert gases in tissues and atmospheric pressure. Divers going immediately to altitude may not have time to achieve this equilibrium. Despite following safe ascent procedures during their dives, divers may put themselves at risk for decompression illness, as decreased atmospheric pressures during flight will result in more free gas formation. The Divers Alert Network (DAN) recommends at least 12 hours between diving and flying.

25. **What is nitrogen narcosis?**
    The amount of each gas that goes into solution in the blood increases with increased pressure (or increased depth, because increased depth causes increased pressure). With nitrogen being the largest component of air, a large amount of nitrogen goes into solution in the blood, ever increasing with increasing pressure. This high concentration of nitrogen causes an anesthetic-like effect that causes lack of motor control and inappropriate behavior, and eventually causes unconsciousness. Nitrogen narcosis usually is seen at depths of 100 ft (4 atm or 33 ft) or more. To avoid nitrogen narcosis, alternative inhaled gas mixtures containing decreased nitrogen are recommended for dives greater than 100 ft (33 ft), such as trimix or heliox.

26. **What is MEBT?**
    MEBT occurs when the pressure of the water on the tympanic membrane during descent is not equalized by the eustachian tube. Usually, a diver will mechanically increase the pressure in his or her middle ear by forcing air

through the eustachian tube to equilibrate the pressure across the tympanic membrane using either a Valsalva or Frenzel maneuver. If this is unsuccessful, the middle ear pressure becomes more negative relative to the ambient pressure. Subsequently, the tympanic membrane is displaced inward, causing pain, and rupture may follow. Risk factors for MEBT include anatomic variation, local edema from allergies or upper respiratory infection, or previous history of eustachian tube dysfunction.

27. How could a diver get a pneumothorax with ascent?
If a diver held his or her breath to go underwater to 10 m (33 ft, or 2 atm), the volume in the lungs would decrease to half the prior volume (1 atm $\times$ normal lung volume = 2 atm $\times$ 1/2 normal lung volume). If upon ascent, the diver did not exhale, the lung volume would increase back to its previous volume, resulting in a drastically increased intrapulmonary pressure. This can lead to rupture of the alveoli, which causes air to enter the mediastinum and the pleural space, producing a pneumothorax.

28. What is AGE?
This condition occurs when expanding gas ruptures an alveolus and the gas is forced into the pulmonary vasculature. The gas is then distributed through the arterial system, which can cause loss of consciousness, apnea, and cardiac arrest. It is the second most common cause of diving-related deaths. Divers with patent foramen ovales are at increased risk given increased exposure to systemic circulation. Closure of the defect significantly decreases risk of AGE. This condition should be suspected in any diver who surfaces and immediately experiences syncope.

29. What about the movies that show people bleeding from their eyes when diving? Does that really happen?
With typical diving masks, an artificial air space is created in front of the eyes. When a diver descends, this air space is subject to the same gas laws as the diver, with the volume of air in the mask decreased by one-half at 1 atm underwater (effectively 2 atm), one-third at an effective 3 atm, and so forth. This pressure change creates a vacuum effect in the mask, which can cause petechial hemorrhage, subconjunctival hemorrhage, and even optic nerve damage, termed *facial barotrauma*. The usual way divers avoid this problem is by wearing a mask that encompasses their nose and then equalizing the pressure by blowing air into their mask.

30. What are the chokes?
The *chokes* is the common term for pulmonary DCS. Pulmonary DCS manifests as cough, shortness of breath, and chest pain resulting from massive venous gas embolism. In addition to mechanically obstructing blood flow through the pulmonary vasculature, bubbles may directly contact the vascular endothelium and activate the inflammatory cascade, which can result in pulmonary edema and acute respiratory distress syndrome (ARDS). Treatment involves high-flow oxygen, support of respiration and circulation, and evacuation to a facility with a hyperbaric chamber.

31. What are the skinny bends?
Skinny bends refers to cutaneous DCS, which is the appearance of a diffuse, reticulated, blotchy rash caused by endothelial damage from bubbles, resulting in blood extravasation. It can also refer to a syndrome of cutaneous itching that only appears in the artificial environment of a hyperbaric chamber.

32. What is spinal cord DCS?
Spinal cord DCS is a syndrome characterized by ascending parestheslas and paralysis, resulting from venous outflow obstruction by venous gas emboli in the epidural plexus of the spinal cord.

33. Is there a CNS form of DCS?
Yes, it commonly presents with headache, blurred vision, dysarthria, diplopia, and inappropriate behavior. The exact mechanism of CNS DCS is poorly characterized.

34. How do I tell the difference between CNS DCS and AGE?
One main point is that loss of consciousness is uncommon with CNS DCS. However, because both are treated the same way, there is little utility in acutely distinguishing between the two.

35. How are dysbarisms treated?
In general, DCS and AGE should be treated with immediate recompression in a hyperbaric oxygen chamber. The longer treatment is delayed, the higher the morbidity and mortality. Until a hyperbaric chamber can be obtained, the patient should be placed on a nonrebreather oxygen mask. Acute pressure-related injuries (e.g., pneumothorax, pneumomediastinum) should be treated with standard therapy, whereas tympanic membrane rupture and inner ear disturbances should be referred to an otolaryngologist. Victims of facial barotrauma should be assessed for more serious injuries, but there usually is no further treatment needed.

36. Is there anything that makes a particular person susceptible to DCS?
Although controversial, there are several studies that have demonstrated increased age and decreased physical fitness as potential risk factors. Other potential risks factors include dehydration, heavy exertion while diving, • hypothermia, hyperthermia, and inexperience.

37. **Who should not dive?**

Individuals who experience seizures or those with insulin-dependent diabetes mellitus are at increased risk for sudden underwater unconsciousness. It is generally recommended that a diving candidate be free of seizures for 4 years prior to attempting to SCUBA dive. Those with diabetes may require specialized training in managing insulin in underwater environments. There has been no demonstrated incidence of increased pulmonary barotrauma in asthmatics. However, a diagnosis of chronic obstructive pulmonary disease (COPD) is generally thought to be associated with significant diving-associated morbidity.

38. **Is there anything that I can do to reduce my risk of DCS?**

Slow ascent driven by an accurate dive table.

BIBLIOGRAPHY

Bartsch P, Swenson ER. Acute high-altitude illnesses. *N Engl J Med.* 2013;368:2294–2302.

Bennet MH, Lehm JP, Mitchell SJ, et al. Recompression and adjunctive therapy for decompression illness. *Cochrane Database Syst Rev.* 2012;(5):CD005277.

Bove A. Diving medicine. *Am J Respir Crit Care Med.* 2014;189:1479–1486.

Hackett PH, Luks AM, Lawley JS, et al. High-altitude medicine and pathophysiology. In: *Auerbach's Wilderness Medicine.* 7th ed. Philadelphia, PA: Elsevier; 2017.

Lechner M, Sutton L, Fishman JM, et al. Otorhinolaryngology and diving – part 1: otorhinolaryngological hazards related to compressed gas scuba diving, a review. *JAMA Otolaryngol Head Neck Surg.* 2018;144:252–258.

Luks AM, McIntosh SE, Grissom CK, et al. Wilderness Medical Society practice guidelines for the prevention and treatment of acute altitude illness: 2014 update. *Wilderness Environ Med.* 2014;25:S4–S14.

Richalet JP, Larmignat P, Poitrine E, et al. Physiological risk factors of severe high altitude illness: a prospective cohort study. *Am J Respir Crit Care Med.* 2012;185:192–198.

Roach RC, Hackett PH, Oelz O, et al. The 2018 Lake Louise Acute Mountain Sickness score. *High Alt Med Biol.* 2018;19:4–6.

Van Hosen KB, Lang MA. Diving medicine. In: *Auerbach's Wilderness Medicine.* 7th ed. Philadelphia, PA: Elsevier; 2017.

EVALUATION OF FEVER IN CHILDREN YOUNGER THAN AGE THREE

Kristine Knuti Rodrigues, MD, MPH and Genie E. Roosevelt, MD, MPH

CHAPTER 62

1. **What is fever?**
   Fever is generally defined as a rectal temperature of 38°C (100.4°F). Whenever possible, have the parents tell you the measured temperature, as some may think temperatures below this threshold are fevers (e.g., 99.2°F).

2. **How should temperature be measured in infants and young children?**
   For infants from birth up to 3 months of age, the most reasonable and accurate method is the rectal temperature. Oral temperatures are generally the preferred method for children who are old enough to cooperate. Tympanic and temporal artery temperatures are less accurate than rectal thermometers; consider confirming with rectal temperature when the exact temperature will change clinical decision making. Axillary temperatures are unreliable and should not be used despite the ease with which they may be obtained.

3. **Is it safe to measure temperatures rectally?**
   Many parents, and even health care providers, are anxious about doing this. British studies investigating safety and efficacy demonstrate an extremely low risk of injury.

4. **What is a serious bacterial infection (SBI)?**
   The most common types of SBIs in children include:
   - urinary tract infection (UTI)
   - bacteremia
   - pneumonia (established by a focal infiltrate on chest radiograph)
   - bacterial meningitis

5. **Does it matter how much fever the child has?**
   Hyperpyrexia (temperature of 40.5°C [104.9°F]) has been associated with higher rates of SBI (4%) in patients 3–36 months of age. However, any child who appears toxic should be evaluated for SBI regardless of the temperature.

6. **What is meant by appearing toxic?**
   Children who appear toxic may be pale, lethargic, or limp. They may show evidence of poor perfusion (such as cyanosis or peripheral vasoconstriction with mottling), or changes in respiratory drive, such as tachypnea or shallow breathing. They may fail to interact with their environment (as evidenced by poor or absent eye contact, poor feeding, or failure to respond to caregivers or objects in their view). These children are generally ill-appearing, often requiring intravenous (IV) fluid administration and immediate resuscitation.

KEY POINTS: SIGNS OF TOXICITY

1. Lethargy
2. Cyanosis
3. Tachypnea
4. Poor tone
5. Failure to respond to caregivers

7. **Which antipyretics work best for children?**
   Studies show that ibuprofen (10 mg/kg; suspension 100 mg/5 mL) and acetaminophen (15 mg/kg; suspension 160 mg/5 mL) have similar efficacy. Because household measuring spoons measure volume inaccurately, parents should be encouraged to use syringes for medication dosing. Ibuprofen is not recommended for children <6 months of age.
   Note: Most children's elixirs contain half the amount of an adult tablet per 5 mL. For example, an adult tablet of ibuprofen contains 200 mg, whereas the children's elixir contains 100 mg/5 mL.

8. **What is the most common cause of antipyretic failure?**
   Underdosing. Parents may not know the child's weight, fail to calculate an appropriate dosage, or be unfamiliar with units of measure (such as *mL*). It is also common for parents to believe that antipyretics should cure the fever, and a parent may say, "I gave her the medicine and it helped for a while, but the fever just came right back." Parental education and provision of an oral syringe are important aspects of caring for pediatric patients with fever.

9. **What is wrong with baby aspirin?**
   Aspirin administration to children with certain viral infections (especially varicella and influenza) has been associated with Reye syndrome (encephalopathy and acute liver failure). This syndrome, although very rare, carries a high mortality rate (20%–40%). Although some pediatric conditions (such as juvenile rheumatoid arthritis and Kawasaki disease) are treated with aspirin, its use in children with fever of unclear etiology should be strictly avoided.

10. **Is there any good reason not to treat a fever?**
    If children are active, playful, and drinking fluids well, there is no reason to treat their fever; fever by itself is not harmful. That said, children with fever often feel ill, drink fluids poorly, and worry their caregivers, and the quickest way to make them feel better is to bring the fever down.

11. **What are febrile seizures?**
    See Chapter 63.

12. **How should tiny babies with fever be evaluated?**
    Febrile infants with a temperature of ≥38°C (100.4°F) who are less than 1 month of age should receive a complete sepsis evaluation.
    - Urinalysis and culture (by catheterization or suprapubic aspiration)
    - Complete blood count with differential and blood culture
    - Lumbar puncture (LP)
    - Chest radiograph (only with respiratory symptoms)
    - Stool analysis for white blood cell (WBC) count and culture (if there is a history of diarrhea)
        Infants should receive IV antibiotics and be admitted to the hospital.
      Note: Age cut-offs for fever evaluation are based on gestational age, not age since birth. This means that a premature infant of 32 weeks' gestation who was born 6 weeks ago is still considered to be younger than 1 month.

13. **What happens after the magic 1-month mark?**
    For infants 1–3 months of age with a fever without a source, risk stratification is recommended. See the algorithm in Fig. 62.1.

14. **What about older infants and young children?**
    For children 3–36 months with a fever without a source, follow the algorithm in Fig. 62.2 (note different temperature cut-off for this older age group).

15. **How do I decide when to do an LP in older babies and young children?**
    A LP should be performed in any child who appears toxic or has signs of meningitis. Be aware that many of the classic signs of meningitis (e.g., Brudzinski sign, Kernig sign, neck stiffness, or bulging fontanelle) are commonly absent and unreliable in young infants and children.

16. **What if the child has a fever source or one is found during the workup?**
    It depends on the source and the age group. A viral source, such as influenza, or recent immunizations (within the last 72 hours) make the risk of bacteremia and meningitis lower. If an identified source completely explains the clinical presentation, no further workup is required. If not, complete the evaluation as previously described. Be aware that UTIs, and rarely bacteremia, may coexist with viral infections such as bronchiolitis and gastroenteritis.

17. **Must I always follow the guidelines, or is there room for clinical judgment in there somewhere?**
    A study of more than 3000 febrile infants seen by almost 600 pediatricians throughout the United States demonstrated that selective testing by experienced clinicians in office-based practice was as effective in identifying and treating SBI as rigid adherence to clinical guidelines. Their findings suggest that if close follow-up monitoring is feasible, experienced clinicians may use clinical judgment in select cases rather than published recommendations in their management strategy of febrile infants. Unfortunately, the emergency department physician may not have the luxury of this close follow-up care.

18. **What if the child looks great; can he or she go home?**
    Children who do not appear toxic, are more than 1 month of age, and meet low-risk criteria may be discharged home with return precautions and closely monitored follow-up care. This decision presumes a child has a reliable caregiver, a tenable social situation, and reasonable access to transportation.

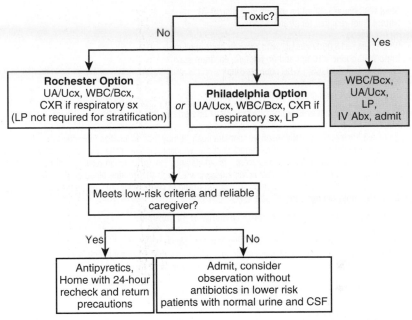

Fig. 62.1 Algorithm for infants 1–3 months of age. *Abx,* Antibiotics; *Bcx,* blood culture; *CSF,* cerebrospinal fluid; *CXR,* chest x-ray; *IV,* intravenous; *LP,* lumbar puncture; *sx,* symptoms; *T,* temperature; *UA,* urinalysis; *Ucx,* urine culture; *WBC,* white blood cell count.

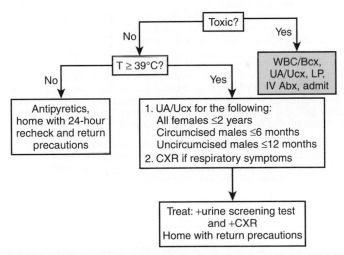

Fig. 62.2 Algorithm for children 3–36 months of age. *Abx,* Antibiotics; *Bcx,* blood culture; *CSF,* cerebrospinal fluid; *CXR,* chest radiograph; *IV,* intravenous; *LP,* lumbar puncture; *sx,* symptoms; *T,* temperature; *UA,* urinalysis; *Ucx,* urine culture; *WBC,* white blood cell count.

19. What are low-risk criteria?
The two sets of low-risk criteria used most often are the Rochester and Philadelphia criteria in infants 1–2 months of age. Both presume the child is previously healthy and appears well at the time of evaluation. If a patient meets low-risk stratification criteria, discharge without antibiotics is recommended with a 24-hour follow-up examination.
Rochester criteria
- WBC between 5000 and 15,000 cells/µL
- Urine WBC count <10/high-power field (hpf)

- Stool WBC count <5/hpf (in infants with diarrhea)
- **Note:** LP not required for stratification

Philadelphia criteria
- WBC count <15,000 cells/μL, with band-to-neutrophil ratio <0.2
- Urine WBC count <10/hpf and no bacteria on Gram stain
- Cerebrospinal fluid (CSF) WBC count <8/hpf
- Negative CSF Gram stain
- Stool and chest radiograph negative (if obtained)

20. **What is the risk of occult bacteremia (presence of bacteria in the blood stream with no apparent focus of infection)?**

Although occult bacteremia usually resolves spontaneously, it may lead to localized infections, such as meningitis, pneumonia, or osteomyelitis. Evidence gathered since the widespread use of the pneumococcal vaccine (13 valent) suggests that the current rate of bacteremia is significantly less than 1% in well-appearing febrile children between the ages of 3 months and 3 years. This risk is low enough that routine blood cultures are no longer recommended for children older than 3 months. The current ratio of contaminant to true positive blood culture is 8:1 in the 3- to 36-month-old age range.

21. **What antibiotic should be used for empiric coverage of bacteremia?**

Under 28 days old
- Cefotaxime (substitute ceftazidime 50 mg/kg IV if unavailable) 50 mg/kg IV (may consider substituting with gentamicin 2.5 mg/kg IV in first week of life to treat group B streptococcal infection or ceftriaxone 50 mg/kg IV if >14 days, >37 weeks corrected gestational age, no hyperbilirubinemia, and no IV calcium administration) plus
- Ampicillin 50 mg/kg IV (to cover for *Listeria*)

Age 28 days to 3 months
- Ceftriaxone 50 mg/kg IV

Age 3–36 months
- Ceftriaxone 50 mg/kg IV or intramuscular (IM; 24-hour dosing)

22. **Which infants should receive acyclovir?**

Risk factors for neonatal herpes simplex virus (HSV) infection include the following:
- Maternal HSV infection at delivery (although two thirds are asymptomatic)
- Maternal history of HSV or other sexually transmitted diseases
- Vesicular rash
- Seizures
- CSF pleocytosis (WBC count typically 20–100 cells/mm^3) with a negative CSF Gram stain

Patients are usually less than 22 days of age. Patients with risk factors should be given acyclovir pending an HSV polymerase chain reaction (PCR) test from the CSF. Clinical judgment should be used in the decision to discontinue acyclovir, given that the initial PCR may be a false negative. The dosage is 20 mg/kg IV every 8 hours (dosage and schedule adjusted for gestational age and renal impairment).

23. **What about children with fever and rapidly progressive petechial rash?**

This is disseminated meningococcemia until proven otherwise. Patients with these types of infection may progress very rapidly. The LP may be deferred until the patient is stable and should not delay antibiotic administration. Dosages below ensure coverage for invasive, resistant pneumococcal meningitis, which also may cause purpura fulminans.
- Ceftriaxone 50 mg/kg IV
- Vancomycin 15 mg/kg IV

Website

Pediatric febrile seizures: http://emedicine.medscape.com/article/1176205-overview; accessed February 1, 2019.

BIBLIOGRAPHY

Krief WI, Levine DA, Platt SL, et al. Influenza virus infection and the risk of serious bacterial infections in young febrile infants. *Pediatrics.* 2009;124:30–39.

Niven DJ, Gaudet JE, Laupland KB, et al. Accuracy of peripheral thermometers for estimating temperature: a system review and meta-analysis, *Ann Intern Med.* 2015;163:768–777.

Odinaka KK, Edelu BO, Nwolisa CE, et al. Temporal artery thermometry in children younger than 5 years: a comparison with rectal thermometry. *Pediatr Emerg Care.* 2014;30:867–870.

Wilkinson M, Bulloch B, Smith M. Prevalence of bacteremia in children aged 3–36 months presenting to the emergency department with fever in the post pneumococcal conjugate vaccine era. *Acad Emerg Med.* 2009;16:220–225.

Wolff M, Bachur R. Serious bacterial infection in recently immunized young febrile infants. *Acad Emerg Med.* 2009;16:1284–1289.

CHAPTER 63

SEIZURES IN INFANCY AND CHILDHOOD

Andrew M. White, MD, PhD

1. **How does one determine if an event in a child is actually a seizure?**
   Many events that appear to be seizures are actually nonepileptic. These events can be classified by the age at which the event occurred (Fig. 63.1).
   Questions helpful in deciding whether an event was or was not a seizure include:
   - Is the movement suppressible? Seizure movements will continue despite someone holding a limb. Tics or stereotypies (a repetitive or ritualistic movement, posture, or utterance) are suppressible.
   - Is the event distractible? Seizures will continue if you call a person's name; daydreaming may not. It may also terminate if the person is pinched or if a finger is placed in their ear.
   - Were the movements jerking or thrashing? Typically, seizures involve rhythmic jerking and not thrashing movements or pelvic thrusting. Side-to-side movements of the head, preserved awareness, eye fluttering, no postictal period, and events only when others are present are clues to a diagnosis of psychogenic nonepileptic spells (PNES). Is the event stereotyped (the same each time)? This favors seizure. A witness or video is helpful.
   - Are the events always provoked? Seizures are generally not provoked; breath-holding spells are always provoked – the child is upset or injured, begins to cry, and stops breathing. There may be associated jerks. (Low iron levels and hematocrit have been associated with breath-holding spells.)
   - Is there tongue biting during the event and, if so, where? During a true seizure, the tongue is usually bitten on the side, and often with a severe laceration. During syncope or conversion disorder, the tongue is usually not bitten, but if so, usually bitten on the tip with a minor injury.
   - Was there urination or loss of stool? This favors a diagnosis of true seizure, although it does not rule out conversion disorder.
   - Does it only happen during exercise? If so, it is more likely to be a cardiac event.
   - What do the eyes do during the event? During most seizures, the eyes remain open. They may roll up or deviate to one side or the other. Forced eye closure should make one consider the diagnosis of PNES.
   - Does it happen only during certain times of day? Seizures will happen at all times of day, but there are certain types that are much more common in sleep (self-limited epilepsy with centrotemporal spikes), and others that are more common during waking hours (self-limited infantile focal seizures). Many types also occur during wake and sleep transition.
   - Does it only happen upon standing? The event is likely to be orthostatic syncope or cardiac in nature.
   - What is the patient like after the event? Except for absence-type or myoclonic seizures, children are usually postictal (tired, confused) after seizures.
   - Does the child retain consciousness during the event? If it is a generalized tonic-clonic seizure (convulsion), this is impossible, because both halves of the brain are involved. Retaining consciousness is possible for focal seizures or brief absences.
   - Does the child remember the event? Typically, the child will not remember a portion of the focal seizure or any part of a generalized tonic-clonic seizure (convulsion). Depending on the length of an absence spell, it is possible that there will be recollection ($<$6 seconds).

2. **What can be learned from the child's history?**
   - Get a step-by-step description of the events before, during, and after the seizure.
   - Learn about activities before the seizure (e.g., provoked breath-holding spells, triggering events such as flashing lights, wake or sleep state of the patient).
   - Get a good description of the seizure itself, including the manner in which it started and evolved, how long it lasted (this is usually significantly overestimated by the parents), and what the patient was like after the event. See if there was unilateral weakness afterwards (Todd's paresis), indicative of a focal seizure.
   - Ask additional questions to establish the cause of the seizure, including any recent illnesses, trauma, and overall progression in development.
   - Obtain past medical history, as well as a family history of seizures.
   - In patients with known epilepsy, inquiries about medication compliance are necessary. Levels can be drawn to ensure compliance.

3. **What things should be sought on physical examination?**
   Perform a complete neurologic examination on any child with a first-time seizure. Components of the neurologic examination include mental status, cranial nerves, motor skills, coordination, reflexes, sensation, and gait. If the patient is febrile, the source of the fever should be sought. A careful search for any evidence of abusive head trauma (retinal hemorrhages, bruising, fractures) should be performed.

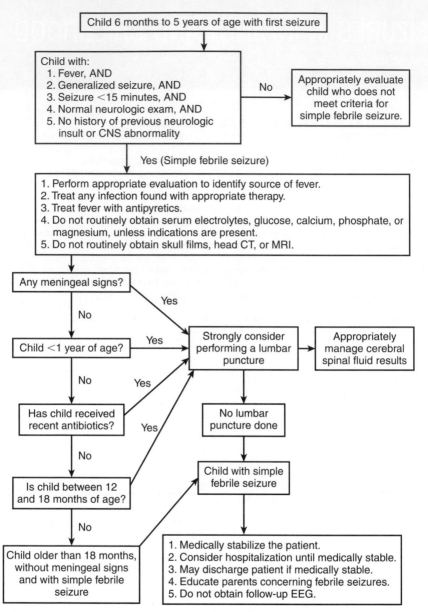

Fig. 63.1 Evaluation of child with simple febrile seizure. *CNS,* Central nervous system; *CT,* computed tomography; *EEG,* electroencephalogram; *MRI,* magnetic resonance imaging. (Modified from Committee on Quality Improvement, Subcommittee on Febrile Seizures, American Academy of Pediatrics. Practice parameter: the neurodiagnostic evaluation of the child with a first simple febrile seizure. *Pediatrics.* 1996;97:769–775.)

4. **How are pediatric seizures classified?**

There are several ways in which a seizure can be classified. The first is by its appearance (focal versus generalized) and how it started (focal versus generalized). If the seizure is focal, it is important to obtain an exact description of where it started and, if possible, what the child experienced before the seizure. This can help significantly in the localization of the epileptic focus. Seizures can also be classified by syndrome, prognosis, and cause. Classification systems have recently been updated. The latest classification system (2010) describes generalized, focal, and unknown seizure types. Focal onset seizures can have impaired awareness and can progress to bilateral tonic-clonic activity. The epilepsy types are similarly described except that they also have a combined general and focal type. They are also classified based on seizure etiology (genetic, structural/metabolic, infectious, immune, or unknown), and can be further categorized based on whether they are part of a syndrome and the corresponding age group.

5. **What are common reasons for a seizure in the neonate?**
   The most common cause for neonatal seizures is hypoxic-ischemic encephalopathy. Additional causes include:
   - Ischemic stroke
   - Intracranial hemorrhage (subarachnoid in full-term infants, germinal matrix in preterm neonates).
   - Metabolic disturbances (hypoglycemia, hypocalcemia, drug withdrawal, amino acidemias, organic acidurias, urea cycle defects).
   - Infection: TORCH infections (toxoplasmosis, rubella, cytomegalovirus, herpes simplex virus), *Escherichia coli, Streptococcus pneumoniae.*
   - Malformations of cortical development.
   - Benign neonatal or infantile familial convulsions.

6. **What tests should be done for a neonate experiencing seizures?**
   Determine serum electrolyte levels, including glucose, calcium, and urine toxicology reports. Request an ammonia level (free-flowing collection), looking for a urea cycle defect. Unless another cause is found, perform a lumbar puncture (LP) for an infectious etiology. Cerebrospinal fluid (CSF) studies should include cell count, protein, glucose, amino acids, lactate, pyruvate, herpes polymerase chain reaction (PCR), and evaluation for xanthochromia (prior bleed). TORCH studies can also be performed. Serum amino acids and urine organic acids can be tested for other inborn errors of metabolism. If there is no clear reason for seizures or a family history of seizures, it is appropriate to obtain an epilepsy panel testing for various genetic mutations (e.g., *KCNQ2, KCNQ3*). These have come down in price significantly, but still require insurance approval and are send outs. Cerebral imaging studies include ultrasound, computed tomography (CT) scan, or magnetic resonance imaging (MRI). Although requiring sedation, MRI is the gold standard and will identify malformations of cortical development. Though easier to obtain, CT has less resolution than MRI and exposes the newborn to radiation. Ultrasound is portable and convenient but does not allow the cortical convexities to be well viewed and may have limited availability. An electroencephalogram (EEG) may be ordered on an inpatient basis.

7. **What medications are used to treat neonatal seizures?**
   There is a dramatic lack of evidence that any drug is useful in the treatment of neonatal seizures. For a long time, phenytoin, phenobarbital, and lorazepam have been used. Newer medications for neonates include topiramate (Topamax), lacosamide (Vimpat), and levetiracetam (Keppra).

8. **What are common reasons for a child to have a seizure?**
   Common reasons include:
   - fever
   - lack of compliance to antiepileptic medication
   - infection
   - trauma
   - metabolic abnormalities
   - toxins
   - tumor
   - genetics (channelopathics, chromosomal abnormalities)
   - structural abnormalities (malformation of cortical development)

9. **What is the definition of a febrile seizure?**
   According to the National Institutes of Health (NIH), a febrile seizure is an event in infancy or childhood usually occurring between 6 months and 5 years of age, associated with fever, but without evidence of intracranial infection or defined cause. Seizures with fever in children who have suffered a previous afebrile seizure are excluded.

10. **Are genetics involved with febrile seizures?**
    Genetic factors are definitely involved with febrile seizures. Two syndromes that include febrile seizures are generalized epilepsy with febrile seizures plus (GEFS+) and Dravet syndrome *SCN1A* mutation. There is a family history of febrile seizures in about one third of patients. Presence of febrile seizures in an older sibling confers a 20% chance of febrile seizures in the younger child.

11. **What are the types of febrile seizures?**
    There are two types of febrile seizures: simple and complex. Complex febrile seizures are those that are focal (4%), prolonged >15 minutes (8%), or occur multiple times during a single day or illness (15%). Approximately one third of all febrile seizures are complex. If a child has a complex febrile seizure, his or her next febrile seizure is also likely to be complex. Simple febrile seizures have none of the complex features.

12. **What factors make the recurrence of febrile seizures more likely?**
    The overall risk of recurrence for febrile seizures is about one third. This is true regardless of whether it was a simple or complex febrile seizure. Risk factors for recurrence include:
    - early occurrence of first seizure
    - history of febrile seizures in first-degree relative
    - family history of epilepsy
    - abnormal neurologic examination
    - lower temperature at onset of seizure
    - brief period of recognized fever
    - more frequent illnesses (daycare)

13. **What tests should be done after a febrile seizure?**
    Children with *simple* febrile seizures should be evaluated and treated based on fever alone, because the concomitant presentation of the seizure does not increase the risk of serious bacterial illnesses above baseline. For *complex* febrile seizures without an obvious source, consider the following:
    - CBC, glucose, electrolytes, calcium, magnesium, urinalysis (UA), and stool culture, particularly for complex febrile seizures. (See Chapter 62 for further discussion on pediatric fever.) Consider LP in patients <18 months with no fever focus.
    - Head CT or, preferably, MRI for focal neurologic features or altered mental status.
    - EEG (as outpatient if patient returns to baseline neurologic status) if complex features or strong family history of epilepsy.
    - Nonemergent outpatient MRI with pediatric neurology follow-up consultation if patient returns to baseline.

14. **Under what conditions should a child having febrile seizures be treated, and what treatments should be used?**
    The two medications shown effective at decreasing subsequent febrile seizures are phenobarbital and valproate. However, phenobarbital may impact cognitive ability in children. Divalproex (Depakote) is not a good drug for children younger than 2 years because of the potential for fatal hepatotoxicity seen with the *POLG1* mutation. Medication should only be started (in consultation with a pediatric neurologist) with the following features: high frequency, prolonged, or a family remote from medical care. Neurologists often recommend levetiracetam.
    Attempts at controlling the fever with agents such as acetaminophen or ibuprofen usually fail; the seizure is typically the first sign of the illness. Use rectal diazepam or intranasal midazolam for children with prolonged (>5 minutes) febrile seizures to treat the seizure and help alleviate parental anxiety.

15. **What is the likelihood that a child suffering febrile seizures will eventually develop epilepsy?**
    The risk of a child with simple febrile seizures developing epilepsy is approximately 1%. This is only slightly above the risk for the general public. The risk of a child with complex febrile seizures developing epilepsy is about 6%.

16. **What are infantile spasms, and what are some common causes?**
    Infantile spasm (West syndrome) occurs in 1/3000 of infants, typically developing between the ages of 3 and 8 months. It involves the triad of epileptic spasms, hypsarrhythmia on EEG, and developmental arrest or regression. Causes include TORCH infections, malformations of cortical development, hypoxic-ischemic injury, genetic disorders (tuberous sclerosis, Down syndrome, neurofibromatosis, incontinentia pigmenti), metabolic disorders (phenylketonuria [PKU], maple syrup urine disease [MSUD], pyridoxine-dependent seizures), and trauma.
    Infantile spasms first present as a jerking movement in which the body may flex or extend suddenly. It is usually a single jerk at first, but multiple clustered jerks lasting several minutes may subsequently occur. The jerking can be unilateral or bilateral, and is often accompanied by crying during the cluster. Developmental regression is a poor prognostic sign. The pattern on the EEG associated with the syndrome is high amplitude and chaotic, termed *hypsarrhythmia*. The actual spasm is associated with an electrodecrement, or flattening of the EEG.

17. **What is the standard treatment for infantile spasms?**
    The standard treatment for infantile spasm is adrenocorticotropic hormone (ACTH) or vigabatrin. ACTH can have severe side effects, including hypertension, osteoporosis, and decreased resistance to infection. ACTH is controversial as it is exceedingly expensive ($100,000 per course). Vigabatrin is a drug that is also available and is the preferred drug if the patient has tuberous sclerosis. It is less expensive ($10,000) and only slightly less effective in studies. Side effects can include permanent visual loss. Because of cost and side effects, practitioners have used high-dose steroids and other antiepileptic drugs such as clobazam, zonisamide, or topiramate as substitutes. These have been shown to be significantly less effective. The ketogenic diet has been shown to be effective in some cases.

18. **What is the prognosis for infantile spasms?**
    The prognosis for infantile spasms is quite poor, with the mortality rate reported as high as 33%. Only 12% of children who survive to adulthood have normal intelligence. There is significant evidence that the earlier treatment is started, and the earlier the cessation of the spasms and hypsarrhythmia, the better the prognosis.

19. **What is epilepsy?**

Epilepsy is described as the tendency to have unprovoked recurring seizures. Operationally, an individual who has had two or more unprovoked seizures is said to have epilepsy. Alternatively, if you have one seizure and a 60% chance of a second (such as would be present in a patient with a single seizure and a stroke), or if you have an epilepsy syndrome, you are operationally said to have epilepsy. Epilepsy can resolve for patients who had an age-dependent epilepsy syndrome and are now past the age where the syndrome causes seizures, or if a patient has been seizure free for 10 years, with no seizure medications for the last 5 years.

20. **What are some common forms of childhood epilepsy?**

- *Childhood absence (nonmotor).* Begins from 4 to 8 years of age. Involves hundreds of seizures per day. Typically associated with normal intelligence and normal imaging. Episodes last 5–10 seconds with no postictal period. It can be safely reproduced with hyperventilation. Treatment is with ethosuximide, or if accompanied by generalized tonic-clonic seizures, valproic acid. In adolescent women, avoid valproate (teratogenicity and multiple side effects). Lamotrigine is a reasonable alternative. Additional drugs used more recently include topiramate, levetiracetam, and clobazam.
- *Self-limited epilepsy with centrotemporal spikes.* Begins from 6 to 10 years of age and involves facial and arm twitching, slurred speech, and drooling. It will occasionally generalize. No treatment is necessary unless seizures generalize or occur during daytime. If that occurs, then carbamazepine or oxcarbazepine are reasonable.
- *Juvenile myoclonic epilepsy.* Begins from 12 to 18 years of age and consists of a triad of morning myoclonic, generalized tonic-clonic, and absence seizures. Seizures are brought on by stress, alcohol, and sleep deprivation. It often requires lifelong treatment with an agent such as valproic acid or lamotrigine. Lamotrigine is preferred in women due to the teratogenicity and side effects of valproic acid.

21. **What workup should be done after an afebrile seizure in an asymptomatic child?**

If the child has returned to normal after a generalized seizure (without focal findings), and has a normal neurologic examination, he or she can go home and then have a follow-up examination with an outpatient EEG and MRI. A neurologic consultation should also be scheduled. If the patient does not return to baseline, had focal seizure findings, or is not significantly improving within 1–2 hours, in addition to standard lab testing (e.g., bedside glucose, CBC, electrolytes, liver function tests [LFTs], ammonia, or urine toxicology), an imaging study (CT or MRI) should be performed emergently. An LP should be performed based on clinical suspicious for meningitis. Occasionally, an acute EEG should also be performed after cessation of clinical symptoms to rule out subclinical status. This is more common in children <1 year old after treatment with benzodiazepines or other antiepileptic drugs.

22. **Under what conditions should afebrile seizures be treated using antiepileptic drugs?**

Treatment of seizures with antiepileptics balances the risk of recurrence with the risks of the medication. Antiepileptics are typically not started until after the second seizure. Patients with a dramatically abnormal EEG, very strong family history, or abnormal neurologic examination may receive seizure prophylaxis in consultation with a pediatric neurologist.

23. **What are the older and newer antiepileptics, and how do they vary?**

Older antiepileptics
- Phenobarbital
- Primidone
- Phenytoin
- Carbamazepine
- Ethosuximide
- Acetazolamide
- Clonazepam
- Valproate

Newer antiepileptics
- Topiramate
- Lamotrigine
- Levetiracetam
- Felbamate
- Gabapentin
- Oxcarbazepine
- Zonisamide
- Pregabalin
- Clobazam
- Tiagabine
- Eslicarbazepine
- Lacosamide
- Vigabatrin
- Perampanel

- Ezogabine – no longer produced
- Rufinamide
- Brivaracetam

Older drugs have the advantage of lower cost and greater experience. Newer drugs have the advantages of better side-effect profiles, decreased monitoring requirements, less frequent dosing regimens, and decreased interaction with other drugs.

24. **What are important side effects of the different antiepileptic drugs?**
Almost all antiepileptics have been linked to suicidal behavior. Specific side effects include:
- Phenobarbital: sedation, hyperkinesis, and cognitive dysfunction
- Carbamazepine (Tegretol): ataxia, dizziness, sedation, and rash
- Valproic acid (Depakote): alopecia, weight gain, and tremor
- Phenytoin (Dilantin): hirsutism, gingival hyperplasia, and ataxia
- Ethosuximide (Zarontin): gastrointestinal (GI) distress, headaches, drowsiness, and hiccoughs
- Levetiracetam (Keppra): psychotic behavior and irritability
- Lamotrigine (Lamictal): rash
- Perampanel (Fycompa): somnolence, headache, fatigue, and irritability
- Topiramate (Topamax): sedation, glaucoma, and kidney stones
- Felbamate (Felbatol): aplastic anemia (can be fatal), insomnia, and anorexia
- Tiagabine (Gabitril): GI intolerance
- Oxcarbazepine (Trileptal): hyponatremia
- Zonisamide (Zonegran): weight loss, kidney stones, headache, and decreased sweating
- Lacosamide (Vimpat): dizziness, headache, nausea, and diplopia
- Carisbamate (Comfyde): dizziness, headache, somnolence, and nausea
- Pregabalin (Lyrica): rhabdomyolysis
- Gabapentin (Neurontin): somnolence, dizziness, ataxia, nystagmus, headache, tremor, weight gain
- Rufinamide (Banzel): somnolence, nausea, and headache
- Clobazam (ONFI): somnolence
- Vigabatrin (Sabril): peripheral vision loss
- Brivaracetam (Briviact): drowsiness, sedation, dizziness, fatigue, nausea, vomiting, irritability

25. **If an individual stopped taking an antiepileptic drug, at what dosage should the medication be restarted?**
If it has been longer than 1 week, the drug must be restarted (often tapered up) as first prescribed. This is especially important for a drug such as lamotrigine, which can cause a rash or Stevens-Johnson syndrome to occur if it is started too quickly.

26. **When should antiepileptic drugs be discontinued?**
Except for a dramatically abnormal EEG or abnormal neurologic examination, an antiepileptic drug can be stopped after 2 seizure-free years. A shorter time can be considered for neonatal seizures; current practice is to stop treatment of neonatal seizures once the seizures have stopped. Most neonates will go home without antiepileptic medications. Approximately two thirds of patients remain seizure free after drug withdrawal; 80% of recurrent seizures present within the first 6 months of treatment cessation.

27. **What happens if a dose of antiepileptic drug is missed?**
If it is time for the next dose, simply continue on without giving additional medication. If it is not time for the next dose, give the missed dose, and slightly delay the subsequent dose.

28. **What if vomiting occurs shortly after taking an antiepileptic drug?**
If >1 hour since the drug was taken, no action is necessary. If 30–60 minutes between the dose and vomiting, give half a dose. If <30 minutes, repeat the dose.

29. **What is status epilepticus?**
Historically, status epilepticus has been defined as continuous or intermittent seizure activity lasting longer than 30 minutes. To provide a more practical definition, status epilepticus has recently been redefined as >5 minutes of seizure activity, indicating a prolonged seizure that requires medical intervention. Beyond 30 minutes of seizure activity, the patient is at risk of suffering neuronal injury.

30. **What is the treatment for status epilepticus?**
Stabilize airway, breathing, and circulation (ABCs) first. Obtain a bedside glucose level, chemistry panel (with calcium, magnesium, and phosphorous), urine toxicology report, and anticonvulsant levels, along with intracranial imaging (usually CT). If possible, a continuous EEG (performed in consultation with a neurologist) is helpful and should establish a burst-suppression pattern if the seizure cannot be stopped. The continuous EEG is especially useful if the patient needs to be paralyzed during intubation. Without this it is not possible to determine if the patient continues seizing.

If there is no intravenous (IV) access, consider either rectal diazepam or intranasal (or intramuscular [IM]) midazolam. After establishing IV access, give a benzodiazepine, such as lorazepam, repeating the dose multiple times if necessary. If seizures persist, give phenobarbital (20 mg/kg), phenytoin (20 mg/kg), valproic acid (40 mg/kg), or levetiracetam (60 mg/kg). If the seizure is still not controlled, the next step is a midazolam drip, ketamine, propofol, or pentobarbital.

31. **What should an onlooker do if the child has another seizure?**
    - Place the child on his or her side.
    - Clear anything near the mouth.
    - Remove anything that may cause injury.
    - Place something soft under the head.
    - Time the event.
        - If it lasts less than 5 minutes, no action is likely needed.
        - If longer than 5 minutes, administer rectal diazepam or intranasal (or IM) midazolam, or take the patient to the emergency department (ED).
        - If rectal diazepam or midazolam has been given and the seizure has lasted longer than 10 minutes, go to the ED.

32. **What cautions should I give to parents of children who have seizures?**
    - No bathing or swimming alone
    - No ladders or activities above shoulder height
    - No activities that may result in harm if there is a temporary loss of consciousness
    - Driving guidelines vary by state.
    - A complete list of recommended activities can be found at the Epilepsy Foundation's website.

KEY POINTS: SEIZURES IN INFANCY AND CHILDHOOD

1. Seizures have characteristic patterns that allow for the differentiation from nonepileptic events. There are typical childhood seizure patterns that guide prognosis and treatment.
2. ED evaluation of a pediatric seizure is dependent on the age, type, and clinical suspicion for infection or nonaccidental trauma.
3. The evaluation of a child in status epilepticus or not returning to baseline neurologic state requires consultation with a pediatric neurologist for treatment and EEG monitoring.

BIBLIOGRAPHY

Berg AT, Berkovic SF, Brodie MJ, et al. Revised terminology and concepts for organization of seizures and epilepsies: report of the ILAE Commission on Classification and Terminology, 2005–2009. *Epilepsia.* 2010;51:676–685.
Berg AT, Scheffer IE. New concepts in classification of the epilepsies: entering the 21st century. *Epilepsia.* 2011;52:1058–1062.
Fenichel GM. *Clinical Pediatric Neurology: A Signs and Symptoms Approach.* 6th ed. Philadelphia: Saunders; 2009.
Fisher RS, Acevedo C, Arzimanoglou A, et al. A practical clinical definition of epilepsy. *Epilepsia.* 2014;55(4):475–482.

CHAPTER 64

ACUTE RESPIRATORY DISORDERS IN CHILDREN

Kristine Knuti Rodrigues, MD, MPH and Genie E. Roosevelt, MD, MPH

1. **What are the signs and symptoms of respiratory distress in a child?**
   The progression of respiratory distress is shown in Fig. 64.1. Tachypnea is often the earliest sign in younger children, because they cannot significantly increase their tidal volume. Normal respiratory rate in children decreases with age; newborns breathe as fast as 60 breaths per minute, whereas a 12-month-old infant averages 30 breaths per minute. Oxygen saturation should not be the sole determinant of severity, with the clinical state primarily dictating any need for intervention. Mental status is often the most important parameter; crying with examination is appropriate. Don't be fooled by a "well-behaved" child that is actually altered.

2. **Why are airway problems more serious in pediatric patients than in adults?**
   There are several important differences between the adult and the pediatric airway. The child's tongue is large and is the most common cause of airway obstruction in the obtunded child. The narrowest portion of the pediatric airway is at the cricoid ring, making obstruction with subglottic pathology more likely than in adults. The small size of the pediatric airway (approximately one-third the diameter of an adult's at birth) means that small changes in diameter cause significant increases in resistance. (Resistance is inversely related to the fourth power of the radius.) Higher oxygen consumption in children contributes to a more rapid decrease in arterial oxygen levels after airway obstruction.

3. **How can I determine where the problem is?**
   All noisy breathing is not asthma; a few seconds of observation often helps differentiate upper and lower airway obstruction. Generally, extrathoracic lesions (e.g., epiglottis, croup) produce inspiratory stridor (i.e., harsh, vibratory sound), whereas intrathoracic lesions (e.g., asthma, bronchiolitis) produce prolonged expiratory wheezing (i.e., high-pitched sound). Regardless of the location, severe pathologic disruption can produce both inspiratory and expiratory sounds.

4. **What are common causes of upper airway obstruction in children?**
   See Table 64.1.

5. **Discuss the signs and symptoms of croup, who gets it, what causes it, and what the physician can do for it.**
   Croup, or laryngotracheitis, is the most common cause of infectious acute upper airway obstruction. The etiology is viral (e.g., parainfluenza, influenza, and respiratory syncytial virus [RSV]) with erythema and swelling of the trachea just below the vocal cords, and patients classically have a "barky" or "seal-like" cough. The mean age of affected patients is 18 months, with an age range of 6 months to 3 years. There is a seasonal increase in autumn and early winter. Patients are often febrile, with a prodrome of mild upper respiratory symptoms that progress to stridor. Symptoms are worse with agitation and at night, classically peaking on day 2 of illness. Because the lungs are not directly affected, oxygen saturation can be maintained even in severe illness. Laboratory data are not helpful. Diagnosis is clinical; radiography is not indicated unless diagnosis is unclear or foreign body obstruction is a consideration.

6. **Who needs nebulized epinephrine?**
   Aerosolized epinephrine decreases airway obstruction. It is indicated for children with stridor at rest or increased work of breathing (e.g., tachypnea, retractions). Racemic epinephrine (0.5 mL of 2.25% solution) is used most commonly, but L-epinephrine alone (5 mL of a 1:1000) is equivalent. Maximal effect is seen within 30 minutes, with potential to return to increased work of breathing and stridor at rest within 3 hours. Patients without resting stridor after 3 hours can be safely discharged home. Criteria for admission include continued stridor at rest, cyanosis, signs of respiratory distress, dehydration, and questionable adherence to follow-up instructions. Intubation is rarely needed but when necessary often requires relatively smaller endotracheal tube (ETT) sizes. A helium-oxygen mixture (heliox) may be considered in children with severe croup and respiratory distress prior to intubation.

7. **What about steroids and croup?**
   Steroids should be considered for any child who comes to the emergency department (ED) with croup. A single oral dose of dexamethasone decreases the need for hospitalization and return ED visits. Dexamethasone has traditionally been given orally at a dose of 0.6 mg/kg (maximum of 10 mg); however, studies have suggested similar

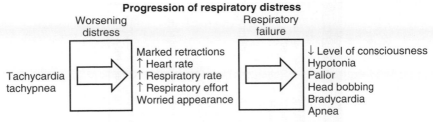

Fig. 64.1 Signs and symptoms of respiratory distress in children.

efficacy with doses of 0.15–0.4 mg/kg. Intramuscular (IM) or intravenous (IV) dexamethasone can also be given for patients who cannot take it orally. There is no evidence to suggest that repeat dosing is indicated, but this might be considered for young patients who seek treatment before the peak of illness (i.e., day 1). Nebulized budesonide shows similar outcomes (rate of return visits, hospital admissions) as dexamethasone and may be considered as another option for patients unable to tolerate oral steroids.

KEY POINTS: CROUP

1. Treatment is with oral dexamethasone 0.6 mg/kg (maximum of 10 mg).
2. Racemic epinephrine is used for patients with moderate to severe respiratory distress or stridor at rest.

---

8. **When should I worry about epiglottitis and bacterial tracheitis?**
   Although both conditions are rare, they warrant careful consideration. Children generally appear toxic with rapid onset of symptoms. Epiglottitis, now rare with universal vaccination against *Haemophilus influenzae* type B, is a bacterial cellulitis of the supraglottic structures, most notably the lingual surface of the epiglottitis. Children display such symptoms as drooling, dysphagia, stridor, and a predilection for the sniffing position. Radiographic evidence includes a swollen epiglottis (the thumb sign), thickened aryepiglottic folds, and obliteration of the vallecula. Bacterial tracheitis, although rare, may be emerging as a more significant problem. Patients have croup-like symptoms but are toxic in appearance, with significant respiratory distress. Radiographs may show shaggy subglottic narrowing and clouding of the trachea. Airway management and broad-spectrum antibiotics (third-generation cephalosporin plus an antistaphylococcal agent, such as vancomycin or clindamycin) are the mainstay of therapy for both disorders.

9. **What is the appropriate initial management of a patient with suspected epiglottitis?**
   Immediately set up for an emergent airway and call an anesthesia, surgical, or ear, nose, throat (ENT) consultant for anticipated emergent airway management in the operating room; do not agitate the child in any way. If epiglottitis is suspected, keep the child in a position of comfort (often on a parent's lap) and defer examination of the pharynx, because direct examination or manipulation of the oropharynx can cause contraction of the pharyngeal muscles and worsen airway obstruction. If the patient will tolerate it without agitation, start high-flow oxygen via a nonrebreather bag reservoir mask (where available, heliox can also be useful). Radiographs, blood work, IV lines, and antibiotics can wait; if a child's airway becomes obstructed, bag-valve-mask ventilation should be attempted first.

10. **What are retropharyngeal space infections?**
    The retropharynx is a potential space located immediately posterior to the pharynx, larynx, and trachea. Infection may arise by direct penetrating trauma or from extension of an acute infection of the ear, nose, or throat, with spread to the lymph nodes in the prevertebral space and subsequent abscess formation. About 90% of patients are younger than 6 years; the affected child usually appears alert (but mildly toxic), with fever. They may have limited range of motion of the neck (particularly unable to extend), upper respiratory symptoms, dysphagia, odynophagia, or neck swelling.

11. **What imaging studies are helpful in the diagnosis of retropharyngeal infections?**
    Lateral neck films are often diagnostic (90% sensitivity) but can be difficult to interpret depending on the phase of respiration and neck position. To avoid false-positive findings, the film should be obtained during inspiration with the neck held in extension. Findings include an increase in the width of the prevertebral space to greater than the anteroposterior width of the adjacent cervical vertebral body, anterior displacement of the airway, and loss of the normal step-off at the level of the larynx. Air-fluid levels may be seen after abscess formation (Fig. 64.2). Computed tomography (CT) scanning is highly sensitive and used to differentiate abscess from phlegmon or soft-tissue cellulitis.

Table 64.1 Causes of Upper Airway Obstruction

	ETIOLOGY	TYPICAL AGE RANGE	ONSET	TOXICITY	DROOLING	TREATMENT
Croup	Parainfluenza type 1, influenza A and B, RSV, rhinovirus, human metapneumovirus, adenovirus, rhinovirus	6 months–3 years	URI prodrome	Mild	Absent	Mist, steroids, aerosolized epinephrine
Epiglottitis	*Haemophilus influenzae* group A, β-hemolytic *Streptococcus, Staphylococcus aureus, Streptococcus pneumoniae,* viruses	3–7 years	Acute	Marked	Common	Airway management, antibiotics
Retropharyngeal abscess	Multiple anaerobes	Infancy–6 years	URI, sore throat	Variable	Variable	Antibiotics, drainage
Bacterial tracheitis	*S. aureus, H. influenzae, S. pneumoniae, Moraxella catarrhalis* (often occurs after viral insult)	Infancy–6 years	"Croup" prodrome	Moderate	Usually absent	Airway management, antibiotics
Foreign body		5 months–3 years	Acute	Variable	Common	Airway management, endoscopic removal of foreign body

RSV, Respiratory syncytial virus; *URI,* upper respiratory infection.

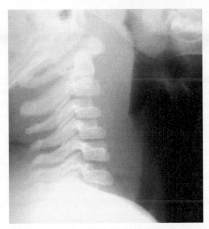

Fig. 64.2 Radiograph of lateral neck showing thickening of prevertebral space.

12. **How are retropharyngeal infections managed?**
    Treatment includes hospital admission, parenteral antibiotic therapy, and incision and drainage if an abscess is present. Most children do not need acute airway management.

13. **When should a foreign body be suspected?**
    Most patients with foreign-body aspiration are males between 5 months and 3 years of age. Although a history of an aspiration event (found in 50%–70%) is the most predictive factor, any sudden onset of cough, dyspnea, or wheezing should raise suspicion. Respiratory signs, such as stridor or focal wheezing, may be absent. Radiographs will only show radiopaque objects. Expiratory or lateral decubitus films have been shown to lack adequate sensitivity or specificity to be useful. Endoscopy is diagnostic.

14. **How are suspected foreign bodies managed in pediatric patients?**
    Immediate management depends on the degree of respiratory distress, but should be minimal unless respiratory failure is imminent. For unconscious patients, call for emergent ENT evaluation and attempt direct laryngoscopy with removal of any visualized foreign object with Magill forceps. If this fails, attempt bag-valve-mask ventilation and intubation to push the offending object into one bronchus. If the child's airway cannot be intubated, perform a needle cricothyroidotomy.

15. **What is bronchiolitis, and who does it affect?**
    Commonly found in children younger than 2 years, bronchiolitis is a predominantly wintertime infection (usually from RSV but less commonly from many other viruses such as rhinovirus, influenza, human metapneumovirus, and paraInfluenza), characterized by inflammation, edema, and mucus accumulation of the bronchioles. Progression of illness leads to lower airway obstruction and, consequently, ventilation/perfusion mismatch. With small bronchioles more prone to mucous plugging and obstruction, peak incidence and severity is at 3–6 months of age.

16. **What are the clinical signs and symptoms of bronchiolitis?**
    Fever, tachypnea, wheezing, and signs of respiratory distress, such as nasal flaring and retractions, are coupled with copious mucus secretions. Symptoms follow a predictive course with a 1- to 2-day prodrome of copious rhinorrhea, cough, and low-grade fever that progresses to lower respiratory signs and respiratory distress. Symptoms peak around days 3–4 of illness. Auscultation reveals diffuse wheezing and crackles that often vary between examinations. Findings of more severe disease include hypoxemia, inability to feed, irritability, and lethargy. Young infants may experience periods of apnea.

17. **Do patients with bronchiolitis need chest radiographs?**
    Infants with bronchiolitis do not need any radiologic evaluation. Chest findings on radiograph are nonspecific and include hyperinflation, a flattened diaphragm caused by air trapping, perihilar peribronchial infiltrates, and atelectasis. Findings can be confused with pneumonia and lead to unnecessary use of antibiotics. Children with atypical presentations or examinations may warrant radiography to rule out other causes of first-time wheezing, including foreign body, congenital airway anomalies, congestive heart failure, and bacterial pneumonia.

18. **When are laboratory tests needed for bronchiolitis?**
    Laboratory tests are generally not indicated for bronchiolitis. Infants older than 1 month with bronchiolitis are at low risk for serious invasive bacterial infection. Routine complete blood count (CBC), lumbar puncture, and blood culture are not warranted. Infants with bronchiolitis and fever continue to be at risk for concurrent urinary tract

infection (UTI) and should have a catheterized urine specimen for culture performed. Management of fever in neonates (<1 month) with bronchiolitis is unchanged and includes a complete sepsis evaluation. Since influenza can cause bronchiolitis, influenza testing may be considered during influenza season for febrile patients with bronchiolitis who fall within influenza treatment recommendation windows (e.g., within 48 hours of onset of symptoms).

19. **What is the treatment for bronchiolitis?**
Bronchiolitis treatment is supportive, and involves supplemental oxygen, nasal suctioning, and hydration. There is no evidence to support the routine use of bronchodilators, steroids, or antivirals in the ED. Recent review of bronchodilators (albuterol or salbutamol) for bronchiolitis for infants with first-time wheezing showed no significant benefit in hospitalized patients, no improvement of oxygen saturation, no reduction in the need for hospitalization, and no reduction in the length of stay in hospital or illness at home. Additionally, albuterol may worsen ventilation/perfusion mismatch and exacerbate hypoxemia. Studies addressing the use of nebulized hypertonic saline suggest that it may improve the clinical severity score, but does not reduce need for hospitalization. Nebulized epinephrine may be slightly more effective, probably because of vasoconstrictive effects. When compared with placebo, epinephrine may be effective for reducing hospital admission but there was no difference found for length of hospital stay in admitted patients.

20. **Who is admitted for bronchiolitis?**
Patients who are hypoxemic, have more than mild respiratory distress, have history of apnea, or are unable to adequately self-hydrate should be admitted. Admission should be strongly considered for all children with risk factors for severe disease (Box 64.1). Some centers use home oxygen therapy protocols for otherwise well-appearing patients requiring less than 0.5 liters per minute (LPM) of oxygen These patients require a 24-hour follow-up visit as well as reliable caretaker oversight. In patients at risk for respiratory failure, the use of heated humidified high-flow nasal cannula therapy (HFNC) has been associated with reduction in work of breathing, improved gas exchange, and decreased rates of intubation. HFNC requires a special circuit that permits high gas flows (up to 8 LPM in neonates, 25 LPM in infants), which are tolerated because of the humidified air. Flow rates ≥6 LPM generate positive expiratory pressure in the range of 2–5 cmH$_2$O throughout the respiratory cycle.

KEY POINTS: BRONCHIOLITIS

1. Bronchiolitis treatment is supportive, involving supplemental oxygen, nasal suctioning, and hydration.
2. Nebulized epinephrine may be helpful in reducing the need for hospital admission.
3. Radiographs and laboratory evaluations are not routinely indicated.

21. **How are bronchodilators used in the management of acute asthma?**
Selective β_2-agonists (e.g., albuterol) are the mainstay of medications to reverse bronchospasm. Delivery of albuterol by nebulizer or meter-dosed inhaler (MDI) with a spacer has been shown to be equally clinically effective, with 4–10 puffs of an MDI equivalent to one nebulizer treatment. Delivery by nebulizer remains the preferred route in the ED setting for young patients, as well as those in too much distress to cooperate with MDI use.
Albuterol is a racemic mixture of the R and S isomers of the compound, with the R isomer having the greatest effect on bronchodilation compared with the S isomer. Levalbuterol, the pure R isomer, may cause less tachycardia but is more costly and has not been demonstrated to be more effective in large clinical trials. In children with moderate to severe asthma, inhaled anticholinergic therapy (ipratropium bromide) decreases severity and hospitalization rates when given in conjunction with β_2-agonists (albuterol) in the ED.

22. **When and how should steroids be administered?**
Controlling inflammation is the cornerstone of asthma treatment. There is lack of consensus regarding the dose and duration of steroid therapy. Generally, a loading dose of prednisone 2 mg/kg (maximum 60 mg) in the ED is followed by a 4-day course of 1 mg/kg/day as a single daily dose or 2 mg/kg/day divided twice daily (maximum 60 mg/day). IV steroids are reserved for children who cannot tolerate oral medications. Dexamethasone, with its

Box 64.1 Bronchiolitis: Risk Factors for Severe Disease

Congenital heart disease
Chronic lung disease (cystic fibrosis, bronchopulmonary dysplasia)
Congenital or acquired immunodeficiency
Major congenital anomalies
Prematurity <37 weeks
Age <6–12 weeks

higher potency and longer half-life, is an appealing alternative. Multiple studies have shown that oral dexamethasone 0.6 mg/kg (maximum 16 mg) given once is not inferior to 5 days of prednisone in children with mild to moderate asthma exacerbations.

23. **When should a chest radiograph be obtained, and what are the typical findings?**
Chest radiography is not indicated in the routine evaluation of a child with asthma but should be obtained if pneumonia, pneumothorax, pneumomediastinum, or foreign body is suspected. Radiography commonly shows hyperinflation, atelectasis, and peribronchial thickening, indicating lower airway obstruction. Pneumothorax is rare. Pneumomediastinum is more common in older children (age >10 years).

24. **Outline the evaluation and treatment of an asthma exacerbation in the ED.**
1. Initial assessment
   - Evaluate vital signs with pulse oximetry, use of accessory muscles, retractions, alertness, auscultation, and peak expiratory flow rate (PEFR) in patients older than 5 years.
   - Consider an asthma score for objective assessment and later reassessment (Table 64.2).
2. Initial treatment
   - Oxygen as needed to keep saturation in the normal range
   - Three consecutive treatments of nebulized albuterol (2.5–5 mg or 0.15 mg/kg per treatment) plus ipratropium 250–500 µg
   - Steroids
3. Repeat assessment
   - Patient should be assessed after initial treatment to determine whether additional treatments are needed or if the patient can be observed for potential discharge. The full effect of albuterol may take 15 minutes.
   - If PEFR is greater than 70% baseline and the patient continues to have no wheezing, retractions, or accessory muscle use at least 2 hours after the last nebulized treatment, the patient can be safely discharged (Step 4a). If symptoms continue, the patient should be given additional therapy (Step 4b).
4a. Discharge
   - Discharge home with a reliable caretaker, patient education, medications, and follow-up instructions.
   - Discharge medications should include albuterol, inhaled or nebulized, every 4 hours as needed for wheezing and oral steroids.
4b. Continued therapy
   - Continuous albuterol by nebulization (7.5–10 mg/h, can increase to 20 mg/h)
   - Ipratropium 500 µg every 4 hours
   - Frequent reassessment of patient
5. Admission criteria
   - Albuterol treatment required every <4 hours
   - Continued hypoxemia by pulse oximetry
   - Continued poor response, requiring escalation of treatment

Table 64.2 Pediatric Asthma Score

	Score		
	1	**2**	**3**
Respiratory Rate			
2–3 years	≤34	35–39	≥40
4–5 years	≤30	31–35	≥36
6–12 years	≤26	27–30	≥31
>12 years	≤23	24–27	≥28
Oxygen requirement	>90% on room air	85%–90% on room air	<85% on room air
Auscultation	Normal or end-expiratory wheeze only	Expiratory wheezes	Inspiratory/expiratory wheezes or decreased breath sounds
Retractions	0–1 site	2 sites	3+ sites
Dyspnea	Speaks in sentences, coos, babbles	Speaks in partial sentences, short cry	Single words, short phrases, grunting

Modified from Kelly CS, Anderson CL, Pestian JP, et al. Improved outcomes for hospitalized asthmatic children using a clinical pathway. *Ann Allergy Asthma Immunol.* 2000;84:509–516.

25. **What about magnesium?**
   Magnesium's effect in asthma is probably the result of the counteraction of calcium ions to prevent bronchial smooth muscle contraction. It may have a role in reducing inflammatory mediators, depressing muscle fiber excitability, and stimulating nitric oxide and prostacyclin synthesis. The benefit in patients with mild to moderate exacerbations is unclear, and its use is often reserved for those patients in severe distress or nonresponsive to albuterol and steroids. In a recent meta-analysis, IV magnesium sulfate improved respiratory function and reduced the number of pediatric hospital admissions. The dosage is a range of 25–75 mg/kg IV (maximum of 2 g).

26. **Does aminophylline have any use?**
   Aminophylline and theophylline do not have a role in the routine management of the pediatric asthma patient in the ED. IV aminophylline has been shown to improve lung function in children with severe asthma exacerbations, but it does not reduce symptoms, number of nebulizer treatments, or length of stay. Several studies have failed to show benefit of theophylline when added to bronchodilators and steroids in noncritically ill patients. There are inconclusive data to suggest that theophylline may be equally effective to terbutaline in patients in the pediatric intensive care unit (PICU).

27. **What about parenteral β-agonists?**
   Use of systemic β-agonists is controversial; few well-designed studies have evaluated their use. They should be considered in patients with severe exacerbations who have failed to respond to maximal inhaled therapy, although significant side effects may include dysrhythmias, hypertension, and myocardial ischemia. Terbutaline, subcutaneous or IV, may be given as an initial bolus of 2–10 µg/kg, followed by a continuous infusion starting at 0.5 µg/kg/min. Epinephrine may also be given subcutaneously. These medications, which should not interrupt inhaled therapy, require monitoring of cardiac function and serum potassium levels.

28. **What should I do if my patient is going into respiratory failure?**
   Consider treatment with magnesium, terbutaline, and epinephrine. Bilevel positive airway pressure (BiPAP; set initially at 10/5) has been shown in small studies to improve respiratory rate and oxygenation in children. If intubation is necessary, ketamine (in conjunction with a paralytic) stimulates the release of catecholamines, causing bronchodilation, making it the inductive agent of choice (at a dosage of 1–2 mg/kg IV). To optimize oxygenation and prevent barotrauma, initial ventilator settings should be set to a reduced rate of 8–12 breaths per minute, allowing for permissive hypercapnia.

KEY POINTS: EVALUATION OF RESPIRATORY DISORDERS

1. Observation before auscultation helps localize and differentiate etiologies of pediatric respiratory complaints.
2. Foreign bodies should be suspected in any child with signs of airway obstruction.
3. Laboratory tests and radiographs are not routinely indicated in many childhood respiratory disorders.

BIBLIOGRAPHY

Carbone P, Capra G, Brigger M. Antibiotic therapy for pediatric deep neck abscesses: a systematic review. *Int J Pediatr Otorhinolaryngol.* 2012;76:1647–1653.
Gadomski AM, Scribani MB. Bronchodilators for bronchiolitis. *Cochrane Database Syst Rev.* 2014;(6):CD001266.
Hartling L, Bialy LM, Vandermeer B, et al. Epinephrine for bronchiolitis. *Cochrane Database Syst Rev.* 2011;(6):CD003123.
Mansbach JM, Piedra PA, Teach SJ, et al. Perspective multicenter study of viral etiology and hospital length of stay in children with severe bronchiolitis. *Arch Pediatr Adolesc Med.* 2012;166:700–706.
Petrocheilou A, Tanou K, Kalampouka E, et al. Viral croup: diagnosis and treatment algorithm. *Pediatr Pulmonol.* 2014;49:421–429.
Ralston SL, Lieberthal AS, Meissner HC, et al. Clinical practice guideline: the diagnosis, management, and prevention of bronchiolitis. *Pediatrics.* 2014;134:e1474–e1502.
Russel KF, Liang Y, O'Gorman K, et al. Glucocorticoids for croup. *Cochrane Database Syst Rev.* 2011;(1):CD001955.
Schwarz ES, Cohn BG. Is dexamethasone as effective as prednisone or prednisolone in the management of pediatric asthma exacerbations? *Ann Emerg Med.* 2015;65:81–82.
Shan Z, Rong Y, Yang W, et al. Intravenous and nebulized magnesium sulfate for treating acute asthma in adults and children: a systematic review and meta-analysis. *Respir Med.* 2013;107:321–330.
Wade A, Chang C. Evaluation and treatment of critical asthma syndrome in children. *Clin Rev Allergy Immunol.* 2015;48:66–83.
Wing R, James C, Maranda LS, et al. Use of high-flow nasal cannula support in the emergency department reduces the need for intubation in pediatric acute respiratory insufficiency. *Pediatr Emerg Care.* 2012;28:1117–1123.
Zhang L, Mendoza-Sassi RA, Wainwright C, et al. Nebulized hypertonic saline solution for acute bronchiolitis in infants. *Cochrane Database Syst Rev.* 2013;(7):CD006458.

CHAPTER 65

PEDIATRIC GASTROINTESTINAL DISORDERS AND DEHYDRATION

Joshua S. Easter, MD, MSc

1. What are the common causes of abdominal pain in children?

Abdominal pain is a common pediatric complaint, and the differential can be guided by age of the patient, history, physical examination, and occasionally diagnostic studies (Table 65.1).

2. What are the strongest indicators of dehydration in children?

Physical examination findings, such as delayed capillary refill time (>3 seconds), abnormal skin turgor, and hyperpnea (deep, rapid breathing without other signs of respiratory distress, suggesting acidosis) are the strongest indicators of **severe** dehydration. Historical factors, such as the number of wet diapers, frequency of vomiting or diarrhea, and amount of oral intake are less predictive. Laboratory studies, such as elevated serum blood urea nitrogen (BUN) and creatinine levels or urine specific gravity are also poor predictors of dehydration. A normal bicarbonate level (>15 mEq/L) reduces the likelihood of dehydration.

3. Do all children with dehydration need intravenous fluids?

For both mild dehydration with minimal clinical signs and moderate dehydration with normal or slightly delayed capillary refill, normal or abnormal skin turgor, or fatigue, the ideal treatment is oral rehydration with breast milk, formula, Pedialyte, or World Health Organization (WHO) solution. Straight water can lead to hyponatremia; highly sugared beverages, such as apple juice and soda, can exacerbate diarrhea. Sports drinks may not contain sufficient salt.

For moderate dehydration, the child should drink approximately 1 mL/kg every 5 minutes for 4 hours. Starting with smaller amounts and gradually increasing the volume over the course of an hour may improve success. If the child vomits, wait 15 minutes and try again. Oral rehydration works as well as intravenous (IV) hydration with shorter times to initiation of therapy and discharge from the emergency department (ED). Despite this, nearly two-thirds of children with moderate dehydration unnecessarily receive IV hydration. As recommended by the Choosing Wisely campaign, IV hydration should be reserved for cases where the child has persistent vomiting or is refusing to drink. Patients that tolerate rehydration can be discharged.

Children with severe dehydration are ill appearing and should receive 30 mL/kg of isotonic crystalloid solutions over the first hour. In children without signs of shock, more rapid IV hydration is not beneficial. Addition of dextrose to IV fluids does not reduce the incidence of hospitalization. Failure to improve with multiple fluid boluses should raise suspicion for concomitant problems, such as sepsis.

4. How are maintenance fluids determined in a child?

Maintenance fluids per hour are calculated based on weight in kilograms using the 4-2-1 rule: 4 mL/kg for the first 1–10 kg; an additional 2 mL/kg for the next 11–20 kg; and 1 mL/kg for every additional kg. For example, a 32-kg child should receive (4 mL/kg $\times$ 10 kg) + (2 mL/kg $\times$ 10 kg) + (1 mL/kg $\times$ 12 kg) = 72 mL/h of maintenance fluids.

5. Should children with vomiting receive antiemetics?

Children receiving oral rehydration therapy should receive an antiemetic medication. Ondansetron reduces vomiting, need for IV fluids, and hospital admission. It can be given orally via a pill, liquid, or disintegrating tablet. It is well tolerated by children of all ages, has a limited side-effect profile, and does not mask other diagnoses such as appendicitis or intussusception.

Young children that are not actively vomiting but refusing fluids may still be nauseated and benefit from ondansetron. Antiemetics such as metoclopramide, promethazine, and prochlorperazine should be used with caution, particularly in children under 5 years of age, who are more likely to experience adverse events.

6. What are the common causes of vomiting in children besides gastroenteritis?

The differential of isolated vomiting is extensive and includes urinary tract infection, appendicitis, pregnancy, diabetic ketoacidosis, otitis media, pneumonia, streptococcal pharyngitis, testicular or ovarian torsion, toxic ingestions, meningitis, and head injury. Do not assume vomiting without diarrhea always represents early gastroenteritis.

7. How do I differentiate between gastroenteritis and more severe abdominal pathology?

This may be difficult and often requires observing the child in the ED for other developing signs or symptoms. Red flags include bilious, bloody, or projectile emesis; focal tenderness in the abdomen; high fever; tachycardia that does not improve with rehydration; and vomiting without diarrhea.

Table 65.1 Differential of Nontraumatic Abdominal Pain by Age

Neonate	**2 Months to 2 Years**
Malrotation	Incarcerated hernia
Necrotizing enterocolitis	Intussusception
Testicular torsion (may be undescended)	Urinary tract infection
2–5 Years	**6–18 Years**
Appendicitis	Appendicitis
Foreign body	Ovarian/testicular torsion
Intussusception	Kidney and gallbladder stones
Ovarian torsion	Diabetic ketoacidosis
Urinary tract infection	Ectopic pregnancy
Streptococcal pharyngitis	Pelvic inflammatory disease
Henoch-Schönlein purpura	Gallbladder disease

8. **Are laboratory tests helpful in evaluating a child with dehydration or gastroenteritis?**
   Most patients require no tests. Laboratory test abnormalities may be present, but their clinical significance is questionable, as abnormalities typically resolve rapidly with oral rehydration. Ill-appearing infants may have depleted their glycogen stores and require bedside glucose testing. Electrolyte studies, looking for hypernatremia or renal insufficiency, should be reserved for ill-appearing children.

9. **What are the causes of infectious diarrhea?**
   Viruses cause 90% of diarrhea in children in the United States. Since the introduction of the rotavirus vaccine, norovirus is the most common pathogen. Viral diarrhea tends to produce voluminous watery diarrhea with diffuse abdominal cramping lasting for less than 1 week. Bacterial diarrhea typically causes lower abdominal pain and bloody or mucous stool. Parasites rarely cause diarrhea in immunocompetent children.

10. **Which children with diarrhea require diagnostic studies?**
    Most children do not require testing. Physicians should consider obtaining stool cultures from patients with significant comorbidities, ill appearance, bloody stools, severe cramping, recent antibiotic use (also obtain *Clostridium difficile* toxin assay), travel to a developing country, diarrhea lasting longer than 1 week (also obtain ova and parasite screen), exposure to a patient with a known bacterial diarrhea, or age <3 months with fever.

11. **What medications and diet should be prescribed for children with diarrhea?**
    Most cases of infectious diarrhea are self-limited, and drugs can be harmful. Antimotility agents may lead to central nervous system (CNS) depression or toxic megacolon. Antibiotics should not be administered empirically to well-appearing, healthy children. A recent randomized controlled trial demonstrated that probiotics do not impact severity or duration of symptoms for pediatric gastroenteritis. Children can eat solid foods. Lactose avoidance in young children may mitigate transient lactose intolerance.

12. **How does hemolytic uremic syndrome (HUS) typically present?**
    Within 1–3 weeks of a bloody diarrheal illness caused by enterohemorrhagic *Escherichia coli* or *Shigella dysenteriae,* children may develop **ART**:
    Anemia
    Renal failure leading to fatigue, pallor, and oliguria
    Thrombocytopenia
    Half of patients with HUS require dialysis and 5% die. Several studies suggest treatment with antibiotics when children have diarrhea caused by enterohemorrhagic *E. coli* may increase the risk of HUS.

KEY POINTS: DEHYDRATION AND GASTROENTERITIS

1. Vomiting in the pediatric population has a broad differential, and gastroenteritis should not be assumed.
2. Ill-appearing children require IV hydration and diagnostic testing, but most children can be successfully managed with ondansetron and oral rehydration only.
3. Diarrhea is typically caused by viruses, and even when there is concern for bacterial etiologies, antibiotics should not be given empirically to well-appearing children.

13. **How do I examine the abdomen of a crying child?**
    The abdominal examination can be difficult in young children but provides useful diagnostic information. First, it is helpful to determine if crying arises from anxiety or pain by observing the child from across the room while obtaining the history. A child who cries or lays still throughout the entire interview, despite soothing from a

caregiver, may have peritonitis. For the examination, begin with a part of the body that is not hurt and slowly progress to gentle palpation of the abdomen. Having the child flex their legs relaxes the abdominal muscles and facilitates the examination. If the child cries with palpation of the entire abdomen, it may be helpful to have the caregiver distract or hold the child. The caregiver can also be enlisted to palpate the abdomen to identify tenderness. Always examine the scrotum of young children with abdominal pain.

14. **Will opioids mask the examination for children with serious etiologies for their abdominal pain?**
No. Multiple studies have shown that diagnostic accuracy from physical examination increases when patients' pain is controlled. Opioids have been shown to improve the diagnostic accuracy of ultrasound.

15. **Does appendicitis present similarly in young and older children?**
Appendicitis is the most common atraumatic surgical emergency in children. Young children present atypically, leading to misdiagnosis and perforation in nearly all infants and half of preschool-age children. Young children may present with vomiting, abdominal pain, fever, diarrhea, irritability, or right hip pain. Similarly, young children's physical examinations commonly reveal diffuse abdominal tenderness or abdominal distention, whereas pain localized to the right lower quadrant is less common.

16. **What physical examination findings are found in older children with appendicitis?**
The most common findings are tenderness in the right lower quadrant over McBurney's point (two thirds of the distance along a line from the umbilicus to the anterior superior iliac spine). Rovsing sign (pain in the right lower quadrant with palpation of the left lower quadrant), obturator sign (pain with internal rotation of the flexed hip), and psoas sign (pain with extension of the right thigh) have not been shown to be particularly sensitive or specific for appendicitis in children.

17. **Do clinical prediction rules accurately identify appendicitis in children?**
The Alvarado Score, Low Risk Appendicitis Rule, and Pediatric Appendicitis Score do not perform better than experienced clinician judgment, but may be used with clinical judgment.

18. **Can the white blood cell count, C-reactive protein, or urinalysis be used to rule out appendicitis?**
Laboratory testing is of little value in the evaluation of appendicitis. A white blood cell (WBC) count of more than 10,000/mm^3 has a sensitivity of 88%, but a specificity of 53%; a WBC count of more than 15,000/mm^3 improves specificity to 60%, but the sensitivity declines to 19%. An elevated C-reactive protein (CRP) level has similar sensitivity and specificity to a WBC count of more than 10,000/mm^3. A positive urinalysis cannot exclude appendicitis; 30% of children with appendicitis have pyuria or bacteriuria.

19. **How does ultrasound help with evaluating children with potential appendicitis?**
Ultrasound (US) is the initial study of choice in children; it does not expose children to radiation and has high sensitivity (92%) and specificity (98%). False negatives may arise with obesity, <48 hours of symptoms, tip appendicitis, or atypical locations of the appendix. Accuracy is also operator dependent. EDs with limited pediatric US experience should consider transferring stable children with concern for appendicitis to centers with ultrasound expertise. There are several possible outcomes of ultrasound:
   • Appendicitis with an appendiceal diameter >6 mm, wall thickness >2 mm, obstruction of the appendiceal lumen, appendicolith, high echogenicity surrounding the appendix, or pericecal free fluid.
   • Identification of a normal appendix should prompt physicians to consider alternate etiologies for the patient's abdominal pain.
   • Nonvisualization of the appendix does not rule out disease; 10%–25% of these children will have appendicitis. These patients should be observed (in the ED or as outpatients) or undergo computed tomography (CT) or magnetic resonance imaging (MRI), depending on the level of concern. Patients with ongoing focal tenderness in the right lower quadrant should not be discharged without additional evaluation.

20. **What other imaging modalities can diagnose appendicitis?**
CT is more sensitive than US for appendicitis, but has higher cost, potential need for sedation, and radiation exposure. Oral contrast increases length of stay and patient discomfort without improving diagnostic accuracy and should not be routinely administered. A rapid-duration, limited MRI demonstrates similar diagnostic accuracy to CT, but has higher cost and may be more difficult to obtain. It is increasingly utilized as a radiation-free alternative to CT for patients with nondiagnostic ultrasounds.

21. **What is the treatment for appendicitis?**
Appendectomy: for uncomplicated appendicitis, laparoscopic appendectomy reduces the risk of postoperative wound infection and shortens recovery time compared with open appendectomy. In contrast, for perforated appendicitis, open appendectomy reduces the risk of postoperative abscess formation. With abscess formation, appendectomy is delayed until after a course of IV antibiotics. Broad-spectrum perioperative antibiotics should be administered in the ED, because they reduce the risk of operative complications. There is evidence that uncomplicated appendicitis may be managed nonoperatively with antibiotics. About 10% of children managed nonoperatively will have a recurrence of appendicitis, and the presence of an appendicolith increases this risk.

KEY POINTS: APPENDICITIS

1. Appendicitis is rare in young children. It presents atypically, resulting in increased frequency of misdiagnosis and perforation.
2. Laboratory tests are not helpful in evaluating a patient with appendicitis.
3. US should be the first imaging study in children with suspected appendicitis.

22. What is the classic triad for intussusception and how common is it?

Intussusception, an invagination of one portion of bowel into a distal segment (most commonly at the ileocecal junction), afflicts children most commonly between infancy and 3 years of age. The classic triad of colicky abdominal pain with the child pulling their knees up to their chest, vomiting, and bloody stool is present in less than 25% of children. Intermittent irritability is often the only symptom, and, on presentation, 30% of children will not have ongoing pain. Currant jelly stools are a late, rare, and ominous finding from bowel ischemia. Younger children may exhibit nonspecific findings, such as altered mental status or lethargy.

23. How do I diagnose intussusception?

US may identify a donut or target sign. With sensitivity and specificity of nearly 100%, it remains the initial test of choice. CT and abdominal x-ray should not be routinely employed to diagnose intussusception. Air enema may be utilized to both diagnose and treat intussusception.

24. How is intussusception managed?

Air enemas successfully reduce 90% of intussusceptions and provide less radiation exposure and lower risk of perforation compared with contrast enemas. Lower rates of successful reduction occur in: children <3 months and >5 years; symptoms lasting longer than 48 hours; hematochezia; or signs of obstruction on radiography. Inpatient observation after the procedure is not routinely required; it does not decrease rates of return to the hospital, recurrence, need for operative intervention, or mortality.

25. Why is bilious emesis in a neonate a surgical emergency until proven otherwise?

Bilious emesis in a neonate could represent malrotation with midgut volvulus. Congenital malrotation of the midgut predisposes the bowel to twisting on itself, leading to bowel obstruction and vascular compromise, with bowel necrosis of the entire involved segment developing in as little as 2 hours. All neonates with bilious emesis, irrespective of their appearance, require emergent pediatric surgical consultation.

Midgut volvulus classically presents with sudden onset of bilious emesis, abdominal pain, and later bloody stools; however, early in the course of illness, more than half of patients have only bilious emesis with normal abdominal examinations. Thus, all infants with bilious emesis should undergo diagnostic testing regardless of their abdominal examinations. Although plain radiography can show small bowel obstruction, a double-bubble sign, or paucity of distal bowel gas with volvulus, plain films are often normal and cannot be used to rule out disease. An upper gastrointestinal (UGI) series with contrast is the gold standard and will show a cork screwing of contrast or the duodenojejunal junction not crossing to the left of the vertebral column. If volvulus is suspected, IV fluids should be given, a nasogastric tube inserted, and broad-spectrum antibiotics administered. Patients require emergent surgical detorsion of the bowel.

26. What characteristics of a patient's history help differentiate pyloric stenosis from other causes of vomiting in infants?

True projectile emesis, where the vomitus shoots away from the patient, is most commonly found with pyloric stenosis. A hypertrophy of the pylorus develops between 2 and 8 weeks of age. Infants vomit at the end of feeds or within 30 minutes. Unlike more severe conditions, such as malrotation, emesis is usually nonbilious because the stenosis is proximal to the duodenum. In addition, the patient will remain hungry and continue attempting to feed. The classically described palpable "olive" on right upper quadrant examination arising from the hypertrophied pylorus is rarely identified early in the disease or when the child is awake.

27. What diagnostic findings arise with pyloric stenosis?

The diagnostic study of choice is a US, which has a sensitivity and specificity of nearly 100%. In pyloric stenosis, the pyloric wall is over 3 mm wide or over 12 mm long. If the US is equivocal, then obtain UGI radiography, which will show a string sign as contrast travels through the narrowed pylorus. Vomiting leads to loss of hydrogen ions from the stomach. The kidneys attempt to conserve sodium in a response to dehydration, spilling potassium into the urine, and resulting in a hypokalemic, hypochloremic metabolic alkalosis. Patients with pyloric stenosis require rehydration and surgical correction with pyloromyotomy.

28. What is the significance of air in the bowel wall visualized on plain radiographs of a neonate with vomiting?

Pneumatosis intestinalis, i.e., air in the bowel wall, is pathognomonic for necrotizing enterocolitis (NEC). NEC is much more common in premature neonates and often presents with vomiting and abdominal distention, while neonates are still in the NICU. If not treated, neonates may develop bowel necrosis and perforation. All neonates with concern for NEC should undergo plain radiography as well as acquisition of blood and urine cultures, emergent consultation with a pediatric surgeon, and empiric treatment with IV fluids and broad-spectrum antibiotics.

KEY POINTS: SURGICAL EMERGENCIES IN YOUNG CHILDREN

1. Intussusception often presents with only intermittent irritability or vomiting, and US is the diagnostic study of choice.
2. Bilious emesis in a neonate is a surgical emergency until proven otherwise, requiring a UGI radiographic series and surgical consultation.
3. Infants with pyloric stenosis have projectile nonbilious emesis but remain hungry and interested in feeding. US is the diagnostic study of choice.

29. **Why is jaundice concerning in a neonate?**
Jaundice becomes apparent when serum bilirubin exceeds 5 mg/dL. Although newborns often have physiologic jaundice that is self-limited, levels of unconjugated bilirubin >20 mg/dL can lead to bilirubin-induced neurologic dysfunction (BIND) and, long term, to kernicterus, with resulting deafness, developmental delay, or death. Elevated levels can arise from a myriad of causes, including Rh or ABO incompatibility, prematurity, polycythemia, intestinal obstruction, sepsis, or dehydration.

30. **Which patients with jaundice require laboratory evaluation?**
All patients with visible jaundice need measurement of bilirubin, and, if elevated, a fractionated level of direct and indirect bilirubin. For indirect hyperbilirubinemia, patients with jaundice in the first day of life, beyond the first week of life, with hepatomegaly, or who appear ill, require additional testing, including obtaining a blood type (child and mother), Coombs test, and complete blood count (CBC).

31. **Which patients with jaundice require treatment?**
Patients with elevated age-specific bilirubin levels above the threshold of American Academy of Pediatrics photo-therapy nomogram require phototherapy. Online calculators such as BiliTool (https://bilitool.org/) can help direct management. Healthy term infants, who are feeding well, with bilirubin levels 2–3 mg/dL below the threshold for hospital phototherapy, can receive home phototherapy. Treated infants have excellent prognoses. Exchange trans-fusion should be reserved for marked elevations (>25 mg/dL) or signs of encephalopathy.

32. **Will phototherapy help with a direct hyperbilirubinemia?**
Direct bilirubin itself is not toxic, and there is no role for phototherapy. However, elevation of direct bilirubin is always pathologic. It arises from sepsis or hepatic and biliary tree problems, including hepatitis, disorders of metabolism, and biliary atresia. Blood and urine cultures, liver function tests, and hepatic ultrasound should be obtained.

33. **What is the treatment of gastroesophageal reflux disease (GERD) in infants in the ED?**
GERD is a frequent cause of vomiting in infants. Standard ED management should focus on encouraging smaller, more frequent feeds followed by burping and maintaining the patient in a semi-upright or left lateral position after feeding. Ranitidine should not routinely be prescribed from the ED, as there is limited evidence it provides any benefit.

34. **Is it normal for a child to have constipation?**
It is normal for infants to strain during bowel movements and have varied amounts of time between bowel movements. Bottle-fed infants can often pass as few as one stool every other day. Breastfed infants may pass a stool with each feed or as infrequently as once every 7–10 days. As infants age, it is typical for stool frequency to decrease; by 4 years of age, children average 1.2 bowel movements per day. Constipation should not be diagnosed solely based on the frequency of stooling. Instead, the diagnosis of constipation should be based on difficulty or pain with passage of a hard bowel movement. This is complicated in infants, who normally cry and strain with stooling; in a healthy infant the stool should be soft.

35. **What are potential life-threatening causes of constipation in an infant?**
The most concerning cause is Hirschsprung disease, where contraction of a segment of the colon creates a blockage. Children often do not pass meconium within the first 24 hours of life. Rectal examination displays a tight anal canal with no stool. Diagnosis is made with a barium enema showing a transition zone in the bowel. Infants with Hirschsprung disease can develop megacolon, leading to enterocolitis with bowel perforation and sepsis. Hypothyroidism, diabetes insipidus, cystic fibrosis, and severe dehydration can also present with constipation in infants.

36. **What is the most common cause of constipation in school-age children?**
Functional constipation is the most common cause. Older children attempt to avoid stooling by tightening their buttocks. Stool remains in the rectum longer, leading to further absorption of water and creation of harder stool. This stool is painful to expel, encouraging the child to avoid stooling further. Eventually this causes rectal dilation and loss of the sensation of the need to defecate. Loose stool may then leak around the harder stool, leading to encopresis.

37. **What is the role of abdominal radiographs in the evaluation of constipation in a school-age child?**
Radiographs are not typically helpful, as they are not specific or sensitive. Children with no symptoms of constipation may have extensive fecal material on radiograph.

38. **How can you treat constipation in the ED?**
A trial of a soy-based formula may relieve constipation in infants with suspected cow's milk intolerance. In older infants and school-age children, prune, pear, and white grape juice can help soften stool. If this is not successful, polyethylene glycol (MiraLAX; 1 g/kg/day) or lactulose can be administered in the short term. A one-time glycerin suppository or enema can occasionally help relieve rectal impaction, but hypertonic phosphate enemas (Fleet) should only be administered to children over 1 year old. Soap suds and tap water enemas may cause water intoxication and should be avoided. Long-term management includes increasing fluid intake and adding fiber to the diet. Patients with severe constipation refractory to these measures may require hospital admission for more aggressive therapy.

40. **What are the most common causes of lower gastrointestinal bleeding in children?**
See Table 65.2.

41. **What foods can cause nonbloody red or black stools?**
Red stools are common after consumption of red drinks (Gatorade, Kool-Aid, etc.), beets, tomatoes, gelatin, and cefdinir. Black stools may arise after consumption of licorice, blueberries, grape juice, spinach, bismuth, and iron. Red meat, iron, broccoli, cauliflower, grapes, cantaloupe, and turnips may cause false-positive results on stool guaiac testing.

42. **What is a Meckel diverticulum?**
It is a remnant of the omphalomesenteric duct in children. It is the most significant cause of painless rectal bleeding in children and can lead to massive bleeding, diverticulitis, or intussusception. If suspected, a technetium-99m Meckel scan can identify the characteristic ectopic gastric mucosal tissue.

43. **How do I manage an ingested gastrointestinal foreign body?**
The management of foreign bodies depends on the foreign body and its location. Any patient with a known ingestion and hematochezia, melena, or signs of an acute abdomen requires immediate surgical consultation (Table 65.3).

44. **What are the possible complications of an esophageal foreign body?**
Airway obstruction, esophageal stricture, esophageal perforation, aorta-esophageal fistula, mediastinitis, or paraesophageal abscess can arise with esophageal foreign bodies.

Table 65.2 Differential of Lower Gastrointestinal Bleeding by Age

Neonate	**2 Months to 2 Years**
Swallowed maternal blood	Anal fissure
Allergic colitis	Allergic or infectious colitis
Infectious colitis	Intussusception
Volvulus	Meckel diverticulum
Necrotizing enterocolitis	Inflammatory bowel disease
2–5 Years	**6–18 Years**
Anal fissure	Anal fissure
Infectious colitis	Infectious colitis
Intussusception	Hemorrhoids
Polyps	Inflammatory bowel disease
Meckel diverticulum	Polyps
Inflammatory bowel disease	Angiodysplasia

Table 65.3 Management of Gastrointestinal Foreign Bodies

EMERGENT ENDOSCOPY	**CONSULTATION WITH GASTROENTEROLOGIST**
Sharp objects in the esophagus	Button battery past the esophagus
Button battery in the esophagus	Sharp objects past the pylorus
Objects causing difficulty controlling secretions or breathing	Long objects past the pylorus (>5 cm)
Objects in the esophagus for >24 hours	Multiple magnets

Table 65.4 Radiographic Findings in Pediatric Abdominal Pain

FINDING	RADIOGRAPHIC DESCRIPTION	DISEASE PROCESS
Double bubble	Paucity of gas with air bubble in stomach and duodenum	Volvulus
Crescent	Curvilinear mass often found near transverse colon beyond hepatic flexure	Intussusception
Pneumatosis intestinalis	Air in bowel wall	Necrotizing enterocolitis
Enlarged pylorus or gastric bubble	Wall of pylorus >4 mm thick Canal >14 mm	Pyloric stenosis

45. **How can I determine the location (trachea versus esophagus) of a coin in the pharynx?**
    Coins in the esophagus typically appear in the coronal plane (face on or round) on anteroposterior radiograph, whereas coins in the trachea appear in the sagittal plane ("on end"). However, this is not always accurate. If there is concern that the coin is in the trachea and operative intervention is intended, a lateral view should be obtained to confirm the tracheal position of the coin.

46. **Why is ingestion of a button battery or multiple magnets problematic?**
    Button batteries lodged in the esophagus may cause necrosis or perforation, and should be removed emergently. Button batteries are round, up to 20 mm in diameter, and thus may be similar in size to pennies and nickels. It is easy to confuse these objects on a radiograph. Unlike coins, button batteries are bilaminar and thus have a double ring or halo on a radiograph. On a lateral radiograph, button batteries have a step-off that is not present with coins.

    Magnets may be attracted across the bowel wall, leading to obstruction or perforation. Children who ingest multiple magnets require observation or endoscopic removal.

47. **What gastrointestinal diseases have classic radiographic finding?**
    See Table 65.4.

BIBLIOGRAPHY

Ferguson CC, Gray MP, Diaz M, et al. Reducing unnecessary imaging for patients with constipation in the pediatric emergency department. *Pediatrics.* 2017;140(1):e20162290.
Freedman SB, Parkin PC, Willan AR, et al. Rapid versus standard intravenous rehydration in paediatric gastroenteritis: pragmatic blinded randomised clinical trial. *BMJ.* 2011;343:d6976.
Freedman SB, Williamson S, Farion KJ, et al. Multicenter trial of a combination probiotic for children with gastroenteritis. *N Engl J Med.* 2018;379(21):2015–2026.
Huang L, Yin Y, Yang L, et al. Comparison of antibiotic therapy and appendectomy for acute uncomplicated appendicitis in children: a meta-analysis. *JAMA Pediatr.* 2017;171(5):426–434.
Litz CN, Amankwah EK, Polo RL, at al. Outpatient management of intussusception: a systematic review and meta-analysis. *J Pediatr Surg.* 2019;54(7):1316–1323.
Repplinger MD, Pichkardt PJ, Robbins JB, et al. Prospective comparison of the diagnostic accuracy of MR imaging versus CT for acute appendicitis. *Radiology.* 2018;288(2):467–475.
Steiner MJ, DeWalt DA, Byerley JS. Is this child dehydrated? *JAMA.* 2004;291:2746–2754.
Sturm JJ, Hirsh DA, Schweickert A, et al. Ondansetron use in the pediatric emergency department and effects on hospitalization and return rates: are we masking alternative diagnoses? *Ann Emerg Med.* 2010;55:415–422.
Williamson K, Sherman JM, Fishbein JS, et al. Outcomes for children with a nonvisualized appendix on ultrasound. *Pediatr Emerg Care.* 2018. doi:10.1097/PEC.0000000000001672.

CHAPTER 66

PEDIATRIC INFECTIOUS DISEASES

Joshua S. Easter, MD, MSc

1. **What are the stages of pertussis infection?**
   Pertussis presents in three stages:
   1. Catarrhal (1–2 weeks): cough and coryza are present, but there is no fever.
   2. Paroxysmal (2–8 weeks): prolonged bursts of coughing with minimal inspiratory effort in between coughs develop: 25%–75% of children display the classic whoop. Children may gag, vomit, or develop cyanosis.
   3. Convalescent (3 weeks–5 months): the cough gradually subsides.

2. **How does pertussis in infants compare to that in older children?**
   Children under 1 year of age only experience a brief catarrhal stage. Twenty-five percent of infants with pertussis experience complications, including apnea, pneumonia, and seizures. Given this risk, physicians should suspect pertussis in infants, particularly those with apnea, whooping, prolonged cough with paroxysms, or post-tussive emesis.

3. **How is pertussis diagnosed and treated?**
   Pertussis is a clinical diagnosis. Polymerase chain reaction (PCR) and culture of specimens obtained from the posterior pharynx provide confirmation of the diagnosis, but require several days to result. When given within 7 days of symptom onset, macrolides shorten the duration of illness and decrease infectivity. Antibiotics should not be held pending laboratory results. Infants under 4 months of age with high suspicion for pertussis should be admitted for observation. Older children should not return to school until they complete their antibiotic course.

4. **Should you administer antivirals to children with chickenpox?**
   Acyclovir should be reserved for adults or immunosuppressed children, who are at higher risk for severe disease. In healthy children, acyclovir decreases the duration of fever and number of lesions but does not reduce complications.

5. **How is mononucleosis diagnosed?**
   It is primary a clinical diagnosis with laboratory testing providing confirmation. The heterophile antibody test (monospot) provides excellent specificity and moderate sensitivity in older children. It has poor sensitivity in children <5 years of age, and Epstein-Barr virus (EBV) antibody titers should be obtained in these children.

6. **What are the concerning complications of mononucleosis?**
   Less than 0.2% of children will experience splenic rupture, which can be life threatening. Trauma increases the risk of rupture, and children with mononucleosis should refrain from contact sports for 3–4 weeks. Children can also develop airway obstruction and rarely encephalitis.

7. **Are steroids helpful for children with mononucleosis?**
   Studies report conflicting results about the benefit of steroids. Given their potential adverse effects, steroids should be reserved for patients with severe dehydration or airway obstruction.

8. **What emergent vasculitis should be considered in a child with fever for $\geq$5 days?**
   Kawasaki disease is a vasculitis of the small and medium-sized vessels, which may lead to the development of coronary aneurysms several weeks after the illness begins. These aneurysms may produce occlusion and myocardial infarction. Treatment with intravenous immunoglobulin (IVIG) and high-dose aspirin within 10 days of the onset of illness decreases aneurysm formation.

9. **Describe the clinical features of Kawasaki disease.**
   In addition to fever $\geq$5 days, children must display four of the five following features described by the CRASH mnemonic:
   1. **C**onjunctivitis: bilateral, nonexudative, bulbar conjunctival injection
   2. **R**ash: polymorphous, generalized rash
   3. **A**denopathy: cervical node >1.5 cm
   4. **S**trawberry tongue: pharyngeal erythema, or red and cracked lips
   5. **H**ands and feet: erythema and swelling

10. **What should you do if a child has $\geq$5 days of fever but only two or three clinical features of Kawasaki disease?**
    Children with <4 of the features may have incomplete Kawasaki disease and still develop coronary artery aneurysms. Children with <4 features but a C-reactive protein (CRP) >3 mg/dL or erythrocyte sedimentation rate (ESR) >40 mm/h should undergo echocardiography to identify coronary aneurysms as well as additional

laboratory work to identify other signs of Kawasaki disease, such as anemia, leukocytosis, thrombocytosis, hypoalbuminemia, sterile pyuria, or elevated alanine aminotransferase (ALT).

11. **Do infants with fever after receiving their vaccinations require diagnostic testing?**
While the risk of serious bacterial infection is lower in infants vaccinated within the past 24 hours, these infants still have significant risk of urinary tract infection (UTI) and should undergo, at minimum, urine catheterization. Although low-grade fever may persist beyond 24 hours after their vaccinations, because a high-risk population, these infants should be managed the same as infants that have not been recently immunized.

12. **How does the time of onset of neonatal conjunctivitis help predict the etiology?**
Table 66.1 describes the different forms of neonatal conjunctivitis.

13. **Which infectious rashes have characteristic appearances?**
Table 66.2 compares different rashes.

14. **What is the significance of a petechial rash in a child with fever?**
The combination of a fever and petechiae can arise with several emergent diseases, including meningococcemia, disseminated intravascular coagulation (DIC), Rocky Mountain spotted fever, pneumococcal bacteremia, or leukemia. A complete blood cell (CBC) count, CRP, coagulation studies, and blood culture should be obtained on nearly all children with fever and petechiae. Well-appearing patients with normal laboratory values can be discharged with close follow-up. Children with a single petechial lesion or petechiae distributed only above the nipple after coughing or vomiting are less likely to have serious bacterial infections and do not require testing, if they are well appearing.

15. **What potentially life-threatening infections present with maculopapular rash and fever?**
The differential includes measles, erythema multiforme, Kawasaki disease, Rocky Mountain spotted fever, ehrlichiosis, and dengue.

16. **What are the stages of measles?**
Measles has three primary stages:
1. Incubation (1–3 weeks): children are asymptomatic but become contagious at the end of this period.
2. Prodrome (2–4 days): fever, cough, coryza, and conjunctivitis predominate. At the end of this stage, most children develop Koplik spots, 1–3 mm white/gray spots on an erythematous base along the buccal mucosa, appearing similar to grains of salt on a pink surface.
3. Rash (4–7 days): the rash begins as an erythematous, maculopapular, blanching rash that begins on the head and spreads downwards. After 3–4 days, the rash darkens, then fades, and finally desquamates. Fever and infectivity resolve within 3–4 days of the onset of the rash. Persistent fever suggests a complication.

17. **What is the treatment for measles?**
Treatment is supportive, and well-appearing children can be discharged home. Isolate infected children from other people as much as possible for 4 days after their rash develops. Children may develop bacterial infections that require antibiotics, such as pneumonia, or other viral complications, including encephalitis.

18. **How do you differentiate between bacterial and viral parotitis?**
Most cases of parotitis in children arise from viral infections, including mumps, influenza, EBV, and adenovirus. Children with viral infections tend to present with several days of fever, malaise, and myalgias followed by parotid gland swelling. This swelling may start unilaterally but typically becomes bilateral. Treatment is supportive.

Table 66.1 Neonatal Conjunctivitis

	Age		
	<24 HOURS	1–5 DAYS	5–14 DAYS
Etiology	Reaction to erythromycin prophylaxis	*Neisseria gonorrhoeae*	*Chlamydia trachomatis*
Presentation	Mild injection	Copious discharge Chemosis	Moderate discharge
Diagnosis	Clinical	Nucleic acid amplification Gram stain and culture	Nucleic acid amplification Gram stain and culture
Treatment	None	Ceftriaxone Admission	Topical erythromycin Oral erythromycin once laboratory confirmed
Complications		Corneal ulcer Sepsis	Pneumonia Rare corneal scarring

Table 66.2 Infectious Rashes in Children

RASH	ETIOLOGY	CLASSIC APPEARANCE	ASSOCIATED FEATURES	TREATMENT
Bacterial				
Impetigo	Staph, Strep	Vesicles on face, rupture with golden crust	Well appearing	Mupirocin
Scarlet fever	Strep	Generalized, erythematous sand-paper rash, later desquamates	Circumoral pallor, strawberry tongue	Penicillin
Staphylococcal scalded skin	Staph	Diffuse blanching erythroderma not involving mucous membranes, later bullae that rupture		Nafcillin and vancomycin, IV fluids
Toxic shock syndrome	Staph	Diffuse erythroderma, later hands and feet desquamate	Ill appearing with fever	Clindamycin and vancomycin, IV fluids
Meningococcemia	*Neisseria meningitidis*	Petechiae, purpura	Ill appearing with fever	Empiric ceftriaxone
Viral				
Measles	Measles	Maculopapular rash spreads from face down, Koplik spots, later fades and desquamates	Cough, coryza, conjunctivitis, fever	None
Chicken pox	Varicella	Macules to papules to vesicles on erythematous base to crusting, spreads from scalp down, lesions in all stages	Fever, pruritus	None
Mononucleosis	EBV	Morbilliform on trunk and extremities	Palatal petechiae, exudative pharyngitis, lymphadenopathy	None
Hand, foot and mouth	Coxsackie	Vesicles on palate, uvula, later on hands, feet, and groin		Pain control, hydration
Rubella	Rubella	Maculopapular rash spreads from face down	Fever is rare	None
Erythema infectiousum	Parvovirus B19	Slapped cheek, then lacy rash on extremities		None
Exanthem subitum	Human herpes 6	Pink macules on trunk and spread peripherally	Fever prior to rash	None
Other				
Rocky Mountain spotted fever	*Rickettsia rickettsii*	Maculopapular rash on wrists and ankles, later petechiae and purpura	Fever, headache, myalgias	Doxycycline
Lyme disease	*Borrelia burgdorferi*	Large target lesion		Doxycycline
Ehrlichiosis	*Ehrlichia*	Nonspecific rash (can be petechiae) anywhere on body	Fever, arthralgia, altered mental status	Doxycycline

EBV, Epstein-Barr virus; *IV,* intravenous; *Staph, Staphylococcus; Strep, Streptococcus.*

Less commonly, bacterial infections may lead to parotitis. These children frequently have unilateral parotitis with purulence found at the exit of Stensen's duct along the buccal mucosa across from the second mandibular molar. Treatment of bacterial parotitis is with cephalexin or dicloxacillin.

19. **What are the complications of mumps?**
Most pediatric mumps infections resolve without issue. Children can develop orchitis, although this is more common in adults, or rarely, encephalitis or meningitis.

20. **Are mumps and measles still found in developed countries?**
Outbreaks are becoming more frequent in developed countries. Measles tends to afflict unvaccinated or partially vaccinated children between 1 and 5 years of age. Meanwhile, recent mumps outbreaks have afflicted both vaccinated and unvaccinated children.

21. **How does the presentation of rubella compare to measles?**
Both infections present with erythematous, maculopapular rashes that begin on the face and spread downwards. However, the rash of rubella spreads more rapidly. Patients with rubella may have tiny red macules on the soft palate but no Koplik spots. They do not appear ill.

22. **What patients are at increased risk of complications from rubella?**
In pregnant women, rubella increases the risk of fetal demise and congenital defects.

23. **What diagnostic studies should you obtain on patients with measles, mumps, or rubella?**
These viral infections are diagnosed clinically. Antibody or PCR testing can be utilized to confirm the diagnosis and are may be helpful from a public health perspective.

24. **What are the potential infectious etiologies of stridor?**
Table 66.3 describes diseases leading to stridor.

25. **What infectious diseases in children should be reported to the Department of Public Health?**
States have unique requirements for disease reporting. The Centers for Disease Control and Prevention (CDC) provides a list of reportable conditions, which includes, amongst others, botulism; diphtheria; ehrlichia; hepatitis; influenza leading to death; Lyme disease; malaria; measles; meningococcus; mumps; pertussis; rubella; salmonella; Shiga toxin–producing *Escherichia coli*; Rocky Mountain spotted fever; toxic shock; and varicella.

26. **Does administration of antibiotics before lumbar puncture impact the results?**
Prior antibiotic administration may lead to sterile cerebrospinal fluid (CSF) with negative Gram stain and culture within as little as 1 hour of antibiotic administration. Antibiotics do not normalize cell counts as quickly. Regardless, antibiotic administration should not be delayed for lumbar puncture in ill children.

27. **Are there any children with meningitis that can be safely discharged?**
Well-appearing children with viral meningitis can be discharged with close follow-up. The bacterial meningitis score indicates that patients with CSF pleocytosis but a peripheral absolute neutrophil count (ANC) <10,000 cells/μL, CSF

Table 66.3 Infectious Causes of Stridor in Children

	GROUP	BACTERIAL TRACHEITIS	RETROPHARYN-GEAL ABSCESS	EPIGLOTTITIS
Epidemiology	<6 years	<6 years	<4 years	6–12 years
Etiology	Viral	*Staph, Strep*	*Strep, Staph*	*Strep., Staph., H. flu*
Presentation	Barky cough Fever ±Stridor	Prior URI Stridor Respiratory distress	Fever Dysphagia Limited neck extension ±Stridor	Rapid onset Fever Dysphagia, drooling Stridor Tripod position
Neck radiograph findings[a]	X-ray not needed Steeple sign (sub-glottic tracheal narrowing)	Irregular margins of trachea below glottis	Widening of preverte-bral soft tissue (>7 mm at C2, or 14 mm at C7)	Thumbprint (swollen epiglottis)
Treatment	Dexamethasone Racemic epinephrine if stridor at rest	Position of comfort ORL/anesthesia to OR	Position of comfort ORL/anesthesia to OR	Position of comfort ORL/anesthesia to OR

[a]Diagnostic imaging should be deferred if it causes distress in toxic children, as this can lead to airway compromise.
H. flu, Haemophilus influenzae; OR, operating room; ORL, otorhinolaryngology; Staph., Staphylococcus; Strep., Streptococcus; URI, upper respiratory tract infection.

ANC <1000 cells/μL, negative CSF Gram stain, CSF protein <80 mg/dL, and no report of seizure have viral meningitis. This prediction model should not be applied to children that are ill appearing, received antibiotics prior to lumbar puncture, or are <2 months of age.

28. **How does otitis media present in children?**
Otalgia is the most common presenting complaint in children >2 years of age with otitis media. Younger children present with nonspecific symptoms such as irritability, fever, or ear pulling. On examination, children will also have a middle ear effusion, with opacification of the tympanic membrane, decreased mobility of the tympanic membrane, or an air-fluid level.

29. **What is "watchful waiting" for otitis media?**
The majority of cases of otitis media are caused by viruses and do not require antibiotics. Children >2 years of age with otalgia for <48 hours and temperature <39°C (102.2°F) can undergo watchful waiting. Children only receive antibiotics if they do not improve after a 48- to 72-hour period of observation, during which they receive ibuprofen or acetaminophen for pain and fever.

30. **How is the presentation of sepsis different in children than adults?**
Early signs of septic shock are more difficult to identify in children. Both children and adults with sepsis display tachycardia and tachypnea; however, these signs are less specific in children, who are often tachycardic and tachypneic with more benign febrile illnesses or anxiety. Children are also adept at maintaining their blood pressure until late in their illness. Finally, children more commonly develop cold shock with increased systemic vascular resistance, delayed capillary refill, and mottled extremities, compared to adults. As a result, physicians must remain vigilant in recognizing pediatric sepsis, relying on other signs such as altered mental status, delayed capillary refill, or poor skin turgor. Similar to adults, elevation of serum lactate is associated with development of organ dysfunction.

31. **Which children are most likely to develop sepsis?**
Nearly half of children that develop sepsis have a significant comorbidity; for example, chronic lung disease or congenital heart disease in infants; neuromuscular disease in older children; and cancer in adolescents. Children with these comorbidities also experience the greatest morbidity and mortality from sepsis.

32. **How should children with septic shock be managed?**
There are limited data in children to guide the treatment of septic shock, and most guidelines are extrapolated from adults. Early recognition and prompt administration of isotonic fluids and antibiotics are crucial. Guidelines now recommend epinephrine for cold shock and norepinephrine for warm shock, refractory to fluid resuscitation.

33. **Which children with influenza-like symptoms should undergo diagnostic testing to confirm the diagnosis?**
Children at high risk for complications from influenza should be tested with PCR or nucleic acid amplification tests, including children <5 years of age, receiving aspirin, or with significant comorbidities, such as asthma, congenital heart disease, sickle cell disease, cancer, diabetes, seizures, or developmental delay. In addition, testing should be performed if it will alter management; for example, obviate the need for a full sepsis workup or antibiotic administration. Testing is not helpful in otherwise healthy children with high pre-test probability of influenza. Rapid diagnostic tests with immunoassays have poor diagnostic accuracy and should not be routinely employed.

34. **Which children with influenza-like symptoms should receive antiviral treatment; that is, neuraminidase inhibitors?**
Children with severe disease requiring hospital admission or with the high-risk features described above as necessitating testing should receive antivirals. Limited evidence in children suggests that antivirals may reduce the duration of hospitalization and need for mechanical ventilation. For otherwise healthy children, the role of antivirals is unclear. Limited evidence suggests that they may reduce the duration of illness by 1–2 days when administered within 48 hours of symptom onset. However, they may induce a host of adverse effects, including neuropsychiatric events, arrhythmias, hypersensitivity reactions, and gastrointestinal upset.

KEY POINTS

1. Consider Kawasaki's disease in all children presenting with fever ≥5 days, as early recognition and treatment reduces morbidity from coronary artery aneurysm formation.
2. While tachycardia and tachypnea may be present with sepsis, they are also common in children with more benign, self-limited febrile illnesses.
3. Most viral illnesses, including influenza, can be diagnosed clinically. Diagnostic testing is appropriate when the results will alter management or impact public health (e.g., isolation of patients with highly virulent diseases).
4. Young infants with pertussis are at high risk of complications, such as apnea, and should be admitted to the hospital.
5. Outbreaks of measles and mumps are becoming more common, and these previously rare diseases should be considered.

BIBLIOGRAPHY

Abrams JY, Belay ED, Uehara R, et al. Cardiac complications, earlier treatment, and initial disease severity in Kawasaki disease. *J Pediatr.* 2017;188:64.

Cherry JD, Wendorf K, Bregman B, et al. An observational study of severe pertussis in 100 infants ≤ 120 days of age. *Pediatr Infect Dis J.* 2018;37:202.

Davis AL, Carcillo JA, Aneja RK, et al. American College of Critical Care Medicine clinical practice parameters for hemodynamic support of pediatric and neonatal septic shock. *Crit Care Med.* 2017;45:1061.

Evans IVR, Phillips GS, Alpern ER, et al. Association between the New York Sepsis Care Mandate and in-hospital mortality for pediatric sepsis. *JAMA.* 2018;320:358.

McCrindle BW, Rowley AH, Newburger JW, et al. Diagnosis, treatment, and long-term management of Kawasaki disease: a scientific statement for health professionals from the American Heart Association. *Circulation.* 2017;135:e927.

Phadke V, Bednarczyk R, Salmon D, et al. Association between vaccine refusal and vaccine-preventable diseases in the United States: a review of measles and pertussis. *JAMA.* 2016;315(11):1149–1158.

Ramaswamy KN, Singhi S, Jayashree M, et al. Double-blind randomized clinical trial comparing dopamine and epinephrine in pediatric fluid-refractory hypotensive septic shock. *Pediatr Crit Care Med.* 2016;17:e502.

Spurling GK, Del Mar CB, Dooley L, et al. Delayed antibiotic prescriptions for respiratory infections. *Cochrane Database Syst Rev.* 2017;9:CD004417.

Uyeki TM, Bernstein HH, Bradley JS, et al. Clinical practice guidelines by the Infectious Diseases Society of America: 2018 update on diagnosis, treatment, chemoprophylaxis, and institutional outbreak management of seasonal influenza. *Clin Infect Dis.* 2019;68(6):e1.

CHAPTER 67

EMERGENCY DEPARTMENT EVALUATION OF CHILD ABUSE

Daniel Lindberg, MD and Gunjan Tiyyagura, MD

1. **What is child abuse?**
   Per the Federal Child Abuse Prevention Treatment Act. 42, United States Code 5106g, it is "the physical or mental injury, sexual exploitation, negligent treatment, or maltreatment of a child by a person who is responsible for the child's welfare under circumstances which indicate harm or threatened harm to the child's health or welfare." Specific definitions of abuse can vary across cultures, since they are influenced by community norms and values. This definition distinguishes child abuse from maltreatment by someone without responsibility for the child (e.g., strangers). This distinguishes sexual abuse from rape and physical abuse from assault. While this distinction may have minimal impact on the medical evaluation of injured children, it can become important when it comes to reporting the situation to Child Protective Services (CPS) or law enforcement.

KEY POINTS

1. **Physical abuse** is any physical injury to a child as a result of acts (or omissions) on the part of the caregivers.
2. **Sexual abuse** is engaging any child in sexual activities that the child cannot comprehend, for which he or she is developmentally unprepared and cannot give informed consent, or which violate the sexual and legal taboos of society. This includes all forms of oral-genital, genital, or anal contact by or to the child. It also includes exhibitionism, voyeurism, and child pornography.
3. **Neglect** occurs when the child's basic needs are not met. This includes denial of basic needs such as medical/dental care, food, shelter, clothing, emotional support, education, or protection.
4. **Emotional abuse** is a repeated pattern of caregiver behavior that conveys to the child that he or she is worthless, flawed, unloved, unwanted, endangered, or only of value in meeting another's needs. This may include name-calling, intimidation, and harassment.

PHYSICAL ABUSE

2. **When should I think about physical abuse?**
   Physical abuse can be difficult to detect and is commonly missed. We recommend using a combination of **age** and **sentinel injuries** to prompt consideration of abuse.

   Age—serious physical abuse is most common in preverbal children <3 years old, and is dramatically increased for those <6 months old, where almost any injury should prompt consideration of abuse.

   Sentinel injuries—where the risk of abuse is high enough that screening should be considered in most cases, regardless of the history given, except in cases with obvious, severe, readily verifiable trauma such as a motor vehicle crash. Sentinel injuries are defined by age and include:

   - *For children <24 months old:* intracranial injuries such as subdural hematoma, subarachnoid hemorrhage, and cerebral contusion; intra-abdominal injury; rib fractures, or unexplained long-bone fractures; multiple fractures in different stages of healing; burns with an immersion pattern; bruising to the torso, ears or neck, frenulum injuries, bruising to the angle of jaw, cheeks, or eyelids or subconjunctival hemorrhages; or bruising that is in the shape of an implement or bite marks.
   - *For children <12 months old:* any of the injuries noted above, and any long-bone fracture or classic metaphyseal ("bucket-handle" or "corner") fracture.
   - *For children <6 months old:* any injury above and any oral injury or bruise.

   The **Pittsburgh Infant Brain Injury Score (PIBIS)** can improve recognition of subtle brain injuries in afebrile infants (31–364 days old) who present with nonspecific signs of head injury and no history of trauma. Nonspecific signs include:
   - vomiting without diarrhea
   - ALTE/BRUE
   - seizure-like activity
   - bruising or scalp swelling
   - neurologic symptoms such as lethargy, fussiness, or poor feeding

For children presenting with these complaints, the PIBIS score assigns 1 point for: age 3–12 months; head circumference >85th percentile; and hemoglobin <11.2; and 2 points for an abnormal cutaneous examination (like bruising). Children with scores ≥2 have a high rate of abnormal neuroimaging.

Other Factors
An approach based on sentinel injuries will not identify all cases of abuse, and you should consider other red flags, including:
- injury unexplained by history or inconsistent with child's developmental age;
- absent, changing, or evolving history;
- delay in seeking care with obvious signs of injury;
- unrealistic expectations, or negative descriptions of the child;
- multiple episodes of significant trauma or multiple injuries of different ages.

Social Factors
At a population level, poverty and other social factors such as substance use disorders, a nonrelated caregiver in the home, or signs of family stress have been associated with increased risk of abuse. Other factors such as the provider's affect, or their interaction with the child, have been suggested by some experts to aid in abuse recognition. While each of these things may be useful, data are spotty, none are particularly sensitive, and they may allow the introduction of racial or socioeconomic bias. The absence of these factors should not affect your treatment or workup.

3. **What about violence in a home?**
   Violence occurring within a family should be considered a sentinel injury for all other household members, and should trigger consideration and testing for physical abuse in a child. In a large multicenter study, approximately 12% of siblings or household contacts sharing a home with an abused child had occult injuries detected on skeletal survey. Many different types of violence are likely to co-occur with child physical abuse within a home (intimate partner violence, elder abuse, and animal abuse). Although there are no currently accepted screening recommendations when children are identified in homes with violence, these children deserve a thorough physical examination.

4. **Why do we do so much more testing for abusive injuries than we do for noninflicted trauma?**
   Unlike nonabusive trauma, it is important to identify abusive injuries to help protect a child from future abuse. Finding a grade I liver laceration is unlikely to help a child who was hit by a car; it is likely to heal on its own, and finding it doesn't prevent another car crash. But for an abused child, finding additional injuries can affect whether the offered history makes sense, and can improve the ability to protect the child (and others) from future abuse.

5. **When I'm concerned for abuse, what parts of the physical examination are most important?**
   All children with concern for abuse should have a careful physical examination, even though some injuries can be missed by even the best examination. The examination for abuse should include:
   - Oropharynx: examine the lips, frenula (labial and lingular), teeth, palate, tongue, and pharynx.
   - Ears: including inside and behind the pinna.
   - Fontanelle: when present. Look for bulging as a sign of increased intracranial pressure.
   - Eyes: look for subconjunctival hemorrhage, blue sclera, and retinal hemorrhages.
   - Skin: all the skin—all surfaces.
   - Genitalia: take off the diaper!
   - Growth chart: if available, especially the head circumference. Make sure to chart a good height, weight, and head circumference.

6. **Which kids need a skeletal survey?**
   A skeletal survey is a series of x-rays designed to identify occult fractures. To be effective, a skeletal survey requires more than 20 separate high-resolution films (at least two views of the skull and spine, anteroposterior [AP], lateral and obliques of the ribs, plus at least one view of the humeri, forearms, hands, femora, tibias, and feet), and should be interpreted by an experienced radiologist. A "babygram" (a single view of the baby's body, or a handful of films) is *not* an adequate skeletal survey. The skeletal survey should be routine for children <2 years old when there is concern for abuse, and many children up to 36 months old should have them when there is moderate or strong concern for abuse, or if there is moderate or strong concern for abuse, or if the child's communication or mobility is impaired. Skeletal surveys are not very useful in children over the age of 5 years, unless the child has decreased mobility or communication. A repeat skeletal survey in 2 weeks often shows healing fractures not seen acutely on the original skeletal survey.

7. **What are "classic" metaphyseal fractures?**
   Also called bucket handle, corner, or metaphyseal chip fractures, classic metaphyseal fractures in young children strongly suggest physical abuse. These fractures occur at the junction between the metaphysis and epiphysis, and they are caused by biomechanical forces rarely produced by accidental trauma in infants. They are thought to be caused by rotational or shearing forces (from shaking or pulling/twisting). No single fracture is pathognomonic for abuse, and nonabusive classic metaphyseal fractures have been described after difficult deliveries,

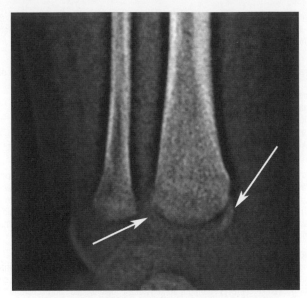

Fig. 67.1 Metaphyseal bucket-handle or corner fractures *(arrows).*

clubfoot surgery, and other events with significant traction on the limbs. Nevertheless, identification of a classic metaphyseal fracture should prompt a thorough evaluation for other signs of abuse (Fig. 67.1)

8. **Which kids need neuroimaging (computed tomography [CT] or magnetic resonance imaging [MRI])?**
Brain injuries are common in abused children, and can be easy to miss in the youngest ones. In children <6 months old who are being evaluated for physical abuse, occult brain injury occurs in 20%–35%. Neuroimaging should be obtained for infants <6 months and considered for infants <12 months who have:
- signs of head injury, bulging fontanelle, altered mental status, or seizure
- history of direct head trauma or being shaken
- facial bruising
- multiple fractures
- rib fractures
    CT is the most commonly used imaging technique, but MRI is a reasonable alternative if there is a concern for radiation. Ultrasound is not an acceptable substitute.

9. **Which kids need dilated retinal examination?**
Children with head injuries and concern for abuse should have a retinal examination by an ophthalmologist. In children with negative neuroimaging (or an isolated simple skull fracture), a retinal examination is not required. While it is noninvasive to look at a child's retina, significant retinal hemorrhages are rare for children without brain injury.
Note: The converse is not true—a retinal examination should not be used to determine which children need neuroimaging; an important fraction of children with abusive head trauma have no retinal hemorrhages.

10. **Which children need screening for occult abdominal injury?**
Clinical signs (abdominal bruising or tenderness) are very specific, but not sensitive for abdominal injuries. We recommend obtaining aspartate aminotransferase (AST) and alanine aminotransferase (ALT) levels for all children with concern for physical abuse and a significant injury (e.g., a long-bone fracture), and an abdominal CT for children where the AST or ALT is >80 IU/L, or for those with abdominal bruising, tenderness, or distention, or with a report of abusive abdominal trauma. The yield of CT using this protocol is >20%, and outweighs the risk from radiation. AST and ALT normalize over hours or days, regardless of whether an injury is present, so rechecking these tests is not a good alternative. Ultrasound has limited sensitivity and should not be used in place of CT.

11. **What are the most common myths about physical abuse?**

    Myth #1: Spiral fractures are especially concerning for abuse.
    Spiral fractures imply a twisting or torqueing force about the axis of the bone, but are not more concerning than other fracture morphology. In fact, one of the most common accidental fractures (the toddler's fracture) is often a

spiral fracture of the proximal tibia. Age, history, and mechanism can help guide decision making about accident versus abuse.

Myth #2: A bruise's age can be determined by its color.
While this is biochemically intuitive, it's just not true. In fact, when it was studied, providers often don't even agree on what colors are present in a bruise. Differences in a bruise's location, depth, and the patient's complexion may account for this. Providers are notoriously bad at estimating a bruise's age, so be careful if you write that in the chart.

Myth #3: Mixed-density subdural hematomas (SDHs) imply multiple episodes of trauma.
While this has been commonly believed, more recent data suggest it is also just not true. Studies of children who have SDH as a result of motor vehicle collisions show that mixed-density (bright and dark blood) subdurals can occur after a single episode of trauma. This might be because the cerebrospinal fluid (CSF) mixes with the blood, or because there is an area of hyperacute bleeding. Whatever the reason, avoid speculating about the age of a subdural based on its CT density alone.

12. **Which conditions can mimic injuries seen in child abuse?**
    - *Accidental injuries*: obtain a detailed history and check for signs of other injuries.
    - *Coagulation disorders*: start with a prothrombin time/partial thromboplastin time (PT/PTT) and platelets if bruises, retinal hemorrhages, and intracranial bleeding are key injuries.
    - *Birth trauma*: the clavicle and skull are most commonly injured during delivery; delivery-associated fractures usually have radiologic healing by 10 days.
    - *Cardiopulmonary resuscitation (CPR)*: rarely causes rib fractures or minor intrathoracic injury and very rarely causes posterior rib fractures; also, uncommonly causes retinal hemorrhages.
    - *Osteomyelitis*: can look a lot like a metaphyseal fracture. Obtain an MRI if a child with odd fractures or possible classic metaphyseal fracture has a fever—even a mild fever.
    - *Bone fragility syndromes* (e.g., osteogenesis imperfecta, rickets, osteopenia of prematurity, Menkes disease): start with calcium, phosphorus, 25OH vitamin D if fractures are the key injuries. Do an examination to look for blue sclera or sparse, fragile hair.
    - *Collagen disorders* (e.g., Ehlers-Danlos): a good physical examination and family history helps rule these out.
    - *Other dermatologic conditions* (e.g., purpurae/petechiae from infection, congenital dermal melanocytosis): bruises should quickly evolve and fade over a matter of days, while other "birthmarks" should be more stable.
    - *Phytophotodermatitis*: looks like a severe burn, but this condition is caused in some people when citrus/plant juices on the skin are exposed to the sun. Get a good history.
    - *Healing practices* (e.g., coining, cupping): these are more common in textbooks than real life these days, but (you knew this was coming), get a good history.

13. **What about an infant who presents dead on arrival without external signs of injury?**
    Any child who presents in this way should be termed an unexplained infant death and should be referred to the coroner's office for further evaluation and investigation. Once a thorough assessment (including a complete autopsy, a review of clinical history, and a death scene investigation) is completed and does not uncover another cause of death, the death may be ruled a sudden unexplained death in infancy (SUDI). This term has largely replaced sudden infant death syndrome (SIDS). The family should still be treated with respect and compassion, as further information may not uncover any other cause for the death or the cause may be a previously unidentified medical illness.

14. **What should I do about siblings and other children in the home?**
    Violence is often a disease that affects the entire household. Routinely ask whether other children share the home of a child with high levels of concern for abuse. For children <24 months old who share a home with a child where there is a high level of concern for abuse and at least one serious injury (fracture, brain injury, etc.), a skeletal survey is recommended. Older children may benefit from a physical examination or interview. CPS can assist with arranging examinations of other children if they do an evaluation of the home.

15. **How do I broach this topic with caregivers?**
    Many clinicians are hesitant to raise their concern for abuse with parents or caregivers, especially since initial information is always limited, and when these caregivers seem caring and sympathetic. Use a nonjudgmental and transparent approach, and avoid accusatory language—after all, your ability to determine the perpetrator of any abuse is extremely limited. When there is concern for abuse, the goals of testing are to identify occult injuries as well as other, nonabusive explanations for concerning findings. One approach is to say: "We have identified [concerning finding] in [the child]. Based on the history we have so far, this is unexpected, and we need to be sure that we are not missing something else that could explain it, like more serious trauma, or a rare medical condition. Whenever we see this, we perform [recommended tests] to be sure we are not missing something that we would need to do to prevent a bad outcome."

SEXUAL ABUSE

16. **If a child has not reported sexual abuse, what should make me think about it?**
   Most ED evaluations for sexual abuse are the result of concern by a caregiver or a report of abuse by the child. However, the possibility of abuse should also be considered for children who present with:
   - genital injury or bleeding (excluding hemorrhagic cystitis in a child with a urinary tract infection);
   - genital discharge;
   - new behavior changes (enuresis, nightmares, behavioral regression, mood swings);
   - siblings or other children who share a household with another child who has been sexually abused;
   - sexualized behaviors—while several surprising behaviors (touching genitals, masturbating, even in public) are actually often normal in children, asking to engage in sexual acts, inserting objects into the genitalia, imitating intercourse, touching animal genitals, or behavior that is persistent, resistant to distraction, or that causes emotional or physical distress are abnormal and should prompt concern for abuse.

17. **When there is a report of abuse, how should I take a history?**
   In order to be useful for medical and legal purposes, forensic interviews require training, experience, and ongoing peer review beyond the resources of most emergency physicians. However, it is appropriate to obtain a history from the child's caregiver separated from the child to determine the reason for the concern and how (and if) the concept of abuse was raised to the child. Most emergency physicians should limit questioning of the child to the information necessary to determine if there is a need for acute intervention: Is the child in pain? Are there other symptoms or signs of infection or injury? Is there recent contact and possible body fluid exposure prompting need for evidence collection or infection/pregnancy prophylaxis? Providers should familiarize themselves with local processes and resources where a full forensic interview may be obtained later (e.g., child abuse team at a referral center, CPS, and/or children's advocacy center). A spontaneous outcry of abuse by the child should be carefully documented, using the child's own words whenever possible.

18. **How should I question a child in order to obtain history and direct my evaluation?**
   Questioning should be based upon the developmental abilities of the child. Interviews are rarely possible with children <3 years old. Children <6 years old frequently have the most difficulty with "when" questions, but do better with "what" or "who" questions. For example, a 5-year-old child will be unlikely to tell you that an assault happened on Saturday, but would be more likely to tell you that it happened at their friend's birthday party, or that the football game was on television at that time. Questioning should take care to use concepts and vocabulary familiar to the child, and should emphasize open-ended, nonleading questions. Providers may find it helpful to ascertain the child's vocabulary for genitalia and other body parts.

19. **Which children need a genital examination immediately?**
   Children with acute physical complaints in the setting of possible sexual abuse (bleeding, pain, dysuria, hematuria, discharge, etc.) or those who report sexual abuse within the past 72 hours should have an examination at the time of presentation. Other children are unlikely to have acute findings and could reasonably be referred for examination in a clinic setting by a child abuse pediatrician, child advocacy center, or their primary care physician. *Never* force a genital examination on a resistant child. For children with concern of major, acute injury (substantial bleeding, ill appearing), arrange for an examination under sedation or anesthesia.

20. **How should I do the genital examination?**
   Most children do not find genital examinations to be uncomfortable. Integrating the examination into the rest of the physical examination and using a matter-of-fact tone can reassure the child. Helpful phrases: "I am going to check all of your body from the tip of your head to the tip of your toes and all your parts in between" and "This is OK because I'm a doctor, and because mom is here and because mom says it is OK."
   Most examinations can be completed in the supine frog-leg position with heels together and knees on the table. Many small children are more comfortable in their parent's lap. For girls, grasp the labia majora between the thumb and the distal interphalangeal joint of the index finger. Pull the labia towards yourself (as opposed to pulling laterally) with the same amount of force one would use to retract someone's lip or cheek to examine their teeth. By convention, findings are described using a clock face, where the navel is at 12 o'clock and the anus is at 6 o'clock. Prepubertal children will have a hymen that is smooth and thin. This tissue is exquisitely sensitive, and the examiner should take care not to contact it with swabs, probes, or other foreign bodies. The speculum is rarely useful in the forensic medical examination and should *never* be used for the prepubertal child without anesthesia. By contrast, pubertal children will have a thickened, redundant hymen that is less sensitive to contact. A cotton-tipped swab can be used to move the redundant hymen and examine all areas for bleeding, lacerations, or abrasions. Some providers recommend a few drops of saline to "float" the hymen and facilitate the examination (Fig. 67.2).

21. **What examination findings are most significant for sexual abuse?**
   In most cases, the history given by the child, a witness to the sexual abuse, or evidence found at the scene will be the determinative factor for the confirmation of sexual abuse. Even in cases where abuse has occurred, the vast majority of examinations, especially outside of the acute phase, will be normal or include normal variants. In this situation, the documentation can reflect "a normal examination does not rule out sexual abuse." In the

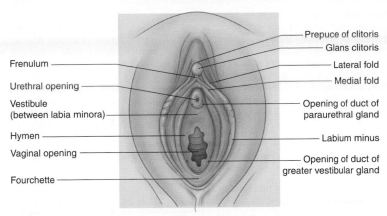

Fig. 67.2 Normal female genitalia anatomy. (From Padmanbhan P. 108 – Surgical, radiographic, and endoscopic anatomy of the female pelvis. In: Peters, CA, Kavoussi LR, Dmochowski RR. *Campbell-Walsh-Wein Urology*. 3-volume set, 12th ed. Elsevier; 2021: Fig. 108.14.)

emergency setting, it is most important to note acute bleeding, contusion, or abrasion of the genitalia or anus. In this situation, if a child abuse specialist or team is available, they should be contacted for further documentation and assistance. Other non-acute findings, such as hymen transections, should be referred to a regional child abuse specialist to be seen nonacutely. No finding can conclusively differentiate between consensual and abusive sexual activity (in patients capable of providing consent).

22. **How can a child who has been sexually abused have a normal examination?**
This question comes up a lot, and some caregivers are reluctant to say it out loud, so you might say it proactively. There are several reasons that the vast majority of sexually abused children (including 90% of pregnant adolescents in one series) have normal genital examinations.
- Mucosal tissues heal quickly. Think how long it takes for your cheek to return to normal when you accidentally bite it.
- Mucosal tissues stretch. The anus, for example, is commonly able to pass large stool without becoming abnormal on examination.
- Some abusive activities are unlikely to affect the tissue. Rubbing a child's genitals over their clothes is certainly abusive, but unlikely to change the tissue.

23. **Which children need evidence collection (rape kit)?**
- Child victims need a full physical examination (looking for trauma) and possibly evidence collection, depending on the incident. Children with history of sexual contact in the last 72–120 hours that may have included secretion of bodily fluids (saliva, semen, blood) should be offered the chance for evidence collection. This time window depends on the policies and practices used by the forensic laboratory in each jurisdiction, and may extend to 7 days. Eligible children should have evidence collected as soon as possible, as the utility of the kit decreases within the time window. State laws inform practice related to who should consent for forensic evidence collection (patient or caregiver). However, no patient should ever be forced against his/her will to undergo sexual assault evidence collection.
- Young children rarely need a full rape kit performed, and collection should be specific to the allegation and examination and guided by an expert team to minimize further trauma to the child. The highest yield component of the kit is the child's undergarments (even if they are not the same as the garments worn at the time of the assault). Some children who do not assent to the kit as a whole may consent to collection of their undergarments.

24. **Which children need testing for sexually transmitted infections (STIs)?**
Because the presence of an STI can dramatically affect the recognition of sexual abuse, testing for gonorrhea or *Chlamydia* is recommended for prepubertal children with discharge and pubertal children in whom a genital examination is undertaken. Additional testing for hepatitis B and C (HBV and HCV), HIV, and syphilis may be considered. Testing is especially useful with:
- a history of multiple assailants;
- known disease or risk factors in the assailant;
- acute physical findings;
- known disease in another child suspected to have been abused by the same perpetrator;
- presence of another sexually transmitted infection (even those that are less specific, such as human papillomavirus [HPV] or herpes simplex virus [HSV]);
- patient or parental concern.

Nucleic acid amplification tests (NAATs; e.g., amplicon or Gen-Probe) using "dirty catch" urine have been shown to have increased sensitivity relative to culture and are much easier to obtain in toilet-trained children.

25. **Which children need empiric treatment for STIs?**
While empiric/prophylactic treatment for gonorrhea and *Chlamydia* is reasonable for many adolescents and young adults, *do not* empirically treat prepubescent children for gonorrhea or *Chlamydia*. Whereas early treatment can prevent ascending pelvic infections (e.g., pelvic inflammatory disease [PID], tuboovarian abscess) in older children, physiologic differences make these ascending infections rare in prepubescent children and empiric treatment may eliminate the chance to complete confirmatory or repeat testing which may be needed in high-stakes decisions about the child's safety or custody if initial test results are inconclusive.

Post-exposure prophylaxis (PEP) for HIV is more complicated. The risk of transmission of HIV by sexual abuse is currently unknown, and depends on the specific factors related to the child, the assailant, and details of the assault. It is reasonable to consult with a child abuse specialist/team and/or infectious diseases before initiating PEP in the setting of a possible sexual assault. In the United States, the Centers for Disease Control and Prevention (CDC) has established a 24-hour hotline for post-exposure prophylaxis (PEPline: 1-888-HIV-4911 [888-448-4911] that can give expert advice about the need for PEP for HIV, hepatitis B, and hepatitis C.

26. **Which children need pregnancy testing/prophylaxis?**
Pubertal children who have experienced sexual assault within 120 hours (5 days) should be offered pregnancy prophylaxis using levonorgestrel (Plan B) 1.5 mg or ulipristal (Ella) 30 mg as a single dose. A repeat dose may be used if vomiting occurs within 2 hours. A pregnancy test should be obtained in pubertal or near-pubertal victims of sexual assault. Because the mechanism of action is suppression of ovulation, patients may be reassured that these treatments do not terminate established pregnancies. In the United States, levonorgestrel can be obtained over the counter by women 17 years of age and older, but ulipristal requires a prescription.

27. **What should ED providers do when caring for victims suspected of being trafficked?**
Human trafficking/commercial sexual exploitation impacts children around the world and places victims at substantial risk for physical and psychologic injury. Medical providers may encounter adolescent victims in EDs where they may seek care for various problems like sexual assault, trauma, infection, mental health problems, or reproductive care. Though victims rarely self-identify as being trafficked and most have no obvious indicators, a history of running away from home, truancy, child maltreatment, involvement with CPS or the law enforcement system, multiple sexually transmitted infections, pregnancy, or substance use places youth at higher risk.

Evaluation can be challenging but should include a complete history related to injuries/abuse, reproductive issues, substance use, and mental health symptoms conducted in a nonjudgmental and empathic manner. Helpful questions include:
1. Has anyone ever asked you to have sex in exchange for something you wanted or needed (e.g., money, food, expensive presents)?
2. Has anyone ever asked you to have sex with another person?
3. Has anyone ever taken sexual pictures of you?

Many states consider human trafficking to be child maltreatment and providers must refer to CPS in these cases. In states where trafficking is not considered maltreatment, providers can contact national trafficking organizations, law enforcement, or local child advocacy centers for additional help.

28. **Which findings can mimic sexual abuse?**
A broad range of infectious and inflammatory diseases and normal variants can cause genital findings in children and raise the concern for sexual abuse. Among the most common are:
- In boys who stand to urinate, a falling toilet seat can cause bruising to the tip of the penis that may mimic a bite mark.
- In children, excessive or colored (e.g., yellow or green) vaginal discharge should prompt concern for sexual abuse, but bacterial infections (e.g., *Streptococcus, Escherichia coli, Enterococcus, Salmonella,* among many others), yeast, foreign bodies, or poor hygiene can also cause discharge.
- In children, mild erythema in the genital area or urinary tract infections are nonspecific findings and may be related to common issues such as bathing, improper wiping, and poor hygiene.
- Vaginal ulcers or vesicles can prompt a concern for HSV, but also can result from Epstein-Barr virus (EBV), cytomegalovirus (CMV), inflammatory bowel diseases, or vaginal aphthosis.
- Straddle injuries can cause bruising and abrasion to the external genitalia, or to the area between the labia majora and minora, but rarely cause injury to the hymen, fossa navicularis, or internal genitalia.
- Urethral prolapse can cause dysuria and vaginal bleeding. The genital examination should always take care to visualize the urethral orifice to determine if the mucosa appears beefy red and inflamed.
- Venous pooling about the perianal plexus is commonly interpreted as bruising. This finding should rapidly resolve over a few minutes, especially if the patient defecates.

29. **What information should I give to parents?**
Concern for sexual abuse can result in information overload for a caregiver. Parents may be unable or reluctant to ask some basic questions. Anticipatory guidance or discharge instructions might emphasize the following information:
- Parents should not attempt to perform their own forensic interview, since this can interfere with other investigations. Parents should, however, create a safe and open atmosphere if the child approaches them about the

event. Outcomes have been shown to be improved for children with at least one caregiver who believes and supports them.
- In the vast majority of cases, the genital examination will be normal, will have normal variants, or will show findings that will heal completely. In these cases, it is helpful to inform the patient and caregiver that they are completely normal and healthy, and that, even when the examination does not prove that abuse has occurred, it certainly doesn't exclude the possibility of abuse either.
- Many caregivers are worried about whether their child is still a virgin—even if they are reluctant to ask the question. In addition to the advice above, we find it useful to share our belief that a person stops being a virgin when they *choose* to have sex.
- Provide contact information to local CPS and/or child protection teams. If counseling referrals are not available through the ED, parents may be counseled to discuss this with their primary care physician or child protection team.

REPORTING CONCERNS FOR CHILD ABUSE

30. How reliable is a child's disclosure of physical or sexual abuse?
ED providers should take children's disclosures of abuse seriously. Assume the child is telling the truth and respond accordingly. The health care provider's job is to notify authorities for suspicion of abuse, not to judge or prove a child is being abused. It is seldom possible, and never necessary to conclusively determine whether abuse has occurred during an ED visit.

31. When should I report my concerns to CPS?
In the United States, physicians have a legal mandate to report any reasonable concern for child maltreatment to public CPS agencies. The definition of a "reasonable concern" for child maltreatment is not black and white, and doctors who consider and reject the diagnosis of abuse are not mandated to report. In some cases, a physician may be faced with a high level of parental concern for abuse, despite a lack of other signs of abuse on their own history, examination, or testing. In these situations, it is important to remember that CPS reports may be made by anyone, not just physicians. Doctors who do not feel that they have identified a reasonable concern for abuse might provide CPS contact information to concerned parents.

32. How do I go about reporting?
Each jurisdiction has a different procedure for reporting concerns for child maltreatment, but in most cases, a report involves a phone call to a public hotline, followed by a written summary of the key information that caused concern for abuse. Because the hotline will have to determine the jurisdiction of the case, doctors may need the following information at the time of the report:
- Child's identifying information (name, birthdate, address)
- Parent/caregiver's information (names, birthdates, addresses, phone numbers)
- Location of the alleged abuse (if known)
- Any information about the alleged perpetrator (name, address, age)
- Presence of other children in the home or exposed to the alleged perpetrator

33. Can I be sued for reporting when the child is not found to be abused?
The Federal Child Abuse Prevention and Treatment Act (CAPTA) provides immunity from civil and criminal liability for those making reports in good faith. Remember that failure to find sufficient evidence to prosecute does not necessarily mean the physician's suspicions were incorrect. Privacy laws, specifically *Health Insurance Portability and Accountability Act* (HIPAA), provide specific exemptions for sharing information specific to the situation while making a good faith report to authorities. Researchers operating under a certificate of confidentiality are usually not exempt from the duty to report reasonable concerns for child maltreatment. For more information on local and national resources for reporting, responding to, and preventing child abuse, visit the Child Welfare Information Gateway website (http://www.childwelfare.gov/index.cfm), a service of the Children's Bureau, Administration for Children and Families, US Department of Health and Human Services.

KEY POINTS

1. This highest risk for physical abuse is in children who are not old enough to provide their own history (<3 years old), especially in children who are immobile (<6 months old).
2. Obtain a skeletal survey for children <2 years old with concern for physical abuse. If your center does not routinely perform skeletal surveys, this may require transfer.
3. *Never* force a genital examination on a reluctant child. The vast majority of examinations will be normal, even when abuse has occurred.
4. Do not give empiric treatment for gonorrhea or *Chlamydia* in prepubertal children. Wait until the diagnosis has been confirmed.
5. Whenever there is a reasonable concern for abuse, US physicians have a legal mandate to report these concerns to CPS.

BIBLIOGRAPHY

Berger RP, Fromkin J, Herman B, et al. Validation of the Pittsburgh Infant Brain Injury Score for abusive head trauma. *Pediatrics.* 2016;138(1): e20153756.

Crawford-Jakubiak JE, Alderman EM, Leventhal JM, et al. Neglect, committee on a care of the adolescent after an acute sexual assault. *Pediatrics.* 2017;139(3):e20170958.

Flaherty EG, Perez-Rossello JM, Levine MA, et al. Evaluating children with fractures for child physical abuse. *Pediatrics.* 2014;133(2): e477–e489.

Kaltiso SO, Greenbaum VJ, Agarwal M, et al. Evaluation of a screening tool for child sex trafficking among patients with high-risk chief complaints in a pediatric emergency department. *Acad Emerg Med: Official J Soc Acad Emerg Med.* 2018. doi:10.1111/acem.13497.

Kellogg ND, Committee on Child Abuse and Neglect, American Academy of Pediatrics. Clinical report – the evaluation of sexual behaviors in children. *Pediatrics.* 2009;124(3):992–998.

Kleinman PK, Di Pietro MA, Brody AS, et al. Diagnostic imaging of child abuse. *Pediatrics.* 2009;123(5):1430–1435.

Levin AV, Christian CW. The eye examination in the evaluation of child abuse. *Pediatrics.* 2010;126(2):376–380.

Lindberg DM, Beaty B, Juarez-Colunga E, et al. Testing for abuse in children with sentinel injuries. *Pediatrics.* 2015;136(5):831–838.

Sheets LK, Leach ME, Koszewski IJ, et al. Sentinel injuries in infants evaluated for child physical abuse. *Pediatrics.* 2013;131(4): 701–707.

Wood JN, Fakeye O, Feudtner C, et al. Development of guidelines for skeletal survey in young children with fractures. *Pediatrics.* 2014;134(1):45–53.

Wooten-Gorges SL, Soares BP, Alazraki AL, et al. ACR Appropriateness Criteria (R) Suspected Physical Abuse-Child. *J Am Coll Radiol.* 2017;14(5S):S338–S349. doi:10.1016/j.jacr.2017.01.036.

CHAPTER 68

PROCEDURAL SEDATION AND ANALGESIA OF THE PEDIATRIC PATIENT

Chelsea McCullough, MD, MPH and Sasha Gubser, MD, MPH

1. Why is it called procedural sedation and analgesia (PSA)?

What used to be called *conscious sedation* is now more accurately referred to as *PSA*. This is described as using sedatives, dissociative agents, and analgesics alone or in combination to assist patients in tolerating unpleasant procedures, while maintaining cardiorespiratory function. An analgesic treats pain, whereas a sedative or anxiolytic relieves fear and anxiety. Some analgesics, particularly opioids, have sedative and analgesic properties, which make them useful in certain procedures. If a procedure is painful and frightening (e.g., fracture reduction), the child would benefit from both sedation and analgesia.

2. Do I need sedation and analgesia when performing procedures on children?

Frightening or painful procedures can be better tolerated by children with the use of sedatives or analgesics, but not all patients need both. These procedures include reduction of fractures or dislocations, laceration repair, incision and drainage of abscesses, burn care, examinations after sexual assault, and diagnostic procedures, such as lumbar puncture, computed tomography (CT), or magnetic resonance imaging (MRI). Systemic sedatives or analgesics may not be needed in older children who can remain calm, or in situations where local anesthetics provide adequate pain control. A comforting staff or family member can be essential to the success of the procedure. Many EDs have also employed child life advocates for this very purpose.

KEY POINTS: WHAT PSA DOES

1. Relieves fear and anxiety.
2. Provides needed analgesia.
3. Provides amnesia for an unpleasant procedure.
4. Facilitates timely and optimal outcome of the procedure.
5. Provides a standard of care now expected and appreciated by most parents.

---

3. What are the different levels of sedation?

- *Analgesia* is the relief of pain without intentionally producing a sedated state. Depending on the medication and dosage used, alteration in mental status may occur as a secondary effect.
- *Minimal sedation (anxiolysis)* refers to a drug-induced state in which patients respond normally to commands, but may have mild impairment of coordination or cognitive function. Patients receiving anxiolysis may better tolerate a procedure about which they are scared or nervous, and may have partial or total amnesia to the event when asked about it in the future.
- *Moderate sedation/analgesia,* previously considered *conscious sedation,* is a drug-induced, depressed level of consciousness in which patients respond purposefully to verbal or light tactile stimulation while protecting their airway reflexes. The child is still awake but with droopy eyes and slurred speech. No intervention is needed to maintain the child's airway.
- *Deep sedation/analgesia* is a depressed level of consciousness from which the child is not easily aroused. The child may need assistance to maintain a patent airway or adequate ventilation.
- *General anesthesia* is at the end of this continuum, and many sedatives can achieve it if given in sufficient doses. The patient cannot be aroused, needs assistance with ventilation, and may have cardiovascular impairment. This level of anesthesia is reserved for the operating room.

4. What is the "continuum of sedation" and why is it important?

Sedation and analgesia is a continuum: patients receiving medication for PSA can easily move from one level of sedation to the next as there is variability in individual response to medication doses. A patient receiving moderate sedation for a procedure can easily progress to deep sedation, or from deep sedation into general anesthesia. Therefore the provider responsible for administering the sedating medication must be able to manage patients who have one level deeper than their target level of sedation, including airway, ventilatory, and cardiovascular support. See Table 68.1.

Table 68.1 Continuum of Depth of Sedation

	MINIMAL SEDATION (ANXIOLYSIS)	MODERATE SEDATION/ANALGESIA	DEEP SEDATION/ANALGESIA	GENERAL ANESTHESIA
Responsiveness	Normal response to verbal stimulation	Purposeful[a] response to verbal or tactile stimulation	Purposeful[a] response to verbal or tactile stimulation	Unarousable even with painful stimulus
Airway	Unaffected	No intervention required	Intervention may be required	Intervention often required
Spontaneous ventilation	Unaffected	Adequate	May be inadequate	Frequently inadequate
Cardiac function	Unaffected	Usually maintained	Usually maintained	May be impaired

[a]Reflex withdrawal from painful stimulus not considered a purposeful response.

Definitions from Apfelbaum J, Gross J, Connis R, et al. Practice Guidelines for Moderate Procedural Sedation and Analgesia 2018: a report by the American Society of Anesthesiologists Task Force on Moderate Procedural Sedation and Analgesia, the American Association of Oral and Maxillofacial Surgeons, American College of Radiology, American Dental Association, American Society of Dentist Anesthesiologists, and Society of Interventional Radiology. *Anesthesiology.* 2018;128:3.

5. **List the ideal characteristics of an agent used for PSA?**
   - Produces effective anxiolysis, even during painful procedures
   - Produces a predictable degree of sedation for a given dose with minimal effect on airway and cardiorespiratory status
   - Provides amnesia for the procedure
   - Produces no adverse interactions with other agents that may be used concurrently
   - Is reversible
   - Can be administered painlessly
   - Is titratable
   - Has rapid onset, short duration, and rapid recovery

6. **What routes of administration are available for administering a sedative?**
   There are several potential routes available for administration of PSA. These include oral, transmucosal (i.e., intranasal [IN], oral mucosal, rectal), intramuscular (IM), intravenous (IV), or inhalational. IV and inhalational routes allow for the important quality of titrating to effect. If it is difficult to obtain IV access and moderate or deep sedation is needed, the IM route may be ideal (e.g., IM ketamine). Likewise, if anxiolysis or mild sedation is needed, oral or IN midazolam may be sufficient. For mild to moderately painful procedures, IN fentanyl is useful.

7. **What is key information to obtain in the medical history before beginning PSA?**
   Focused history uses **SAMPLE:**
   - **S**igns/symptoms. Respiratory infections or obstruction (snoring/stridor), heart disease, reflux?
   - **A**llergies. To any sedatives or analgesics, egg, soy, or latex?
   - **M**edications. Concurrent use of medications (e.g., narcotics; additive or resistant effects)?
   - **P**ast medical and sedation history. Chronic medical issues (seizures, chronic lung disease), prior sedation, or anesthesia problems?
   - **L**ast meal, liquid intake (for documentation). When were the last liquids and solids?
   - **E**vents leading to sedation. Head injury, ingestion, or fall?

8. **Are there guidelines for presedation fasting?**
   There are official guidelines for elective procedures per the American Society of Anesthesiologists (ASA). However, adherence to these presedation fasting guidelines in the ED has not been shown to alter the rate of adverse events. The majority of ED procedures with indications for PSA are urgent or emergent with variable prearrival fasting times. For urgent or emergent procedures, the ASA practice guidelines state that PSA should not be delayed "based on fasting time alone" (2018). The risk of aspiration in pediatric patients undergoing PSA for an elective procedure is about 1 per 10,000 sedations.

9. **What physical examination findings are important to note before providing PSA?**
   It is important to undergo a full airway assessment as if you were preparing to intubate the patient. This includes, but is not limited to, the following:
   - Evaluating for the presence of airway abnormalities, such as large tonsils or adenoids; congenital abnormalities that may cause a floppy or anatomically susceptible airway (Down syndrome, Pierre Robin syndrome, Treacher Collins syndrome); or lower respiratory findings, such as wheezing and rales.
   - Noting obesity that may be associated with sleep apnea and an increased risk of adverse respiratory events.
   - Performing a visual inspection of the open mouth, including Mallampati score (a visual assessment of the distance between the tongue base and the roof of the mouth), loose teeth, or dental hardware (retainers).

Children with a Mallampati score of III or IV are likely to have an increased need for repositioning to maintain airway patency during procedural sedation.
• Performing a careful cardiac and neurologic examination.

10. **Are there any children who should not receive PSA?**
Relative contraindications to procedural sedation in the ED relate to the risk of complications, including aspiration and potential difficulty in managing the airway. Children who may be better candidates for operating room procedures under more controlled conditions include:
• Infants <6 months old
• Children with craniofacial malformations
• Children with cerebral palsy (abnormal swallowing mechanisms)
• Children with snoring, stridor, apnea, or abnormal breathing regulation
• Children with poorly controlled seizure disorders
• Children with vomiting or gastroesophageal reflux
• Children with severe systemic disease
• Children with anticipated complicated and lengthy procedural needs best performed in the operating room

11. **What monitoring should occur with PSA?**
The level of monitoring can parallel the degree of sedation. A patient receiving medication only for anxiolysis may be monitored with pulse oximetry alone, whereas patients undergoing moderate or deep sedation require more intensive monitoring. The best monitor is a skilled, dedicated observer who is not involved in the procedure and who can observe the child's level of consciousness, response to verbal and physical stimulation, airway patency, respiratory function, and perfusion. Sedated children should not be left unobserved.

12. **What is the equipment needed for PSA?**
See Box 68.1.

13. **What are the agents used for pediatric PSA?**
Knowledge of specific medications and comfort with their use is critical to safe PSA practice. See Table 68.2.

14. **When and how can I use nitrous oxide?**
Nitrous oxide (N_2O) is an anesthetic gas that is blended with oxygen to produce a 50%–70% mixture of N_2O that can be used for a variety of procedures. When inhaled, it results in mild analgesia, sedation, amnesia, and anxiolysis. Children need to be able to hold the mask to their own face when N_2O is used with a demand-valve mask, generally aged 4 or older. If a continuous flow system is used, N_2O can be given to children younger than 4 years, but the risk of side effects such as vomiting is higher than with the demand-valve mask. N_2O administration requires special equipment such as a portable or wall-mounted N_2O delivery system, emergency oxygen safety devices, and a scavenger system. Contraindications include nausea, vomiting, trapped gas within the body cavity (middle ear infection, pneumothorax), and pregnancy.

15. **What agents would I use if I need to obtain a CT scan on a young child?**
Often, sedatives alone are adequate, as imaging is not painful. Potential agents via the IV route include propofol, dexmedetomidine, etomidate, ketamine, as well as the short-acting benzodiazepines pentobarbital, methohexital, and midazolam. Sedation is effective in greater than 95% using these agents; however, sedation with benzodiazepines is associated with a higher risk of respiratory depression with transient oxygen desaturation. If the patient does not have IV access, options include oral or IN midazolam, IM ketamine, or IN dexmedetomidine.

16. **Would the agents used for obtaining a CT scan work for an MRI?**
MRIs require that the child remain motionless for a longer period of time; therefore, ultrashort-acting sedatives would not be the best choice. Instead, agents that can be continuously infused such as propofol or dexmedetomidine would be preferred. In many institutions these are administered by a sedation service or anesthesia department because of long monitoring times.

17. **What are the advantages and disadvantages of propofol for PSA?**
See Table 68.3.

Box 68.1 Equipment Needed for PSA – SOAP-ME

Suction: hooked up, turned on, with Yankauer attached
Oxygen: nasal cannula on patient prior to procedure, appropriate-sized bag valve mask (BVM) available and attached to oxygen prior to procedure
Airway: appropriate-sized oral and nasopharyngeal airways as well as intubating equipment (endotracheal tubes and laryngoscope) should be immediately available
Pharmacy: medications for sedation and reversal agents should be drawn up at appropriate weight-based doses prior to procedure
Monitoring: patient should be hooked up to cardiorespiratory monitor and continuous pulse oximetry with record and vital signs, including blood pressure, every 5 minutes
End-tidal CO_2 monitoring –for all patients undergoing moderate or deep sedation for the early detection of hypoventilation

Table 68.2 Procedural Sedation, Analgesia, and Reversal Agents

AGENT	DOSAGE	ROUTE	COMMENT
Anxiolytics			
Midazolam	0.1 mg/kg	IV, IM	Titrate to effect Max. dose IM = 10 mg Max. dose IV = 6 mg for children 6 months to 5 years, 10 mg for children 6 years and older
	0.2–0.4 mg/kg	IN	10 mg max. (mucosal atomizer needed for administration)
	0.5 mg/kg	PO, PR	15 mg max.
Sedative Analgesics			
Fentanyl	1–2 µg/kg	IV	Avoid rapid or high-dose infusion
	1–2 µg/kg	IN	
Morphine	0.05–0.1 mg/kg	IV, IM	
Ketamine (sub-dissociative dose)	0.1–0.3 mg/kg	IV	Max. dose 30 mg
Ketamine sub-dissociative dose	0.5–1 mg/kg	IN	Max. dose 50 mg
Dissociative Agents			
Ketamine (PSA dose)	1–2 mg/kg	IV	Give IV dose over 1–2 minutes
	2–4 mg/kg	IM	Longer recovery, increase vomiting
Pure Sedatives			
Pentobarbital	2–6 mg/kg	IM	Max. dose 100 mg
	1–2 mg/kg mg/kg	IV	Additional doses of 1–2 mg/kg every 3–5 min to desired effect; total max. dose 1–6 mg/kg; max. dose 100 mg
Etomidate	0.1–0.2 mg/kg	IV	Ultrashort, pain with injection
Propofol[a]	0.5–1 mg/kg	IV	Rapid onset and offset, follow initial dose with 0.5 mg/kg every 3–5 min as needed until desired effect
Dexmedetomidine	0.5–2 µg/kg/dose loading dose	IV	Give over 10 minutes; may be repeated if sedation not adequate. May be given in conjunction with continuous infusion.
Methohexital	0.5–1 mg/kg	IV	Ultrashort, limited studies
Ketofol	0.5–0.75 mg/kg (1:1 mixture of ketamine:propofol)	IV	Titrate to effect, limited pediatric studies
Inhalational Agents			
Nitrous oxide (N₂O)	30%–70% N₂O	Inhalation	Cooperative child, scavenger system
Reversal Agents			
Naloxone	0.01–0.1 mg/kg/dose, up to 2 mg max. single dose	IV, IM, IO ETT	Reverses opioids. Can repeat every 5 minutes, 4 mg max. dose
Flumazenil	0.01 mg/kg, up to 0.2 mg max. single dose	IV	Reverses benzodiazepines. Titrate to max. of 0.05 mg/kg or 1 mg, whichever is lower

[a]Can be given as a continuous infusion: 25–150 µg/kg/min or in additional boluses of 0.5 mg/kg IV every 3 minutes as needed.
ETT, Endotracheal tube; *IM*, intramuscular; *IN*, intranasal; *IO*, intraosseous; *IV*, intravenous; *N₂O*, nitrous oxide; *PO*, by mouth; *PR*, per rectum.

Table 68.3 Propofol for Procedural Sedation and Analgesia: Considerations

ADVANTAGES	DISADVANTAGES
Sedative hypnotic qualities	Risk of apnea
Rapid onset and offset	Hypoxia-hypoventilation, 2%–31%
High efficacy	Dose-related hypotension
Amnesia	Lipophilic suspension = pain at injection
Constant infusion for longer procedures	Needs opioid for painful procedures
	Contraindicated with egg or soy allergy

18. **What medications can be utilized for a 2-year-old child with a facial laceration?**
For older children, local anesthetic such as topical lidocaine, epinephrine, and tetracaine (LET), or local injection with lidocaine is sufficient. For younger children requiring anxiolysis, effective sedation can be provided with midazolam, administered IV, IN, or by mouth. When this does not provide adequate sedation and motion control for a difficult repair (e.g., laceration crossing the vermillion border of the lip), an agent such as ketamine either intravenously or intramuscularly works well.

19. **What medications can be utilized for a 6-year-old child needing reduction of an angulated forearm fracture?**
Fracture reduction requires treatment of both pain and anxiety. Several options can be effective, including the following:
- Fentanyl or morphine plus midazolam
- Ketamine
- Propofol plus an opioid
- "Ketofol" (a 1:1 mixture of ketamine and propofol)
- Nitrous oxide with a hematoma block
    Ketamine has been shown to have fewer adverse respiratory events when compared with fentanyl and midazolam.

20. **What makes ketamine useful as a PSA agent?**
Ketamine, a dissociative agent causing a trancelike cataleptic state, is a commonly used medication for pediatric PSA. It provides strong sedation, analgesia, and amnesia while maintaining cardiovascular stability and protective airway reflexes. Ketamine onset is within a few minutes IV and 5–10 minutes IM. Ketamine can increase salivation; however, coadministration with an antisialagogue, such as atropine, is no longer recommended because it does not decrease adverse respiratory events. Recovery agitation or emergence phenomenon consisting of vivid dreams, hallucinations, or delirium may occur. Coadministration of midazolam has not been shown to reduce its occurrence, but can be used to treat severe emergence phenomenon that occurs in 1.4% of patients. These patients are typically older or have a history of psychiatric illness. Ondansetron has been shown to reduce recovery emesis associated with ketamine that occurs in approximately 8% of patients. Ketamine, although protective of airway reflexes, is associated with such airway or respiratory complications as oxygen desaturation or airway obstruction in 2.8%, transient apnea in 0.8%, and transient laryngospasm in 0.8%.

21. **What is subdissociative dose or "pain dose" ketamine and how is it used?**
Ketamine can be given to patients ≥1 year IV or ≥3 years IN as an alternative to narcotics to treat acute severe pain. It is given at a much lower dose than ketamine for PSA, and does not cause the dissociative amnesia. The dosage is as follows:
- 0.1–0.3 mg/kg IV (maximum 30 mg)
- 0.5–1 mg/kg IN (maximum 50 mg)
    If a second dose needs to be given via either route, consider giving half of the original dose. Patients receiving subdissociative dose ketamine should still be monitored for respiratory depression, although the risk is much less than for PSA-dose ketamine.

22. **What are the contraindications for ketamine?**
Absolute contraindications include age younger than 3 months or schizophrenia/psychosis. Relative contraindications include:
- procedures stimulating the posterior pharynx (e.g., endoscopy; although there is no contraindication for typical ED oropharyngeal procedures);
- airway instability (e.g., tracheal surgery or stenosis);
- active pulmonary infection or disease (e.g., including upper respiratory infection);
- cardiovascular disease;
- hypertension;
- porphyria;
- previous adverse reaction;

- central nervous system masses or obstructive hydrocephalus (mild association with increasing intracranial pressure; however, head trauma is not a contraindication);
- glaucoma or increased intraocular pressure (conflicting evidence).

23. What complications are seen with PSA?
Below is a list of the most frequent complications. Complications of PSA are infrequent, but because they may be life-threatening, verbal or written consent must be obtained and documented.
- Respiratory events: aspiration (from vomiting and loss of airway reflexes), hypoventilation, hypoxia, laryngo-spasm, and apnea
- Cardiovascular events: hypotension, bradycardia
- Vomiting
- Emergence phenomenon: during the postsedation recovery period, children may vomit, become agitated, ataxic, or dysphoric

24. What are the complications associated with fentanyl?
Fentanyl is a commonly used narcotic in the ED, because it provides analgesia and sedation with a rapid onset and recovery. However, when given rapidly or in high dosages, it can cause rigid-chest syndrome (thoracic and abdominal wall rigidity) that may require ventilation support.

25. Are some agents safer than others?
With proper monitoring, most agents can be used and any adverse events promptly treated; reversal agents are seldom needed. Certain drug types used are associated with different adverse event profiles (Table 68.4). Ultimately, the best agent is based on the duration and type of procedure to be performed, patient characteristics, and provider comfort with a given agent.

KEY POINTS: HOW TO AVOID ADVERSE EVENTS WITH PEDIATRIC PSA

1. Beware of infants, children with systemic disease processes, obstructive airway disease, severe obesity, or active respiratory infections.
2. Become acquainted and comfortable with PSA drug regimens.
3. Verify the weight is in kilograms, not pounds, before dosing.
4. Monitor carefully, both with equipment and a dedicated medical staff per American Academy of Pediatrics (AAP) and American College of Emergency Physicians (ACEP) guidelines.
5. Be attentive to the end of the procedure when the painful stimulus is over and the child is more prone to developing respiratory depression.
6. Before starting PSA, have advanced airway equipment ready, including suction, oxygen, and a properly sized bag-valve-mask.
7. Use of local or regional anesthesia (e.g., lidocaine) after a first PSA dose (e.g., ketamine) can decrease the need for additional PSA doses

---

26. What other options do I have to help with analgesia in pediatric patients?
1. *LET* is a topical solution made of lidocaine, epinephrine, and tetracaine. It can be applied directly to open wounds to provide anesthesia for laceration repair. It is most effective in highly vascular areas (e.g., face and scalp) and often makes the use of injected local anesthetic unnecessary. LET cannot be used on mucosal surfaces or to areas of end-arterial supply (e.g., tips of digits, nose, ears, or penis).
2. *"J-tip" needle-free injection system* uses a CO_2 gas cartridge to push aerosolized lidocaine into the subcutaneous tissue. It can be used to provide local anesthesia for IV starts, lumbar punctures, digital blocks or other painful injections. The device is contraindicated in patients receiving chemotherapy.

27. What about acetaminophen with codeine (Tylenol #3)?
Although acetaminophen with codeine was previously frequently used for analgesia for pediatric patients, this is no longer recommended. The drug is absolutely contraindicated in children <12 years old and in children aged 12–18 years old who have recently undergone tonsillectomy or adenoidectomy, or who have other risk factors associated with codeine (obstructive sleep apnea, obesity, severe pulmonary disease). Codeine has been associated with life-threatening or fatal respiratory depression in children and teens. This is primarily because they may be unrecognized ultra-rapid converters of codeine to morphine.

28. What reversal agents are available for children?
See Table 68.2.

29. When can I discharge a child home after performing PSA?
The child should have normal vital signs, be reasonably alert, able to sit without assistance or maintain head control if they are still in a child seat, and respond to commands given in a normal voice.

Table 68.4 Adverse Events by Drug Type		
SEDATION DRUGS	RESPIRATORY EVENTS[a] (%, OR)	VOMITING (%, OR)
Ketamine alone	6%, 1	10%, 1
Ketamine/midazolam	10%, 1.7	5%, 0.5
Fentanyl/midazolam	19%, 3.7	2%, 0.2
Midazolam alone	6%, 0.9	0.8%, 0.07

[a]Respiratory events include hypoxia, laryngospasm, and apnea.
OR, Odds ratio.

Website
Agency for Healthcare Research and Quality. National guideline clearinghouse: www.guideline.gov; accessed February 23, 2019.
https://jtip.com/; accessed January 23, 2019.

BIBLIOGRAPHY

Beach ML, Cohen DM, Gallagher SM, et al. Major adverse events and relationship to nil per os status in pediatric sedation/anesthesia outside the operating room: a report of the Pediatric Sedation Research Consortium. *Anesthesiology.* 2016;124(1):80–88.

Graudins A, Meek R, Egerton-Warburton D, et al. The PICHFORK (Pain in Children Fentanyl or Ketamine) trial: a randomized controlled trial comparing intranasal ketamine and fentanyl for the relief of moderate to severe pain in children with limb injuries. *Ann Emerg Med.* 2015;65(3):248–254.

Green SM. Clinical practice guideline for emergency department ketamine dissociative sedation: 2011 update. *Ann Emerg Med.* 2011;57:449–461.

Iyer MS, Pitetti RD, Vitale M. Higher Mallampati scores are not associated with more adverse events during pediatric procedural sedation and analgesia. *West J Emerg Med* 19(2):430–436. 2018.

Practice guidelines for moderate procedural sedation and analgesia 2018. A report by the American Society of Anesthesiologists Task Force on Moderate Procedural Sedation and Analgesia, the American Association of Oral and Maxillofacial Surgeons, American College of Radiology, American Dental Association, American Society of Dentist Anesthesiologists, and Society of Interventional Radiology. *Anesthesiology.* 2018;3(128):437–479.

Shah A, Mosdossy G, McLeod S, et al. A blinded, randomized controlled trial to evaluate ketamine/propofol versus ketamine alone for procedural sedation in children. *Ann Emerg Med.* 2011;57:425–433.

Siddappa R, Riggins J, Kariyanna S, et al. High-dose dexmedetomidine sedation for pediatric MRI. *Paediatr Anaesth.* 2011;21(2):153–158.

Tobias JD, Green TP, Coté CJ. Codeine: time to say "no." *Pediatrics.* 2016;138(4):e20162396.

Zier JL, Liu M. Safety of high-concentration nitrous oxide by nasal mask for pediatric procedural sedation: experience with 7802 cases. *Pediatr Emerg Care.* 2011;26:1107–1112.

CHAPTER 69

PEDIATRIC AND NEONATAL RESUSCITATION

Brooke Watson, RN, BSN and Taylor McCormick, MD, MSc

1. **What is the Pediatric Assessment Triangle and how can it be used in the initial evaluation of a child?**

   The Pediatric Assessment Triangle (PAT) is a tool used to rapidly determine clinical status ("sick vs. not sick") and illness category in children. It can be performed in 30–60 seconds by observation alone and can help guide triage decisions and resuscitation priorities. The three components of the PAT are appearance, work of breathing, and circulation. Assess the child's appearance using the TICLS pneumonic (tone, interactiveness, consolability, look/gaze, and speech/cry); work of breathing, noting abnormal airway sounds, retractions or nasal flaring, or positioning; and circulation to the skin, looking for pallor, mottling, or cyanosis. An abnormality of any arm of the PAT suggests a potentially unstable child and should prompt immediate assessment of the airway, breathing, and circulation (ABCs) and concurrent intervention as needed (Table 69.1).

2. **How should you prepare the ED for a pediatric cardiac arrest?**

   Maintain a list of pediatric resuscitation equipment to be stocked and checked regularly. Practice often with mock resuscitations to identify gaps in equipment, medications, knowledge, and processes:

   - Assign roles: chest compressions and plan for rotating, intravenous/intraosseous (IV/IO) access and medication delivery, monitor, airway management, documentation/timing, team leader (depending on staffing, one team member may fill multiple roles).
   - Review equipment sizing and medication dosing:
     - The use of age- or length-based medication dosing and equipment systems reduces time to medication delivery, dosing errors, and provider anxiety.
   - Review compression ratio, and plan for airway management (including a difficult airway) and other potential interventions (e.g., IO/central line placement).
   - Summon appropriate ancillary staff (e.g., respiratory therapy, pharmacy, social work).
   - Remind the team that family will be given the option to remain present during their child's resuscitation.

3. **What equipment should be readily available for a pediatric resuscitation?**

   An example of an age-based equipment system is shown in Table 69.2.

4. **List the medications (and pediatric doses) commonly used in pediatric resuscitation.**

   Given IV/IO unless otherwise indicated (Table 69.3).

5. **What is the survival rate from pediatric cardiopulmonary arrest?**

   Studies of pediatric out-of-hospital cardiac arrest report survival rates ranging from 4% to 38%, with favorable neurologic outcomes in 1%–16% of children. Shockable rhythms, witnessed arrest, bystander cardiopulmonary resuscitation (CPR), and age >1 year are associated with improved survival.

Table 69.1 Components of the Pediatric Assessment Triangle and the General Impression

ILLNESS CATEGORY	APPEARANCE	WORK OF BREATHING	CIRCULATION
Stable	Normal	Normal	Normal
Respiratory distress	Normal	Abnormal	Normal
Respiratory failure	Abnormal	Abnormal	Normal
Shock	Normal or Abnormal	Normal or Abnormal	Abnormal
Central nervous system or metabolic disorder	Abnormal	Normal or Abnormal	Normal
Cardiopulmonary failure	Abnormal	Abnormal	Abnormal

Adapted from Horeczko T, Enriquez B, McGrath NE, et al. The Pediatric Assessment Triangle: accuracy of its application by nurses in the triage of children. *J Emerg Nurs*. 2013;39(2):182–189.

Table 69.2 An Age-Based Equipment System

	PREMIE/ NEWBORN	6 MONTHS	1 YEAR	2 YEARS	3–4 YEARS	5–6 YEARS	7–8 YEARS	9–13 YEARS
BVM	Infant/Child	Infant/Child	Child/Adult	Child/Adult	Child/Adult	Child/Adult	Child/Adult	Adult
Blade	1 Miller	1 Miller	1 or 1.5 Miller	1.5 or 2 Miller	1.5 or 2 Miller	2 Miller or Mac	2 Miller or Mac	3 Miller or Mac
ETT	25 weeks—2.5 30 weeks—3.0 ≥35 weeks—3.5 Uncuffed Newborn—3.0 Cuffed	3.5 Uncuffed	3.5 Cuffed 4.0 Uncuffed	4.0 Cuffed 4.5 Uncuffed	4.5 Cuffed 5.0 Uncuffed	5.0 Cuffed 5.5 Uncuffed	6.0 Cuffed	6.5–7.0 Cuffed
Stylet	6 Fr	6 Fr	6 Fr	6 Fr	10 Fr	10 Fr	14 Fr	14 Fr
Suction catheter	6–8 Fr	6–8 Fr	10 Fr	10 Fr	10 Fr	10 Fr	10 Fr	10–12 Fr
ETT depth	6+wt(kg) cm	10 cm	12 cm	13.5 cm	15 cm	16.5 cm	18 cm	18.5–22 cm
LMA	1	1.5	2	2	2	2 or 2.5	2.5	3 or 4
NG tube	5 Fr	8 Fr	8 Fr	10 Fr	10 Fr	12 Fr	14 Fr	16 Fr
Chest tube	10 Fr	12 Fr	16 Fr	18 Fr	20 Fr	22 Fr	24 Fr	28 Fr
Foley	5 Fr	8 Fr	8 Fr	10 Fr	10 Fr	12 Fr	12 Fr	14 Fr
Central line	3 Fr 8cm	4 Fr 12 cm	4 Fr 12 cm	4 Fr 12 cm	5 Fr 12 cm	5 Fr 12 cm	5 Fr 12 cm	5 Fr 12 cm
Glidescope blade/baton	#0 (2 kg) #1 (3 kg) #2 (4 kg) Small	#2 Small	#2 or 2.5 Small	#2.5 Small	#2.5 Small	#2.5 Small	#2.5 or 3 Small	#3 Large

BVM, Bag-valve-mask; *ETT,* endotracheal tube; *LMA,* laryngeal mask airway; *NG,* nasogastric.
Reproduced and adapted, with permission, from the customizable Handtevy Pediatric System.

Table 69.3 Medications (and Pediatric Doses) Commonly Used in Pediatric Resuscitation; Given IV/IO Unless Otherwise Indicated

Epinephrine 0.01 mg/kg 1:10,000 (max 1 mg) q3–5min; if no IV/IO can give 0.1 mg/kg 1:1000 via ETT; for anaphylaxis 0.01 mg/kg IM 1:1000 (max 0.5 mg)	Ketamine 2 mg/kg, 4 mg/kg IM Propofol 2 mg/kg Succinylcholine 1.5 mg/kg
Amiodarone 5 mg/kg (max 300 mg) bolus for VT/VF; over 30 min for SVT/VT with pulse	Rocuronium 1.2 mg/kg 3% NaCl 5 mL/kg
Lidocaine 1 mg/kg (max 150 mg)	Mannitol 0.5–1 g/kg
Magnesium 50 mg/kg (max 2 g)	Adenosine 0.1 mg/kg (max 6 mg) rapid push
Defibrillation 2 J/kg, then 4J/kg up to 10 J/kg	0.2 mg/kg (max 12 mg) second dose (IO ineffective)
Synchronized cardioversion 0.5–2 J/kg	Procainamide 15 mg/kg (max 1 g, over 30 min)
Sodium bicarbonate 1 mEq/kg	Atropine 0.02 mg/kg (min 0.1 mg, max 0.5 mg) IV
Calcium chloride 20 mg/kg (max 1 mg)	Norepinephrine 0.05–2 mcg/kg/min
PGE_1 0.1 mcg/kg/min	Epinephrine 0.1–1 mcg/kg/min
Dextrose: 1 mL/kg D50; 2 mL/kg D25; 5 mL/kg D10	Dopamine 5–20 mcg/kg/min
Normal saline/lactated Ringer's 20 mL/kg	Dobutamine 5–20 mcg/kg/min
Packed red blood cells 10 mL/kg	Milrinone 50 mcg/kg load over 30 min
Naloxone 0.1 mg/kg	then 0.25–0.75 mcg/kg/min gtt
Etomidate 0.3 mg/kg	Hydrocortisone 25 mg (for CAH)

CAH, ; *ETT*, endotracheal tube; *gtt*, ; *IM*, ; *IV/IO*, intravenous/intraosseous; *PGE₁*, ; *SVT*, ; *VF*, ventricular fibrillation; *VT*, ventricular tachycardia.

6. **What are the most common underlying etiologies and initial rhythms in pediatric cardiac arrest?**
Respiratory failure, leading to pulseless electrical activity (PEA), followed by asystole, is the most common cause of cardiopulmonary arrest in children, although cardiac and traumatic causes are not uncommon. Over 90% of pediatric out-of-hospital cardiac arrests will have PEA or asystole as the initial rhythm, while the minority of pediatric cardiac arrests present with ventricular fibrillation (VF) or ventricular tachycardia (VT). VF/VT arrest is more common in older children and those with underlying congenital cardiac anomalies; though rare, they have the highest potential for survival, with reported neurologically favorable survival rates exceeding 50%.

7. **When should CPR be initiated in a child and how should it be performed?**
Chest compressions and rescue breaths should be initiated when an unresponsive child is pulseless with absent/abnormal breathing *OR* if a child's heart rate is less than 60 beats per minute (bpm) with evidence of end-organ hypoperfusion (e.g., depressed mental status). Chest compressions should be performed at a rate of 100–120 bpm and a depth of approximately one-third the diameter of the chest. For infants, the compressor should use two thumbs with the hands encircling the chest; the two-finger method is less effective. For children >1 year old, traditional compressions should be delivered using one or two hands on the sternum, depending on the size of the child. The compression to breath ratio is 15:2 (assuming at least two rescuers) until a definitive airway is in place. As with adults, high-quality, uninterrupted chest compressions and early defibrillation should be prioritized. Of note, compression-only CPR is not recommended for children; CPR with compressions and rescue breaths should be performed for infants and children in cardiac arrest. While it can be uncomfortable, allow parents the opportunity to be present during CPR. Multiple studies show most parents would like the opportunity to be present for their child's resuscitation; it can help with grieving, and most would recommend it to another family.

8. **After return of spontaneous circulation (ROSC), what are the management priorities for post-arrest care?**
   1. Avoid hypotension with norepinephrine or epinephrine.
   2. Optimize ventilator settings to achieve normal oxygen saturation (target 94%) and carbon dioxide levels (target partial pressure of CO_2 [$PaCO_2$] 35–45 mmHg).
   3. Avoid hyperthermia.

9. **What is the role of targeted temperature management (i.e., therapeutic hyperthermia) in pediatric post-arrest care?**
The Therapeutic Hypothermia After Pediatric Cardiac Arrest Out-of-Hospital (THAPCA-OH) trial randomized 295 pediatric post-arrest patients to therapeutic hypothermia (target temperature, 33°C) and therapeutic normothermia

(target temperature, 36.8°C), and showed no statistically significant difference in the primary outcome of survival with favorable functional status at 1 year between groups (20% vs. 12%; relative likelihood, 1.54; 95% CI, 0.86–2.76; $P = 0.14$). These results are consistent with the adult trial of 33°C versus 36°C for out-of-hospital cardiac arrest by Nielsen et al, despite expected differences in etiology of the arrest being predominantly respiratory in children and cardiac in adults. There were no significant differences in safety outcomes between the groups, but there was a trend toward benefit in the 33°C group in the primary and all secondary outcomes; it is reasonable to suspect a larger trial may have detected a statistically significant treatment effect. Based largely on THAPCA-OH and previous observational trials, the 2015 American Heart Association Pediatric Advanced Life Support (AHA PALS) guideline recommends either maintaining normothermia (36°C–37.5°C) for 5 days or 2 days of mild hypothermia (32°C–34°C) followed by normothermia for 3 days for infants and children who remain comatose after out-of-hospital cardiac arrest.

10. **What are the fundamental differences between the pediatric and adult airway?**
Compared to adults, the pediatric glottis is more anterior and cephalad. Tonsillar hypertrophy, a relatively large tongue, excess submental/submandibular tissue, and underdeveloped cartilage and supporting structures make the pediatric airway very susceptible to obstruction; proper positioning and the bag-valve-mask ventilation technique facilitated by naso- or oropharyngeal airways are paramount to maintain a patent airway. A towel roll or stack of sheets under a young child's shoulders will overcome the cervical flexion caused by their prominent occiput and help align the oral, pharyngeal, and laryngeal axes. While the narrowest point of the adult airway is the inlet of the cords, the narrowest point of a child's airway is below the vocal cords at the cricoid cartilage. Care should be taken to avoid excessive cuff pressures and downsize the endotracheal tube (ETT) if significant resistance is met just beyond the cords. The pediatric epiglottis is bigger, floppier, and more omega-like in shape than the adult epiglottis and can obstruct cord visualization and ETT passage when a laryngoscope blade is placed in the vallecula. While appropriate to use either a straight (Miller) or curved (Macintosh) blade to intubate children, many experts recommend a straight blade in young children to lift the epiglottis out of view. Alternatively, a curved blade can be used in the same manner or can be advanced further into the vallecula to engage the hypo-epiglottic ligament. Finally, it is important to keep in mind during any intubation attempt that children have higher oxygen consumption rates and lower functional residual capacity than adults, leading to shorter safe apnea times and precipitous desaturation.

11. **Should cricoid pressure be applied during pediatric intubation?**
Cricoid pressure during intubation is not necessary and can interfere with airway management. If needed to visualize the vocal cords, the intubating provider can perform bimanual laryngoscopy, using his or her own hand to manipulate either the cricoid or the thyroid cartilage to provide better visualization. At that point, another provider can take over the placement of pressure to facilitate intubation. In the event that positive pressure bag-valve-mask ventilation is needed between intubation attempts, cricoid pressure can be gently applied to help prevent gastric insufflation. When applying cricoid pressure, providers should be careful not to obstruct the very malleable pediatric upper airway.

12. **How is ETT size determined?**
In children between the ages of 1 and 8 years, the simple formula (age/4) + 4 can be used for uncuffed tube sizes, and (age/4) + 3.5 for cuffed tubes. More and more evidence suggests that past the neonatal period, cuffed tubes are preferred to prevent air leaks that can require risky tube changes and limit effective ventilation (particularly in children requiring high ventilator pressures). Cuff pressures must be checked with a manometer and should not exceed pressures >20 cmH$_2$O, as even 30 minutes of higher pressures can lead to permanent airway injury.

13. **Should atropine be given prior to rapid sequence intubation in children?**
The 2015 AHA PALS recommendation states, "the available evidence does not support the routine use of atropine preintubation of critically-ill infants and children" but "it may be reasonable … when there is higher risk of bradycardia," such as infants <1 year old or when given succinylcholine as the paralytic agent.

14. **What are the difficult airway options for children?**
After a failed endotracheal intubation, bag-valve-mask ventilation using proper technique and an appropriately sized oropharyngeal airway should be attempted and will often temporize the situation until backup personnel or equipment are available. Gastric decompression with a naso-/orogastric tube may be necessary. In a "cannot intubate, cannot ventilate" situation, a supraglottic airway should be placed. The laryngeal mask airway (LMA), for example, is available in multiple weight-based sizes for infants and children.

15. **Can a cricothyrotomy be performed on a child?**
The cricothyroid membrane is too small for an open cricothyrotomy in children under ~10 years old; needle cricothyrotomy is recommended for infants and children after failed endotracheal intubation and supraglottic airway placement. This is a temporizing measure to provide some oxygenation while awaiting definitive operative intervention; ventilation is passive through the mouth, and not effectively provided through needle cricothyrotomy.

16. **How should vascular access be obtained in the pediatric patient?**
Peripheral IV access should be attempted for most children who require vascular access in the ED. If a child is cardiac arrest, or after two unsuccessful IV attempts in a child who requires resuscitation, the provider should immediately obtain IO access. The anterior proximal tibia is the preferred site for IO access in children, followed by the distal femur, then medial malleolus. Central venous access is rarely needed in the ED for children, and when performed, should be obtained under ultrasound guidance.

17. **What is the earliest gestational age that a newborn has been successfully resuscitated after birth?**
In 2014, at 21 weeks and 4 days gestational age, and weighing 410 g, Lyla Stensrud became the youngest premature baby in the world. According to Wikipedia, in 2018 she was attending preschool with a slight speech delay, but there were no other known medical problems.

18. **You receive a call from paramedics who are bringing a woman in labor to the ED. What information about the pregnancy will help guide your management? List the equipment you'll need to have ready.**
1. Gestational age?
2. How many babies?
3. Any pregnancy complications?
Equipment checklist:
a. Infant warmer and monitoring equipment
b. Warm blankets
c. Bulb and deep suction
d. Medications: epinephrine, normal saline, dextrose (D10)
e. Oxygen blender
f. Flow inflating bag and mask
g. Intubation supplies
h. Umbilical vein catheter supplies
i. Plastic bag

19. **Describe the essential components of the initial assessment once the baby is born.**
1. Term gestation?
2. Breathing or crying?
3. Good tone?
    If the answer is *yes* to all three, only routine care is recommended: cord clamping, suction only if needed, dry, and warm. If the answer is *no* to any of the three questions, take no more than 30 seconds to clamp the cord, suction the mouth, then nose, dry, and warm the infant prior to initiating resuscitative measures if necessary. Place two clamps on the umbilical cord and cut between them. The proximal clamp should be at least 6 cm from the baby to allow for umbilical venous cannulation if needed. The Neonatal Resuscitation Program (NRP), 7th edition, recommends delaying cord clamping 30–60 seconds in most vigorous term and preterm infants. There is no recommendation for infants who require resuscitation at birth. The infant must be dried and warmed immediately to prevent evaporative heat loss. Remove wet linens and place the newborn under a radiant warming unit or skin-to-skin with the mother covered with a warm blanket to lessen loss of radiant heat. Infants can lose a substantial amount of heat from their head, so remember to put on a stocking cap early in resuscitation, especially for premature infants. These initial steps take only seconds to accomplish and may prevent significant metabolic derangements. These steps should be taken even before the initiation of CPR. Cold babies respond poorly to even the best resuscitation efforts.

20. **Does the presence of meconium-stained amniotic fluid change management?**
Approximately 10%–15% of births are complicated by meconium-stained amniotic fluid. Meconium is more common in post-term infants but can occur with any birth and can lead to pulmonary injury. Previous editions of NRP recommended intubation and tracheal suctioning in the setting of meconium-stained fluid for all infants, then only for nonvigorous infants. However, the latest edition does not recommend routine intubation for tracheal suctioning even in nonvigorous infants; they should be treated like any infant in respiratory distress, first with positive pressure ventilation. Vigorous newborns with normal respiratory effort and muscle tone can stay with mom for routine care even if born through meconium-stained fluid.

21. **What is the normal blood oxygen saturation (SpO$_2$) in a newborn?**
Healthy newborns undergoing normal transition to extrauterine life may take several minutes to increase their SpO$_2$ from approximately 60% in utero to more than 90%. This transition can take up to 10 minutes (see Fig. 69.1 and Fig. 69.2). Preductal oxygen saturations (measured on the right wrist or hand) should be monitored to guide the amount of oxygen provided. Term babies should be resuscitated initially with room air, preterm babies with 30% oxygen. Peripheral cyanosis involving the hands and feet, referred to as *acrocyanosis*, may persist and usually has no clinical significance.

Pediatric Cardiac Arrest

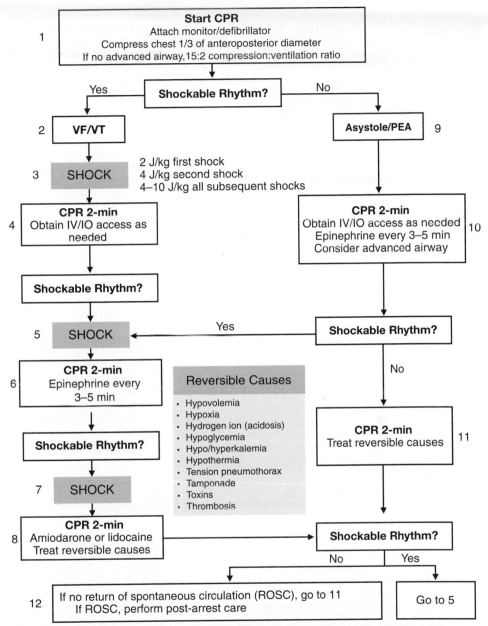

Fig. 69.1 Pediatric cardiac arrest. *CPR*, Cardiopulmonary resuscitation; *IV/IO*, intravenous/intraosseous; *PEA*, pulseless electrical activity; *VF/VT*, ventricular fibrillation/ventricular tachycardia. (Source: American Heart Association, Inc, PALS Algorithm.)

22. **After the initial steps of warming, drying, and stimulating the baby, how do I determine if further intervention is needed?**
    Approximately 10% of newborns require additional intervention, and only about 1% will require advanced life support efforts. If the infant is active, crying, and has a heart rate >100 bpm, further intervention is seldom necessary. If the infant demonstrates apnea, bradycardia (<100 bpm), or central cyanosis, then the use of positive pressure ventilation is indicated. Ideally, this should be accomplished using a device

Neonatal Resuscitation Algorithm

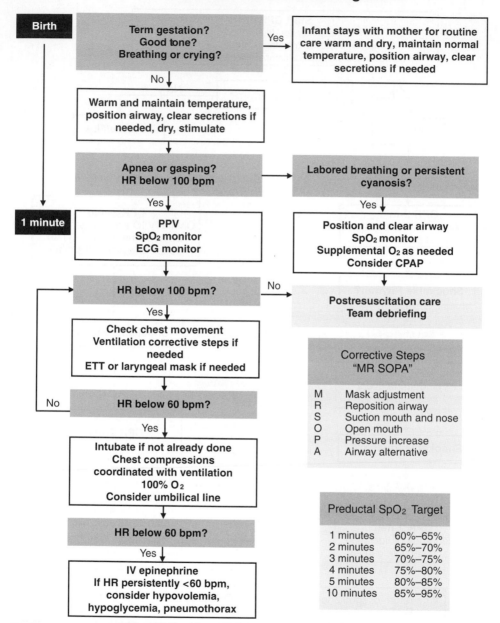

Fig. 69.2 Neonatal resuscitation algorithm. *Bpm,* Beats per minute; *CPAP,* continuous positive airway pressure; *ECG,* electrocardiogram; *ETT,* endotracheal tube; *HR,* hear rate; *IV,* intravenous; *PPV,* positive pressure ventilation; *SpO2,* blood oxygen saturation. (Source: American Heart Association, Inc, NRP Algorithm.)

that is equipped with a manometer and can deliver positive end expiratory pressure (PEEP), such as a flow-inflating bag, with starting ventilation pressures of 20–25 cmH2O and PEEP of 5 cmH2O. Bilateral chest rise and an increase in heart rate are the best indicators that ventilations are adequate. The heart rate often improves immediately with a few effective assisted breaths. Start with room air (21% oxygen) for full term babies and 30% oxygen for preterm babies; respiratory insufficiency is usually a ventilation problem, rather than oxygenation. If the heart rate has not improved after providing 30 seconds of effective respiratory support, consider whether your ventilation technique is correct, and remember the mnemonic *MR SOPA*.

Mask adjustment: this may require one person to hold the mask and one to squeeze the bag

Reposition the airway

Suction the mouth with bulb or deep suction

Open the mouth and lift the jaw forward

Pressure increase (5–10 cmH$_2$O at a time to a max of 40 cmH$_2$O)

Airway alternative: consider intubation or an LMA

If the heart rate is >100 bpm but labored breathing or hypoxia persists, free flow oxygen and begin a trial of continuous positive airway pressure (CPAP). If the heart rate remains at <100 bpm, positive pressure ventilations (PPVs) should be continued. If the heart rate is <60 bpm after corrective measures, the patient should be intubated.

23. **When should chest compressions be initiated and how should they be performed?**
Compressions should be started if the heart rate is <60 bpm after the child has been intubated. The compressor should stand at the head of the warmer and the person delivering PPV should stand to the side. Compressions should be delivered by encircling the baby's chest with the hands and placing thumbs side by side or on top of each other in the center of the sternum at the nipple line. Compress approximately one-third the anterior-posterior diameter of the chest at a rate of 90 compressions per minute. Coordinate compressions with ventilations by repeating out loud "one-and-two-and-three-and-breath." Allow recoil of the chest during the "ands." Increase the fraction of inspired oxygen (FiO$_2$) to 100% after the infant is intubated and compressions initiated. Recheck the heart rate using a cardiac monitor every 60 seconds, and stop compressions if the heart rate reaches 60 bpm. If the heart rate does not improve, prepare for umbilical vein catheter placement and epinephrine.

24. **At what point during a neonatal resuscitation should vascular access be obtained? How?**
When the decision has been made to intubate the patient, vascular access should be obtained. An umbilical venous catheter (UVC) is the preferred method of vascular access, but IO is an acceptable alternative. Use a 3.5 Fr catheter for preterm infants and a 5 Fr catheter for term infants; if an umbilical catheter is not available, a feeding tube may be used. Gather your supplies and use the following steps for UVC placement:
    1. Don sterile gloves.
    2. Flush the catheter with saline.
    3. Loosely tie an umbilical tie at the base of the cord tight enough to prevent bleeding but loose enough to allow passage of the catheter.
    4. Clean the cord and cut as close to the clamp as possible to leave extra cord for future procedures.
    5. Insert catheter into single large umbilical vein (the cord also contains two smaller arteries).
    6. Advance gently while aspirating until there is blood return.
    7. Secure to the abdomen.

25. **What medications are used during neonatal resuscitation?**
    - Epinephrine 1:10,000 should be given if the heart rate is still <60 bpm after 30 seconds of adequate ventilation with 100% oxygen through an ETT or LMA *and* 60 seconds of coordinated chest compressions and PPV. The dose is epinephrine 0.01–0.03 mg/kg (0.1–0.3 mL/kg) via UVC or IO every 3–5 minutes.
    - Normal saline or O negative blood should be given for suspected hypovolemia or hemorrhage at a dose of 10 mL/kg over 5–10 minutes.
    - Dextrose 2 mL/kg of 10% dextrose solution may be given to newborns suspected of having symptomatic hypoglycemia based on clinical findings and blood glucose levels <40 mg/dL. Although the normal nadir can be as low as 30 mg/dL, glucose consumption is increased when a newborn is distressed. Sodium bicarbonate should not be routinely given to treat metabolic acidosis during neonatal resuscitation.
    - Naloxone is not recommended for the resuscitation of newborns, even those born to opioid-dependent mothers. Sudden opioid withdrawal can be dangerous for the infant, causing seizures and unnecessary distress. Focus should be on support of the airway and breathing.

KEY POINTS: PEDIATRIC AND NEONATAL RESUSCITATION

1. Use the Pediatric Assessment Triangle to identify children in need of immediate assessment and intervention.
2. In preparation for a critically ill child, all ED providers should be familiar with pediatric resuscitation algorithms (PALS and NRP), equipment, and resources.
3. Use a weight-, length-, or age-based system for medication dosing and equipment size to offload cognitive burden and anxiety among providers.
4. Allow the family the opportunity to be present for the resuscitation of their child.

BIBLIOGRAPHY

Atkins DL, Berger S, Duff JP, et al. Part 11: Pediatric basic life support and cardiopulmonary resuscitation quality: 2015 American Heart Association guidelines update for cardiopulmonary resuscitation and emergency cardiovascular care. *Circulation.* 2015;132(18 Suppl 2):S519–S525.

de Caen AR, Berg MD, Chameides L, et al. Part 12: Pediatric advanced life support: 2015 American Heart Association guidelines update for cardiopulmonary resuscitation and emergency cardiovascular care. *Circulation.* 2015;132(18 Suppl 2):S526–S542.

deCaen AR, Garcia Guerra G, Maconochie I. Intubation during pediatric CPR: early, late, or not at all? *JAMA.* 2016;316(17):1772–1774.

Horeczko T, Enriquez B, McGrath NE, et al. The Pediatric Assessment Triangle: accuracy of its application by nurses in the triage of children. *J Emerg Nurs.* 2013;39(2):182–189.

McCormick T, McVaney K, Pepe PE. No small matter: pediatric resuscitation. *Curr Opin Crit Care.* 2017;23(3):193–198.

Moler FW, Silverstein FS, Holubkov R, et al. Therapeutic hypothermia after out-of-hospital cardiac arrest in children. *N Engl J Med.* 2015;372(20):1898–1908.

Wyckoff MH, Aziz K, Escobedo MB, et al. Part 13: Neonatal resuscitation: 2015 American Heart Association guidelines update for cardiopulmonary resuscitation and emergency cardiovascular care. *Circulation.* 2015;132(18 Suppl 2):S543–S560.

GENERAL APPROACH TO POISONINGS

Nicklaus Brandehoff, MD

1. List the 10 most common causes of death from acute poisoning reported to poison centers.

Sedative/hypnotics/antipsychotics, 12%

Opioids, 10%

Stimulant and street drugs, 9%

Alcohols, 6%

Calcium antagonists, 5%

Acetaminophen combinations, 4%

Acetaminophen alone, 4%

Beta blockers, 4%

Antidepressants, 3%

Unknown drug, 3%

Note: Despite a high incidence of involvement, these substances are not the most toxic, but rather the most readily accessible. Often, multiple substances are involved in fatal exposures. Percentages are based on total number of human exposures rather than total number of substances.

2. What is the role of activated charcoal?

Activated charcoal is the most widely used method of gastrointestinal (GI) decontamination. While it has been shown to decrease drug absorption, it has not been shown to change clinical outcomes. It is most effective if administered within 1 hour of ingestion, but may be useful beyond 1 hour after ingestion of modified release formulations, or very large ingestions in which absorption may be prolonged. Some drugs are not absorbed by activated charcoal; these include lithium, potassium, iron, most metals, and alcohols. Activated charcoal is contraindicated after ingestion of hydrocarbons, acids, or alkalis. Adverse effects include aspiration, especially in patients with depressed mental status or vomiting. The decision to administer activated charcoal should take into consideration the potential benefit and risk of administration. It should not be routinely administered to all patients. Patients with inconsequential ingestions do not require activated charcoal.

3. What is the role of gastric lavage in treating acute poisonings?

Gastric lavage has a limited role in overdose. It may be considered in the treatment of patients with large, recent ingestions of substances with the potential to cause life-threatening toxicity, for which reliable treatment options are limited though it has not been shown to alter clinical outcome in a large series of patients with overdose. Although serious sequelae of gastric lavage are rare, it carries the risk of aspiration, laryngospasm, and esophageal injury. The risk of injury appears to be greater in uncooperative patients. Endotracheal intubation should precede gastric lavage in patients with altered mental status or inability to protect their airway. Although lavage can be accomplished without prior tracheal intubation in awake patients, airway equipment, including suction, should be immediately available at the bedside. Placing the patient on the left side in mild Trendelenburg position helps prevent aspiration if vomiting occurs. Whenever gastric lavage is done, a large-bore tube (36 French [Fr] or 40 Fr in adults) should be placed through the mouth with a bite-block to prevent the patient from biting the tube. A nasogastric tube may be placed to remove liquids preparations within 30 minutes of ingestion. Proper location of the lavage tube in the stomach must be verified clinically or radiographically before lavage or administration of fluid or charcoal. Deaths have been reported resulting from charcoal instillation into the trachea by nasogastric tube. Gastric lavage use is rare and generally reserved for a small number of patients with potentially life-threatening overdose who come to the emergency department within 1–2 hours after ingestion.

4. What about the asymptomatic overdose patient?

The role of simple observation versus active management such as giving activated charcoal prior to the onset of symptoms is controversial. Although observation is safe for many patients who have ingested substances with limited toxicity, if a patient ingested something life threatening, an opportunity to prevent absorption may be lost if nothing is done until symptoms develop. Administering a dose of activated charcoal to a patient with a history of recent deliberate drug overdose involving a substance with the potential to cause moderate to severe toxicity may reduce toxicity. If a reliable history indicates ingestion of substances with minimal toxicity, or the time since ingestion is long, activated charcoal is unnecessary.

5. **Is there a role for cathartics in treating acute poisoning?**
   Cathartics are thought to increase GI transit time, potentially decreasing drug absorption. Cathartics have not been shown to reduce drug absorption or improve outcome significantly after overdose. Cathartics can cause vomiting, abdominal pain, and electrolyte abnormalities. Use of cathartics is not recommended.

6. **What is the role of whole-bowel irrigation in the treatment of acute poisoning?**
   Whole-bowel irrigation uses a polyethylene glycol electrolyte solution, such as GoLYTELY or CoLyte, which is not absorbed, and flushes drugs or chemicals rapidly through the GI tract. This procedure seems to be most useful when radiopaque tablets or chemicals have been ingested, because their progress through the GI tract can be monitored by radiography. It should also be considered when toxic amounts of substances that are not well absorbed by activated charcoal (i.e., iron, lithium, heavy metals) are ingested. This procedure also is commonly used when multiple packets of intricately packaged street drugs, such as heroin or cocaine, have been ingested and need to be passed through the GI tract as quickly as possible. It should also be considered after overdose of sustained-release products. The limitations of the procedure are that, unless the patient is awake, cooperative, and able to sit on a commode, there is a risk of electrolyte disturbance, vomiting, and aspiration, in addition to the logistical problem of having an unconscious patient in bed with massive diarrhea.

7. **What is the role of multiple-dose activated charcoal (MDAC) in the treatment of acute poisoning?**
   MDAC, also known as GI dialysis, may enhance the elimination of a select number of drugs. It has been shown to be effective for theophylline and possibly phenobarbital poisoning. Numerous other drugs have been shown to have pharmacokinetics altered by MDAC, but it is not clear if this makes a difference in clinical outcome. Many of these drugs have large volumes of distribution, and increasing elimination of the small amount present in the blood is unlikely to be of benefit. MDAC is used commonly after overdose of dapsone, theophylline, phenobarbital, phenytoin, carbamazepine, and quinidine.

8. **Is forced diuresis of benefit in the treatment of acute poisoning?**
   Few drugs are excreted unchanged in the urine; therefore, increasing urine flow significantly above baseline is unlikely to be of benefit. By manipulating the pH of the urine with infusions of bicarbonate solution along with enhanced urine flow, however, drug elimination can be increased for specific drugs. This most commonly is used for salicylates and phenobarbital. By placing three ampules of sodium bicarbonate in 1 L of dextrose 5% in water (D_5W) along with potassium chloride and infusing this solution at rates sufficient to produce at least a normal urine flow and a urine pH of 7.5 or greater, the elimination of salicylate and phenobarbital can be increased. Intake and output and urine pH should be monitored hourly. In the presence of pulmonary or cerebral edema, which may occur in severe salicylate intoxication, or known severe congestive heart failure, alkaline diuresis is dangerous and should generally be avoided.

   The use of high-volume normal saline to treat lithium intoxication is common, but it is important to maintain adequate urine output and serum sodium in this scenario. It is not clear if forced saline diuresis for lithium intoxication is of extra benefit over simply ensuring normal renal flow.

9. **When are extracorporeal techniques, such as hemodialysis or hemoperfusion, indicated?**
   Drugs can be removed successfully by extracorporeal maneuvers if they have a small molecular size, relatively small volumes of distribution, and are found in significant quantities in the circulation. In practice, the toxins most commonly dialyzed after overdoses include salicylate, lithium, methanol, and ethylene glycol. Dialysis has the advantage over charcoal hemoperfusion in that it is usually easier and faster to get started, and it can correct metabolic acidosis and fluid and electrolyte abnormalities as it removes toxins. Because protein binding may be saturated in overdose, hemodialysis may be effective for treatment of severe overdose of some highly protein-bound toxins at therapeutic concentrations. As protein binding is saturated, increasing quantities of drug are present as free, unbound drug in the serum, and may be removed by hemodialysis (e.g., valproic acid).

   Charcoal hemoperfusion may be more effective at removing drugs that are highly bound to plasma proteins, because the affinity for charcoal may be higher than the affinity for the protein carrier. Disadvantages of hemoperfusion are it is minimally available, and causes hypocalcemia, thrombocytopenia, and results in canister clotting.

10. **How can the diagnosis of a drug overdose be made when the patient is unconscious and the history is unavailable?**
    The diagnosis of acute overdose is often difficult and requires detective work. All unconscious patients should receive a rapid bedside serum glucose concentration. Administration of naloxone should be considered if the presentation is consistent with opioid overdose (central nervous system [CNS], respiratory depression, and miosis). Whenever possible, examine pill bottles available, review medical records, and interview family and friends to elucidate exposure. It may be useful to call the pharmacies where the prescriptions were filled. Discovering which xenobiotics were available to the patient, including street drugs, is always important. If needle track marks are seen, consider street drugs commonly used intravenously (IV), such as opioids, cocaine, and/or amphetamines. The physical examination is useful in narrowing the diagnosis. Reactions to specific classes of drugs are commonly called *toxic syndromes* (Table 70.1) or *toxidromes*.

Table 70.1 Most Common Toxic Syndromes

SYNDROME	COMMON SIGNS	COMMON CAUSES
Anticholinergic	Agitated delirium, often with visual hallucinations and mumbling speech, tachycardia, dry flushed skin, dilated pupils, myoclonus, temperature slightly elevated, urinary retention, decreased bowel sounds. Seizures and dysrhythmias may occur in severe cases	Antihistamines, antiparkinsonism medication, atropine, scopolamine, amantadine, antipsychotics, antidepressants, antispasmodics, mydriatics, skeletal muscle relaxants, many plants (notably jimson weed)
Sympathomimetic	Delusions, agitation, paranoia, tachycardia, hypertension, hyperpyrexia, diaphoresis, piloerection, slight mydriasis, hyperreflexia. Seizures and dysrhythmias may occur in severe cases	Cocaine, amphetamine, methamphetamine (and derivatives MDA, MDMA, MDEA), over-the-counter decongestants (phenylpropanolamine, ephedrine, pseudoephedrine). Caffeine and theophylline overdoses cause similar findings secondary to catecholamine release, except for the organic psychiatric signs
Opioid/sedative	Coma, respiratory depression, miosis, hypotension, bradycardia, hypothermia, acute lung injury, decreased bowel sounds, hyporeflexia, needle marks	Narcotics, barbiturates, benzodiazepines, ethchlorvynol, glutethimide, methyprylon, methaqualone, meprobamate
Cholinergic	Confusion/central nervous system depression, weakness, salivation, lacrimation, urinary and fecal incontinence, GI cramping, emesis, diaphoresis, muscle fasciculations, pulmonary edema, miosis, bradycardia (or tachycardia), seizures	Organophosphate and carbamate insecticides, physostigmine, edrophonium, some mushrooms (Amanita muscaria, Amanita pantherina, Inocybe, Clitocybe), some Alzheimer medications
Serotonin	Fever, tremor, incoordination, agitation, mental status changes, diaphoresis, lower extremity myoclonus, diarrhea, rigidity	Fluoxetine, sertraline, paroxetine, venlafaxine, clomipramine; the preceding drugs in combination with monoamine oxidase inhibitors

GI, Gastrointestinal; MDA, methylenedioxyamphetamine; MDEA, methyl diethanolamine; MDMA, 3,4-methylenedioxymethamphetamine (Ecstasy).

11. **How can a toxicology screen and other ancillary laboratory tests make the diagnosis of acute poisoning?**
    The urine toxicology screen has a limited role in the evaluation of overdose patients. Toxicology screens often are inexact and commonly do not give all the information expected by the clinician. It is important to interpret toxicology screens carefully and know which drugs or chemicals were excluded from the screen. Multiple studies have demonstrated that urine toxicology screening rarely impacts clinical decision making; routine use is not warranted. Screening may be useful in evaluating young children where there is concern for abuse and patients with persistent altered mental status or significant vital sign abnormalities.
    Urine immunoassays are commonly used and relatively easy to perform; however, they screen for limited classes of drugs (primarily drugs of abuse), and both false-positive and false-negative results are common. In addition, these tests are qualitative and often screen for metabolites rather than the parent drug; thus the presence of a substance does not necessarily indicate intoxication. Many of the newer drugs of abuse are not detected on current assays.
    Comprehensive urine toxicology screens can detect a wider variety of toxins; however, they are time consuming to perform, and the accuracy of results is dependent on the skill and experience of the technician performing the assay. Alternatives to a full toxicology screen include testing discrete serum concentrations of suspected toxins based on the patient's clinical presentation and/or the substances known to be available to the patient.

12. **What other studies are useful in the evaluation of a poisoned patient?**
    An acetaminophen concentration level should be obtained in patients with deliberate overdose. It is a substance which is widely available, commonly involved in overdose, and causes little in the way of initial symptoms. Treatment with N-acetylcysteine is most effective if begun within 8 hours of ingestion. A salicylate level should be obtained in patients with deliberate overdose as well. Acute salicylate poisoning is usually not quiescent; however, chronic exposures can be challenging to diagnose.

An electrocardiogram (ECG) should be obtained on all patients with intentional ingestions to assess for potential toxicity from tricyclic antidepressants or other cardiac medications. A chest radiograph in patients with pulmonary symptoms or hypoxia may help in the diagnosis of acute lung injury from agents like salicylates, hydrocarbons, or opioids.

Rarely, a kidney, ureter, and bladder (KUB) x-ray, looking for radiopaque material, may be beneficial when assessing for the ingestion of heavy metal, iron, phenothiazines, chloral hydrate, or chlorinated hydrocarbon solvents. Liver enzyme levels are not necessary after most overdoses: exceptions include ingestion of hepatotoxins, such as acetaminophen, *Amanita phalloides*, or carbon tetrachloride later in the course of poisoning. A urinalysis is rarely beneficial as a screening tool.

The acid-base status of the patient is important and should be evaluated in all patients with deliberate overdose. Persistent unexplained metabolic acidosis should prompt suspicion for ingestion of salicylates, iron, methanol, or ethylene glycol. Many other drugs can cause a persistent, unexplained metabolic acidosis, including the ingestion of acids, cyanide, carbon monoxide, theophylline, and others. Keep in mind that acid-base changes generally develop only after a toxin has been absorbed and metabolized. A specimen obtained shortly after ingestion may show a normal acid-base status despite ingestion of significant amounts of a toxin that can cause metabolic acidosis.

In the workup of persistent metabolic acidosis, a serum osmolality test done by freezing point depression can be useful if it is elevated. A difference between the measured osmolality and the calculated osmolality of greater than 10 is significant, though not diagnostic. A normal osmolal gap does not rule out toxic alcohol ingestion. A pregnancy test should be considered, because unintended pregnancy may be the precipitant for an overdose and pregnant patients may need counseling regarding the potential effects of the drugs ingested on the fetus.

KEY POINTS: MANAGEMENT OF SUSPECTED TOXIC INGESTION

1. Activated charcoal in the correct clinical setting is sufficient decontamination for most overdose patients.
2. Routine urine toxicology screens are not recommended.
3. Serum electrolytes, ECG, salicylate, and an acetaminophen concentration should be obtained in deliberate overdose.
4. Although there are a few antidotes for specific toxins, most poisoned patients recover with supportive care.

13. **Discuss some other useful antidotes for common poisonings.**
Naloxone and dextrose are the most common antidotes. Any patient with altered mental status in whom a bedside blood glucose measurement cannot be rapidly performed should receive IV dextrose. Administration of naloxone that results in awakening of a patient is diagnostic of acute opioid overdose. Small, incremental doses of 0.2 mg should be used if it is suspected that the patient may be opioid dependent, because large doses will precipitate withdrawal. Naloxone can be administered intravenously, intramuscularly, intranasally, or via nebulization. Continuous infusion of naloxone is likely to be necessary after long-acting or modified-release opioid ingestion.

Physostigmine is an antidote for the anticholinergic syndrome. Physostigmine can be used diagnostically and therapeutically when the diagnosis of the anticholinergic syndrome is suspected. It should not be used to treat tricyclic antidepressant poisoning (or in patients with ECG changes suggestive of tricyclic antidepressant poisoning, such as QRS widening or a large R wave in AVR). Seizures and bradydysrhythmias have been reported when used in this setting, although their occurrence is extremely rare. A dose of 1–2 mg given over 2 minutes IV is recommended.

Digoxin immune Fab (Digibind, DigiTAb) is a safe and effective antidote for digitalis glycoside poisoning and can rapidly reverse dysrhythmias and hyperkalemia, which can be life threatening. In contrast to naloxone, digoxin immune Fab does not work immediately, and a full response to therapy may not be seen until approximately 20 minutes after administration. For a life-threatening digitalis overdose when the dose and the serum level are unknown, 10 vials of Digibind should be given. For overdoses where the serum concentration or dose taken is known, there are several online calculators to help determine the appropriate dose along with your local poison center.

Atropine and pralidoxime (Protopam) are antidotes used for cholinesterase inhibitor toxicity. This group of pesticides includes organophosphates and carbamates, which commonly are found in household insecticides. Atropine should be titrated to dry up pulmonary and oral secretions. Pralidoxime is used primarily to reverse the skeletal muscle toxicity of these agents, including weakness and fasciculations.

Flumazenil is a benzodiazepine antagonist used thoughtfully in cases of acute benzodiazepine overdose resulting in significant toxicity. Its use may precipitate benzodiazepine withdrawal, including seizures; it should not be used in patients who have seizures, chronically use benzodiazepines or tricyclic antidepressants, or have coingested other proconvulsants. The usual adult dose is 0.2 mg over 30 seconds; if there is an inadequate response after 30 seconds, administer 0.3 mg IV over 30 seconds. Additional doses of 0.5 mg IV over 30 seconds may be given at 1-minute intervals if needed, up to a maximum total of 3 mg.

Ethanol is preferentially metabolized by alcohol dehydrogenase, and fomepizole is an alcohol dehydrogenase blocking agent. Both are used to treat methanol and ethylene glycol poisoning. They prevent the metabolism of methanol and ethylene glycol to their toxic metabolites. IV ethanol is less expensive than fomepizole but can be very difficult to titrate to recommended concentration. The initial IV dose is 8 mL/kg of 10% ethanol over 30 minutes, followed by an infusion of 0.8 mL/kg/h in a nondrinker and 1.5 mL/kg/h in a chronic ethanol user. Blood ethanol concentration should be measured immediately after the loading dose and repeated every hour initially. The dosage should be adjusted to maintain a blood ethanol of 100–125 mg/dL. The loading dose of fomepizole is 15 mg/kg IV over 30 minutes, with subsequent doses of 10 mg/kg every 12 hours. The dose of both agents must be increased in patients undergoing dialysis.

N-acetylcysteine is extremely effective in preventing acetaminophen-induced liver injury. It is most effective if administered within 8 hours of ingestion but reduces morbidity and mortality even in patients with acetaminophen-induced acute liver failure. It can be administered orally (loading dose 140 mg/kg, subsequent doses 70 mg/kg every 4 hours) or IV (initial dose 150 mg/kg in 200 mL D_5W over 15 minutes, followed by 50 mg/kg in 500 mL D_5W over 4 hours, followed by 100 mg/kg in 1 L D_5W infused over 16 hours; please note various two-bag protocols are commonly used at multiple institutions).

ACKNOWLEDGMENT

A special thank you to Katherine M. Hurlbut, MD for her work on the previous version of this chapter.

BIBLIOGRAPHY

Benson BE, Hoppu K, Troutman WG, et al. Position paper update: gastric lavage for gastrointestinal decontamination. *Clin Toxicol (Phila).* 2013;51(3):140–146. doi:10.3109/15563650.2013.770154.

Chyka PA, Seger D, Krenzelok EP, et al. Position paper: single-dose activated charcoal. *Clin Toxicol (Phila).* 2005;43(2):61–87. doi:10.1081/Clt-200051867.

Gummin DD, Mowry JB, Spyker DA, et al. 2017 Annual Report of the American Association of Poison Control Centers' National Poison Data System (NPDS): 35th Annual Report. *Clin Toxicol (Phila).* 2018;56(12):1213–1415.

Proudfoot AT, Krenzelok EP, Vale JA. Position paper on urine alkalinization. *J Toxicol Clin Toxicol.* 2004;42:1–26.

Thanacoody E, Caravati EM, Troutman B, et al. Position paper update: whole bowel irrigation for gastrointestinal decontamination of overdose patients. *Clin Toxicol.* 2015;53(1):5–12.

Vale JA, Krenzelok EP, Barceloux GD. Position statement and practice guidelines on the use of multi-dose activated charcoal in the treatment of acute poisoning. *J Toxicol Clin Toxicol.* 1999;37:731–751.

CHAPTER 71

THE ALCOHOLS: ETHYLENE GLYCOL, METHANOL, ISOPROPYL ALCOHOL, AND ALCOHOL-RELATED COMPLICATIONS

Travis D. Olives, MD, MPH, MEd and Louis J. Ling, MD

ETHYLENE = GLYCOL AND METHANOL

1. **Why is it important to understand the metabolism of ethylene glycol?**

   Ethylene glycol (EG) is not toxic; however, it is metabolized by alcohol dehydrogenase (ADH) and aldehyde dehydrogenase (AIDH) to metabolites that are VERY TOXIC. Ethanol and fomepizole, antidotes, competitively inhibit and block ADH, greatly slowing the metabolism of EG to toxic metabolites. Magnesium, pyridoxine (vitamin B_6), and thiamine are cofactors in the final steps of EG metabolism that are thought to shift metabolism toward nonharmful end products. Oxalate crystals appear late in the course of EG poisoning (Fig. 71.1).

2. **What is the toxicity of ethylene glycol?**

   Initially, there is central nervous system (CNS) intoxication and gastrointestinal (GI) irritation, followed by metabolic acidosis. Renal failure unresponsive to fluid repletion occurs frequently and typically is delayed in presentation. Cranial nerve deficits are a rare complication; they are more commonly encountered with other toxic alcohols like diethylene glycol.

3. **Why does antifreeze have such a bright color?**

   Fluorescein causes the bright color in antifreeze. It is added to antifreeze so that leaks from auto radiators are more easily detected. If the mouth and the urine are examined with ultraviolet light (UV) light (e.g., a Wood's lamp), fluorescein can be detected in about 30% of patients' urine after ingestion; this is a very nonspecific test, as many foods can also cause the urine to fluoresce.

4. **How does the metabolism of methanol direct treatment?**

   Methanol (MeOH) undergoes the same metabolism as EG, so ethanol and fomepizole, respectively, competitively inhibit and block ADH conversion of methanol into formic acid, a toxic metabolite. Folate is a cofactor in the breakdown of formic acid in monkeys (and other primates) and is thought to decrease toxicity (Fig. 71.2).

5. **What are the signs and symptoms of MeOH poisoning?**

   GI symptoms include nausea, vomiting, and abdominal pain. CNS toxicity includes headache, confusion, and decreased level of consciousness. Retinal edema, hyperemia of the disc, and decreased visual acuity (like looking through a snowstorm or through clouds) are signs of ocular toxicity. Metabolic acidosis is an important indicator of serious toxicity and suggests a poor prognosis.

6. **Why are the symptoms of ethylene glycol and methanol overdose often delayed?**

   It may take 6–12 hours for sufficient quantities of the toxic metabolites to accumulate and cause symptoms. The delay in symptoms is even greater with concurrent ethanol intoxication because ethanol stops or slows the rate of MeOH and EG metabolism, delaying the appearance of the toxic metabolites.

7. **How do methanol and ethylene glycol cause similar laboratory findings?**

   Both poisons result in metabolic acidosis, with an anion gap due to the production of organic acid byproducts of metabolism. Because of their low molecular weight, both toxins contribute to an elevated osmolar gap.

8. **What is an anion gap?**

   A normal anion gap is the difference between measured (Na^+) and unmeasured anions (e.g., various proteins, organic acids, phosphates) and measured (HCO_3^-, Cl^-) and unmeasured cations (e.g., potassium, calcium, and magnesium).

   $$\text{Anion gap} = (Na^+) - (Cl^- + HCO_3^-)$$

9. **What causes an increased anion gap?**

   When metabolic acidosis results from an ingestion of nonvolatile acids, there are increased hydrogen ions with positive charges. Because there is an equal increase in unmeasured negatively charged anions but no increase in chloride, the difference between the measured cations and measured anions is increased, causing an increased anion gap. The normal anion gap is about 6–10 mEq/L but varies by laboratory.

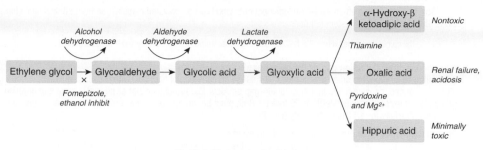

Fig. 71.1 Ethylene glycol metabolism.

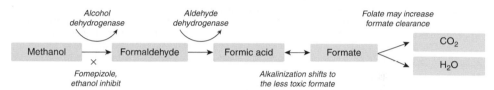

Fig. 71.2 Methanol metabolism.

10. **How can an increased anion gap help in a differential diagnosis?**
    The causes of increased anion gap can be remembered by the mnemonic **MUD PILE CATS**:
    M = Methanol and Metformin
    U = Uremia
    D = Diabetic ketoacidosis
    P = Paraldehyde, Paracetamol, and Phenformin
    I = Iron, Isoniazid (INH), and Inborn errors of metabolism
    L = Lactate
    E = Ethylene glycol
    C = Cyanide, Carbon monoxide
    A = Analgesics (massive acetaminophen and nonsteroidal anti-inflammatory drugs [NSAIDs]), Alcohol (via lactate accumulation), and Alcoholic ketoacidosis
    T = Toluene
    S = Salicylates, Starvation ketoacidosis

    Other mnemonics include **KULT**:
    Ketones
    Uremia
    Lactate
    Toxins

11. **What is an osmolal gap?**
    You may recall from Chemistry 101 that small atoms and molecules in solution are osmotically active, and this activity can be measured by a depression in the freezing point or an elevation in the boiling point of the solution. If there is an increase in low-molecular-weight molecules, such as acetone, MeOH, ethanol, mannitol, isopropyl alcohol (isopropanol), or EG, the osmolality is greater than what is calculated from the measured serum molecules. The difference between the actual measured osmoLALity (Lab) and the calculated osmoLARity (aRithmetic) is the osmol gap, and a gap greater than about 10 mOsm is considered abnormal. WARNING! "Normal" osmol gaps are based on different studies, which include different "measured" osmoles, and different "normal" osmol gaps of between −2 and 15. A high osmolal gap is suggestive of, but a normal osmolal gap does not exclude, toxic levels of MeOH or EG.

12. **How is an osmolal gap calculated?**
    One formula is:

    $$\text{osm gap} = 2 \times \text{Na}^+ \text{ (mEq/L)} + \text{glucose (mg/dL)}/18 + \text{blood urea nitrogen (BUN) (mg/dL)}/2.8 + \text{ethanol (mg/dL)}/4.6.$$

The inclusion of the ethanol level excludes patients who have an elevated osmolal gap from ethanol ingestion alone. Using International System (SI) units,

$$\text{the calculated osmolality} = 2 \times \text{Na}^+ \text{(mEq/L)} + \text{glucose (mmol/L)} + \text{BUN (mmol/L)} + \text{ethanol (mmol/L)}$$

13. **What comes first, the anion gap or the osmol gap?**
    With initial absorption, the small parent molecules cause an early osmol gap, but, with metabolism, acidic metabolites are formed, causing a late metabolic anion-gap acidosis. But remember that a "normal" osmol gap or anion gap does not exclude serious MeOH or EG toxicity. Both must be interpreted in the context of time from ingestion or followed serially for evidence of toxicity (Fig. 71.3).

14. **How much methanol or ethylene glycol is dangerous?**
    Unfortunately, an accurate history of ingestion amount is rarely available. While MeOH is reportedly lethal at approximately 1 g/kg, and EG at 1–2 mg/kg, limited data calls these figures into question. Measured blood levels greater than 20 mg/dL should be treated; CNS, renal (EG), and ocular (MeOH) toxicity, as well as metabolic acidosis, become more likely with increasing blood levels. Large ingestions may fare well with early ADH blockade, while smaller ingestions may fare poorly without prompt care.

15. **How should patients with methanol and ethylene glycol poisoning be treated?**
    As always, airway protection is paramount in patients with decreased level of consciousness or respiratory depression. Small volumes and rapid absorption limit the effectiveness of gastric lavage and charcoal. Acidosis (pH < 7.2) should be treated with sodium bicarbonate. Fomepizole can be given before laboratory results arrive for patients with a heightened suspicion of ingestion. Pyridoxine and thiamine should be given for EG, and folate for MeOH.

16. **How do you use fomepizole?**
    Fomepizole is loaded with an intravenous (IV) dose of 15 mg/kg, followed by 10 mg/kg doses every 12 hours for the first four doses. If continued, the dose is increased to 15 mg/kg every 12 hours—because of autoinduction of ADH. The dose is increased to every 4 hours during dialysis. Typical treatment is for 48 hours, although this varies based on the initial blood concentration. Ethanol can be used if fomepizole is unavailable, but dosing is more complex.

17. **What are the indications for hemodialysis?**
    Dialysis should be considered in cases of severe metabolic acidosis, renal failure, MeOH-induced changes in vision, or when blood concentrations exceed 50 mg/dL.

18. **What if dialysis is unavailable?**
    Patients with EG poisoning can be treated successfully with fomepizole alone without dialysis if there is no acidosis or renal failure. Because the half-life of EG is prolonged to 17 hours, the treatment may be extended, but avoids the invasive treatment of dialysis. With MeOH poisoning, using fomepizole alone increases the half-life of MeOH to 30–52 hours, obligating a less appealing, prolonged hospital stay.

KEY POINTS: ETHYLENE GLYCOL AND METHANOL

1. Symptoms and acidosis are often delayed for both.
2. Urinary oxalate crystals, fluorescence, early osmolal gap, and delayed metabolic acidosis all suggest (but don't exclude when absent) EG poisoning.
3. Measuring visual acuity is key, but often forgotten on MeOH cases.
4. Fomepizole, ethanol, and dialysis can all be used to treat both. Do not forget the adjuncts (bicarbonate and folate for MeOH, thiamine, magnesium, and pyridoxine for EG).

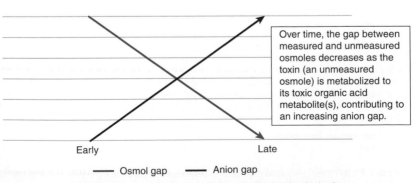

Over time, the gap between measured and unmeasured osmoles decreases as the toxin (an unmeasured osmole) is metabolized to its toxic organic acid metabolite(s), contributing to an increasing anion gap.

Early   Late

⸺ Osmol gap   ⸺ Anion gap

Fig. 71.3 Osmol gap and anion gap in ethylene glycol and methanol poisoning.

ISOPROPYL ALCOHOL

19. **How is isopropyl alcohol poisoning different from methanol and ethylene glycol poisoning?**
Isopropyl or rubbing alcohol is metabolized in the liver to acetone, which results in measurable ketonemia in the serum. Acetone is excreted by the kidney, resulting in ketonuria, and is exhaled through the lungs, giving the breath an acetone aroma. Because acetone is not acidic, isopropyl alcohol poisoning does not cause metabolic acidosis and is far less toxic than either MeOH or EG, although it may still result in depressed mental status, gastritis, or GI bleeding.

20. **What are the symptoms of isopropyl alcohol ingestion?**
Isopropyl alcohol has a three-carbon chain rather than the two-carbon chain of ethanol, so it crosses the blood–brain barrier faster and is more intoxicating than ethanol. Because it is commonly found in concentrated solutions and is more potent than ethanol, the CNS depression can occur rapidly and may continue from residual poison in the stomach. Isopropyl alcohol is much more irritating to the gastric mucosa than ethanol and often causes abdominal pain, vomiting, and hematemesis.

21. **Why is isopropyl alcohol so frequently abused?**
Isopropyl alcohol is easy and legal to obtain; rubbing alcohol is 70% isopropyl alcohol. Unlike consumable beer, wine, and liquor, it is not taxed and is very inexpensive.

22. **What is the treatment for isopropyl alcohol poisoning?**
Patients need observation to watch for respiratory depression, similar to patients intoxicated with ethanol. An isopropyl alcohol level is roughly equivalent to an ethanol level twice as high, but levels do not add value to real-time clinical observation. In the rare instance of coma or hypotension, intubation and ventilation may be necessary. Hemodialysis removes isopropyl alcohol but is rarely needed. There is no antidote.

KEY POINTS: ISOPROPYL ALCOHOL

1. Symptoms and toxicity are completely different from methanol and ethylene glycol.
2. Ketosis occurs, but acidosis does not.
3. There is an osmolar gap without an anion gap.
4. Supportive treatment is adequate in almost all cases.

OTHER GLYCOL ETHERS: DIETHYLENE GLYCOL

23. **Why worry about this?**
Brake fluid contains up to 60% diethylene glycol (DEG) (DOT 3, 4, and 5.1), which may cause seizures, depressed mental status, renal failure, and profound metabolic acidosis. It is not metabolized to EG, there is no common laboratory assay, and no clearly agreed upon treatment, toxic threshold, or diagnostic pathway. One should contact a medical toxicologist or regional Poison Center (1-800-222-1222).

ETHANOL-RELATED COMPLICATIONS

24. **What complications arise from ethanol?**
Alcohol greatly increases the chances that a person will become an emergency department patient. While ethanol increases the risk for many diseases, its use has even more direct effects. The most lethal effect is respiratory depression and asphyxia, but trauma resulting from incoordination or bad judgment is also deadly.

25. **What is the most dangerous alcohol consumption?**
Binge drinking (defined by SAMHSA as >4 drinks for females or >5 drinks for males over a several hour period, or drinking to a BAC of ≥0.08 g/dL) is much more dangerous than a drink (or two) a day. Your stomach serves as a reservoir, so that even after you pass out, you are still absorbing ethanol and increasing your blood level to the point of asphyxia.

26. **When should an acutely intoxicated patient be intubated?**
Hypopnea and hypoventilation sometimes require airway management, but inability to adequately protect the airway is much more common. For patients who are heavily intoxicated but not requiring intubation, lateral decubitus positioning is preferred to avoid aspiration of vomit.

27. **Which medications are best for management of alcohol withdrawal?**
Benzodiazepines, usually diazepam or lorazepam, can be given orally, IV, or in combination and titrated to clinical response. While IV treatment is faster and more easily titrated, oral medication is less expensive. Sometimes huge doses are needed and are given under close observation. If benzodiazepines alone fail (and in the context of common, ongoing benzodiazepine shortages), barbiturates are also well-supported as primary agents to treat withdrawal symptoms, acknowledging the potential risks of hypotension and respiratory depression. Haloperidol is a reasonable adjunct for hallucinosis. Adjuncts such as dexmedetomidine are reported, with less robust data to support their use in the primary setting.

28. What is an appropriate workup for repeat alcohol withdrawal seizures (AWDS)?

AWDS occur in up to 10% of patients withdrawing from alcohol and demand scrupulous history and physical examination to ensure there is no other cause. If the presentation and examination match prior episodes, no other workup, including computed tomography (CT), is necessary. Lingering postictal confusion warrants a check of glucose and electrolytes. If the history or examination has changed significantly or is worrisome, you should start from scratch with a broader differential diagnosis.

29. How should AWDS be managed?

- *Acute.* Benzodiazepines in the immediate and 2-day postseizure period decrease the incidence of additional seizures during this time. Phenobarbital is an additional treatment option.
- *Chronic.* Patients whose seizures have an epileptogenic focus (e.g., old subdural) should have an anticonvulsant, such as levetiracetam, administered. In the patient with pure AWDS, long-term anticonvulsant therapy is contraindicated.

30. Can AWDS be prevented?

Benzodiazepines in the acute withdrawal period, particularly in patients with a history of AWDS, can decrease the frequency of AWDS.

31. Who is at risk for alcohol-induced hypoglycemia (AIH)?

Because of alcohol-induced impairment of gluconeogenesis, a combination of low glycogen stores and limited caloric intake place three groups at risk for AIH: (1) those with long-term alcohol use disorder; (2) binge drinkers; and (3) young children.

32. How is AIH managed?

The management of AIH is with repletion of dextrose. AIH may occur during intoxication or up to 20 hours after the last drink. Symptoms of neuroglycopenia (e.g., headache, depressed mental status, seizure, or coma) predominate. Evidence of catecholamine excess, typical of insulin-induced hypoglycemia (tremulousness, diaphoresis, anxiety), is unusual. Seizures are a frequent presentation in children. Localized CNS signs, including a stroke-like picture (alcohol-induced hypoglycemic hemiplegia), often occur in adults. Although thiamine is commonly co-administered in cases concerning for Wernicke's encephalopathy, it should not delay dextrose in cases of severe AIH.

33. How does alcoholic ketoacidosis (AKA) develop?

AKA commonly occurs early after heavy binge drinking with starvation and vomiting, and occasionally, shortness of breath (Kussmaul respirations) and abdominal pain. Ketoacidosis results from accumulation of acetoacetate and, particularly, β-hydroxybutyrate. Because the latter is not measurable on routine blood and urine tests, the patient may have traces or absent ketones at presentation. As the patient improves and β-hydroxybutyrate is metabolized to acetoacetate, there may be a paradoxical spike in urine and serum ketones.

Average serum pH and bicarbonate are 7.1 and 10, respectively, but these values vary with frequently overlapping ketoacidosis (metabolic acidosis), withdrawal-related hyperventilation (respiratory alkalosis), and protracted emesis (metabolic alkalosis). Decreased body stores of potassium and phosphate are typical. In AKA, serum glucose is usually normal or low.

34. How should you manage AKA?

Treatment consists of rehydration with dextrose-containing crystalloid, antiemetics, benzodiazepines for withdrawal, and potassium and phosphate as indicated. Metabolic abnormalities usually resolve within 12–16 hours.

35. Why do you need to give an AKA patient dextrose-containing crystalloids?

AKA patients are in a redox state that favors the formation of lactate from pyruvate. Dextrose-containing fluids reduce fatty acid oxidation (thus limiting acetoacetate generation) and provide another source of adenosine triphosphate (ATP), shifting the nicotinamide adenine dinucleotide/reduced nicotinamide adenine dinucleotide (NAD^+/NADH) ratio to reduce lactate generation.

36. What is the relationship between different alcohols and metabolic acidosis?

- *Ethanol.* Acute ethanol ingestion results in a mild increase in the lactate-to-pyruvate ratio without a clinically significant metabolic acidosis, but many secondary complications of ethanol (trauma, hypopnea) may cause metabolic derangements.
- *AKA.* The ethanol abstinence syndrome results in increased acetoacetate and β-hydroxybutyrate. From this, an occasionally profound increased anion-gap metabolic acidosis may occur. During the correction phase, a nonanion gap, hyperchloremic picture often develops (because some of the bicarbonate-bound ketoacids are excreted in the urine).
- *EG and MeOH.* Toxic metabolites of these compounds produce increased anion-gap metabolic acidosis. A concomitant osmolal gap, which exceeds 25 mOsm/kg, is 88% specific for the presence of EG or MeOH.
- *Isopropyl alcohol.* This is metabolized to acetone, a ketone but not a ketoacid, causing ketosis and ketonuria but not acidosis.

37. **How is coagulation affected in a chronic alcoholic?**
Bone marrow suppression from ethanol, folate deficiency, and hypersplenism secondary to portal hypertension result in thrombocytopenia, but platelet counts <30,000/mL are uncommon. Qualitative platelet defects also occur. Liver disease from chronic alcohol abuse depletes all coagulation factors except VIII, particularly II, VII, IX, and X.

38. **When is vitamin K useful?**
Chronic drinkers often have inadequate vitamin K, a requisite cofactor for the production of factors II, VII, IX, and X. When faced with GI hemorrhage in a chronic drinker, IV vitamin K supplementation is worthwhile. Vitamin K does not begin to restore factor levels for 2–6 hours, so for emergent scenarios, fresh frozen plasma provides immediate factor supplementation.

39. **Must thiamine be administered before glucose in the hypoglycemic patient?**
Wernicke-Korsakoff syndrome develops over hours to days, while the consequences of neuroglycopenia begin within 30 minutes and are easily prevented. In alcohol-dependent patients with known or suspected hypoglycemia, prompt glucose is given with thiamine as soon afterward as possible. Because magnesium is a cofactor of thiamine, and because alcohol-dependent patients are frequently hypomagnesemic, 2 g of IV magnesium should be given with suspicion of Wernicke-Korsakoff syndrome.

40. **Is it dangerous to administer thiamine intravenously?**
Orally administered thiamine is often absorbed poorly in the alcohol-dependent patient. The intramuscular (IM) route is painful and can result in hematomas or abscesses. Experience with IV thiamine is extensive and supports its safety. Thiamine may be given as part of fluid hydration or by bolus.

KEY POINTS: ALCOHOL-RELATED DISORDERS

1. Whether an acutely intoxicated patient requires intubation for airway protection is based on the clinician's physical assessment. Long-term antiepileptics should only be given to patients with clear indication of an epileptogenic focus. Levetiracetam and phenytoin have no role in the prevention of AWDS.
2. Large doses of benzodiazepines may be needed for treating withdrawal, followed by barbiturates if needed.
3. Time and IV hydration with dextrose-containing crystalloids improves AKA; dextrose need not await the administration of thiamine.

BIBLIOGRAPHY

Klein LR, Driver BE, Miner JR, et al. Intramuscular midazolam, olanzapine, ziprasidone, or haloperidol for treating acute agitation in the emergency department. *Ann Emerg Med.* 2018;72(4):374–385.
Kraut JA, Mullins ME. Toxic alcohols. *N Engl J Med.* 2018;378(3):270–280. doi:10.1056/nejmra1615295.
Lin M. Paucis Verbis: toxic alcohols—ethylene glycol. January 29, 2019. Retrieved June 3, 2019, from https://www.aliem.com/paucis-verbis-toxic-alcohols-ethylene-glycol/.
Lin M. Paucis Verbis: toxic alcohols—isopropyl alcohol. August 2, 2017. Retrieved June 3, 2019, from https://www.aliem.com/paucis-verbis-toxic-alcohols-isopropyl-alcohol/.
Lin M. Paucis Verbis: toxic alcohols—methanol. January 29, 2019. Retrieved June 3, 2019, from https://www.aliem.com/paucis-verbis-toxic-alcohols-methanol/.
McMartin KE, Sebastian CS, Dies D, et al. Kinetics and metabolism of fomepizole in healthy humans. *Clin Toxicol.* 2012;50(5):375–383.
Robinson CN, Latimer B, Abreo F, et al. In-vivo evidence of nephrotoxicity and altered hepatic function in rats following administration of diglycolic acid, a metabolite of diethylene glycol. *Clin Toxicol.* 2017;55(3):196–205.

CHAPTER 72

ANTIPYRETIC POISONING

James C. Mitchiner, MD, MPH

SALICYLATE POISONING

1. What's new with salicylate toxicity?
Not much. Given the myriad presentations of salicylism, the challenge still lies in its detection.

2. What are the causes of salicylate overdose?
A salicylate overdose may be intentional or accidental. Parental administration of adult doses of aspirin to a child may cause toxicity. Bismuth subsalicylate (Pepto-Bismol), which contains 262 mg/tablespoon of salicylate, is occasionally the culprit. In adults, concurrent ingestion of aspirin-containing prescription or nonprescription medications may lead to unintentional overdose with possible formation of gastric concretions. Liquid methyl salicylate (oil of wintergreen) is especially toxic because of its high salicylate content (1 teaspoon = 7 g of salicylate) and rapid absorption. Dermal application of salicylic acid ointment is a rare cause of acute salicylism. The minimal acute toxic ingestion is 150 mg/kg.

3. What are the characteristics of a patient who is experiencing an acute salicylate overdose?
Early diagnosis is essential. Patients may have nausea, vomiting, tinnitus, vertigo, fever, diaphoresis, and confusion. Patients may present with hyperventilation, which may be erroneously ascribed to anxiety. Patients also may have headache or chronic pain, which prompted the excess ingestion of salicylate. Clinical features are summarized in Table 72.1.

4. Describe the acid-base disturbances associated with salicylate toxicity.
Acute respiratory alkalosis, without hypoxia, is caused by salicylate stimulation of the cerebral respiratory center. If the patient is hypoxic, coingestion of a sedative or salicylate-induced noncardiogenic pulmonary edema should be considered. Within 12–24 hours after ingestion, the acid-base status in an untreated patient shifts toward an anion-gap metabolic acidosis as a result of accumulation of lactic acid and ketoacids. A mixed respiratory alkalosis and metabolic acidosis typically is seen in adults. In patients with respiratory acidosis, concomitant ingestion of a central nervous system (CNS) depressant should be suspected. Metabolic acidosis is the predominant acid-base disturbance in children, patients who ingest massive amounts of salicylates, hemodynamically unstable patients, and patients of all ages who have chronic salicylate toxicity.

5. What are some of the other metabolic disturbances seen in acute salicylate poisoning?
The patient may be dehydrated secondary to vomiting, the diuretic effects of increased renal sodium excretion, or diaphoresis in response to the hyperpyretic state. Insensible losses are increased in patients with hyperventilation. Hypokalemia is caused by renal potassium excretion and respiratory and metabolic alkalemia (secondary to bicarbonate therapy).

6. I thought aspirin was an antipyretic. How does it cause a fever?
At a cellular level, salicylate poisoning leads to the uncoupling of oxidative phosphorylation. When this occurs, the energy obtained from oxygen reduction and reduced nicotinamide adenine dinucleotide (NADPH) oxidation that is normally captured in the form of adenosine triphosphate (ATP) instead is released as heat.

7. Name some of the hematologic abnormalities.
These are rare in an acute overdose. Features include decreased production of prothrombin (factor II) and factor VII, an increase in capillary endothelial fragility, and a decrease in the quantity and function of platelets (i.e., decreased adhesiveness). However, significant hemorrhage is unusual.

8. How is the severity of salicylate overdose assessed?
Salicylate levels should be obtained at the time of initial ED evaluation and repeated at least 2 hours apart, while the patient is still under observation in the ED, so that the severity of poisoning can be trended. Most patients show signs of intoxication at salicylate levels of 40 mg/dL or higher. A nomogram is not used for salicylate toxicity.

9. Which laboratory tests are indicated?
Serial serum salicylate levels should be obtained initially and every 2 hours in the ED, until a decreasing trend in the level is established, the most recent level is below 20 mg/dL, and the patient is asymptomatic with a normal respiratory rate. Additional tests include a complete blood cell count; serum electrolytes, blood urea nitrogen

Table 72.1 Common Features of Acute Salicylate Toxicity

GENERAL	HYPERTHERMIA, DEHYDRATION
Respiratory	Hyperventilation (may be mistaken for anxiety), noncardiogenic pulmonary edema
Central nervous system	Tinnitus, confusion, delirium, seizures, coma
Gastrointestinal	Nausea, vomiting, diarrhea, gastrointestinal hemorrhage
Dermatologic	Eyelid petechiae
Laboratory	Acid-base disturbances, azotemia, hyperkalemia or hypokalemia, hypoglycemia (children), elevated creatine kinase levels (rhabdomyolysis), coagulopathy

(BUN), creatinine, and glucose levels; and a urinalysis. Prothrombin time (PT), international normalized ratio (INR), and arterial blood gases should be considered. A quantitative acetaminophen level is also recommended to exclude acetaminophen cotoxicity.

10. **What is the initial ED treatment for an acute salicylate overdose?**
If poisoning is through dermal contact, the skin should be washed copiously with tap water. For acute ingestions, intravenous (IV) normal saline should be given initially, with conversion to alkaline diuresis if the patient is toxic. A slurry of activated charcoal, 1 g/kg, mixed with a cathartic (sorbitol or magnesium sulfate) should be given orally or by gastric lavage tube if the patient is intubated. Lavage may be useful even if the patient comes to the ED several hours after ingestion, because large amounts of aspirin may form gastric concretions with ongoing absorption.

11. **What else needs to be done in the ED?**
After the patient has responded with diuresis, potassium losses should be replaced with potassium chloride at a dosage of 20–40 mEq/L. Patients with hyperthermia should be cooled with a cooling blanket. Hypoglycemia should be treated with IV dextrose 50% in water ($D_{50}W$). Patients with aspirin-induced noncardiogenic pulmonary edema should be treated with oxygen and noninvasive ventilation (continuous positive airway pressure [CPAP] or bilevel positive airway pressure [BiPAP]). If intubation is required, minute ventilation should be preserved.

12. **Is there a role for repetitive dosing of activated charcoal?**
Because of aspirin release from the aspirin-charcoal complex in the gastrointestinal tract and subsequent reabsorption, salicylate levels may not decline significantly after a single dose of activated charcoal. Repeated doses of charcoal after an initial dose of 50–100 g (every 2 or every 4 hours at a dose equivalent to 12.5 g/h) may be indicated to enhance elimination.

13. **What is the rationale for alkaline diuresis?**
Because aspirin is an organic acid, administration of IV bicarbonate raises the pH of the blood and traps salicylate ions, limiting the amount of salicylate crossing the blood–brain barrier. Similarly, an alkalotic urine retains salicylate ions, preventing their reabsorption by the renal tubules. Isotonic alkaline diuresis is achieved by adding three ampules of sodium bicarbonate ($NaHCO_3$) to 1 L of dextrose 5% in water (D_5W), with infusion at a rate of 2–3 mL/kg/h. The patient should be monitored for the development of pulmonary edema or signs of fluid overload.

14. **Explain the paradox of a decreasing serum salicylate concentration and increasing clinical toxicity.**
The serum salicylate level by itself does not reflect tissue distribution of the drug. If the patient's blood is acidemic, salicylate acid remains unionized and penetrates the blood–brain barrier, resulting in CNS toxicity. Salicylate levels should be interpreted in light of the patient's clinical condition and a concurrent blood pH; an acidotic pH may be associated with toxicity, regardless of the salicylate level.

15. **What are the indications for hemodialysis?**
Standard indications include persistent, refractory metabolic acidosis (arterial pH <7.10), renal failure with oliguria, cardiopulmonary dysfunction (e.g., pulmonary edema, dysrhythmias, cardiac arrest), CNS deterioration (e.g., seizures, coma, cerebral edema), and a serum salicylate level greater than 100 mg/dL at 6 hours postingestion in the acute setting. Because ingestion of more than 300 mg/kg predicts severe toxicity, a nephrologist should be consulted early in anticipation of the possible need for dialysis.

16. **What are the most common findings in chronic salicylate poisoning?**
In contrast to acute salicylate poisoning, chronic salicylism is usually accidental. The principal diagnostic feature is a change in mental status manifested by weakness, tinnitus, lethargy, confusion, drowsiness, slurred speech, hallucinations, agitation, or seizures. Because these signs are common to many other disorders, the diagnosis commonly is missed, resulting in a mortality rate of 25%. Most patients are tachypneic, which is a compensatory response to an anion-gap metabolic acidosis. The serum salicylate level may be normal or minimally elevated;

however, given the body burden, this patient population may benefit from more aggressive therapy such as hemodialysis if they cannot tolerate a fluid load.

ACETAMINOPHEN POISONING

17. Is there anything new in acetaminophen toxicology?
Yes. Acute ingestion of acetaminophen-diphenhydramine preparations requires ongoing monitoring due to the risk of altered absorption. The IV form of the antidote *N*-acetylcysteine (NAC) is often preferred over the oral formulation, and should be continued as long as serum acetaminophen levels are detectable, hepatic transaminases are elevated, or the patient reminds altered.

18. What are the characteristics of acetaminophen overdose?
Taken in large doses, acetaminophen is a hepatotoxin. As the most widely used analgesic and antipyretic, it is ubiquitous, either as a single agent or in combination with various cough, cold, or pain remedies. Prompt diagnosis of acute acetaminophen toxicity is important, because early symptoms may be subtle or absent and the onset of hepatotoxicity is delayed by several days after ingestion. A delay in diagnosis can thus result in the development of liver failure, with a mortality rate of up to 28%. Acetaminophen toxicity should always be considered in any ED patient with an unexplained acute elevation in hepatic transaminase levels.

19. What are the initial CNS manifestations of acetaminophen poisoning?
Trick question! In the early stages, there are none, and abnormalities in mental status or level of consciousness should be attributed to coingestion of CNS depressants (e.g., opioids, sedatives), other drugs alone (e.g., ethanol), or to other disease states.

20. Describe the pathophysiology of acetaminophen toxicity.
Acetaminophen is rapidly absorbed in the gastrointestinal tract, although absorption may be delayed in the presence of food or drugs that delay gastric emptying (e.g., anticholinergics), or in the case of extended-release preparations. It is metabolized primarily by the liver. About 90% is conjugated with glucuronic or sulfuric acid to form nontoxic compounds that are excreted in the urine. About 2% of the drug is excreted unchanged in the urine. The remainder is metabolized by the cytochrome P-450 mixed-function oxidase system. This involves formation of a toxic intermediary compound, which is conjugated rapidly with hepatic glutathione. The resulting conjugate is metabolized further, and its by-products are excreted in the urine. Because the liver normally has a fixed amount of glutathione, this compound is depleted rapidly in an acute overdose. The toxic intermediary then accumulates, unmetabolized, and binds to the sulfhydryl groups of hepatic enzymes. The result is irreversible centrilobular hepatic necrosis. Certain drugs, such as cimetidine, compete with acetaminophen for metabolism by the P-450 pathway and theoretically offer protection from hepatotoxicity. Other drugs, such as phenytoin and phenobarbital, may induce P-450 enzymes and facilitate metabolism to the toxic intermediary, thereby increasing the risk of toxicity.

21. How is hepatotoxicity predicted?
An acute ingestion of 7.5 g or 150 mg/kg (whichever is less) is generally predictive of hepatotoxicity. However, the most accurate predictor of hepatotoxicity is the timed serum acetaminophen level obtained between 4 and 24 hours after *acute* ingestion, and plotted on the Rumack-Matthew nomogram. Levels above the nomogram's treatment line confirm risk of hepatic injury and prompt the initiation of NAC therapy. If the initial acetaminophen level is close to the treatment line on the nomogram, check another level in 2 hours. Note that the nomogram is not useful for *chronic* overdose or ingestion.

22. Are serial serum acetaminophen levels helpful?
If an accurate estimate of the time of ingestion cannot be obtained, the nomogram cannot be used. Treat patients with a credible history of acetaminophen exposure and unknown ingestion time by checking a single acetaminophen level and liver enzymes; if the acetaminophen level is greater than 20 µg/mL or hepatic transaminases are elevated, treat with NAC for 12 hours and then repeat the laboratory tests. If acetaminophen is undetectable and liver function has improved, NAC can be halted; otherwise, continue NAC and contact the regional poison control center (call 1-800-222-1222).

23. Why is hepatotoxicity in children rare?
No one knows for sure. Toxicity in children is rare, even when toxic levels of acetaminophen are found. One theory holds that acetaminophen metabolism in children shows a preference for alternative pathways other than the P-450 system; childhood ingestions in the form of a solution may also be a factor. The conversion from juvenile to adult metabolism is believed to occur between 6 and 9 years of age.

24. Which laboratory tests are helpful?
If a serum acetaminophen level is in the toxic range on the nomogram in an acute overdose, or detectable at any level in a suspected chronic overdose, a complete blood cell count, electrolytes, BUN, glucose, PT, INR, ethanol, and liver function tests should be obtained. Serial acetaminophen and transaminases are important.

25. **Outline the general treatment of acetaminophen poisoning.**
The main issue in treatment is prevention of hepatotoxicity. Activated charcoal (1 g/kg) mixed with a cathartic (e.g., sorbitol or magnesium sulfate) can be considered and administered orally or by gastric lavage tube (if the airway is protected); however, NAC is an extremely effective antidote if given early and the risk of aspiration secondary to activated charcoal must be considered. The specific antidote is NAC. This agent is a glutathione substitute with a high therapeutic-to-toxic safety ratio. Although it can be given orally, it is often given by the IV route. It should be started as early as possible, but within 8 hours after an acute overdose when the serum acetaminophen level is above the treatment line on the nomogram. NAC also should be administered to patients with hepatic failure where acetaminophen poisoning is suspected, regardless of time after ingestion or acetaminophen level.

KEY POINTS: ED APPROACH TO ANALGESIC TOXICITY

1. Salicylate levels must be interpreted in light of the patient's clinical condition, the formulation of the drug (pills, capsules, or liquids), and a concurrent blood pH.
2. Acetaminophen toxicity should always be considered in the ED patient with unexplained elevation in liver enzymes.
3. The primary goal in the treatment of acetaminophen toxicity is the prevention of hepatotoxicity.
4. The antidote for acetaminophen overdose is NAC. It is most effective when administered as soon as possible, but within 8 hours after an acute overdose.

26. **How is NAC administered?**
Although NAC was traditionally given orally, toxicologists often recommend the IV formulation (Acetadote) because of ease of use, less risk of vomiting, and faster infusion time. The standard 20-hour protocol is 150 mg/kg in D_5W over 60 minutes, followed by 12.5 mg/kg/h over 4 hours, then 6.25 mg/kg/h over 16 hours. Other dosing regimens have been described. A repeat acetaminophen level and transaminases should be drawn after 18 hours of NAC infusion, with NAC continued beyond 20 hours (at 6.25 mg/kg/h) if serum acetaminophen is detectable, transaminases are elevated, or the patient is not clinically well. In all cases, consultation with the local poison control center (call 1-800-222-1222) is advised. Recent accumulating evidence in medical toxicology literature has explored a two-bag regimen (200 mg/kg over 4 hours followed by 100 mg/kg over 16 hours), which has been shown to reduce the risk of adverse reactions.

27. **Is there a critical window in time to administer NAC?**
Yes, whenever possible, NAC should be given within 8 hours of acute acetaminophen overdose. NAC still may be of benefit if given more than 8 hours after overdose, particularly in patients who have taken extended-release formulations or staggered ingestions, and in patients with persistently toxic acetaminophen levels or elevated liver enzymes.

28. **If the patient has hepatic encephalopathy, is it too late for NAC therapy?**
No, NAC should be given by at the usual dose, followed by a steady infusion of 6.25 mg/kg/h until the patient is clinically better, the acetaminophen level is undetectable, the transaminases decreasing, and the INR is less than 2. Failure to improve suggests possible referral to a liver transplant center. The regional poison control center (call 1-800-222-1222) should be consulted.

29. **What are the potential adverse reactions to IV NAC?**
The incidence of hypersensitivity reactions is 10%–20%, and they tend to occur during infusion of the loading dose (see above regarding two-bag regimen). Typical symptoms not requiring therapy include transient nausea, vomiting, and flushing; mild urticaria can be treated with diphenhydramine. Interruption of NAC therapy is not necessary, but the initial infusion rate should be slowed. Serious reactions, such as bronchospasm, angioedema, and hypotension, require aggressive therapy with antihistamines, steroids, albuterol, and epinephrine, and discontinuation of the IV NAC. Oral NAC may be substituted.

30. **What is the acetaminophen-alcohol syndrome?**
Acute alcohol coingestion is said to be protective, because alcohol competes with acetaminophen as a substrate for cytochrome P-450, thus limiting the production of the toxic metabolite. In contrast, chronic alcohol abuse affects acetaminophen detoxification in two ways:
1. It lowers hepatic glutathione stores, resulting in a reduced capacity to detoxify the toxic metabolite.
2. It induces the cytochrome P-450 system, increasing the proportion of ingested acetaminophen that is converted to the toxic metabolite.
    Diagnostic findings include a history of acetaminophen ingestion and elevated aspartate transaminase (AST) levels in patients with known or occult alcohol abuse who regularly take acetaminophen in supratherapeutic doses. The diagnosis initially is missed in one-third of cases, and the mortality rate is greater than 30%. Treatment is supportive, including NAC, and liver transplantation is an option.

31. **What is the treatment for chronic acetaminophen toxicity?**
    NAC is recommended for patients with detectable acetaminophen levels greater than 20 µg/mL and evidence of liver injury. Treat for 12 hours, and then repeat acetaminophen level and liver function tests. If acetaminophen is not detectable, liver function has decreased or normalized, and the patient is clinically well and treatment may be stopped; otherwise, continue and contact the regional poison control center (call 1-800-222-1222) for guidance.

IBUPROFEN POISONING

32. **What are the characteristics of ibuprofen overdose?**
    Ibuprofen is readily available as an over-the-counter medication used in the treatment of mild to moderate pain and fever. Rapid absorption leads to peak drug levels within 2 hours. Symptoms usually are seen within 4 hours of ingestion and are more likely to be serious in children. Toxicity is limited in patients who ingest less than 100 mg/kg, whereas patients, primarily children, who ingest more than 400 mg/kg may be at risk for more severe symptoms.

33. **List the primary symptoms of ibuprofen toxicity.**
    - Gastrointestinal toxicity is manifested by nausea, vomiting, abdominal pain, and hematemesis.
    - Nephrotoxicity results in acute renal failure.
    - CNS toxicity (seen mostly in children) includes somnolence, apnea, seizures, and coma.
    - Severe metabolic acidosis and thrombocytopenia have also been described.

34. **Should a serum ibuprofen level be obtained?**
    No. Because the serum ibuprofen level does not correlate with clinical symptoms, there is no role for this test in medical decision making.

35. **Describe the treatment for ibuprofen toxicity.**
    Treatment is directed at alleviating symptoms and providing supportive care, primarily with IV fluids and anti-emetics. If hematemesis is present, there should be further investigation. A limited toxicology screen to search for other readily treatable toxins (i.e., salicylates, acetaminophen, opioids, barbiturates, cyclic antidepressants, and ethanol) is recommended if the patient is centrally depressed. Seizures should be treated with IV diazepam. Renal and hepatic function tests should be ordered for massive ingestions. Children with ingestions of greater than 400 mg/kg should be observed in the hospital. Forced diuresis, alkalization, and hemodialysis are not indicated.

BIBLIOGRAPHY

Green JL, Heard KJ, Reynolds KM, et al. Oral and intravenous acetylcysteine for treatment of acetaminophen toxicity: a systematic review and meta-analysis. *West J Emerg Med.* 2013;14:218–226.

Greenberg MI, Hendrickson RG, Hofman M. Deleterious effects of endotracheal intubation in salicylate poisoning. *Ann Emerg Med.* 2003;41:583–584.

Levine M, Khurana A, Ruha AM. Polyuria, acidosis, and coma following massive ibuprofen ingestion. *J Med Toxicol.* 2010;6:315–317.

Schmidt LE, Rasmussen DN, Petersen TS, et al. Fewer adverse effects associated with a modified two-bag intravenous acetylcysteine protocol compared to traditional three-bag regimen in paracetamol overdose. *Clin Toxicol.* 2018;56:1128–1134.

Wong A, Graudins A. Risk prediction of hepatotoxicity in paracetamol poisoning. *Clin Toxicol.* 2017;55:879–892.

CHAPTER 73

BITES AND STINGS

Shawn M. Varney, MD, FACEP, FAACT, FACMT and Sophia Ahmed, MD

KEY POINTS: BITES AND STINGS SECRETS

1. *Centruroides* scorpion stings are most dangerous for small children. Severe envenomation manifests as salivation, tachycardia, roving eye movements, involuntary muscle jerking, opisthotonos, and tongue fasciculations.
2. Dog and cat bites are common, but rabies is uncommon. Nevertheless, administer rabies immune globulin, and the vaccine series (on days 0, 3, 7, and 14) to patients experiencing bites from high-risk animals.
3. Treatment for marine envenomation:
   a. In stinging attacks, pour vinegar over wound for 30 seconds.
   b. In spine attacks, immerse affected area in hot water (45°C [113°F]) for 60 minutes.
4. Crotaline (pit viper) venom contains toxins that cause local tissue destruction, as well as systemic findings and coagulopathy. In contrast, elapids possess a neurotoxin that may cause weakness and respiratory paralysis, but no tissue destruction.
5. Two antivenoms exist for crotaline (pit viper) bites: CroFab (Crotalidae Polyvalent Immune Fab [Ovine]) and Anavip (Crotalidae Immune F(ab')2 [Equine]).
6. Antivenom is administered and can be repeated until initial control is achieved. Maintenance doses are sometimes debated with CroFab but are not required with Anavip.

ARACHNIDA (CHIGGERS, SCABIES, SCORPIONS, AND SPIDERS)

1. What is the difference between poisonous and venomous?
Poisonous refers to a substance that may cause toxicity or death if absorbed, ingested, or inhaled (e.g., touching a poison dart frog, licking a *Bufo* toad). *Venomous* implies a mechanism of delivering the poison to the victim (e.g., snakes bite, scorpions sting). The key distinction is the delivery mechanism.

2. What is a tarantula?
It is a large spider of the family Theraphosidae. The largest is the South American *Grammostola mollicoma,* with a leg span of up to 27 cm and a body length of up to 10 cm. Tarantula venom contains a family of voltage-gated sodium channel modulators that paralyze its insect prey, but tend to cause little toxicity in humans, namely, localized pain, numbness, and lymphangitis. The bites usually do not cause necrosis or serious sequelae. More commonly, the spider has tiny urticating barbed hairs which can cause skin and mucous membrane irritation with edema and pruritus that can last for weeks (Table 73.1). Eye exposure can cause a severe keratoconjunctivitis and ophthalmia nodosa.

3. What spider bites are likely to be an issue?
Although all spiders possess venom, there are two spiders of particular clinical importance in the United States: *Latrodectus* (black widow) and *Loxosceles* (brown recluse or fiddle back). In 2017 the American Association of Poison Control Centers (AAPCC) reported 1346 bites from *Latrodectus* and 898 from *Loxosceles.* There were no deaths and only nine major reactions attributed to *Latrodectus* bites (0.6%). Similarly, 1 death and 15 major reactions (1.6%) were attributed to *Loxosceles.* The envenomation syndromes and treatment of these two spiders are distinct (Tables 73.1 and 73.2).

4. What is "mustov disease?"
It is a play on words. It is mistakenly attributing nonbite skin lesions (especially community-acquired methicillin-resistant *Staphylococcus aureus* abscesses) to spiders or other animals, as in, "Doc, I woke up with this. I *must've* been bitten by a spider in my sleep." Although there were 5255 spider bites reported to the AAPCC in 2017, this number underestimates the true incidence, because these are only the cases reported to poison centers.

5. A 5-year-old boy has genital itching that started several hours after sitting on the lawn watching a fireworks display. His examination reveals intensely pruritic, erythematous papules around his groin. What caused this, and what is the treatment? (Clue: he had been wearing shorts.)
Chiggers are tiny mite larvae (0.3 mm) that cause intense pruritus. The diagnosis is based on identifying the characteristic skin lesions in a person with an outdoor exposure in a chigger-prone area. Itching begins within a few hours of exposure, and the papules can enlarge to form nodules in 1–2 days. Treat with topical (calamine) or

Table 73.1 General Overview of Bites/Stings and Treatments

BITE OR STING	SYMPTOMS	TREATMENT
Tarantula	Localized pain, edema, pruritis, numbness, lymphangitis	Supportive
Latrodectus (black widow)	Localized pain, diffuse muscle cramping ("peritonitis"), headache, nausea/vomiting, facial muscle spasm, lacrimation, periorbital edema. If severe—dysphagia, hypertension, respiratory failure, shock, coma.	Wound care Opioids, benzodiazepines Horse IgG or F(ab')2 fragment antivenom
Loxosceles (brown recluse)	Fever, chills, vomiting, arthralgias, myalgias, hemolysis, coagulopathy. If severe—may result in renal failure and death.	Wound care Analgesics Surgical debridement Transfusion or dialysis
Chiggers	Severe pruritus at bite site	Calamine lotion Antihistamines Steroids Wash clothes with hot water or treat them with permethrin
Scabies	Pruritus, predominantly to web spaces between fingers and toes	Permethrin cream Oral ivermectin
Scorpion	Localized pain If systemic—salivation, tachycardia, roving eye movements, involuntary muscle jerking, tongue fasciculations	Wound care Opioid analgesia Benzodiazepines Scorpion-specific F(ab')2 antivenom
Formicidae (ants)	Intensely pruritic papules	Cool compresses Oral antihistamines Steroids
Killer bees	Localized pain	Stinger removal If allergic—EpiPen, antihistamines, steroids
Mexican beaded lizard and the Gila monster	Localized pain, swelling, discoloration, enlarged lymph nodes, weakness, diaphoresis, tinnitus, hypotension, rarely angioedema	Remove retained teeth Analgesics Supportive care
Culicidae (Mosquitoes)	Depends on disease transmitted—encephalitis, malaria, yellow fever, dengue fever, filariasis, West Nile virus, Ross River virus, chikungunya fever, Rift Valley fever	Treatment is disease dependent
Dog bite	Localized pain	Antibiotics in high-risk wounds (amoxicillin-clavulanate) High-pressure irrigation and cleansing Suture for cosmesis
Cat bite	Localized pain	Antibiotics (amoxicillin-clavulanate)
Raccoon, skunk, bat, fox, woodchuck bite (rabies transmission)	Low-grade fever, malaise, myalgias, vomiting, paraesthesias, encephalitis, hydrophobia, aerophobia, agitation, opisthotonos, paralysis	Human rabies immunoglobulin Human rabies vaccine
Human bite	Localized pain Risk of invasion to deep fascia and joint capsule	Antibiotics If infected, surgical debridement
Jellyfish (sea jellies)	Localized pain and swelling Certain species—severe pain, skin necrosis, cardiac arrest, respiratory arrest, limb paralysis, anaphylaxis	Pour salt water over wound; (use vinegar outside the United States) Immerse in hot water Remove nematocysts Antivenom (for Australian box jellyfish)

Table 73.1 General Overview of Bites/Stings and Treatments *(Continued)*

BITE OR STING	SYMPTOMS	TREATMENT
Stingray, lionfish, scorpionfish, stonefish, cat-fish, weever fish	Localized pain, tissue injury and necrosis Occasionally nausea, vomiting, headache, sweating, hypotension, and syncope	Remove barbs or spines Place wound in hot water (45°C) for 60 minutes to deactivate toxin Antivenom for stonefish envenomation
Crotalinae (rattle-snakes, copper-heads, water moccasins)	Local destruction, edema, severe burning pain, compartment syndrome	Polyvalent Fab or F(ab')2 specific antivenom Elevate extremity Avoid NSAIDs
Elapidae (coral snakes, cobras)	Nausea, vomiting, headache, abdominal pain, diaphoresis, pallor, weakness, respiratory paralysis	Coral Snake Antivenin Coralmyn

IgG, Immunoglobulin G; *NSAID,* nonsteroidal anti-inflammatory drug.

Table 73.2 Comparison of Black Widow and Brown Recluse Spiders

LATRODECTUS: BLACK WIDOW	*LOXOSCELES:* BROWN RECLUSE
Markings Red hourglass shape on ventral abdomen (female)	Dark, violin-shaped spot anterodorsally
Presentation Pain at the bite site within 1 hour Target-shaped erythema, swelling, localized diaphoresis • Diffuse large muscle cramping, including the back, chest, and abdomen (may mimic peritonitis) • Latrodectism: characteristic facial muscle spasm, lacrimation, photophobia, and periorbital edema • Headache • Lightheadedness • Nausea and vomiting	Mild erythematous bite Becomes necrotic over 2–4 days Systemic reaction may occur in 1–2 days: • Fever • Chills • Vomiting • Arthralgia, myalgia • Hemolysis, coagulopathy
Severe envenomations may result in dysphagia, hypertension, respiratory failure, shock, and coma	May result in renal failure and death
Treatment • Wound care • Opioid analgesics, benzodiazepines for spasm • Tetanus prophylaxis • Horse-serum IgG antivenom: administer one vial IV or horse *Latrodectus* immune F(ab')2 antivenom. If no improvement, a second and third vial can be given at hourly intervals	 • Wound care • Analgesics • Tetanus prophylaxis • Surgical debridement and possible grafting • Transfusion or dialysis • Consider hyperbaric oxygen therapy, corticosteroids, or dapsone • No available antivenom

IgG, Immunoglobulin G; *IV,* intravenous.

oral antihistamines (hydroxyzine, diphenhydramine) and steroids for the symptoms (see Table 73.1). Wash the clothes in hot water or treat them with permethrin. Mites do not burrow into the skin, and the pruritic reaction does not develop until the mites have already detached. Symptoms resolve completely within 2 weeks.

6. What are the distinguishing features of scabies?
Scabies bites are typically in the web spaces between the fingers and toes (also the penis, face, and scalp in children) and are intensely pruritic, often preventing patients from sleeping. In contrast to chiggers, scabies create burrows of pruritic, white, threadlike patterns with small gray spots at the closed end, where the parasite rests. Treat with a thorough application of permethrin 5% cream from the neck down and wash off after 8–14 hours (repeat 1 week later), or take oral ivermectin 200 µg/kg once and repeat 2 weeks later (see Table 73.1).

7. How dangerous are scorpion stings?

North American scorpions are generally not dangerous except for the bark scorpion *(Centruroides)*, which is capable of producing systemic toxicity usually only in small children. They do not hunt for prey, but rather hide and wait. They hold their prey with their pincers, arch their tail over their body, and sting (not bite) the victim. The venom causes an increase in the sodium permeability of presynaptic neurons, which leads to continuous depolarization. In North America, *Centruroides exilicauda* are found in Baja California, while *Centruroides sculpturatus* are found in Sonora, Mexico, and in the southwestern United States (Arizona, Utah, New Mexico, Nevada, and California). They can hitch a ride in unsuspecting travelers' luggage. In 2017, the AAPCC reported 12,669 patients with scorpion stings, with 4.4% moderate morbidity, 0.2% major morbidity, and no deaths.

8. What are the signs of scorpion envenomation?

The sting is acutely painful. Systemic manifestations are rare and mainly occur in small children, where a larger venom-to-body weight ratio exists. The principal signs of systemic toxicity are salivation, tachycardia, roving eye movements, involuntary muscle jerking, opisthotonos, and tongue fasciculations in awake patients (see Table 73.1).

9. What is the treatment for a scorpion sting?

Supportive care with local wound care, opioid analgesia, and benzodiazepines for the neuromuscular symptoms is the mainstay of treatment. A relatively new US Food and Drug Administration (FDA)-approved scorpion-specific fragment antigen–binding F(ab')2 antivenom (Anascorp, Rare Disease Therapeutics, Franklin, TN) is available in the United States and costs about $3500 per vial, for the standard three-vial treatment dose. In critically ill children with neurotoxic effects, the antivenom has been shown to resolve the clinical syndrome within 4 hours, to reduce the need for concomitant sedation with benzodiazepines, and to reduce the levels of circulating unbound venom.

FORMICIDAE (ANTS)

10. I have a patient who received multiple stings from fire ants. What do I do?

Do not panic. Fire ants belong to the order Hymenoptera, which includes wasps and bees. Treatment is the same as for a bee sting. Fire ants swarm during an attack, and each sting contributes to the total antigen load. The individual stings result in intensely pruritic papules that may evolve to sterile pustules within 24 hours. Local necrosis and scarring may occur. Cool compresses, oral antihistamines, and topical steroids for local stings suffice. For multiple stings, use a similar approach, along with oral corticosteroids, if systemic allergic manifestations are present (see Table 73.1).

HYMENOPTERA (BEES AND WASPS)

11. What types of reactions occur from Hymenoptera stings (bees and wasps)?

There are four types of reactions:

1. The toxic reaction is a nonantigenic response to the venom, characterized by local irritation at the sting site and, potentially, vomiting, diarrhea, light-headedness, and syncope. There may also be headache, fever, drowsiness, involuntary muscle spasms and edema without urticaria. Local toxic reactions are treated with supportive care, including cool packs and analgesics.
2. Anaphylactic reactions are most commonly seen in Vespidae stings (i.e., wasps, hornets, yellow jackets). These reactions can range from mild to fatal and occur from 15 minutes to 6 hours after the sting. These reactions are treated like any other allergic reaction.
3. Delayed reactions present as a serum sickness–like syndrome (type III hypersensitivity) 10–14 days after the sting and are treated with antihistamines and corticosteroids.
4. Unusual reactions reported after Hymenoptera stings include encephalitis, neuritis, vasculitis, and nephritis.

12. How does a bee sting differ from a wasp sting?

Bees have barbed stingers that usually remain in the victim, pulling the venom sac off of the bee. Whereas the bee dies after a single sting, a wasp is capable of stinging multiple times. In addition, Hymenoptera can release defense pheromones that attract other Hymenoptera and induce them to sting. It is better to remove the stinger from a bee by scraping it out with a credit card rather than by pinching and plucking it with fingers or tweezers and risking the inadvertent injection of more venom. Stinger removal should be done as soon as possible, because the venom sac continues to pulse venom over the first minute after it has detached from the bee.

13. What about killer bees?

Africanized honeybees *(Apis mellifera scutellata)* were introduced into Brazil in 1956 as a potential honey producer in the tropical environment. They have migrated to the United States. Africanized bees and European bees are similar in appearance, venom toxicity, amount of venom they carry, and number of times they can sting— once. The difference lies in their aggressive defensive behavior. They swarm in larger numbers, pursue victims over greater distances (up to 1 km), and have a lower threshold for stinging. Hence, victims typically receive multiple stings during an attack and therefore a greater venom burden. For this reason, the Africanized honeybees have been called *killer bees* (see Table 73.1).

14. **After a patient has survived an anaphylactic reaction to a bee sting, what should be done to prepare the patient in case he or she is stung again in the future?**
First, tell the patient to avoid bees and wasps. Second, have them carry medical identification describing the bee sting allergy, such as a medical alert bracelet. Third, the patient should carry and learn to use an epinephrine self-injector (e.g., Adrenaclick or EpiPen).

HELODERMA (LIZARDS)

15. **Are there any venomous lizards (Heloderma) in the world?**
Yes, there are two species: the Mexican beaded lizard *(Heloderma horridum)* and the Gila monster *(Heloderma suspectum)*. Both lizards live in the desert areas of the southwestern United States and in Mexico. The venom is somewhat similar to crotaline snake venom, although the clinical course is typically milder. The more serious problem with these reptiles is their powerful jaws and the tendency to hold onto their victims. They deliver their venom by chewing tissue and dripping the venom into the lacerations created by their teeth. Their teeth also commonly break off in the wounds and become a nidus for infection if not removed (see Table 73.1). The teeth are difficult to visualize on radiographs. Envenomation is present in about 70% of bites. Cases of angioedema of the oropharynx have also been reported.

16. **How do I open the jaws of a Gila monster?**
A few ways to disengage the powerful jaws are to submerge the lizard underwater, wrap a towel around its head to frighten it, pour alcohol on it, or pry open its mouth with a stick or crowbar.

CULICIDAE (MOSQUITOES)

17. **What is the major clinical significance of mosquito (Culicidae) bites?**
There are about 3500 species of mosquitoes, and they are found on every continent except Antarctica. Responsible for more bites than any other blood-sucking organism, mosquitoes are attracted by carbon dioxide, lactic acid, body heat, and sweat. Children younger than 1 year of age rarely show a skin reaction to the bite; however, by age 5 years, almost all children react. Both immediate and delayed hypersensitivity reactions can occur. The major significance is the role of the mosquito as a disease vector. They can transmit malaria, encephalitis, yellow fever, dengue fever, filariasis, West Nile virus, Ross River virus, chikungunya fever, and Rift Valley fever. They transmit disease to more than 700 million people annually, with at least 1 million reported deaths in Africa, South and Central America, Mexico, and Asia (see Table 73.1).

MAMMALS (BATS, DOGS, CATS, FOXES, HORSES, HUMANS, RACCOONS, SKUNKS, AND WOODCHUCKS)

18. **How many dog and cat bites are there annually in the United States, and what is the risk of infection?**
The majority of mammalian bites that require medical attention are from dogs. It is estimated that 4.7 million dog bites occur annually, causing approximately 800,000 victims to seek medical attention. The annual incidence of cat bites is about 400,000. The risk of infection from a bite is determined by multiple factors, including the location of the bite (hands are worse), the type of wound (crush injury from dogs and punctures from cats are worse), the biting species, and host factors (immunocompromising comorbidities). Dog bites to the hand have a risk of infection as high as 30%. Cat bites carry up to an 80% rate of infection, which may be the result of the deep inoculation of bacteria in the wound (see Table 73.1).

19. **Should I give prophylactic antibiotics to the victim of a dog or cat bite?**
This is controversial. Meticulous wound care is the most effective means of reducing infection potential. In a 2001 *Cochrane Database Review,* prophylactic antibiotics showed no benefit in low-risk wounds. However, prophylactic antibiotics should be used for high-risk wounds (immunocompromised patients, puncture wounds, crushed tissue, hand, genitalia, or face involvement, or wounds requiring closure). Wounds infected with *Pasteurella multocida* generally manifest symptoms and signs of infection within 12–24 hours of the bite. When choosing antibiotics, consider the polymicrobial nature of these infections (*Staphylococcus, Streptococcus, P. multocida*, anaerobes). Amoxicillin-clavulanate (Augmentin, or "Dog-mentin") is the drug of choice. We recommend treating all cat bites. We also recommend treating dog bites to the hand, or other areas of comprised tissue vascularization and high risk of infection.

20. **Can dog bites be closed primarily (sutured)?**
Yes, dog bites can be sutured with a few caveats. Favorable conditions include wounds <8 hours old and treating with copious high-pressure irrigation. Wound infection rates are similar between sutured and nonsutured dog bites, and comparable among all age groups, but sutured wounds have better cosmesis scores. We recommend considering primary closure of dog bites, when cosmetic outcome is the primary concern (e.g., facial bites). We *do not* recommend suturing dog bites to the hand, foot, genitalia, or areas of possible compromised tissue (e.g., crushed tissue).

21. **What is *Capnocytophaga canimorsus*?**
    Capnocytophaga canimorsus (dysgonic fermenter [DF2]) is a gram-negative rod that requires special growth media and can cause sepsis after a dog bite. Eighty percent of the patients who become seriously ill from this infection are immunocompromised (e.g., splenectomy, hematologic malignancy, cirrhosis, human immunodeficiency virus/acquired immunodeficiency syndrome [HIV/AIDS], or long-term steroids). It is a rare infection that carries a 25%–36% mortality rate. Always ask if a patient with a dog bite has his or her spleen.

22. **What types of bites are at risk for the transmission of rabies?**
    Rabies is a disease caused by an RNA rhabdovirus transmitted by inoculation with infectious saliva. The virus primarily affects the central nervous system and is almost always fatal. In the United States, animal bites from raccoons, skunks, bats, foxes, and woodchucks should be considered a risk (see Table 73.1). Exposures from livestock, rodents, and lagomorphs rarely require postexposure prophylaxis, because the host dies before the rabies virus can replicate sufficiently. Consult your state health department for local recommendations.

23. **What is postexposure prophylaxis for rabies?**
    Postexposure prophylaxis means trying to prevent the disease before it manifests after a high-risk exposure. It begins with a thorough cleansing of the wound. Then administer 20 IU/kg of human rabies immunoglobulin (as much as possible injected in and around the wound, the remainder given intramuscularly [IM] in the gluteal muscle). Inject 1 mL of human rabies vaccine into the deltoid muscle (or the anterolateral thigh in young children) on days 0, 3, 7, and 14. Do not administer the rabies vaccine and the immunoglobulin in the same site. Also inquire about tetanus immunization status.

24. **What is a fight bite?**
    A fight bite or clenched fist injury is a human bite when a fist strikes the teeth of an opponent and usually involves the knuckles of the dominant hand. The laceration can involve the extensor tendon and its bursa, the superficial and deep fascia, and the joint capsule. These structures are contaminated with oral flora at the time of injury, with the fingers in flexed position, and are notorious for infection. The most commonly cultured organism from human saliva in fight bites is *Streptococcus,* followed by *S. aureus* (usually penicillin resistant); 31% of these wound infections are caused by gram-negative organisms, and 43% are the result of mixed gram-negative and gram-positive organisms. Up to 29% of these infections may be caused by a facultative anaerobic gram-negative rod, *Eikenella corrodens.* This harmful organism is typically resistant to the semisynthetic penicillins, clindamycin, and the first-generation cephalosporins. However, it is usually sensitive to penicillin and ampicillin. These wounds require meticulous care with thorough exploration and irrigation. Consider the polymicrobial nature of these infections when choosing antibiotics. If a patient has an infected wound, give broad-spectrum intravenous (IV) antibiotics and obtain a surgical consult for possible debridement (see Table 73.1).

MARINE FAUNA (SEA JELLIES, SHARKS, AND VENOMOUS FISH)

25. **How do I treat jellyfish or other coelenterate stings?**
    Jellyfish are invertebrate marine animals with a gelatinous, umbrella-shaped body that does not possess cartilage or scales, and are not fish. A more accurate term is *jelly* or *sea jelly.* Jellies possess thousands of nematocysts on their tentacles and envenomate by injecting small harpoon-shaped spines into their prey, releasing venom (Fig. 73.1). The discharge is triggered by either physical contact or chemical stimulation (e.g., fresh water, ethanol, or urine – so don't use as a treatment!). Frequently, undischarged nematocysts in the tentacles remain in contact with the victim's skin and may inadvertently be stimulated and inject additional venom. Treatment is controversial and depends on species and geography. In North America, administer opioids and antihistamines, apply salt (sea/ocean) water, and place the affected area in warm (43.3°C–45°C) water for 60 minutes. With a gloved hand, carefully remove nematocysts using forceps or scraping with a blunt straight-edged tool (e.g., credit card). In other areas of the world (e.g., Indo-Pacific), pour acetic acid (vinegar) over the affected area for 30 seconds to inhibit nematocyst discharge in most sea jellies. The same treatment can be used for the stings from sea anemones or fire coral. There is an Australian box jellyfish *(Chironex fleckeri)* antivenom available. The recommended dosage for the antivenom is one to three ampules (see Table 73.1).

26. **Name some venomous fish, and state what their venoms have in common. How can that feature of their venom be used in treatment?**
    Venomous fish have spines that inject a heat-labile poison (heat destroys the toxin). Examples of venomous fish are stingray, lionfish, scorpionfish, stonefish, catfish (i.e., freshwater catfish, sea catfish, coral catfish), and weever fish. Barbs and spines may remain embedded in the wound and should be promptly removed. The venoms can be rendered nontoxic by placing the affected extremity of the victim into hot water (45°C) for 60 minutes. There is an antivenom for stonefish envenomation. Give one to three vials IM (see Table 73.1).

27. **How do I acquire antivenom for exotic snake or marine envenomations?**
    Call your local or regional poison center in the United States (call 1-800-222-1222) for assistance. They will have the most success in obtaining antivenom from the local zoo or aquarium. Note that although zoos and aquaria may possess antivenom for exotic envenomations, the supply is primarily intended for their workers in case of an emergency. They may choose to release specific antivenom under a compassionate use clause, but they are not obligated to do so.

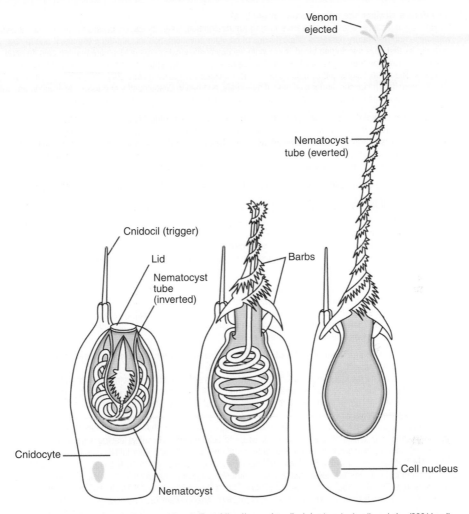

Venom
ejected

Nematocyst
tube (everted)

Cnidocil (trigger)

Lid

Nematocyst
tube
(inverted)

Barbs

Cnidocyte

Cell nucleus

Nematocyst

Fig. 73.1 Diagram of a cnidocyte ejecting a nematocyst. (From https://manoa.hawaii.edu/sealearning/media_colorbox/3221/media_original/en. Accessed January 26, 2019.)

28. **How many people are killed by sharks worldwide annually?**
    In 2017, there were a total of 88 unprovoked shark attacks, of which 5 were fatal. None of the fatalities occurred in the United States.

CROTALINAE (RATTLESNAKES, COPPERHEADS, WATER MOCCASINS) AND ELAPIDAE (CORAL SNAKES)

29. **What are distinguishing physical features of crotaline (pit vipers) and elapid snakes?**
    Pit vipers include rattlesnakes, copperheads, and water moccasins (or cottonmouths), and are distinguished by a heat-sensing pit located between the nostril and the elliptical pupil on their triangular head. The heat-sensing pit enables the snakes to sense the direction and size of their prey. Elapids include coral snakes (the main indigenous elapid in North America) and cobras, and have round heads and round pupils. Not all pit vipers have rattles, and not all rattlesnakes use their rattles.

30. **What is a dry snakebite?**
    A dry snakebite is a bite in which no venom was introduced. About 20%–25% of all US pit viper bites do not result in envenomation. Coral snakes, lacking long fangs, mainly envenomate by chewing the skin, but also puncture with shorter fangs at the rear of the mouth. Up to 50% of their bites are dry.

31. How does a pit viper bite differ from an elapid bite?

Pit viper venom contains toxins that cause local tissue destruction, whereas elapids possess a neurotoxin causing weakness and respiratory paralysis. Clinical signs of pit viper envenomation include the presence of one to two fang marks that ooze nonclotting blood, surrounding ecchymosis, local edema, and severe burning pain. In coral snake envenomation there is usually little local tissue damage, and systemic signs may be delayed for as long as 12 hours. The earliest signs and symptoms of neurotoxic venom effect from coral snake envenomation include nausea, vomiting, headache, abdominal pain, diaphoresis, and pallor. Coagulopathy and tissue destruction are not features of coral snake envenomation, but respiratory paralysis is the feared outcome (see Table 73.1).

32. True or false: snakebites are uncommon but highly lethal in the United States.

This statement is both true and false. In the United States, indigenous snakebites are uncommon, and mortality is rare. Snakebite is a problem of morbidity, not mortality. The 2017 AAPCC report documented 4071 crotalid snakebites and 80 coral snakebites but only 2 deaths. An additional 2567 snakebites occurred from nonpoisonous and unknown types of snakes and caused 1.1% major outcomes and no deaths.

33. List some of the epidemiologic characteristics of snakebites in the United States.

- 75% occur from April to October.
- 45% occur between 2:00 p.m. and 6:00 p.m.
- Male-to-female victim ratio is 7:1.
- 55% of victims are age 17–27 years.
- 85% of bites are on the fingers or hand; 15% involve the foot or ankle.
- 30%–60% of victims were intoxicated with ethanol (especially if pet snakes were involved).
- 15% had previous snakebites.

34. List the three main clinical effects of crotaline (pit viper) envenomation.

1. Local (e.g., pain, edema, ecchymosis, bullae, oozing blood)
2. Systemic (e.g., nausea, weakness, hypotension, fasciculations, or multiorgan dysfunction syndrome)
3. Coagulopathy (e.g., low platelets, elevated international normalized ratio [INR], low fibrinogen)

Patients may manifest all, some, or none of these effects.

35. What FDA-approved antivenoms are available in the United States for crotaline (pit viper) envenomation and how are they dosed?

Two antivenoms are FDA approved: CroFab (Crotalidae polyvalent immune Fab [ovine]) approved in 2000, and Anavip (Crotalidae immune F(ab')2 [equine]) approved in 2018. Note that the goal of antivenom is to attain *initial control* (described as halting progression of all components of envenomation, including local effects, systemic effects, and coagulopathy).

    CroFab is produced from pooled sheep serum immunized against North American crotaline snake venoms (western diamondback, eastern diamondback, Mojave, and cottonmouth). The initial loading dose is four to six vials within 6 hours of the bite and can be repeated until symptoms are controlled. After initial control, additional two-vial maintenance doses are infused at 6, 12, and 18 hours. Each vial of CroFab costs the hospital approximately $2300.

    Anavip is produced from pooled horse serum immunized against South American crotaline snake venoms (*Bothrops asper* [fer-de-lance] and *Crotalus durissus*). The initial loading dose is 10 vials and can be repeated until symptoms are controlled. No maintenance dosing is required. Anavip costs $220 per vial.

36. Which patients should receive Fab-specific antivenom?

Antivenom is indicated for any patient with progressive local tissue effects, hematologic effects (significantly abnormal prothrombin time [PT], platelet count, and fibrinogen level) or systemic signs (nausea, vomiting, hypotension, localized fasciculations) caused by the venom. Antivenom is not indicated for localized pain and edema that do not progress over 4–6 hours.

37. Is the antivenom maintenance dosing always required?

This is debated. Some affirm giving maintenance doses because they were included in the study data that the FDA approved for CroFab. Others state that antivenom dosing should be tailored to the severity of the envenomation and that achieving initial control may be adequate. Some physicians report that copperhead bites are less severe in general and may not require maintenance dosing or, possibly, any antivenom. A recent trial found that treatment with FabAV for mild copperhead envenomation reduced limb disability at 14 days, but all patients recovered by 4 months, regardless of treatment (https://www.ncbi.nlm.nih.gov/pubmed/28601268).

38. Can a crotaline bite cause compartment syndrome?

Compartment syndrome rarely results from crotaline envenomation, because venom is usually deposited in the subcutaneous tissue, not in fascial compartments. Children, however, with the smaller body mass and potential for relatively deeper envenomations, are more prone to develop compartment syndrome, but it is still rare. Compartment syndrome cannot be diagnosed reliably without directly measuring intracompartmental pressures, because the signs and symptoms (e.g., paresthesias, pain on motion, and decreased pulses) are similar to signs and symptoms of envenomation. Antivenom is the treatment for compartment syndrome, as opposed to traditional fasciotomy. In addition, elevate the extremity.

39. **What is the importance of the coloring of coral snakes, and what are the active components of its venom?**
Coral snakes are small (usually up to about 18 inches), thin, brightly colored venomous snakes. The king snake has similar coloration in a different pattern, but is nonvenomous.

Red on yellow, kill a fellow (coral snake). Red on black, venom lack (harmless snake).

This rhyme helps only with identifying North American coral snakes. Coral snake venom contains a neurotoxin that irreversibly binds to presynaptic nerve terminals and blocks acetylcholine receptors. It may take weeks to regenerate the receptors. The clinical effects are slurred speech, ptosis, dilated pupils, dysphagia, and myalgias. Death results from progressive paralysis and respiratory failure. There is virtually no local tissue destruction.

40. **How is coral snake envenomation treated?**
Coral Snake Antivenin is no longer manufactured in the United States. Any remaining supply has exceeded its initial shelf life, but the FDA continues to extend the expiration date. Supportive care with good wound care and attention to impending muscle paralysis are the treatment. Coralmyn, a coral snake antivenom produced by the Mexican pharmaceutical company Instituto Bioclon, effectively neutralizes clinically important coral snake venom, but is not FDA approved.

41. **Which prehospital treatments for crotaline bites are now considered to be ineffective or harmful?**
Incising the wound and attempting to extract the poison by oral suction (cut and suck), venom extraction devices, electric shock to denature the toxin proteins, carbolic acid, strychnine, enemas, urine, cauterization, prophylactic antibiotics, ice packs (cryotherapy), and arterial tourniquets are ineffective and, in some cases, harmful. Venom extraction devices do not remove a significant amount of venom (0.04%–2% in one study). Although controversial, nonsteroidal anti-inflammatory drugs (NSAIDs) may compound a crotaline venom–induced thrombocytopenic bleeding diathesis and should be avoided.

42. **Which prehospital non-antivenom treatments are reasonable?**
Remain calm, avoid activity, remove jewelry or constricting items, immobilize the extremity, follow good basic life support principles, and transport the patient rapidly to the ED. A lymphatic constriction band (broad and flat band as opposed to a ropelike tourniquet) is controversial but can be applied to exert a pressure great enough to occlude superficial veins and lymphatic channels (typically 20 mmHg) but loose enough to admit one or two fingers. It delays the systemic absorption of venom and may have use in cases with prolonged transport time. Despite the American Heart Association's adoption of this practice in its 2010 guidelines, many toxicologists recommend against using constriction bands. Local tissue damage may occur, and people have difficulty applying the correct amount of pressure.

43. **What about exotic snakes (at least exotic by North American standards)?**
In 2017 the AAPCC reported 74 exotic snake exposures (i.e., poisonous, nonpoisonous, and unknown if poisonous). There were two major medical outcomes (2.7%) and no deaths. An antivenom index exists that includes a catalog of all of the antivenoms stocked by North American zoos and aquariums. The law may restrict possession of exotic venomous snakes, and these cases should be reported to the authorities.

44. **What are other general guidelines for crotaline (pit viper) snakebite patient care?**
Antibiotics for snakebite are not indicated. Elevation and immobilization of the affected extremity, along with antivenom, reduce pain. Avoid nonsteroidal analgesics (NSAIDs) due to the antiplatelet effect from snake venom. Remove constricting bands/jewelry from patient's extremities. Administer the same dose of antivenom to adults and children, because dosages are based on the amount of venom injected, not the size of the patient. Finally, avoid fasciotomy.

BIBLIOGRAPHY

Africanized Honeybees. http://labs.biology.ucsd.edu/nieh/TeachingBee/eds_africanized.htm. Accessed January 7, 2019.
Centers for Disease Control and Prevention: *Rabies.* www.cdc.gov/rabies/medical_care/index.html; accessed January 7, 2019.
Chigger bites. www.uptodate.com/contents/chigger-bites?source=search_result&search=chiggers&selectedTitle=1~6. Accessed January 7, 2019.
Clinical manifestations and initial management of bite wounds. https://www.uptodate.com/contents/clinical-manifestations-and-initial-management-of-bite-wounds. Accessed January 7, 2019.
Evaluation and management of Crotalinae (rattlesnake, water moccasin [cottonmouth], or copperhead) bites in the United States. https://www.uptodate.com/contents/evaluation-and-management-of-crotalinae-rattlesnake-water-moccasin-cottonmouth-or-copperhead-bites-in-the-united-states. Accessed January 7, 2019.
Gerardo CJ, Quackenbush E, Lewis B, et al. The efficacy of Crotalidae polyvalent immune Fab (ovine) antivenom versus placebo plus optional rescue therapy on recovery from copperhead snake envenomation: a randomized, double-blind, placebo-controlled, clinical trial. *Ann Emerg Med.* 2017;70(2):233–244.e3. doi:10.1016/j.annemergmed.2017.04.034.
Gummin DD, Mowry JB, Spyker DA, et al. 2017 Annual report of the American Association of Poison Control Centers' National Poison Data System (NPDS): 35th Annual Report. *Clin Toxicol(Phila).* 2018;56(12):1213–1415.
Lavonas EJ, Ruha AM, Banner W, et al. Unified treatment algorithm for the management of crotaline snakebite in the United States: results of an evidence-informed consensus workshop. *BMC Emerg Med.* 2011;11:2.
Medeiros I, Saconato H. Antibiotic prophylaxis for mammalian bites, *Cochrane Database Syst Rev* (2):CD001738, 2001. https://www.ncbi.nlm.nih.gov/pubmed/11406003. Accessed January 7, 2019.
Scorpion envenomation. https://emedicine.medscape.com/article/168230-overview. Accessed January 7, 2019.
Widow spider envenomation. http://emedicine.medscape.com/article/772196-overview. Accessed January 7, 2019.

CHAPTER 74

SMOKE INHALATION

Richard E. Wolfe, MD

1. Where is a fire most likely to cause a death?

Every 24 seconds, a fire department in the United States responds to a fire. A home fire occurs every 88 seconds; 77% of all fire deaths occur in homes.

2. What is the most common way to die in a fire?

Although there are many ways to die in a fire, smoke inhalation is by far the most common cause. It accounts for as much as 80% of fire-related deaths, with many of these due to hypoxia. In those that survive the initial fire, the presence of smoke injury increases mortality by nearly 24 times in patients with a burned surface area <20%. Twenty percent of these patients have an inhalation injury. The prevalence of smoke-related lung injury increases with the burn surface area, but significant pulmonary complications secondary to smoke inhalation occur even without cutaneous burns.

3. Is smoke inhalation so lethal because it causes thermal injury to the lungs?

Not usually; although flames can cause direct thermal burns to the upper airway, this type of injury is rare. Air has such a low heat-carrying capacity that it rarely produces lower airway damage. The upper respiratory tract generally cools hot air before it reaches the vocal cords. Injuries from superheated air are thus generally limited to the upper airway. Lung injury from smoke inhalation is usually caused by a wide variety of toxic substances that cause direct chemical injuries, and inflammatory responses from the trachea to the alveoli. Steam is the exception. With 4000 times the heat-carrying capacity of air, steam can cause severe upper airway burns with fatal glottic edema, as well as bronchial mucosal destruction and alveolar hemorrhage.

4. Why is smoke inhalation so dangerous?

Carbon dioxide (CO_2) and carbon monoxide (CO), the major components of smoke, are responsible for a decrease in the concentration of ambient oxygen from 22% to 5%–10%. CO and, more rarely, hydrogen cyanide block the uptake and use of oxygen, leading to severe tissue cellular hypoxemia and metabolic acidosis. Depending on the fuel, temperature, and rate of heating, smoke contains a wide variety of toxins. Soot may act as a vehicle in transporting these toxic gases to the lower respiratory tract, where they dissolve to form acids and alkali. Removal of soot is impaired by the action of certain of these toxins on respiratory cilia, with noxious smoke components causing the release of neuropeptides that induce inflammation. Ultimately, direct tissue toxicity and inflammation lead to severe, delayed pneumonia.

5. Name the four clinical stages of smoke inhalation.

1. Acute respiratory distress begins 1–12 hours postinjury, and is caused by bronchospasm, laryngeal edema, and bronchorrhea.
2. Noncardiogenic pulmonary edema (adult respiratory distress syndrome) begins 6–72 hours post-injury secondary to increased capillary permeability.
3. Strangulation occurs 60–120 hours post smoke injury from eschar formation in patients with circumferential neck burns.
4. Onset of pneumonia occurs 72 hours after injury, usually from *Staphylococcus aureus, Pseudomonas aeruginosa,* or gram-negative organisms.

6. How should smoke inhalation victims be managed in the field?

All victims should be given a 100% nonrebreather mask, even if they are asymptomatic. Oxygen administration dramatically accelerates the washout of CO, shortening the half-life from 4 hours at room air to about 90 minutes. Endotracheal intubation is indicated for patients in respiratory distress. When the patient's airway has been externally controlled, it should be suctioned to remove inhaled soot. Patients with a loss of consciousness or altered mental status should be transported to a facility capable of providing hyperbaric oxygen (HBO) therapy.

7. What should I ask the emergency medical technicians (EMTs) about the fire?

Ask if the patient was trapped in a closed space, because significant inhalation injury would be less likely in an open area. Try to determine what material was burning. The fuel is of primary importance in determining the composition of smoke and risk to the patient.

8. Name some toxins produced by smoke, and the materials from which they derive.

- Hydrogen cyanide: combustion of wool, silk, nylons, and polyurethanes found commonly in furniture and paper
- Aldehydes, acrolein: wood, cotton, paper, and plastic materials

- Hydrogen chloride, phosgene: pyrolysis of chlorinated polymers; polyvinyl chloride (wire insulation materials); chlorinated acrylics; and wall, floor, and furniture coverings
- Oxides of nitrogen: nitrocellulose film
- Sulfur dioxide, hydrogen sulfide: rubber

9. **What are the earliest clinical manifestations of acute inhalation injury after smoke exposure?**
Inflamed nares, cough, sputum production, and hoarseness are the first signs of injury. This is because the nasopharynx and larynx are exposed to the highest concentration of inhaled toxins, leading to the most severe chemical burns. Furthermore, the proximal airway is usually the only part of the airway subjected to thermal burns. However, even when injured, nasopharyngeal and laryngeal edema may be delayed in some cases. Furthermore, rapid progression to complete airway obstruction may occur in patients with mild symptoms. For this reason, close observation followed by early airway management is often necessary to ensure patient safety.

10. **Besides damage to the airway and the cutaneous burns, what occult life threats do you need to rule out?**
Systemic effects of CO, cyanide, and, more rarely, hydrogen sulfide can cause multisystem tissue damage through mitochondrial respiratory chain poisoning. In addition, CO displaces oxygen by combining with hemoglobin, preventing the blood from carrying oxygen. Methemoglobinemia may occur due to heat denaturation of hemoglobin, oxides produced in fire, and methemoglobin-forming materials such as nitrites.
    Finally, always carefully assess any fire victim for associated traumatic injuries.

11. **Why is HBO therapy thought to be beneficial for smoke inhalation?**
    - HBO therapy provides increased oxygen to poorly functioning mitochondrial enzymes inhibited by CO and cyanide.
    - HBO therapy at 3 atm decreases the half-life of CO to 23 minutes.
    - HBO therapy has been shown to reduce smoke-induced pulmonary edema.
    - At a cellular level, HBO therapy decreases the formation of intercellular adhesion molecules on the endothelial membrane, which prevents neutrophils from infiltrating the central nervous system and causing a damaging inflammatory reaction and permanent neurologic sequelae.

    Despite these theoretic benefits, there has not yet been sufficient evidence to obtain consensus on the use of HBO therapy for smoke inhalation.

12. **How do I make the diagnosis of smoke inhalation injury?**
Bronchoscopy is needed to confirm the presence of inhalation injury. Soot deposition in the airway, extensive edema, mucosal erythema, hemorrhage, and ulceration confirm smoke inhalation has occurred. The initial bronchoscopy may be relatively normal, because hyperemia and edema formation may take some time to evolve. A normal proximal airway does not rule out more distal injury.

13. **How should asymptomatic patients be managed?**
Observe the patient in the ED for a few hours first. If still asymptomatic, provide comprehensive discharge instructions on when to return if the patient is reliable. Although the physical examination cannot reliably rule out all complications, such as delayed noncardiogenic pulmonary edema or pneumonia, ED or in-hospital observation are not cost effective. The patient should be instructed to return to the ED if shortness of breath, chest pain, or fever occurs.

14. **If the patient's pulse oximetry is normal, would arterial blood gas analysis yield additional information?**
In the presence of carboxyhemoglobin (COHb), pulse oximetry may yield a falsely elevated (normal) reading. Arterial blood gases may be helpful only if the oxygen saturation is measured directly and not derived from the arterial partial pressure of oxygen (PaO_2) measurement. Although an increased alveolar-arterial gradient may correlate with smoke inhalation injury, it does not predict the severity of injury. Arterial blood gases are most useful in determining hypoventilation (increased partial pressure of carbon dioxide [PCO_2]) and the presence of a metabolic or respiratory acidosis.

15. **Should I get a chest radiograph on all patients with a history of smoke inhalation?**
Chest radiographs are usually normal immediately after smoke inhalation injury, and abnormalities usually appear on a delayed basis. A chest radiograph is not indicated in asymptomatic patients and, in most instances, it is useful only as a baseline in symptomatic patients. A decision to obtain a radiograph should be made on a case-by-case approach, pending clinical presentation.

16. **Can I use the standard burn formula for intravenous (IV) fluids if smoke inhalation is present?**
Patients with cutaneous and inhalation injuries pose a difficult problem because their fluid requirements are usually greater, but because of leaky capillaries, they are much more likely to develop membrane permeable pulmonary edema. IV fluids must be guided by regular clinical reevaluation (i.e., breath sounds, oxygen saturation, urinary output, vital signs) rather than by formulas. Swan-Ganz monitoring may be required.

17. **Is HBO therapy the only available therapy for cyanide poisoning?**
No, the hydroxocobalamin (CYANOKIT) can be used for victims of cyanide toxicity. When this is not available, the sodium thiosulfate component in the Lilly cyanide antidote kit should be used. The military is currently evaluating the efficacy of other agents which can be administered intramuscularly.

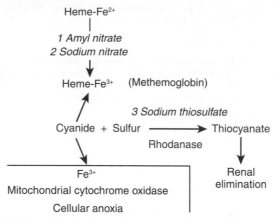

Fig. 74.1 Mechanism of the Lilly cyanide antidote kit. Fe^{2+}, Ferrous; Fe^{3+}, ferric (iron).

18. **Tell me about hydroxocobalamin.**
    Hydroxocobalamin (vitamin B_{12}) reduces cyanide concentrations by combining with cyanide to form cyanocobalamin. It should be considered for patients who are comatose, in cardiac arrest, or have clear signs of cardiovascular extremis. If hydroxocobalamin is used, it should be given as early as possible. The usual dose is 5 g IV. Unlike the cyanide antidote kit, it does not cause methemoglobinemia and may be redosed as needed. Hydroxocobalamin interferes with many standard colorimetric and co-oximetric laboratory assays; therefore, if feasible, send labs prior to administration.

19. **How does the Lilly cyanide antidote kit work?**
    Cyanide binds to the ferric ions (Fe^{3+}), blocking the mitochondrial cytochrome oxidase pathway and cellular respiration. The cyanide antidote kit acts in two ways to limit this:
    1. Nitrites generate methemoglobin, creating heme-ferric ions to compete with cyanide with mitochondrial ferric ions.
    2. Sulfur transferase (rhodanese) binds cyanide molecules to sulfur-forming thiocyanate, which is nontoxic and eliminated in the urine. Thiosulfate accelerates this process by increasing available sulfur molecules (Fig. 74.1).

20. **When should I use the cyanide antidote kit?**
    Symptomatic patients can have CO or cyanide toxicity. Nitrites can cause more prolonged asphyxia in patients with hypoxemia and elevated COHb fractions. They can also worsen underlying methemoglobinemia. These drugs should be reserved for patients in extremis or who remain critically ill after intubation and 100% oxygenation. The sodium thiosulfate portion of the kit can be used safely even when the measured oxygen saturation is low. High lactate levels can help distinguish cyanide from CO, because elevations in serum lactate correlate well with cyanide toxicity.

KEY POINTS: SMOKE INHALATION

1. Obtain CO level and treat any patient who has inhaled smoke in an enclosed space with nonrebreather high-flow mask oxygen.
2. Consider cyanide poisoning when the patient in extremis inhaled smoke from burning furniture fabric (e.g., wool, silk, or polyurethanes).

---

21. **How do I make the diagnosis of CO poisoning in the ED?**
    The obvious history is any exposure to fire or smoke in a confined space. The more subtle presentation is early morning headache, which improves after exiting a residence with a defective heating system, often affecting family members as well. A CO level should be obtained from all patients in whom the diagnosis is considered.

CONTROVERSY

22. **Is the early respiratory failure seen in smoke inhalation victims worsened by aggressive crystalloid resuscitation?**
    Respiratory failure from interstitial fluid accumulation is a rare event. When it occurs, it is caused by capillary leakage caused by inflammation of pulmonary tissue. The amount of crystalloid used during resuscitation does

not increase the risk or the severity of the resultant pulmonary edema. Fluids should not be withheld in a patient with severe cutaneous and respiratory burns.

23. How do I treat CO poisoning?

All patients should be given high-flow O_2 via a nonrebreather bag reservoir mask, which will reduce the half-life of CO from 4 to 5 hours on room air to approximately 1 hour. Although the long-term benefit of HBO therapy has been called into question with conflicting published studies, most still recommend its use in the following patients:

- A pregnant woman with a CO level greater than 15%
- Any patient with a neurologic abnormality (i.e., coma or altered mentation)
- Any patient with cardiac ischemia or instability

BIBLIOGRAPHY

Dries DJ, Endorf FW. Inhalation injury: epidemiology, pathology, treatment strategies. *Scand J Trauma Resusc Emerg Med.* 2013;21:31.
Enkhbaatar P, Pruitt BA, Suman O, et al. Burns 3. Pathophysiology, research challenges, and clinical management of smoke inhalation injury. *Lancet.* 2018;388:1437–1446.
Kaita Y, Tarui T, Shoji T, et al. Cyanide poisoning is a possible cause of cardiac arrest among fire victims, and empiric antidote treatment may improve outcomes. *Am J Emerg Med.* 2018;36:851–853.
Miller AC, Elamin ME, Suffredini AF. Inhaled anticoagulant regimen for the treatment of smoke inhalation and associated acute lung injury: a systematic review. *Crit Care Med.* 2014;42:413–419.
Nguyen L, Afshari A, Kahn SA, et al. Utility and outcomes of hydroxocobalamin use in smoke inhalation patients. *Burns.* 2017;43:107–113.
Wolf SJ, Maloney GE, Shih RD, et al. Clinical policy: critical issues in the evaluation and management of adult patients presenting to the emergency department with acute carbon monoxide poisoning. *Ann Emerg Med.* 2017;69(1):98–107.

CHAPTER 75

COMMON DRUGS OF ABUSE

Caitlin F. Bonney, MD and Vikhyat S. Bebarta, MD

1. **How are the rates of US drug overdoses and deaths changing?**
   The Centers for Disease Control and Prevention (CDC) has reported data showing a steep increase in the rate of drug overdose deaths since 2000, including a 200% increase in the rate of overdose deaths involving opioids. Analgesics (opioids and non-opioids) are the most common agents involved in mortality of pharmaceuticals since 1995. Opioids represent approximately half of those deaths each year. Since 2008, the CDC has reported that unintentional overdose, mostly from opioids, is the most common cause of unintentional death, superseding traumatic deaths from motor vehicle accidents. Fortunately, preliminary data from the CDC from 2017 and 2018 show that drug overdoses may be leveling off or decreasing.

2. **What are body packers and stuffers?**
   - **Body packers** are individuals who transport large amounts of illegal drugs carefully packaged to maintain integrity while in the gastrointestinal tract. Packets are usually composed of wax, plastic, rubber, or foil, sealed and ingested by the human carrier along with an antimotility agent. Alternatively, the individual may insert the containers into the rectum or vagina. The individual then travels by plane or other vehicle to another location. Body packing is used to transport illegal drugs, such as heroin or cocaine, to other countries. The individual then defecates the vials and delivers them to the recipient. The packets are designed to prevent rupture, but can be life threatening if they do rupture.
   - **Body stuffers** are individuals who quickly ingest (stuff) poorly wrapped illegal drugs while attempting to evade law enforcement. The wrapping containing the drug is usually referred to as a *baggie*. Commonly, it is a much smaller amount of drug than body packers handle and is loosely wrapped. The drug is typically absorbed quickly, and the patient usually develops symptoms shortly after ingestion.

3. **How should body stuffers and body packers be managed?**
   Urine drug screening is not helpful for determining which drug, if any, was ingested. In addition, the patient's history for timing, content, and amount of ingested substance is often unreliable.
   - Body stuffers should receive activated charcoal and be observed in a monitored setting for at least 6 hours. Radiographs are not helpful. If the patient develops symptoms or vital sign abnormalities, admit the patient for observation.
   - The packets from body packers may be seen on plain abdominal radiographs, radiographs with oral contrast material (Gastrografin), or require abdominal computed tomography (CT) to visualize. Based on limited data, contrasted radiographs and CT scans are the most sensitive. Body packers should receive activated charcoal and polyethylene glycol electrolyte solution (e.g., CoLyte, GoLYTELY) to enhance elimination through the colon. Polyethylene glycol may be administered through a nasogastric tube at approximately 2 L/h until all packets have cleared. Clear rectal effluent is not a sufficient end point to end decontamination. Repeat radiologic testing with abdominal CT or a radiograph with oral contrast should be used to determine whether all packets have cleared. Surgery is rarely needed to remove retained packets. Occasionally, packets may take days to evacuate. Body packers are at risk of intestinal obstruction from the large amount of foreign bodies in the bowel. Packet rupture can cause bowel wall necrosis or life-threatening toxicity, which requires urgent surgical intervention for packet removal.

OPIOIDS

4. **What do the terms opium, opiate, opioid, and narcotic mean?**
   - **Opium** is a mixture of alkaloids, including morphine and codeine, extracted from the opium poppy.
   - An **opiate** is a drug derived from opium (e.g., heroin, codeine, and morphine).
   - An **opioid** is any drug that has opium-like activity, including the opiates and all synthetic and semisynthetic drugs that interact with opioid receptors in the body (e.g., fentanyl, hydrocodone, and oxycodone).
   - The term **narcotic** is nonspecific; it refers to any addictive drug that reduces pain, alters mood and behavior, and usually induces sleep or stupor, and is more specific to law enforcement than medicine.

5. **What is the typical clinical presentation of opioid poisoning?**
   The classic triad of opioid poisoning is central nervous system (CNS) depression, respiratory depression, and miosis. Patients who overdose on opioids are hyporeflexic and have decreased bowel sounds. They may be hypothermic, cyanotic, and mildly hypotensive and bradycardic.

Table 75.1 Common Causes of Non–Opioid-Related Miosis	
Sympatholytic agents	Clonidine, antipsychotics, oxymetazoline, and tetrahydrozoline
Cholinergic agents	Organophosphates, carbamates, nicotine, pilocarpine, phencyclidine, and similar congeners
Miscellaneous	Pontine infarct and Horner syndrome

6. Do all patients with opioid intoxication cases have miosis?
No, mydriasis or normal pupils can occur in the following cases:
- Intoxication of specific synthetic opioids (i.e., meperidine [Demerol], propoxyphene, or pentazocine)
- Diphenoxylate-atropine (Lomotil) use
- After naloxone use
- With hypoxia
- With mydriatic eye drops use
- Coingestion of other mydriatic drugs (e.g., anticholinergics)
- Occasionally, phenylephrine, instilled into the patient's nares by paramedics for nasal intubation, may spill into the patient's eyes, causing mydriasis (Table 75.1)

7. How should a patient with respiratory compromise from opioid overdose be treated?
Resuscitation takes precedence over naloxone administration. Support the patient's ventilation with a bag mask until the opioid antagonist is administered. Intubate the apneic or cyanotic patient's airway if the patient does not awaken after naloxone, but make sure to give him or her enough time to respond to naloxone. Obtain a serum glucose level and administer oxygen.

8. What is the appropriate naloxone dose?
For children younger than 5 years or less than 20 kg, administer 0.01 mg/kg intravenously (IV) for respiratory depression initially. If there is no response, then attempt 0.1 mg/kg IV. In an adult patient who has coma and respiratory depression (severe bradypnea or hypoxia), infuse an initial dose of 0.2–0.4 mg IV. If there is no response to this dose, repeated doses up to 2 mg can be given. Administer 1–2 mg IV initially for the apneic or cyanotic adult or child. For patients who abuse opioids or who use opioids for chronic pain, infuse 0.05–0.1 mg to wake the patient without inducing opioid withdrawal. Additional doses should be given judiciously to patients who consume opioids chronically. Opioid withdrawal is unpleasant to the patient, but is not life threatening.

9. Can naloxone be administered by other routes besides IV?
Yes, if venous access cannot be accomplished, administer the naloxone intramuscularly (IM) or subcutaneously. A dose of 0.8 mg IM has an equal time to effect as 0.4 mg IV. Naloxone can also be administered via an endotracheal tube, intranasally via an atomizer, intraosseously, or via sublingual injection. Naloxone is not effective orally because of significant first-pass metabolism.

10. Do all patients respond to a standard dose of naloxone?
No, larger doses of naloxone may be required to reverse the effects of synthetic opioids, such as codeine, diphenoxylate-atropine (Lomotil), propoxyphene (Darvon), pentazocine (Talwin), dextromethorphan, and the fentanyl derivatives. If an opioid overdose is suspected and the patient does not respond to an initial naloxone dose, repeat additional doses until a response is noted or until 10 mg has been given. Consider concomitant ingestions or alternative diagnoses in patients requiring more than 10 mg naloxone.

11. How long does the clinical effect of naloxone last?
The duration of action of IV naloxone is 40–75 minutes, although the serum half-life is shorter. Many oral and some injected opioids produce clinical effects that last for 3–6 hours. Although the duration of action of most opioids is much longer than that of naloxone, resedation is uncommon, particularly with short-acting parenteral opioids (e.g., heroin). Most oral opioids, particularly long-acting agents (e.g., methadone or sustained-release morphine), last several hours and may require additional naloxone and hospital admission. Caution should be taken with overdoses of methadone, which has a duration of action that can last 40 hours.

12. How should recurrent sedation and respiratory depression resulting from a long-acting opioid be treated?
Treat most patients with boluses of naloxone as needed, along with hospital admission, supplemental oxygen, and close monitoring in an intensive care setting. On occasion, patients require several doses of naloxone over a short time interval to maintain normal oxygenation. In these cases, a continuous naloxone infusion may be started. A naloxone infusion is administered at an hourly rate that provides two-thirds of the dose needed to reverse the respiratory depression. The infusion can be adjusted based on the patient's symptoms of withdrawal or sedation.

13. Who should I observe in the ED, and for how long?
It depends. The duration of action of naloxone is 30–80 minutes, so patients who have injected or insufflated (snorted) opioids should be observed for at least 2 hours after a dose of naloxone to monitor for resedation. Most physicians consider observation for up to 4 hours after the last dose of naloxone in an asymptomatic patient to

be more than adequate. This extended period may allow for recognition of coingestants and recurrent respiratory depression. Unfortunately, quality control is lacking and many agents billed as heroin actually may contain agents which may cause prolonged respiratory depression, ultimately requiring longer observation periods. Occasionally, patients who have inadequate ventilation, which necessitates treatment, or who develop complications of opioid use must be admitted. Observe for 8 hours or admit the patient who ingested short-acting oral opioids, such as oxycodone or hydrocodone. Admit patients who have ingested or injected long-acting opioids, such as methadone or long-acting preparations of oxycodone, for 12–24 hours or longer. Admit patients who develop signs of non-cardiogenic pulmonary edema (see Question 18, later). Patients should have normal oxygen saturations, be awake, and be ambulatory before discharge. The patient should preferably be discharged into the care of a competent adult and with home naloxone for emergent therapy.

14. What are the signs of opioid withdrawal?
Signs of withdrawal include anxiety, yawning, lacrimation, rhinorrhea, diaphoresis, mydriasis, nausea and vomiting, diarrhea, piloerection, abdominal pain, and myalgias. Opioid withdrawal typically occurs approximately 12 hours after last heroin use and 30 hours after last methadone use. Seizures, altered mentation, dysrhythmias, and other life-threatening complications are not usually consistent with opioid withdrawal.

15. How is opioid withdrawal best treated?
Treatment is symptomatic. Treat with IV fluids, sedation, antiemetics, and antidiarrheal agents. Oral clonidine 0.1–0.2 mg may also be helpful. However, published cases describe a concomitant abuse of clonidine, because the user feels it enhances the opioid euphoria. Discharge patients with symptomatic medications as well. If naloxone is administered, the most severe withdrawal symptoms commonly resolve in 45–75 minutes. More commonly, EDs are equipped to transition patients in opioid withdrawal to buprenorphine maintenance therapy to reduce withdrawal and illicit opioid dependence.

16. How useful are toxicology screens for opioids, and which opioids are not often detected?
Toxicology screens are not generally helpful in acute management. Not only are the results delayed but also clinical presentation is also more helpful than an insensitive test. Opioid screens do not detect methadone or other synthetic opioids, such as fentanyl, pentazocine, loperamide, meperidine, oxymorphone, oxycodone, and propoxyphene. Ingestion of poppy seeds does not commonly cause a positive screen, because the lower limit threshold has been raised. However, with further testing, this erroneous cause of positive screens can be excluded. Fluoroquinolones can cause a false-positive result for opioids.

17. Are there any other tests that should be checked in patients with opioid ingestions?
Obtain acetaminophen levels in all patients because it is often combined with hydrocodone, oxycodone, propoxyphene, and codeine. Also obtain a metabolic panel, salicylate level, and electrocardiogram (ECG).

18. What is the most common pulmonary complication of opioid use?
Noncardiogenic pulmonary edema occurs in 3% of opioid overdoses. The mechanism is unclear, but it may be a result of capillary permeability and fluid leak, or from breathing deeply and quickly against a closed glottis after a period of apnea. The patient has pink frothy sputum, cyanosis, and rales. Bilateral alveolar infiltrates are seen on the chest radiograph. Naloxone does not reverse the process, and some patients will need assisted mechanical ventilation.

19. Can opioids cause seizures?
Seizures are rare in patients with therapeutic doses of opioids, but they have been reported with use of synthetic opioids (i.e., meperidine, tramadol, pentazocine, and propoxyphene) and chronic use of morphine.

20. Is it safe to give dextromethorphan or meperidine to patients taking antidepressant medications?
No. The combination of these opioids with antidepressants may precipitate serotonin syndrome. Meperidine and dextromethorphan inhibit serotonin reuptake similar to selective serotonin reuptake inhibitors. A combination of these opioids and monoamine oxidase inhibitors (MAOIs) is also contraindicated, because MAOIs decrease serotonin metabolism.

21. Why should I avoid prescribing meperidine (Demerol)?
The duration of action of meperidine is only 2–3 hours, shorter than morphine or hydromorphone. In contrast to morphine, meperidine's half-life is prolonged by hepatic disease or concomitant use of cytochrome P450 3A4 inhibitors (e.g., amiodarone, tetracycline antibiotics, antifungals, protease inhibitors, grapefruit juice), resulting in toxic effects after repeated doses. Seizures are an adverse effect of normeperidine, a renally cleared metabolite of meperidine. Normeperidine levels are elevated with repetitive administration of oral meperidine, renal failure, and concomitant use of drugs that induce hepatic enzymes, such as phenytoin, phenobarbital, and chlorpromazine. Normeperidine causes CNS agitation, tremors, and psychosis. Meperidine produces serotonin syndrome when combined with other serotonergic agents.

22. Which antidiarrheal agents can cause significant toxicity if ingested?
Diphenoxylate 2.5 mg plus atropine 0.025 mg (Lomotil) can be toxic. Most toxic cases occur in children. Classically, the overdose is a two-phase toxicity: phase 1, with anticholinergic symptoms (flushing, dry mouth); and

phase 2, with opioid effects. However, this pattern is uncommon. Delayed presentations have been reported, and all children should be observed in a monitored setting for at least 24 hours.

Loperamide (Imodium) is a nonprescription antidiarrheal agent derived from diphenoxylate. Acute overdoses typically produce only mild drowsiness, but individuals using high doses of loperamide off-label to prevent opioid withdrawal may exhibit QRS prolongation, QTc prolongation, arrhythmias, and cardiac arrest.

23. **Which opioids can produce ventricular dysrhythmias, a wide QRS complex, mydriasis, and seizures?**
Propoxyphene and loperamide have quinidine-like effects that blocks sodium channels, similar to cyclic antidepressants. Large doses of naloxone (10 mg) may reverse the CNS depression but not the cardiotoxic effects. Sodium bicarbonate has been used successfully for propoxyphene-induced dysrhythmias. Propoxyphene is no more effective for analgesia than salicylates, acetaminophen, or codeine.

24. **What are "designer drugs," and what are the two most notorious designer drugs that have been used?**
Designer drugs are substitutes for other chemicals or drugs that are popular with illicit drug users. They are made inexpensively in clandestine laboratories. 3-Methylfentanyl is an analog of fentanyl known as *China white* or *Persian white*. It is 2000 times more potent than morphine and 20 times more potent than fentanyl. It can cause respiratory compromise quickly. It does not cause the abbreviated rush of heroin, but instead causes a longer duration of euphoria.

1-Methyl-4-phenyl-1,2,5,6-tetrahydropyridine (MPTP) is a compound that was produced accidentally during the synthesis of desmethylprodine or 1-methyl-4-phenyl-4-propionoxypiperidine (MPPP), a meperidine analog. MPTP is cytotoxic to dopaminergic neurons in the substantia nigra. It produces a permanent parkinsonian-like syndrome and occurs after a single ingestion of MPTP. The symptoms do not respond to typical antiparkinsonism medications.

25. **What over-the-counter cold remedy is sometimes abused by teenagers?**
Dextromethorphan (DM) is the D-isomer of levorphanol, a potent opioid agonist. Its metabolite stimulates the release of serotonin and acts at the phencyclidine receptor site, which accounts for its abuse as a hallucinogen. Although Coricidin is its most well-known trade name, DM is available in many other cough medications. It is also known as *ROBO, DEX, red devils, triple C, CCC,* and *skittles*. DM toxicity may present with symptoms of opioid toxicity (miosis, sedation, and respiratory depression) but more commonly presents with slurred speech, nystagmus, hyperexcitability, vomiting, and ataxia. Not all individuals can metabolize DM to its psychoactive metabolite. Naloxone does not usually reverse the symptoms of toxicity. DM does cause false-positive phencyclidine results on urine screening, but it usually does not produce positive results for opioids. Coingredients may cause a predominance of another clinical syndrome (anticholinergic or sympathomimetic toxidrome). Acetaminophen is a common coingredient and should be screened for in all patients abusing DM.

26. **What are some examples of synthetic opioids?**
- Fentanyl, carfentanil, remifentanil
- Methadone
- Tramadol

Fentanyl, carfentanil, and remifentanil are extremely potent (effective at very low doses) short-acting opioids. Fentanyl is about 100 times more potent than morphine, and carfentanil is around 10,000 times stronger. These drugs are often used to increase the potency of heroin and may result in unintentional overdose in an otherwise opioid-tolerant patient. Methadone is an oral opioid used for maintenance therapy in opioid addiction. It has a very long duration of action of 40 hours. Tramadol (Ultram) is a synthetic opioid. The usual effects with overdose are mild sedation and opioid effects. Overdoses have occasionally been associated with seizures, hypertension, respiratory depression, and agitation. The seizures do not respond to naloxone. Although the drug has a low abuse potential, it is not recommended for patients with an opioid dependence history.

SEDATIVE-HYPNOTICS

27. **What is a sedative-hypnotic drug?**
Sedative-hypnotic drugs primarily cause relaxation and tranquilization, and induce drowsiness and sleep. There is no consistent structural relationship among the agents of this group. In sufficient quantities, all drugs of this group result in CNS depression.

28. **What medications fall into this category?**
There are four groups: benzodiazepines, barbiturates, the "Z-drugs" (zolpidem, zopiclone, zaleplon, and eszopiclone), and the miscellaneous group. Some examples of miscellaneous sedative-hypnotics are chloral hydrate, ethanol, and γ-hydroxybutyrate (GHB). Many of the miscellaneous agents are also pharmaceutical agents. For example, ethanol is used in the treatment of methanol and ethylene glycol toxicity, GHB (Xyrem) is used for narcolepsy, and nitrous oxide is used for anesthesia. These drugs are also commonly abused.

29. **What are the Z-drugs?**
Zolpidem, zopiclone, zaleplon, and eszopiclone are drugs that are prescribed for insomnia. While they are not structurally related to benzodiazepines, they have a similar mechanism by binding at the α-1 subunit of the

γ-aminobutyric acid (GABA)-A receptor, and are useful as a sleep aids. Because of its specific affinity for the α-1 subunit, zolpidem has minimal muscle relaxant, anxiolytic, and anticonvulsant properties. Therefore, intoxication presents with CNS depression, and respiratory depression is uncommon. Under rare circumstances, the Z-drugs can be reversed with flumazenil in patients who are neither addicted nor have a history of seizures. Hallucinations and psychosis are rare, but unusual, adverse effects of some of these drugs. The Z-drugs can impair driving and alertness for up to 8 hours after taking a dose. Women may be more affected by the sedation than men, and thus a lower dose is advised in women.

30. **What is a typical presentation of sedative-hypnotic intoxication?**
    Mild intoxication presents with slurred speech, ataxia, and loss of coordination. Moderate to severe intoxication presents with greater CNS depression. Respiratory depression may occur with large ingestions and is compounded by other agents which suppress respiratory drive, such as opioids or ethanol. Pupils are usually midsize and reactive, and may be disconjugate. There are also symptoms specific to individual drugs. Some examples are choral hydrate (pear odor), ethchlorvynol (pulmonary edema, vinyl odor), and glutethimide (anticholinergic effects) (Table 75.2).

31. **Many overdoses seem to present this way, so how are sedative-hypnotics different?**
    Many overdoses present with CNS depression. However, some intoxications also present with a pattern of symptoms known as a *toxidrome* (Table 75.3). Signs of antipsychotic intoxication include sedation and are similar to sedative-hypnotics, but also commonly include tachycardia, mild hypotension, and occasionally, miosis. CNS depression is also a common presentation of illness other than intoxication. Maintain a broad differential when evaluating these patients for such illnesses as meningoencephalitis, intracranial hemorrhage, hypoglycemia, shock, and sepsis.

32. **How do sedative-hypnotics cause CNS depression?**
    Most sedative-hypnotics, particularly benzodiazepines and barbiturates, cause CNS depression by enhancing the effects of GABA, an inhibitory neurotransmitter in the brain. Benzodiazepines increase the rate of the opening of chloride channels associated with GABA. Propofol and barbiturates directly open the chloride channels, potentially causing greater sedation and respiratory suppression. Propofol may also inhibit excitatory brain neurotransmitters, adding to the GABA effects.

33. **How do I make the diagnosis of sedative-hypnotic overdose in a patient with undifferentiated CNS depression?**
    Making the diagnosis can be difficult. Elicit help from friends, family, and involved prehospital providers and police. Review the patient's medical records for previous visits and search his or her belongings for paraphernalia and empty bottles. Often a specific agent will not be identified; rather, only a constellation of symptoms seen with

Table 75.2 Clinical Presentations of Less Common Sedative-Hypnotics

Chloral hydrate	Vomiting and ventricular dysrhythmias
Ethchlorvynol	Vinyl-like odor on breath, prolonged coma, and noncardiogenic pulmonary edema
Glutethimide	Cyclic coma, anticholinergic symptoms (tachycardia uncommon), and thick secretions
Methaqualone	Hyperreflexia, clonus, and muscle hyperactivity
Meprobamate/carisoprodol	Euphoria and concretions in stomach may be seen on radiographs

Table 75.3 Clinical Presentation of Toxidromes Resulting in Depressed or Altered Mental Status

TOXIDROME	PRESENTATION
Opioid	Central nervous system depression, miosis, respiratory depression, hypothermia, and mild bradycardia
Sympathomimetic	Psychomotor agitation, mydriasis, hypertension, tachycardia, diaphoresis, hyperthermia, and seizure
Cholinergic	Bradycardia, bronchorrhea, miosis, salivation, lacrimation, urination, diaphoresis, diarrhea, vomiting, altered mental status, and seizures
Anticholinergic	Delirium, sedation, mydriasis, dry/flushed skin, tachycardia, decreased/absence of bowel sounds, seizures, and mild pyrexia

sedative-hypnotic intoxication may be recognizable. Routine laboratory and radiologic studies, including chemistries, cerebrospinal fluid analysis, and cranial CT scans, may assist in ruling out metabolic, infectious, and CNS disorders as the cause. Urine drug screens are available but typically are not helpful or timely.

34. Is there a role for drug screens or specific drug levels?
Routine drug screens are often not useful in acute management of these patients. The sensitivities and specificities of the assays for detecting specific drugs are variable. For example, the assay for benzodiazepines in the most commonly used urine drug screen is designed only to detect the metabolite of some older, long-lasting benzodiazepine medications. Many newer benzodiazepines will not be detected. The same is true for many barbiturates. Most sedative-hypnotics are not tested for on the routine urine drug screen, and thus their use cannot be excluded. If the screen is positive, it only indicates use within the past several days and may not correlate with clinical presentation. Other agents cause a false-positive result and lead to missing the true etiology for the altered mental status. In addition, many other chemicals and drugs cause altered mental status but will not be present on urine toxicology screening (e.g., jimson weed, isopropanol, inhalant toxicity, lithium, ketamine, chloral hydrate, and bromides). Because the most important treatment in sedative-hypnotic intoxication is supportive care, recognizing the intoxication pattern is more helpful than toxicology testing.

35. What is the treatment for sedative-hypnotic overdose?
Rapid resuscitation is the initial treatment. Manage the patient's airway, assess the respiratory effort and oxygenation, evaluate the circulation and perfusion, and examine for neurologic deficits (ABCDs). After resuscitation, consider gastrointestinal decontamination with activated charcoal and then exclude other causes for altered mentation, acid-base disturbances, or unstable hemodynamics. Do not use flumazenil in undifferentiated intoxication.

36. How do patients die of sedative-hypnotic overdose?
Respiratory depression and resultant hypoxia is the cause of most deaths.

37. Are there specific antidotes for sedative-hypnotic intoxication?
Flumazenil can be used for overdose of benzodiazepine and related medications such as zolpidem.

38. How does flumazenil work?
Benzodiazepines and zolpidem act as GABA-A receptor agonists. Flumazenil antagonizes the effects of these drugs by competitively inhibiting the GABA receptor. This antagonism can cause seizures in benzodiazepine-tolerant individuals. Administer 0.2–0.5 mg of flumazenil IV in increasing doses to a generally accepted maximum dose of 5 mg. Most patients respond to 0.6–1 mg; infuse at a rate of 0.2 mg/min. If there is no response with 5 mg, consider another intoxication, coingestant, or other source for the patient's mental status.

39. Should flumazenil be given empirically to all patients with depressed mental status?
No, flumazenil may be used for a patient with iatrogenic toxicity during procedural sedation or in an unintentional ingestion by a benzodiazepine-naive child or adult. Consider it with a sole benzodiazepine overdose causing significant CNS depression. It has no role in undifferentiated or mixed overdose, because it can induce seizures, unmask the effects of a coingestant, and, rarely, cause life-threatening dysrhythmias. Flumazenil may also induce seizures and withdrawal symptoms in chronic benzodiazepine users. The onset of flumazenil is 1–5 minutes, and the duration of effect is 1–4 hours. Sedation will resume after its effects have worn off. Most patients with a benzodiazepine overdose only require supportive care and do not require flumazenil.
    The ideal patient for flumazenil use would be one with iatrogenic oversedation who does not have the following:
- prior seizure history
- ECG evidence of tricyclic antidepressants
- chronic benzodiazepine use
- abnormal vital signs, including hypoxia
- coingestants that provoke seizures or dysrhythmias (e.g., Z-drugs; see Question 29)

40. What is GHB?
GHB is a naturally occurring human neurotransmitter similar in structure to GABA. GHB has been used as a sleep aid, anesthetic, and muscle builder. Sold online, GHB is abused for its sedating and euphoric effects. Although restricted by the US Food and Drug Administration (FDA) in the 1990s, GHB is available (trade name Xyrem) as a tightly controlled treatment for narcolepsy. However, it is easily synthesized; recipes and materials are widely available. Congeners, including γ-butyrolactone and 1,4-butanediol, are metabolized to GHB and have the same effects and are common.

41. How does a GHB overdose present?
Most ingestions of GHB are mild and produce minimal sedation and euphoria. Rarely, patients overdose on GHB and come to the ED with a decreased level of consciousness. In contrast to other sedative hypnotic intoxications, the level of consciousness tends to fluctuate between mild agitation and severe CNS depression. Airway reflexes are usually intact and often hypersensitive. An attempt at direct laryngoscopy may cause the patient to quickly sit

up and be agitated for several minutes. Because the clinical effects of GHB usually last less than 6 hours, decisions about airway management should be based on the patient's respiratory status and the ability to monitor oxygenation closely in the ED. Although naloxone, flumazenil, and physostigmine have been described as reversal agents in GHB intoxication, no antidote has consistently been shown to be effective. Death is generally from respiratory failure.

42. What are the effects of GHB withdrawal?
Recreational users of GHB manifest withdrawal symptoms of anxiety, insomnia, disorientation, tachycardia, hypertension, and visual and auditory hallucinations. GHB withdrawal is similar to benzodiazepine withdrawal, but can be more intense.

43. What are date rape drugs?
Date rape drugs, which encompass a vast array of agents, are often used to induce CNS depression, causing the victim to lose consciousness, and facilitating an assault (see Chapter 79).

44. What are some effects of inhalant abuse?
Household and automotive products may be abused by sniffing (inhaling directly from the container), huffing (inhaling from a rag that has been sprayed or soaked with the material), or bagging (inhaling from a bag that has been filled with the material). Inhalants cause euphoria and CNS depression. Most substances used as inhalants are aerosolized hydrocarbons such as brake cleaner or keyboard cleaner. Toluene, found in brake cleaner, causes type I renal tubular acidosis (RTA), characterized by metabolic acidosis, hypokalemia, and acute kidney injury. Prolonged use of inhalants can cause leukoencephalopathy, confusion, and ataxia.

45. What is sudden sniffing death syndrome?
Inhalational abuse of halogenated hydrocarbons, commonly found in keyboard cleaners, can cause a condition where a sudden event, such as being startled by police, causes cardiac arrest. The theory is that the halogenated hydrocarbon causes myocardial sensitization that is prone to dysrhythmia after an adrenergic surge. These patients may not respond to epinephrine in cardiac arrest. Esmolol and overdrive pacing should be considered adjuncts to advanced cardiac life support when inhaled halogenated hydrocarbons are suspected.

46. What are "whip-its?"
The practice of inhaling nitrous oxide (N_2O) directly from whipped cream canisters is known as "whip-its." Nitrous oxide is commonly known as laughing gas or nitrous and is used as an inhalational anesthetic. It may also be sold at raves in balloons filled with N_2O gas. Nitrous oxide causes euphoria via CNS hypoxia. Regular and prolonged use of N_2O causes a pseudo-B_{12}-deficiency syndrome with subacute combined degeneration of the spinal cord with progressive weakness, numbness, and tingling of the extremities.

HALLUCINOGENS

47. What are hallucinogens?
Typically, the term *hallucinogen* refers to agents that are used recreationally for their mind-altering effects.

48. List some examples of hallucinogens.
- Ayahuasca
- 4-Bromo-2,5-dimethoxyphenethylamine (2C-B)
- *N,N*-Dimethyltryptamine (DMT), 5-methoxy-*N,N*-dimethyltryptamine (5-MeO-DMT)
- *N,N*-Diisopropyl-5-methoxytryptamine (Foxy-Methoxy)
- Ketamine
- Lysergic acid diethylamide (LSD), lysergic acid amide (LSA)
- Marijuana
- Mescaline (peyote)
- 3,4-Methylenedioxymethamphetamine (MDMA, ecstasy, Molly)
- 3,4-Methylenedioxypyrovalerone (MDPV)
- Methoxetamine (MXE)
- 1-(1-Phenylcyclohexyl) piperidine (PCP or phencyclidine)
- Psiolocybin, psilocin (active components in *Psilocybe* mushrooms)

49. List the life-threatening effects of hallucinogens.
Common effects are seizures, hyperthermia, metabolic acidosis, hypertension, and dysrhythmias. Rhabdomyolysis can develop subsequently. The effects of hallucinogens are unpredictable and different with each use. Trauma commonly occurs as a result of the disinhibition and aggressiveness caused by hallucinogen abuse.

50. Why would someone "lick a toad"?
Hallucinations are produced by bufotenine, the substance in the skin secretions of *Bufo (Bufo vulgaris, Bufo marinus)* toads. Bufotenine and many other natural toxins have been used for years for hallucinogenic effects. However, *Bufo* toad secretions also contain cardiac glycosides and patients who have ingested toad venom may present with life-threatening cardiac glycoside toxicity (see Chapter 76). Mescaline is the toxin in peyote, a cactus

found in the southwestern United States and Mexico. Psilocybin (4-phosphoryloxy-*N,N*-dimethyltryptamine) is found in some species of mushrooms; DMT is in many plants and seeds. Natural agents (such as these) and their synthetic derivatives are used for hallucinogenic purposes.

51. What is the treatment for hallucinogen toxicity?
Reassurance, a calm environment, avoidance of further trauma, and good supportive care are important. Administer a benzodiazepine to calm agitated patients or to treat seizures. Consider physical restraint and antipsychotics for patients experiencing hallucinations and psychosis.

STIMULANTS

52. What are examples of stimulants?
- Cocaine
- Crack cocaine
- Amphetamines
- Methamphetamine
- Ecstasy (MDMA)
- Caffeine
- Cathinone

53. What is the difference between cocaine and amphetamines?
Both drugs are stimulants, and both work by increasing release of norepinephrine, epinephrine, dopamine, and serotonin. Cocaine has direct vasoconstrictive effects, blocks nervous system and cardiac sodium channels, and has a shorter duration of action than amphetamines.

54. How should I screen for cocaine use?
The best way to screen for recent cocaine use is with a urine drug screen. Cocaine is metabolized rapidly, and detection of the parent compound in blood indicates recent use. However, blood tests for cocaine are rarely used. Cocaine undergoes nonenzymatic degradation to benzoylecgonine and ecgonine methyl ester. These metabolites are excreted renally and may be detected in the urine for several days after the initial exposure.

55. What are freebase and crack cocaine?
Cocaine is extracted from the leaves of the coca plant and usually arrives in the United States as a white powder, cocaine hydrochloride (CHCl). This powder is highly water soluble and therefore crosses mucous membranes and intestinal mucosa very quickly. High temperatures destroy cocaine hydrochloride, so the powder is not suitable for smoking. The powder can be dissolved with sodium bicarbonate (baking soda) or ammonia and water. This solution may subsequently be treated with diethyl ether, decanted, and dried to form freebase, or it can be boiled, ice added to reduce the temperature, and dried to form crack (so called because of the popping sound that occurs during heating). Freebase and crack are resistant to pyrolysis and can be smoked.

56. What is the significance of chest pain after using cocaine?
Pneumothorax or pneumomediastinum may occur after a Valsalva maneuver when cocaine has been smoked. Aortic dissection is rare. Myocardial infarction and acute coronary syndrome have followed intranasal, IV, and smoked cocaine, even in young patients with normal coronary arteries. Benzodiazepine is the initial treatment of choice for cocaine-induced chest pain.

57. Does concomitant ingestion of ethanol change the effects of cocaine?
Yes, in the presence of ethanol, cocaine is metabolized to cocaethylene (ethylbenzoylecgonine), a metabolite that retains cocaine's vasoconstrictive properties. Cocaine and ethanol cause synergistic depression of ventricular contraction and relaxation. Simultaneous ethanol ingestion and intranasal cocaine increase peak plasma concentration of cocaine by 20%, compared with intranasal cocaine alone. The increased cocaine concentration increases euphoria, and thus concomitant abuse.

58. What is "ice"?
Ice is the smokable form of methamphetamine, named for its appearance of transparent crystals. In contrast to CHCl, this pure base form of methamphetamine HCl evaporates easily at room temperature and is absorbed rapidly from the lungs. Similar to IV methamphetamine, it causes an immediate euphoric effect, but without the risks of IV drug administration. The clinical manifestations of methamphetamine are secondary to heightened catecholamine activity and are the same, regardless of the route of administration. Potential adverse effects include hypertension, dysrhythmias, intracranial hemorrhage, seizures, and hyperthermia.

59. What are "ecstasy," "Eve," and "Molly"?
Adam, ecstasy, Molly, E, and *XTC* are street names for MDMA. *Eve* is a street name for 3,4-methylenedioxyethylamphetamine (MDEA) and is less commonly used. These are designer drug analogs of amphetamines and are illegal. These drugs increase serotonin release and reduce degradation more potently than other amphetamines. Their

unique chemical structure results in greater euphoria and less sympathomimetic toxicity. MDMA causes long-term neurotoxic damage in the brains of experimental animals. Large overdoses of MDMA or MDEA, both phenylethylamines, can resemble amphetamine toxicity. Hyperthermia (caused by the drug, high skeletal muscle activity, and hot, crowded conditions at raves) and seizures are associated with death. In addition, ecstasy use has been associated with severe hyponatremia related to increased water intake during raves and drug-induced increased secretion of antidiuretic hormone. Ecstasy and other designer drugs may not be detected on routine urine drug screens for amphetamines and methamphetamine.

60. How should I treat someone with toxicity from stimulants?
The triple C method:
- **C**alm them.
- **C**ool them.
- Uncover **C**omplications.

Treat agitation and seizures with a benzodiazepine. Large and repeated doses may be required. Treat hyperthermia aggressively by reducing psychomotor agitation with sedation, by adding cooling measures (i.e., evaporation, cooling blanket, and cool IV fluids), or by paralysis. Stimulant complications include rhabdomyolysis, pyrexia, acidosis, intracranial hemorrhage, pneumomediastinum, abdominal ischemia, and injection-related complications (i.e., abscess, endocarditis, and cellulitis). Cocaine is more likely to cause complications, because it directly causes vasoconstriction in addition to the secondary effects of increased release and decreased uptake of norepinephrine, epinephrine, serotonin, and dopamine.

61. How do I treat stimulant-induced hypertension?
Most cases are short lived and can be treated with benzodiazepines. A true hypertensive emergency, although rare, can be treated with benzodiazepines and nitroglycerin. Phentolamine, nitroprusside, and calcium channel blockers are rarely needed, and supportive data are limited. Nitroglycerin and other cardiac interventions may be used in patients with ischemic chest pain from vasoconstriction or myocardial infarction. β-Blockers, such as propranolol, should be avoided in the patient with cocaine toxicity, because they allow unbridled α-agonism, which can result in elevated blood pressure and coronary artery vasoconstriction.

62. What are "bath salts"?
Bath salts are designer drugs that are synthetic β-ketone cathinones, which are similar to amphetamines in structure. They are a white crystalline solid that is similar in appearance to Epsom salt and other actual bath salts. They are often sold as potpourri or plant food "not for human consumption" to avoid the laws prohibiting these products. Effects are similar to amphetamines (tachycardia, hypertension, psychomotor agitation), and psychosis, hallucinations, and aggression may be more common with these drugs. Common examples are mephedrone, methedrone, MDPV, methylone, and pyrovalerone.

63. What are synthetic cannabinoids?
Synthetic cannabinoids are chemically altered analogs to tetrahydrocannabinol (THC), cannabidiol (CBD), and cannabinol (CBN). The chemicals are sprayed onto inert plant material and then consumed by smoking or ingestion. Common names are *spice, space, K2,* and *chill out.* They are sold in shops as materials such as potpourri or plant food "not consumable for humans," similar to bath salts. Effects are widely variable, and include symptoms typical of marijuana use—eye injection, euphoria, hunger, tachycardia, and paranoia—as well as sympathomimetic symptoms such as psychomotor agitation and hypertension. In addition, these drugs can cause psychosis, seizures, hallucinations, and acute kidney injury. They are not detected on the drug screen for THC. Treatment is supportive; benzodiazepines are often used for agitation.

64. Can consumable (edible or drinkable) marijuana cause a patient to come to the ED?
Yes, consumable (edible or drinkable) THC products are concentrated and contain 5–50 times more THC than THC designed for smoking. Children, in particular, can develop sedation, hallucinations, and altered mentation with accidental ingestions. Adults can develop similar symptoms with large ingestions or with intentional "overdose" of concentrated edible products.

65. I had a patient with ear and nose ischemia from cocaine use. Why did that happen?
Cocaine is a potent vasoconstrictor and may cause nasal septal ischemia. However, cocaine itself should not cause ischemia distal from the site of use. Often, cocaine is adulterated or contaminated, and one of the most common adulterants is levamisole. Levamisole is an anthelminthic and immunomodulator. It can cause vasculitis and neutropenia. Surgical management may be required for debridement and skin grafting of ischemic areas.

66. What is the stimulant-induced occult triad of death (OTD)?
OTD is the occult triad of death: acidemia, rhabdomyolysis, and pyrexia. These three occult effects occur often, can be easily missed in the agitated patient, and, if not detected early, can lead to death. With the moderately or severely agitated patient, obtain an arterial or venous blood pH level. Also, obtain a creatine kinase level and repeat it if the patient continues to be physically agitated or it is notably elevated.

ANTICHOLINERGIC AGENTS

67. What are anticholinergic agents, and how do they present?

Common anticholinergic agents include antihistamines, classically diphenhydramine, along with other over-the-counter cough and cold products. Another profoundly anticholinergic agent is jimson weed, a plant that can be found ubiquitously across the United States, which is often steeped for tea to be ingested or smoked; it is profoundly anticholinergic. The anticholinergic toxidrome consists of altered mentation, but not aggression, dry flushed skin, mydriasis, hypertension, hyperthermia, tachycardia, urinary retention, and seizure.

68. How should patients with the anticholinergic toxidrome be managed?

Initiate supportive care and IV fluids. Insert a Foley catheter if urinary retention is suspected; this may be a source of agitation, but patients may not be able to communicate their feeling of discomfort. Check an ECG for QRS widening, as some anticholinergics can cause sodium channel blockade. Treat agitation and seizures with benzodiazepines. If symptoms are not controlled with benzodiazepines, physostigmine may be given. Do not give physostigmine to patients with a history of asthma, aspirin allergy, or suspected ingestion of tricyclic antidepressants. The dose of physostigmine is 0.02 mg/kg to a max of 2 mg, given as a slow IV push over 5 minutes. Prior to administration, place the patient on a monitor and have atropine at the bedside in case of bradycardia. Adverse effects of physostigmine include bradycardia, bronchospasm, and bronchorrhea. Patients with true anticholinergic toxicity should rapidly improve within 5–10 minutes of physostigmine infusion. The effects of physostigmine last only 20–45 minutes, but this medication can be used as a diagnostic tool, or to calm a patient at harm to themselves or staff due to agitation. Although anticholinergic symptoms will likely return, they are often less profound.

KEY POINTS: COMMON DRUGS OF ABUSE

1. The classic triad of opioid poisoning is CNS depression, respiratory depression, and miosis.
2. In patients with respiratory compromise secondary to opioid intoxication, patient resuscitation takes precedence over administration of opioid antagonists, such as naloxone.
3. Flumazenil is an antidote to benzodiazepine intoxication, and it is a specific antagonist to the GABA-A receptor. It has no role in the undifferentiated or mixed overdose.
4. The use of routine toxicology screens in undifferentiated overdose is generally not helpful because of the false-positive results, limited number of drugs screened, lack of correlation to clinical presentation, and prolonged length of time to obtain the results.
5. Simultaneous cocaine and ethanol use depresses myocardial contractility.
6. Ecstasy (MDMA) can cause hyponatremia and hyperthermia.

Websites
https://www.datafiles.samhsa.gov/study-series/drug-abuse-warning-network-dawn-nid13516. Accessed January 9, 2019.
www.aapcc.org. Accessed January 9, 2019.
https://www.erowid.org/. Accessed January 9, 2019.

BIBLIOGRAPHY

Boyer EW. Management of opioid analgesic overdose. *N Engl J Med.* 2012;367(2):146–155.
Dawson AH. Naloxone, naltrexone, and nalmefene. In: Dart RC, ed. *Medical Toxicology.* 3rd ed. Philadelphia, PA: Lippincott Williams & Wilkins; 2004:228–230.
Ernst T, Chang L, Leonido-Yee M, et al. Evidence for long-term neurotoxicity associated with methamphetamine abuse. *Am Acad Neurol.* 2000;54:1344–1349.
Kirages TJ, Sule HP, Mycyk MB. Severe manifestations of Cloricidin intoxication. *Am J Emerg Med.* 2003;21:473–475.
Lange RA, Hillis LD. Cardiovascular complications of cocaine use. *N Engl J Med.* 2001;345:351–358.
Lee DC. Sedative-hypnotics. In: Hoffman RS, Howland MA, Lewin NA, et al., eds. *Goldfrank's Toxicologic Emergencies.* 10th ed. New York, NY: McGraw-Hill; 2014:1002–1012.
Snead OC, Gibson KM. Gamma hydroxybutyric acid. *N Engl J Med.* 2005;352:2721–2736.
Traub SJ, Hoffman RS, Nelson LS. Body packing – the internal concealment of illicit drugs. *N Engl J Med.* 2003;349(26):2519–2526.
Wolfe T, Barton E. Nasal drug delivery in EMS: reducing needlestick risk. *JEMS.* 2003;28:52–63.

CHAPTER 76

CARDIOVASCULAR TOXICOLOGY

Alexa Camarena-Michel, MD and Ryan Chuang, MD

KEY POINTS: CARDIOVASCULAR TOXICOLOGY

1. For sodium channel blocking agents, give sodium bicarbonate boluses if there is QRS widening and clinical signs of toxicity.
2. There is no single proven successful treatment for calcium channel blocker (CCB) and β-blocker (BB) overdose. Severe ingestions often require multiple interventions. Start with symptomatic and supportive care first (ABCs), IV fluids, and pressors. Remember atropine, glucagon, calcium, and high-dose insulin. Think of high-dose insulin early, as it often takes time to prepare.
3. There is no serum digoxin level that is considered an absolute indication for digoxin immune Fab.

1. **How do different poisons affect heart rate, blood pressure, and QRS duration?**
   See Table 76.1.

2. **What drugs cause cardiovascular toxicity by blocking cardiac sodium channels?**
   The major clinical manifestations of sodium channel blockade are QRS prolongation and ventricular dysrhythmias.
   - Drugs with primary toxic effects on sodium channels include quinidine, flecainide, mexiletine, disopyramide, propafenone, and procainamide.
   - Drugs with sodium channel effects and other serious effects include tricyclic antidepressants (TCAs), propranolol, cocaine, diphenhydramine, carbamazepine, lidocaine, chloroquine, and norpropoxyphene (a metabolite of propoxyphene). Patients poisoned with these agents have other symptoms but should be observed and treated if prolonged QRS duration or arrhythmias develop.

3. **What is the antidote for drugs that cause sodium channel blockade?**
   Sodium bicarbonate 1–2 mEq/kg as a bolus is used for the treatment of dysrhythmias or prolongation of the QRS duration. If the QRS duration does not narrow after administration of sodium bicarbonate, a second bolus should be given. Hyperventilation should be initiated to induce a serum pH of 7.5–7.55. Hypertonic saline can also be administered in a dose of 200 mL of 7.5% solution or 400 mL of a 3% solution. In addition to sodium bicarbonate, patients with cardiovascular toxicity often require fluids and vasopressors for hypotension, benzodiazepines for seizures, and endotracheal intubation for altered mental status.

4. **What symptoms do patients with a CCB overdose experience?**
   CCBs decrease calcium influx into cardiac tissue and vascular smooth muscle. The heart depends on calcium for automaticity, conduction through the atrioventricular node, and contractility. Vascular smooth muscle requires calcium to maintain tone. Patients with CCB overdose have hypotension, bradycardia, and atrioventricular blocks. If hypotension is significant, patients may have altered mental status, organ ischemia, and acidosis. These patients may also be hyperglycemic.

5. **What is the treatment for CCB overdose?**
   Begin treatment by addressing airway, breathing, and circulation (ABCs). Gastric decontamination (e.g., gastric lavage, activated charcoal, and whole bowel irrigation) may be indicated after the airway is adequately protected. Hypotension is treated initially with fluid boluses (i.e., 2 L normal saline), and symptomatic bradycardia can be transiently treated with atropine or pacing. Inotropic agents, such as norepinephrine or epinephrine, often at high doses, are used next.

   Calcium is an adjunctive treatment in toxicity. The recommended dose is 1–2 g of calcium chloride or 3–6 g of calcium gluconate IV, which may be repeated every 10 minutes, three to four times. Calcium chloride requires a central line or large IV line because of risk for vein necrosis, but it delivers three times the amount of elemental calcium compared with calcium gluconate. An infusion of calcium may be used to keep the serum calcium at the upper limit of normal.

   Glucagon (5–10 mg IV push) may be given; if improvement is noted, a drip at 5–10 mg/h diluted in 5% dextrose should be initiated. Glucagon may cause vomiting; therefore, patients must be able to maintain their own airway or be intubated in order for the drug to be administered.

   If the bedside cardiac ultrasound shows decreased contractility, hyperinsulinemia euglycemia (HIE) therapy or high-dose insulin, an inotropic therapy (1 unit/kg bolus, followed by 0.5 unit/kg/h with supplemental dextrose and

Table 76.1 Cardiovascular Effects of Different Poisons

Bradycardia With Hypertension
- Centrally acting presynaptic α_2-agonists (clonidine, guanfacine, oxymetazoline, and tetrahydrozoline): patients progress to bradycardia and hypotension by arrival to the hospital; the initial hypertension and bradycardia is transient

Bradycardia With Hypotension and Narrow-Complex QRS
- Centrally acting presynaptic α_2-agonists (same as above): Inhibit sympathetic outflow in the CNS, resulting in hypotension, bradycardia, pinpoint pupils, and somnolence
- BBs without sodium channel effects
- CCBs
- Cardiac glycosides
- Sedative-hypnotics, opioids, benzodiazepines, and barbiturates decrease CNS sympathetic outflow. Hypotension and bradycardia are usually minimal.
- Organophosphates and carbamates by increasing vagal tone

Bradycardia With Hypotension and Wide-Complex QRS
- Lidocaine, tocainide (class 1b antiarrhythmics)
- BBs with sodium channel effects (i.e., propranolol, acebutolol, or metoprolol)
- CCBs (severe toxicity causes ventricular escape rhythms)
- Cardiac glycosides (severe toxicity causes ventricular escape rhythms)
- Propafenone and flecainide (class 1c antiarrhythmics that cause sodium channel blockade)
- Quinidine, procainamide, and disopyramide (class 1a antiarrhythmics that cause sodium channel blockade, prolonged QRS and QT intervals)
- Hyperkalemia from cardiac glycosides, BBs, and potassium-sparing diuretics

Tachycardia With Hypertension
- Sympathomimetics (amphetamines, cocaine, ephedrine, pseudoephedrine): stimulate the sympathetic nervous system
- Anticholinergics (diphenhydramine and atropine): from decreased vagal tone and agitated delirium

Tachycardia With Hypotension
- Monoamine oxidase inhibitors: inhibit the breakdown of catecholamines in CNS synapses, tachycardia with hypotension and narrow-complex QRS. In overdose, hypertension can also be profound
- α_1-Antagonists (i.e., prazosin, terazosin, doxazosin): vasodilatation and reflex tachycardia
- Phenothiazines: result of α_1-antagonism causing vasodilatation and reflex tachycardia
- Diuretics: tachycardia and hypotension usually mild secondary to dehydration
- Nitrates: vasodilatation and reflex tachycardia
- Theophylline and caffeine: inhibition of adenosine receptors, β-adrenergic stimulation from catecholamine release, resulting in tachycardia and hypotension

Tachycardia With Hypotension and Wide-Complex QRS
- Tricyclic antidepressants (amitriptyline and imipramine), cyclobenzaprine, and diphenhydramine: sodium channel blockade causing widening of the QRS complex. (In severe toxicity, this can lead to hypotension despite tachycardia from anticholinergic effects.)
- Cocaine: sodium channel effects that, late in the course, override the ability to maintain blood pressure from tachycardia and vasoconstriction

BB, β-Blocker; *CCB,* calcium channel blocker; *CNS,* central nervous system.
Compiled using sources listed in the Bibliography.

potassium) should be administered if hypotension is refractory to IV fluids, calcium, and inotropic agents. Many toxicologists consider this first-line therapy in CCB overdose and will escalate doses of insulin as needed if patient is not responsive to lower doses. Heroic measures, such as using IV lipid emulsion (1.5 mL/kg of a 20% lipid emulsion, followed by an infusion of 0.25 mL/kg/min for 30–60 minutes), extracorporeal membrane oxygenation, intraaortic balloon pump, and cardiopulmonary bypass, may be used in severe refractory cases. Other experimental therapies to mention include methylene blue (1–2 mg/kg bolus and 0.5–1 mg/kg/h infusion of 1% solution), the calcium sensitizer inotrope levosimendan (6–12 µg/kg bolus over 10 minutes and then a continuous infusion of 0.05–0.2 µg/kg/min), and L-carnitine (6 g IV bolus and then 1 g IV every 4 hours).

6. **What are the symptoms in patients with β-blocker (BB)?**
   BBs compete with endogenous catecholamines for receptor sites; this blunts the normal adrenergic response, leading to bradycardia, atrioventricular blocks, and hypotension from decreased contractility. Patients suffering from BB toxicity experience symptoms similar to those of patients with CCB overdose. There can be a few differences,

however, depending on which BB is involved. Some BBs, such as propranolol, are lipid soluble. This allows entry into the central nervous system, leading to seizures and altered mental status unrelated to blood pressure. Some BBs (i.e., propranolol, acebutolol, alprenolol, and oxprenolol) antagonize sodium channels, leading to a widened QRS. Sotalol also blocks potassium channels, causing a prolonged QT interval that can result in torsades de pointes.

7. What is the treatment for BB toxicity?
Treatment is similar to that for CCB overdose. Glucagon may be used for treatment after fluids, vasopressors, and atropine. The dose of glucagon is the same as for CCB overdose. High-dose insulin therapy may be beneficial as well. Calcium has not been well studied for treatment of BB overdose. Seizures unrelated to hypotension should be treated with benzodiazepines; sodium bicarbonate is used for QRS widening. Refractory sympathetic bradycardia should be treated with external cardiac pacing. There are case reports of using dialysis for atenolol overdoses, because it has relatively low protein binding and volume of distribution.

8. How do acute and chronic digoxin poisonings manifest?
- Acute digoxin toxicity occurs after accidental or intentional ingestion of a supratherapeutic amount of digoxin-containing products. A dose of more than 1 mg in a child and more than 3 mg in an adult is potentially toxic. Patients with acute digoxin toxicity often develop gastrointestinal symptoms, such as nausea or vomiting. The most common cardiac effects are bradycardia and heart block. After acute digoxin ingestion, blockade of the cellular sodium-potassium exchange pump leads to systemic hyperkalemia. Severe hyperkalemia (serum level >5.5 mEq/L) is associated with a mortality rate of greater than 90% if untreated.
- Chronic digoxin toxicity occurs when there is a change in the dosage or clearance of digoxin in a patient who is receiving digoxin therapy. Initiation of treatment with quinidine, amiodarone, spironolactone, or verapamil may change the steady-state clearance of digoxin and result in toxicity. Decreased clearance of digoxin may occur when patients develop renal insufficiency. Symptoms of chronic digoxin toxicity are often subtle and nonspecific, including confusion, anorexia, vomiting, visual changes, and abdominal pain. The patient is often bradycardic with varying degrees of heart block. Patients may develop premature atrial and ventricular contractions, supraventricular tachycardia, ventricular tachycardia, or ventricular fibrillation. In contrast to acute digoxin toxicity, serum potassium is often normal or depressed, unless the patient has hyperkalemia from renal insufficiency.

9. What are the indications for digoxin immune antibody fragments (Fab)?
The most common indications are symptomatic bradycardia, complete heart block, ventricular tachycardia, or ventricular fibrillation. Often, digoxin immune Fab must be administered to critically ill patients without laboratory confirmation of elevated digoxin levels. Fab should be administered to patients who seek treatment after an acute ingestion with hyperkalemia or hemodynamically significant dysrhythmias. The indications for Fab therapy in patients with chronic digoxin toxicity are not well defined. Because serum digoxin levels correlate poorly with symptoms, there is no specific serum digoxin level that is considered an absolute indication for digoxin Fab. Additionally, digoxin Fab interferes with digoxin immunoassay measurement.

10. How is digoxin Fab administered?
Digoxin Fab may be administered in one of several ways, depending on the information available to the clinician:
- If the patient is critically ill, 10–20 vials should be given empirically.
- If the amount of digoxin ingested is known, the following formula should be used: Milligrams of digoxin ÷ 0.5 mg of digoxin bound per vial = Number of vials needed to treat.
- If the steady-state serum level is known, the following formula should be used: Serum digoxin level (ng/mL) × Ideal patient weight (kg)/100 = Number of vials. (This normally results in a patient with chronic toxicity receiving one to three vials.)

ACKNOWLEDGMENT

We would like to thank Jennie Buchanan who authored this chapter in previous editions and contributed substantially to this edition.

BIBLIOGRAPHY

Hack JB. Cardioactive steroids. In: Hoffman RS, Howland MA, Lewin NA, et al., eds. *Goldfrank's Toxicologic Emergencies*. 10th ed. New York, NY: McGraw-Hill; 2014: 895–903.

Kerns W. Management of beta blocker and calcium channel antagonist toxicity. *Emerg Med Clin North Am.* 2007;25:309–331.

St-Onge M, Dube PA, Gosselin S, et al. Treatment for calcium channel blocker poisoning: a systematic review. *Clin Toxicol.* 2014; 52:926–944.

Wax PM. Sodium bicarbonate. In: Hoffman RS, Howland MA, Lewin NA, et al., eds. *Goldfrank's Toxicologic Emergencies*. 10th ed. New York, NY: McGraw-Hill; 2014:528–535.

Yuan TH, Kerns WP, Thomaszewski CA, et al. Insulin-glucose as adjunctive therapy for severe calcium channel antagonist poisoning. *J Toxicol Clin Toxicol.* 1999;37:463–474.

CHAPTER 77

PEDIATRIC INGESTIONS

Laurie Seidel Halmo, MD and George Sam Wang, MD, FAAP, FAACT

KEY POINTS: PEDIATRIC INGESTIONS

1. Most pediatric ingestions and exposures are low risk and do not cause significant toxicity.
2. However, pediatric patients can easily become toxic from exposures to small volumes of common medications.
3. Because the precise amount ingested is often difficult to determine in small children, prolonged observation is often required to rule out a potentially toxic ingestion.
4. Although the range of toxicity may vary, treatment for children usually mirrors that for adults with similar ingestions.

1. **How common are pediatric ingestions?**

   Approximately 60% of ingestions reported to US poison centers occur in children, with 75% of those occurring in children younger than 6 years. The epidemiology of pediatric ingestions is bimodal, with the majority of ingestions occurring in children younger than 6 years and then a second smaller peak in adolescence. Children younger than 6 years exhibit exploratory hand-to-mouth behavior and have not yet developed cognitive capacity to understand the potential danger of ingestion. The increase in adolescence is largely the result of self-harm or abuse purposes. The vast majority of pediatric ingestions result in minimal or no clinical effects, with an overall mortality rate less than 0.1%. Approximately 4% of pediatric exposures reported to US poison centers result in moderate or major outcomes or death, with approximately two thirds of those being in the adolescent age group.

2. **How do children differ from adults with respect to ingestions and exposures?**

   Fortunately, most pediatric ingestions are lick, sip, or taste in nature and thus are small volume, which minimizes toxicity and translates to low morbidity and mortality rates. However, small amounts of highly concentrated products or a therapeutic adult dose of some medications can be very dangerous. Children are often more vulnerable to dense gas and vapor exposures because they are shorter in stature and thus lower to the ground, have less capability to remove themselves from a dangerous environment, and have higher minute ventilation. They also have a large body surface area-to-weight ratio, making them more vulnerable to dermal exposures and hypothermia. Adolescent ingestions are similar to adult ingestions, because they are typically the result of drug abuse or self-harm gestures.

3. **What are some dangerous household agents?**

   Accidental exposures or ingestions of most household products are benign. However, the following substances can be dangerous: caustics, hydrocarbons, products that contain ethanol or toxic alcohols, button or disc batteries, magnets, and camphor.

4. **What products contain caustics?**

   Many cleaning detergents, such as bathroom and kitchen cleaners, bleach, rust remover, and automotive cleaners, can contain either alkali or acidic caustic ingredients.

5. **What are concerning signs after caustic ingestion?**

   Most caustic products have a low enough concentration that small exposures do not cause significant injury. However, large-volume exposures, or highly concentrated products, can cause significant esophageal burns. Dangerous symptoms include stridor or dyspnea, persistent vomiting, dysphagia or refusal to eat or drink, and drooling. Some products, such as hydrofluoric acid, can cause systemic symptoms as well, such as hypocalcemia, leading to life-threatening dysrhythmias.

6. **Which children who have ingested a caustic substance require endoscopy?**

   The role of endoscopy after ingestion of a caustic substance is to evaluate for the presence and degree of esophageal injury, as the presence or absence of oropharyngeal lesions is a poor predictor of esophageal findings. As such, endoscopy should be considered for any symptomatic patient; patients who are completely asymptomatic and can tolerate eating and drinking without difficulty or emesis are unlikely to have significant esophageal injury, and thus generally do not require endoscopy.

7. **What products contain hydrocarbons, and what are the symptoms of exposure?**

   Hydrocarbons include essential oils, kerosene, and petroleum distillates. Some can cause sedation and central nervous system (CNS) depression, but the most concerning exposure is aspiration, leading to pneumonitis.

8. **How should hydrocarbon exposures be managed?**
   Most children who are asymptomatic with normal chest radiography findings after 6 hours will not go on to develop serious pulmonary toxicity; others may require hospital admission for hypoxia or respiratory distress. Antibiotics and steroids have not been shown to be of significant benefit after acute exposure. Complications include respiratory failure, CNS depression, pneumonia, and pneumatocele formation. Significant toxicity requiring intubation as a result of respiratory distress, acute respiratory distress syndrome (ARDS), or poor oxygenation has been successfully treated with high-frequency ventilation, extracorporeal membrane oxygenation, and surfactant.

9. **What products contain ethanol and the toxic alcohols?**
   Many products contain high concentrations of ethanol, including hand sanitizer solutions, perfumes, hair sprays, and food extracts (e.g., vanilla and lemon). Methanol is typically found in windshield wiper fluid, isopropanol is in rubbing alcohol, and ethylene glycol is in antifreeze. Pediatric patients can develop more profound CNS depression and possibly hypoglycemia after small amounts of ethanol and at lower serum ethanol concentrations compared with adults. Isopropanol may also cause notable gastritis and CNS depression in children. Children can also develop metabolic acidosis and subsequent end-organ toxicity from smaller volumes of methanol and ethylene glycol than adults would because of their smaller body size.

10. **Why are button battery and magnet ingestions dangerous?**
    Button or disc batteries that are retained in the esophagus even for just a few minutes can cause significant burns and erosions through the entire esophageal wall, leading to potentially massive bleeding, perforation, fistula formation, mediastinitis, and death. While the definitive management for button batteries lodged in the esophagus is endoscopic removal, administration of honey or sucralfate has been shown to decrease injury severity in a porcine model and should be considered for patients awaiting endoscopic removal. Do not utilize honey as a measure to avoid emergent evaluation. Magnets can also be dangerous, because ingestion of more than one can trap gastric or intestinal mucosa between them, leading to bowel wall ischemia, necrosis, and perforation.

11. **Are there any over-the-counter (OTC) products that can be dangerous?**
    Analgesics, such as acetaminophen and salicylates, are very common and can lead to liver failure and acidosis, respectively. Oil of wintergreen contains very high amounts of methyl salicylate (see Question 37). Lomotil (atropine/diphenoxylate, see Question 19) can also lead to dangerous toxicity. Iron is found in many OTC multivitamins, though it is often (but not always) omitted in gummy vitamins. Many cough and cold medications contain acetaminophen, dextromethorphan, and an antihistamine (diphenhydramine, doxylamine, chlorpheniramine, brompheniramine), all of which can lead to serious toxicity. Imidazolines found in eye drops and nasal decongestants can cause toxicity similar to clonidine (see Question 32).

12. **How much iron is needed to cause significant toxicity, and what are the symptoms?**
    Ingestions of more than 20 mg/kg of elemental iron typically lead to symptoms. Common formulations include iron fumarate (33% elemental iron), iron gluconate (12%), and ferrous sulfate (20%). Symptoms classically progress through five stages:
    1. Gastrointestinal (GI) symptoms (vomiting and diarrhea, which may be hemorrhagic secondary to corrosive effects of iron)
    2. Latent (apparent improvement in GI symptoms, which belies ongoing occult toxicity)
    3. Metabolic acidosis/shock (usually 12–24 hours after ingestion)
    4. Hepatic failure (usually 1–3 days after ingestion)
    5. Gastric outlet obstruction (secondary to scarring from the original corrosive injury)

13. **What are symptoms of OTC cough and cold medication overdose?**
    Dextromethorphan can lead to psychosis, agitation, hallucinations, sedation, and, rarely, seizures and serotonergic toxicity. Diphenhydramine can lead to somnolence, anticholinergic toxicity, and, in large overdoses, seizures and cardiac dysrhythmias, similar to tricyclic antidepressant (TCA) toxicity. Acetaminophen is found in many combination cough and cold preparations.

14. **Why are children more predisposed to methemoglobinemia?**
    Patients younger than 4 months are at higher risk for developing methemoglobinemia because their ability to reduce ferric iron to ferrous iron is limited. Common causes of methemoglobinemia include nitrites/nitrates (well water and foods), local anesthetics (benzocaine, lidocaine), dapsone, sulfonamides, naphthalene, and silver nitrate.

15. **How is methemoglobinemia treated?**
    Indications to treat include symptomatic patients with methemoglobin concentrations greater than 20%–25%. The dose for methylene blue is 1 mg/kg intravenously (IV) of a 1% solution.

16. **Are there any plants that can cause serious illness?**
    Most plants in small amounts will not cause significant toxicity. However, there are some plants that can be dangerous, such as foxglove, lily of the valley, oleander (digoxin-like toxicity), jimson weed/moon flower (anticholinergic toxicity), poison hemlock (respiratory paralysis), and water hemlock (seizures).

17. What comprises the pediatric "one pill can kill" list?
This is a list of pharmaceuticals that may be lethal in a toddler at a therapeutic adult dosage. In actuality, the literature may not support the fact that one pill can kill. Regardless, any ingestion by a child from this list should be considered to have the potential to produce serious toxicity at low doses.

18. What drugs may be found on the "one pill can kill" list?
Although not a consensus list, these drugs are often mentioned:
- Diphenoxylate and atropine (Lomotil)
- TCAs
- Calcium channel blockers (CCBs)
- β-Blockers
- Sulfonylureas
- Clonidine
- Camphor
- Salicylates
- Phenothiazines
- Opioids
- Benzonatate

19. What are the mechanisms of action of the components of Lomotil, and what is the clinical presentation associated with its ingestion?
Lomotil is an antidiarrheal agent composed of diphenoxylate (an opioid) and atropine (an anticholinergic agent).
   Classically, Lomotil ingestions were considered to have a two-phase presentation. The first phase consists of an anticholinergic toxidrome, followed by an opioid toxidrome. This classic presentation is unusual, and Lomotil ingestion should be thought of as ingestion of a long-acting opioid that may include features of atropine toxicity. Lomotil ingestions should be observed for 24 hours.

20. How low a dose of a TCA is potentially lethal in a child?
Ingestions of 10–20 mg/kg can lead to significant toxicity, with fatalities occurring from as little as 250 mg of amitriptyline in pediatric patients.

21. What electrocardiogram (ECG) finding in TCA ingestions is helpful in predicting toxicity in children?
The terminal 40-msec QRS axis has been shown in adults to be a useful marker in identifying TCA overdose. In a retrospective study of 35 children with TCA ingestions, the terminal 40-msec QRS axis was not helpful in predicting TCA ingestions. In a study of children and adolescents, increasing QRS duration was associated with serum tricyclic levels, which suggested that QRS duration could be of prognostic value in a similar manner to TCA ingestions in adults.

22. Have deaths been reported in single ingestions of dihydropyridine (e.g., nifedipine) ingestions in children?
Yes. Although ingestions of dihydropyridines are considered to be less serious than ingestions of phenylalkylamine (e.g., verapamil) and benzothiazepines (e.g., diltiazem) because of the relative lack of direct cardiotoxicity in dihydropyridine ingestions, there is a report of a death in a 14-month-old child from a single 10-mg ingestion of nifedipine.

23. What is the pediatric dosage of calcium for CCB ingestions?
Calcium is one of the first-line treatments for CCB toxicity and can improve inotropy and hypotension. In children, bolus 0.1–0.2 mL/kg of 10% calcium chloride or 0.3–0.5 mL/kg of 10% calcium gluconate and repeat every 10–20 minutes, up to three to four doses. In severely poisoned patients, however, calcium's effects are often negligible or short-lived. Furthermore, calcium chloride can sclerose veins, an issue when dealing with the smaller-caliber veins in children. In severely poisoned patients, it is prudent to begin other treatments, such as vasopressors and inotropes, simultaneously with calcium administration.

24. What other therapy is used in treatment of CCBs and β-blockers?
Hyperinsulinemia/euglycemia has shown to be effective in animal models of CCB toxicity. There are no human clinical trials, but experience published in human case reports and case series supports improved hemodynamics with insulin/dextrose administration in both children and adults. The typical suggested starting dose is 1 U/kg insulin bolus, followed by a continuous infusion of 1 U/kg/h titrated to effect, with reports as high as 10 U/kg/h of insulin. Dextrose should be administered to maintain euglycemia.

25. What is a potential side effect of β-blocker and CCB ingestions other than cardiovascular toxicity in children?
There have been reports of severe hypoglycemia associated with propranolol ingestions, including in children taking therapeutic doses for management of infantile hemangiomas. A prospective series of 208 children, however, suggested that exposure to one or two β-blocker pills is very unlikely to result in any toxicity, and a systematic review of the safety of oral propranolol for treatment of infantile hemangioma identified that most of the cases of hypoglycemia in this population occurred during times of illness or fasting. CCB toxicity often precipitates hyperglycemia, because the release of insulin is calcium-dependent.

26. **For how long should a child with a sulfonylurea ingestion be observed?**
A child should be observed for 12–24 hours, depending on the sulfonylurea type and preparation. There are case reports of hypoglycemia occurring up to 21 hours after the initial ingestion. Ingestions of single tablets of glipizide have caused hypoglycemia in children, as well as in sulfonylurea-naive adults.

27. **How often should blood sugars be monitored?**
Initially, blood sugars should be monitored hourly, with additional checks as needed for symptoms of hypoglycemia.

28. **After a sulfonylurea ingestion in a child, should prophylactic dextrose or maintenance fluids with dextrose be given?**
No, dextrose may potentiate the insulin release caused by sulfonylureas. In many reports of delayed hypoglycemia, the child received prophylactic dextrose. The child should be allowed to eat a normal diet free of concentrated sweets. If the child's blood sugar drops, then dextrose should be administered.

29. **What is the rule of 50?**
The *rule of 50* is a mnemonic for calculating a dextrose dosing for pediatric resuscitation. When the concentration of the dextrose solution multiplied by the dose in mL/kg equals 50, 0.5 g/kg bolus of dextrose is provided. For example, either a 10% dextrose solution at 5 mL/kg or a 25% dextrose solution at 2 mL/kg provide 0.5 g/kg.

30. **What is the antidote for sulfonylurea ingestions?**
Octreotide is the antidote. Glucose metabolism (and sulfonylureas) close a potassium efflux channel on beta islet cells, which depolarizes the cell and leads to the opening of voltage-gated calcium channels, which in turn triggers insulin secretion via intracellular signaling. Octreotide independently closes the calcium channel, resulting in decreased insulin secretion. It is important to note that octreotide does not raise the serum blood sugar, but only stops further insulin secretion. Dextrose is still needed to normalize blood sugar when giving octreotide.

31. **How is octreotide administered in pediatric sulfonylurea ingestions?**
The appropriate dosing, frequency, and side-effect profile of octreotide in pediatric sulfonylurea ingestions have not been rigorously studied. Adults typically receive 50–100 μg subcutaneously every 6–12 hours. A suggested pediatric dose is 1 μg/kg subcutaneously with an initial dosing interval of every 6 hours. Octreotide IV infusions can also be used.

32. **What are the cardiovascular effects that may be seen with clonidine ingestions?**
Bradycardia and hypotension are most commonly reported. However, early transient hypertension has also been reported in children. This likely occurs from activation of peripheral α_2-receptors and does not usually require specific treatment. Other commonly reported effects are CNS depression, respiratory depression, hypothermia, and miosis. No specific antidote exists; treatment is generally focused on general respiratory and hemodynamic support. Most unintentional ingestions do well.

33. **Can naloxone be used in pediatric clonidine ingestions?**
The experience with naloxone in pediatric clonidine ingestions largely parallels the experience with adult ingestions; it only works a fraction of the time. In a review of pediatric ingestions receiving variable doses, naloxone was observed to have a positive response in 16% of patients. Although clonidine ingestions often present similar to opioid ingestions, naloxone's effect is not completely understood.

34. **What are some common OTC products that contain pharmaceuticals with similar mechanisms of action to clonidine?**
Oxymetazoline, naphazoline, xylometazoline, and tetrahydrozoline are imidazolines with the same mechanism of action as clonidine. They are found in ophthalmic solutions and nasal decongestants. Ingestion of these products can cause significant toxicity. As little as 2.5–5 mL of a 0.05% tetrahydrozoline solution caused drowsiness, bradycardia, respiratory depression, cool extremities, and miotic pupils in a 1-year-old girl. Onset of symptoms is typically rapid, occurring in 15–30 minutes.

35. **How do ingestions of camphor present?**
Ingestions initially cause GI symptoms, such as burning of the mouth and throat and vomiting. Severe toxicity manifests as neurologic symptoms, such as seizures, hyperreflexia, myoclonic jerks, and coma. The onset of symptoms tends to be rapid, occurring 5–90 minutes after the exposure. There is no specific antidote, and treatment is primarily symptomatic and supportive. A 2009 case series suggested that camphor should be considered as a cause of undifferentiated seizures in children from communities with widespread use of the substance. Camphor is found in products such as Campho-Phenique, Vick's Vaposteam, Vick's VapoRub, Tiger Balm, Anbesol Cold Sore Therapy Ointment, BenGay Ultra Strength, and many other OTC topical creams. The US Food and Drug Administration (FDA) limits products sold in the United States to no more than 11% camphor. Foreign products, however, may contain much higher percentages of camphor. Five hundred milligrams can cause serious toxicity in a child. In an 11% solution, this would equal approximately 4.6 mL.

36. At what salicylate dose do children begin to manifest toxicity in an acute ingestion?
Both children and adults manifest acute toxicity at approximately 150 mg/kg. Serious toxicity is likely to occur at 300 mg/kg.

37. How does the potency of methyl salicylate compare to aspirin (acetyl salicylate)?
One milligram of methyl salicylate is roughly as potent as 1.4 g of aspirin (acetyl salicylate). Methyl salicylate is found in oil of wintergreen, many topical OTC creams, and many Asian herbal remedies.

38. Approximately how much aspirin (or acetylsalicylate) is equal to 5 mL of 100% methyl salicylate?
Five milliliters (or 1 teaspoon) of 100% methyl salicylate is equal to approximately 7000 mg of acetyl salicylate, or almost 22 regular-strength adult aspirin tablets. In a 10-kg child, this would be 700 mg/kg, easily a life-threatening ingestion. Oil of wintergreen often contains 98%–100% methyl salicylate, and ingestions of 4 mL have been fatal in children.

39. Which phenothiazine is believed to be the most dangerous in pediatric accidental ingestions?
Chlorpromazine (Thorazine) is responsible for nearly every serious documented pediatric phenothiazine ingestion. As little as 280 mg resulted in the death of a 2-year-old child. Phenothiazine toxicity manifests as CNS depression, hypotension, and anticholinergic symptoms. Fatal pediatric cases of neuroleptic malignant syndrome have been reported after acute ingestions of phenothiazines. Serious morbidity or mortality has not been reported from isolated ingestions of small doses of the antiemetic phenothiazines, promethazine (Phenergan) and prochlorperazine (Compazine).

40. What is the pathophysiology of chloroquine and hydroxychloroquine ingestions?
These drugs are believed to exhibit quinidine-like effects and thus inhibit cardiac sodium and potassium channels, so toxicity may manifest with QRS prolongation, atrioventricular block, ST- and T-wave depression, and QTc prolongation. Chloroquine is generally not found in US households because of its primary use as malarial prophylaxis or treatment. However, hydroxychloroquine is increasingly being used as an anti-inflammatory agent. Although hydroxychloroquine is considered safer than chloroquine, both have the potential to cause serious toxicity, including cardiotoxicity, respiratory depression, CNS depression, and seizures.

41. What other drug besides standard therapy has been used to treat chloroquine poisoning?
Other than sodium bicarbonate for QRS widening, high-dose diazepam (2 mg/kg IV over 30 minutes) may be tried. Although its mechanism of action is unclear and one randomized controlled trial failed to demonstrate a clear benefit, diazepam may be considered in severe poisonings.

42. What newer opioid can result in significant toxicity with ingestion of one pill?
Buprenorphine is an opioid that is often marketed as Suboxone, a preparation that contains naloxone, and is most often used to treat opioid addiction. It is typically given as a dissolving sublingual tablet, increasing the potential for toxicity in children. Despite the fact that it is a partial (rather than full) agonist at the opioid receptor, ingestions of one pill have been associated with significant respiratory depression in children; as such, children should be observed for 24 hours after exposure. Children with opioid toxicity (whether from buprenorphine or any other opioid) should receive naloxone 0.01 mg/kg IV for respiratory depression and 0.1 mg/kg IV (up to 2 mg) for apnea.

43. What symptoms develop after benzonatate (Tessalon) perle ingestion?
Young children can become symptomatic after ingestion of only a few benzonatate perles. Toxicity is similar to local anesthetic toxicity and can lead to seizures, CNS depression, and cardiac dysrhythmias.

ACKNOWLEDGMENT

The editors and authors of this chapter would like to acknowledge and thank Dr. Shan Yin for his previous contributions to this chapter.

BIBLIOGRAPHY

Anfang RR, Jatana KR, Linn RL, et al. pH-neutralizing esophageal irrigations as a novel mitigation strategy for button battery injury. *Laryngoscope.* 2019;129:49–57.
Centers for Disease Control and Prevention. Injuries from batteries among children aged <13 years, United States, 1995–2010. *MMWR Morb Mortal Wkly Rep.* 2012;61:661–666.
Dart RC, Paul IM, Bond GR, et al. Pediatric fatalities associated with over the counter (nonprescription) cough and cold medications. *Ann Emerg Med.* 2009;52:411–417.
Dougherty PP, Lee SC, Lung D, et al. Evaluation of the use and safety of octreotide as antidotal therapy for sulfonylurea overdose in children. *Pediatr Emerg Care.* 2013;29:292–295.
Engebretsen DK, Kacsmarek KM, Morgan J, et al. High-dose insulin therapy in beta-blocker and calcium channel-blocker poisoning. *Clin Toxicol (Phila).* 2011;49:277–283.

Green JL, Wang GS, Reynolds KM, et al. Safety profile of cough and cold medication use in pediatrics. *Pediatrics.* 2017;139(6):e20163070. doi:10.1542/peds.2016-3070.

Gummin DD, Mowry JB, Spyker DA, et al. 2017 annual report of the American Association of Poison Control Centers' National Poison Data System (NPDS): 35th annual report *Clin Toxicol.* 2018;56(12):1213–1415.

Jolliff HA, Fletcher E, Roberts KJ, et al. Pediatric hydrocarbon-related injuries in the United States: 2000–2009. *Pediatrics.* 2013;131:1139–1147.

Klein-Schwartz W, Stassinos GL, Isbister GK. Treatment of sulfonylurea and insulin overdose. *Br J Clin Pharmacol.* 2016;81(3):496–504. doi:10.1111/bcp.12822.

Leaute-Lebreze C, Boccara O, Degrugillier-Chopinet C, et al. Safety of oral propranolol for the treatment of infantile hemangioma: a systematic review. *Pediatrics.* 2016;138(4):e20130353.

Lowry JA, Brown JT. Significance of the imidazoline receptors in toxicology. *Clin Toxicol (Phila).* 2014;52:454–469.

McLawhorn MW, Goulding MR, Gill RK, et al. Analysis of benzonatate overdoses among adults and children from 1969–2010 by the United States Food and Drug Administration. *Pharmacotherapy.* 2013;33:38–43.

Toce MS, Burns MM, O'Donnell KA. Clinical effects of unintentional pediatric buprenorphine exposures: experience at a single tertiary care center. *Clin Toxicol (Phila).* 2017;55(1):12–17. doi:10.1080/15563650.2016.1244337.

Tormoehlen LM, Tekulve KJ, Nañagas KA. Hydrocarbon toxicity: a review. *Clin Toxicol (Phila).* 2014;52(5):479–489. doi:10.3109/15563650.2014.923904.

Wang GS, Le Lait MC, Heard K. Unintentional pediatric exposures to central alpha-2 agonists reported to the National Poison Data System. *J Pediatr.* 2014;164:149–152.

PELVIC INFLAMMATORY DISEASE

David B. Richards, MD, FACEP and Jamal Taha, MD

CHAPTER 78

1. What is pelvic inflammatory disease (PID)?

PID is a spectrum of acute infectious disorders involving the female upper genital tract. PID may include any of the following: endocervicitis, endometritis, salpingitis, oophoritis, tubo-ovarian abscess, or peritonitis. The sexually transmitted organisms *Neisseria gonorrhoeae* and *Chlamydia trachomatis* are often causative agents, although vaginal flora has also been implicated.

2. What are the risk factors for PID?

Young women of reproductive age with multiple sexual partners have the greatest risk for PID. Other risk factors include earlier age at first intercourse, intrauterine devices (IUDs; only in the first 3 weeks after insertion, not simply the presence of the device itself), and sexual activity during or immediately after menses. Older sex partners, prior involvement with a child protection agency, prior suicide attempts, alcohol use before intercourse, cigarette smoking, and concurrent *C. trachomatis* infection have also been identified as risk factors for the development of PID.

3. What are the signs and symptoms of PID?

There are no specific signs or symptoms that are diagnostic for PID. Lower abdominal pain is a common presenting symptom, although it may be subtle. Dyspareunia, abnormal vaginal discharge, abnormal uterine bleeding, or dysuria can be the only presenting symptoms. On examination, patients may have lower abdominal tenderness, cervical motion tenderness (CMT), or bilateral adnexal tenderness.

4. What are the microbiologic causes?

PID is an ascending infection typically initiated by a sexually transmitted agent, most notably *N. gonorrhoeae* or *C. trachomatis*, although in many cases the etiology of PID is unknown. It is thought that a number of community-acquired agents are capable of disturbing the normal endocervical mucosal barrier, allowing vaginal flora access to the female upper genital tract. Clinically, PID should be viewed as a mixed (facultative and anaerobic) polymicrobial infection after an initiating event. Microbes found in these infections include pelvic anaerobes, endogenous pelvic flora, gram-negative rods, group B streptococci, *Mycoplasma genitalium, Mycoplasma hominis, Staphylococcus aureus, Gardnerella vaginalis,* and *Haemophilus influenzae.*

5. What are the diagnostic criteria for PID?

There is no gold standard for the diagnosis of PID, and laboratory testing adds little to the diagnosis. A low threshold for the diagnosis should be maintained as delay in treatment leads to substantial morbidity. The Centers for Disease Control and Prevention (CDC) recommends empiric treatment of PID when CMT, uterine tenderness, or adnexal tenderness is associated with lower abdominal or pelvic pain, when occurring in sexually active women of reproductive age, or other women at risk for sexually transmitted infections (STIs). The diagnosis should be considered in any female patient presenting with fever, vaginal discharge, abnormal bleeding, dyspareunia, or dysmenorrhea.

Additional criteria used to support presumptive treatment of PID include the presence of one or more of the following features:

- oral temperature greater than 38.3°C (100.9°F);
- abnormal cervical or vaginal mucopurulent discharge;
- presence of increased white blood cells on microscopy of vaginal secretions;
- elevated erythrocyte sedimentation rate (ESR);
- elevated C-reactive protein (CRP);
- laboratory documentation of cervical infection with *N. gonorrhoeae or C. trachomatis.*

The most specific criteria for diagnosing PID include the following:

- endometrial biopsy demonstrating endometritis;
- imaging demonstrating thickened, fluid-filled tubes with or without pelvic free fluid or tubal hyperemia;
- laparoscopic abnormalities consistent with PID.

6. Which diagnostic tests should be performed in patients suspected of PID?

- A pregnancy test is necessary to rule out complications associated with pregnancy.
- A catheter-obtained urinalysis may reveal a urinary tract infection.

- Nucleic acid amplification for *C. trachomatis* and *N. gonorrhoeae* should be obtained,
- Ultrasound for all pregnant patients to exclude ectopic pregnancy, patients being considered for admission because of systemic symptoms, or for those with a possible tubo-ovarian abscess.

  Short of laparoscopy, there is no reliable test to exclude PID. Although abnormal laboratory results may provide supportive evidence, all laboratory studies may be normal in a patient with PID. The CDC also recommends testing for human immunodeficiency virus (HIV) in women diagnosed with PID.

7. **What other diseases should be considered?**
   The differential diagnosis includes:
   - cervicitis
   - endometriosis
   - ovarian cyst
   - ovarian torsion
   - spontaneous abortion
   - septic abortion
   - ectopic pregnancy
   - uterine fibroids
   - cholecystitis
   - appendicitis
   - diverticulitis
   - gastroenteritis
   - cystitis
   - pyelonephritis
   - renal colic
   - HIV

   In some patients, the cause of pelvic pain is never diagnosed, despite extensive testing.

8. **What are the consequences of PID?**
   PID is associated with a number of serious short-term and long-term complications. Acutely, PID can result in tubo-ovarian abscess, perihepatitis (Fitz-Hugh–Curtis syndrome), or peritonitis. Long-term sequelae include chronic pelvic pain, tubal factor infertility, and increased risk of ectopic pregnancy. Chronic pelvic pain may occur in up to 33% of patients with PID. The incidence of infertility and ectopic pregnancy substantially increase with each episode of PID. This is thought to be primarily the result of tubal occlusion from scar and adhesion formation within tubal lumens. The rate of an ectopic is 12%–15% higher in women who have had PID.

9. **Who should be considered for hospitalization?**
   In women with PID of mild to moderate clinical severity, outpatient therapy is reasonable. Some criteria for hospitalization suggested by the CDC include the following:
   - Pregnant patients.
   - When a surgical emergency (e.g., appendicitis) cannot be excluded.
   - Patients who do not respond clinically to oral antimicrobial therapy.
   - Patients who are unable to follow or tolerate an outpatient oral regimen.
   - Patients with severe illness, nausea and vomiting, or high fever.
   - Patients with tubo-ovarian abscess.

10. **Summarize the recommended antibiotic regimens for PID treatment.**
    See Table 78.1. Note there may be regional variation in treatment recommendations.

11. **Are there alternative outpatient treatment regimens for cervicitis?**
    Yes, cefixime 800 mg PO × 1 may be substituted for ceftriaxone if ceftriaxone is unavailable or if patient declines IM therapy, but it is not the preferred agent because of risk for treatment failure when treating *N. gonorrhea*. Doxycyline 100 mg PO bid × 7 days maybe used to treat chlamydia.

12. **How does management of PID differ in women with IUDs?**
    The risk of PID in IUD users is limited to the first 3 weeks after insertion. If a patient with an IUD is diagnosed with PID, the IUD does not need to be removed, unless there is no clinical improvement after 48–72 hours following initiation of antibiotics. Continued symptomatology after 48–72 hours may necessitate removal of the IUD.

13. **Does the presence of an intrauterine pregnancy effectively rule out PID?**
    PID can occur in pregnant women, although it is extremely rare. Suppurative salpingitis during the first trimester has been described in case reports, where the infection is thought to be transmitted concurrently with fertilization.

Table 78.1 Treatment of Pelvic Inflammatory Disease

Recommended Outpatient Regimen

Ceftriaxone 500 mg IM and 1 g for patients weighing $\geq$ 150 kg per 2020 CDC recommendations in a single dose
Plus
Doxycycline 100 mg PO bid for 14 days
with or without
Metronidazole, 500 mg PO bid for 14 days
OR
Cefoxitin 2 g IM plus probenecid 1 g PO in a single dose concurrently once, or other parenteral third-generation
   cephalosporin (e.g., ceftizoxime or cefotaxime)
Plus
Doxycycline 100 mg PO bid for 14 days
with or without metronidazole 500 mg PO bid for 14 days

Recommended Inpatient Regimen A

Cefotetan, 2 g IV every 12 hours, or cefoxitin 2 g IV every 6 hours
Plus
Doxycycline 100 mg IV or PO every 12 hours
Note: Because of pain associated with infusion, doxycycline should be given orally when possible, even when the patient is hospitalized. Oral and intravenous administration of doxycycline provide similar bioavailability. If intravenous
   administration is necessary, lidocaine or another short-acting local anesthetic, heparin, or steroids with a steel needle or extension of the infusion time may reduce infusion complications. Parenteral therapy may be discontinued 24
   hours after a patient improves clinically, and oral therapy with doxycycline (100 mg bid) should continue for 14 days.
   When tubo-ovarian abscess is present, clindamycin or metronidazole may be used with doxycycline for continued
   therapy, rather than doxycycline alone, because it provides more effective anaerobic coverage.

Recommended Inpatient Regimen B

Clindamycin 900 mg IV every 8 hours
Plus
Gentamicin loading dose IV or IM (2 mg/kg body weight), followed by a maintenance dose (1.5 mg/kg) every 8 hours.
   Single daily dosing may be substituted
Note: Although use of one daily dose of gentamicin has not been evaluated for the treatment of PID, it is efficacious in analogous situations. Parenteral therapy may be discontinued after 24 hours. Doxycycline 100 mg PO
   bid or clindamycin 450 mg PO qid, after a patient improves clinically, should be used to complete a 14-day
   course of therapy. When tubo-ovarian abscess is present, clindamycin may be used for continued therapy
   rather than doxycycline, because clindamycin provides more effective anaerobic cover

bid, Twice a day; *IM*, intramuscularly; *IV*, intravenously; *PID*, pelvic inflammatory disease; *PO*, per os, orally; qid, four times a day.
Modified from Centers for Disease Control and Prevention. Sexually transmitted diseases treatment guidelines 2015. *MMWR Recomm
   Rep.* 2015;64:1–137.

14. **Does a history of tubal ligation preclude the diagnosis of PID?**
   No, tubo-ovarian abscesses have been reported up to 20 years after tubal ligation.

15. **What is the appropriate follow-up care for patients with PID?**
   Patients treated as outpatients should be assessed within 3 days. For reliable patients, a follow-up phone call
   may suffice. For all patients, a test of cure by repeat examination and cervical nucleic acid amplification tests for
   C. trachomatis and *N. gonorrhoeae* is recommended 3–6 months after the initial intervention.

16. **How should sex partners of patients diagnosed with PID be managed?**
   Men who have had intercourse with woman diagnosed with PID during the 60 days preceding symptom onset
   should be tested and treated empirically for *C. trachomatis* and *N. gonorrhoeae*. For women whose last sexual
   contact was more than 60 days prior to presentation, their most recent sexual partner needs to be treated. Patients should abstain from sexual activity until completion of therapy and resolution of symptoms.

17. **Summarize the principles of management of acute PID.**
   - Rule out pregnancy and surgical emergencies.
   - Maintain a high level of suspicion for PID, because the consequences of untreated PID include infertility and
     chronic pelvic pain.
   - Treat early with antibiotics if PID is suspected.
   - Recommend all patients with PID be tested for other STIs, particularly HIV, syphilis, hepatitis B and C.
   - Inform the patient that her partner(s) also needs to be treated to prevent reinfection.

KEY POINTS: PID

1. Consider PID in sexually active patients with pelvic pain.
2. There are no historical, physical, or laboratory findings that conclusively diagnose PID.
3. PID requires antibiotics for treatment.
4. Abnormal uterine bleeding may be the only sign of PID.
5. Neither pregnancy nor tubal ligation excludes a diagnosis of PID.
6. Rule out surgical emergencies and complications of pregnancy before empirically treating for PID.

ACKNOWLEDGMENT

The editors and authors of this chapter would like to acknowledge and thank Leslie L. Armstrong, MD, Susan Brion, MD, and Bartholomew B. Paull, MD for their previous contributions to this chapter.

BIBLIOGRAPHY

Centers for Disease Control and Prevention. Sexually transmitted diseases treatment guidelines 2015. *MMWR Recomm Rep.* 2015;64:1–137.

Haggerty CL, Peipert JF, Weitzen S, et al. Predictors of chronic pelvic pain in an urban population of women with symptoms and signs of pelvic inflammatory disease. *Sex Transm Dis.* 2005;32:293–299.

Haggerty CL, Totten PA, Tang G, et al. Identification of novel microbes associated with pelvic inflammatory disease and infertility. *Sex Transm Infect.* 2016;92:441–446.

Mitchell C, Prabhu M. Pelvic inflammatory disease: current concepts in pathogenesis, diagnosis, and treatment. *Infect Dis Clin North Am.* 2013;27:793–809.

Savaris RF, Teixeira LM, Torres TG, et al. Comparing ceftriaxone plus azithromycin or doxycycline for pelvic inflammatory disease: a randomized controlled trial. *Obstet Gynecol.* 2007;110:53–60.

Soper DE. Pelvic inflammatory disease. *Obstet Gynecol.* 2010;116(2 Pt 1):419–428.

Wiesenfeld HC, Hiller SL, Meyn LA, et al. Subclinical pelvic inflammatory disease and infertility. *Obstet Gynecol.* 2012;120:37–43.

CHAPTER 79

SEXUAL ASSAULT

Michelle Metz, RN, BSN, SANE-A, CEN, and Sarah Tolford Selby, DO, FACEP

1. What is the definition of sexual assault?
Sexual assault generally refers to any deliberate sexual contact of another person without that person's explicit consent. This act may be facilitated by coercion, abuse of authority, or threatening physical abuse. Special consideration must be given to individuals incapable of giving consent due to mental incapacity or impaired mental function due to intoxicants. The legal definitions and penalties of sexual assault vary from state to state. The more traditional term *rape* is defined by the Federal Bureau of Investigation's (FBI's) Uniform Crime Report Summary Reporting System as "the penetration, no matter how slight, of the vagina or anus with any body part or object, or oral penetration by a sex organ of another person, without the consent of the patient." The definition of *sexual assault* is inclusive of gender, age, and sexual preference.

2. How common is sexual assault?
Sexual assault is one of the most underreported crimes; only 40% of sexual assaults are reported to law enforcement. Every 2 minutes someone in the United States is sexually assaulted. One in six women and one in 33 men will report a completed or attempted rape during their lifetime. Women ages 16–19 years are four times more likely to be sexually assaulted. Of women who report being raped, 44% were younger than 18 years. Women who are sexually assaulted as children and adolescents are at greater risk of being sexually assaulted as an adult. Although most victims of sexual assault are women, men can be assaulted by other men, and conversely, women can perpetrate sexual assaults against other women or men. Nearly three-quarters of perpetrators of sexual assault are someone the victim knows, and only 3% are sentenced to imprisonment.

3. What role does a medical provider have in cases of sexual assault?
The emergency department (ED) is the most common place for a victim of sexual assault to come for acute medical care and forensic evidence gathering. Thirty-two percent of women older than 18 years who are sexually assaulted report being injured in the assault, and 36% seek some type of medical treatment, which includes care for traumatic injuries. The physician's primary responsibility is to care for the patient's physical and psychological well-being. Patients should be encouraged to undergo a medical forensic examination as soon as possible, because critical evidence may be lost if this examination is delayed. Collection of forensic evidence does not commit the patient to seek prosecution through the criminal justice system, as victims have a nonreport option, in which evidence is stored, allowing the victim time before deciding to file a report.

Many hospitals now have sexual assault nurse examiners/sexual assault forensic examiners (SANE/SAFE) who have been specially trained to care for these patients. These SANE/SAFEs are educated and trained to complete a comprehensive medical-legal examination. If a SANE/SAFE is not available, each ED should have a comprehensive sexual assault protocol that addresses medical care and evidentiary collection either in-house or upon transfer.

4. What information should be elicited in the patient history?
- A comprehensive medical and surgical history, current medications, medication allergies, and social history, including a complete gynecologic history with birth control use, date and time of last consensual intercourse, last menstrual period, and history of recent gynecologic symptoms prior to the assault. Body surface injuries which occurred prior to the assault should also be documented.
- A directed history of the assault includes the date, time, and location of the assault; information concerning the relation the victim had with the assailant; the type and details of sexual acts, including type of force or threats used; and details of any physical assault including strangulation. The history must be obtained in a private setting without the presence of law enforcement personnel.

5. What should be included in the physical examination?
The purpose of the physical examination is to detect injuries requiring treatment and to record and gather forensic evidence. A complete head-to-toe medical examination should be performed by the SANE/SAFE. General body trauma occurs more commonly than genital trauma. Injuries may include, but are not limited to, abrasions and bruises on the arms, head, face, mouth, and neck; signs of restraint (such as rope burns or mouth injuries); broken teeth, fractured nose or jaw from being punched or slapped; ligature marks or signs of nonfatal strangulation; muscle soreness; or stiffness from restraint in positions allowing sexual penetration. These injuries should be documented (i.e., size, color, and shape) on a body diagram, with photographic documentation if possible.

The gynecologic examination should include a thorough search for contusions, abrasions, lacerations, tears, bleeding, or tenderness. Semen or saliva may fluoresce under an alternative light source. Toluidine blue dye can be applied to external genitalia to highlight genital injuries, such as tears or abrasions that might be difficult to see with the naked eye. A colposcopic examination may help identify anogenital and cervical injuries, and if possible, photographs of the genital area should be taken. A careful rectal examination should be done in cases of rectal penetration, and if blood is present, anoscopy or sigmoidoscopy may be necessary to identify internal injuries. It is imperative to remember that lack of visible injury does not mean an assault did not occur.

6. **What evidence is gathered as part of the forensic examination?**
   The forensic evidence may be divided into four categories: control samples from the victim; evidence that might identify the assailant; evidence for proof of recent sexual contact; and evidence for proof of force or coercion (Table 79.1).

7. **What laboratory studies are indicated?**
   A urine or serum pregnancy test will rule out a preexisting pregnancy. If pregnant, the patient should be reassured that this pregnancy was not likely the result of the assault. The routine collection of sexually transmitted infection (STI) cultures is debatable. From a medicolegal perspective, positive cultures, indicating preexisting STIs, have been used by the perpetrator's defense attorneys as evidence of the victim's sexual promiscuity. A preexisting STI is present in approximately 5% of assault victims, the same rate as in the general population. It is reasonable to only culture those patients with signs or symptoms of infection and presumptively treat all victims for their exposure. If the patient does not wish to receive prophylactic antibiotics in the ED, follow-up STI cultures should be obtained in 2 weeks.

8. **What about blood alcohol levels and tests for drug use?**
   In general, urine drug screens and blood alcohol levels are not recommended. Proof of intoxication or drug use may or may not be used against the patient in court. Alternatively, the results may help prove the patient was too intoxicated to give informed consent for a medical forensic examination. If drug testing is medically indicated based on history and physical examination findings and will influence medical management, then laboratory testing may be indicated.

9. **What historical features might indicate a drug-facilitated rape?**
   A history of amnesia or suddenly feeling very intoxicated at a social event should raise concerns about a drug-facilitated sexual assault (DFSA). Sometimes the patient simply relates a history of waking up without clothes on, unsure of what occurred, with genital or pelvic soreness. In these situations, urine and blood samples should be obtained for drug testing. The samples can be collected in the ED by the SANE/SAFE and handed directly to law enforcement to preserve the chain of evidence. The samples should be refrigerated after receipt by law enforcement to preserve the detection of drugs of abuse. Patients should also be informed that any previous volitional, recreational drug use (such as cocaine or marijuana) may also be revealed in toxicologic screening. Conviction of DFSA increases legal penalties in a sexual assault case.

Table 79.1 Forensic Evidence Kit Contents: Based on Jurisdiction

Control Samples From Patient
- Head hair samples
- Saliva sample
- Pubic hair samples

Samples to Identify Assailant
- Skin swabbing for assailant's saliva or sperm
- Fingernail scrapings or clipping (from patient)
- Pubic hair combing
- Trace evidence (such as stray hair, bits of clothing, foreign matter)

Evidence for Proof of Recent Sexual Contact
- Oral, vaginal, or anal swabs for semen
- Skin swabbing for saliva or semen
- Any tampons, vaginal pads, or condoms left in vaginal vault if present

Evidence for Proof of Force or Coercion
- Documentation and photographs of injuries found on examination
- Fingernail scrapings or clippings
- Urine or blood for toxicologic testing (if drug-facilitated sexual assault is suspected)
- All clothing

Modified from Patel M, Minshall L. Management of sexual assault. *Emerg Med Clin North Am.* 2001;19:817–831. Feldhaus KM, Tintinalli JE, Kellen GB, et al. Female and male sexual assault. In: Tintinalli JE, Kellen GB, Stapcznski JS, eds. *Emergency Medicine: A Comprehensive Study Guide.* 6th ed. New York: McGraw-Hill; 2004:1851–1854.

10. **What are the most common STIs that may be contracted as a result of a sexual assault?**
    Sexual assault patients are at highest risk of contracting gonorrhea, chlamydial infection, trichomoniasis, and bacterial vaginosis. The risks of contracting these infections as the result of sexual assault are hard to estimate given their prevalence in the population; risk varies according to geographic area and type of assault. In general, the risk of contracting chlamydial infection or gonorrhea is 4%–17%, and the risk of developing bacterial vaginosis is slightly higher. Victims are also at higher risk of contracting hepatitis B virus (HBV), hepatitis C virus (HCV), human papilloma virus (HPV), and human immunodeficiency virus (HIV) through sexual contact.

11. **Is empiric antibiotic treatment of STIs for sexual assault patients indicated?**
    Because of historically poor follow-up rates by sexual assault patients, along with the significant risk of contracting a new STI, prophylaxis should be offered to all patients. Effective treatment for gonorrhea and chlamydial infection is ceftriaxone 250 mg intramuscularly (IM) and azithromycin 1 g orally. If there is a documented cephalosporin allergy, an alternative regimen for treating gonorrhea and chlamydial infections includes gentamicin 240 mg IM and azithromycin 2 g orally. Treatment of trichomoniasis consists of a single 2 g oral dose of metronidazole. The Centers for Disease Control and Prevention (CDC) also recommends the same regimen for pregnant patients. Quinolones and tetracyclines should be avoided in pregnancy. Contracting bacterial vaginosis during pregnancy carries a risk of premature rupture of membranes, preterm labor, and chorioamnionitis; pregnant women should be encouraged to seek follow-up care (approximately 4–6 weeks) with a gynecologist and receive treatment if they develop bacterial vaginosis.

12. **What other postexposure prevention is recommended after sexual assault?**
    The CDC recommends treatment and prevention of HBV, HPV, and HIV.
    Hepatitis B is transmitted by percutaneous and mucous membrane exposure to HBV-infected blood or body fluids (semen, vaginal secretions, and saliva). Hepatitis B prevention includes HBV vaccination and, if indicated, hepatitis B immune globulin (HBIG). HBIG provides temporary antibody protection from HBV infection for 3–6 months while the HBV vaccination series is being administered. Sexual assault patients previously vaccinated against HBV need no further treatment if the source of exposure's infectious status is unknown. However, if the source is known to have hepatitis B infection, then the patient should receive a single HBV vaccine booster dose. If the sexual assault patient has been unvaccinated, or is known to be a vaccination nonresponder, HBV vaccination should be administered and follow-up should be arranged to complete the vaccination series (1–2 more doses, depending on patient age and manufacturer). HBIG should be administered to unvaccinated sexual assault patients if the source of exposure is known to have hepatitis B infection. Remember to review the CDC guidelines for the most up-to-date recommendations.
    HPV vaccination is recommended for patients from 9 to 45 years old, and follow-up doses should be administered 1–2 months and 6 months after the first dose.
    HIV nonoccupational postexposure prophylaxis (nPEP) to prevent transmission is individualized, based on risk, and is discussed later.

13. **What is HIV postexposure prophylaxis (PEP) and how do I initiate it for my patient?**
    HIV PEP means taking antiretroviral medicines after a potential exposure to HIV to prevent becoming infected. HIV PEP guidelines are based on studies on health care workers with percutaneous exposures to HIV-infected blood. These findings have been extrapolated to nonoccupational injection and sexual HIV exposures, and thus nPEP guidelines were developed.
    Sexual assault patients should have baseline HIV testing, preferably with a serum HIV-1/2 antigen/antibody test. nPEP should begin within 72 hours of exposure. If more than 72 hours have lapsed since the assault, the risks of antiretroviral therapies may outweigh the benefit. The decision to give nPEP for patients within 72 hours of exposure depends upon the HIV status of the assailant. If the assailant is known to be HIV positive, nPEP is recommended. If the HIV status is unknown, as will be the case for most sexual assaults, nPEP is determined on a case-by-case basis. The current preferred regimen is a 28-day course of a combination pill of emtricitabine (200 mg) plus tenofovir disoproxil fumarate (300 mg once daily), plus dolutegravir (50 mg once daily) or raltegravir (400 mg twice daily). It is recommended to provide the patient with at least a 3- to 7-day starter pack of the selected medication regimen and schedule a follow-up visit to review the results of HIV testing, review baseline laboratory data, discuss medication side effects, and change therapies if needed.

14. **My patient is terrified of contracting HIV after her sexual assault. What do I do now?**
    Provide counseling regarding transmission risks and offer nPEP. The estimated risk is dependent on the HIV status of the assailant, the type of sexual contact, the amount of mucosal trauma involved, the time elapsed after the assault, and the potential benefits and risks associated with the nPEP regimen. The HIV status of the assailant is often unknown; known high-risk behaviors include injection drug use, sex workers, men who have sex with men (MSM), or prisoner status. Studies in prison populations reveal that HIV infection rates are higher in male sexual assailants than in the general male population (1% versus 0.3%). The type of sexual contact is important to know, as anal penetration has the highest risk of HIV transmission, whereas oral sex transmission is quite low. Overall, the frequency of HIV seroconversion in sexual assault is low given the per-act risk for HIV transmission ranges from 4 per 10,000 exposures for insertive penile-vaginal intercourse to 138 per 10,000 for receptive anal intercourse. In comparison, a percutaneous needle stick from an infected source carries a 23 per 10,000 exposures

risk of contracting HIV. Genital trauma, bleeding, inflammation, and presence of STIs or genital lesions associated with sexual assault increase the risk of HIV transmission. To optimize the benefit of nPEP, it should be initiated within 72 hours of exposure. The clinical side effects of HIV nPEP medications include headache, nausea, vomiting, and fatigue, along with laboratory abnormalities like elevated liver function tests.

15. **What is the risk of pregnancy after sexual assault?**
    Although the risk of pregnancy after an isolated sexual encounter during nonfertile periods of the menstrual cycle is thought to be less than 1%, it is significantly higher at mid-cycle, with approximately 5% of all sexual assault victims becoming pregnant as a result of the assault. The presence of a preexisting pregnancy must be identified in the ED.

16. **What are the current options for pregnancy prevention?**
    When a preexisting pregnancy has been ruled out, emergency contraceptives can be used to prevent pregnancy by inhibiting or disrupting ovulation or inhibiting fertilization or implantation. Emergency contraception is not effective once implantation has occurred, and it will not disrupt an existing pregnancy. The two most common oral emergency contraceptives are Plan B One-Step (levonorgestrel) and Ella (ulipristal acetate). Products may be taken up to 5 days after sexual contact, but ideally within 72 hours. Common side effects include nausea, vomiting, and vaginal spotting. If taken within 24 hours of the sexual assault, Plan B One-Step is 95% effective at preventing pregnancy, and if taken within 72 hours of the sexual assault, it is 89% effective. A copper intrauterine device (IUD) can also be inserted by qualified providers as emergency contraception up to 5 days after the sexual assault and is 99.9% effective at preventing pregnancy. If a dedicated emergency contraceptive product is not available, a levonorgestrel-containing oral contraceptive pill may be utilized.

17. **What are special characteristics of the male sexual assault victim?**
    The male sexual assault victim should be treated similarly to a female victim. Special attention should be paid to the mouth, genitalia, anus, and rectum. Men represent approximately 5% of reported sexual assault victims. It is estimated that one in six men experience sexual violence.

18. **Discuss the special characteristics of pediatric sexual assault.**
    In pediatric sexual assault, the assailant is often known to the victim, and sometimes has a history of repetitive actions. In addition to documenting signs of acute trauma, the examiner should look for signs of previous trauma, such as healed hymenal tears/transections, posterior fossa or fossa navicularis lacerations, and healed anal injuries. It is important to look for pathologic vaginal discharge, vulvovaginitis, or a foreign body. The anogenital examination should take into account the disclosure of events. In prepubertal children, the estrogen-sensitive tissue of the vaginal introitus and hymen are exquisitely sensitive to touch, so any contact (e.g., speculum or vaginal swabs) should not be attempted without sedation. A speculum examination is only necessary if there is concern for active vaginal vault bleeding, and is best supervised by a gynecologist or a physician specializing in child abuse, neglect, and assault, and may require procedural sedation. The diagnosis of sexually transmissible infections beyond the neonatal period suggests sexual abuse. If one STI is diagnosed, testing for all STIs should be performed. In children, chlamydial and gonorrhea testing on the urine is better tolerated than vaginal swabs. Lastly, health care providers are mandatory reporters for suspected child abuse and assault and are required to notify the local child protection service agency.

19. **Should pediatric patients be given prophylactic antibiotics?**
    Prophylactic antibiotics are not always indicated for prepubertal children who have been sexually abused. The risk of a child acquiring an STI from sexual abuse or assault has not been well studied. However, presumptive treatment for STIs is not recommended because the incidence of most STIs in children is low after abuse/ assault, prepubertal girls appear to be lower risk for developing ascending vaginal infections than adolescents or adults, and medical follow-up usually can be ensured to evaluate for developing infections. Prophylactic treatments should not be given until all appropriate testing is completed. HIV prophylaxis should be considered based on level of risk and in consultation with a pediatric infectious disease specialist. Repeat evaluation and possible STI testing should be performed 2 weeks after exposure, and antibiotic treatment can also be readdressed at that time.

20. **State the important aspects of follow-up care for any victim of sexual assault.**
    Follow-up medical care should ensure that any physical injuries have healed properly (follow-up photographs may be taken), adequate pregnancy prophylaxis has been administered, STIs have been treated, vaccination regimens have been completed, follow-up serology has been obtained for HBV and HIV, and the victim has accessed supportive counseling. Provision of written aftercare instructions and information on community resources is essential.

21. **What types of emotional trauma might sexual assault victims experience?**
    The development of a posttraumatic stress disorder, manifested by sleep disturbances, feelings of guilt, memory impairment, and detachment from the world and others may occur in the days to weeks after the assault. Long-term psychological sequelae in the form of rape trauma syndrome may also occur. Many communities have rape crisis centers with social workers and volunteers who are trained to provide counseling for sexual assault survivors.

Sexual assault response teams (SARTs) have been organized in other areas to provide a coordinated approach to the sexual assault victim, including emotional support after the event. Physicians should be aware of the availability of such services so that they can recommend them to their patients.

KEY POINTS: CARE OF THE SEXUAL ASSAULT VICTIM

1. First and foremost, care for the victim's medical and emotional needs.
2. Collection of forensic evidence may not be performed without the patient's consent.
3. Victims must be told of the options they have as to reporting and evidence collection: they can report to law enforcement and have evidence collected; they can decline to report to law enforcement but still have evidence collection; or they can decline to report and decline evidence collection.
4. All patients should be offered prophylactic antibiotics for STIs, vaccinations, and nPEP as indicated.
5. Women of child-bearing age should be informed about emergency contraception; if it is not offered to the patient at the hospital, a referral should be made so that the patient may receive it in a timely manner.
6. Written referral to community resources for post-assault counseling is critical.

WEBSITES

Antiretroviral postexposure prophylaxis. Available at www.cdc.gov/hiv/basics/pep.html; accessed February 11, 2019.

Centers for Disease Control and Prevention: 2015 sexually transmitted disease treatment guidelines. Available at www.cdc.gov/std/tg2015/sexual-assault.htm; accessed February 12, 2019

Facts about sexual assault. Available at www.rainn.org/statistics; accessed February 11, 2019.

HIV Risk Behaviors: https://www.cdc.gov/hiv/risk/estimates/riskbehaviors.html; accessed February 5, 2019.

National Crime Victimization Survey 2014. Available at http://ovc.ncjrs.gov/ncvrw2014/pdf/StatisticalOverviews.pdf; accessed February 20, 2015.

Sexual Assault and Abuse and STDs: https://www.cdc.gov/std/tg2015/sexual-assault.htm; accessed February 5, 2019.

Sexual violence fact sheet. Available at www.cdc.gov/ncipc/factsheets/svfacts.htm; accessed February 12, 2019.

ACKNOWLEDGMENT

The editors gratefully acknowledge the contributions of prior authors of this chapter, notably Jennie A. Buchanan, MD.

BIBILIOGRAPHY

Cheng L, Gulmezoglu AM, Oel CJ, et al. Interventions for emergency contraception. *Cochrane Database Syst Rev.* 2004;(3):CD001324.

Feldhaus KM, Tintinalli JE, Kellen GB, et al. Female and male sexual assault. In: Tintinalli JE, Kellen GB, Stapcznski JS, eds. *Emergency Medicine: A Comprehensive Study Guide.* 6th ed. New York: McGraw-Hill; 2004:1851–1854.

Patel M, Minshall L. Management of sexual assault. *Emerg Med Clin North Am.* 2001;19:817–831.

Patel P, Borkowf CB, Brooks JT, et al. Estimating per-act HIV transmission risk: a systematic review. *AIDS.* 2014;28(10):1509–1519.

CHAPTER 80

SPONTANEOUS ABORTION, ECTOPIC PREGNANCY, AND VAGINAL BLEEDING

Alexander Guillaume, MD and Mindi Guptill, MD, FACEP

1. **What are the important causes to consider in the emergency department (ED) evaluation of first-trimester vaginal bleeding or pain?**
   - Spontaneous abortion
   - Ectopic pregnancy (EP)
   - Gestational trophoblastic disease (molar pregnancy)
   - Subchorionic hemorrhage/hematoma (SH)
   - Vaginal or cervical trauma
   - Sexually transmitted infections
   - Nongenital (e.g., urinary or gastrointestinal) sources of bleeding

---

KEY POINTS: APPROACH TO THE PATIENT WITH A POSITIVE PREGNANCY TEST AND FIRST-TRIMESTER VAGINAL BLEEDING OR PAIN

1. Recognize immediately that this clinical scenario may represent EP. These patients are at risk for precipitous hemodynamic deterioration and should be approached with a high index of suspicion.
2. Establish appropriate intravenous (IV) access. Two large-bore (18-gauge or larger) IV lines are recommended if there is any concern for hemodynamic instability.
3. Obtain a measurement of hemoglobin and/or hematocrit or complete blood count (CBC). A blood type and screen should be sent if the patient may require a blood transfusion.
4. Establish maternal rhesus (Rh) type to determine the need for Rh immunoglobulin (RhoGAM).
5. Quantitative serum β-human chorionic gonadotropin (β-HCG) assay will help in assessing ectopic risk and coordinating follow-up care.
6. Treat hypotension or tachycardia with IV fluids or transfusion of blood products, as indicated by patient condition.
7. Perform a speculum and bimanual pelvic examination to assess the source of bleeding, and examine the cervical os to assess for the presence of products of conception in the cervix or vaginal vault.
8. If there is active bleeding, remove any visualized tissue using gentle traction with ring forceps; this may help abate ongoing bleeding.
9. Determine whether an intrauterine pregnancy (IUP) has been previously documented, preferably by bedside ultrasound. If no IUP is documented, consultative ultrasound should be performed to evaluate for a possible EP. Unstable patients should not be allowed to leave the ED for diagnostic studies. Consider also performing a bedside FAST (focused assessment with sonography for trauma) examination, looking for free fluid that raises concern for ruptured EP.
10. Consult a specialist in obstetrics and gynecology (OB/GYN) for an open cervical os (suggesting inevitable or incomplete abortion), ongoing profuse bleeding, hypovolemic shock, or continued decreasing hemoglobin or hematocrit in the ED.

---

2. **What is spontaneous abortion or miscarriage?**
   Miscarriage is spontaneous termination of IUP before achieving fetal maturity compatible with survival outside the uterus (<24 weeks' gestation).

3. **State the incidence and timing of spontaneous abortion.**
   Ten percent to 20% of clinically recognized pregnancies <20 weeks' gestation will miscarry; 80% of these occur in the first 12 weeks' gestation. The rate of miscarriage may even be higher, as many miscarriages occur before a pregnancy is clinically detected.

4. **What are the different types of miscarriage or abortion?**
   - Threatened abortion: a pregnant patient within the first half of pregnancy with vaginal bleeding and a closed internal cervical os on bimanual examination. Cramping abdominal, pelvic, or back pain may also be present.
   - Inevitable abortion: Findings of a threatened abortion, but with an open internal cervical os.

- Incomplete abortion: a miscarriage in progress. Only parts of the products of conception have passed and may be visible in the cervical os or vaginal canal.
- Complete abortion: all products of conception have been passed. Pain and significant bleeding should stop after a completed abortion. Typically, the cervical os is closed. The uterus is small, empty, and well-contracted.
- Missed abortion: retention of a nonviable IUP within the uterus. Products of conception are demonstrable, but fetal development has ceased, no cardiac activity is visible, the cervical os is closed, and spontaneous passage has not occurred.

5. **Identify important questions to consider during the examination and treatment of spontaneous abortion.**
   - Is the patient hemodynamically stable?
   - Is there abdominal tenderness, guarding, or rebound, concerning for possible EP?
   - Are products of conception visible in the cervical os or vaginal canal?
   - Is the cervical os open or closed?
   - Is the patient febrile, indicating a possible septic abortion?
   - What is the patient's Rh factor?

6. **What is a septic abortion?**
   A septic abortion is a spontaneous abortion complicated by infection of the products of conception (fetus and placenta) with possible spread to the endometrium, myometrium, and peritoneum.

7. **What are the signs and symptoms of a septic abortion?**
   - Malodorous discharge from the cervix or vagina
   - Pelvic and abdominal pain
   - Uterine tenderness
   - Fever
   - Sepsis or septic shock

8. **How is a septic abortion managed?**
   Stabilize the patient with IV fluid. Obtain blood and cervical cultures. Begin broad-spectrum antibiotics with anaerobic coverage. Consult obstetrics emergently for dilation and curettage.

9. **What is the prognosis and management for patients with threatened abortion?**
   Patients with bleeding and a closed internal os have ~50% risk of miscarriage. There is no treatment regimen that influences the course of a threatened abortion, including pelvic rest, bed rest, or exercise avoidance. Patient should generally follow up with an obstetrician within 72 hours for light bleeding or within 48 hours for moderate bleeding.

10. **Which types of abortion require obstetric consultation in the ED?**
    Inevitable and incomplete abortions generally require obstetric consultation in the ED for management options. Missed abortions may be sent home if vital signs are stable and labs do not reveal coagulopathy. Expectant management at home for women in early pregnancy failure with stable vital signs is becoming an increasingly popular option, and up to 80% of patients complete their abortions without intervention in the first trimester.

11. **What factors are associated with spontaneous abortion?**
    In the first trimester, the most significant factor is chromosomal abnormalities causing abnormal development of the zygote, seen in 50%–85% of spontaneous abortions. Maternal diseases such as diabetes mellitus, thyroid disorders, antiphospholipid syndrome, and inherited thrombophilias (antithrombin deficiency, protein C and protein S deficiency, factor V Leiden mutation) also play a lesser role. Other factors include increasing maternal age, uterine structural abnormalities, and drugs (high alcohol use, cocaine, certain prescription agents).

12. **What is implantation bleeding?**
    Implantation bleeding is scant pink or brownish discharge that occurs in up to one third of pregnant women when a fertilized egg implants and invades the wall of the endometrial cavity. It is usually both lighter and shorter than a typical menstrual period, and is usually not accompanied by additional symptoms such as cramping or backaches. Implantation bleeding occurs approximately 4 weeks after a woman's last menstrual period.

13. **Is minor trauma a significant factor associated with spontaneous abortion?**
    No, fetuses are well protected by maternal structures and amniotic fluid from minor falls or blows; however, penetrating trauma, such as a gunshot or stab wound, is dangerous to the fetus.

14. **Name the drug used to prevent Rh alloimmunization.**
    RhoGAM; any pregnant woman who is experiencing vaginal bleeding must have an Rh type checked. If she is Rh negative and the fetus is less than 12 weeks' gestation, she should receive a minidose of RhoGAM, 50 μg intramuscularly. If she is Rh negative and the fetus is greater than 12 weeks' gestation, administer the full dose of RhoGAM, 300 μg.

15. **What follow-up instructions should be given for a threatened abortion?**
    Careful instructions are given to return for an increase in pain, bleeding, or signs of hemodynamic instability, such as syncope or near-syncopal episodes. In practice, patients are commonly instructed to return if bleeding exceeds

saturation of 1 pad per hour for 4–6 hours, regardless of symptomatology. Instruct patients to bring any passed tissue to the ED or primary care physician (PCP). Make arrangements for repeat quantitative β-HCG measurements and ultrasound within 48–72 hours.

16. What about the emotional aspects of an early miscarriage?
Miscarriage is associated with a significant amount of psychological stress and grieving. Many patients and their partners experience guilt about things they perceive as contributing to their pregnancy loss. Important therapeutic messages include informing the patient that early miscarriages are common, and that miscarriages are usually the result of spontaneous chromosomal abnormalities and not the patient's own actions.

17. What is an EP?
An EP is a pregnancy in which implantation of the gestational sac occurs outside of the uterus. In 90% of cases, the pregnancy is located in the fallopian tubes, but EPs can occur in a cesarean scar (1%–3%), intra-abdominally (1%), on the ovary (1%–3%), or within the cervix (1%). EP occurs in approximately 2% of all pregnancies, and is the leading cause of maternal first trimester deaths. By some reports, up to 18% of pregnant women presenting to the ED with vaginal bleeding or abdominal pain in the first trimester are diagnosed with EP. Patients with EP may have abdominal pain, syncope, amenorrhea, or vaginal bleeding. However, many women with EP are asymptomatic before tubal rupture, and 50% do not have a single risk factor for EP.

18. Name common risk factors for EP.
- Prior EP
- Pelvic inflammatory disease
- Tubal surgeries (including ligation)
- Pelvic surgery
- Infertility and fertilization treatments
- Cigarette smoking
- Age >35

19. Define heterotopic pregnancy. What is the main risk factor for this condition, and what is its incidence?
A heterotopic pregnancy is the simultaneous implantation of an embryo at two or more sites, most commonly manifesting as an IUP and EP. The most significant risk factor is assisted fertility treatment. With natural conception in the general population, the incidence is thought to be low, and has been historically cited as 1 in 30,000; however, this is thought to be increasing, with some estimating the incidence as 1 in 4000 or higher. The incidence is much higher among patients undergoing fertility treatments: ≥1 in 100.

20. How reliable are routine serum and urine pregnancy tests in a patient with EP?
Sensitive serum or urine pregnancy tests are almost always positive in EP. β-HCG is secreted from the time of implantation, and is detectable about 7–8 days after implantation of the fertilized ovum. Qualitative pregnancy tests that can detect β-HCG levels between 10 and 50 mIU/mL are positive in 99% of patients with EP. Home pregnancy tests and less sensitive tests with higher thresholds may have false-negative results. Serum and urine tests provide similar accuracy for qualitative testing when their thresholds are similar.

21. What clinical signs and symptoms are useful to increase suspicion of an EP?
The classic picture of EP consists of vaginal bleeding, pelvic or abdominal pain, prior missed menses, and an adnexal mass. However, this picture is neither sensitive nor specific. A recent systematic review determined that all historical and symptomatic components had positive likelihood ratios of less than 1.5. When progesterone levels fall as a result of insufficient HCG from the abnormal EP, endometrial integrity breaks down, producing uterine bleeding. Sometimes the decidua cast (not true pregnancy) is passed and may be clinically confused with a spontaneous abortion. Otherwise, symptoms such as vaginal bleeding and pain may occur only later, when the growing EP begins to fail or overstretch its abnormal implantation site, potentially leading to intra-abdominal bleeding after rupture occurs. Physical examination findings such as peritoneal signs, severe pain on pelvic examination, adnexal masses, and cervical motion tenderness increase suspicion for a ruptured EP. There is, however, no constellation of historical factors or physical examination findings that confirms or excludes EP with sufficient reliability to obviate the need for sonography.

22. Define paradoxical bradycardia in relation to a ruptured EP.
This refers to absolute or relative bradycardia in the setting of significant intra-abdominal hemorrhage, as seen in ruptured EP. Although the mechanism is not fully understood, vagal stimulation may contribute to this phenomenon. ED clinicians should avoid relying on "stable" vital signs in the setting of potential ruptured EP.

23. Why are corpus luteum cysts commonly confused with EPs?
The corpus luteum of the ovary supports the pregnancy with secretion of progesterone during the first 6–7 weeks' gestation and may become cystic and relatively large. Cyst rupture can occur in the first trimester, presenting in a patient in early pregnancy as sudden pain, unilateral peritoneal findings, and adnexal tenderness.

24. What is the most efficient way to evaluate for EP in the ED?
Ultrasound evaluation of early pregnancy is the best first ancillary study. Normal IUPs can be seen by trans-vaginal sonography by 4–5 weeks' gestational age, depending on equipment resolution and sonographer

proficiency. EPs can be seen on occasion, but an empty uterus may be the only finding. The risk of EP can be defined further by obtaining a quantitative β-HCG level if the ultrasound is inconclusive. IUP, if present, should be detected on ultrasound when the β-HCG concentration is above the discriminatory zone (see No. 27).

25. **Describe the role of bedside ultrasonography in the ED evaluation of the patient with first-trimester complaints.**
    Emergency physician performed–point-of-care ultrasound (POCUS) has become an increasingly common modality in the evaluation of patients with complaints of pain or bleeding in the first trimester. When used appropriately, POCUS can more rapidly confirm the diagnosis of IUP, and has been shown to decrease the ED length of stay, as compared with ultrasound performed in the radiology department. In this setting, the goal of bedside ultrasonography should not be to rule out EP, but rather to *rule in* IUP. In the absence of risk factors for, or signs and symptoms suggestive of, heterotopic pregnancy, definitive identification of IUP by POCUS makes the diagnosis of EP unlikely. It can also be used to assess the abdomen for the presence of free fluid, suggestive of hemoperitoneum, when concern for ruptured EP exists.

26. **Identify the early sonographic findings in a healthy pregnancy.**
    - Gestational sac: one of the earliest findings of normal pregnancy, first seen at about 4 weeks' gestational age by transvaginal ultrasound. This is a well-circumscribed fluid collection within the endometrial cavity. A true gestational sac is surrounded by two layers of tissue, forming the "double decidual" sign: an inner layer, called the *decidua capsularis,* and an outer layer, called the *decidua vera.* This sign distinguishes a true gestational sac from a pseudosac, a poorly defined fluid collection within the endometrial cavity that may be seen with an EP.
    - Yolk sac: seen at about 5 weeks' gestational age by transvaginal ultrasound. This is a well-defined echogenic ring seen within the gestational sac. For the purposes of emergency bedside ultrasound, this is considered by many authors to be the most reliable early finding that confirms the presence of an IUP, and is easily recognized at all skill levels.
    - Embryo: fetal pole visible within the gestational sac, seen at about 5–6 weeks' gestational age by transvaginal ultrasound.
    - Fetal cardiac activity: generally recognizable by about 6–7 weeks.

27. **Describe the concept of the discriminatory zone as it applies to the serum β-HCG level.**
    In the early stages of a normal pregnancy, β-HCG levels increase at a predictable rate, correlating to expected stages of fetal development. The discriminatory zone is that β-HCG level at which a normally developing IUP, if present, should be visible by ultrasound. For transvaginal ultrasonography, the discriminatory zone is generally considered to be between 1000 and 2000 mIU/mL, depending on institutional protocols. If a patient has a serum β-HCG level above the discriminatory zone, but no IUP can be seen by ultrasound, the suspicion for EP increases significantly. In recent years, the American College of Obstetricians and Gynecologists (ACOG) has recommended a discriminatory zone (as high as 3500 mIU /mL) to avoid accidental termination of a desired IUP misdiagnosed as EP. After a consultative ultrasound has excluded the presence of EP, stable patients with β-HCGs higher than the discriminatory zone and pregnancies of unknown location may be discharged with close obstetrics follow-up,

28. **How else is quantitative β-HCG used?**
    In normal IUPs, levels of β-HCG double every 2–3 days during the first 7–8 weeks. Because many women do not know the date of their last menstrual period, quantitative levels may be useful to estimate gestational age and correlate with expected sonographic findings. With β-HCG above the discriminatory zone, a healthy IUP should be visible by transvaginal sonography. Failure to double normally during the first 7 weeks indicates a failed pregnancy, either within the uterus or at an ectopic site. EP is more likely if the ultrasound is indeterminate and the quantitative β-HCG is above the discriminatory zone or rising on serial measurements.

29. **Does every patient with bleeding or pain in the first trimester require ultrasound before discharge from the ED?**
    All first-trimester complaints are treated as "rule out EP" until the diagnosis of IUP is established. In general, an ultrasound should be performed in all patients with a positive pregnancy test and vaginal bleeding or pain. Unstable patients or those with peritoneal signs, severe pain, or heavy ongoing bleeding should have their ultrasound performed in the ED.

30. **What are the ultrasound findings in patients with suspected EP?**
    An EP is confirmed when a gestational sac with a yolk sac or fetal pole is visualized outside the uterus. Sonographic findings that are highly suspicious for ectopic pregnancy include free fluid, adnexal masses, and tubal rings. Although small amounts of free fluid visualized in the posterior cul-de-sac may be physiologic, increasing amounts of fluid raise the likelihood of EP. Free fluid does not necessarily indicate ruptured EP, as early in EP blood can leak back from the end of the fallopian tube, or an ovarian cyst may have ruptured. Adnexal masses are not specific for EP; additional possible diagnoses include ovarian cysts and neoplasms.

31. **Define pseudogestational sac and note its importance.**
These are intrauterine, blood-filled sacs seen in 10% of EPs. Because pseudogestational sacs can mimic the early gestational sac of an IUP, clinicians should avoid diagnosing an IUP until an intrauterine yolk sac or fetal pole is visualized.

32. **Which patients with EP can be discharged from the ED?**
Women who are unstable with severe pain or signs of significant blood loss require admission. ED or inpatient observation may be useful in stable patients with worrisome symptoms, risk factors, or expected poor adherence to facilitate rapid sonography, quantitative β-HCG interpretation, or specialist consultation. Stable patients with indeterminate ultrasound results (rule out EP) may be monitored on an outpatient basis. Expectant management or chemotherapy for women with few symptoms and low hormonal levels should be determined in consultation with an obstetrician. The role of the ED physician is to make every effort to exclude or confirm the diagnosis of EP, educate the patient on the signs that should be of concern to her, and ensure access to close follow-up care for this potentially fatal condition.

33. **Describe the role of methotrexate in treating EP.**
Medical treatment is often less expensive than laparoscopic surgery, and single-dose methotrexate is effective in 88% of patients. Methotrexate, a folate antagonist that inhibits DNA synthesis and cell reproduction, targets rapidly growing cells and has replaced surgery for many hemodynamically stable patients with EPs and no contraindications. Because of significant failure rates, patients must be monitored closely. Failure rates are higher when the EP is >4 cm, has fetal cardiac activity, or the β-HCG is greater than 5000. Patients commonly have significant pain with or without peritoneal signs several days after treatment with methotrexate. The decision to use this medication should be made in discussion with an OB/GYN specialist.

KEY POINTS: CANDIDATES FOR MEDICAL TREATMENT OF EP WITH METHOTREXATE

1. Hemodynamically stable
2. No evidence of ectopic rupture
3. The ability and willingness to adhere to post-treatment monitoring
4. No significant hepatic or renal dysfunction
5. No significant anemia, leukopenia, or thrombocytopenia
6. Ectopic gestational sac <4 cm*
7. No fetal cardiac activity on ultrasound examination*

*Sac size >4 cm or presence of cardiac activity are relative, not absolute, contraindications.
Modified from American College of Obstetricians and Gynecologists. ACOG Practice Bulletin No. 193: tubal ectopic pregnancy. *Obstet Gynecol.* 2018;131:e91–e103.

34. **What are absolute contraindications to methotrexate therapy for EP?**
   - Hemodynamic instability
   - Ruptured EP
   - Breastfeeding
   - Immunodeficiency
   - Inability to participate in follow-up
   - Hepatic or renal dysfunction
   - Significant leukopenia, anemia, or thrombocytopenia
   - Active pulmonary disease
   - Active peptic ulcer disease
   - Methotrexate sensitivity

35. **What is gestational trophoblastic disease?**
Gestational trophoblastic disease, also known as *molar pregnancy,* is a disease spectrum that develops in placental trophoblastic cells. Signs and symptoms include painless first- or second-trimester vaginal bleeding, hyperemesis, hypertension that develops before the third trimester, and uterine size that is larger than expected for gestational age. Serum β-HCG measurements are commonly significantly higher than predicted for gestational age based on time since last menstrual period. Ultrasound shows a "snowstorm" appearance, with hypoechoic areas scattered throughout a hyperechoic background within the uterus. Due to the need for uterine evacuation and the risk of malignancy, obstetric consultation should be obtained for suspected molar pregnancies.

36. **What is SH?**
SH is bleeding that occurs between the chorionic layer and the uterine wall. It is the most common sonographic abnormality seen with a live embryo. The cause is unclear because it may develop spontaneously, or be seen following blunt trauma. Large SH may increase the risk of miscarriage, but small ones are thought to not significantly affect the course of pregnancy.

37. **Name the sources and causes of third-trimester vaginal bleeding.**
    The sources are the vagina, cervix, and uterus. In the following list, life-threatening causes are indicated by an asterisk:
    - *Placenta previa
    - *Placental abruption
    - *Uterine rupture
    - Vasa previa (life-threatening to fetus)
    - Bloody show
    - Local trauma
    - Cervical polyps and lesions

38. **What is placenta previa?**
    Seen in 0.3%–0.5% of pregnancies, placenta previa occurs when the placenta overlies the cervical os to any degree. A low-lying placenta, in contrast, occurs when the placental edge approaches but does not cover any of the os. Because transvaginal ultrasound can provide precise spatial measurements, the terms "marginal" and "partial" are no longer used to describe the degree of previa. Placenta previa can be life threatening because vaginal penetration or manipulation of the cervix during a pelvic examination may rupture placental blood vessels and cause massive hemorrhage.

39. **Describe the presentation and diagnosis of placenta previa.**
    Placenta previa should be suspected when a patient in the second half of pregnancy presents with bright red vaginal bleeding. Bleeding is classically painless, but can be associated with abdominal pain and uterine contractions. Previa is best diagnosed via transvaginal ultrasound, which is safe when performed by properly trained sonographers. Previa may be diagnosed incidentally during routine prenatal sonography and, if asymptomatic, may be followed with serial ultrasounds until delivery; up to 90% of cases diagnosed before 20 weeks' gestational age spontaneously resolve.

40. **How is placenta previa treated?**
    Early consultation with an OB/GYN specialist should occur when the diagnosis is suspected. Administer supplemental oxygen, obtain two large-bore IV lines, and perform maternal and fetal monitoring. Obtain a CBC, coagulation levels, and blood type and screen for anticipated transfusion. Place the patient in the left lateral decubitus position to prevent compression of the inferior vena cava by the gravid uterus. Because life-threatening bleeding may occur with placental manipulation, do not perform a pelvic examination if the diagnosis is known. Definitive management is cesarean delivery by an OB/GYN specialist.

41. **What is placental abruption (abruptio placentae)?**
    Placental abruption is the premature separation of the placenta from its insertion on the uterine wall. Depending on the amount of placental separation and subsequent bleeding, the presentation of abruption may range from asymptomatic to maternal shock and fetal demise. Abruption occurs spontaneously or after abdominal trauma. Common symptoms include dark red vaginal bleeding, uterine contractions, uterine tenderness, and significant abdominal pain. Vaginal bleeding occurs in about 80% of patients, and correlates poorly with the degree of abruption. This presentation is in contrast to the classically painless, bright red bleeding of placenta previa.

42. **How is placental abruption diagnosed?**
    Abruption is diagnosed clinically. In stable patients with an uncertain diagnosis, an ultrasound may be obtained, although it is only diagnostic for abruption in 15%–25% of cases; when a clot is visualized on ultrasound, however, the positive predictive value for abruption is 88%. Laboratory results such as the Kleihauer-Betke test are not sensitive enough to diagnose abruption.

43. **Describe the treatment of placental abruption.**
    Immediately consult a specialist in OB/GYN. ED management is similar to placenta previa. Start two large-bore IV lines, and administer oxygen. Monitor fetal heart tones and maternal vital signs. Obtain a CBC, type and screen blood for anticipated transfusion, and perform coagulation studies. Monitor for hemorrhagic shock and disseminated intravascular coagulation (DIC). If the mother and fetus are stable, arrange an immediate ultrasound. Unstable patients should be transferred directly to the operating room or obstetrics suite for emergent delivery.

44. **What is uterine rupture, and why is it dangerous?**
    This is a grave complication of late pregnancy in which the uterus ruptures, usually during contractions. It can produce massive, intra-abdominal hemorrhage that threatens the lives of both mother and fetus. Uterine rupture presents with sudden abdominal pain, change in pattern of uterine contractions, loss of fetal station, and shock late in pregnancy. There may be scant vaginal bleeding, but the abdomen is extremely tender. The most significant risk factor for uterine rupture is a scarred uterus from prior cesarean section or other uterine surgery.

45. **How is uterine rupture treated?**
    Start two large-bore IV lines, administer oxygen, and support respiration and hemodynamics as necessary. Emergent OB/GYN consultation is required, because the treatment is emergent laparotomy and possible hysterectomy. Ultrasound may be useful in selected cases to distinguish uterine rupture from placental abruption.

46. **Define vasa previa.**

Vasa previa occurs when unprotected fetal vessels course over or near the endocervical os. Tearing of these vessels during rupture of membranes or labor can lead to rapid fetal exsanguination. Occurring in between 1 in 2500 and 1 in 5000 pregnancies, this condition is associated with up to a 60% rate of perinatal mortality if not diagnosed during prenatal ultrasonography. Treatment is typically an early, planned cesarean delivery. ED management of vaginal bleeding due to suspected vasa previa consists of stabilizing the mother as needed, maternal and fetal monitoring, and emergent OB/GYN consultation.

47. **Describe the non–life-threatening causes of third-trimester vaginal bleeding.**

- Bloody show is a pink mucous discharge caused by cervical changes that precedes labor by several hours to a week.
- The cervix is prone to hemorrhage during late pregnancy, and local trauma from vaginal penetration, including intercourse, may cause bleeding.
- Cervical erosions or preexisting polyps produce limited bleeding.

ACKNOWLEDGMENT

The editors gratefully acknowledge the contributions of Brandon H. Backlund, MD, FACEP and Dane M. Chapman, MD, previous edition authors.

BIBLIOGRAPHY

American College of Obstetricians and Gynecologists. ACOG Practice Bulletin No. 193: tubal ectopic pregnancy. *Obstet Gynecol.* 2018;131):e91–e103.
Avitabile NC, Kaban NL, Siadecki SD, et al. Two cases of heterotopic pregnancy: review of the literature and sonographic diagnosis in the emergency department. *J Ultrasound Med.* 2015;34(3):827–530.
Crochet JR, Bastian LA, Chireau MV. Does this woman have an ectopic pregnancy? The rational clinical examination systematic review. *JAMA.* 2013;309(16):1722–1729.
Eschenbach DA. Treating spontaneous and induced septic abortions. *Obstet Gynecol.* 2015;125(5):1042–1048.
Hsu S, Euerle BD. Ultrasound in pregnancy. *Emerg Med Clin North Am.* 2012;30(4):849–867.
Huancahuari N. Emergencies in early pregnancy. *Emerg Med Clin North Am.* 2012;30(4):837–847.
Jurkovic D, Overton C, Bender-Atik R. Diagnosis and management of first trimester miscarriage. *BMJ.* 2013;346:f3676.
Meguerdichian D. Complications in late pregnancy. *Emerg Med Clin North Am.* 2012;30(4):919–936.
Mendez-Figueroa H, Dahlke JD, Vrees RA, et al. Trauma in pregnancy: an updated systematic review. *Am J Obstet Gynecol.* 2013;209(1):1–10.
Robertson JJ, Long B. Emergency medicine myths: ectopic pregnancy evaluation, risk factors, and presentation. *J Emerg Med.* 2017;53(6):819–828.
Silver RM. Abnormal placentation: placenta previa, vasa previa, and placenta accreta. *Obstet Gynecol.* 2015;126(3):654–668.

CHAPTER 81

THIRD-TRIMESTER COMPLICATIONS AND DELIVERY

Deborah Vinton, MD

1. **What are the major hypertensive disorders in pregnancy?**
   - Chronic hypertension
   - Gestational hypertension
   - Preeclampsia
   - Preeclampsia superimposed on chronic hypertension

2. **What is preeclampsia?**
   Preeclampsia is a multisystem progressive disorder of pregnancy that occurs most often after 20 weeks' gestation. The condition may also develop postpartum. It is characterized by new-onset hypertension with either proteinuria or significant end-organ dysfunction due to widespread maternal and placental vascular endothelial malfunction. The spectrum of disease can range from mild to severe.

3. **What is gestational hypertension, and how does it differ from chronic hypertension?**
   Gestational hypertension is a systolic blood pressure (SBP) greater than 140 mmHg or a diastolic blood pressure (DBP) greater than 90 mmHg on two occasions, more than 4 hours apart, after 20 weeks' gestation in a previously normotensive woman. Gestational hypertension is considered severe when SBP reaches 160 mmHg or DBP reaches 110 mmHg. Chronic hypertension predates a patient's pregnancy and is detected before 20 weeks' gestation.

4. **Which conditions must be present to diagnose preeclampsia?**
   - Hypertension: new-onset SBP >140 mmHg or a DBP >90 mmHg on two occasions, at least 4 hours apart; or an SBP >160 mmHg and a DBP >110 mmHg on a single occasion. (Criteria for a woman who has preexisting hypertension: an SBP increased by 30 mmHg or a DBP increased by 15 mmHg.)
     And one of the following:
   - Proteinuria: excretion of ≥300 mg protein in the urine in a 24-hour period or a protein/creatinine ratio of 0.3 mg/dL
   - Thrombocytopenia: <100,000 platelets/µL
   - New renal insufficiency: elevated serum creatinine >1.1 mg/dL or a doubling of the serum creatinine in the absence of renal disease
   - Impaired liver function: elevated transaminases at least twice normal concentrations
   - Pulmonary edema
   - Visual symptoms or new-onset headache not accounted for by alternative diagnoses
     Note: Prior to 2013, the diagnosis of preeclampsia required the presence of proteinuria to meet criteria for the condition. Proteinuria is no longer required to make the diagnosis if hypertension and other end-organ dysfunction are present.

5. **What are the diagnostic criteria for preeclampsia with features of severe disease?**
   The presence of *one or more* of the following constitutes preeclampsia with features of severe disease:
   - SBP > 160 mm Hg or DBP > 110 mmHg on two occasions 4 hours apart (unless antihypertensive therapy has been initiated)
   - Pulmonary edema
   - Thrombocytopenia (<100,000 platelets/µL)
   - New-onset headache unexplained by alternative diagnoses
   - Visual disturbances
   - Transaminase concentration greater than twice the upper level of normal or severe persistent upper abdominal pain not accounted for by alternative diagnoses
   - Progressive renal insufficiency with creatinine greater than 1.1 or doubling of creatinine

6. **How is a diagnosis of preeclampsia superimposed on chronic hypertension made?**
   This diagnosis is made in a patient who has chronic hypertension diagnosed in early pregnancy, who then has a sudden onset of proteinuria, increased hypertension, or new onset of signs and symptoms of preeclampsia after 20 weeks' gestation.

7. **What causes preeclampsia?**
   Several mechanisms have been proposed, but the exact pathophysiology is unknown. Research suggests there may be placental vasculature abnormalities that contribute to chronic uteroplacental hypoperfusion, hypoxia, and

ischemia. The placenta then releases inflammatory substances into the maternal circulation, resulting in widespread endothelial dysfunction and end-organ damage.

8. **Are there risk factors for preeclampsia?**
Preeclampsia is primarily a complication of first pregnancies and often occurs in healthy women without obvious risk factors. Risk factors that have been identified include a personal or family history of preeclampsia, conception before age 20 years, multifetal pregnancies, advanced maternal age, high body mass index, assisted reproductive technology, and adverse outcome in previous pregnancy. There are also several preexisting medical conditions that increase the risk for preeclampsia, including antiphospholipid antibody syndrome, systemic lupus erythematosus, insulin-dependent diabetes, connective tissue disease, renal disease, and hypertension.

9. **How common is preeclampsia?**
Worldwide, 2%–8% of pregnancies are complicated by preeclampsia. In the United States, the prevalence is ~3%, with the majority of these occurring after 34 weeks.

10. **What is the definitive treatment for preeclampsia?**
Delivery of the fetus is definitive treatment for preeclampsia. The decision to initiate delivery is based on gestational age, severity of disease, and well-being of the mother and fetus.

11. **When is immediate delivery indicated?**
Immediate delivery is indicated in any patient with greater than 34 weeks' gestation who meets criteria for preeclampsia with features of severe disease, or when maternal or fetal condition is considered to be unstable, regardless of gestational age. In these cases, delivery should not be delayed for the administration of steroids in the late preterm period. For preeclampsia without features of severe disease, expectant management is appropriate up to 37 weeks.

12. **What is the treatment for preeclampsia in the ED?**
   - Magnesium sulfate should be administered immediately for patients who present with preeclampsia with severe features to reduce the risk of seizure and eclampsia. Magnesium slows neuromuscular conduction and decreases central nervous system (CNS) irritability, but does not lower BP or reduce the risk of disease progression. The magnesium loading dose is 4–6 g over 15–20 minutes, followed by a 1–2 g/h continuous infusion.
   - For patients with sustained SBP > 160 mmHg or DBP > 110 mmHg, antihypertensives should be used in consultation with an obstetrician.
   - Administer corticosteroids to patients between 24 and 34 weeks' gestation to enhance fetal lung maturity.

13. **Which antihypertensive medications can be used?**
   - Labetalol 20 mg intravenously (IV); then 20–80 mg every 10–30 min to a maximum cumulative dose of 300 mg, or constant infusion of 1–2 mg/min IV. Avoid in women with asthma.
   - Hydralazine 5–10 mg IV over 2 minutes, then 5–10 mg IV every 20–40 minutes to a maximum cumulative dose of 30 mg; or constant infusion of 0.5–10 mg/h.
   - Nifedipine 10–20 mg orally, repeat in 20 minutes, then 10–20 mg every 2–6 hours with maximum cumulative dose of 180 mg.

14. **Which antihypertensive medications should be avoided in pregnancy?**
   - Angiotensin-converting enzyme (ACE) inhibitors, angiotensin II receptor blockers (ARBs), and direct renin inhibitors are associated with fetal renal abnormalities and should be avoided in pregnancy.
   - Sodium nitroprusside is also best avoided, because of risk for fetal cyanide poisoning.

15. **How should patients treated with magnesium be monitored?**
A clinical examination, including assessment for patellar reflexes and respiratory rate, should be performed every 1–2 hours in patients receiving a magnesium infusion. It is not necessary to check magnesium levels routinely unless signs or symptoms of toxicity develop.

16. **What are the findings of magnesium toxicity?**
The first sign of symptomatic hypermagnesemia is loss of patellar reflexes, followed by respiratory rate <12 breaths/min, increased somnolence, slurred speech, and flushing. Loss of deep tendon reflexes occurs at 7–10 mEq/L. At levels of 10–13 mEq/L, respiratory paralysis may occur. Cardiac arrest is seen at levels of >25 mEq/L. If signs of magnesium toxicity develop, administer 1 g of calcium gluconate IV over 2–5 minutes. In patients with severe magnesium toxicity or cardiac arrest, administer 1.5–3 g of calcium gluconate IV over 2–5 minutes.

17. **What are the maternal complications of preeclampsia?**
Ten to fifteen percent of maternal deaths are associated with preeclampsia. Additional serious complications include eclampsia, intracerebral hemorrhage, hemolysis with elevated liver enzymes and low platelets (HELLP) syndrome, renal failure, and posterior reversible encephalopathy syndrome (PRES). Women with preeclampsia are also at increased risk for future cardiovascular disease.

18. **What complications to the fetus can occur?**
Fetal growth restriction, oligohydramnios, preterm delivery, abruptio placentae, and stillbirth occur with preeclampsia.

19. **Is there a way to prevent preeclampsia?**
New evidence suggests that low-dose aspirin can prevent preeclampsia in women at high risk for developing disease.

20. **What is eclampsia?**
Eclampsia is the new onset of focal or generalized seizure, or unexplained coma in a patient with signs and symptoms of preeclampsia without other causative conditions, such as epilepsy, drug use, or intracranial hemorrhage. Symptoms may occur any time after the second trimester or in the postpartum period. Eclampsia is often preceded by severe persistent frontal or occipital headache, visual disturbances, photophobia, or altered mental status. However, eclampsia may also present without warning signs before, during, or after labor. Eclampsia occurs in 2%–3% of patients with preeclampsia with severe features.

21. **What is the treatment for eclampsia?**
- Immediate stabilization of airway, breathing, and circulation (ABCs) with administration of oxygen, placement of IV lines, and continuous monitoring of mother and fetus. The patient should be rolled into the left lateral decubitus position to prevent compression of vena cava and aspiration.
- Administer magnesium sulfate: 4–6 g IV over 15–20 minutes, followed by a magnesium drip run at 1–2 g/h. Administration of a benzodiazepine, such as diazepam or lorazepam, may be considered if the patient has a second seizure. However, magnesium is superior to benzodiazepines in preventing recurrent seizures. Most eclamptic seizures are self-limited, so efforts should be focused on preventing recurrence rather than arresting the seizure.
- BP should be controlled with hydralazine or labetalol.
- Evaluate for prompt delivery following maternal hemodynamic stabilization. Eclampsia is considered to be an absolute contraindication for expectant management of pregnancy, and definitive treatment is delivery.

22. **What are the most common complications of eclampsia?**
Up to 70% of women with eclampsia develop complications, including abruption, disseminated intravascular coagulation (DIC), pulmonary edema, acute renal failure, HELLP syndrome, and preterm birth. Maternal mortality rates range from 0% to 14%, with the most common cause of death related to CNS complications, such as cerebral edema, hemorrhages, and infarctions, as well as pulmonary edema.

23. **Does a woman have to be pregnant to have preeclampsia or eclampsia?**
No, 20% of cases occur in the postpartum period, when the most common presenting symptoms include headache, shortness of breath, blurry vision, nausea or vomiting, edema, or epigastric pain.

24. **What is HELLP syndrome?**
HELLP is an acronym referring to a syndrome characterized by **h**emolysis, **e**levated **l**iver enzymes, and a **l**ow **p**latelet count. HELLP syndrome probably represents a severe form of preeclampsia. Patients with HELLP syndrome most often present with epigastric or right upper abdominal pain. Additionally, patients may report nausea and vomiting or generalized malaise, which can be mistaken for a viral syndrome or viral hepatitis. Less common signs and symptoms include headache, visual disturbances, jaundice, or ascites.

25. **How is HELLP syndrome diagnosed?**
Laboratory findings are helpful in distinguishing:
- Microangiopathic hemolytic anemia: evidence of schistocytes on blood smear or other findings indicative of hemolysis, such as elevated indirect bilirubin or low serum haptoglobin level (<25 mg/dL)
- Thrombocytopenia <100,000 platelets/µL
- Total bilirubin >1.2 mL/dL
- Serum aspartate transaminase (AST) >70 IU

26. **How is HELLP syndrome treated?**
Prompt delivery is the only curative and effective treatment for HELLP syndrome. Therefore in a patient >34 weeks' gestation or a patient with severe maternal or fetal distress, immediate delivery is the treatment of choice after diagnosis confirmation and initial steps have been taken to stabilize the mother.
A short delay may be considered in patients between 23 and 34 weeks' gestation, but only when both maternal and fetal status are clinically reassuring. In these cases, corticosteroids are administered for fetal lung development, and delivery is recommended within 48 hours of evaluation and stabilization. Antihypertensive medications similar to those used to manage preeclampsia should be administered to treat severe hypertension. IV magnesium to prevent convulsions should also be administered.
Prior to 23 weeks' gestation, prompt delivery is indicated after maternal stabilization.

27. **What are the complications of HELLP syndrome?**
DIC is the most common complication of HELLP syndrome, occurring in 21% of patients. This is followed by abruptio placentae (16%), acute renal failure (8%), and pulmonary edema (6%). While less common, severe postpartum hemorrhage (PPH), rupture of a subcapsular liver hematoma, intracranial hemorrhage, or infarction may also occur. Fifty-five percent of patients require blood transfusions.

28. **What are the maternal and fetal mortality rates associated with HELLP?**
    - The maternal mortality rate is approximately 1.1%, although some studies have reported the mortality rate to be as high as 25%. The leading causes of maternal death are intracerebral hemorrhage, cerebral infarction, and hepatic rupture.
    - Fetal mortality rates range from 7% to 20%, with improved survival after 32 weeks' gestation. The most common causes of neonatal death with HELLP syndrome are abruptio placentae, placental insufficiency, and prematurity.

KEY POINTS: PREECLAMPSIA AND ECLAMPSIA

1. Preeclampsia is characterized by new-onset hypertension with or without proteinuria and signs of end-organ dysfunction that can present any time from 20 weeks' gestation to 4 weeks' postpartum.
2. Hydralazine or labetalol, in addition to magnesium sulfate, are the first-line agents to treat hypertension, and reduce the risk of convulsions associated with preeclampsia and eclampsia.
3. Delivery of the fetus is the definitive and curative treatment for preeclampsia, eclampsia, and HELLP syndrome.

29. **What do I do when a pregnant patient presents to the ED with concern for active labor?**
    When a pregnant patient arrives in the ED with concern for active labor, obtain vital signs and the chief complaint, and then proceed immediately to establish IV access (14 or 16 gauge needle catheter). If transport of a pregnant patient is required, she should be transported in the left lateral recumbent position to reduce pressure on the vena cava. For imminent deliveries, call obstetrics and pediatric specialists to assist in caring for both mother and infant.

30. **What information do I need to care properly for the pregnant patient?**
    Quickly obtain the patient's gestational age or estimated due date, medical history, and delivery history. Ask her if she feels the baby moving, and if she is having contractions, vaginal bleeding, or leakage of fluid from the vagina. Inquire about any problems with the current pregnancy or prior pregnancies, including gestational diabetes, gestation hypertension, or preeclampsia. Clarify whether she is only carrying one baby. In addition to identifying her current medications and allergies, ask about illicit drug use. Women who have had prior vaginal deliveries or precipitous births are known to have more rapid labors.

31. **How are the baby and pregnancy evaluated?**
    Fetal heart tones should be obtained as soon as the mother's condition is stabilized. A normal fetal heart rate is between 120 and 160 beats per minute. For women who do not know their due date, or are unable to communicate, palpate the top of the uterine fundus. Fundal height (the distance in centimeters from the symphysis pubis to the top of the pregnant uterus) should then be measured to estimate gestational age. After 20 weeks' gestation, the fundal height in centimeters will roughly correspond with the week gestation. Gestational age will impact the type of pediatric care required for the fetus, as babies delivered <37 weeks' gestation are considered preterm, with anticipated respiratory problems and difficulty maintaining temperature. If time permits, a bedside ultrasonography can be helpful in determining fetal position, number of fetuses, presence of cardiac activity, and quantity of amniotic fluid.

32. **How do I check cervical dilation?**
    Under sterile conditions, perform a digital pelvic examination. The diameter of the cervical opening in front of the baby's head is estimated in centimeters. The measurements vary from closed to 10 cm. Never perform a digital pelvic examination in any patient who has vaginal bleeding in the late second or third trimester. A digital examination can exacerbate bleeding from placenta previa.

33. **What should be in an emergency delivery pack?**
    Each emergency delivery pack, at minimum, should contain:
    - sterile gloves and gowns
    - sterile towels to dry off the baby and keep the baby warm (newborn beanie hat, if available)
    - four Kelly clamps for the umbilical cord, or vaginal or perineal bleeders
    - Mayo scissors to cut the umbilical cord
    - small bulb syringe to clear the baby's nose and mouth
    - three packs of 4 × 4 sponges
    - container for the placenta and blood-stained sheets/clothing
    - sanitary napkin

34. **How can I determine whether a delivery is imminent?**
    If the fetus is visible and beginning to emerge from the vagina (crowning), delivery is imminent. Additional signs of imminent delivery include rupture of the amniotic sac, or the urge to push or bear down. The patient may be visibly bearing down or pushing with contractions. If digital examination of the patient reveals the cervix is 6 cm or more dilated, delivery may occur before or during transport to labor and delivery. If contractions

are regularly occurring 1–2 minutes apart and lasting 45–60 seconds, this is also a good indication that delivery is imminent.

35. **I have a laboring pregnant patient in the ED, and the baby can be seen distending the mother's perineum. What do I do now?**
The goal is to control the head and support the perineum to prevent sudden expulsion and allow for gradual stretching of the perineum so as to reduce the risk of maternal or fetal trauma. Provide slight downward pressure against the presenting part. As the head emerges, check if the cord is around the neck. On delivery of the head, suction the baby's mouth, then nose. Apply very gentle guidance of the head downward to deliver the anterior shoulder; then provide very gentle traction upward to deliver the posterior shoulder. Once both shoulders have been delivered, the remainder of the delivery will usually occur very quickly. Keep a strong grip because the baby may be slippery. When the feet are out, rotate the baby 180 degrees and again suction the nose and mouth. Double clamp the umbilical cord 7–10 cm from the baby, and cut the cord between the clamps. Dry and stimulate the baby, remembering to keep the baby warm. Place a beanie hat on the newborn to prevent heat loss.

36. **The baby is part way out. Should I pull on the baby to help the delivery?**
In most cases, the mother will push the baby out without help. Pulling on the baby may interrupt the normal delivery process and contribute to brachial plexus injuries. The best way to help with the delivery is to use your hands to help control the head and guide the delivery of the rest of the baby's body to reduce risk of trauma.

37. **What is shoulder dystocia?**
Shoulder dystocia occurs when the baby's anterior or posterior shoulder becomes impacted behind the pubic symphysis or sacral promontory. It is a clinical diagnosis that should be suspected when the fetal head emerges and then retracts against the perineum, commonly referred to as the "turtle sign," and routine, gentle, downward traction of the fetal head fails to deliver the anterior shoulder. The impaction of the fetal shoulders and thorax can lead to inadequate respiration and compression of the umbilical cord. Shoulder dystocia is often associated with post-term pregnancy, fetal macrosomia, diabetes mellitus, maternal obesity, and multiparity.

38. **What maneuvers are available to resolve shoulder dystocia during delivery?**
The McRoberts maneuver is a noninvasive proven-effective maneuver that should be attempted first. To perform, have two assistants flex and abduct each of the mother's thighs back against her abdomen, which increases the inlet diameter. Then, have the patient continue to push. The McRoberts maneuver reduces 40% of shoulder dystocia. Other options include applying suprapubic pressure while continuing downward traction, delivering the posterior arm, or performing the Woods screw maneuver, in which the fetus is rotated 180 degrees by exerting pressure on the anterior clavicular surface of the posterior shoulder. Excessive neck rotation/traction and fundal pressure should be avoided, because this can lead to increased shoulder impaction, brachial plexus injuries, or uterine rupture.

39. **What do I do if the umbilical cord is wrapped around the neck during a delivery?**
If the umbilical cord is noted to be around the baby's neck, attempt to slip the cord over the baby's head, so that it does not tighten as the baby is being born. If the cord is too tight to do so, lift over the head, carefully apply two clamps to the cord and cut the cord between the clamps. Then unwind the cord from around the neck and deliver the baby.

40. **The placenta has not delivered. What should I do now?**
There is no hurry to deliver the placenta unless there is heavy bleeding. If there is heavy bleeding, urge the mother to push out the placenta vaginally. Provide very gentle traction using ring forceps on the distal end of the cord. Wind the cord around the forceps, as the placenta is delivered; never forcibly pull on the cord, as doing so can cause the uterus to involute. If the placenta delivers by itself, gently, but firmly, massage the uterus until it has contracted into a firm ball. As long as the uterus stays firmly contracted, bleeding should be minimal (up to 500 mL is considered within the normal range).

41. **How do I manage a breech presentation?**
Vaginal breech delivery occurs in approximately 4% of deliveries and is associated with increased neonatal morbidity and mortality due to risk of head entrapment. If the fetus is breech, call for immediate obstetric and pediatric assistance. For imminent deliveries, rotate the fetus to deliver the arms and legs. If the head becomes entrapped during delivery, apply suprapubic pressure to push the baby down into the pelvis and insert fingers to draw the fetal chin down to the chest. Unlike cephalic deliveries, the head must be flexed in a breech delivery. Applying suprapubic pressure has been reported to reduce perinatal mortality from 3.2% to 0%.

42. **How do I recognize postpartum hemorrhage (PPH)?**
PPH is defined as (1) cumulative blood loss >1000 mL or (2) bleeding associated with signs or symptoms of hypovolemia within 24 hours of the birth (though this number may vary depending upon source used to define PPH). Bleeding may not be visible externally, or blood in collection may be mixed with amniotic fluid, making the diagnosis problematic. Therefore physicians should be monitoring patients for signs and symptoms associated with blood loss, including pallor, confusion, syncope, lightheadedness, palpitations, and confusion.

43. **What are the most common causes of PPH?**

Uterine atony (lack of effective contractions) is the most common cause, contributing to 75% of cases of PPH. Atony is most common in the setting of uterine overdistention, secondary to multiple gestations or polyhydramnios. Additionally, atony may occur in the setting of infection, prolonged or induced labor, uterine inversion, or retained placenta. Lacerations caused by trauma or underlying coagulation defects, such as von Willebrand disease, can also contribute to PPH.

44. **How is PPH managed?**

Establish large-bore IV access and place the patient on oxygen. Begin fluid resuscitation with crystalloid. If the patient has persistent hypotension despite 2–3 L of crystalloid, administer blood products, beginning with 2 units of packed red blood cells. Inspect the vagina and cervix for obvious lacerations to repair. While fluids are infusing, if uterine atony is suspected, perform uterine massage by placing one hand on the vagina, pushing against the body of the uterus, while the other hand compresses the uterus through the abdominal wall. Evacuate any retained products of conception. If uterine atony continues despite massage, administer uterotonic drugs, beginning with oxytocin 10–40 MU/min. Adjust the infusion rate to maintain uterine contraction. Misoprostol (400 µg sublingually) may be given if other uterotonic medications are unavailable. Also consider tranexamic acid 1 g IV

KEY POINTS: CHILDBIRTH IN THE ED

1. If a precipitous delivery does begin in the ED, remember to control the head and support the perineum to prevent sudden expulsion. Provide gentle downward traction on the head to first deliver the anterior shoulder, followed by gentle traction upward to deliver the posterior shoulder.
2. Shoulder dystocia should be suspected immediately if the "turtle sign" is present. The McRoberts maneuver should be performed first.
3. If PPH is suspected due to uterine atony, perform immediate uterine massage and administer uterotonic drugs to initiate uterine contraction.

BIBLIOGRAPHY

American College of Obstetricians and Gynecologists Committee on Obstetric Practice. Practice Bulletin No. 202: Gestational hypertension and preeclampsia. *Obstet Gynecol.* 2019;133:e1–e25.

American College of Obstetricians and Gynecologists Committee on Obstetric Practice. Committee Opinion No. 767: Emergent therapy for acute-onset, severe hypertension during pregnancy and the postpartum period. *Obstet Gynecol.* 2019;133(2):409–412.

Bartsch E, Medcalf KE, Park AL, et al. Clinical risk factors for pre-eclampsia determined in early pregnancy: systematic review and meta-analysis of large cohort studies. *BMJ.* 2016;353:i1753.

Bernstein PS, Martin JN Jr, Barton JR, et al. National partnership for maternal safety: consensus bundle on severe hypertension during pregnancy and the postpartum period. *Obstet Gynecol.* 2017;130:347–357.

Committee on Practice Bulletins – Obstetrics. Practice Bulletin No. 183: Postpartum hemorrhage. *Obstet Gynecol.* 2017;130:e168–e186.

Committee on Practice Bulletins – Obstetrics. Practice Bulletin No. 178: Shoulder dystocia. *Obstet Gynecol.* 2017;129:e123–e133. Reaffirmed 2019.

Marshall AL, Durani U, Bartley A, et al. The impact of postpartum hemorrhage on hospital length of stay and inpatient mortality: a national inpatient sample-based analysis. *Am J Obstet Gynecol.* 2017;217:344.e1–344.e6.

Nyfløt LT, Sandven I, Oldereid NB, et al. Assisted reproductive technology and severe postpartum haemorrhage: a case-control study. *BJOG.* 2017;124:1198–1205.

MULTIPLE TRAUMA

Lee Shockley, MD, MBA and Eric Legome, MD

1. **What is the leading cause of death in the United States for people age 1–45 years?**
   Trauma. It is also a worldwide problem, with motor vehicle crashes killing 1.2 million people annually worldwide.

2. **What is multiple trauma?**
   Multiple trauma or polytrauma means injuries to several organ systems or body parts. The risk of mortality and morbidity can be greater than would be expected from the individual injuries.

3. **How do paramedics decide who to take to a trauma center?**
   Paramedics use physiologic and anatomic criteria, mechanism of injury, and special circumstances to decide which patients to take to a facility providing the highest level of care in the defined trauma system.
   Physiologic criteria
   - Glasgow Coma Scale (GCS) score ≤13, or
   - Systolic blood pressure (SBP) of <90 mmHg, or
   - Respiratory rate of <10 or >29 breaths per minute (<20 in <1 year of age), or need for ventilatory support
   Anatomic criteria
   - Penetrating injuries to head, neck, torso, and extremities proximal to elbow or knee
   - Chest wall instability or deformity (e.g., flail chest)
   - Two or more proximal long-bone fractures
   - Rushed, degloved, mangled, or pulseless extremity
   - Amputation proximal to wrist or ankle
   - Pelvic fractures
   - Open or depressed skull fractures
   - Paralysis
   Mechanism of injury criteria
   - Motorcycle crash >20 mph
   - Automobile versus pedestrian/bicyclist thrown, run over, or high speed >20 mph
   - Falls
     - Adults: >20 feet (one story = 10 feet)
     - Children: >10 feet or two to three times the height of the child
   - High-risk auto crashes
     - Intrusion, including roof: >12 inches occupant site; >18 inches any site
     - Ejection (partial or complete) from automobile
     - Death in same passenger compartment
     - Vehicle telemetry data consistent with a high risk for injury
   Special circumstances
   - Older adults (risk for injury/death increases after age 55 years)
     - SBP <110 mmHg might represent shock after age 65 years
     - Low-impact mechanisms (e.g., ground-level falls) might result in severe injury
   - Children: should be triaged preferentially to pediatric-capable trauma centers
   - Anticoagulants and bleeding disorders: patients with head injury are at high risk for rapid deterioration
   - Pregnancy >20 weeks
   - Burns
     - Without other trauma mechanism: triage to burn facility
     - With trauma mechanism: triage to trauma center

4. **Which criteria are most sensitive to capture severely injured patients?**
   The *overall* sensitivity and specificity of the field triage criteria for identifying major trauma patients is 86% and 69%, respectively. Physiologic criteria such as vital sign abnormalities or altered mental status, which account for the patient's response to serious injury, are the best predictors of the need for operative intervention or intensive care, notwithstanding obvious anatomic findings such as gunshot wounds to the thorax or head. Mechanism of injury in the triage may increase sensitivity (more seriously injured patients are captured) at the expense of specificity (more uninjured or minor injured patients are sent to trauma centers than needed).

5. **How is the multiply injured trauma patient evaluated?**

Steps in management include primary survey, resuscitation, and secondary survey. The primary survey focuses on identifying causes of early trauma death, which include airway obstruction, respiratory failure, shock from hemorrhage, and brain injuries.

Primary Survey (**ABCDE** examination or ABCs of trauma):

A: Airway with cervical spine protection

B: Breathing and ventilation

C: Circulation with hemorrhage control

D: Disability (assessing neurologic status)

E: Exposure and environmental control

Military medics frequently use a **CABC** approach to trauma, where the first **C** stands for "catastrophic hemorrhage," which may require immediate application of a tourniquet prior to securing the airway. An expansion on **CABC** is the **MARCH** mnemonic.

M: Massive hemorrhage

A: Airway

R: Respiratory

C: Circulation

H: Head injury/Hypothermia

Most important is to have a standard consistent approach in the management of trauma. In the primary survey, when a life-threatening problem is identified, it is addressed immediately. For example, a patient with an obstructed airway needs the airway secured before breathing is assessed. Early resuscitation efforts include vascular access, volume resuscitation, transfusion, and monitoring; initial diagnostics are started once the primary survey is completed. The secondary survey is performed next, obtaining a thorough but focused history and head-to-toe physical examination with the purpose of identifying all injuries and comorbidities. The greatest risk of missing or underappreciating an injury is to do a hurried, incomplete, or inadequate secondary survey.

6. **What are the key elements of a well-functioning trauma team?**

While trauma teams vary in size and composition, a clearly defined team leadership is critical. At a minimum, there will be one physician who is the leader. On bigger teams, there may be shared leadership occurring sequentially, not simultaneously. For example, a senior emergency medicine resident may be the leader (under supervision); however, if they are needed to assist with a procedure, they may hand off the role to a surgical resident while they are occupied, or vice versa. The leader focuses the efforts of the team on prioritization of critical tasks and diagnostics, provides strategic direction in decision making, and makes sure there is available support to carry out necessary tasks. Thought processes and plans must be verbalized, and orders clearly communicated with feedback, to guarantee compliance. While it is preferred for the leader to solely direct the resuscitation, in smaller centers, the leader may need to provide direct patient care.

7. **How should the team prepare for arrival of a trauma patient?**

Preparation is based on expected type of patient and their immediate needs, if known. Regardless, each individual team member's role and responsibilities should be delineated and agreed upon. There should be verbal confirmation of plans for major interventions, including diagnostic and therapeutic. Other things to prepare or have readily available include:

1. Drugs for analgesia, sedation, and rapid sequence intubation
2. Blood products
3. Intubation equipment and ventilator
4. Procedure trays
5. Monitoring equipment
6. Imaging equipment (portable x-ray and ultrasound)

8. **What is a massive transfusion?**

A massive transfusion is defined as the transfusion of 10 units of red cells in 24 hours or more than three units over an hour in a patient with ongoing blood loss. A massive transfusion protocol (MTP) is the delivery of a prespecified ratio of blood and blood products (platelets and fresh frozen plasma). Blood that is universally compatible is type O (Rh− should be reserved for childbearing-aged females; otherwise, use Rh+). Blood should be transfused in a 1:1:1 ratio (one unit of blood, one unit of platelets, and one unit of fresh frozen plasma, infused at the same time if possible). In practice, a cooler for trauma may contain six units PRBCs, four to six units of thawed plasma, and six units of pooled platelets or one apheresis unit. Tranexamic acid (TXA) is an antifibrinolytic agent often transfused with MTP, as it may decrease mortality when given within 3 hours of injury. MTP is activated based on obvious severe hemorrhage, or a combination of factors that predict the need for significant blood transfusion. While clinical judgment may be used, objective scoring systems may be best to activate the protocol. The ABC (assessment of blood consumption) scale is a scoring system that gives points for penetrating mechanism, hypotension, tachycardia, and a positive focused assessment with sonography for trauma (FAST). Scoring ≥2 predicts increasing likelihood to require the protocol. Using the shock index (heart rate [HR]/SBP) ≥1 is also common.

9. **What is damage control resuscitation?**
Damage control resuscitation (DCR) is used in the critical and actively bleeding trauma patients. Components include:
- avoidance of hypothermia
- early transfusion (MTP with ratios approaching 1:1 or 1:2)
- permissive hypotension (to prevent clot disruption)
- surgical control of bleeding *with*
- delayed surgery for definitive treatment

10. **What if an unstable pelvic fracture is identified on secondary examination?**
Mortality from pelvic fractures ranges from 5% to 30%, and is as high as 42% in patients with closed pelvic fractures and hypotension. These fractures can cause catastrophic retroperitoneal bleeding. Early stabilization with a tightly tied sheet encircling the pelvis, commercial pelvic binder, or mechanical device may help control hemorrhage. This is more effective in the "open-book" pelvic fracture caused by an anterior-posterior compression. Consult surgery early to determine need for pelvic packing in the operating room, or interventional radiology for embolization. Have a low threshold to activate MTP.

11. **What are the indications for intubation?**
Absolute indications
- GCS <8
- Evidence of immediate inability to protect the airway:
  - Massive facial trauma
  - Injury to the airway itself (i.e., inhalation burns)
  - Hematoma causing airway distortion
  - Uncontrolled oral or posterior nasal hemorrhage after trauma
- Inability to maintain oxygenation or ventilation

Relative indications
- Patient safety and facilitation of workup
- High potential to deteriorate, requiring intubation in a less controlled setting

12. **How can I predict the difficult intubation?**
It is hard to predict a difficult airway. A small percentage of intubations are unsuccessful, despite several attempts, requiring a surgical airway. Factors contributing to the difficulty of the trauma airway include:
- full stomachs
- presence of blood, vomitus, or secretions in the airway
- anatomic distortions from the injury
- hypovolemia and hypotension

The accuracy of prediction rules to suggest who will be difficult is less than optimal in the trauma population. Additionally, due to the emergent nature and ability of the patient to cooperate, they often cannot be fully instituted. However, if applied they may suggest when difficulty may be encountered. Common systems include the modified Mallampati classification and the **LEMON**. The modified Mallampati provides an estimate of intubation space by evaluating the relationship between the tongue and pharyngeal size. The **LEMON** (**L**ook–**E**valuate–**M**allampati–**O**bstruction–**N**eck mobility) score offers more information, although it is neither fully sensitive nor specific.

13. **How can the risk of a difficult intubation be mitigated?**
Preparation is critical. Bag valve mask (BVM), endotracheal (ET) tubes, and difficult airway equipment should be readily available. Backup plans may include a bougie, laryngeal mask airway (LMA), or surgical airway. All participants must be aware of the plan in case it must be rapidly instituted. The most experienced intubator should intubate the most complex or obviously challenging airways, as the likelihood of success decreases on subsequent attempts. The preferred use of direct laryngoscopy (DL) versus video laryngoscopy (VL) remains unclear. While there are very strong proponents for both, especially VL, the absolute benefits on outcomes and success remains unproven.

14. **Which patients are at risk for decompensation during intubation?**
Cardiovascular collapse may occur during intubation in patients that are elderly, hypotensive, or hemorrhaging. In these high-risk patients, consider lower dose induction agents, ketamine instead of opioids or etomidate, blood prior to intubation (when safe), and push-dose peri-intubation pressors.

15. **What are the benefits and risks of "pan-scanning" all trauma patients?**
One common strategy in the multiple trauma patient is the use of the head-to-pelvis scan (i.e., "pan scan"). Its use is controversial due to cost, potential for unnecessary imaging, time, and radiation exposure. The other downside may be the discovery of unimportant incidental findings that may lead to cost-intensive follow-ups. Pan scan compared with standard workup has been shown to decrease time to diagnosis and treatment (about 10 minutes), without an impact on mortality.

16. **What is the role of ultrasound in the trauma resuscitation room?**
Ultrasound is a useful adjunct in the initial resuscitation of the trauma patient. FAST and an extended, or E-FAST, evaluation are used in trauma. The FAST involves obtaining views of the right upper quadrant, left upper quadrant, suprapubic region, and cardiac subxyphoid region. The abdominal views assess for free fluid and the cardiac view assesses for evidence of a pericardial effusion, volume depletion, and overall function. The E-FAST includes a bilateral anterior/lateral evaluation of both lungs, looking for hemothorax, pneumothorax, or effusions. By looking for several well-described findings, for example, sliding lung sign and comet tail artifacts, it can be rapidly performed and has significantly improved sensitivity with similar specificity to the chest radiograph for pathologic findings. Ultrasound can also be used for a variety of other interventions and diagnostics, including ultrasound-guided vascular access, foreign body localization, ET tube confirmation, evidence of retinal detachment, and estimate of cerebral pressure by optic nerve sheath diameter.

17. **How can ultrasound findings guide management?**
Blunt trauma
- Positive free fluid and unstable → operating room
- Positive free fluid and stable → CT scan
- Negative free fluid and unstable → consider other causes of hypotension (e.g., other bleeding sites and spinal shock), diagnostic peritoneal lavage, or early repeat ultrasound
- Negative free fluid and stable → computed tomography (CT) if suspicion for intra-abdominal injury, or observation and repeat ultrasound in lower-risk patients

Penetrating trauma
- Free fluid has a highly positive predictive value for a therapeutic laparotomy
- Negative ultrasound is unable to rule out a clinically significant injury
- Pericardial effusion with tamponade on ultrasound mandates intervention

18. **How should vascular access be obtained in a multiple trauma patient?**
Vascular access is a critical intervention. First-line treatment: a large-bore (14- or 16-gauge) peripheral intravenous (IV) catheter is placed in the antecubital fossa. With obvious fractures or deformity, place the IV above the injury or elsewhere. If IV access is not rapidly obtained, move to another option. Second-line options are a central venous line (using a single, large-bore lumen) placed in the femoral, internal jugular, or subclavian vein, or an interosseous needle. Saphenous venous cut-down is another option.

19. **How do I change my approach if my trauma patient is pregnant?**
Some factors to consider in pregnancy include:
- During the last half of pregnancy, the gravid uterus can compress the inferior vena cava in the supine position, leading to hypotension. This "supine hypotension syndrome" is prevented and treated by placing the patient in the left lateral decubitus position or manually displacing the uterus to the left.
- Placental abruption is the most common cause of fetal loss. Early and continuous cardiotocographic monitoring is indicated for pregnant women who are more than 20 weeks, even if asymptomatic.
- Administer Rhogam for Rh-negative pregnant women with trauma.
- Uncrossmatched transfusion should be Type O Rh− until blood type is known.

20. **How do I change my approach if my trauma patient is obese?**
Obesity is a risk factor for increased mortality in trauma. The odds ratio risk of 30-day mortality after a motor vehicle collision in patients between 100 and 119 kg is 2.6, and rises to 4.5 in those ≥120 kg.
Considerations in the obese trauma patient include:
Airway
- Decreased desaturation time and safe apnea period
  - Provide oxygen by nasal cannula during apneic phase to improve oxygenation
- Poor visibility of the airway
  - Intubate in the reverse Trendelenburg and ramped up position

Breathing
- Hypoventilation due to chest wall mass (obesity hypoventilation syndrome)
- Low chest wall compliance – may require PEEP after intubation and higher airway pressures, increasing risk for barotrauma

Injury patterns
- Thoracic, pelvic, extremity injuries → increased
- Abdominal injuries → decreased (cushioning effect)

Procedures
- Thick chest walls make needle decompression ineffective, and conventional chest tubes may be too short

Diagnostic studies
- Traditional CT scanners → gantry diameter of 70 cm and table capacity of 450 pounds; newer generation scanners → gantry diameter of 90 cm and table capacity of 680 pounds; 18 cm of a CT's gantry may be taken up by the table itself

- Traditional magnetic resonance imaging (MRI) → bore diameter of 60 cm and table capacity of 350 pounds; newer generation MRIs → bore diameter of 70 cm and table capacity of 550 pounds

Drugs
- Dosages based on lean body weight or real body weight, depending on drug pharmacokinetics
- Use ideal body weight for narcotics, etomidate, and succinylcholine
- Use real body weight for dosing heparin
- Use ideal body weight + 30%–40% for dosing lipophilic drugs (i.e., antibiotics)
- Lean body weight (in kg) =
  - Men: patient's height (in cm) − 100
  - Women: patient's height (in cm) − 105

21. How do I change my approach for an elderly trauma patient?

Aging is a risk factor for increased mortality and morbidity after trauma. For minor trauma, age greater than 60 years increases morbidity threefold and mortality fivefold. For major trauma, age greater than 60 years doubles morbidity and increases mortality fourfold. Therefore many experts recommend that patients older than 60 years of age should receive the highest level of trauma activation for any significant traumatic injury.

Considerations in the elderly include:

Airway
- Nasal mucosa may be friable, leading to bleeding
- Edentulous patients may have a poor mask seal
- Cervical spine may lack mobility
- Rapid sequence intubation drug dosages may need adjusting:
  - Etomidate: 0.1–0.2 mg/kg, instead of 0.3 mg/kg
  - Versed (midazolam) and fentanyl: decrease by 20%–40%
  - Succinylcholine → no adjustment

Injury
- Osteoporosis may increase risk of rib fractures, sternal fractures, and pulmonary contusions.
- Rib fractures → incidence as high as 60% in the elderly. Each additional rib fracture increases mortality rate by 19% and the risk of pneumonia by 27%.
- The elderly may have blunted responses to hypoxia, hypercarbia, and acidosis. More frequent monitoring in an intensive care setting, use of frequent blood gas or CO_2 monitoring and early intubation may be prudent.

Medications
- Many medications require dosage reduction based on glomerular filtration rate (GFR).
- Opioid analgesics should be carefully titrated, starting with low dosage.

22. What about the pediatric trauma patient?

Motor vehicle collisions (occupant, pedestrian, or cyclist) are the most common cause of traumatic death in children. Due to their lighter body mass, the same amount of energy from an impact or fall results in a greater force applied per body area in children. Combined with their lesser body fat, lesser connective tissue, and closer proximity of multiple organs, children have a higher rate of multiple organ injuries (see Chapter 92).

23. What is the approach to a multiple trauma patient in a rural hospital with limited resources?

The approach includes:
1. Recognizing the severely injured patient who benefits from a higher level of service.
2. Arranging a safe and expeditious transfer to a trauma center.
3. Providing life-saving stabilization while arranging the transfer.
4. Performing as leader of the trauma team and active participant in direct patient care.
5. Making rational decisions about diagnostic testing.

Prearranged transfer agreements and streamlined communication channels help expedite the transfer of trauma patients. A single transfer call with direct clinician-to-clinician communication is very important. The call serves to transfer information and discuss the plan. While a medical helicopter may be the most efficient in some circumstances, it may not be the best choice for short transports (ground ambulance may be faster), long transports (fixed-wing aircraft from airport to airport may be faster), or when bad weather is an issue. Obese patients may exceed the load limits of some helicopters.

24. What's new in trauma care since the last edition of this book?

New changes in trauma care include:
- DCR is focused on stopping hemorrhage, reversing shock, and preventing coagulopathy. The approach includes a MTP, tranexamic acid, limiting crystalloid use, permissive hypotension, early operative intervention focusing only on controlling bleeding and contamination, and continued intensive care unit (ICU) resuscitation to correct metabolic derangements, hypothermia, and coagulopathy.
- The use of thromboelastography (TEG) and rotational thromboelastography (ROTEM) allows measurement of viscoelastic changes in blood, adding information about clot strength and fibrinolysis to direct replacement of clotting factors. Replacement is started with the standard MTP ratio (1:1:1), and subsequently guided by the assays.

- CT angiography has supplanted angiography in the evaluation of peripheral and craniocervical vascular injuries. Formal catheter-directed angiography still has a diagnostic role in the patient with high suspicion who could potentially be treated with angioembolization.
- Resuscitative endovascular balloon occlusion of the aorta (REBOA) can be applied to help control bleeding from noncompressible sites. Although the indications are still being defined, it appears to be most beneficial in the hypotensive patient with a pulse who has either abdominal or pelvic hemorrhage. Using the Seldinger technique, a large catheter sheath is inserted in the common femoral artery. A balloon catheter is threaded through the sheath and, using landmarks, ultrasound, or fluoroscopy, placed into position. The position or zone is dependent on the likely source of bleeding (e.g., zone 1 in the infrarenal aorta to control pelvic and lower extremity bleeding). The balloon is inflated and secured, and the team proceeds with the next immediate steps to control hemorrhage.

KEY POINTS: MULTIPLE TRAUMA

1. Trauma care is a team sport involving prehospital providers and emergency physicians and surgical staff.
2. All trauma patients should be completely undressed and examined, front and back.
3. All trauma victims must be assessed for occult bleeding in the cranial vault, chest, and abdomen.
4. When indicated by mechanism of injury, symptoms, or signs, spinal precautions must be maintained until the spine is cleared.

BIBLIOGRAPHY

Cannon JW, Khan MA, Raja AS, et al. Damage control resuscitation in patients with severe traumatic hemorrhage: a practice management guideline from the Eastern Association for the Surgery of Trauma. *J Trauma Acute Care Surg.* 2017;82(3):605–617.

Centers for Disease Control and Prevention. Guidelines for field triage of injured patients recommendations of the National Expert Panel on Field Triage, 2011. *MMWR Recomm Rep.* 2012;61:1–2.

Morrison JJ, Galgon RE, Jansen JO, et al. Systematic review of the use of resuscitative endovascular balloon occlusion of the aorta in the management of hemorrhagic shock. *J Trauma Acute Care Surg.* 2016;80(2):324–334.

Newgard CD, Zive D, Holmes JF, et al. A multisite assessment of the American College of Surgeons Committee on Trauma field triage decision scheme for identifying seriously injured children and adults. *J Am Coll Surg.* 2011;213(6):709–721.

Saul T, Rose G, Tansek R, et al. Utilizing ultrasound. In: Legome E, Shockley LW, eds. *Trauma in Emergency Trauma Care: Current Topics and Controversies.* Vol. 3. Norcross, GA: EB Medicine; 2018.

Sierink JC, Treskes K, Edwards MJ, et al. and REACT-2 study group. Immediate total-body CT scanning versus conventional imaging and selective CT scanning in patients with severe trauma (REACT-2): a randomised controlled trial. *Lancet.* 2016;388(10045):673–683.

CHAPTER 83

MAXILLOFACIAL TRAUMA

Daniel J. Berman, MD and Carlo L. Rosen, MD

1. What are the facial bones?
The facial bones are the frontal, temporal, nasal, ethmoid, lacrimal, palatine, sphenoid bones, vomer, zygoma, maxilla, and mandible.

2. What is the initial approach to a patient with maxillofacial trauma?
The initial management of patients with facial trauma should follow the ABCs (airway, breathing, and circulation) of trauma resuscitation. The airway is the primary concern and can be challenging to manage in these patients. Significant facial trauma may cause distortion of the airway as a result of bleeding, edema, loose teeth, or fractures. In patients with mandibular fractures, the tongue loses its support and can occlude the airway.

3. How should the airway be managed in patients with maxillofacial trauma?
Early endotracheal intubation should be considered in patients with significant midface or mandibular trauma, especially if they exhibit any signs of airway distress. Standard methods of intubation, such as rapid-sequence intubation using direct or video laryngoscopy, should be attempted first. However, airway distortion resulting from facial trauma may lead to a difficult airway situation that necessitates a cricothyrotomy. All patients with facial and head trauma should be assumed to have a cervical spine injury. In-line cervical spine stabilization should be used during intubation. In patients with facial fractures, up to 24% will have an associated cervical spine fracture. The risk increases with severity and number of facial fractures.

4. Which procedure is contraindicated in patients with maxillofacial trauma?
Nasogastric tube placement should not be performed because of the risk of inadvertent intracranial placement through a fracture in the cribriform plate. The small size and flexibility of the nasogastric tube allow it to be misdirected through such a fracture into the brain. However, there is literature to support that inadvertent nasotracheal tube placement into the brain through the cribriform plate is extremely low. This is likely due to the nasotracheal tube being larger and more rigid than the nasogastric tube.

5. What is a blow-out fracture, and what is the entrapment syndrome?
A blow-out fracture is a pure internal fracture of the orbit that results from a direct blow. The sudden increase in intraorbital pressure causes rupture of either the floor of the orbit or the median orbital wall. This can cause entrapment of the inferior rectus muscle through the bony defect. This entrapment syndrome can cause diplopia and paralysis of upward gaze. A physical examination should include assessing for infraorbital nerve injury by testing sensation of the cheek, upper gums, upper lip, and teeth. Enophthalmos is posterior displacement of the globe into the orbit, causing a sunken eye appearance. Exophthalmos may be caused by proptosis from retrobulbar hematoma. Patients may also have tenderness or palpable step-offs at the infraorbital rim or subcutaneous emphysema secondary to a fracture into the maxillary sinus. Ophthalmologic evaluation should be considered for associated ocular trauma (e.g., globe rupture, hyphema, retinal tear or detachment), even despite an initially normal visual acuity and funduscopic examination.

6. What is ocular compartment syndrome and what is the treatment?
If a patient sustains trauma to the orbit, resulting in a retrobulbar hematoma, the buildup of pressure behind the globe can lead to ischemia of the optic nerve and retina, and permanent blindness in as little as 90 minutes after injury. It can present as proptosis, impaired extraocular movement, decreased vision, and increased intraocular pressure; retrobulbar hematoma can be confirmed by a computed tomography (CT) scan. In order to prevent optic nerve or retinal ischemia, a lateral canthotomy is performed by incising the lateral canthal ligaments of the orbit to relieve intraocular pressure, in conjunction with emergent ophthalmology consultation.

7. What are Le Fort fractures?
The Le Fort classification is used to describe maxillary fractures (Fig. 83.1). Midface fractures can often be diagnosed by grasping the upper alveolar ridge and noting which part of the midface moves.

It is rare for these fracture types to occur in isolation; they usually occur in combination (one type on one side of the face and another on the other side).
- *Le Fort I.* A transverse fracture just above the teeth at the level of the nasal fossa that allows movement of the alveolar ridge and hard palate. Patients usually report malocclusion.
- *Le Fort II.* A pyramidal fracture with its apex just above the nasal bridge and extending laterally and interiorly through the infraorbital rims that allows movement of the maxilla, nose, and infraorbital rims.
- *Le Fort III.* Complete craniofacial disruption that involves fractures of the zygoma, infraorbital rims, and maxilla. This is a severe injury and can be associated with a cerebrospinal fluid (CSF) leak.

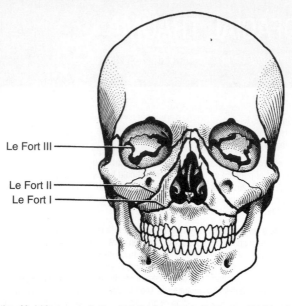

Le Fort III

Le Fort II
Le Fort I

Fig. 83.1 Le Fort classification of facial fractures. Le Fort I: palatofacial disjunction. Le Fort II: pyramidal disjunction. Le Fort III: craniofacial disjunction. (From Cantrill SV. Face. In: Marx JA, Hockberger RS, Walls RM, et al., eds. *Rosen's Emergency Medicine: Concepts and Clinical Practice.* 5th ed. St. Louis: Mosby; 2002:325.

8. **Which patients would benefit from screening for blunt cerebrovascular injury?**
   Blunt cerebrovascular injury (BCVI) to the carotid or vertebral artery is found in nearly 0.5% of all blunt cranio-maxillary facial trauma patients and may cause significant morbidity if left untreated. These injuries may initially be silent, without focal neurologic deficits noted. Computed tomography angiography (CTA) should be performed in patients suspected of having a BCVI based on signs or symptoms, or focal neurologic deficits. High-risk patients that should be screened include those with a Le Fort II or III fracture, mandibular fractures, certain cervical spine fracture patterns (subluxation, fractures extending into the transverse foramen, vertebral body fractures of C1, C2, or C3), basilar skull fracture with carotid canal involvement, traumatic brain injury with Glasgow Coma Scale (GCS) scores <6, near-hangings with anoxic brain injury, or seatbelt sign of the neck.

9. **Does an isolated nasal fracture require imaging?**
   Almost never. Nasal fractures typically are a clinical diagnosis without the need for routine imaging. Physical examination may reveal swelling, angulation, bony crepitus, deformity, pain on palpation, epistaxis, and periorbital ecchymosis. As long as the pain is isolated to the nares, the patient can breathe from either nostril, there is no septal deviation, and you do not have any suspicion for other craniofacial injuries, imaging is not needed.

10. **What is a septal hematoma, and why is it important?**
    All patients with nasal trauma and suspicion of a nasal fracture require inspection of the nasal septum for a septal hematoma. This is a collection of blood between the mucoperichondrium and the cartilage of the septum. It appears as a grapelike swelling over the nasal septum. If left undrained, it may result in septal abscess, necrosis of the nasal cartilage, and permanent saddle nose deformity. If a septal hematoma is identified, incision and drainage, with suction and irrigation, is indicated in the emergency department (ED). This is followed by nasal packing (similar to epistaxis), antistaphylococcal antibiotics (prophylaxis for toxic shock syndrome), and urgent referral to otolaryngology.

11. **When should a consultation be obtained for a nasal fracture?**
    Most nasal fractures do not require immediate reduction unless there is significant deformity and malalignment. After anesthetizing the nose with lidocaine or tetracaine-soaked gauze or pledgets, early closed reduction of an angulated fracture can be performed by exerting firm, quick pressure toward the midline with both thumbs. However, reduction is associated with significant pain, and systemic analgesia should be considered. Patients should be referred to an otolaryngologist or a maxillofacial or plastic surgeon for follow-up care in 4–7 days. Immediate consultation is indicated for nasal fractures with associated facial fractures, CSF rhinorrhea, nasolacrimal duct injury, and sustained epistaxis.

12. **How is a frontal sinus fracture diagnosed?**
Frontal sinus fracture should be suspected in any patient with a severe blow to the forehead. There is often an associated brain injury (e.g., frontal lobe contusions and dural tears). The clinical signs include supraorbital nerve anesthesia, anosmia, CSF rhinorrhea, subconjunctival hemorrhage, crepitus, and tenderness to palpation. The preferred diagnostic modality is CT to determine whether there is involvement of the anterior or posterior walls of the sinus or intracranial hemorrhage.

13. **How are frontal sinus fractures treated?**
After surgical consultation, patients with nondisplaced anterior wall fractures may be discharged on prophylactic antibiotics, with instructions to avoid Valsalva maneuvers and to follow up in 1 week with the surgical consultant to ensure that a mucocele hasn't formed. Patients with displaced anterior wall and sinus floor fractures require surgical consultation, admission, and antibiotic therapy. Patients with posterior wall fractures require antibiotics and immediate neurosurgical consultation.

14. **What are zygoma and zygomaticomaxillary complex fractures?**
The zygoma is one of the most commonly fractured facial bones. Zygoma fractures are classified into three basic types:
1. *Arch.* The bone may be nondisplaced or displaced typically medially. Pain and trismus are caused by bony arch fragments abutting the coronoid process of the mandible. Because the masseter muscle originates on the zygoma, any movement causes further arch disruption. Surgical intervention depends on displacement and potential aesthetic deformities. These are typically diagnosed with a CT scan to evaluate for other midface trauma.
2. *Tetrapod.* A tetrapod fracture is much more serious and similar to a blowout fracture. It is composed of frontal bone at the frontozygomatic attachment, maxilla at the zygomaticomaxillary attachment, temporal bone at the zygomaticotemporal attachment, and the sphenoid at the zygomaticosphenoid attachment. A maxillofacial CT scan is typically indicated to better define the extent of these fractures. These usually necessitate surgical consultation by either plastic or maxillofacial surgery, and probably require admission. Patients may present with malar flattening (flatness of the cheek). Given its close proximity to the infraorbital wall there is high incidence of intraocular injury, as well as infraorbital nerve injury, and inferior rectus muscle entrapment causing diplopia on upward gaze. Bedside tests include visual acuity, extraocular movements, and evaluating for paresthesias, specifically over the V2 segment.
3. *Body.* Fracture of the body of the zygoma, which involves the clinical signs and symptoms of the tripod fracture, results from severe force and leads to exaggerated malar depression.

15. **What are the typical findings of a mandible fracture?**
Patients with mandible fractures have mandibular tenderness and deformity, sublingual hematoma, and malocclusion on physical examination. The jaw appears asymmetric, with deviation toward the side of the fracture. There may also be lacerations under the chin and intraoral, as well as potential for alveolar nerve paresthesias.

16. **What is the tongue blade test?**
The tongue blade test is performed by asking the patient to bite down strongly on a tongue depressor and keep the tongue depressor clenched between the teeth. The tongue blade should be twisted by the examiner. If there is no fracture of the mandible, the examiner should be able to break the blade. In the presence of a mandible fracture, the patient opens their mouth because of pain from the fracture, and the tongue blade remains intact. This has a sensitivity of approximately 95%.

17. **What are the most commonly fractured areas of the mandible?**
The most commonly fractured areas are the body (36%), angle of the mandible (31%), and the condyle (18%). The symphyses, ramus, and coronoid process make up the rest of the fractures.

18. **What is the mechanism for a temporomandibular joint dislocation, and how is it treated?**
Anterior temporomandibular joint (TMJ) dislocation can result from blunt trauma to the mandible or from exaggerated opening or closing of the jaw, such as after a seizure or with yawning. Patients with a TMJ dislocation have jaw deviation away from the side of the dislocation if it is a unilateral dislocation. Bilateral TMJ dislocations are more common and typically present with the mandible pushed forward (underbite). There are multiple options for reduction, some of which may require procedural sedation for analgesia and anxiolysis:
- The classic approach is to use the emergency physician's gauze-wrapped thumbs to place pressure on the posterior molars while standing above and behind the patient or in front of the seated patient. The mandible is then pushed downward and posterior.
- The syringe method (Fig. 83.2) is performed by placing a 5 or 10 cc syringe within the mouth cavity between the upper and lower teeth or gums on the affected side. Site selection is done to maximize the engagement of both the upper and lower molars. The patient is instructed to gently bite down on the syringe and roll it forward and backward between the teeth. This is then attempted on the other side in the same manner.
- In the extraoral reduction technique the mandible is pulled forward on one side while using the ipsilateral zygoma as a fulcrum, thus further dislocating that side anteriorly to allow for contralateral TMJ reduction. On the contralateral side, the practitioner is placing pressure on the coronoid process to push the coronoid and TMJ back. This process is then reversed for the other side.

Superior and posterior dislocations of the TMJ are extremely rare. They usually result from high-energy trauma and are associated with severe facial traumas.

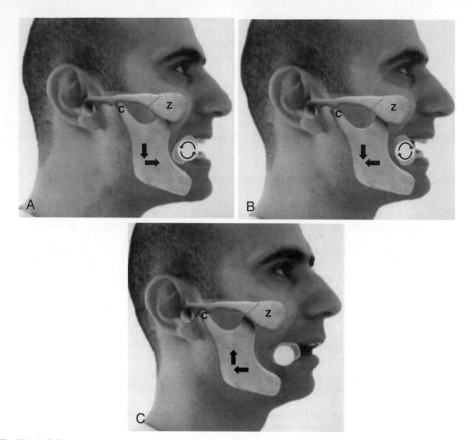

Fig. 83.2 (A–C) The syringe technique. (Gorchynski J, Karabidian E, Sanchez M. The "syringe" technique: a hands-free approach for the reduction of acute nontraumatic temporomandibular dislocations in the emergency department. *J Emerg Med.* 2014;47(6):676–681; Figure 1.)

19. What is the best imaging modality in the evaluation of maxillofacial trauma?

In patients with physical findings that are highly suggestive of facial fractures (tenderness, step-offs, crepitus, or evidence of entrapment), a CT scan is the preferred imaging modality of choice over plain films. While noncontrast head CT can be used to evaluate for maxillofacial trauma, it is still recommended to consider a maxillofacial CT scan, as this provides high resolution and thin cuts to better elucidate bony and soft-tissue injuries. This is especially true if tripod, orbital, or midface fractures are suspected, as these may be missed with a noncontrast head CT.

20. How do I recognize an injury to the Stensen duct?

The Stensen (parotid) duct arises from the parotid gland and courses from the level of the external auditory canal (superficial) through the buccinator muscle to open at the level of the upper second molar (Fig. 83.3). Any laceration along this pathway may involve the parotid gland, parotid duct, or buccal branch of the facial nerve. Laceration of the parotid system is recognized by a flow of saliva from the wound or bloody drainage from the duct orifice. Careful exploration reveals whether the flow is from the parotid gland or duct. In addition, the buccal branch of the facial nerve travels in close proximity to the Stensen duct. Injury to the nerve leads to drooping of the upper lip, which indicates a possible parotid duct injury. To assess for parotid duct patency, the parotid gland should be milked to see if saliva is expressed from the intraoral opening of the parotid duct. Damage to the duct requires consultation with a plastic surgeon and repair over a stent.

21. When should closure of a facial laceration be deferred?

Closure of facial lacerations in the ED depends on the severity of facial and systemic injuries. Complex lacerations in patients needing operative intervention should be cleansed with normal saline, covered with moist gauze, and deferred for intraoperative closure. Closure of the highly vascular tissues of the face may be delayed for up to 24 hours. Wounds involving the facial nerve, lacrimal duct, parotid duct, and avulsions should be referred on

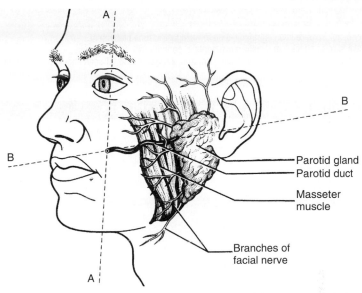

Fig. 83.3 Parotid gland and parotid duct with nearby branches of the facial nerve. Line *B* demonstrates approximate course of the parotid duct from the parotid gland, entering the mouth at the junction of lines *A* and *B*. (From Cantrill SV. Face. In Marx JA, Hockberger RS, Walls RM, et al., eds. *Rosen's Emergency Medicine: Concepts and Clinical Practice.* 5 ed. St. Louis: Mosby; 2002:323.)

presentation to the appropriate surgeon for definitive care. Given the high vascularity of the face, dog bites are at low risk of infection, and physician judgment may be used to decide whether to close a facial laceration from a dog bite and whether to use prophylactic antibiotics.

22. **How is the ear anesthetized?**
A regional auricular block (Fig. 83.4) is a way to anesthetize the entirety of the ear. This is performed by using 1% lidocaine with epinephrine as long as it is not injected into the cartilage. It is performed by aiming the needle and inserting at the point of the inferior ear and then going posteriorly, aiming towards the mastoid process to reach the greater auricular nerve and lesser occipital nerve. This can also be extended to the anterior portion without removal of the needle from the skin, done over the superior portion of the ear in a similar manner to have complete circumferential local anesthesia of the ear.

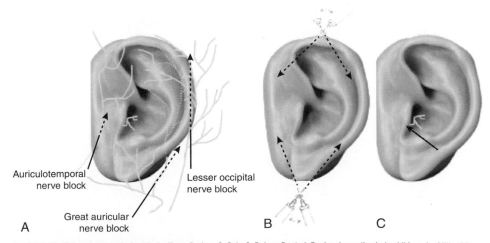

Fig. 83.4 (A–C) A regional auricular block. (From Dadure C, Sola C, Dalens B, et al. Regional anesthesia in children. In: Miller RD, ed. *Miller's Anesthesia.* 8th ed. Philadelphia: Elsevier; 2015:2706–2756, Figure 92-60.)

KEY POINTS: MAXILLOFACIAL TRAUMA

1. Concern for facial fracture is a contraindication to nasogastric tube placement.
2. Always make sure to check extraocular movements in patients with facial trauma.
3. If there is significant concern for maxillofacial fractures, a maxillofacial CT scan should be performed.

KEY POINTS: CLINICAL SIGNS OF ORBITAL FRACTURES

1. Eyelid edema
2. Endophthalmos
3. Proptosis
4. Limitation of upward gaze
5. Diplopia
6. Infraorbital anesthesia
7. Subcutaneous emphysema

BIBLIOGRAPHY

Bromberg WJ, Collier BC, Diebel LN, et al. Blunt cerebrovascular injury. Eastern Association for the Surgery of Trauma guideline. *J Trauma.* 2010;68:471–477.

Chukwulebe S, Hogrefe C. The diagnosis and management of facial bone fractures. *Emerg Med Clin N Am.* 2019;37:137–151.

Gorchynski J, Karabidian E, Sanchez M. The syringe technique: a hands-free approach for the reduction of acute nontraumatic temporomandibular dislocations in the emergency department. *J Emerg Med.* 2014;47(6):676–681.

Huang LK, Wang HH, Tu HF, et al. Simultaneous head and facial computed tomography scans for assessing facial fractures in patients with traumatic brain injury. *Injury.* 2017;48(7):1417–1422.

CHAPTER 84

CERVICAL SPINE AND SPINAL CORD TRAUMA

Erin Lindsay, MD and Maria Moreira, MD, FACEP

1. **What is the annual incidence of spinal cord injury (SCI) in the United States?**
   There are about 17,700 new cases per year, with SCI ~2% of injuries presenting to emergency departments (EDs); the proportion of sports-related injuries have been decreasing and the proportion related to falls have been increasing.

2. **Name the most common causes of SCI from most common to least.**
   - Vehicular crashes
   - Falls
   - Violence, primarily gunshot wounds
   - Sports
   - Medical/surgical
   - Other

3. **What are the most common levels of injury?**
   The most common level of injury in adults is C4 and C5, followed by C6, C7, T12, and L1. Overall, about half of all spine injuries are cervical injuries. In children under the age of 8 years, fractures of C3 and higher are more common due to a higher fulcrum of neck movement.

4. **Who gets SCIs?**
   SCI primarily affects young, healthy adults, and thus is a devastating and life-altering injury. Average age of injury is 42.9 years old; however, 47.6% of all SCIs occur between the ages of 16 and 30. There is a significant male predominance – 80.5% of all SCIs. Alcohol intoxication is also present in over a quarter of traumatic SCIs.

5. **In patients discharged from the hospital with neurologic impairment, what percentage has paraplegia and what percentage has tetraplegia (quadriplegia)?**
   People with paraplegia have injuries to the thoracic, lumbar, or sacral regions. Since the 1970s, the percentage of persons with incomplete tetraplegia has increased, whereas complete paraplegia and complete tetraplegia have decreased.
   - Incomplete tetraplegia 47%
   - Incomplete paraplegia 20%
   - Complete paraplegia 20%
   - Complete tetraplegia 12%
       Less than 1% of patients have complete recovery by discharge.

6. **Why should we worry about spinal injuries?**
   The management of any spinal injury is important, because improper care can result in permanent neurologic injury. It is important to maintain a high index of suspicion for SCI, as well as ensure proper immobilization and handling of the patient. It is equally imperative to have good-quality diagnostic imaging, and to choose the appropriate imaging modality, because inadequate studies and interpretation errors can lead to permanent injury.

7. **What is the financial impact of an SCI?**
   It is huge. The health care and living costs can vary greatly, depending on the severity of injury sustained and the age of the individual at the time of injury. The estimated yearly costs (including only costs related to health care and living expenses) can range from $43,700 to $191,436, depending on the severity of the injury. This does not include the first-year costs, which range from $359,783 to $1,102,403. These costs also do not include indirect costs such as wages and productivity lost, which approaches another $75,000 per year.

8. **Name the two main causes of reduced life expectancy in patients with SCI.**
   Pneumonia and sepsis.

9. **Are there any underlying conditions that could precipitate or heighten the chance of an SCI?**
   Less force is required to cause fractures in the elderly. Rheumatoid arthritis can lead to subluxation problems at C1 and C2. Normal development of the odontoid may not occur in a patient with Down syndrome, leading to increased risk of atlantoaxial instability. Osteoporosis and metastatic cancer may also lead to a fracture with insignificant trauma.

10. **How do I immobilize the patient with a potential spinal injury?**
    Historically, when spinal injury was suspected, the entire spine was immobilized with a long board, along with placement of a rigid collar to immobilize the cervical spine. Patients brought in by emergency medical services (EMS) may also have their forehead taped to the board with towels or other bolsters to prevent further neck movement. While cervical spine immobilization with a collar remains standard practice for suspected cervical spine injury, total spinal immobilization with a backboard has never been shown to have benefit in preventing secondary neurologic injury, and has in fact shown evidence of harm in some situations. Cervical collars should also be removed as soon as it is safe to do so, as they have been found to contribute to skin breakdown and ulcers, as well as increased intracranial pressure in patients with traumatic brain injury.

11. **Why is using a backboard considered a problem?**
    Patients who are placed on a backboard should be removed from them as soon as practical. Immobilization on a backboard causes significant discomfort to the patient and has also been demonstrated to potentially compromise ventilatory status in some patients and increase difficulty of intubation. Patients who are allowed to remain on the board for prolonged periods have developed skin breakdown and decubitus ulcers.

12. **If the backboard causes all of these problems, should it ever be used?**
    The backboard should continue to be used for specific purposes. It is an excellent device to help extricate patients, or when patients need to be carried over large distances.

13. **How should I approach the patient with potential spinal injury?**
    There are several mnemonics for the initial stabilization of any trauma patient. Advanced trauma life support (ATLS) teaches the *ABCDE* mnemonic:
    Airway
    Breathing
    Circulation
    Disability
    Exposure
        According to another mnemonic, a proper history is *A MUST*:
    Altered mental state: Check for drugs or alcohol.
    Mechanism*: Does the potential for injury exist?
    Underlying conditions: Are high-risk factors for fractures present?
    Symptoms: Is pain, paresthesia, or neurologic compromise part of the picture?
    Timing: When did the symptoms begin in relation to the event?

14. **What should be assessed on a physical examination?**
    There are two key areas: the spine itself and the neurologic examination. The spine is palpated to assess for tenderness, deformity, and paraspinous muscle spasm. The neurologic examination should include motor function, sensory function, some aspect of posterior column function (position and vibration), and a rectal examination to assess sphincter tone and sensation. The assessment of light touch examines the integrity of the posterior neurologic columns, and pinprick testing assesses the anterior spinothalamic tracts. In an unconscious patient, the only clues to an SCI may be poor rectal tone, priapism, absence of deep tendon reflexes, or diaphragmatic breathing.

15. **What is neurogenic shock, and how is it treated?**
    Neurogenic shock is a syndrome resulting from loss of neurologic function and accompanying sympathetic tone, leading to unopposed parasympathetic tone. Neurogenic shock can occur in the setting of any cervical or high thoracic spine injury (above T6). This is usually exhibited by flaccid paralysis, with loss of reflexes and loss of urinary and rectal tone. Accompanying this are hypotension, bradycardia, hypothermia, and ileus. Neurogenic shock is a diagnosis of exclusion after other forms of shock, particularly hemorrhagic, have been addressed or eliminated. Hypotension is treated with rapid infusion of crystalloid. If intravenous fluids are not adequate to maintain organ perfusion, norepinephrine is the preferred vasopressor, as it can address both hypotension and bradycardia. Bradycardia can be treated with atropine or glycopyrrolate. In refractory bradycardia, a pacemaker may be required. In most cases of neurogenic shock, hypotension resolves within 24–48 hours.

16. **What are the general principles of emergency treatment in the patient with spinal cord trauma?**
    First, do no harm: that means proper immobilization, coordinated extrication, and movement of the patient only when absolutely necessary. Any patient with an SCI higher than C5 should be considered for intubation, as the roots of the phrenic nerve emerge between C3 and C5, and injury to the phrenic nerve can result in respiratory failure due to diaphragm paralysis. Rapid-sequence intubation (RSI) with manual in-line stabilization is considered

---

*Fall injuries are common. In the case of a fall, the physician should get information as to the height of the fall and any preceding events, such as syncope, chest pain, or seizure.

the safest way to intubate these patients. Typically, the goal mean arterial pressure (MAP) for patients with SCI is between 85 and 90 mmHg to maintain adequate perfusion to the spinal cord, although this has not been proven to lead to better clinical outcomes. Early gastric and bladder decompression are also indicated. The absence of pain below the level of the spine injury can mask other injuries.

17. Which patients need cervical spine imaging?
There are two validated decision rules available to the emergency physician. One is the National Emergency X-Radiography Utilization Study (NEXUS) decision rule. The other is the Canadian C-Spine Rule (CCR). Both have been shown to reduce the number of imaging studies ordered in patients at low risk for cervical spine injury.

18. What are the NEXUS criteria?
- No midline cervical tenderness
- No focal neurologic deficit
- Normal alertness
- No intoxication
- No painful distracting injury

   If patients meet these criteria, they have a low probability of injury and cervical spine imaging is not needed. In this large multicenter study, the overall rate of missed cervical spine injuries was less than 1 in 4000 patients. Note that there are specific definitions of the previous five criteria that must be reviewed when applying the NEXUS criteria. There is also concern that this rule may not be as sensitive in patients over the age of 65, so caution is required in this population. Overall, this rule was 99.6% sensitive and 12.9% specific for significant injury.

19. What is the CCR?
The CCR study had a sensitivity of 100% and a specificity of 42.5% for identifying clinically important cervical spine injuries. The CCR asks three questions:
1. Is there any high-risk factor that mandates radiography? These are:
   - age older than 65 years;
   - significant mechanism of injury (i.e., fall from >1 m, axial loading injury, high-speed motor vehicle accident [MVA]/rollover/ejection, bike collision);
   - the presence of paresthesias.
2. Can the patient be assessed safely for range of motion (simple mechanism, sitting position in the ED, ambulatory at any time, delayed onset of neck pain, or absence of midline cervical spine tenderness)?
3. Can the patient actively rotate the neck 45 degrees to the left and the right?

20. What are distracting injuries?
- *NEXUS.* Includes a long list, such as long bone fractures, large lacerations, visceral injury, and burns
- *CCR.* Injuries such as fractures that are so severely painful that the neck examination is unreliable

21. Can these decision rules be applied to children?
NEXUS and CCR have not been validated in the pediatric population, though some studies have found adequate sensitivity in older children. The American Association of Neurologic Surgeons currently recommends applying NEXUS criteria to patients >9 years of age. There is no validated set of criteria for determining need for imaging in children <9 years of age, so decisions regarding imaging must be made on a case-by-case basis. While a computed tomography (CT) scan is the preferred imaging modality in adults, plain radiographs are often a reasonable first test in pediatric patients who require imaging.

22. Which radiographs should be obtained?
The standard three views of the cervical spine are anteroposterior (AP), lateral, and open-mouth (odontoid) views. If obtaining cervical radiographs during the initial evaluation, a cross-table lateral radiograph should be taken, because it does not require any movement on the part of the patient. Cervical spine precautions should not be discontinued based solely on the cross-table lateral view. Multiple studies have shown that plain radiographs alone lack the sensitivity to rule out clinically important cervical spine injury. The most commonly missed injuries are at C1 to C2, followed by the lower C6–C7–T1 junction. In the elderly, C1 and C2 fractures account for approximately 70% of cervical spine fractures. Some series include oblique and pillar views of the vertebrae as well.

23. How do I interpret the lateral cervical spine radiograph?
The first rule is to make sure that the radiograph is technically adequate, that all seven cervical vertebrae are seen, and that the top of T1 is visible on the film. Next, follow the mnemonic *ABCS*:
Alignment. Check for a smooth line at the anterior and posterior aspect of the vertebral bodies and the spinolaminar line from C1 to T1 (Fig. 84.1).
Bones. Evaluate each vertebral body to ensure that the anterior and posterior heights are similar (>3 mm difference suggests fracture); follow the vertebrae out to the laminae and spinous processes. Look carefully at the upper and lower cervical segments where fractures are likely to be missed. Examine the "ring" of C2, which can show a fracture through the upper portion of the vertebral body of C2.

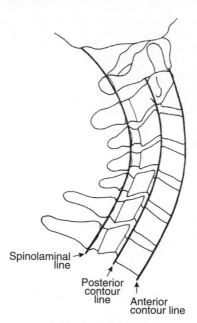

Spinolaminal
line
Posterior
contour
line
Anterior
contour line

Fig. 84.1 Curve of alignment.

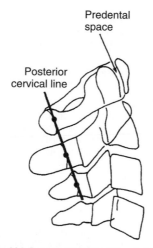

Predental
space

Posterior
cervical line

Fig. 84.2 Posterior cervical line and predental space.

Cartilage. Check the intervertebral joint spaces and the facet joints.
Soft-tissue spaces. Look for prevertebral swelling, especially at the C2 to C3 area (>5 mm) and check the predental space (Fig. 84.2), which should be less than 3 mm in adults and less than 5 mm in children. From C4 to C7 the soft-tissue thickness should not be greater than 22 mm.

24. **What are the indications for flexion-extension views of the cervical spine?**
   Based on the NEXUS study, flexion-extension imaging is unnecessary in the acute evaluation of patients with blunt trauma. If a patient has persistent neck pain after a CT scan, flexion-extension films can be considered to evaluate for cervical spine instability, though there is not conclusive data to suggest that these have adequate sensitivity to rule out this type of injury. Magnetic resonance imaging (MRI) is the preferred modality to evaluate for non-bony spinal cord injury.

25. **When should a CT or MRI be ordered?**

   With the advent of rapid helical scanning, a CT scan is the preferred imaging modality due to increased sensitivity of CT for bony injury. CT is also indicated when plain radiographs are obtained and are inconclusive or difficult to interpret. A CT scan is good for detection of bony injury and to identify surgical conditions, such as hematoma or disk fragments within the spinal canal. A CT scan is also needed for the clearance of the cervical spine in a comatose or obtunded patient. In a study of patients with traumatic brain injury, 5.4% of the patients had C1 or C2 fractures and 4% had occipital condyle fractures that were not visualized on the three-view radiography series. (The current Eastern Association of Trauma-EAST guidelines recommend that CT be the primary screening tool for cervical spine injury in high-risk patients.)

   MRI is useful to identify injury to the spinal cord itself in the face of neurologic deficit. As a result of its greater sensitivity for evaluating soft tissue, MRI can show areas of contusion and edema within the spinal space. MRI can also detect rupture of intervertebral disks and ligamentous injury. CT is better than MRI for the identification of vertebral fractures.

26. **What is SCIWORA?**

   It is **S**pinal **C**ord **I**njury **W**ithout **R**adiographic **A**bnormalities. Children are thought to be more susceptible to SCIWORA because of the greater elasticity of their cervical structures, but many cases have been found in adults as well. Usually a rapid deceleration injury leads to transient spinal column subluxation and stretching of the spinal cord. These patients may have a brief episode of upper extremity weakness or paresthesias with delayed development of neurologic deficits that appear hours to days later. Neurologic deficits related to SCIWORA may be transient or permanent. MRI should be obtained on all patients with suspected SCIWORA.

KEY POINTS: SPINAL CORD TRAUMA

1. It is important to have a high index of suspicion for injury and ensure proper immobilization and handling of the patient.
2. Use clinical decision rules, such as NEXUS or CCR, to minimize cervical spine imaging.
3. The use of steroids in blunt spinal cord trauma is not standard of care.
4. Special populations, such as pediatric and geriatric patients, require thoughtful consideration for more intensive workup, as they may not present with the typical signs and symptoms that an adult patient might.
5. A CT scan is the preferred imaging modality for initial evaluation of cervical spine injury. If there is concern for cervical spine instability due to soft-tissue or ligamentous injury, MRI is preferred, but flexion-extension films can be considered.

---

27. **Describe the Jefferson, Hangman, Clay shoveler, and Chance fractures.**
   - Jefferson fracture is a burst fracture of the ring of C1 that occurs from axial loading.
   - Hangman fracture is a disruption of the posterior arch of C2 with anterior subluxation of the body of C2 on C3, typically due to a hyperextension injury.
   - Clay shoveler fracture is a stable fracture of the spinous process that is classically caused by forceful cervical flexion combined with contraction of the paraspinous muscles causing significant force through the interspinous ligament.
   - Chance fracture is a vertebral fracture, usually in the lumbar segment, involving the posterior spinous process, pedicles, and vertebral body. It is caused by the flexion forces on the spinal column. This is associated with the use of lap belts.

28. **Describe the incomplete cord syndromes or injuries.**
   - **Anterior cord syndrome** results in loss of function in the anterior two thirds of the spinal cord from damage to the corticospinal and spinothalamic pathways. Findings include loss of voluntary motor function as well as pain and temperature sensation below the level of the injury, with preservation of the posterior column functions of proprioception, pressure, and vibration. The key issue is the potential reversibility of this lesion if a compressing hematoma or disk fragment can be removed. This condition requires immediate neurosurgical evaluation.
   - **Central cord syndrome** results from injury to the central portion of the spinal cord. Because more proximal innervation is placed centrally within the cord, this lesion results in greater involvement of the upper extremities than of the lower extremities. Bowel or bladder control is usually preserved. The mechanism of injury is hyperextension of a cervical spine with a cord space narrowed by congenital variation, degenerative spurring, or hypertrophic ligaments. This syndrome can occur without actual fracture or ligamentous disruption.
   - **Brown-Séquard syndrome** is an injury to a hemisection of the spinal cord, usually from penetrating trauma. Contralateral sensation of pain and temperature is lost, and motor and posterior column functions are absent on the side of the injury.

- **Cauda equina syndrome** is an injury to the lumbar, sacral, and coccygeal nerve roots, causing a peripheral nerve injury. There can be motor and sensory loss in the lower extremities, bowel and bladder dysfunction, and loss of pain sensation at the perineum (saddle anesthesia).

29. What is the significance of sacral sparing and spinal shock?

Sacral sparing refers to the preservation of any function of the sacral roots, such as toe movement or perianal sensation. If sacral sparing is present, the chance of functional neurologic recovery is good. Spinal shock is a temporary concussive-like condition in which voluntary movement, sensation, and cord-mediated reflexes, such as the anal wink, are absent. Spinal shock also may result in bradycardia and hypotension. While self-limited, symptoms can last for up to several weeks. The extent of underlying cord injury – and prognosis – cannot be determined until these reflexes return.

30. What can emergency physicians do to prevent spinal injuries?

Get involved in injury prevention and education. Because of the predominance of vehicle crashes causing SCIs, one can work to reduce driving under the influence of alcohol and drugs, as well as the use of cell phones or texting while driving. Furthermore, the use of safety belts should be emphasized at discharge in every ED visit, regardless of the reason the person came in for treatment. Diving and sporting injuries can be reduced by proper public education and coaching.

CONTROVERSY

31. What is the status of steroids in spinal cord trauma?

This continues to be a very controversial topic. In 1975, the first National Acute Spinal Cord Injury Study (NASCIS) was established. This was followed by NASCIS 2 (1992) and NASCIS 3 (1998), which evaluated regimens of high-dosage methylprednisolone. NASCIS 2 demonstrated some improvement in motor symptoms at 1 year in patients who received methylprednisolone within 8 hours of the initial injury; however, there was no significant difference in overall functional outcomes between the steroid and placebo groups. Initial support for the use of steroids was encouraging, but multiple critical reviews of the NASCIS study and other literature argued that there is insufficient evidence to support the use of corticosteroids in the treatment of patients with acute SCI. Furthermore, a recent level I study showed that patients treated with high-dosage methylprednisolone had a higher incidence of serious complications, such as gastrointestinal bleeding, pneumonia, and hyperglycemia. While steroids are still used in some institutions, the American Academy of Neurological Surgeons and Congress of Neurological Surgeons recommend that steroids not be used in the first 24–48 hours after SCI. The American Academy of Emergency Medicine and Canadian Association of Emergency Physicians state that steroids may be a treatment option, but are not standard of care. In view of these statements, it seems prudent to consult with the treating neurosurgeon before considering steroid therapy.

Websites

American Academy of Emergency Medicine: www.aaem.org/positionstatements/steroidsinacuteinjury. shtml; accessed October 27, 2019.
Canadian Association of Emergency Physicians: www.caep.ca/; accessed October 27, 2019.
Eastern Association for the Surgery of Trauma: www.east.org; accessed October 27, 2019.
National Spinal Cord Injury Statistical Center: www.spinalcord.uab.edu; accessed October 27, 2019.

BIBLIOGRAPHY

Como J, Diaz J, Dunham C, et al. Practice management guidelines for identification of cervical spine injuries following trauma: update from the Eastern Association for the Surgery of Trauma Practice Management Guidelines Committee. *J Trauma.* 2009;67:651–659.
Easter J, Barkin R, Rosen C, et al. Cervical spine injuries in children. Part I: mechanism of injury, clinical presentation, and imaging. *J Emerg Med.* 2011;41:142–150.
Hurlbert RJ, Hadley MN, Walters BC, et al. Pharmacological therapy for acute spinal cord injury. *Neurosurgery.* 2013;72:93–105.
National Spinal Cord Injury Statistical Center. *2018 Annual Statistical Report for the Spinal Cord Injury Model Systems.* Birmingham: University of Alabama; 2018.
Saadeh Y, Smith BW, Joseph JR, et al. The impact of blood pressure management after spinal cord injury: a systematic review of the literature. *Neurosurg Focus.* 2017;43:E20.

CHAPTER 85

HEAD TRAUMA

Edward Newton, MD and Taku Taira, MD

1. What is the scope of head injury in the United States?

There are more than 1.3 million emergency department (ED) visits and approximately 52,000 deaths as a result of traumatic brain injury (TBI) every year in the United States. Although the incidence of severe head injury is increasing, deaths from TBI are decreasing, most likely because of the preventive benefits of helmets, seat belts, and air bags in automobiles. In spite of this, head trauma remains the most lethal traumatic injury and accounts for a large proportion of patients with permanent disability. The peak incidence of head injury is in the 15- to 24-year-old age group, with males affected twice as often as females. The spectrum of head injury includes relatively minor problems, such as lacerations and scalp contusions, and major, often lethal, intracranial trauma. Distinguishing between minor and potentially lethal head injuries, while using diagnostic resources appropriately, is one of the most difficult tasks facing the emergency physician.

2. What groups of patients are at particular risk from head trauma?

Because assessment of mental status is such an integral part of the evaluation of patients with head injury, patients who are unable to communicate because they are preverbal (e.g., infants), intoxicated, mentally impaired, aphasic, or have a language barrier pose a special challenge. When such communication barriers are present, there should be a lower threshold for obtaining a computed tomography (CT) scan.

Certain age groups are at higher risk for intracranial injury:

- Infants are at higher risk because of their relatively large head size and compressibility of the skull. Infants also are at high risk for nonaccidental trauma (e.g., abusive head trauma, which is also known as *shaken baby syndrome*), in which case an accurate history may be unavailable or deliberately withheld. If the cranial sutures and fontanelles are not closed, the cranium can expand as a result of intracranial bleeding. Infants can bleed sufficiently intracranially to produce hemorrhagic shock, whereas in older children and adults, some other source of bleeding is responsible for hemorrhagic shock.
- Both the elderly and patients with chronic alcoholism are at higher risk of intracranial injury, particularly subdural hematoma (SDH). Cerebral atrophy results in stretching of bridging veins from the dura to the brain parenchyma, making these veins vulnerable to tearing from deceleration forces. Both populations are also at higher risk from the greater incidence of head trauma from falls.
- Patients who are taking anticoagulants or antiplatelet agents or who have intrinsic bleeding diatheses bleed more actively than patients with normal coagulation and have higher mortality from brain injury.

KEY POINTS: PATIENTS AT HIGH RISK FOR HEAD INJURY

1. Very young and very old patients.
2. Patients with chronic alcoholism.
3. Patients with coagulopathy.

3. What is a cerebral concussion?

A cerebral concussion is a sudden, transient loss of central neurologic function secondary to trauma. It is typically characterized by loss of consciousness (LOC; although LOC is not necessary to make the diagnosis), transient amnesia, confusion, disorientation, or transient visual changes, without any gross cerebral abnormalities or neurologic deficits on examination.

4. What is postconcussive syndrome?

Although the patient may have a completely normal neurologic examination after a concussion, there are common sequelae from this type of injury. Patients commonly report migraine-type headaches, dizziness, inability to concentrate, and irritability. Although in 90% of cases these symptoms resolve within 2 weeks, they rarely may persist for up to 1 year. Treatment is supportive, and the long-term prognosis is good.

5. What is second impact syndrome?

Second impact syndrome is when a second head trauma during a vulnerable period after a concussion results in severe and often fatal diffuse cerebral edema. Consequently, athletes should be held out of contact sports until all postconcussive symptoms have resolved and they have completed a gradual, step-wise return to activity without symptoms. Repeated concussions can result in permanent impairment in cognition, speech, balance, and movement.

6. **What complications are associated with basilar skull fractures?**
Basilar skull fractures are often complicated by cranial nerve or cerebrovascular injury. CT angiography is often used to detect vascular injuries associated with basilar skull fracture. A patient with signs of basilar skull fracture (i.e., raccoon eyes, hemotympanum, or Battle sign) with clear drainage from the nose or ear canal, and any patient with posttraumatic rhinorrhea or otorrhea, should be suspected of having leakage of cerebrospinal fluid (CSF). Analysis of the glucose content of the drainage by glucometer or laboratory analysis may distinguish CSF (containing 60% of serum glucose levels) from nasal mucus (0% glucose). In cases in which blood is mixed with CSF, applying a drop of the fluid to filter paper reveals CSF in a target shape, with blood at the center and pink-tinged CSF forming an outer ring. However, bedside tests are neither specific nor sensitive for detecting CSF leaks. CSF leaks may present days to weeks after the initial injury

7. **How are CSF leaks treated?**
CSF leaks through tears in the dura generally are managed conservatively. The use of prophylactic antibiotics is controversial because they have not been shown to significantly reduce the incidence of meningitis, and may instead select for antibiotic-resistant bacteria. Due to the risk for meningitis, patients must be monitored closely until the dural tear heals. Conservative management still includes referral to a specialist, as dural tears that fail to close spontaneously over 2–3 weeks usually require operative or endoscopic repair.

8. **What are signs or symptoms of a patient with epidural hematoma?**
Epidural hematoma occurs in 5%–10% of severe head injuries. In the classic pattern, a patient loses consciousness from the initial trauma, gradually recovers over a few minutes, and enters a lucid interval wherein he or she is relatively asymptomatic and has a normal neurologic examination. During this interval, accumulation of arterial blood in the epidural space, usually from a lacerated middle meningeal artery, eventually causes compression and shift of brain across the midline. This process is accompanied by a second reduction in the level of consciousness and the pupillary and motor signs of herniation. This classic pattern occurs in only about 30% of cases, however. Many patients remain unconscious after the initial impact or have minor hemorrhages, and they may not develop increased intracranial pressure (ICP) at all. The characteristic CT scan appearance of an epidural hematoma is a hyperdense lenticular collection of blood that indents adjacent brain parenchyma and does not extend beyond cranial sutures where the dura is attached.

9. **How does an SDH present?**
An SDH may be acute, subacute (6–14 days), or chronic (>14 days after trauma).
   - An acute SDH is associated with a high incidence of underlying brain injury. The presentation varies with the severity of the underlying injury, but patients commonly have a diminished level of consciousness, headache, and focal neurologic deficits corresponding to the area of brain injury. If sufficient bleeding occurs, ICP increases and herniation may occur. The characteristic appearance of an acute SDH on CT scan is a collection of hyperdense blood in a crescent-shaped pattern conforming to the convexity of the hemisphere and often extending past cranial sutures (Fig. 85.1).
   - At times, the injury causes a minimal amount of bleeding and the patient does not immediately seek medical care. The SDH undergoes lysis over several days and eventually organizes into an encapsulated mass.
   - A subacute or chronic SDH is a difficult clinical diagnosis, because the symptoms are vague, nonspecific, and common (e.g., persistent headache, difficulty concentrating, lethargy), and the trauma may have been forgotten. Even the CT scan diagnosis is difficult, because subacute SDH becomes isodense and may be indistinguishable from surrounding brain unless special contrast-enhanced CT techniques are used. Chronic SDH appears as an encapsulated lucent collection of fluid in the same position as the acute type.

10. **What is axonal shear injury?**
Axonal shear injury, also referred to as diffuse axonal injury (DAI), occurs during abrupt deceleration. The white and gray matter have differing densities and thus differing rates of deceleration. As a result, rapid and severe deceleration produces a shearing force and widespread tearing of the axons at the white-gray interface. In contrast to focal brain injuries, DAI results in severe neurologic derangements, such as prolonged coma or persistent vegetative state. The CT scan may appear completely normal or show only small petechial hemorrhages. Magnetic resonance imaging (MRI) of the brain is a more sensitive tool in detecting these injuries.

11. **What is brain herniation?**
Herniation is caused by increased ICP. Because the cranium is a rigid structure, pressure varies with the volume of its contents. Intracranial volume is made up of 10% blood and 10% CSF, and the remainder is brain parenchyma and intracellular fluid. An increase in any of these compartments by blood, tumor, or edema causes a predictable response. Initially, CSF is forced into the spinal canal, and the ventricles and cisterns collapse. Once this has occurred, ICP rises steeply, and the brain parenchyma shifts away from the accumulating mass or collection and herniates through one of several spaces, eventually causing death by brain stem compression.

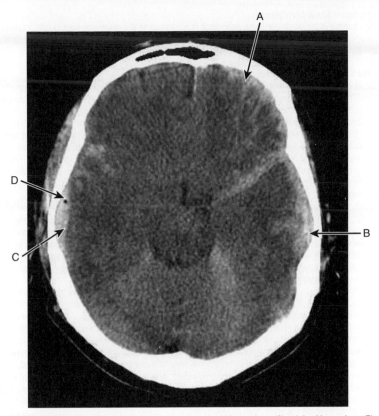

Fig. 85.1 Computed tomography (CT) scan of the head showing subarachnoid hemorrhage (A), subdural hemorrhage (B), and subdural hemorrhage (C) with intracranial free air (D, *black dot*).

12. **List the four types of herniation syndrome.**
    1. Uncal herniation
    2. Central herniation
    3. Cingulate herniation
    4. Posterior fossa herniation

13. **Describe uncal herniation syndrome.**
    The uncus is the most medial portion of the hemisphere and is often the first structure to shift below the tentorium that separates the hemispheres from the midbrain. As the uncus is forced medially and downward, the ipsilateral third cranial nerve is compressed, producing pupillary dilation, ptosis, and oculomotor paresis. As herniation progresses, the ipsilateral cerebral peduncle and pyramidal tract are compressed, resulting in contralateral hemiplegia.
    In approximately 10% of cases, the hemiparesis occurs on the same side as the brain lesion, making this a less reliable finding for localizing the injury. Further progression results in brain stem compression with respiratory and cardiac arrest. Uncal herniation is the most common variety of transtentorial herniation.

14. **What is central herniation syndrome?**
    Occasionally, hematomas located at the vertex or frontal lobes cause simultaneous downward herniation of both hemispheres through the tentorium. Clinical findings can be similar to uncal herniation, except for the presence of bilateral motor weakness and bilateral ocular findings in central herniation.

15. **How does cingulate herniation occur?**
    Rarely, the cingulate gyrus is forced medially beneath the falx by an expanding lateral hematoma, causing compression of the ventricles and impairing cerebral blood flow.

16. **Explain posterior fossa herniation.**
Bleeding or edema in the posterior fossa can result in herniation of the cerebellar tonsils either upward through the tentorium or downward through the foramen magnum. In the latter case, coma and fatal brain stem dysfunction may occur rapidly and with little warning.

17. **What is the ED treatment for increased ICP?**
- The focus is in avoiding the five *Hs* (**h**ypotension, **h**ypoxia, **h**ypercarbia, **h**ypoglycemia, and **h**yperthermia) and seizures. These are conditions that either increase the metabolic demands of the brain or decrease cerebral perfusion, and in turn, worsen the prognosis.
- Early and careful airway management and ventilation are essential to avoid hypoxia. Patients with head injury who experience hypoxia (partial pressure of oxygen [PO_2] <60 mmHg) also have a twofold increase in mortality rate. Given that recent studies have linked hyperoxia with worsening outcomes, providers should aim for normoxia.
- Care should be taken to maintain adequate cerebral perfusion pressure. Patients who experience hypotension (systolic blood pressure <90 mmHg) have a twofold increase in mortality. Although there is often misguided reluctance to hydrate patients with concomitant head and systemic injuries, ED providers should focus on maintaining cerebral perfusion by avoiding hypotension.
- After brain trauma, there is a cascade of secondary neuronal metabolic injuries that are detrimental to recovery of neurologic function. At present, few interventions have proven effective in limiting these changes.
- Coagulopathies should be corrected with fresh frozen plasma (FFP), and platelet transfusion should be considered in patients who have recently taken aspirin or other antiplatelet drugs. Patients with intracranial hemorrhage (ICH) on vitamin K antagonist anticoagulants should be considered for reversal with a prothrombin complex concentrate (PCC). Currently, trials are underway to evaluate the effectiveness of antifibrinolytics – for example, tranexamic acid (TXA) – for the treatment of ICH.
- Hyperventilation: carbon dioxide is one of the main determinants of cerebrovascular tone. High levels produce cerebral vasodilatation; low levels cause vasoconstriction. Hyperventilation decreases carbon dioxide, leading to vasoconstriction, resulting in a decrease in the vascular compartment of the brain. This intervention may prevent worsening herniation long enough for definitive surgical interventions. Unfortunately there is a trade-off: as blood flow to the brain decreases, delivery of oxygen and glucose also decreases, resulting in ischemic injury and worsening edema. This intervention is used only in patients who are rapidly deteriorating neurologically (i.e., herniating), as a bridge to surgery. The optimal level of hypocarbia is uncertain at present, but most clinicians recommend moderate short-term hyperventilation, with a goal partial pressure of carbon dioxide (PCO_2) level no less than 35 mmHg in patients with evidence of herniation. To accomplish this degree of hypocarbia, it is necessary to intubate and mechanically ventilate with settings determined by arterial blood gases. Hyperventilation should never be used prophylactically.
- Diuresis: the use of an osmotic diuretic, such as mannitol 0.5–1.0 g/kg intravenously over 15 minutes, or a loop diuretic, such as furosemide 0.5–1.0 mg/kg intravenously, is effective in reducing brain edema. Infusion of mannitol creates an osmotic gradient between the intravascular space and the extracellular fluid, drawing fluid from the extracellular fluid and reducing brain water content and ICP. Mannitol is filtered by the kidneys, producing systemic dehydration. This diuresis can be problematic in patients with hypovolemic hypotension. Clinical experience and animal studies seem to support the concomitant administration of osmotic diuretics and volume resuscitation in patients with hypovolemic shock.
- Hypertonic saline: various concentrations of hypertonic saline, ranging from 3% to 23%, have been used to simultaneously decrease brain edema, maintain cerebral perfusion pressure, and restore systemic volume. Hypertonic saline has been shown to reduce ICP faster and more effectively than mannitol without changes in mortality. It is preferred over mannitol in hypotensive patients. Patients receiving hypertonic saline will develop significant hypernatremia and hyperosmolarity. Unless serum sodium exceeds 160 mEq/L, these abnormalities should be allowed to correct themselves gradually over a period of several days.
- Ventriculostomy: although generally an intensive care unit (ICU) technique, removal of CSF through an external ventricular drain (EVD) is occasionally implemented in the ED and is perhaps the most effective way of monitoring and rapidly lowering ICP.
- Sedation: conscious patients who are paralyzed for intubation also must be sedated. A short-acting barbiturate, such as thiopental, is the ideal agent for this purpose because it lowers ICP, prevents seizures, and decreases cerebral metabolism. However, barbiturates can cause hypotension and cannot be used in hypotensive patients. When the patient is hypotensive, consider sedation with a reversible agent, such as morphine 0.1 mg/kg, lorazepam 0.05–0.2 mg/kg, or midazolam 0.1 mg/kg followed by an infusion at 0.01–0.2 mg/kg/h. This approach is preferred because adverse effects on blood pressure and cardiac output can be reversed by specific antagonists. There are other options for sedation with various advantages and disadvantages. Etomidate 0.2 mg/kg is a short-acting sedative agent that has the advantage of decreasing ICP without adversely affecting cardiac output, cerebral perfusion pressure, and systemic blood pressure. However, it is known to cause adrenal suppression. Propofol 2–2.5 mg/kg induction dose, followed by an infusion of 0.1–0.4 mg/kg/min is an effective agent for sedation. Because propofol can also cause hypotension, it should be used with caution. Fentanyl 0.1–0.3 µg/kg has the disadvantage of causing a slight increase in ICP and is not the preferred agent for sedation of a patient with head injury.

18. **Is there any role for therapeutic hypothermia in patients with TBI?**

Reducing a patient's body temperature to 32°C–33°C (90°F–93°F) for 24–48 hours has shown some benefit in preserving neurologic function in survivors of cardiac arrest, and it was hoped that it would show the same benefits in patients with brain injury. However, the results of several trials have been conflicting. If any benefit occurs, it is likely in those who have a Glasgow Coma Scale (GCS) score of 5–8, but even in these patients, the treatment should be considered experimental. Fever should be treated aggressively, however, and patients who arrive in the ED with mild hypothermia should be allowed to passively rewarm.

KEY POINTS: TREATMENT OF HEAD INJURY

1. Maintain cerebral perfusion and avoid hypotension.
2. Maintain oxygenation.
3. Secure airway using rapid-sequence intubation (RSI) if the GCS is less than 8.
4. Seizure prophylaxis with phenytoin (15 mg/kg intravenously) or levetiracetam (Keppra).
5. Hyperventilate to pCO_2 of 35 mmHg only if patient has elevated ICP and is clinically herniating.
6. Mannitol or hypertonic saline can be used for osmotic therapy to decrease ICP.
7. Correct coagulopathy with FFP or PCC.

19. **If the patient has a normal CT scan after head trauma, is it completely safe to discharge the patient home?**

Nothing is completely safe. There are well-documented instances of delayed epidural and subdural bleeding many hours after injury. Consequently, although it is generally safe to discharge such patients, head injury instructions should be given to responsible family members, and the patient should be instructed to return immediately if symptoms worsen. If the patient is socially isolated or unreliable, a judgment has to be made regarding the seriousness of the mechanism of injury and the risk of discharge. Intoxicated patients should be kept under observation until their mental status can be evaluated properly.

20. **What are the indications for a repeat head CT scan?**

Some centers routinely schedule a repeat head CT scan after the initial scan is positive for ICH, although this practice is not recommended based on the evidence. The indications for repeat head CT scan are as follows:

- Clinical deterioration, as indicated by worsening mental status, progression of focal neurologic deficits, or declining GCS score should prompt a repeat scan.
- Patients taking Coumadin (warfarin) or other anticoagulant drugs have up to a 2.5% chance of developing a delayed ICH after head trauma, even if the initial head CT is normal. Options for management after an initial normal head CT include: (1) repeat head CT after an observation period of 6–12 hours, or, in reliable patients who don't live alone, (2) documentation of a normal neurologic examination without symptoms after an observation period with strict return precautions. Patients taking antiplatelet agents, such as aspirin or clopidogrel, have a higher overall risk of ICH after head trauma and a worse prognosis if bleeding occurs. However, the hemorrhage is typically present on the initial head CT and patients do not appear to have an increased risk of delayed bleeding; thus, a repeat CT is not necessary in these patients.

BIBLIOGRAPHY

Almenawar SA, Bogza J, Blake Y, et al. The value of scheduled repeat cranial computed tomography after mild head injury: single center series and meta-analysis. *Neurosurgery.* 2013;72:56–64.

Baugnon KL, Hudgins PA. Skull base fractures and their complications. *Neuroimaging Clin N Am.* 2014;24:439–465.

Bauman ZM, Ruggero JM, Squindo S, et al. Repeat head CT? Not necessary for patients with a negative initial head CT on anticoagulation or antiplatelet therapy suffering low-altitude falls. *Am Surg.* 2017;83(5):429–435.

Bey T, Ostick B. Second impact syndrome. *West J Emerg Med.* 2009;10:6–10.

Chauny JM, Marquis M, Bernard F, et al. Risk of delayed intracranial hemorrhage in anticoagulated patients with mild traumatic brain injury: systematic review and meta-analysis. *J Emerg Med.* 2016;51(5):519–528.

Kheirbek T, Pascual JL. Hypertonic saline for the treatment of intracranial hypertension. *Curr Neurol Neurosci Rep.* 2014;14:482–488.

Perry EC, Ahmed HC, Origitano TC. Neurotraumatology. In: Biller J, Ferro JM, eds. *Handbook of Clinical Neurology.* Vol. 121, 3rd series. Amsterdam: Elsevier; 2014.

Stocchetti N, Maas AIR. Traumatic intracranial hypertension. *N Engl J Med.* 2014;370:2121–2130.

Swap C, Sidell M, Ogaz R, et al. Risk of delayed intracranial hemorrhage in anticoagulated patients after minor head trauma: the role of repeat cranial computed tomography. *Perm J.* 2016;20(2):14–16.

CHAPTER 86

TRAUMATIC OPHTHALMOLOGIC EMERGENCIES

W. Gannon Sungar, DO and Jeffrey R. SooHoo, MD

1. List eyelid lacerations requiring expert consultation.
- Full-thickness lid lacerations
- Tarsal plate involvement
- Orbital fat prolapse (concern for penetrating orbital injury and occult globe injury)
- Lid margin laceration
- Superior lid lacerations with associated ptosis (possible levator palpebrae muscle [raises the upper lid] injury)
- Lacerations medial to the punctum (medial canthus), concerning for lacrimal system injury; fluorescein in the wound after instillation in the eye suggests an injury to the lacrimal system
- Any laceration with avulsion or loss of tissue in which the injury or repair may affect the ability of the eyelids to adequately close

2. How often are ocular injuries present in patients with eyelid lacerations?
Two-thirds of eyelid lacerations have associated ocular injuries. Perform a thorough eye examination (slit lamp and fluorescein staining for corneal injury, foreign body, and ruptured globe).

3. What is the treatment for ocular chemical burns?
Immediate copious irrigation for at least 20 minutes should be initiated before transport to the emergency department (ED). A Morgan Lens helps ensure adequate irrigation. Irrigate until the pH of the eye is neutral (7.0). Check pH by inserting a strip of nitrazine paper into the inferior fornix.

4. What chemical burns are most concerning and when is consultation indicated?
Alkali burns (fertilizers, drain cleaners, airbag propellants, cement and plaster components, and some detergents) are more dangerous, quickly penetrating ocular tissues through liquefactive necrosis. Acid burns (car batteries, refrigerants, and pool cleaners) cause coagulation necrosis with depth of penetration limited by eschar formation. Following irrigation, perform a slit lamp and fluorescein examination to evaluate for extent of corneal damage and perforation. If perforation is excluded, measure intraocular pressure, as pressures can spike following chemical injuries. Obtain emergent consultation for severe exposures (pH <2 or >12), severe injuries (corneal perforation or ischemia), and elevated intraocular pressure.

5. What is solar keratitis?
Solar keratitis (e.g., ultraviolet keratitis, flash burns, and snow blindness) is a corneal injury secondary to overexposure to ultraviolet light. Fluorescein staining shows multiple punctate lesions on the cornea, often with discrete horizontal lines marking the superior and inferior borders of eyelid protection. Treat with artificial tears, prophylactic topical antibiotics, and adequate systemic analgesia. Spontaneous resolution is expected in 12–24 hours.

6. List eight injuries that must be considered with blunt injury to the eye.
- Blow-out fractures (inferior and medial orbital wall fracture)
- Corneal abrasion
- Hyphema
- Traumatic iritis
- Lens dislocation
- Vitreous hemorrhage
- Retinal detachment
- Ruptured globe (rare after blunt injuries)

7. What is the most common eye injury seen in the ED?
The most common injury is corneal abrasion.

8. How is corneal abrasion diagnosed?
Corneal defects may be directly visualized on slit-lamp examination. Stain the anesthetized eye with fluorescein and illuminate with the ultraviolet light on the slit lamp; corneal defects fluoresce bright yellow-orange.

9. What is the treatment for a corneal abrasion?
Analgesia with oral analgesics or nonsteroidal anti-inflammatory eye drops is the mainstay of treatment. Given the risk of toxic keratitis with overuse, outpatient topical anesthesia is not recommended, although there are

some data supporting the safety of dilute drops for the first 24 hours. Other treatment includes cycloplegic agents to relieve ciliary spasm, update tetanus prophylaxis, and topical prophylactic antibiotic drops or ointment.

10. **What is the role of an eye patch in treatment of corneal abrasions?**
Patches do not increase healing and may promote infection. They do not prevent eye movement and should not be used.

11. **How does a contact lens–associated corneal abrasion differ from other causes of corneal trauma?**
Contact lens–associated corneal abrasions are more likely to have a bacterial superinfection, especially *Pseudomonas*. Avoid a patch and treat with topical antibiotics effective against *Pseudomonas* organisms (tobramycin or gentamicin). Instruct the patient to avoid contact lens use until symptoms resolve and they are cleared by an ophthalmologist. If unable to perform a slit-lamp examination, refer to an ophthalmologist to evaluate for ulcer.

12. **What is the most common location of an ocular foreign body?**
Foreign bodies are often lodged beneath the upper eyelid along the palpebral conjunctiva. Evert the upper eyelid to examine this area adequately.

13. **What is the proper treatment for a corneal foreign body?**
After applying topical anesthesia (e.g., proparacaine), remove nonembedded foreign bodies with a sterile, moist cotton swab. Remove embedded foreign bodies with the side (not tip) of a 27-gauge needle. Perform the procedure under direct visualization under slit lamp. Most metallic foreign bodies leave a residual rust ring that may require ophthalmologist consultation for removal.

14. **Why is a history of hammering or grinding metal on metal important?**
These mechanisms pose the risk that a small, high-velocity fragment can penetrate the globe with minimal or no physical findings. This injury, which can cause inflammation or infection weeks later, should be suspected in anyone with an eye complaint and concerning history. Perform a computed tomography (CT) scan of the globe and consult an ophthalmologist.

15. **What is the significance of traumatic eye pain not relieved with topical anesthesia?**
Complete symptomatic relief indicates a superficial injury involving only the cornea. Persistent pain after applying anesthetic drops is concerning for an intraocular cause (e.g., traumatic iritis or elevated intraocular pressure).

16. **What is a hyphema?**
A hyphema is a collection of blood in the anterior chamber, seen as a layering of red blood cells, and better identified when a patient is upright. Microhyphemas do not form a discrete layer and can be identified only with a slit-lamp examination.

17. **How is a hyphema treated?**
Most hyphemas are managed on an outpatient basis. Keep the patient upright as much as possible and initiate ophthalmologic consultation to arrange for prompt follow-up treatment. Complications include rebleeding, synechiae, increased intraocular pressure (particularly in patients with sickle cell disease), and corneal blood staining. Indications for ophthalmology consultation and inpatient management include hyphema involving >50% of the anterior chamber, intraocular pressure >30 mmHg, and a history of sickle cell disease or coagulopathy.

18. **What physical findings lead to the suspicion of a blow-out fracture?**
Classic findings of a blow-out fracture (inferior orbital wall fracture with herniation of globe contents into the maxillary sinus) are:
- decreased sensation over the inferior orbital rim, extending to the edge of the nose and ipsilateral upper gums and lip (inferior orbital nerve injury);
- enophthalmos (sunken appearance of the eye), which may be masked by edema; and
- paralysis or limitation of upward gaze (manifested as diplopia), resulting from entrapment of the inferior rectus muscle.

19. **What potentially life-threatening complication can result from entrapment of the inferior rectus muscle?**
The oculocardiac reflex, vagal stimulation from ciliary ganglion via the trigeminal nerve, can cause severe sinus bradycardia, heart block, hemodynamic collapse, asystole, and death. The reflex is exacerbated by strain on the entrapped inferior rectus muscle. Having the patient look down can relieve some of this stimulus. Atropine may be effective in cases of oculocardiac reflex–induced bradycardia. In severe cases, emergent operative intervention is indicated to release the entrapped muscle.

20. **What is traumatic mydriasis?**
Traumatic mydriasis is an efferent pupillary defect manifested by a dilated (and in most instances irregular) pupil, nonreactive to direct or consensual light. Given the risk for more serious eye injuries, a careful eye examination is required. Consider the possibility of uncal herniation secondary to intracranial injury in a patient with a decreased level of consciousness and a perfectly round, nonreactive, unilateral, dilated pupil. With a normal level of consciousness, this is most likely an isolated ocular injury or pre-existing finding.

21. When should penetration of the globe be suspected?
History of direct injury or a high-velocity mechanism (e.g., metal grinding) should raise suspicion for an open globe. The pupil is often misshapen, pointing in the direction of the penetration. With blunt globe trauma, a circumferential subconjunctival hemorrhage should raise concern for a posterior globe rupture, most commonly at the insertion site of the extraocular muscles (the thinnest part of the globe). The globe may appear soft because of decreased intraocular pressure. Diagnosis is confirmed with a CT scan of the orbit and/or with a positive Seidel's sign (stream of aqueous humor flowing out of the site of penetration on fluorescein examination). If globe rupture is suspected, do not test intraocular pressure, as applying pressure may promote extrusion of intraocular contents.

22. What is the treatment for an open globe?
Shield (not patch) the affected eye to avoid any pressure on the globe and extravasation of aqueous humor. Use analgesic and antiemetic agents to avoid increases in intraocular pressure. Administer prophylactic intravenous antibiotics, update the patient's tetanus status, and obtain emergent ophthalmology consultation.

23. What is the significance of a retro-orbital (retrobulbar) hematoma?
Bleeding behind the globe can lead to elevated orbital pressures, known as orbital compartment syndrome. Retinal ischemia can occur if orbital pressures exceed the perfusion pressure of the retina and optic nerve. Perform an emergent lateral canthotomy with cantholysis, releasing the inferior canthal ligament to temporarily relieve the elevated orbital pressure, preserving blood flow to the retina and optic nerve. Indications for lateral canthotomy include proptosis with decreased vision, intraocular pressure >40 mmHg, or a new afferent pupillary defect. Obtain an emergent ophthalmology evaluation.

24. What are the signs and symptoms of lens dislocation?
Traumatic lens dislocation, ectopia lentis, results from direct blunt force trauma to the eye, causing disruption of the zonular fibers that hold the lens in place. Patients may complain of eye pain, vision loss, and monocular diplopia. Iridodonesis, or trembling of the iris, is a common physical finding. The diagnosis is confirmed using slit lamp, ocular ultrasound, or CT imaging, and an ophthalmology consultation is indicated.

25. When should traumatic retinal detachment be suspected?
Traumatic retinal detachment can occur with rapid deceleration injuries to the head, causing a retinal tear with subsequent migration of fluid under the retina. Patients report painless vision loss in a curtain-like distribution. Ocular ultrasound can be useful in confirming the diagnosis once globe penetration has been excluded.

26. List traumatic eye injuries that require immediate ophthalmologic consultation.
- Severe chemical burns of the eye
- Retro-orbital hematoma causing orbital compartment syndrome
- Inferior orbital wall fracture with entrapment and vagal symptoms (bradycardia, heart block, severe nausea)
- Perforation of the globe or cornea
- Lacerations involving the lid margin, tarsal plate, or tear duct

27. Name two ophthalmologic injuries that require urgent ophthalmologic consultation (within 12–24 hours).
- Traumatic hyphema
- Blow-out fracture

KEY POINTS: OPHTHALMOLOGIC EMERGENCIES

1. Preservation of vision in a chemical burn is directly related to the time from exposure to initiation of irrigation; initiate irrigation on patient contact.
2. Never put a patch on a patient with a contact lens–related eye injury; a patch provides a perfect environment for bacterial proliferation. Treat corneal injuries in contact lens wearers with a topical antipseudomonal agent.
3. Diplopia on upward gaze is the hallmark of a blow-out fracture with entrapment of the inferior rectus muscle.

BIBLIOGRAPHY

Blice JP. Ocular injuries, triage, and management in maxillofacial trauma. *Atlas Oral Maxillofacial Surg Clin North Am.* 2013;21:97–103.
Fahling JM, McKenzie LK. Oculocardiac reflex as a result of intraorbital trauma. *J Emerg Med.* 2017;52(4):557–558.
McInnes G, Howes D. Lateral canthotomy and cantholysis: a simple, vision-saving procedure. *CJEM.* 2004;4:49–52.
Quinn SM, Kwartz J. Emergency management of contact lens associated corneal abrasions. *Emerg Med J.* 2004;21:755.
Romaniuk VM. Ocular trauma and other catastrophes. *Emerg Med Clin N Am.* 2013;31:399–411.
Turner A, Rabiu M. Patching for corneal abrasion. *Cochrane Database Syst Rev.* 2006;2:264–270.

CHAPTER 87

NECK TRAUMA

Spencer Tomberg, MD, MA

1. Why is neck trauma a complicated topic?

The neck is the conduit for structures with vital tasks: bringing blood to the brain, air to lungs, nerves to the body, and nutrition to the thorax. These structures can be injured by both blunt and penetrating trauma. The mobility of the neck makes it vulnerable to shear and rotational forces. Some neck injuries can be easily accessed by a surgeon; others are hidden behind bony structures. All of these factors make neck trauma complex.

2. What common findings indicate significant neck injury?

Potentially dangerous signs of injury are broken up into soft and hard signs. The presence of a hard sign is an indication for emergent surgical intervention. Soft signs can be indicators of serious injury and must be thoroughly evaluated (Table 87.1).

3. What are the most urgent concerns in the initial management of neck trauma?

Start with the ABCs:
- *Airway.* Airway management can be straightforward or extremely complex, as outlined in Question 4.
- *Breathing.* Diaphragm function can be compromised by damage to the phrenic nerve or spinal cord. Zone I trauma can cause a pneumothorax. Bubbling wounds should be covered with a petroleum jelly–infused gauze to prevent an air embolism.
- *Circulation.* Bleeding can be severe. Hematomas can expand and compress the airway or other vascular structures. Bleeding should be controlled with localized pressure: apply compression with two or three fingers. If bleeding persists, a Foley catheter inserted into the wound can be used to tamponade bleeding by gently inflating the balloon.
- *Disability.* In addition to an initial neurologic examination, establish if a projectile's path crossed the spine, if there was a blunt mechanism of injury, and if there are vascular or peripheral nerve injuries.
- *Exposure.* All clothing should be removed for evaluation of other occult injuries.

4. What makes airway management especially challenging in patients with neck trauma?

Trauma to the neck poses challenges to oxygenation, ventilation, and performance of cricothyrotomy. The airway can be distorted by an expanding hematoma, foreign bodies in the neck, or from direct trauma to the airway. Some important considerations include:
- If a cricothyrotomy is required and an incision is made, any tamponading force provided by the neck soft tissue is released, which can worsen bleeding and compromise the visual field for the procedure. A hematoma over the cricothyroid membrane is a contraindication to performing a cricothyrotomy, because of the risk of converting a partial cricotracheal separation into a complete separation. In this case, a tracheostomy is the rescue airway method of choice.
- Penetrating trauma can cause false lumens in the neck, which are dangerous if you place an endotracheal (ET) tube into one, but think it is in the trachea. Confirm ET intubation in penetrating neck trauma by a secondary method (bronchoscopy).
- If the trachea is transected and the lumen of the trachea is visible on the neck, intubation can be performed directly into the wound/trachea (confirm that the ET tube is not placed in a false lumen).
- Trauma to the upper airway can cause bleeding and swelling that limits visualization of epiglottis or vocal cords. In these circumstances, consider an early transition to a cricothyrotomy.
- Any patient with blunt cervical trauma will need to remain in a c-collar. This limits cervical motion during intubation.

5. Who should be intubated?

Patients with the following characteristics need emergent intubation:
- Airway obstruction
- Severe injuries with impending obstruction
- Inability to maintain adequate ventilation
- Inability to maintain oxygen saturations of 90% despite supplemental oxygen;
- Spinal cord injuries: generally, for any complete injury at or above C5, and for partial injuries with signs of respiratory distress
- Combative patients: may have concomitant head injury
- Anticipated decline in clinical course

Table 87.1 Hard and Soft Signs of Penetrating Neck Injuries	
HARD SIGNS	**SOFT SIGNS**
Airway compromise/stridor	Significant bleeding on the scene of the injury
Expanding or pulsatile hematoma	Stable hematoma
Massive subcutaneous emphysema or air bubbling out of the wound	Mild subcutaneous emphysema
Active bleeding	Mild dysphasia
Shock	Mild dysphonia
Neurologic deficit	Neck tenderness
Hematemesis	
Audible bruit or palpable thrill	

6. **What is the preferred method to secure the airway?**
   Rapid-sequence intubation (RSI) with oral tracheal intubation should be the initial airway approach in patients who have no damage to, and minimal distortion of, their airway. Video laryngoscopy has been shown to be most advantageous in patients with a predicted difficult airway. The advantage of direct laryngoscopy (DL) is that it does not rely on a camera that can be obscured by blood or vomit in the airway. Choose the tool that fits the patient and the circumstances best. Etomidate and ketamine are the induction agents of choice, as they are both hemodynamically stable agents. Succinylcholine is the paralytic of choice in trauma: it is a safe and reliable drug with few contraindications. In patients with prolonged immobilization, muscular dystrophy, or kidney disease, rocuronium can be used as a substitute. In situations where it is anticipated that bag-mask-ventilation will be difficult, an awake intubation can be attempted, combining a disassociating dose of ketamine with medications to numb the oral pharynx and base of the tongue. This allows intubation while the patient is still breathing. Laryngeal mask airway (LMA) and Combitubes are not recommended if the injury involves the upper airway.

7. **When do you immobilize the cervical spine in neck trauma?**
   Indications for c-spine immobilization in blunt trauma include posterior neck tenderness, pain with motion of the neck, or focal neurologic findings on examination. Since spinal injury is rare in penetrating neck trauma, only place a c-collar in the setting of obtundation, altered mental status, or focal neurologic findings. A c-collar can easily obscure other important injuries. If the patient is presenting with a c-collar in place, make sure to examine the neck by looking under the collar. Take collars off as soon as it is clinically safe.

8. **Penetration of what muscle defines a penetrating neck injury?**
   The platysma muscle. If it is not penetrated, stitch up the wound and you're done.

9. **What are the three anatomic zones of the neck?**
   - Zone I is from the clavicles to below the cricoid cartilage.
   - Zone II extends from the cricoid cartilage to the angle of the mandible.
   - Zone III extends from the angle of the mandible to the base of the skull.
       Fig. 87.1 illustrates the zones of the neck.

10. **How are Zone I injuries managed?**
    Because it is difficult to evaluate injuries in Zone I, all these injuries should receive computed tomography angiography (CTA). Zone I injuries carry a high mortality rate, and patients are frequently initially asymptomatic. The chest wall covers the inferior aspect of Zone I, which makes it challenging to treat these injuries surgically.

11. **What are the current recommendations for the management of Zone II injuries?**
    This is the most surgically accessible zone of the neck. In the 1940s, surgeons began exploring all Zone II penetrating neck injuries. This led to significant reductions in mortality, but the negative exploration rate was 50%. As imaging technology advanced, the treatment of Zone II injuries has been refined. This has decreased the negative exploration rate to 30%, while retaining the sensitivity to pick up morbid injuries. Fig. 87.2 details the current selective approach to the management of penetrating neck injuries. One exception to the rules is transcervical gunshot wounds (GSWs), as they are frequently associated with severe injuries to multiple zones of the neck. Transcervical GSWs mandate surgical exploration, coupled with CTA to evaluate for concomitant Zone I or Zone III injuries.

12. **What are the current recommendations for the management of Zone III injuries?**
    It is also difficult to surgically access Zone III, and imaging is indicated prior to intervention. Zone III is where the majority of blunt cerebrovascular injuries occur. Some Zone III injuries are best treated by endovascular intervention.

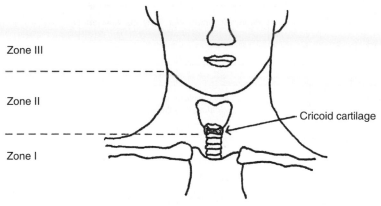

Zone III

Zone II

Cricoid cartilage

Zone I

Fig. 87.1 Zones of the neck.

13. **What is the current algorithm for the workup of penetrating neck trauma?**
    The Western Trauma Association algorithm for managing penetrating neck trauma is shown in Fig. 87.2.

14. **How are vascular injuries from penetrating neck trauma surgically managed?**
    All carotid injuries (except for small pseudoaneurysms without neurologic injuries and small intimal tears) are surgically explored and treated with ligation of the vessel, reconstruction of the vessel, or monitoring of an occluded vessel. Vertebral injuries are generally managed with endovascular repair or observation.

15. **Which diagnostic studies are important in suspected laryngeal injuries?**
    - Flexible laryngoscopy provides information about the integrity of the cartilaginous framework and the function of the vocal cords.
    - Computed tomography (CT) scans can identify the location and extent of laryngeal fractures.
    - Soft-tissue x-rays may show a fractured larynx, subcutaneous air, or prevertebral air.

16. **What are the signs and symptoms that raise concern for an esophageal injury?**
    Approximately 80% of patients with an esophageal injury will have one of the following symptoms: dysphagia, odynophagia, drooling, or hematemesis. Examination findings include neck crepitus or a sucking neck wound.

17. **Which diagnostic studies are important in suspected esophageal injuries?**
    Esophageal injuries are challenging because they frequently have no associated physical examination findings, and if not addressed in the first 24 hours, morbidity significantly increases. Esophagography (contrasted swallow study) and esophagoscopy are combined to evaluate possible esophageal injuries. A positive esophagography is an indication for surgical repair. When esophagography is followed by esophagoscopy, the combined sensitivity for detecting esophageal injury is close to 100%. CT scans, neck x-rays, and chest x-rays may show signs of injury, but are not reliable for ruling out esophageal injuries. CT scans miss up to 50% of clinically important injuries.

18. **What are the signs and symptoms of blunt carotid or vertebral artery trauma?**
    Blunt cerebrovascular injuries (BCVIs) are relatively uncommon (~1% of blunt trauma patients), but create significant morbidity and mortality. The major concern for these injuries is embolic stroke, vessel transection, or vessel occlusion. Neurologic symptoms most frequently occur 12–24 hours after the initial injury, but can present 1 week after the injury. Carotid artery injury signs and symptoms include neck hematoma, audible bruit, Horner syndrome, transient ischemic attack, aphasia, or hemiparesis. Vertebral artery injury signs and symptoms include ataxia, vertigo, nystagmus, hemiparesis, dysarthria, and diplopia.

19. **What are the indications for imaging to evaluate for vascular injury in patients with blunt cervical trauma?**
    The Modified Denver Criteria (updated in 2016) for screening for BCVI recommend imaging patients with the following conditions (this is a long list, and it constantly expands to keep sensitivity close to 100%):
    - Severe cervical hyperextension and rotation, or hyperflexion injury
    - Focal neurologic deficits
    - Neurologic examination that does not fit the injury findings on CT scan
    - High-energy trauma with the following injuries:
      - Le Fort II or III midface fracture
      - Mandible fracture
      - Basilar skull fracture/complex skull fracture/occipital condyle fracture

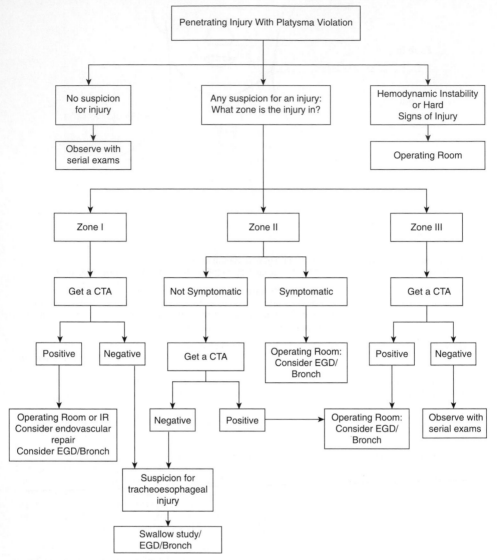

Fig. 87.2 Penetrating neck trauma evaluation algorithm. *CTA,* Computed tomography angiography; *EGD,* esophagogastroduodenoscopy; *IR,* interventional radiology. (Adapted from westerntrauma.org.)

- Closed head injury with Glasgow Coma Scale (GCS) score less than 6
- Any level cervical spine fracture, ligamentous injury, or subluxation
- Near-hanging incident with anoxic brain injury
- Large anterior neck soft-tissue injury or hematoma
- Motor vehicle collision (MVC) with a seatbelt sign across the neck, associated with swelling, pain, or altered mentation
- Traumatic brain injury and a thoracic injury
- Stroke noted on secondary CT scan
- Expanding cervical hematoma
- Scalp degloving
- Thoracic vascular injury
- Blunt cardiac rupture
- Any upper rib fracture

Table 87.2 Denver Grading Scale for Blunt Cerebrovascular Injuries (BCVIs)

GRADE	RADIOGRAPHICAL FINDINGS	TREATMENT
Grade I	Arteriographic appearance of irregularity of the vessel wall or a dissection/intramural hematoma with less than 25% luminal stenosis	Consider systemic anticoagulation
Grade II	Intraluminal thrombus or raised intimal flap is visualized, or dissection/intramural hematoma with 25% or more luminal narrowing	Systemic anticoagulation (initiated 24 hours after hemostasis from other injuries is confirmed), and consideration of surgical or endovascular repair
Grade III	Pseudoaneurysm	Surgical or endovascular repair
Grade IV	Vessel occlusion	Systemic anticoagulation (initiated 24 hours after hemostasis from other injuries is confirmed)
Grade V	Transection with free extravasation	Surgical treatment

20. **What diagnostic testing is preferred in the detection of BCVIs?**
   Angiography or CTA (at least 16 slice) are the studies of choice. The advantage of CTA is that it is readily available in most hospitals and can significantly reduce the time to diagnose injuries. Magnetic resonance angiography (MRA) has limited utility, as some studies have found it to have a sensitivity of 50%. Ultrasound may be useful in Zone II injuries, but is limited in Zone I and Zone III injuries (where the majority of BCVI occur), because of interference from surrounding bony structures.

21. **What is the appropriate management of BCVIs?**
   Blunt carotid injuries are graded and treated according to the Denver Grading Scale (Table 87.2). For patients with an ischemic stroke after BCVI, antiplatelet or anticoagulation therapy should be continued for 3–6 months. Many physicians repeat CT angiography to confirm recanalization of the vessel before stopping anticoagulation.

22. **How are strangulation and hanging injuries different from other blunt neck trauma?**
   Strangulation causes death by restricting jugular venous return, resulting in loss of consciousness. In hanging injuries, once the patient is unconscious, they fall into the ligature, obstructing the airway with more force. Choking generally delivers greater forces and can cause direct occlusion and damage to the carotid arteries.

KEY POINTS: MANAGEMENT OF NECK TRAUMA

1. Secure the airway early for anticipated clinical deterioration.
2. RSI with DL or video laryngoscopy are the preferred initial airway management options.
3. Have plans for surgical airway, which may be cricothyrotomy or tracheostomy, while attempting oral tracheal intubation.
4. Zone II injuries have a defined treatment algorithm based on physical examination and radiographic findings. All Zone I and Zone III injuries should have a CTA.
5. Patients with continued suspicion for occult injury after a negative CTA should undergo ancillary tests, including conventional angiogram, esophagoscopy/esophagography, or laryngoscopy.
6. BVCIs are rare, but potentially devastating injuries, and patients with risk factors should be evaluated by CTA.

BIBLIOGRAPHY

Biffl WL, Cothren CC, Moore EE, et al. Western Trauma Association critical decisions in trauma: screening for and treatment of blunt cerebrovascular injuries. *J Trauma*. 2009;67:1150–1153.
Bromberg WJ, Collier BC, Diebel LN, et al. Blunt cerebrovascular injury practice management guidelines: the Eastern Association for the Surgery of Trauma. *J Trauma*. 2010;68:471–477.
Deshaies EM, Nair AK, Boulos AS, et al. Blunt traumatic injuries to the carotid and vertebral arteries of the neck and skull base. *Contemp Neurosurg*. 2008;30:1–6.
Lewis SR, Butler AR, Smith AF, et al. Videolaryngoscopy versus direct laryngoscopy for adult patients requiring tracheal intubation: a Cochrane Systematic Review. *Br J Anaesth*. 2017;119:369–383.
Nagpal P, Bathla G, Skeete D, et al. Blunt cerebrovascular injuries: advances in screening, imaging, and management trends. *AJNR Am J Neuroradiol*. 2018;39:406–414.
Tisherman SA, Bokhari F, Collier B, et al. Clinical practice guideline: penetrating zone II neck trauma. *J Trauma*. 2008;64:1392–1405.
Upchurch CP, Grijalva CG, Russ S, et al. Comparison of etomidate and ketamine for induction during rapid sequence intubation of adult trauma patients. *Ann Emerg Med*. 2017;69:24–33.e2.

CHAPTER 88

CHEST TRAUMA

Anthony W. Bacon, MD and Eric M. Campion, MD

1. What is the initial approach to the patient with chest trauma?
The initial approach to the patient with chest trauma should follow standard Advanced Trauma Life Support (ATLS) protocol, and includes assessing the airway, breathing, circulation, disability, and exposure (see Chapter 82).

2. What is the proper way to examine the chest during the trauma survey?
Remember to look, listen, and feel.
- *Look (inspect).* Examine the entire chest, including the axillae and back. Roll patients with penetrating injuries early to identify any life-threatening wounds on the back. Gunshot or stab wounds should be identified, and bruises or lacerations noted. Abnormal chest rise or paradoxical movements may indicate rib fractures or a flail segment.
- *Listen (auscultate).* The examiner should listen for bilateral breath sounds. Decreased or absent breath sounds can indicate a pneumothorax, hemothorax, or diaphragm injury.
- *Feel (palpate).* Palpate the chest, specifically looking for any subcutaneous emphysema (potentially an indication of underlying pneumothorax), fractures, or tenderness. The patient should be rolled, using in-line cervical spine stabilization as necessary, and the back and thoracic spine inspected and palpated.

3. What are the immediate threats to life after thoracic trauma, and how are they identified?
The immediate threats to life include airway obstruction, tension pneumothorax, open pneumothorax, flail chest, massive hemothorax, large airway injury, and cardiac tamponade. Airway obstruction, tension pneumothorax, open pneumothorax, and severe flail chest are diagnosed with physical examination. Chest radiography can diagnose massive hemothorax and flail chest. Large airway injury presents with a profound air leak upon treatment of pneumothorax. Definitive diagnosis is made by bronchoscopy or at the time of surgery. The pericardial view of the focused assessment with sonography for trauma (FAST) can diagnose cardiac tamponade.

4. Which major organs may be injured in blunt or penetrating chest trauma?
- Lungs and tracheobronchial tree
- Heart and great vessels (aorta, vena cava, and pulmonary, axillary, and subclavian vessels)
- Esophagus, diaphragm, and thoracic duct
- Chest wall structures, including the ribs, clavicles, scapulae, sternum, and thoracic spine

KEY POINTS: INITIAL ASSESSMENT CHEST TRAUMA

1. Evaluation of thoracic trauma begins with assessment of the airway, breathing, circulation, and disability, and exposure.
2. To fully assess the chest, one must look, listen, and feel.
3. Immediate threats to life that must be identified and treated in the primary survey include airway obstruction, tension pneumothorax, open pneumothorax, flail chest, massive hemothorax, and cardiac tamponade.

5. What is a pneumothorax?
A pneumothorax is air in the pleural space. It is caused by any disruption of the visceral or parietal pleura that allows air into the pleural space via the tracheobronchial tree, lung parenchyma, mediastinum, or chest wall.

6. What are the signs and symptoms of a pneumothorax?
Signs and symptoms of a pneumothorax include shortness of breath, chest pain, hypoxia, tachypnea, tachycardia, diminished breath sounds on the affected side, and subcutaneous emphysema. In some cases, the patient may be asymptomatic.

7. How is a pneumothorax diagnosed?
A pneumothorax is most commonly diagnosed with a chest radiograph as an adjunct to the primary and secondary survey. Computed tomography (CT) scan may diagnose smaller or occult pneumothoraces not appreciated on plain films. Ultrasonography to assess for pneumothorax has been shown to be useful in skilled hands (see Chapters 5 and 82).

8. **How do I treat a pneumothorax?**
   A pneumothorax is treated with tube thoracostomy. Smaller bore chest tubes are adequate for the treatment of a pneumothorax without hemothorax. Small, asymptomatic pneumothoraces may be observed with no intervention. In cases where no intervention is made, follow-up imaging is prudent to ensure stability or resolution of the pneumothorax.

9. **What is a tension pneumothorax?**
   A tension pneumothorax results from the accumulation of pressurized air in the pleural space, as with a sucking wound that closes on expiration. When pressure reaches a critical level, displacement of the heart impairs venous return to the right atrium, leading to decreased pre-load, decreased cardiac output, and imminent cardiovascular collapse.

10. **What are the possible signs and symptoms of a tension pneumothorax?**
    All of the signs of a simple pneumothorax may be present; however, classic signs of a tension pneumothorax include tachycardia, distended neck veins, hypotension, tracheal deviation (a late sign), and cardiovascular collapse.

11. **How should a tension pneumothorax be diagnosed?**
    A tension pneumothorax is a life-threatening emergency and should be diagnosed clinically, by recognizing the above signs and symptoms.

12. **How is a tension pneumothorax treated?**
    It is treated with immediate decompression of the pleural space, which is both diagnostic (with a positive rush of air) and therapeutic. Temporary needle decompression with a large-bore needle is performed in the second or third intercostal space anteriorly, followed by tube thoracostomy. Depending on the setting and availability of equipment, a rapidly placed chest tube may also be an appropriate first choice. In the event of cardiovascular collapse, entering the pleural space sharply with a scalpel can be life-saving.

KEY POINTS: TENSION PNEUMOTHORAX

1. Tension pneumothorax is a clinical diagnosis.
2. Tension pneumothorax presents with absent breath sounds, tachycardia, hypotension, and distended neck veins.
3. Treatment is immediate decompression with a large-bore needle, chest tube, or scalpel.

13. **What is an open pneumothorax, and how is it diagnosed?**
    Also known as a sucking chest wound, an open pneumothorax is an open communication between the pleural space and the atmosphere. An open pneumothorax is an immediate threat to life, compromising oxygenation and ventilation. It is diagnosed on physical examination, and classically requires a wound of at least three-quarters the size of the trachea.

14. **How should an open pneumothorax be treated?**
    In the prehospital setting, emergency medical services (EMS) uses a three-sided, nonocclusive dressing. This prevents the accumulation of pressure in the pleural space and the development of a tension pneumothorax, while improving respiratory dynamics. Purpose-made, vented chest seals may also be used. Upon arrival in the hospital, a chest tube is placed, and the open wound covered with an occlusive dressing.

15. **What is a hemothorax, and how is it diagnosed?**
    A hemothorax is blood in the pleural space. The blood may come from a variety of sources, including trauma to the lung, intrathoracic blood vessels, or heart. A hemothorax is commonly diagnosed with chest radiography or CT scan. Signs and symptoms are similar to those of pneumothorax, including shortness of breath, hypoxia, respiratory compromise, and decreased breath sounds. Large hemothoraces may cause hypotension.

16. **What is the treatment of hemothorax?**
    For the hemodynamically stable patient, tube thoracostomy drainage is the standard treatment. Though there remains some debate as to exactly how large a hemothorax should be to prompt drainage, all moderate to large hemothoraces should be drained. Some advocate that any hemothorax seen on a chest radiograph should be drained. Traditionally, a large-bore ($\geq$32 Fr) chest tube has been used, but recent data suggest that a smaller tube is adequate. For the hemodynamically unstable patient, drainage and volume resuscitation remains the first step in treatment, followed by operative hemorrhage control.

17. **What should I do if my chest tube does not completely drain the hemothorax?**
    While in the past a second chest tube was placed to facilitate evacuation, followed by thoracoscopic washout if adequate evacuation still was not obtained, currently, video-assisted thoracoscopic evacuation has shown improved efficacy over additional chest tubes.

18. **What is a massive hemothorax?**

A massive hemothorax occurs when more than 1500 mL of blood, or one-third of a patient's blood volume, accumulates in the chest. Patients with massive hemothoraces usually show signs of respiratory compromise and hemorrhagic shock. Treatment consists of tube thoracostomy and rapid resuscitation with crystalloid solutions and blood products, followed by definitive operative control of hemorrhage.

19. **How much ongoing blood loss out of the chest tube is an indication for operative exploration?**

Any hemodynamically unstable patient with ongoing chest hemorrhage should be emergently taken to the operating room. In the hemodynamically stable patient having sustained blunt trauma, immediate drainage of 1500 mL of blood with ongoing bleeding is an indication for operative intervention. For penetrating trauma, surgical intervention is indicated after immediate drainage of 1000 mL of blood with ongoing bleeding. Finally, drainage greater than 200 mL/h of gross blood for more than 2 hours is an indication for exploration, mechanism of injury notwithstanding.

20. **What other fluids may fill the pleural space after trauma?**

The most common is serous fluid, although almost any fluid can be present. Other rare examples include chyle, pancreatic fluid, and bile.

21. **What is the best management of an asymptomatic, hemodynamically stable patient after penetrating thoracic trauma with no pneumothorax or hemothorax on initial chest radiography?**

Observe the patient in the emergency department (ED). If no other traumatic injuries are identified, obtain a chest radiograph at 3–6 hours and, if still normal, the patient may be discharged home.

22. **What is a pulmonary contusion, and how is it diagnosed?**

A pulmonary contusion is an injury to the lung parenchyma that causes accumulation of blood and fluid in the macro- and microscopic airspaces. Severity may range from asymptomatic to fulminant respiratory failure. Signs and symptoms include chest pain, shortness of breath, hypoxia, and hemoptysis. Diagnosis is made with a chest radiograph or CT scan. A pulmonary contusion appears as a ground-glass infiltrate or consolidation, not confined to anatomic divisions of the lung. It is common for a pulmonary contusion to "blossom" 24–48 hours after injury, resulting in worsening respiratory status. A pulmonary contusion should be suspected after almost any blunt chest trauma, and is commonly associated with rib fractures and especially with flail segments.

23. **How is a pulmonary contusion managed?**

Observation, continuous pulse oximetry, and expectant management are imperative, as respiratory status may progressively worsen. Pain control, supplemental oxygen, and pulmonary toilet are the mainstays of therapy. Mechanical ventilatory support may be required in severe cases.

24. **What are the signs and symptoms of an intrathoracic tracheobronchial tree injury?**

Patients with injury to the tracheobronchial tree typically present with shortness of breath, hypoxia, persistent pneumothorax despite tube thoracostomy, and a persistent air leak through the chest tube. Small injuries are easily missed and can present in a delayed fashion as pneumonia, pulmonary abscess, mediastinitis, or sepsis.

25. **How are tracheobronchial tree injuries diagnosed and treated?**

Tracheobronchial tree injuries are diagnosed via bronchoscopy or upon surgical exploration, where injuries most commonly occur on the right, within 2.5 cm of the carina. Suggestive radiographic findings include tracheal and bronchial extraluminal air, the fallen lung sign, pneumomediastinum, and subcutaneous emphysema. While imaging studies may indicate a high likelihood of injury, bronchoscopic confirmation is often necessary. Small injuries may be observed. Large injuries require operative repair.

26. **What are the signs and symptoms of cardiac tamponade?**

Cardiac tamponade occurs when the pericardial sac fills with fluid or blood. In its most severe form, cardiac tamponade can cause cardiogenic shock and hemodynamic collapse. Early signs of tamponade include tachycardia, *pulsus paradoxus*, and elevated jugular venous pressure. *Beck's triad* is the combination of muffled heart sounds, jugular venous distention, and hypotension, and is suggestive of cardiac tamponade.

27. **How can cardiac tamponade be diagnosed?**

Cardiac tamponade can be quickly diagnosed in the ED using the FAST examination subxiphoid or transthoracic windows. This test can be quickly repeated with any signs of decompensation and has high sensitivity and specificity.

28. **How is cardiac tamponade treated?**

A positive FAST examination should prompt emergent transfer for operative intervention. Pericardiocentesis is not definitive treatment of the tamponade, but can be a bridge to operative repair. When possible, intubation should be delayed until the patient is prepped and draped in the operating room, as cardiovascular collapse on induction is likely. Tamponade resulting in cardiac arrest is an indication for resuscitative thoracotomy and pericardiotomy.

KEY POINTS: TRAUMATIC CARDIAC TAMPONADE

1. Cardiac tamponade occurs when the pericardial sac fills with blood.
2. Signs and symptoms include dyspnea, tachycardia, elevated jugular venous pressure, and hypotension.
3. Diagnosis can be made quickly at the bedside with the FAST examination.
4. Optimal treatment is operative decompression.

29. **What is blunt cardiac injury (BCI)?**

    BCI occurs when blunt force to the chest results in altered structure or function of the heart. BCI is a spectrum of disease that can include cardiac contusion, coronary artery thrombosis, cardiac rupture, valvular disruption, pericardial rupture, and *commotio cordis* (ventricular tachycardia or fibrillation after a sudden blow to the chest). Clinically, these entities may manifest as chest pain, electrocardiographic changes, or a new dysrhythmia.

30. **What is the appropriate management for suspected BCI?**

    An electrocardiogram (ECG) should be performed on any patient with suspected BCI. The most common ECG findings after BCI are sinus tachycardia or premature contractions. ECG alone does not rule out BCI. However, a normal ECG combined with a normal troponin has a negative predictive value of 100%. If an ECG shows a new dysrhythmia, new heart block, or ischemic changes, the patient should be admitted for continuous cardiac monitoring. Echocardiography (ECHO) should be performed on any symptomatic patient or any patient with any ischemic changes on ECG, new dysrhythmias, or hypotension.

31. **When should a penetrating cardiac injury be suspected, and how is it diagnosed?**

    A penetrating cardiac injury should be suspected with any penetrating injury in proximity to the heart. If the patient is stable, a FAST examination should be performed to evaluate for pericardial fluid. If positive, the patient should undergo operative exploration. A chest radiograph may demonstrate a hemothorax from a cardiac injury that is decompressing into the thorax. Hemodynamic instability should initiate emergent transportation to the operating room for diagnosis and definitive treatment.

32. **How does the management of a suspected transmediastinal gunshot wound differ in a hemodynamically stable patient from the management of an unstable patient?**

    Any patient with a missile trajectory that crosses the midline should be evaluated for potential injury to any of the mediastinal structures.

    - In the hemodynamically stable patient, the primary and secondary surveys are completed and interventions (e.g., tube thoracostomy) performed as needed. Imaging should include a FAST examination, chest radiography with radiolucent markers over wounds to help identify trajectory, and a thoracic CT scan with intravenous (IV) contrast. Depending on missile trajectory, diagnostic adjuncts may include angiography, bronchoscopy, esophagoscopy, or esophagography as indicated.
    - An unstable patient with a suspected transmediastinal gunshot wound should be taken emergently to the operating room. Management in the trauma bay should be limited to only immediate life-saving interventions, such as tube thoracostomy. Delays in transport to the operating room should be minimized. A resuscitative thoracotomy should be performed for a loss of vital signs within 15 minutes of arrival.

33. **What is blunt aortic injury, and how does it occur?**

    Blunt aortic injury occurs when shear, torsion, or compressive forces are applied to the thorax with transmission to the aorta. This occurs most commonly after a large deceleration following a motor vehicle collision. Tears in the intima or media can lead to dissection or pseudoaneurysm, predisposing the aorta to rupture. Aortic rupture is a common cause of death after blunt thoracic trauma prior to arrival in the ED.

34. **At which anatomic location is the aorta most commonly injured after blunt trauma?**

    Blunt aortic injury occurs in areas where the aorta is fixed: the aortic root, the ligamentum arteriosum, and at the diaphragmatic hiatus. The most common location for blunt aortic injury is at the ligamentum arteriosum, just distal to the takeoff of the left subclavian artery.

35. **How do blunt aortic injuries present, and how are they diagnosed?**

    Blunt aortic injuries are often clinically occult, in that the patient may be asymptomatic with no external signs of trauma. Chest pain, shortness of breath, or back pain may be present. Physical examination may reveal tenderness or ecchymosis over the sternum or anterior ribs. An abnormal upper extremity arterial–arterial blood pressure gradient may be present. With the appropriate mechanism of injury, a high index of suspicion is paramount to timely diagnosis.

36. **Which modalities are used to diagnose blunt aortic injury, and what are the radiographic findings?**

    Chest radiography and CT angiography (CTA) are first-line imaging modalities in the workup of any patient with high-mechanism blunt chest trauma. Findings on chest radiography can include a widened mediastinum, an obscured aortic knob, or hemothorax, but these findings are not always present. CTA findings include intravascular contrast extravasation, intimal flap or dissection, pseudoaneurysm, aortic thrombus, and periaortic hematoma. A transthoracic echocardiogram is often a confirmatory adjunct.

37. How are blunt aortic injuries treated?
Repair with endovascular or open surgical techniques is standard. Until definitive repair can be performed, maintain strict hemodynamic control (heart rate <100 bpm and systolic blood pressure <100 mmHg) with short-acting agents such as esmolol or nicardipine.

38. How do penetrating injuries to the great vessels present?
The great vessels include the aorta, subclavian, axillary, and pulmonary arteries and veins, and the superior and inferior vena cavae. Hard signs of vascular injury, prompting emergent repair, include pulsatile bleeding, an expanding hematoma, absent distal pulses, a cold limb, or cardiovascular collapse. Hemoptysis, hemothorax, cardiac tamponade, or hemoperitoneum may be present. Great vessel injuries can present with exsanguinating hemorrhage and loss of vital signs. In these cases, resuscitative thoracotomy is indicated for direct vessel control.

39. How are great vessel injuries evaluated, and what is the treatment?
In stable patients, CTA is the optimal study to evaluate great vessel injuries. CTA may demonstrate contrast extravasation, an intimal flap, dissection, pseudoaneurysm, or hematoma. Great vessel injuries may be treated with endovascular or open operative techniques. Unstable patients should be taken directly to the operating room for definitive surgical repair.

40. What are the goals of ED resuscitative thoracotomy?
A resuscitative thoracotomy is a life-saving procedure that is performed when a patient loses vital signs after trauma. Goals of resuscitative thoracotomy include:
- Decompress a tamponade.
- Gain control of intrathoracic hemorrhage.
- Perform effective cardiac massage.
- Maintain cerebral perfusion pressure with aortic occlusion distal to the subclavian arteries.
- Temporarily control intraabdominal hemorrhage with thoracic aortic occlusion.

41. What are the contraindications for ED resuscitative thoracotomy?
The contraindications for ED resuscitative thoracotomy include:
- Prehospital cardiopulmonary resuscitation exceeding 10 minutes after blunt trauma with no signs of life.
- Prehospital cardiopulmonary resuscitation exceeding 15 minutes after penetrating trauma with no signs of life.
- Isolated penetrating trauma to the head with no signs of life.

42. Which is the more common mechanism for thoracic esophageal injury: blunt or penetrating?
Penetrating injury more commonly causes esophageal injury. Blunt injury to the esophagus is rare, likely due to its relatively protected location in the posterior mediastinum.

43. What are the signs and symptoms of esophageal injury and rupture?
Specific symptoms of esophageal injury are difficult to ascribe. Commonly, patients with esophageal injury have multiple injuries and may be obtunded. However, chest pain is a common symptom. Signs of inflammation and extraluminal air around the esophagus may be seen on cross-sectional imaging. Pleural effusions may be present. With an appropriate mechanism, pneumomediastinum is suggestive and should be further investigated. Following penetrating trauma, a mediastinal trajectory should raise the index of suspicion for esophageal injury. A chest tube placed for pneumothorax or hemothorax may drain enteric contents.

44. How should a suspected thoracic esophageal injury be investigated?
Esophageal injury is best evaluated with contrast imaging via a diatrizoate (Gastrografin) swallow study. If this study is normal, but suspicion persists, repeat imaging using thin barium may be performed. CT imaging findings suggestive of injury include pneumomediastinum, periesophageal air, and a new pleural effusion, and should prompt more sensitive and specific imaging. If a patient must go to the operating room emergently, direct esophagoscopy can be performed, but should not replace a formal swallow study.

45. What is the treatment of esophageal injury?
The treatment of esophageal injury is drainage and prompt surgical repair with open, thoracoscopic or endoscopic techniques. Initial source control is obtained through wide drainage via open or percutaneous tube thoracostomy, with or without ultrasound guidance. Definitive treatment consists of primary repair or resection and reconstruction using open thoracotomy or minimally invasive thoracoscopic surgery. Endoscopic stenting can be used as a temporizing measure or, in the moribund patient, definitive therapy.

46. Why are diaphragm injuries important to recognize?
Diaphragm injuries occur after a sudden increase in intraabdominal pressure against a fixed diaphragm, which leads to rupture. A diaphragm injury is three times more common on the left, because of the protection afforded by the liver on the right. A tear in the diaphragm may allow abdominal contents to herniate into the chest. These injuries have the potential for high morbidity and mortality should herniated intraabdominal organs torse, strangulate, or perforate.

47. How is a diaphragm injury diagnosed?
Diaphragmatic injuries can be clinically silent. Chest pain and shortness of breath may be the only presenting symptoms. Small defects may have no radiographic findings. In larger injuries, chest radiography may demonstrate

a gastric bubble in the chest, a nasogastric tube above the diaphragm, or intraabdominal contents above the diaphragm. When in doubt, definitive diagnosis should be made with laparoscopy or thoracoscopy.

48. **What are the manifestations of a chyle leak resulting from blunt thoracic trauma, and how do I confirm the diagnosis?**
A chyle leak, usually resulting from trauma to the thoracic duct, can present as a painless supraclavicular mass, a cervical fistula, or as a chylothorax. The diagnosis is made by sending a sample of the fluid for triglyceride level.

49. **What are the signs and symptoms of rib fractures, and how are they diagnosed?**
Signs and symptoms of rib fractures include pain and tenderness over the fracture, referred pain to the fracture site upon compression of the fractured rib away from the fracture, mobility of the ribs, bony crepitus, ecchymosis over the ribs, splinting, and hypoventilation. Chest radiography and CT are the imaging studies of choice to confirm the diagnosis.

50. **Name the potential complications after rib fractures.**
    - Pneumonia
    - Empyema
    - Hemothorax
    - Ventilator dependence
    - Chronic pain
    - Decreased exercise tolerance
    - Pneumothorax

51. **How are rib fractures treated?**
Rib fractures are treated with supportive care, including pain control, supplemental oxygen administration, and pulmonary toilet. Major morbidity comes from inadequate pain control with subsequent impairment of pulmonary toilet, resulting in pneumonia. Multimodal pain strategies have shown to be beneficial. Common regimens include simultaneous use of narcotics, nonsteroidal anti-inflammatory drugs (NSAIDs), and muscle relaxing agents. For patients with multiple rib fractures, local and regional anesthetic techniques, including epidural and paracostal pain catheters, can be used. Operative rib plating is becoming increasingly common, and ongoing research studies are attempting to define the appropriate operative indications.

52. **What are the risk factors for increased morbidity and mortality from rib fractures?**
Advanced age and number of fractures are associated with increased morbidity and mortality. Underlying comorbidities also play a role in the clinical significance of these fractures.

53. **What is a flail chest?**
A flail chest occurs when multiple contiguous ribs are broken in more than one location, causing a portion of the rib cage to be completely detached from the remainder of the bony thorax. Paradoxical motion occurs with respiration, compromising pulmonary mechanics and impairing oxygenation and ventilation. Flail chest is often associated with significant underlying pulmonary contusion. As such, nearly half of the patients with flail chest require mechanical ventilation.

54. **What is the treatment of choice for flail chest?**
After initial stabilization, treatment goals center on optimization of pain control and pulmonary toilet. Ongoing investigations into surgical rib fracture stabilization suggest a benefit in repairing certain fracture patterns.

KEY POINTS: RIB FRACTURES AND FLAIL CHEST

1. Rib fractures are common injuries following thoracic trauma.
2. Diagnosis starts with physical examination; signs and symptoms include pain, bony crepitus, chest wall instability, ecchymosis over the ribs, and splinting.
3. A flail chest occurs when multiple contiguous ribs are broken in more than one place, causing a portion of the rib cage to be detached from the remainder of the bony thorax.
4. Treatment for both entities includes pain control, supplemental oxygen administration, and pulmonary toilet.
5. Advanced age and multiple rib fractures are risk factors for increased morbidity and mortality.

55. **What injuries are associated with a posterior sternoclavicular dissociation and scapular fracture?**
Posterior sternoclavicular dissociation may cause injury to the great vessels, the trachea, and the esophagus. Scapular fractures are often associated with a high-energy mechanism; injuries may include hemopneumothorax, a lung contusion or laceration, spinal fractures, subclavian vessel injury, or brachial plexus injury.

56. **What is the significance of a sternal fracture, and how is it diagnosed?**
Similar to first and second rib fractures, sternal fractures are considered markers of high-energy transfer and should raise the concern for blunt cardiac injury and other undiagnosed intrathoracic injuries. Sternal fractures may be seen on lateral chest radiography but are commonly diagnosed with a CT scan.

57. What is the imaging modality of choice for suspected thoracic spine injuries?

A thoracic CT scan is more sensitive than plain radiography in identifying thoracolumbar spine fractures. Patients with back pain, tenderness, altered mental status, distracting injuries, or high-energy mechanisms should undergo a thoracic CT scan with reconstruction of the spine. Imaging of the thoracic spine should be performed in patients with a known cervical or lumbar fracture to rule out a concomitant thoracic spine fracture.

58. What is neurogenic shock, and how does it manifest?

Neurogenic shock occurs after cervical or high thoracic injuries cause impairment of sympathetic stimulation to the heart and peripheral vasculature. Signs and symptoms include vasodilatation resulting in flushing, warm extremities, hypotension, and bradycardia (i.e., absence of compensatory tachycardia). Neurogenic shock is treated with vigorous volume resuscitation and peripheral vasoconstrictors, such as dopamine or norepinephrine.

59. How does thoracic trauma in children differ from thoracic trauma in adults?

Children trauma patients differ from adult trauma patients in many ways. Children are able to compensate and maintain normal vital signs and hemodynamics, despite significant injury. As such, tachycardia and hypotension are late findings that may quickly proceed to cardiopulmonary collapse and arrest. Pediatric bones are more pliable, so any visible rib fractures indicate a high-energy force. Conversely, the absence of rib fractures does not preclude underlying organ injury. The surface area is proportionally larger in a child; therefore, children have a greater predisposition for hypothermia (see Chapter 92).

BIBLIOGRAPHY

American College of Surgeons Committee on Trauma. *Advanced Trauma Life Support.* 10th ed. Chicago: American College of Surgeons; 2018.

Clancy K, Velopulos C, Bilaniuk JW, et al. Screening for blunt cardiac injury. *J Trauma Acute Care Surg.* 2012;73:S301–S306.

Demehri S, Rybicki FJ, Desjardins B, et al. ACR appropriateness criteria blunt chest trauma-suspected aortic injury. *Emerg Radiol.* 2012;19:287–292.

Dennis BM, Bellister SA, Guillamondegui OD. Thoracic trauma. *Surg Clin North Am.* 2017;97(5):1047–1064.

Eddine SBZ, Boyle KA, Dodgion CM, et al. Observing pneumothoraces: the 35-millimeter rule is safe for both blunt and penetrating chest trauma. *J Trauma Acute Care Surg.* 2019;86(4):557–564.

Jones TS, Burlew CC, Stovall RT, et al. Emergency department pericardial drainage for penetrating cardiac wounds is a viable option for stabilization. *Am J Surg.* 2014;207:931–934.

Moore EE, Knudson M, Burlew CC, et al. Defining the limits of resuscitative emergency department thoracotomy: a contemporary Western Trauma Association perspective. *J Trauma.* 2011;70:334–339.

Mowery N, Gunter O, Collier B, et al. Practice management guidelines for management of hemothorax and occult pneumothorax. *J Trauma.* 2011;70:510–518.

Pieracci FM, Majercik S, Ali-Osman F, et al. Consensus statement: surgical stabilization of rib fractures rib fracture colloquium clinical practice guidelines. *Injury.* 2017;48(2):307–321.

Tanizaki S, Maeda S, Sera M, et al. Small tube thoracostomy (20–22 Fr) in emergent management of chest trauma. *Injury.* 2017;48(9):1884–1887.

Waller CJ, Cogbill TH, Kallies KJ, et al. Contemporary management of subclavian and axillary artery injuries – a Western Trauma Association multicenter review. *J Trauma Acute Care Surg.* 2017;83(6):1023–1031.

CHAPTER 89

ABDOMINAL TRAUMA

Alexander P. Morton, MD and Ernest E. Moore, MD

1. **Why is ABCDE (Airway, Breathing, Circulation, Disability, and Exposure) relevant to the evaluation of significant abdominal trauma?**

   This acronym represents the primary survey employed to identify and treat the most life-threatening injuries in a systematic fashion. Airway, breathing, circulation, disability, and exposure are the important elements in the initial evaluation of a trauma patient. Circulation involves evaluating hemodynamics and identifying active hemorrhage. Persistent hemodynamic instability in the setting of abdominal trauma is an indication for emergent laparotomy. Exposure and examination of the abdomen, pelvis, back, buttock, and perineum may yield important findings, including penetrating trauma, active hemorrhage, evidence of significant blunt trauma (e.g., seat belt sign, unstable pelvis), abdominal tenderness, or diffuse peritonitis. Significant disability (i.e., neurologic injury) can render the clinical examination less effective and thus warrant more diagnostic studies. With the increasing use of resuscitative endovascular balloon occlusion of the aorta (REBOA), some have proposed the order A-B-C should be C-A-B in certain patients; ideally, these can be done simultaneously with adequate personnel.

2. **Discuss the key aspects of the secondary survey in the evaluation of abdominal trauma.**

   The secondary survey includes a thorough history and systematic physical examination to inform the sequence and extent of early diagnostic efforts. Prehospital providers can relay invaluable information regarding the mechanism and force of the accident or injury, time from injury, use of seat belts, air bag deployment, ejection from a vehicle, drug and alcohol use, and the trend in a patient's clinical status. Consider lower thoracic and upper abdominal trauma as a unit; suspect abdominal injury in any penetrating wound below the level of the nipple anteriorly or tip of the scapula posteriorly. Abdominal tenderness and guarding may be early signs of significant injury, but rebound tenderness and rigidity are relatively uncommon early after injury. Initially, 20% to 40% of patients with serious intraabdominal injury may appear asymptomatic. Imaging during the secondary survey should include repeated extended focused assessment with sonography for trauma (E-FAST) examinations of the chest and abdomen. Chest and pelvis radiographs are often included in cases of major blunt trauma, and can provide valuable information that allows for timely intervention in the emergent setting. In hemodynamically stable patients, plain x-rays can be omitted, as computed tomography (CT) will diagnose the vast majority of intraabdominal injuries, although diaphragmatic, ureteral, and hollow viscous injuries are not always apparent.

3. **What are some of the biomechanical principles in blunt and penetrating trauma?**

   The severity and location of blunt trauma depends on the type of impact (e.g., compression versus shear forces), direction of impact, momentum of the involved objects, and properties of the affected tissues (Fig. 89.1). In penetrating trauma, damage is caused by the dissipation of energy as the knife, bullet, or other object traverses tissues. The injury pattern is dependent both on the momentum of the projectile and its trajectory through the body. Because of significantly increased momentum and unpredictable intracavitary trajectories, gunshot wounds can produce extensive damage with unexpected injury patterns when compared with stab wounds. Therefore penetrating abdominal gunshot wounds typically require laparotomy, and maintenance of a broad differential for sources of intraabdominal hemorrhage or injury, whereas stab wounds can often be managed selectively (Fig. 89.2).

KEY POINTS: INDICATIONS FOR EMERGENT LAPAROTOMY

1. Diffuse peritonitis.
2. Hemodynamic instability with evidence of abdominal injury.
3. Penetrating gunshot wounds with peritoneal violation, with the possible exception of the right upper quadrant.
4. Penetrating stab wounds with evisceration or uncontrolled bleeding.

---

4. **What are the most commonly injured abdominal organs?**

   The liver and spleen are the most commonly injured abdominal solid organs. The stomach and small bowel are the most commonly injured abdominal hollow viscera. CT allows for the grading of injuries from I to VI using Organ Injury Scales, which aid in treatment and prognosis. The vast majority of blunt solid organ injuries can be managed nonoperatively, but patients must be watched carefully for signs of clinical deterioration and ongoing hemorrhage, necessitating intervention (Tables 89.1 and 89.2).

Blunt Abdominal Trauma

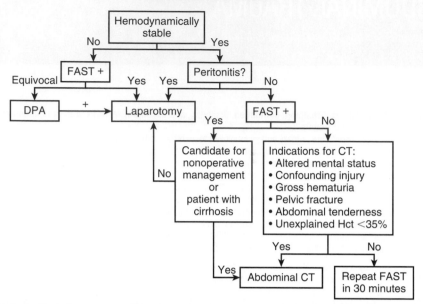

Fig. 89.1 An algorithm for the management of blunt abdominal trauma. Peritonitis and hemodynamic instability with positive FAST or DPA are indications for immediate laparotomy. *CT,* Computed tomography; *DPA,* diagnostic peritoneal aspiration; *FAST,* focused assessment with sonography for trauma; *Hct,* hematocrit.

5. **What is a seat belt sign?**
   It is an ecchymotic imprint of the seat belt or shoulder strap on the anterior chest or abdomen of a restrained passenger, indicating rapid deceleration from a motor vehicle crash. The presence of a seat belt sign is associated with a 20% incidence of intraabdominal injury; patients have an increased risk of blunt injury to the hollow viscus, often not apparent on initial FAST or CT. Unexplained free fluid in an otherwise stable patient with blunt trauma to the abdomen is an important finding. These patients should be observed for clinical deterioration or the development of peritonitis, and explored in the operating room when symptoms worsen. Virtually 100% of patients with hollow viscus injury will become clinically apparent within 12 hours after injury.

6. **Lower rib fractures are typically associated with what intraabdominal injuries?**
   Lower rib fractures are associated with injuries to the liver and spleen. In children, trauma to the lower ribs may not result in fracture; however, lack of fractures does not preclude the possibility of major solid organ injury after blunt trauma.

7. **What is a Chance fracture?**
   A Chance fracture is a transverse fracture of a low thoracic or lumbar vertebra caused by flexion of the back, and is associated with lap-belt only use. The incidence of associated intraabdominal injuries with a Chance fracture approaches 50%, and includes the small bowel and aorta.

8. **What abdominal injuries are associated with pelvic fractures?**
   Pelvic fractures are associated with injuries to the solid (11%) and hollow (4%) intraabdominal organs, the diaphragm (2%), and the bladder or urethra (6%).

9. **In the setting of trauma, what is the significance of gross hematuria?**
   Hematuria suggests injury to the genitourinary system, including the kidneys, ureters, bladder, or urethra. Physical examination can provide key information regarding the location of injury, such as flank ecchymosis, penetrating injuries near the kidneys or bladder, perineal laceration, or a high-riding prostate. Important diagnostic modalities include retrograde cystourethrography to identify bladder rupture and urethral injuries, as well as CT with contrast, including the excretory phase to identify renal and ureteral injuries.

10. **Describe the incidence of diaphragmatic rupture in trauma and how it can be diagnosed on a chest radiograph.**
    Diaphragm injuries occur in 1%–7% of blunt trauma and 10%–15% of penetrating trauma. A displaced nasogastric tube representing the stomach through the left hemithorax indicates a diaphragm rupture. However, the chest radiograph is normal in up to half of patients with left diaphragmatic injury and is often normal with right-sided injuries.

Penetrating Abdominal Injuries

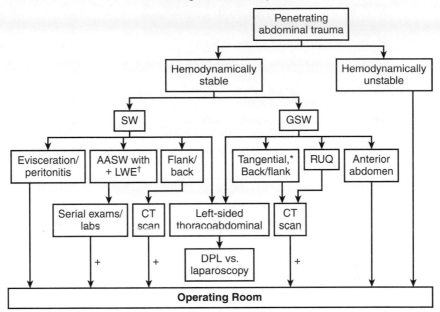

*Tangential GSWs may also be evaluated with diagnostic laparoscopy.
†A positive local wound exploration LWE is defined as violation of the peritoneum.

Anterior abdomen: From inguinal ligaments to costal margin, from anterior axillary line to anterior axillary line
Flank/back: From anterior axillary line around posteriorly to opposite anterior axillary line below costal margin and above pelvis
LWE: Positive if there is peritoneal penetration
Serial examinations: Documented by upper level every 2 hours
　Consider CT A/P if Hgb drops without peritonitis in stable patient
　Consider CT A/P if RUQ SW to evaluate isolated liver injury

Fig. 89.2 An algorithm for the management of penetrating abdominal trauma. Penetrating trauma with hemodynamic instability, anterior abdominal gunshot wounds, and abdominal stab wounds with evisceration are indications for immediate laparotomy. *AASW,* Anterior abdominal stab wound; *A/P,* abdomen/pelvis; *CT,* computed tomography; *DPL,* diagnostic peritoneal lavage; *GSW,* gunshot wound; *Hgb,* hemoglobin; *LWE,* local wound exploration; *RUQ,* right upper quadrant; *SW,* stab wound.

Left-sided injuries are more common following blunt trauma than right-sided injuries, because the liver absorbs more energy during right-sided injuries, protecting the diaphragm. High clinical suspicion for diaphragm injury should be maintained in the setting of any penetrating thoracoabdominal trauma.

11. **Does a normal serum amylase test exclude pancreatic injury?**
No, the initial serum amylase test is neither a sensitive nor specific pancreatic injury indicator (i.e., a normal amylase result does not exclude pancreatic injury), and an elevated amylase may be the result of an increase in salivary amylase. Pancreatic injuries are found in 3%–6% of patients undergoing laparotomy for trauma. Because of its close association with many vital structures, penetrating pancreatic injury is associated with other injuries in more than 90% of cases.

KEY POINTS: INJURY PATTERNS IN BLUNT ABDOMINAL TRAUMA

1. Certain injuries should increase suspicion for intraabdominal injury after blunt trauma, including a seat belt sign, lower rib fractures, pelvic fractures, and Chance fractures.
2. The most commonly injured solid organs are the liver and spleen. The most commonly injured hollow viscera are the stomach and small bowel.
3. Gross hematuria is a sign of genitourinary trauma, including the urethra, bladder, ureters, and kidneys.

Table 89.1 Organ Injury Scale: Liver

		Liver Injury Scale (1994 revision)		
GRADE[a]	TYPE OF INJURY	DESCRIPTION OF INJURY	ICD-9	AIS-90
I	Hematoma	Subcapsular, <10% surface area	864.01 864.11	2
	Laceration	Capsular tear, <1 cm parenchymal depth	864.02 864.12	2
II	Hematoma	Subcapsular, 10%–50% surface area Lntraparenchymal, <10 cm in diameter	864.01 864.11	2
	Laceration	Capsular tear 1–3 parenchymal depth, <10 cm in length	864.03 864.13	2
III	Hematoma	Subcapsular, >50% surface area of ruptured subcapsular or parenchymal hematoma; intraparenchymal hematoma, >10 cm or expanding		3
	Laceration	>3 cm parenchymal depth	864.04 864.14	3
IV	Laceration	Parenchymal disruption involving 25%–75% hepatic lobe or 1–3 Couinaud's segments	864.04 864.14	4
V	Laceration	Parenchymal disruption involving >75% of hepatic lobe or >3 Couinaud's segments within a single lobe		5
	Vascular	Juxtahepatic venous injuries (i.e., retrohepatic vena cava/central major hepatic veins)		5
VI	Vascular	Hepatic avulsion		6

[a]Advance one grade for multiple injuries up to grade III.
From Moore EE, Cogbill TH, Jurkovich GJ, et al. Organ injury scaling: spleen and liver (1994 revision). *J Trauma.* 1995;38(3):323–324.

Table 89.2 Organ Injury Scale: Spleen

		Spleen Injury Scale (1994 Revision)		
GRADE[a]	INJURY TYPE	DESCRIPTION OF INJURY	ICD-9	AIS-90
I	Hematoma	Subcapsular, <10% surface area	865-01 865.11	2
	Laceration	Capsular tear, <1 cm parenchymal depth	865.02 865.12	2 2
II	Hematoma	Subcapsular, 10%–50% surface area Intraparenchymal, < 5 cm in diameter	865.01 865.11	
	Laceration	Capsular tear, 1–3 cm parenchymal depth that does not involve a trabecular vessel	865.02 865.12	2
III	Hematoma	Subcapsular, >50% surface area or expanding; ruptured subcapsular or parenchymal hematoma; intraparenchymal hematoma ≥5 cm or expanding		3
	Laceration	>3 cm parenchymal depth or involving trabecular vessels	865.03	3
IV	Laceration	Laceration involving segmental or hilar vessels producing major devascularization (>25% of spleen)	865.13	4
V	Laceration Vascular	Completely shattered spleen Hilar vascular injury with devascularized spleen	865.04 865.14	5 5

[a]Advance one grade for multiple injuries up to grade III.
From Moore EE, Cogbill TH, Jurkovich GJ, et al. Organ injury scaling: spleen and liver (1994 revision). *J Trauma.* 1995;38(3):323–324.

12. What is the initial imaging modality of choice to evaluate for evidence of abdominal trauma?

FAST is the initial test of choice in the evaluation of blunt abdominal trauma. Performed by emergency medicine physicians and trauma surgeons, FAST is a rapid, painless, and sensitive test for identifying intraabdominal fluid (Fig. 89.3). If the test is initially negative, repeating the examination in an unstable patient is imperative; more than 250 mL of blood must accumulate within Morrison's pouch before a fluid stripe will appear on the FAST. A single negative FAST cannot rule out abdominal injury.

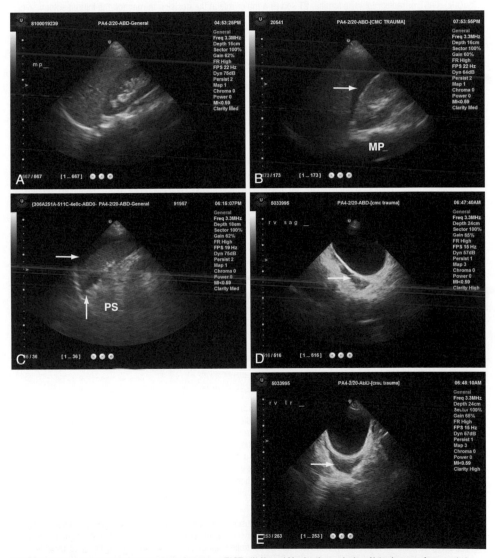

Fig. 89.3 Focused assessment with sonography for trauma (FAST). (A) Normal Morrison's pouch view. Note absence of an anechoic stripe, which would represent a fluid collection between the liver and kidney. (B) Positive Morrison's pouch *(MP)* view. Note presence of an anechoic stripe representing a fluid collection between the liver and kidney *(arrow)*. (C) Positive perisplenic *(PS)* view. Note anechoic fluid around spleen *(arrows)*. (D) Positive fluid in the sagittal retrovesicular view *(arrow)*. Note anechoic stripe indicative of retroperitoneal fluid. (E) Positive transverse retrovesicular view. Note anechoic area indicative of retroperitoneal fluid *(arrow)*. (From Nichols JR, Puskarich MA. Abdominal trauma. In: Walls RM, ed. *Rosen's Emergency Medicine: Concepts and Clinical Practice*. 9th ed. Philadelphia, PA: Elsevier; 2018:404–418.)

13. **What are the four locations evaluated with the FAST examination?**
    1. *Pericardium.* Presence of pericardial fluid could indicate cardiac tamponade as a source of hypotension.
    2. *Right upper quadrant.* Morrison's pouch is the most common location of a positive FAST, regardless of injury location.
    3. *Left upper quadrant.* Splenorenal space and subphrenic space.
    4. *Suprapubic area.* Bladder and rectovesical space.

14. **What is the role of CT scanning in blunt abdominal trauma?**
    Abdominopelvic CT is the test of choice for evaluating the abdomen of hemodynamically stable patients with significant blunt abdominal trauma. Indications include signs or symptoms of abdominal injury; patients with significant disability or distracting injury (e.g., femur fracture); and injuries detected on diagnostic peritoneal lavage (DPL), FAST, or radiography. Abdominal CT serves a major role in the decision to manage the injured spleen, liver, or kidney nonoperatively, by allowing for injury grading and identification of active arterial extravasation.

15. **What is the role of DPL?**
    The major advantage of DPL is a sensitivity rate greater than 95% for the identification of intraperitoneal hemorrhage. Because the technique is invasive and fails to identify the source of bleeding, its use has declined as FAST has become routine. For hemodynamically unstable patients, FAST is a more rapid, less invasive test, but is operator dependent. DPL is used predominantly if the composition of the free fluid is in question (e.g., ascites vs. blood) or the FAST results are negative, but there is no other source to account for a patient's acute blood loss. The DPL is often done without the infusion of fluid (i.e., diagnostic peritoneal aspirate [DPA]). If the patient is hemodynamically unstable because of intraabdominal hemorrhage, a gross blood sample should be retrieved on insertion of the catheter.

16. **How are DPL results interpreted?**
    DPA is considered positive if more than 10 mL of free blood, or any enteric contents, are aspirated. Otherwise, 1 L of warmed normal saline is infused. A minimal recovery of 75% of lavage effluent is required for the test to be considered valid. The fluid is analyzed for red blood cell (RBC) counts, white blood cell (WBC) counts, lavage amylase, alkaline phosphatase, and bilirubin, and inspected for particulate material. The test is positive for the following results:
    - Greater than 100,000 RBCs/mL
    - Greater than 500 WBCs/mL
    - Greater than 175 IU/mL amylase
    - Any bile, bacteria, or food particles
      A positive DPL is an indication for laparotomy.

KEY POINTS: DIAGNOSTIC TOOLS FOR BLUNT TRAUMA

1. FAST examination should be done as soon as possible and repeated when necessary.
2. CT scanning is preferred in the hemodynamically stable patient, even if the FAST reveals free fluid.
3. DPL is used to exclude major abdominal injuries in unstable patients with a normal FAST.
4. Serial physical examination is an important aspect of initial management, and peritonitis warrants laparotomy without confirmatory CT.

---

17. **Do all abdominal stab wounds need exploratory laparotomy?**
    No. In patients with anterior stab wounds lacking an indication for emergent laparotomy (stab wound with evisceration, hemodynamic instability, peritonitis, or uncontrolled hemorrhage), a local wound exploration can be performed in the emergency department. The area is anesthetized and the wound widened enough for adequate evaluation of the fascia. The patient can be discharged if hemodynamically stable, the fascia is not penetrated, and there are no other identified injuries. If the fascia *is* violated, the patient is admitted for close observation. The majority of these patients will not require an operation, and the delay to operation created by the observation period is generally due to small bowel injury, and is not clinically significant.

18. **What is REBOA?**
    REBOA stands for resuscitative endovascular balloon occlusion of the aorta. This is a relatively new procedure being studied and performed in trauma centers for the temporary control of noncompressible torso hemorrhage. By occluding the aorta proximal to the injury, blood loss can be controlled similar to thoracic cross-clamping via resuscitative thoracotomy. Hemodynamic stabilization with a REBOA allows for additional diagnostic imaging (using CT) to identify the location of injury, and facilitate transport to the operating room (OR) or interventional radiology (IR) suite for definitive management.

19. **What are the unique concerns in a pregnant patient with abdominal trauma?**
    Physiologic changes occur in the pregnant patient, including hypervolemia, a decrease in peripheral vascular resistance, venous return, and blood pressure, which can mask signs of shock or lead to supine hypotensive syndrome.

Pregnant patients' blood becomes hypercoagulable, leading to increased risks of venous thromboembolism, and they have displacement of their abdominal organs, making the physical examination less reliable. Optimal care of the mother ensures the best outcome for the fetus. Conservative management of blunt abdominal injuries is the treatment of choice in stable, pregnant trauma patients. Hemodynamic instability, uterine rupture, placental abruption, and other injuries requiring immediate repair are indications for abdominal exploration. Patients requiring laparotomy have an increased risk of preterm labor, which increases with gestational age.

20. **What are the general principles of trauma in the elderly population?**
The combination of chronic medical conditions, limited organ reserve, and atherosclerosis makes elderly patients especially vulnerable to trauma. Preinjury β-blocker use inhibits the physiologic response to hemorrhagic shock and is associated with increased mortality. Anticoagulant use (e.g., warfarin and thrombin inhibitors) prolongs hemostasis, and is associated with increased mortality in patients with head injuries. Age-related cardiac dysfunction can result in a relatively fixed cardiac output and heart rate, with vasoconstriction as the sole response to hypovolemia.

    Because of the masking of traditional signs of hemorrhagic shock, elderly patients are more susceptible to failure of conservative management and have a higher mortality rate than younger patients with similar injuries. Traditional markers of hypovolemia may not be accurate, necessitating extended observation or imaging.

21. **In the management of abdominal trauma, are children really just small adults?**
No, injury patterns are different in children because of their size and tissue elasticity. They can have minimal external signs of injury, even in the setting of significant blunt trauma and intraabdominal injuries. A thin abdominal wall and close proximity of organs leaves children at increased risk of multiple organ injuries even from a single blow. External signs of injury, such as a seat belt sign or abdominal tenderness, significantly increase the likelihood of abdominal injury. Although blunt injuries to solid abdominal organs tend to be self-limited in children, those with hemodynamic instability or ongoing blood loss should undergo prompt operative management. Additionally, pediatric blood pressure and heart rate can be falsely reassuring while compensatory mechanisms remain intact. Hemodynamic instability can be masked until hemorrhagic shock becomes severe and cardiovascular collapse occurs. As with any pediatric injury, clinical suspicion for abuse should be maintained in the setting of a discrepant history or a physical examination that shows signs of abuse, such as bruises in multiple stages of healing, evidence of old fractures, or abdominal organ injury without a history of abdominal trauma. Finally, the risk of delayed radiation-associated malignancy from CT scanning underscores the importance of selective scanning for children.

KEY POINTS: ABDOMINAL TRAUMA

1. Patients who have persistent hemodynamic instability with free intraabdominal fluid or peritonitis after abdominal trauma require emergent laparotomy.
2. A detailed history and physical examination are key elements in the evaluation of the lucid trauma patient.
3. A single negative FAST examination does not reliably exclude significant intraperitoneal bleeding.
4. Observing a trauma patient is an active process, including serial physical examinations and repeat abdominal ultrasonography.
5. Pregnant, elderly, and pediatric trauma patients have unique anatomy and physiology that affects injury patterns, physiologic response to trauma, and treatment algorithms.

BIBILIOGRAPHY

Bensard D, Wesson D. The pediatric patient. In: Moore EE, Feliciano DV, Mattox KL, eds. *Trauma*. 8th ed. New York, NY: McGraw-Hill Professional; 2017: Chapter 43.

Biffle WL, Fox CJ, Moore EE. The role of REBOA in exsanguinating torso hemorrhage. *Am Surg*. 2017;83(11):1193–1202.

Brenner M, Hicks C. Major abdominal trauma: critical decisions and new frontiers in management. *Emerg Med Clin North Am*. 2018; 36(1):149–160.

Ciesla D, Kerwin A, Tepas III J. Trauma systems, triage, and transport. In: Moore EE, Feliciano DV, Mattox KL, eds. *Trauma*. 8th ed. New York, NY: McGraw-Hill Professional; 2017: Chapter 4.

Feliciano D. Abdominal trauma revisited. *Am Surg*. 2017;83(11):1193–1202.

Ho VP, Patel NJ, Bokhari F, et al. Management of adult pancreatic injuries: A practice management guideline from the Eastern Association for the Surgery of Trauma. *J Trauma Acute Care Surg*. 2017;82(1):185–199.

Jones EL, Stovall RT, Jones TS, et al. Intraabdominal injury from blunt trauma becomes apparent within 9 hours. *J Trauma Acute Care Surg*. 2014;76(4):1020–1023.

Notrica DM, Eubanks JW, Tuggle D, et al. Nonoperative management of blunt liver and spleen injury in children: Evaluation of the ATOMAC guideline using GRADE. *J Trauma Acute Care Surg*. 2015;79(4):683–693.

Rhee PM, Moore EE, Joseph B, et al. Gunshot wounds: a review of ballistics, bullets, weapons, and myths. *J Trauma Acute Care Surg*. 2016;80(6):853–867.

Yeung LL, McDonald AA, Como JJ, et al. Management of blunt force bladder injuries: A practice management guideline from the Eastern Association for the Surgery of Trauma. *J Trauma Acute Care Surg*. 2019;86(2):326–336.

CHAPTER 90

PELVIC FRACTURES AND GENITOURINARY TRAUMA

Philip F. Stahel, MD, FACS and Darryl A. Auston, MD, PhD

KEY POINTS: PELVIC FRACTURES

1. High-energy pelvic ring disruptions represent a major cause of preventable trauma deaths due to major occult blood loss in the retroperitoneal space.
2. Resuscitative endovascular balloon occlusion of the aorta (REBOA) provides temporary bleeding control in the emergency department (ED) for hypotensive patients with bleeding pelvic fractures.
3. Injury mechanism-based classification systems are essential for understanding the severity of pelvic ring disruptions and to guide therapeutic decision making.
4. Open pelvic fractures are associated with increased mortality and must be diagnosed during the initial assessment.
5. A protocolized approach of pelvic packing and external fixation, with consideration for delayed angioembolization if indicated, reduces mortality from high-energy pelvic fractures.

1. **What are the pitfalls in patients with pelvic fractures?**

   High-energy pelvic ring disruptions are associated with a high mortality rate (>30%) from associated retroperitoneal hemorrhage, traumatic-hemorrhagic shock, and post-injury coagulopathy. The main bleeding sources in >90% of all pelvic fractures are of venous origin, from venous presacral and paravesical plexuses and cancellous bone bleeding from sacral fractures, none of which are amenable to angioembolization. Open fractures are frequently missed during the initial assessment, due to occult vaginal or rectal lacerations that occur in about 5% of all patients with high-energy pelvic ring disruptions. The early recognition and proactive management of open pelvic fractures by perineal debridement and fecal diversion is paramount in preventing septic complications and high post-injury mortality rates.

2. **How are pelvic fractures classified?**

   Pelvic injuries are graded by anatomic (AO/OTA or Tile) and mechanistic (Young and Burgess) classification systems (Fig. 90.1).

   A-Type

   Stable fractures, with a stable pelvic ring (APC-1, LC-1)*

   B-Type

   Rotationally unstable, but vertically stable injuries (APC-2, LC-2)*

   C-Type

   Rotationally AND vertically unstable fractures (APC-3, LC-3, VS, CM)*

   The World Society of Emergency Surgery (WSES) classification system provides a combination of the anatomic/mechanistic classification in conjunction with hemodynamic stability and response to resuscitation:

   1. *Minor* pelvic ring injuries (**WSES grade 1**): mechanically (APC-1, LC-1) and hemodynamically stable injury patterns.
   2. *Moderate* pelvic ring injuries: mechanically unstable (**WSES grade 2**: LC-2, LC-3, APC-2, APC-3; **WSES grade 3**: VS or CM) with hemodynamic stability and/or adequate response to resuscitation ("responders").
   3. *Severe* pelvic ring injuries (**WSES grade 4**): any hemodynamically unstable injury pattern with patients at risk for acute exsanguinating hemorrhage, independent of the mechanistic fracture classification.

3. **How are patients with pelvic fractures assessed on initial presentation?**

   The initial diagnostic workup in the ED is guided by Advanced Trauma Life Support (ATLS) protocol, and requires a coordinated multidisciplinary approach. Many patients with pelvic fractures have significant associated thoracic, intraabdominal, neurologic, and genitourinary injuries. An anteroposterior (AP) pelvis radiograph can be obtained as an adjunct to the primary survey. Advanced imaging includes dedicated inlet/outlet views and computed tomography (CT) scan. Open fractures must be ruled out by a physical examination. Presence of blood in the vaginal vault

---

*APC, Anteroposterior compression; *LC,* lateral compression; *VS,* vertical shear; *CM,* combined mechanism.

AO/OTA (Tile)	Description/examples	Young & Burgess
A-type: **Stable pelvic ring.** 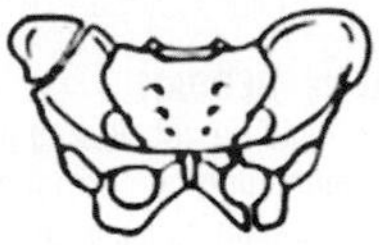 	Iliac wing fractures, pubic rami fractures, pubic symphysis sprain	• APC-1 • LC-1
B-type: **Rotationally unstable,** **vertically stable.** 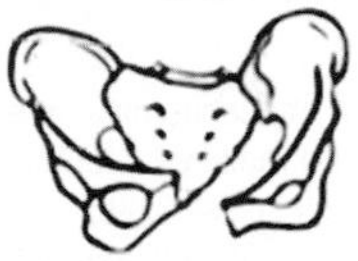 **Antero-posterior** **compression**	Pubic symphysis >2.5 cm (stress exam if equivocal) *"Open book" injury*	• APC-2
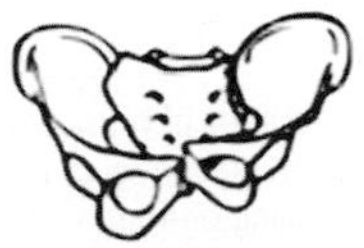 **Lateral** **compression**	Unstable lateral compression injuries *"Crescent fracture"* *"Bucket handle fracture"*	• LC-2
C-type: **Rotationally AND** **vertically unstable.** 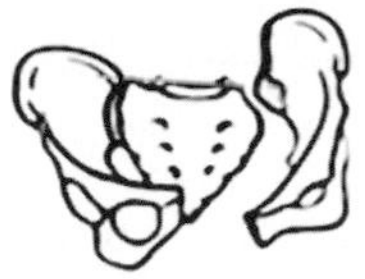 	Complete detachment of hemipelvis, unilateral or bilateral, posterior injury through SI-joint or sacrum *"Vertical shear" injury* *"Combined mechanism"*	• APC-3 • LC-3 • VS • CM

Fig. 90.1 Comparison of the prevalent classification systems for pelvic ring injuries, based on injury mechanism and pelvic ring stability. *APC,* Anteroposterior compression; *CM,* combined mechanism; *LC,* lateral compression; *SI-joint,* sacroiliac joint; *VS,* vertical shear.

or on a digital rectal examination should prompt direct visualization with speculum and rectal endoscopy. The early presence of postinjury coagulopathy is best assessed by bedside point-of-care testing modalities—for example, thromboelastography (TEG) or rotational thromboelastometry (ROTEM)—for a targeted resuscitation from traumatic-hemorrhagic shock and coagulopathy.

4. **Which laboratory parameters help detect "hidden shock" in pelvic fractures?**
Serum lactate and base deficit are sensitive tests for the early recognition of traumatic-hemorrhagic shock, and for monitoring of the response to resuscitation in patients with pelvic ring disruptions.

5. **What is the role of pelvic binders?**

The application of pelvic binders is recommended as an early measure to stabilize the pelvic ring and decrease the amount of acute hemorrhage in the prehospital and hospital setting. By reducing the pelvic volume and preventing further fracture motion, binders promote tamponade of bleeding bone fragments and vessels. Pelvic binders are available as commercial products, and can alternatively be created using standard bedsheets and clamps. These should be removed as soon as possible once a patient's vital signs are adequately monitored and resuscitative measures have been initiated.

6. **What is the role of resuscitative endovascular balloon occlusion of the aorta (REBOA)?**

REBOA has recently been advocated as an alternative to ED thoracotomy and should be considered as a temporary, minimal invasive measure of acute bleeding control in patients with exsanguinating hemorrhage *in extremis* and refractory hypotension (systolic blood pressure <80 mmHg). The REBOA technique consists of a percutaneous femoral arterial cannulation with a size 7 French gauge balloon catheter. The approximate distance of catheter insertion is measured externally, with the tip of the balloon located at the umbilicus. The balloon catheter is advanced to zone III of the aorta, that is, just proximal to the aortic bifurcation and distal to the most caudal renal artery (Fig. 90.2). The balloon is gradually inflated using a mixture of saline and contrast dye, with a maximal inflation volume of 24 mL. Documentation includes vital signs, catheter insertion depth, and time of balloon inflation. Radiographic imaging is recommended to confirm proper catheter placement in aortic zone III.

7. **How does pelvic packing work?**

The concept of pelvic packing was initially described in Europe as a technique of transabdominal open pelvic packing through an explorative laparotomy. The pelvic packing technique has been modified with the "Denver protocol," by direct preperitoneal pelvic packing (PPP) through a suprapubic midline incision, which provides an effective tamponade of retroperitoneal bleeding sources. Of note, the modern PPP technique allows for a simultaneous midline laparotomy through a separate incision, if indicated, for management of associated intraabdominal injuries. The pelvic packing protocol-incorporated as part of a standardized institutional guideline-has been shown to decrease blood product utilization and improve patient outcomes and to decrease the historic mortality rate of >30% to 2%.

8. **When should angioembolization be considered?**

Less than 10% of patients with high-energy pelvic ring disruptions have arterial sources of retroperitoneal hemorrhage. A ngioembolization does not represent the first modality of choice for bleeding control in hemodynamically unstable pelvic fractures, as only about 2% of all patients have successful coiling of arterial bleeding sources. The interventional procedure requires 2–3 hours for completion, which is an excessive time during the

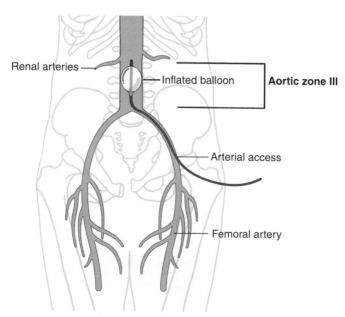

Renal arteries — Inflated balloon **Aortic zone III**

Arterial access

Femoral artery

Fig. 90.2 Schematic depiction of resuscitative endovascular balloon occlusion of the aorta (REBOA) for temporary bleeding control in hemodynamically unstable pelvic fractures. (© Phil Stahel 2017.)

critical "golden hour" of trauma. Angioembolization should be reserved for selected patients with a positive blush on initial CT scan, or as a secondary procedure after pelvic packing in cases of persistent hemorrhage with ongoing blood product requirements.

9. **When and how is the pelvis externally fixed?**
   Any unstable pelvic fracture of the B- or C-type (see Fig. 90.1) with associated hemodynamic instability must be considered for temporary external pelvic fixation as a resuscitation tool by retaining closure and temporary stability of the pelvic ring. In unstable pelvic fractures, the effectiveness of packing relies on adjunctive external fixation for counterpressure to the retroperitoneal lap sponges. Anterior external pelvic fixation is applied as a "resuscitation frame" for unstable pelvic ring injuries of the B-type, either through the conventional iliac crest route or the fluoroscopy-guided supraacetabular route. For selected C-type injuries with complete sacroiliac joint disruption, the posterior pelvic "C-clamp" represents an effective measure of acute hemorrhage control. However, the use of a C-clamp is technically challenging and must be restricted to selected indications and experienced surgeons due to the risk of potentially serious complications.

10. **What are evidence-based guidelines for patients with high-energy pelvic fractures?**
    The WSES published an encompassing international expert consensus guideline. The recommended algorithm is based on the WSES classification and addresses the role of pelvic binders, REBOA, angioembolization, and pelvic packing (Fig. 90.3).

KEY POINTS: UROLOGIC TRAUMA

1. Urethral injury or a bladder rupture must be presumed and ruled out in any patient with a high-energy pelvic ring disruption.
2. Gross hematuria or persistent microhematuria warrants further evaluation.
3. Renal injury represents the most common urologic trauma.
4. Renal pedicle injuries can lead to significant retroperitoneal hemorrhage.

11. **Describe a significant urologic traumatic injury.**
    Most genitourinary trauma is not acutely life threatening and can be worked up and managed after stabilization of vital functions and associated injuries. However, renal pedicle injury can lead to uncontrolled hemorrhage or acute renal ischemia. The kidneys are not anatomically fixed and move to a limited degree on the vascular pedicle. Complete transection of the pedicle can lead to exsanguination, whereas lesser injury to the renal vessels can cause thrombosis and renal ischemia. Early diagnosis and surgical intervention are crucial for hemorrhage control and salvage of the affected kidney.

12. **What clinical signs may indicate injury to the kidney?**
    - Flank ecchymosis
    - Lateral abdominal tenderness or mass
    - Hematuria
    - Fracture of lumbar posterior ribs or lumbar vertebrae and transverse processes

13. **What is the general management strategy for renal injury?**
    Nonoperative management is appropriate in the large majority of patients, because most renal injuries will heal spontaneously. Surgery is indicated for hemodynamic instability, ongoing bleeding, or urinary extravasation.

14. **What diagnostic tools can be used to evaluate renal trauma?**
    CT is the preferred modality for the evaluation of blunt abdominal trauma which allows for comprehensive evaluation of all intraabdominal structures. Helical CT has increased the sensitivity for ureteral injury. Intravenous pyelography (IVP) is less sensitive and does not allow for evaluation of nonurologic injuries. However, it may still be used in cases of suspected renal or ureteral injury when CT is unavailable, or if urologic imaging is required in the operating room. Renal angiography may be indicated in the presence of a suspected vascular injury. Magnetic resonance imaging (MRI) may be useful in stable patients with contrast allergies.

15. **When should a urethral injury be suspected?**
    A urethral injury should be suspected in any patient with a high-energy pelvic ring disruption. Blood is visualized at the urethral meatus in almost 90% of all cases. Additional clinical signs include penile, scrotal, or perineal hematoma. The historic notion of a "high-riding prostate" on rectal examination is no longer part of the current ATLS algorithm. A suspected urethral injury must be worked up by a retrograde urethrogram. Insertion of a Foley catheter is contraindicated in the presence of a urethral injury and temporizing ED management consists of a percutaneous suprapubic cystostomy.

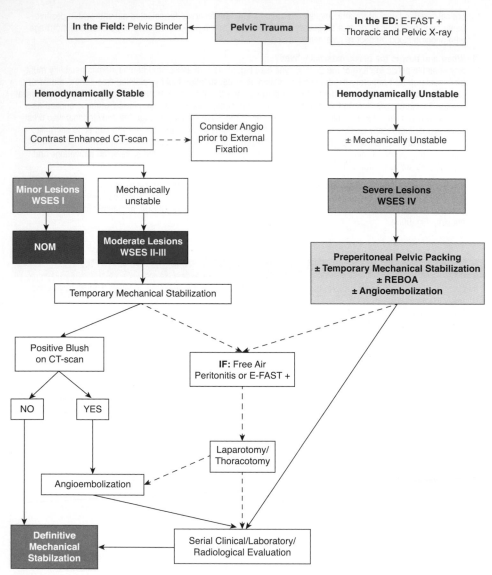

Fig. 90.3 International consensus algorithm for the management of acute pelvic ring injuries by the World Society for Emergency Surgery (WSES). *CT*, Computed tomography; *E-FAST*, extended focused assessment with sonography for trauma; *IV*, intravenous; *REBOA*, resuscitative endovascular balloon occlusion of the aorta. (Adapted with permission from Coccolini F, Stahel PF, Montori G, et al. Pelvic trauma: WSES classification and guidelines. *World J Emerg Surg.* 2017;12:5. Creative Commons 4.0 International License.)

16. **How is a retrograde urethrogram performed?**
    The urethrogram is obtained using a 12-French urinary catheter secured in the meatal fossa by inflating the balloon to approximately 3 mL. Alternatively, a catheter-tipped syringe may be used. Under fluoroscopic guidance, about 25 mL of standard water-soluble contrast material is injected under gentle pressure as AP, oblique, and lateral views are obtained.

17. **Describe the diagnostic workup for asymptomatic microhematuria.**
    Asymptomatic microscopic hematuria in adults is not a sensitive predictor of significant urologic injuries in patients with blunt abdominal trauma and the amount of blood in the urine does not correlate with the severity of injury. Repeat urinalyses are recommended, with advanced imaging for persisting hematuria.

18. **When to suspect a ureteral injury?**
    Ureteral injuries are very rare. Penetrating injuries in proximity to the ureter should raise a high level of suspicion. Hematuria may be absent even when the ureter is completely transected. The diagnostic workup consists of a CT or IV pyelogram. Ureteral injuries are invariably managed surgically.

19. **When to suspect a bladder injury?**
    Traumatic bladder rupture most often occurs in conjunction with a high-energy pelvic fracture and can also be seen with lower abdominal compression injuries caused by lap belt or steering wheel injuries. Gross hematuria is present in more than 95% of patients.

20. **How is a bladder injury evaluated?**
    The two main diagnostic modalities for evaluation of a bladder injury are CT cystography and conventional retrograde cystography. The accuracy of either method depends on adequate distention of the bladder. Bladder imaging is mandatory in the setting of gross hematuria associated with a pelvic fracture. Penetrating trauma in the vicinity of the bladder should be evaluated with a cystogram, even in absence of hematuria.

21. **What is a penile fracture?**
    A penile fracture is a sudden tear in the tunica albuginea with subsequent rupture of the corpora cavernosum which can occur in the erect penis and usually is associated with falls or sudden unexpected moves during sexual intercourse. It has also been reported with direct blunt trauma. A sudden intense pain associated with a snapping noise and immediate detumescence are typical symptoms. Most authors support surgical intervention in an attempt to restore normal function and prevent a chronic deformity. Inability to urinate, bleeding from the urethral meatus, or extravasation of urine may indicate injury to the corpora spongiosum and urethra.

22. **What is the role of ultrasound in the evaluation of testicular trauma?**
    Testicular injuries are most often caused by a fall or a kick to the scrotal area. Ultrasound is a valuable tool in assessing the integrity of the testicles. Clinical examination may be equivocal due to hematoma formation. Ultrasound can distinguish between simple hematoma and disruption of the parenchyma. Failure to suspect and diagnose testicular rupture may result in subsequent loss of the testicle.

BIBLIOGRAPHY

Burlew CC, Moore EE, Stahel PF, et al. Preperitoneal pelvic packing reduces mortality in patients with life-threatening hemorrhage due to unstable pelvic fractures. *J Trauma Acute Care Surg.* 2017;82:233–242.

Chiara O, di Fratta E, Mariani A, et al. Efficacy of extra-peritoneal pelvic packing in hemodynamically unstable pelvic fractures: a propensity score analysis. *World J Emerg Surg.* 2016;11:22.

Coccolini F, Stahel PF, Montori G, et al. Pelvic trauma: WSES classification and guidelines. *World J Emerg Surg.* 2017;12:5.

Costantini TW, Coimbra R, Holcomb JB, et al. Current management of hemorrhage from severe pelvic fractures: Results of an American Association for the Surgery of Trauma multi-institutional trial. *J Trauma Acute Care Surg.* 2016;80:717–723.

Gamberini E, Coccolini F, Tamagnini B, et al. Resuscitative endovascular balloon occlusion of the aorta in trauma: a systematic review of the literature. *World J Emerg Surg.* 2017;12:42.

Hou Z, Smith WR, Strohecker KA, et al. Hemodynamically unstable pelvic fracture management by advanced trauma life support guidelines results in high mortality. *Orthopedics.* 2012;35:e319–e324.

Kashuk JL, Moore EE, Sawyer M, et al. Postinjury coagulopathy management: goal-directed resuscitation via POC thrombelastography. *Ann Surg.* 2010;251:604 614.

Kim FJ, Pompeo A, Molina WR, et al. Early effectiveness of endoscopic posterior urethra primary alignment. *J Trauma Acute Care Surg.* 2013;75:189–194.

Stahel PF, Burlew CC, Moore EE. Current trends in the management of hemodynamically unstable pelvic ring injuries. *Curr Opin Crit Care.* 2017;23:511–519.

Stahel PF, Hammerberg EM. History of pelvic fracture management: a review. *World J Emerg Surg.* 2016;11:18.

Stahel PF, Mauffrey C, Smith WR, et al. External fixation for acute pelvic ring injuries: decision making and technical options. *J Trauma Acute Care Surg.* 2013;75:882–887.

CHAPTER 91

TRAUMA IN PREGNANCY

Melissa Parsons, MD and Jedd Roe, MD, MBA, FACEP

1. What is the most important concept I need to remember from this chapter?

Fetal outcome is largely related to maternal morbidity. The best fetal resuscitation is maternal resuscitation.

2. How common is trauma in pregnancy?

An estimated 6%–8% of pregnancies are complicated by trauma. In blunt abdominal trauma, the most common causes include motor vehicle accidents (MVAs), falls, and intimate partner violence. Immediate complications are seen in 3.2% of pregnant trauma patients, most commonly preterm labor and placental abruption. One study showed that serious MVAs accounted for a 7% maternal mortality rate, whereas the fetal mortality rate was 15%. Of falls, 80% occur after 32 weeks' gestation. In hospitalized fall patients, there are eight times the number of placental abruptions, and more than four times as many women with preterm labor.

3. Is physical or sexual abuse often seen in pregnant patients?

Yes. Intimate partner violence is reported to occur in 4%–8% of all pregnancies. One large study reported a 32% prevalence of abuse in pregnant women presenting from urban settings. Of physically abused women, 60% will be victims of multiple episodes of assault. When pregnant patients are physically abused, there is a higher incidence of low-birth-weight infants, low maternal weight gain, maternal anemia, and substance abuse. Homicides account for one-third of maternal trauma deaths. The maternal and fetal mortality rates associated with domestic violence are 3% and 16%, respectively.

4. Given the impact of domestic violence, what can be done in the emergency department (ED)?

Effective screening is essential and can be done in an abbreviated fashion. One study showed that three screening questions can detect the majority of patients who are victims of intimate partner violence, which suggests that screening for domestic violence should be pursued with all pregnant trauma patients (see Chapter 99).

5. What are the implications of MVA mechanisms of injury for pregnant patients?

MVAs are one of the leading causes of maternal and fetal mortality, and 87% of pregnant women in an MVA receive medical care. Blunt trauma from an MVA can result in abruptio placenta, uterine rupture, fetomaternal hemorrhage (FMH), amniotic fluid embolism, and direct fetal injury. One of the major risk factors for adverse outcomes is improper seat belt placement. Approximately 75% of pregnant women are noncompliant with seat belt usage during pregnancy, despite studies showing that unrestrained patients are more likely to have major complications, including adverse fetal outcomes. Proper seat belt placement is critical to decreasing injury. If the lap belt is placed too high, instead of low across the bony pelvis, it will allow the uterus to flex over the belt, increasing the risk of abruption, uterine rupture, and direct fetal injury. Use of the shoulder restraint with the lap belt will prevent excessive flexion, decreasing maternal injury and improving fetal outcomes. Only half of patients reported receiving prenatal counseling from their provider regarding appropriate seat belt placement. Another risk factor is the use of alcohol and other intoxicants, because 40%–45% of pregnant patients in an MVA test positive for such substances. Even without significant injuries to the mother, the fetus is still at risk. Placental abruption may be seen in up to 8.5% of uninjured pregnant women involved in an MVA, and 13% of those who are severely injured.

6. How do physiologic changes in pregnancy affect the evaluation of the trauma victim?

While tachycardia and hypotension may indicate hypovolemic shock in a nonpregnant woman, in pregnancy, these vital sign "abnormalities" may merely reflect physiologic changes or supine positioning. The maternal blood volume increases by 50% by the end of the second trimester, and as a result, signs of shock may not be clinically apparent until 2000 mL or 30%–40% of maternal blood volume is lost. Furthermore, uterine flow comprises 20% of cardiac output, approximately 600 mL/min. Given the markedly increased blood flow, the uterus is a potential source of blood loss that requires investigation. Because physiologic changes also result in increased oxygen demand and decreased oxygen reserve, tissue hypoxia develops more rapidly in response to a traumatic insult. In addition, placental blood flow has no autoregulation, and thus small changes in blood pressure can result in fetal distress. Finally, decreased gastric emptying increases the aspiration risk in pregnant women.

7. How do physiologic changes of pregnancy affect laboratory values?

A physiologic anemia is seen as the plasma volume rises by more than twice the amount of red blood cells. Hematocrit levels are typically 32%–34% by the third trimester. Fibrinogen levels are double those seen in other trauma patients; therefore, normal fibrinogen levels in a pregnant patient should raise suspicion of disseminated intravascular coagulation (DIC). Because of hormonal stimulation of the central respiratory drive, the partial pressure of carbon dioxide (PCO_2) falls to between 27 and 32 mmHg, and injury sufficient to cause a respiratory acidosis might be manifested by what ordinarily would be considered a normal PCO_2 of 40 mmHg.

8. **Are serious maternal injuries required for fetal injury to be present?**
   Not always. Although in utero damage is often associated with maternal pelvic fractures, 7% of maternal cases with minor trauma have poor fetal outcome. Even with only minor trauma to the mother, significant placental abruption can occur without obvious symptoms, requiring fetal monitoring. Direct injuries to the fetus in utero are unusual, but given the size of the fetal head, when direct trauma occurs, fetal head injury is the most common injury.

9. **Name the most common causes of fetal death.**
   - Maternal death
   - Maternal shock
   - Placental abruption

10. **How does placental abruption occur?**
    Abruption results from the separation of the relatively inelastic placenta from an elastic myometrium of the uterus secondary to a shearing or deceleration force. There may be vaginal bleeding, uterine contractions, or fetal heart rate abnormalities. Conversely, there may be little or no external evidence of injury. Although abruption may be present in 50% of patients with life-threatening injuries, it also exists in 2%–4% of those with a minor mechanism of injury.

11. **What are the findings of abruption after trauma?**
    Classically, the clinical findings of abruption have included vaginal bleeding and abdominal and uterine tenderness. In many cases, fetal distress may be the only presenting sign, because the reduction in placental blood flow to the fetus causes hypoxia and acidosis. DIC may occur with placental injury, and evaluation for DIC can be performed by screening for a serum fibrinogen level, with low or low–normal levels being the indication for obtaining a complete DIC panel (prothrombin time, partial thromboplastin time, fibrinogen, and fibrin degradation products).

12. **How often does ultrasound detect placental abruption?**
    Because a large separation must be present for an ultrasound to be diagnostic, it detects only about half of all cases. In many instances, fetal distress is present before clear visualization of an abruption by ultrasound. The fetal mortality rate from abruption is reported to be 30%–68%. Usually, an abruption large enough to place the fetus at risk becomes apparent within 48 hours, and detection of fetal distress mandates prompt delivery of the fetus.

13. **Are radiologic investigations harmful to the fetus?**
    The fundamental effects of radiation on the developing fetus are intrauterine growth retardation, defects in the central nervous system (microcephaly, mental retardation), and risk of cancer. The most vulnerable period is between 2 and 15 weeks' gestation. Cumulative exposure of less than 5 rads (50 mGy) during pregnancy has been shown to have negligible risk to the fetus. In general, all ***necessary*** radiographic studies should be undertaken regardless of any radiation concerns. Pelvic shielding should be employed as often as possible. Additionally, there have been no reported adverse effects on neonatal thyroid function with the use of iodinated contrast, and it should be administered if required. Evaluation should begin with the nonradiographic alternative of ED ultrasound (focused assessment with sonography for trauma [FAST]) to rapidly determine the presence of intraperitoneal hemorrhage, pericardial effusion, or pneumothorax.

14. **How should these patients be managed in the field?**
    Given the reduced maternal oxygen reserve and increased fetal oxygen demand, oxygen therapy is crucial. Intravenous volume resuscitation with crystalloid should proceed as with other trauma patients. Avoid uterine compression of the inferior vena cava by manually displacing the uterus to the left, transporting the patient on her left side, or, if the patient is immobilized, elevating the right side of the backboard to 15 or 20 degrees. Aside from early transport, the most important aspect of prehospital management is to notify the ED so that the appropriate obstetric consultants may participate on the trauma team.

15. **What are the priorities for ED management?**
    The prehospital therapies mentioned previously should be continued. Of particular importance is the history of this pregnancy with attention directed at estimating gestational age and fetal viability. After the usual primary and secondary survey, a sterile speculum examination should be performed to evaluate for the presence of vaginal fluid or blood, opening of the cervical os, and genital tract trauma. Continued aggressive resuscitation with warmed lactated Ringer solution (less acidotic, more physiologic than normal saline) and blood is especially important, given the physiologic changes mentioned previously.

16. **How do I begin to evaluate the fetus?**
    First, determine the size of the uterus and the presence or absence of abdominal and uterine tenderness. Uterine size, measured in centimeters from the pubic symphysis to fundus, provides a rough estimate of gestational age and potential viability. At 20 weeks' gestation, the fundus should be at the level of the umbilicus. At 24 weeks'

gestation, which is considered viable, the fundus should be three finger breadths above the umbilicus. At 36 weeks' gestation, the fundus is approximately at the xiphoid process. Next, carefully inspect the vaginal introitus for evidence of vaginal bleeding, and assess for fetal distress, which is the earliest indication of maternal hypovolemia. Abnormal fetal heart rates are greater than 160 beats per minute (bpm) and less than 120 bpm. As soon as possible after patient arrival, continuous electronic fetal monitoring (EFM) should be initiated to ascertain early signs of fetal distress (e.g., decreased variability of heart rate or fetal decelerations after contractions). Ultrasound should be done promptly thereafter to confirm gestational age, fetal viability, and the integrity of the placenta.

17. What is fetomaternal hemorrhage (FMH)?

FMH is hemorrhage of fetal blood into the usually distinct maternal circulation. The incidence of FMH in trauma patients has been reported to be 30% (four to five times the incidence of noninjured controls). With FMH, the complications of maternal Rhesus factor (Rh) sensitization, fetal anemia, and fetal death can occur. Laboratory techniques, specifically the Kleihauer-Betke (KB) test, which detects fetal erythrocytes in the maternal circulation, is not sensitive enough to diagnose FMH accurately.

18. How is FMH managed?

The prudent course is to give Rh immunoglobulin (RhIG) to all Rh-negative patients who are suspected of having abdominal trauma, because RhIG given within 72 hours of antigenic exposure prevents Rh isoimmunization. In the first trimester, 50 µg of RhIG is the dosage used. This dosage is increased to 300 µg after 12 weeks' gestation. Massive transfusion (>30 mL) into the maternal circulation can occur with severe abdominal trauma. Although the KB test cannot rule out FMH, it can be used to determine whether the patient requires more than 300 µg of RhIG in the setting of massive hemorrhage. A standard dose of 300 µg neutralizes 30 mL of fetal blood, so the KB test will show if additional doses of RhIG are necessary.

19. When is emergency cesarean section indicated?

The first factor to be considered is the stability of the mother. Given the fact that uteroplacental blood flow may require up to 30% of a mother's cardiac output, staging of the perimortem cesarean section with other necessary procedures in a mother who has sustained multiple serious injuries is critical, as emptying the uterus improves maternal physiology. The next factor to consider is gestational age. Fetuses whose gestational age is 24 weeks, or whose weight is estimated to be greater than 750 g, are predicted to have a 50% survival rate in the neonatal intensive care unit (NICU) setting and are considered viable. The most common indication for cesarean section is fetal distress. Other indications are uterine rupture and malpresentation of the fetus.

20. When should perimortem cesarean section be performed?

Perimortem cesarean section should be done when ultrasound or uterine size suggests viability (i.e., above the umbilicus) and maternal death is imminent. Resuscitation should be instituted within 4 minutes of loss of pulses, but fetal survival with normal neurologic outcome has been reported 30 minutes after maternal decompensation. Delivery of the near-term fetus improves maternal cardiac output by 30%–80%, relieves aortocaval compression and improves the effectiveness of cardiopulmonary resuscitation (CPR). Thus maternal outcomes have been shown to improve with perimortem delivery as well.

21. Which pregnant patients with abdominal trauma require admission for fetal monitoring?

Any viable (>23–24 weeks' gestation) fetus requires continuous electronic fetal monitoring. EFM is recommended even for patients without external evidence of trauma, because it has been well documented that these patients are at risk from placental abruption. Current guidelines suggest that these patients be observed for a minimum of 4 hours with a cardiotocograph. If any abnormalities are discovered – including contractions, amniotic membrane rupture, vaginal bleeding, serious maternal injury, significant abdominal pain, and concerning fetal heart rate variability – the patient should be hospitalized and monitored for 24 hours.

KEY POINTS: TRAUMA IN PREGNANCY

1. Aggressive maternal resuscitation is the best therapy for the fetus.
2. The fetus may be in acute distress with little or no maternal manifestation of injury.
3. Ultrasound is the investigation of choice to evaluate the maternal abdomen and the fetus.
4. All clinically necessary radiologic investigations should be performed regardless of radiation concerns.

Website
www.perinatology.com/exposures/Physical/Xray.htm; accessed March 2, 2015.

BIBLIOGRAPHY

Benrubi GI. *Handbook of Obstetric and Gynecologic Emergencies.* Philadelphia, PA: Wolters Kluwer; 2020.

Huls CK, Detlefs C. Trauma in pregnancy. *Semin Perinatol.* 2018;42(1):13–20.

Jain V, Chari R, Maslovitz S, et al. Guidelines for the management of a pregnant trauma patient. *J Obstet Gynaecol Can.* 2015; 37(6):553–574.

Luley T, Fitzpatrick B, Grotegut CA, et al. Perinatal implications of motor vehicle accident trauma: identifying populations at risk. *Am J Obstet Gynecol.* 2013;208:466e1–466e5.

Melamed N, Aviram A, Silver M, et al. Pregnancy course and outcome following blunt trauma. *J Matern Fetal Neonatal Med.* 2012; 25(9):1612–1617.

Mendez-Figueroa H, Dahlke JD, Vrees RA, et al. Trauma in pregnancy: an updated systematic review. *Am J Obstet Gynecol.* 2013;209(1):1–10.

Pearce C, Martin SR. Trauma and considerations unique to pregnancy. *Obstet Gynecol Clin North Am.* 2016;43(4):791–808.

Roe E, Hang BS, Lyon D, et al. Perimortem cesarean delivery. eMedicine from WebMD. Updated May 23, 2017. http://emedicine.medscape.com/article/83059-overview. Accessed October 9, 2014.

Sakamoto J, Michels C, Eisfelder B, et al. Trauma in pregnancy. *Emerg Med Clin North Am.* 2019;37(2):317–338.

CHAPTER 92

PEDIATRIC TRAUMA

Patrick Joynt, MD, MA and Taylor McCormick, MD, MSc

1. **How common is pediatric trauma?**

   There are ~10 million emergency department (ED) visits and ~10,000 deaths in children and adolescents from traumatic injuries each year. Though in the United States, trauma is the leading cause of death and disability in children, most cases of pediatric trauma are minor, single-system injuries. Timely recognition and management of severe injury is critical for optimal outcomes. Every ED, regardless of trauma center designation, must be prepared to stabilize a severely injured child.

2. **What are the most common injuries in children?**

   Blunt trauma accounts for ~90% of pediatric injury, and can lead to multisystem injuries as force is widely distributed through a child's small body. Head injury is the most common cause of death in pediatric trauma. Common mechanisms of severe injury include motor vehicle collisions, auto versus pedestrian encounters, falls, and firearm injuries. Unfortunately, nonaccidental trauma (NAT) is common and must always be considered; 40% of deaths from child abuse occur in children less than 12 months of age (see Chapter 67).

3. **What can be done to ease the cognitive burden when caring for injured children?**

   The use of length, age, and weight-based dosing and equipment systems have been shown to reduce time to medication delivery, quantitative errors, and anxiety among emergency care providers. Transfer agreements and protocols should be established in advance.

4. **Name the anatomic and physiologic differences between children and adults that should be considered in the initial evaluation and management of a pediatric trauma patient?**

   While the initial assessment and simultaneous stabilization of injured children does not differ from adults, the following anatomic and physiologic differences should be recognized:

   Airway
   - The pediatric glottis is high and anterior, and the prominent occiput causes neck flexion; elevate the shoulders and back with a towel roll or stack of sheets to align the oral, pharyngeal, and laryngeal axes and maintain a neutral spine.
   - The cricothyroid membrane in young children is too small for an open cricothyrotomy; needle cricothyrotomy is recommended for infants and children after failed endotracheal intubation and supraglottic airway placement.
   - The cricoid cartilage is the narrowest portion of the airway in children <8 years; downsize the endotracheal tube if unable to advance once past the vocal cords.

   Breathing
   - High oxygen consumption rates and low physiologic reserve lead to short safe apnea times and precipitous desaturation during pediatric intubation; apneic oxygenation can reduce hypoxemia at the following age-based flow rates:
     - 4 L for ≤2 years
     - 6 L for >2 years to ≤12 years
     - 8 L for >12 years
   - Compliant chest walls make pulmonary contusions without rib fractures common in children.
   - Gastric insufflation with bag-valve-mask ventilation can compromise ventilation; avoid excessive volumes and place a nasogastric or orogastric tube as soon as possible.

   Circulation
   - Compensatory mechanisms (tachycardia and vasoconstriction) may maintain blood pressure in pediatric trauma patients until loss of ~40% of blood volume, at which time decompensation abruptly occurs; do not rely on hypotension alone to identify shock.
   - There are no documented survivors from ED thoracotomy following blunt traumatic arrest in children <15 years old; withholding ED thoracotomy should be considered in children.
   - Anterior tibia, then distal femur, and medial malleolus are preferred sites for interosseous access in children if peripheral intravenous (IV) placement is unsuccessful.

   Disability
   - Young children with open sutures and large fontanelles may have delayed signs of increased intracranial pressure after significant head injury.
   - Use the pediatric Glasgow Coma Scale (GCS) score or AVPU (alert, verbal, painful, unresponsive) scale for mental status assessment of preverbal children; an AVPU score of V or better correlates to a GCS score of ≥9.

- Due to their relatively large head and high cervical fulcrum, children <8 years are prone to upper cervical spine injuries. Ligamentous cervical injuries without fracture are common in children due to horizontally situated facet joints, incomplete spinal ossification, and immature ligamentous support structures.

Exposure

- Children have a large surface area to volume ratio and greater metabolic demand, placing them at higher risk for hypothermia and coagulopathy.

5. **Does the FAST examination help in the diagnosis or management of pediatric trauma?**
   The focused assessment with sonography for trauma (FAST) should not be used in isolation to screen for intraabdominal injury (IAI) in children or adults. FAST is less accurate in children than adults, with reported sensitivities ranging from 20% to 80% and specificities of 80%–95%. FAST (or more accurately, extended FAST [E-FAST], which includes evaluation for pneumothorax) is still recommended in the evaluation of an unstable child following trauma, and may be considered in the evaluation of the stable patient along with other clinical factors.

6. **Where is free fluid most likely to be found on the pediatric FAST examination?**
   In the pelvis, followed by the right upper quadrant.

7. **What is the survival rate after ED thoracotomy in pediatric traumatic arrest?**
   The survival rate after ED thoracotomy for pediatric penetrating thoracic trauma is ~14%, similar to that of adults. For blunt trauma, while the survival rate for 15- to 18-year-olds undergoing thoracotomy mirrors adults at 1%–2%, there are no documented survivors from ED thoracotomy in children less than 15 years old. For children under 15 years old with no signs of life after blunt trauma, withholding ED thoracotomy should be considered.

8. **When should a massive transfusion protocol (MTP) be activated for an injured child? What blood product ratio should be used?**
   The limited evidence in pediatric trauma supports initiating MTP once 40 mL/kg of blood product have been, or are expected to be, transfused. The optimal ratio of blood products for children is unknown, but 1:1:1 or 1:1:2 of plasma, platelets, and packed red blood cells (pRBCs) is reasonable. Thromboelastography (TEG) is a whole blood measure of clot formation under physiologic conditions that allows for a goal-directed approach to the management of acute traumatic coagulopathy using plasma, platelets, cryoprecipitate, and pRBCs to target specific coagulation defects. A TEG-based transfusion strategy may also be considered as an alternative to fixed ratio MTP if available.

9. **What is tranexamic acid (TXA) and should it be given for hemorrhage control in pediatric trauma?**
   TXA inhibits plasminogen, leading to the prevention of clot breakdown, and ultimately, hemorrhage control. Preliminary evidence for TXA shows a reduction in mortality for children with ongoing severe hemorrhage, and should ideally be guided by TEG results.

10. **How are pRBCs, plasma, platelets, cryoprecipitate, and TXA dosed in children?**
    - pRBCs 10 mL/kg
    - plasma 10 mL/kg
    - platelets 10 mL/kg
    - cryoprecipitate 10 mL/kg
    - TXA <12 years old: 15 mg/kg over 10 minutes within 3 hours; then, 2 mg/kg/h over 8 hours
    - TXA ≥12 years old: 1 g over 10 minutes within 3 hours; then, 1 g over 8 hours

11. **What is the role of permissive hypotension in injured children?**
    Permissive hypotension is a controversial tenet of damage control resuscitation in adults. There are no data to support the use of permissive hypotension in children. On the contrary, volume expansion with 10–40 mL/kg of crystalloid until blood products are available is recommended for children in compensated shock.

12. **How do I recognize shock in a pediatric patient?**
    Children have increased physiologic reserve and robust hemodynamic compensatory mechanisms. As a result, they often maintain a blood pressure in the normal range even in the presence of significant blood loss (this is referred to as *compensated shock*). Young children are less able to increase their cardiac contractility, and therefore maintain their cardiac output and blood pressure in the presence of blood loss by increasing their heart rate and systemic vascular resistance (SVR). In addition to the vital sign abnormalities listed below, it is critical to evaluate children for other signs of hemodynamic instability, such as poor skin perfusion (mottling of the skin, cool extremities, capillary refill greater than 2 seconds), decreased pulse pressure, increased work of breathing, and abnormal mental status (depressed level of consciousness or agitation).
    - Tachycardia may be the result of pain or emotional distress in the injured child, but should always alert the provider to possible blood loss.
    - Bradycardia in an injured child is an ominous sign that can result from head injury, spinal cord injury, respiratory failure, or profound shock; bradycardia can herald cardiac arrest.

- Hypotension may be a late or perimortem sign of shock in a child. Quickly estimate the lower limit of normal blood pressure (fifth percentile) based on a child's age:
  - <1 year old: >60 mmHg
  - 1–10 years old: [70 + (2 × Age in years)] mmHg
- Consider calculating the shock index: heart rate divided by systolic blood pressure. Values >1.2 for 4–6 years old, 1.0 for 7–12 years old, and 0.9 for 13–19 years old should prompt concern, as they have been associated with greater need for operation, intubation, and transfusion, when compared with hypotension alone.

13. What is a child's normal blood volume?
Approximately 80 mL/kg: a 5-year-old child weighing 20 kg has a total blood volume of 1.6 L.

14. What is Waddell's triad?
Waddell's triad consists of a femur fracture, intraabdominal or intrathoracic injury, and head injury, which can occur when a child is struck by an automobile at high speed. It is an example of the propensity toward multisystem injury in children, when significant blunt force is applied to a small body mass.

15. What is a handlebar injury?
The term *handlebar injury* refers to a direct blow to the abdomen from a bicycle handlebar with or without significant external signs of trauma. Handlebar injuries carry a high risk for solid organ injury, hollow viscous injury, and abdominal wall hernias.

16. What is the seat belt syndrome?
Seat belt syndrome, or lap belt syndrome, is the classic triad of abdominal wall ecchymosis, hyperflexion-distraction injury of the lumbar spine (Chance fracture), and IAI. It is usually associated with motor vehicle collisions, in which a child is wearing a seat belt improperly (lap belt positioned high over the abdomen rather than low over the pelvis, or the shoulder belt positioned behind the child's back). A seat belt sign alone is highly associated with IAI. Proper installation and use of car seats, including booster seats, are essential for reducing morbidity and mortality rates among children in motor vehicle collisions.

17. What are some considerations regarding intraosseous (IO) line placement in children?
IO lines can be inserted easily and quickly. IO line insertion should be considered in any critically ill patient if a peripheral line cannot be established immediately. IO lines are safe for administration of virtually any fluid, blood product, or drug. Infusion rates are comparable to a 21-gauge IV. While most serum laboratory testing can be sent from an IO aspirate, the white blood cell count, potassium, calcium, and aspartate transaminase/alanine transferase (AST/ALT) may not be accurate. The preferred site is the proximal tibia below the tibial tuberosity. Other potential sites include the distal femur and medial malleolus. The proximal humerus should be avoided until late adolescence when a child has reached skeletal maturity. For the conscious child experiencing pain with IO infusion, 0.5 mg/kg of 2% lidocaine (20 mg/mL) may be administered with a maximum dose of 40 mg (2 mL). IO lines should not be placed distal to a fracture and should be aimed away from the physis to prevent growth plate damage. They should be removed within 24 hours once peripheral or central IV access is secured. Complications are rare but include cellulitis, osteomyelitis, growth plate injury, fat embolism, compartment syndrome, and iatrogenic fractures.

18. What is the leading cause of trauma-related death and disability in children?
Traumatic brain injury.

19. Name the different types of traumatic brain injury and risk factors for poor outcomes.
Focal brain injuries include subdural hematoma, epidural hematoma, intraparenchymal hemorrhage, subarachnoid hemorrhage, and cerebral contusion. Diffuse brain injuries range in severity from mild concussion to diffuse axonal injury, which results from shearing forces at the gray–white matter junction. Low initial GCS score, younger age (<4 years old), hypotension, coagulopathy, and hyperglycemia are associated with poor outcomes.

20. Which children need computed tomography (CT) imaging after minor head trauma?
The Pediatric Emergency Care Applied Research Network (PECARN) decision rules are used to guide clinician's use of imaging by identifying children at very low risk for clinically important traumatic brain injury (ciTBI). The rules (below) have been shown in multiple validation studies to be highly sensitive (99%–100%) and moderately specific (55%–69%) for ciTBI.
- <2 years old: normal mental status, no scalp hematoma (except frontal), no loss of consciousness or loss of consciousness <5 seconds, nonsevere mechanism, no palpable skull fracture, and acting normally per parents.
- ≥2 years old: normal mental status, no loss of consciousness, no vomiting, nonsevere mechanism, no signs of basilar skull fracture, and no severe headache.

  Not all children that do not meet the low-risk criteria defined in PECARN require neuroimaging; consider a period of observation for all children with normal mental status and no evidence of skull fracture. It should be noted that clinician judgement has also been shown to be highly sensitive, and perhaps more specific in determining which children need a CT.

21. **What is a concussion? How should patients and parents be counseled on returning to activity?**
    Concussion is defined as trauma-induced brain dysfunction without structural injury on standard neuroimaging. Concussions may occur with initial loss of consciousness, but loss of consciousness is not required for diagnosis. Initially, a child may have amnesia, headache, dizziness, nausea/vomiting, blurry vision, or confusion. CT imaging, if obtained, will be normal, but subtle diffuse axonal abnormalities may be seen on magnetic resonance imaging (MRI). Recent guidelines recommend against "brain rest," instead advocating for a graded, but immediate return to some physical and cognitive activity. Athletes should be immediately removed from competition and strenuous activity, but can be permitted to walk briskly if minimally symptomatic. Special accommodations for schoolwork should be tailored to each child. Complete cessation of screen time can lead to social isolation and worsen mood symptoms; screen time should be limited based on symptoms. Consider reducing brightness, duration, and increasing font size. Sequelae can include headaches, cognitive impairment, disrupted sleep, and behavioral or psychological issues. The average length of symptoms from a concussion is 5–7 days, but in some children, especially younger children, symptoms may last weeks to months. Parents and children should be counseled on this possibility and arrange clear follow-up with a primary care provider.

22. **How do cervical spine injures in children differ from those in adults?**
    - The anatomic fulcrum of the cervical spine moves caudally from C2-3 at birth to C5-6 at 8 years old, predisposing young children to higher cervical spine injuries than older children and adults.
    - Pediatric cervical spine injuries are often associated with severe brain injury and respiratory arrest, often leading to death at the scene of the accident.
    - Children often sustain ligamentous cervical injuries without fractures as a result of more horizontally oriented facet joints, spinal elasticity, incomplete ossification, and immature ligamentous support structures.

23. **What is SCIWORA?**
    SCIWORA stands for Spinal Cord Injury WithOut Radiographic Abnormality. Before the widespread availability of thin-slice CT and MRI, the term SCIWORA was used to describe children with normal x-rays or CT scans and significant spinal cord injuries (most commonly cervical). We now know these injuries are actually more common in adults than children and can be identified on MRI. Both adults and children with neurologic symptoms (radicular or myelopathic), but normal x-rays or CT scans, should be further evaluated with MRI in the ED. Patients with transient spinal cord symptoms that quickly resolve should also undergo MRI, as this may represent spinal cord stretching that can herald delayed cord edema and recurrent spinal cord pathology. Patients without neurologic symptoms, but persistent spinal pain or tenderness, may be discharged in a rigid cervical collar with outpatient follow-up and MRI if pain persists.

24. **Which children should undergo cervical spine imaging after trauma?**
    Children with neck pain, midline bony tenderness, decreased range of motion, torticollis, altered mental status (GCS score <14), focal neurologic abnormality, predisposing conditions, or transient spinal cord symptoms should have their cervical spine imaged. Plain radiographs (anteroposterior [AP], lateral, and odontoid views) are preferred for most patients. Patients with abnormal plain radiographs or concerning physical examination findings should undergo CT or MRI, and often require both.

25. **What is pseudosubluxation of the cervical spine, and how common is it?**
    Pseudosubluxation of the cervical spine in which the C2 vertebral body is slightly anteriorly displaced relative to the C3 body (C2 on C3 pseudosubluxation) is a normal anatomic variant in children. It is due to the normal mobility of the vertebral bodies in young children, and is seen in about 40% of children under age 7, and 20% up to age 16. It can be differentiated from true subluxation by evaluating Swischuk's line, which is drawn along the anterior edge of the spinous processes of C1 and C3. Injury is suspected if the line passes at a distance greater than 1.5 mm from the anterior spinous process of C2 (Fig. 92.1).

26. **Should all pediatric trauma patients get routine chest and pelvis x-rays?**
    Chest x-ray is indicated for an abnormal thoracic examination, hemodynamic instability, severe mechanism, or after endotracheal intubation or thoracostomy tube placement. Pelvic fractures are uncommon in young children and x-ray is seldom useful in hemodynamically stable children of all ages; significant pelvic pain or instability warrants CT imaging.

27. **How common are mediastinal (great vessel) injuries in children?**
    Mediastinal injuries are very rare in children. Because of the high compliance of the chest wall and laxity of the ligamentous structures of the mediastinum, aortic injuries are exceedingly rare in children compared with adults. Chest CT should be avoided in children without a high pre-test probability for a blunt thoracic aortic injury; the estimated cancer risk from a chest CT in children has been shown to exceed the positive rate of chest CTs in this cohort.

28. **What are predictors of pediatric IAIs?**
    High-risk mechanisms for IAI should be taken into consideration, including high-speed motor vehicle collisions, pedestrians struck by automobiles, bicycle accidents (including handlebar injuries), lap belt usage, and direct

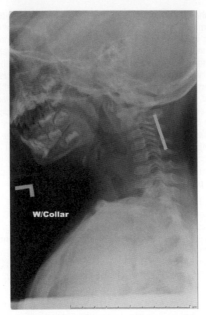

Fig. 92.1 Pseudosubluxation of C2 on C3 – 2 mm of anterolisthesis of C2 on C3 is apparent. Swischuk's line *(solid line)* shows the anterior aspect of the C2 spinous process is within 2 mm of this line, suggesting this is pseudosubluxation and not a dislocation of C2 on C3. (From Easter JS, Barkin R, Rosen CL, et al. Cervical spine injuries in children, part II: management and special considerations. *J Emerg Med.* 2011;41(3):252–256.)

blows to the abdomen. A clinical decision rule has been validated for identifying children at very low risk for clinically important IAI (defined as requiring therapeutic laparotomy, angiographic embolization, blood transfusion for abdominal hemorrhage, or IV fluid for ≥2 nights for pancreatic/gastrointestinal injuries). In patients with the following examination findings, CT can safely be avoided:

1. No evidence of abdominal wall trauma or seat belt sign
2. GCS score 14–15
3. No abdominal tenderness
4. No evidence of thoracic wall trauma
5. No complaint of abdominal pain
6. No absent or decreased breath sounds
7. No vomiting

KEY POINTS: PEDIATRIC TRAUMA

1. While most cases of pediatric trauma are minor, single-system injuries, trauma is the leading cause of death and disability in children in the United States.
2. The use of length, age, and weight-based dosing and equipment systems have been shown to reduce time to medication delivery, quantitative errors, and anxiety among emergency care providers.
3. The evaluation of pediatric trauma patients mirrors that of adults with special consideration of pediatric anatomy and physiology.
4. Hypotension is a late and ominous finding in the pediatric trauma patient. Tachycardia and signs of poor perfusion are earlier clues.
5. Clinical decision rules can help identify children at low risk for clinically important brain and intraabdominal injuries.
6. Chest CT is rarely useful in the evaluation of a pediatric trauma patient; the risk of radiation exceeds the likelihood of great vessel injury in most injured children.

BIBLIOGRAPHY

American College of Surgeons Committee on Trauma. *Advanced Trauma Life Support (ATLS) Student Course Manual.* 9th ed. Chicago, IL: American College of Surgeons; 2012.

Arbuthnot M, Onwubiko C, Osborne M, et al. Does the incidence of thoracic aortic injury warrant the routine use of a chest computed tomography in children? *J Trauma Acute Care Surg.* 2019;86(1):97–100.

Golden J, Isani M, Bowling J, et al. Limiting chest computed tomography in the evaluation of pediatric thoracic trauma. *J Trauma Acute Care Surg.* 2016;81(2):271–277.

Halstead ME, Walter KD, Moffatt K. Sport-related concussion in children and adolescents. *Pediatrics.* 2018;142(6):1–24.

Holmes JF, Kelley KM, Wootton-Gorges SL, et al. Effect of abdominal ultrasound on clinical care, outcomes, and resource use among children with blunt torso trauma: a randomized clinical trial. *JAMA.* 2017;317(22):2290–2296.

Holmes JF, Mao A, Awasthi S, et al. Validation of a prediction rule for the identification of children with intra-abdominal injuries after blunt torso trauma. *Ann Emerg Med.* 2009;54(4):528–533.

Kupperman N, Holmes JF, Dayan PS, et al. Identification of children at very low risk of clinically-important brain injuries after head trauma. *Lancet.* 2009;374(9696):1160–1170.

National Center for Health Statistics: *CDC using WISQARS,* 1999–2018. https://www.cdc.gov/injury/wisqars/LeadingCauses.html. Accessed February 28, 2019.

Nordin A, Coleman A, Shi J, et al. Validation of the age-adjusted shock index using pediatric trauma quality improvement program data. *J Pediatr Surg.* 2017;S0022-3468(17)30645-0. doi:10.1016/j.jpedsurg.2017.10.023.

Springer E, Frazier SB, Arnold DH, et al. External validation of a clinical prediction rule for very low risk pediatric blunt abdominal trauma. *Am J Emerg Med.* 2018;37(9):1643–1648. doi:10.1016/j.annemergmed.2012.11.009.

CHAPTER 93

MUSCULOSKELETAL TRAUMA, CONDITIONS OF THE EXTREMITY, AND HAND INJURIES

Kyros Ipaktchi, MD, FACS and Sean Morell, MD

1. What are immediate treatment priorities in open fractures?

Open fractures warrant an immediate orthopedic consultation. After ruling out associated vital organ injuries, open fractures are assessed during the secondary survey. Any skin break near a fracture site should be presumed to communicate with the fracture until proved otherwise. After careful examination, including neurologic and vascular assessment, clean the wound of gross contamination, and apply a sterile dressing. Unless needed to control hemorrhage, wound probing in the emergency department (ED) is discouraged. Whenever possible, direct pressure should be used for hemorrhage control. Axial realignment and splinting immobilize the bone, decreasing blood loss, and protecting the soft tissue from further damage. Avoid wound cultures, extensive irrigation, and multiple examinations of the wound, because of the increased potential for secondary contamination and soft-tissue damage. Administer tetanus prophylaxis and intravenous (IV) antibiotics. A first-generation cephalosporin, such as cefazolin, is used most commonly for antibiotic prophylaxis. In more severe open fractures, Gustilo-Anderson 3, and grossly contaminated fractures, consider piperacillin/tazobactam or adding an aminoglycoside. Fig. 93.1 depicts the institutional multidisciplinary protocol for the initial management of open fractures.

2. What percentage of polytrauma patients have unrecognized fractures at time of admission?

Up to 20% of all multiply injured patients have unrecognized fractures at the time of initial assessment. These occult injuries are located most commonly around the wrist, hand, ankle, and foot. This important fact highlights the need for a tertiary survey of multiply injured patients. The patient's family should be informed from the beginning of the patient's care about the potential that initially unrecognized injuries and fractures may be found in later surveys.

3. What is compartment syndrome?

Acute compartment syndrome (ACS) develops when the pressure within the confined space of the muscle compartment exceeds capillary filling pressures, resulting in muscle ischemia and edema. Muscle ischemia, in turn, increases intracompartmental pressure and leads to a vicious cycle, resulting in muscle and nerve necrosis. Any progressive mismatch between size of a compartment and its contents can result in ACS.

4. What causes compartment syndrome?

Common causes include fractures, crush injuries, extravasated IV fluids, hemorrhage, postischemic swelling after vascular injury repair, tight-fitting casts or dressings, and circumferential burns. Importantly, ACS can result from minor injury mechanisms as well. Have a high level of suspicion for ACS in the following scenarios:

- Pain out of proportion to clinical findings after a soft-tissue injury, with or without associated underlying fracture or joint dislocation.
- Peripheral ischemic events secondary to vascular injuries by direct trauma or indirectly by kinking of a critical vascular structure (e.g., popliteal artery kinking after prolonged surgical procedures in lithotomy position, prolonged travels by airplane or motor vehicle with flexed knees, superficial femoral artery [SFA] injuries associated with femur fractures).
- Exercise-induced compartmental pain and swelling that resolves with rest. "Exertional compartment syndrome" is a rare variant. It is most typically seen in horseback riders, cyclists, and runners.

  As a general rule of thumb, it is prudent to exclude the presence of ACS in any patient with painful extremities of uncertain etiology.

5. What are the clinical signs and symptoms of ACS?

The classic five Ps to reflect symptoms of ACS (**p**ain, **p**aresthesia, **p**allor, **p**ulselessness, **p**aralysis) should be revisited to exclusively reflect the main cardinal symptom of ACS: *Pain, pain, pain, pain, pain!* In fact, pain out of proportion to the clinical examination represents the earliest and most common symptom associated with ACS. Pain is typically exacerbated when passively stretching the muscles of the involved compartment (e.g., passive extension of great toe and ankle for assessment of suspected lower limb ACS). Pain is typically ischemic in nature and often not relieved by narcotics. The other four Ps represent late symptoms of a "missed" compartment syndrome and typically reflect the extent of an irreversible ischemic injury.

  Although there are various methods of measuring intracompartmental pressures, the diagnostic gold standard is represented by a positive clinical examination in conjunction with pain out of proportion and a plausible history (as outlined).

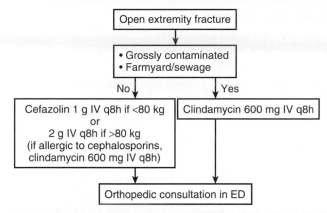

Fig. 93.1 Emergency department *(ED)* management of open fractures. *IV,* Intravenous; *q8h,* every 8 hours. (Modified from Mauffrey C, Bailey JR, Bowles RJ, et al. Acute management of open fractures: proposal of a new multidisciplinary algorithm. *Orthopedics.* 2012;35: 877–881. Healio.com. Accessed April 10, 2015.)

6. **What are the most common sites for compartment syndrome?**
   The leg is the most common anatomic location for ACS, most often associated with proximal tibia fractures and tibia shaft fractures. The anterior compartment of the leg is most commonly affected, and the deep posterior compartment of the leg is the site that is most often missed. Thigh compartment syndrome is less common, and therefore more at risk for being missed. Similarly, upper extremity ACS requires a high level of suspicion, because volar compartment (carpal tunnel syndrome) and forearm compartment syndromes are often missed. These are often associated with both-bone forearm fractures, high-energy distal radius fractures, radiocarpal dislocations, and pediatric supracondylar humerus fractures.

7. **How do I treat compartment syndrome?**
   Detailed documentation and timing of physical findings are of essential importance. The only valid and curative treatment option for ACS is the immediate surgical release of all involved compartments by fasciotomies. Non-operative measures are justified for monitoring suspected compartment syndrome in equivocal cases. Removal of all circumferential dressings and maintenance of normal limb perfusion by maintaining a normotensive blood pressure are important adjuncts to managing limbs at risk. When in doubt, surgical compartment release by fasciotomies represents the treatment of choice. Rare exceptions to this rule include the presence of crush syndrome and nonviable compartments, and this difficult judgment requires a decision by a qualified surgeon.

8. **Describe the joint fluid analysis consistent with septic arthritis.**
   See Chapter 55.

9. **How do I diagnose a traumatic arthrotomy (open joint)?**
   Probing of a wound in proximity to a joint is inadvisable, because this may increase the risk of a spreading deep infection and septic arthritis. Radiographs of the involved joint may reveal an air arthrogram. A saline challenge will help in diagnosing a traumatic arthrotomy. Larger joints, such as the knee joint, may be injected with up to 170 mL sterile saline. The traumatic wound is inspected for egress of the injected fluid. A positive saline challenge mandates a formal surgical washout of the traumatic open joint, with exploration and closure of the joint capsule. Traumatic arthrotomy can also be diagnosed by computed tomography (CT) scan.

10. **When should I order radiographs, and how many should I order?**
    Radiographic diagnostics should not delay resuscitation in a multiply injured patient. Whenever existing limb deformity results in vascular compromise or may devitalize overlying skin, radiographs should be delayed, pending emergent realignment and splinting or application of traction to the involved extremity. Radiographs should be ordered based on physical examination findings. Three-way view radiographs should include the joints above and below the area of injury.

KEY POINTS: MUSCULOSKELETAL TRAUMA – GENERAL PRINCIPLES

1. Open fractures require immediate orthopedic consultation and must be recognized and managed urgently.
2. ACS must be identified early and managed by urgent surgical fasciotomies because of the risk of irreversible long-term sequelae with loss of function and potential loss of limb.
3. Suspected septic joints require immediate diagnostic workup and surgical management for positive cases.

HAND AND FOREARM INJURIES

11. **What is the incidence of hand injuries seen in EDs?**
    At least one of every 8–10 injury-related ED visits is for a hand or wrist injury.

12. **List the essential elements of the history in hand injuries.**
    - Age
    - Handedness
    - Occupation
    - Injury details (how, when, where)
    - Tetanus status
    - Prior hand injury
    - Preexisting disability

13. **List the elements of a complete hand examination.**
    Inspect skin, soft-tissue, and skeletal components, assess neurovascular function, and examine tendon function. Detailed documentation and timing of physical findings are of essential importance.

14. **What is the best method to control bleeding in lacerations of the hand and forearm?**
    Apply direct pressure. Tourniquets are rarely necessary. Blood vessels are in close anatomic association with nerves in neurovascular bundles; blindly placing surgical clamps or ligation sutures into the wound is discouraged secondary to the risk of damaging adjacent nerves.

15. **What is the normal posture of the hand at rest, and what is the tenodesis test?**
    When the wrist is held in slight extension, the fingers cascade progressively with a more flexed position from index to small finger. Passive wrist extension will cause tension in the flexor tendons and more cascading; in contrast, wrist flexion will extend the fingers as the flexor tendons relax. Any alteration in this normal posture should raise suspicion for the diagnosis of a tendon injury.

16. **Does dorsal hand swelling always signify a dorsal hand injury or infection?**
    No, most of the palmar lymphatics drain to lymph channels and lacunae located in the loose areolar layer on the dorsum of the hand. Always check for a palmar pathology when a patient has dorsal swelling.

17. **What is the Allen test, and how is it performed?**
    The Allen test verifies patency of the radial and ulnar arteries and is performed as follows:
    - Occlude radial and ulnar arteries at the wrist by applying firm finger pressure.
    - Have the patient hold the hand in a tight fist for about 5 seconds.
    - Ask the patient to open the hand while holding compression. The palmar aspect of the hand will be blanched.
    - Release the ulnar artery; this should lead to full digital and thenar reperfusion within 5 seconds.
    - Repeat the test, releasing the radial artery instead of the ulnar artery, and look for any delay in reperfusion.

18. **How is function of the flexor digitorum superficialis (FDS) tendon tested?**
    The FDS inserts on the middle phalanx and flexes only the proximal interphalangeal (PIP) joint. The flexor digitorum profundus (FDP) inserts on the distal phalanx; its contraction flexes both the PIP (by contribution only) and the distal interphalangeal (DIP) joints. The FDS muscle-tendon units are independent of one another, whereas the FDP tendons (with the exception of the index finger, which may have an independent muscle-tendon) arise from a common muscle belly. To test FDS function of a finger, the patient is asked to flex the PIP joint of an isolated finger while blocking the other fingers in extension, thereby disabling the FDP flexion contribution. Because the FDP to the index finger can be independent of the other profundi, the FDS test is unreliable in the index finger.

19. **How do I test the extrinsic extensor tendons?**
    The extrinsic extensors extend the metacarpophalangeal (MCP) joints. They combine with interosseous and lumbrical tendons to form the extensor mechanism for the interphalangeal (IP) joints. To test the extrinsic extensor, ensure that the patient can extend at the MCP joint.

20. **Can extensor function to a finger be intact despite complete laceration of the extensor digitorum communis (EDC) to that finger?**
    Yes, the juncturae intertendineum connect the EDC tendons at the mid-metacarpal level. If the EDC to a finger is completely lacerated on the dorsum of the hand, proximal to the juncturae, extension at the MCP joint can still be possible. Careful and complete wound exploration is necessary to identify this injury.

21. **How do I test sensory nerve function?**
    Assess and document, in writing, motor and sensory nerve function before injecting local anesthetic. Test digital nerves by checking two-point discrimination on the volar pad, using calipers or self-fabricated opened paper clips. The two points should be less than 5 mm apart.

22. **Describe the sensory distributions of the median, ulnar, and radial nerves**
    See Fig. 93.2.

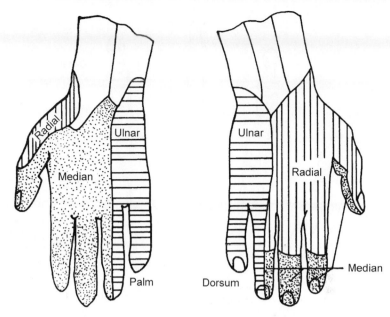

Fig. 93.2 Sensory distribution of the median, ulnar, and radial nerves.

23. **How is the motor function for the median, ulnar, and radial nerves tested?**
    - Median (abductor pollicis brevis [APB]): abduct the thumb against resistance while palpating the APB muscle belly; touch the tip of the small finger with the thumb ("OK" sign).
    - Ulnar (first dorsal interosseous): abduct the index finger against resistance.
    - Radial (no intrinsics; extensor pollicis longus [EPL]): extend the thumb IP joint against resistance.

24. **Name the carpal bones, including the most commonly dislocated carpal bone?**
    The proximal carpal row contains, from radial to ulnar side, the following bones:
    - Scaphoid
    - Lunate
    - Triquetrum
    - Pisiform

    The distal carpal row consists of:
    - Trapezium
    - Trapezoid
    - Capitate
    - Hamate
        The lunate bone is most commonly dislocated, such as in perilunate injury patterns.
        See Figs. 93.3 and 93.4.

25. **Which is the most commonly fractured carpal bone?**
    The scaphoid is the most commonly fractured carpal bone. Its predominant distal blood supply increases the likelihood of avascular necrosis (AVN) in the proximal segment after a proximal pole fracture.

26. **How much deformity can be tolerated in metacarpal fractures?**
    Rotational deformity does not correct itself and is an indication for surgery. Metacarpal neck or shaft rotation may cause finger scissoring when attempting to make a fist. Apex dorsal flexion deformity is common and usually functionally well tolerated: 20, 30, 40, and 50 degrees of flexion in the index through small fingers can be accepted without functional deficiency in most patients. A greater degree of deformity is tolerated at the small finger, because of the increased motion at the carpometacarpal (CMC) and MCP joints. The same is true for a thumb metacarpal fracture, in which 40 degrees of angular deformity can be accepted.

27. **What are Rolando and Bennett fractures?**
    These eponyms describe intraarticular fractures of the base of the first metacarpal bone. A Rolando fracture is seen after axial trauma and results in a three-part Y pattern, whereas a Bennett fracture is seen in eccentric shear injuries, where the volar beak of the metacarpal tears off as an avulsion piece held by the volar oblique ligament. Both fractures require surgery. Prognosis of Rolando fractures is worse than for Bennett fractures.

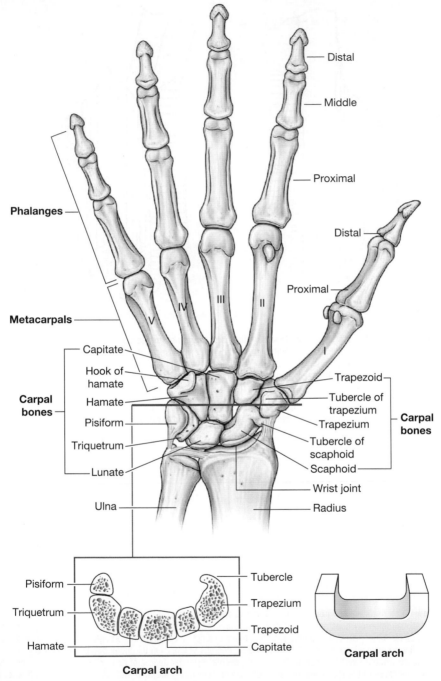

Fig. 93.3 Carpal bones of the wrist. (From Drake R, Vogl AW, Mitchell A. *Gray's Anatomy for Students*. Philadelphia, PA: Saunders; 2005: Fig. 7–91.)

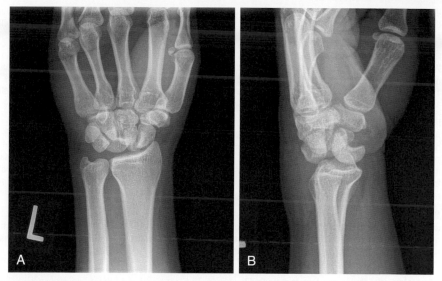

Fig. 93.4 Perilunate transscaphoid fracture dislocation with associated lunate fracture. (From Marx J, Hockberger R, Wall R. *Rosen's Emergency Medicine – Concepts and Clinical Practice. 8th ed.* Philadelphia, PA: Saunders; 2013:Fig. 51–22B.)

28. **What is the appropriate treatment for a patient with pain in the snuffbox of the wrist and normal radiographs after a traumatic event to the wrist?**
    The scaphoid lies at the floor of the anatomic snuffbox of the wrist, which is bordered by the EPL and the extensor pollicis brevis tendons. Tenderness in this area is suggestive of a scaphoid fracture, which can be undetectable on initial radiographs. Trabecular resorption at the fracture site aids secondary radiographic detection approximately 10–14 days after injury. Patients with a concern for a possible occult scaphoid fracture should be immobilized in a thumb spica splint or cast and referred to an orthopedist for evaluation. Bone scans and magnetic resonance imaging (MRI) are not indicated in the acute setting.

29. **What is the difference between a "nightstick" fracture and a Monteggia fracture?**
    Proximal-third ulna fractures with associated radial head dislocation are usual presentations of a Monteggia fracture. This fracture can occur from a fall on an outstretched hand with associated valgus force on the extremity. The treatment requires internal fixation of the ulnar fracture. Nightstick fractures of the ulna result from a direct blow to the ulnar shaft. There is no associated injury to the proximal radioulnar joint. In most cases, these injuries can be treated by closed means and early range of motion. Nightstick fractures with significant comminution, greater than 10 degrees of angulation, or greater than 50% displacement, may be considered for operative fixation.

30. **What nerve can be injured in a Monteggia fracture?**
    The posterior interosseous nerve (PIN) lies in close proximity to the neck of the radius. The PIN can be acutely stretched during dislocation or sustain a chronic traction neuroma in persisting dislocations. The patient usually has an inability to extend the thumb or wrist.

31. **Why are high-pressure injections serious hand injuries?**
    High-pressure injection injuries (from paint or grease guns) may initially seem innocuous. Whereas there is usually only a small entry point, the underlying tissue destruction can be extensive and disastrous. Emergent surgical debridement and release is indicated. Loss of function, even loss of the finger, is well described in the literature.

32. **List Kanavel's four cardinal signs of flexor tenosynovitis.**
    1. Flexed finger posture
    2. Fusiform finger swelling
    3. Pain on passive IP joint extension
    4. Percussive tenderness along the flexor tendon sheath
       Flexor tenosynovitis requires urgent surgical management.

33. **What is a paronychia, and how is it treated?**
    Paronychia is a common infection involving the nail fold. Although *Staphylococcus aureus* is the usual pathogen in acute presentations, fungal infections are common pathogens in chronic infections. In the absence of visible pus or fluctuance, treatment consists of warm moist compresses, elevation, and antistaphylococcal antibiotics.

If there is fluctuance or pus present, irrigation and debridement is indicated. This may consist of simply elevating the eponychial fold or making a small longitudinal incision over the area of fluctuance. Removal of a longitudinal section of the nail plate may be necessary.

34. How is whitlow different from a paronychia?
Whitlow is a herpes simplex virus infection with burning pain and erythema, followed by a vesicular rash with serous drainage on the distal phalanx. Whitlow can be seen more commonly in health care workers and in preschoolers. A Tzanck smear can be diagnostic. The patient also may have perioral cold sores. The treatment consists of observation and acyclovir administration. Surgery is not necessary or indicated.

35. What is a felon, and how is it treated?
A felon is a painful and potentially disabling infection of the fingertip pulp. The finger pulp anatomy features fibrous septae. These structures complicate treatment of the infection and preclude full drainage unless properly debrided. Mid-lateral incisions, including J-shaped incisions, are favored. Older fish-mouth or double-longitudinal incisions have fallen out of favor because of excessive scarring and tissue necrosis risk. Care must be taken not to convert a felon into a flexor tendon sheath infection by opening up the flexor sheath. Cultures should be obtained, and wounds kept open by a wick to facilitate drainage, followed by daily soaks.

36. What is a jersey finger, and how is it treated?
Jersey finger describes a rupture of the FDP in sudden forceful flexion against resistance, such as occurs when a football player snags a finger on an opponent's jersey. The tendon is avulsed from its insertion at the palmar base of the distal phalanx and can take a bone fragment along. Surgical repair within the next several days is indicated.

37. What is a mallet finger, and how is it treated?
A mallet finger may be seen as an opposite of the jersey finger. In this case the insertion of the extensor tendon is avulsed from the dorsum of the distal phalanx, often pulling off a bone fragment. Appropriate treatment is to splint the DIP joint in neutral position for 8–10 weeks in a DIP blocking (Stack) splint while allowing PIP joint motion to prevent a swan neck deformity. A hand specialist should do the follow-up consultation and aftercare of this injury.

38. Describe a subungual hematoma. How is it treated?
Subungual hematomas are painful collections of blood under the nail plate. Relieving the pressure by nail trephination will result in immediate pain relief. Use a cautery device or an 18-gauge needle to trephinate the nail, allowing for drainage of accumulated blood. One must insure that there is no underlying fracture with an x-ray of the digit. If there is a fracture, a hand surgery consultation is recommended. Removal of an intact nail plate is almost never indicated.

39. What is a gamekeeper's thumb, and how is it diagnosed?
Gamekeeper's thumb describes a torn ulnar collateral ligament (UCL) of the thumb's MCP joint, resulting from forceful abduction of the thumb. The name arose from an initial description in 24 Scottish game wardens who sustained UCL injuries while breaking the necks of wounded rabbits. The injury, also called *skier's thumb,* can be disabling because of chronic instability of the thumb at the MCP joint and ensuing arthritis. One way to test for injury to the UCL of the thumb MCP joint is to hand the patient a heavy can or bottle. If the MCP joint is unstable, the patient will be unable to hold the object without supinating to balance the object in the palm or dropping it. Complete rupture of the ligament usually requires surgical repair. ED treatment consists of application of a thumb spica splint and referral. A Stener lesion occurs when the aponeurosis of the adductor pollicis muscle is trapped between the ruptured UCL and its site of insertion, at the base of the proximal phalanx. This interposition prevents UCL healing and requires surgical repair.

40. What is a boxer's fracture?
Boxer's fractures of the small or ring finger metacarpal neck typically occur as a result of a fist fight. Because of increased small- and ring-finger metacarpal mobility in the CMC joint and greater MCP joint motion, fracture deformities up to 60 degrees flexion can be well tolerated, especially in the small finger. Nevertheless, attempts to correct significant angulation of an acute boxer's fracture are indicated. Of particular importance is that any rotational deformity must be corrected. A laceration accompanying a boxer's fracture is assumed to be a fight bite.

41. What is a fight bite?
As the name implies, the injury occurs when a punch is thrown at an opponent's mouth, resulting in the hand striking the teeth. Because of the close proximity of the underlying MCP joint, any resulting skin laceration must be assumed to be a traumatic arthrotomy. All suspected fight bites require formal irrigation and debridement in the operating room to prevent septic arthritis. This includes extending the skin laceration to visualize tendon and joint injuries. Underlying cartilaginous injuries can be present and escape radiographic detection. Associated tendon injuries and metacarpal fractures must be ruled out. Incisions are loosely approximated or left open to allow drainage. Patients should be admitted for overnight hospitalization for IV antibiotics and wound care.

42. **Name six hand emergencies.**
    1. Partial or complete amputations with acute vascular compromise
    2. ACS
    3. Third-degree and circumferential burns
    4. High-pressure injection injury
    5. Flexor tenosynovitis
    6. Septic joint

43. **Name indications and contraindications for a microvascular replantation.**
    Indications:
    - All pediatric amputations
    - Multiple finger amputations
    - Thumb amputation proximal to the nail fold
    - Whole-hand or midhand amputation
    - Any major upper extremity limb amputation
    Contraindications:
    - Patients who have experienced multiple trauma
    - Severe crush or avulsion injuries
    - Multilevel injuries
    - Heavy contamination
    - Single-finger amputations in adults
    - Severe associated medical problems
      The ultimate decision should be deferred to a hand or microvascular surgeon, including discussion of options and outcomes with patient and family.

44. **How should an amputated part be handled and stored for transport?**
    - Remove gross contamination with saline irrigation.
    - Wrap the part in a saline-moistened (not soaked) sterile gauze.
    - Place the wrapped part into a sealed plastic bag or container.
    - Place the bag or container into an ice water bath.
      Never put the amputated part directly onto ice or immerse it in disinfection solution.

45. **What should be done with a devascularized, but still partially attached, digit?**
    Leave the part attached (preserves veins for replantation), gently wrap it in moist gauze, and apply an immobilizing bulky dressing.

KEY POINTS: HAND AND FOREARM INJURIES

1. Scaphoid fractures can escape radiographic detection in the acute setting. Assume the patient with snuffbox tenderness has an occult scaphoid fracture, apply a thumb spica, and repeat evaluation in 1–2 weeks.
2. The extensive tissue destruction of high-pressure injections can be missed because of an innocuous entry wound. These injuries require urgent surgery.
3. Any laceration over the dorsal MCP joint is suspicious for a fight bite. Fight bites require meticulous exploration and wound care in the operating room. If the wound penetrates the extensor hood, thorough joint washout and IV antibiotics are required.
4. Bleeding from a wound is best controlled with direct pressure and not clamps or a ligature stitch.
5. Never place an amputated part directly on ice or immerse in water; always double bag amputated parts.

SHOULDER AND UPPER ARM INJURIES

46. **How can I detect anterior and posterior shoulder dislocations on radiographic film?**
    Anteroposterior (AP) radiographs may show an inferomedial bony overlap in anterior dislocations. In AP radiographs, a posterior shoulder dislocation can be diagnosed by a vacant glenoid sign, because the humeral head fails to fill most of the glenoid. There is also a positive rim sign, with space between the anterior rim of the glenoid and the humeral head exceeding 6 mm. A true axillary lateral, or a Velpeau view, is necessary to rule out a dislocation.

47. **What is the incidence and what are common causes of posterior shoulder dislocations?**
    Posterior dislocations account for 5% of shoulder dislocations. The usual mechanism is a fall onto the outstretched hand. Other causes include tonic-clonic seizures, electrical shock, and direct anterior shoulder trauma. Reduction can be accomplished with flexion of the arm to 90 degrees and adduction to disimpact the humeral head, followed by external rotation of the arm until the humeral head has cleared the glenoid rim. A sling should be applied in neutral position to 5–10 degrees of external rotation and slight abduction.

48. **What percentage of patients with anterior shoulder dislocations experience recurrences?**
In patients ≤30 years of age, 90% experience a recurrent dislocation; in older patients, the percentage is lower and more variable, depending on the injury mechanism.

49. **What are potential complications of anterior shoulder dislocations?**
The axillary nerve can be injured at the time of dislocation. Examination of the deltoid muscle motor function and sensation to the lateral aspect of the shoulder are mandatory. Additionally, rotator cuff tears can occur, especially in first-time dislocations in patients older than 40 years.

50. **How is a rotator cuff tear diagnosed?**
Pain with overhead activity, night pain, and pain with abduction of the arm are typical symptoms of a rotator cuff injury. Patients have difficulty abducting the arm, and are often unable to lift the arm above the level of the shoulder. With the shoulder in 90-degree abduction, 30-degree forward flexion, and maximal internal rotation, the patient cannot resist against downward pressure (supraspinatus strength test). A drop test is done in the same manner with the arm simply at 90-degree abduction. The patient is not able to lower the arm slowly from 90-degree abduction. If injecting 10 mL of 1% lidocaine into the subacromial space relieves these findings, then subacromial impingement rather than a pure rotator cuff tear is more likely.

51. **What is the most common neurologic deficit seen with humeral shaft fractures?**
The radial nerve may be contused, stretched, or, rarely, lacerated. This condition typically occurs with fractures involving the distal third of the humerus, where the radial nerve passes through the intermuscular septum (Holstein-Lewis fracture) and is prone to injury. Disability includes inability to extend the wrist and fingers at the MCP joints and numbness on the dorsum of the radial side of the hand. IP extension may be preserved, because of normal ulnar and median nerve function. Triceps function is usually intact, because radial nerve branches exiting proximal to the radial groove power it.

52. **What about clavicle fractures?**
Clavicle fractures result mainly from indirect trauma forces as the most common etiology, typically from a fall onto the shoulder or on the outstretched hand (e.g., bicycle accident). Direct trauma, such as a blow to the clavicle during contact sports, represents a less common cause of clavicle fractures. Clavicle fracture is the most common fracture in pediatric patients. The most common site is the middle third of the clavicle, in approximately 75% of all cases.

53. **How are clavicle fractures treated?**
Most clavicle fractures are treated in the ED with a sling for comfort and pain control. The historic "figure-of-8" bandage is outdated and considered obsolete. Orthopedic consultation is appropriate for fractures that may require operative repair. These include completely displaced fracture ends, fractures with greater than 2 cm of shortening, displaced fractures causing skin tenting, open fractures, and fractures associated with neurovascular injuries.

54. **What is a shoulder separation, and how does it occur?**
The term *shoulder separation* more properly refers to a separation at the acromioclavicular (AC) joint. AC separations typically result from a direct blow to the point of the shoulder, such as occurs in high-energy contact sports (football). AC separations are divided into different types, depending on the degree of damage to the AC ligament and the amount of displacement of the clavicular end.

55. **How is an AC separation treated?**
The large majority of AC separations are managed conservatively with a sling, ice packs, and analgesics. Surgery is usually reserved for significant displacement in young patients with high demands on their shoulders.

KEY POINTS: SHOULDER AND UPPER ARM

1. Shoulder dislocations can be associated with rotator cuff injuries in first-time dislocations in patients older than 40 years.
2. Document motor and sensory function of the axillary nerve in shoulder dislocations.

LOWER EXTREMITY AND PELVIC FRACTURES

56. **Name major complications seen in pelvic fractures.**
   - Hemorrhagic shock
   - Death from exsanguinating hemorrhage
   - Urogenital and rectal injuries (see Chapter 89)

57. **What is the mortality rate for patients with open pelvic fractures?**
Mortality has decreased from 60% in the 1990s to 10%–25% now, because of multidisciplinary approaches, proactive concepts of early hemorrhage control (including retroperitoneal pelvic packing), and advances in critical care.

58. What is the incidence and injury mechanism in posterior hip dislocation?

Around 80% of all hip dislocations are posterior dislocations; the mechanism is usually a posterior directed force applied to a flexed knee, as occurs when the knee strikes the dashboard in a head-on motor vehicle crash.

59. What complications can be seen in posterior hip dislocations?

Sciatic nerve injuries are found in 10% of patients, resulting in weakness or loss of hamstring function in the thigh and leg.

AVN of the femoral head is seen in 10%–15% of patients. The risk of AVN increases to 50% if reduction is delayed beyond 12 hours. Even with prompt reduction, 20% of patients develop osteoarthritis. The risk of recurrent dislocation is increased during early rehabilitation.

60. How are posterior hip dislocations clinically differentiated from femoral neck fractures?

Both result in lower extremity shortening. In posterior hip dislocation, the hip is flexed, adducted, and internally rotated. With a femoral neck or intertrochanteric fracture, the lower extremity is not flexed but shortened, abducted, and externally rotated.

61. How much blood loss can be expected from a femoral shaft fracture?

Patients typically lose 1500–2000 mL of blood.

62. How are femoral shaft fractures best stabilized in the ED?

Stabilization is best achieved with immediate application of longitudinal traction, using a self-contained traction unit. Most emergency medical service providers carry these and can apply them in the field or ambulance. Another option in the hospital is placement of a distal femoral traction pin and in-line traction connected to the bed or gurney. Conventional splinting is ineffective and contraindicated. Femoral traction dramatically reduces the mortality and risk of remote organ injury (brain, lungs) from femoral shaft fractures.

63. Why can patients with pathologic conditions of the hip experience knee pain?

A patient with a hip problem may complain only of pain to the anterior distal thigh and medial aspect of the knee. The knee and the hip share innervation through the obturator nerve. Always suspect a hip problem in a patient who complains of knee pain without corresponding findings on physical examination. Careful examination of the knee and hip, with appropriate radiographs of the hip, is necessary to complete the evaluation.

64. Name the most common injury associated with traumatic hemarthrosis of the knee joint.

Anterior cruciate ligament (ACL) ruptures are most commonly causes for knee hemarthrosis. If fat globules are noted in the joint aspirate, the possibility of an associated intraarticular fracture should be pursued.

65. Name the most commonly injured ligament seen in an inversion-type ankle sprain.

The most commonly injured ligament is the anterior talofibular ligament (ATFL). The calcaneofibular ligament can also be injured in more severe sprains.

66. Describe the treatment for ankle sprains.

Ankle sprains are treated by the RICE protocol: **R**est, **I**ce, **C**ompression, and **E**levation. Early protected weight bearing with crutches and an early range-of-motion program should be instituted. More severe sprains may require a short period of immobilization.

67. What is a locked knee, and what are the most common causes?

The patient is unable to extend the knee actively or passively beyond 10- to 45-degree flexion. True locking and unlocking occur suddenly. The most common causes are medial meniscus tears, a loose body such as an osteochondral fragment in the knee joint, or a dislocated patella.

68. What is the most common direction of a knee dislocation?

The direction is determined by the position of the tibia relative to the femur. Anterior dislocations are seen in around 40% of cases, followed by posterior dislocations in 25%. Hyperextension trauma causes anterior dislocations, and dashboard mechanisms often result in posterior dislocations: 40%–50% of all anterior/posterior dislocations are associated with a popliteal artery injury. Post-reduction angiography should be considered for all patients with abnormal distal pulses or ankle-brachial index (ABI).

69. What direction is associated with irreducible knee dislocations?

Posterolateral dislocations are irreducible. Here the medial femoral condyle produces a dimple sign as it buttonholes through the anteromedial joint capsule, thus becoming entrapped. An open reduction in the operating room is required.

70. How is the ABI calculated?

The ABI is calculated by dividing the Doppler systolic arterial pressure measured in the injured leg by the pressure measured in an uninjured arm. An ABI value of greater than 0.9 is considered normal. The ABI measurement may be inaccurate in patients with risk factors for peripheral arterial disease, such as diabetes and hypertension. Vessel calcification in the elderly can also increase the risk of a false-positive result. An ABI less than 0.9 must trigger immediate further diagnostic workup or surgical exploration in the operating room.

71. What injuries are often associated with calcaneal fractures?
Depending on injury mechanism and type of calcaneal fracture, up to 50% of patients may have an associated compression fracture of the lumbar or lower thoracic spine. Ten percent of all calcaneal injuries are bilateral, and about 25% are associated with other lower extremity injuries.

KEY POINTS: LOWER EXTREMITY AND PELVIS

1. A multidisciplinary approach is required for the successful management of acute traumatic pelvic hemorrhage.
2. ACL injuries are common causes for a hemarthrosis of the knee.
3. All knee dislocations require a thorough vascular examination, including ABI measurement, to rule out an associated vascular injury.

PEDIATRIC ORTHOPEDICS

72. What is a torus or buckle fracture?
This fracture is typically seen in the radial metaphysis. Torus, or buckling, describes the pediatric plastic bone deformity, resulting in a round swelling or protuberance, which happens when bone fails in compression, while the opposite cortex remains intact. Because the opposite cortex remains intact, these fractures are stable and require cast immobilization for 4 weeks.

73. What is a greenstick fracture?
Children's bones have increased elasticity. An angular force applied to a long bone of a child causes a greenstick fracture. One cortex fails in tension, while the opposite cortex bows but does not fail or fracture in compression. The fracture is similar to what occurs when one attempts to break a green branch of a tree. This fracture pattern is common in the forearm and may require reduction, in which case the fracture should be completed to achieve an adequate reduction. Immobilization in a cast is required for 6 weeks.

74. What is the Salter-Harris classification?
Fractures involving the physeal zone may result in growth disturbance, and parents must be informed accordingly. About 80% of these injuries are Salter-Harris types I and II, both of which have a low complication rate. Salter-Harris types III, IV, and V injuries have a worse prognosis. Displaced Salter-Harris types III and IV fractures may require open reduction to restore the normal anatomic physeal relationship.
    The five types of fracture according to the Salter-Harris classification are (Fig. 93.5):
- *Type I.* Physeal separation; this may appear as a widening of the radiolucent area representing the growth plate.
- *Type II.* Fracture traverses the physis and exits on the metaphyseal side.
- *Type III.* Fracture traverses the physis and exits on the epiphyseal side.
- *Type IV.* Fracture traverses through epiphysis, physis, and metaphysis.
- *Type V.* Physeal crush injury; this may be difficult to determine on plain radiographs.

75. Which vascular complication is associated with pediatric supracondylar humerus fractures?
Displaced pediatric supracondylar humerus fractures have a 5% incidence of vascular injuries. The brachial artery can be compressed or lacerated by the anteriorly displaced humeral shaft. Posterolateral displacement of the supracondylar fracture is the pattern most likely to result in vascular injury. Children with pink, pulseless hands should undergo prompt reduction and fracture fixation in the operating room, with subsequent reexamination and vascular surgery consultation.

76. Describe the neurologic complications associated with pediatric supracondylar humerus fractures.
The anterior interosseous nerve (AIN; branch of the median nerve) is the most commonly injured nerve. It innervates muscles in the deep flexor compartment of the forearm: radial part of the FDP, the pronator quadratus, and flexor pollicis longus (FPL). AIN function is tested, evaluating FPL and FDP function at the thumb and index finger IP joint

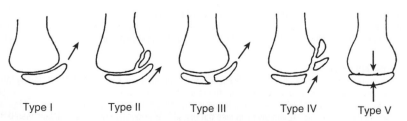

Type I   Type II   Type III   Type IV   Type V

Fig. 93.5 Salter-Harris classification of physeal injuries.

(OK sign). The radial nerve is the next most commonly injured nerve, followed by the ulnar nerve. A thorough physical examination must be done to identify these injuries, a difficult task in the small child.

77. **What is a nursemaid's or pulled elbow, and what is its management?**
A longitudinal pull on the outstretched arm of a small child may subluxate the cartilaginous radial head out of the annular ligament. The child typically experiences pseudoparalysis of the injured extremity. Radiographs are negative for fracture or radial head dislocation. The two techniques most commonly used for reduction are supination-flexion or hyperpronation. A click over the radial head signifies reduction. The child often begins using the extremity within minutes of reduction. The parent or caregiver should be educated to avoid longitudinal traction on the arm to prevent this from reoccurring.

78. **Describe the potential implications of long bone fractures in a small child.**
In nonambulating children with long bone fractures, nonaccidental trauma (child abuse) must be considered (see Chapter 67).

79. **Which nontraumatic hip disorders cause a limp in a child?**
- Septic arthritis
- Transient synovitis
- Slipped capital femoral epiphysis (SCFE)
- Idiopathic AVN
- Perthes disease
- Juvenile rheumatoid arthritis

    Among these uncommon diagnoses, transient synovitis is probably the most prevalent cause of a nontraumatic limp in a child and a diagnosis of exclusion. Symptomatic treatment is prescribed for transient synovitis, including nonsteroidal anti-inflammatory drugs and non–weight bearing or bed rest. Untreated or delayed treatment of septic arthritis can irreversibly damage articular cartilage. Infection in a child with atraumatic hip pain must be ruled out. The white blood cell count, erythrocyte sedimentation rate, and body temperature commonly are elevated in cases of infection. If doubt persists, a hip aspiration is the gold standard and is usually performed in the operating room. Standard AP and lateral radiographs of the hip help differentiate between Perthes disease and an SCFE.

80. **What are the early radiographic findings of an SCFE?**
Any asymmetry of the relationship of the femoral head to the femoral neck should raise the suspicion of SCFE, even if evident on only one radiographic view. If AP and lateral radiographs are normal, frog-leg views should be obtained. Comparison of the two hips may not be helpful in discerning subtle changes, because SCFE is bilateral in 20% of cases. Further diagnostics, such as MRI, can diagnose pre-slip conditions if radiographs are negative. MRI examinations are usually ordered through a pediatric orthopedic consultation.

81. **What is the ED management of a child with injury and tenderness over an open epiphysis but a normal radiograph?**
In this circumstance, assuming there is an occult physeal injury is prudent. Splint the extremity and keep the child non–weight bearing if the lower extremity is involved. Parents should be notified of the possibility of this type of injury and the potential for growth disturbance. The need for prompt follow-up consultation with a specialist must be emphasized and is best arranged before discharging the child from the ED. A nondisplaced physeal fracture that becomes displaced because of lack of immobilization can have significant long-term consequences. Short-term extremity immobilization in an appropriately applied splint or cast is well tolerated. When in doubt, immobilize.

KEY POINTS: PEDIATRIC ORTHOPEDICS

1. Rule out septic arthritis in a child with hip pain independent of a history of trauma, because septic seeding of a joint can be facilitated by a preceding trauma.
2. Consider nonaccidental trauma (child abuse) in nonambulating children with long bone fractures.

BIBLIOGRAPHY

Berwald N, Khan F, Zehtabchi S. Antibiotic prophylaxis for ED patients with simple hand lacerations: a feasibility randomized controlled trial. *Am J Emerg Med.* 2014;32(7):768–771.
Bexkens R, Washburn FJ, Eygendaal D, et al. Effectiveness of reduction maneuvers in the treatment of nursemaid's elbow: a systematic review and meta-analysis. *Am J Emerg Med.* 2017;35(1):159–163.
Bloom JM, Hammert WC. Evidence-based medicine: metacarpal fractures. *Plast Reconstr Surg.* 2014;133(5):1252–1260.
Cannon TA. High-pressure injection injuries of the hand. *Orthop Clin North Am.* 2016;47(3):617–624.

Cepela DJ, Tartaglione JP, Dooley TP, et al. Classifications in brief: Salter-Harris classification of pediatric physeal fractures. *Clin Orthop Relat Res*. 2016;474(11):2531–2537.

Georgiadis AG, Zaltz I. Slipped capital femoral epiphysis: how to evaluate with a review and update of treatment. *Pediatr Clin North Am*. 2014;61(6):1119–1135.

Halawi MJ, Morwood MP. Acute management of open fractures: an evidence-based review. *Orthopedics*. 2015;38(11):e1025–e1033.

Ipaktchi K, Demars A, Park J, et al. Retained palmar foreign body presenting as a late hand infection: proposed diagnostic algorithm to detect radiolucent objects. *Patient Saf Surg*. 2013;7(1):25.

Ipaktchi K, Livermore M, Lyons C, et al. Current concepts in the treatment of distal radial fractures. *Orthopedics*. 2013;36(10):778–784.

Karimkhani C, Amir M, Dellavalle RP, et al. Current concepts for oil decontamination of crush injuries: a review. *Patient Saf Surg*. 2014;8:22.

Konda SR, Davidovitch RI, Egol KA. Computed tomography scan to detect traumatic arthrotomies and identify periarticular wounds not requiring surgical intervention: an improvement over the saline load test. *J Orthop Trauma*. 2013;27(9):498–504.

Malahias M, Jordan D, Hughes O, et al. Bite injuries to the hand: microbiology, virology and management. *Open Orthop*. 2014;8: 157–161.

Ryan DD. Differentiating transient synovitis of the hip from more urgent conditions. *Pediatr Ann*. 2016;45(6):e209–e231.

Schmidt AH. Acute compartment syndrome. *Orthop Clin North Am*. 2016;47(3):517–525.

Seigerman DA, Choi D, Donegan DJ, et al. Upper extremity compartment syndrome after minor trauma: an imperative for increased vigilance for a rare, but limb-threatening complication. *Patient Saf Surg*. 2013;7:5.

Toker S, Oak N, Williams A, et al. Adherence to therapy after flexor tendon surgery at a level 1 trauma center. *Hand (N Y)*. 2014;9(2): 175–178.

Yaffe MA, Kaplan FT. Agricultural injuries to the hand and upper extremity. *J Am Acad Orthop Surg*. 2014;22(10):605–613.

CHAPTER 94

BURNS

Jean Hoffman, MD and Daniel Adams, MD

KEY POINTS

1. Physicians should be facile in estimating burn depth and percentage of total body surface area (%TBSA) involved, as these drive early resuscitation, management, and referral decisions.
2. Airway compromise can evolve quickly in the burned patient. Historical features of the injury, subjective symptoms, and objective signs suggesting significant airway involvement inform the decision to intubate.
3. Consider consultation and transfer to a burn center in patients with larger, deeper burns, extremes of age, circumferential burns, burns of the hands or genitalia, patients with complex social needs or comorbidities, or burns complicated by significant trauma.
4. A majority of burns can be managed in the outpatient setting. Outpatient management must include pain control, wound care, close initial follow-up care, return criteria, and, in pediatric patients, a reliable and safe home environment.

1. What first aid should be offered after a thermal injury?

First, stop the burn process (i.e., remove from heat source, extinguish the flame, dilute chemicals). Next, cool thermal burns for a minimum of 20 minutes with cool tap water. This may have positive effects when applied up to 3 hours after the burn. Ice may provide analgesia but can extend tissue damage through tissue necrosis and is not recommended. After pain management, initial wound care may involve debridement, depending on the provider's level of comfort and access to burn resources. A suture removal kit, skin cleansing solution, and sterile gauze may be used to gently remove peeling or blistering tissue.

2. How is the burn patient evaluated?

Begin with a trauma evaluation, including primary and secondary survey, with careful attention to airway patency, ventilation, and oxygenation. Evaluate the burn depth and distribution of involved areas. Early intubation should be considered in cases of respiratory insufficiency or severe inhalation injury. Hypothermia can rapidly develop, particularly in patients with large burns. Initiate extrinsic warming measures. Obtain at least two large-bore intravenous (IV) or intraosseous (IO) access sites. While it is preferable to insert IV and IO catheters through unburnt tissue, resuscitation takes priority, and access can be through burnt areas when necessary.

3. What if there is both trauma and burns?

Concomitant trauma and burns increase the chances of morbidity and mortality. These patients require early fluid resuscitation with trauma evaluation and stabilization. Coordination of care is important, and transfer to a burn center should be strongly considered after stabilization.

4. What factors are important in assessment of the burn patient's airway?

It is difficult to predict who will develop laryngeal edema and airway obstruction. Concerning history includes an enclosed space burn. Additionally, there is an increased risk with larger burns, typically greater than 40%. Physical examination findings suggestive of airway injury include soot around the mouth or nares, hoarseness or stridor, facial burns, or carbonaceous sputum. Since not all patients with carbonaceous sputum, oral or nasal soot, and/or facial burns have significant inhalation injury, clinical judgment must be used to decide on the need for intubation. Stridor, increased work of breathing, and hypoxemia are more reliable indicators of significant inhalational injury. However, decreased oxygen saturation occurs late in patients with significant airway injury. Patients who present with facial burns from smoking on oxygen have a low risk of significant inhalation injury, and normally have a baseline oxygen requirement.

5. List the criteria for transfer to a burn center.

- Partial-thickness burns greater than 10% of total body surface area (10%TBSA)
- Burns involving the face, hands, feet, genitalia, perineum, or major joints
- Full-thickness burns (early grafting improves outcomes)
- Electrical burns, including lightning injury
- Chemical burns
- Inhalation injury
- Burns in patients with preexisting medical disorders (especially diabetes) complicating management, prolonging recovery, or affecting mortality

- Patients with burns and concomitant trauma, in which the burn injury poses the greatest risk of morbidity or mortality
- Burn injury in children at hospitals without qualified personnel or equipment to care for children
- Burn injury in patients requiring social, emotional, or long-term rehabilitative intervention needs

6. **What informs the decision to intubate a burn patient?**
   The likelihood of a patient's injury progressing to airway compromise is difficult to reliably estimate. Historical features of injury (confined space exposure, loss of consciousness, advanced age) or physical examination findings (early oropharyngeal edema, facial or circumferential neck involvement, or stridor) can be important clues to impending airway obstruction. Increased cyanide or carbon monoxide (CO) levels should raise suspicion for significant inhalation injury. Nasopharyngoscopy may yield supporting evidence of upper airway injury that can threaten airway patency in minutes or hours. Even in the absence of signs of inhalation injury, providers must evaluate for evolving airway obstruction that, if occurring during transport, can have catastrophic consequences.

7. **What dangers might be encountered with airway intubation of the burn patient?**
   Facial or oropharyngeal edema portends a difficult airway. Intubation, with a surgical airway should difficulties with oxygenation or ventilation occur, should be performed by the most skilled provider. Cautious consideration of paralytic agent use is important, to avoid the paralyzed, apneic patient who is subsequently unable to be ventilated. Additionally, since a patient with significant burns can be hypovolemic, profound hypotension can occur after administration of sedative or paralytic medications employed in rapid-sequence intubation. Full-thickness neck burns can also limit neck mobility during intubation.

8. **Can succinylcholine be used safely to intubate the burn patient?**
   The concern about succinylcholine use in burn patients is secondary to changes in muscle receptors that can cause hyperkalemia. These changes generally take place over the first 7–10 days after the burn. *This is not a concern in the acute burn patient.* Therefore succinylcholine is safe to use up to 48 hours after the burn injury.

9. **How is the burn depth categorized?**
   Classification of burns as first-, second-, or third-degree burns has transitioned to a more functional descriptive terminology. The currently accepted terminology is *superficial burns, superficial partial-thickness burns, deep partial-thickness burns,* and *full-thickness burns.* This terminology is useful in the assessment, management, and referral of burn patients.

10. **What do superficial burns look like?**
    Superficial burns (previously *first-degree burns)* are characterized by blanching red coloration, dry surface, and absence of blisters. Previously described as epidermal burns, the dermal–epidermal interface is the downward limit of damage, though irritation of dermal vessels and nerve endings projecting upward result in erythema and pain. Edema may result, particularly in sensitive areas such as the surrounding soft tissues of the eyes. This is the typical burn suffered after sun exposure, developing over hours and resolving in 3–5 days. This type of burn is NOT included in the %TBSA calculation.

11. **Describe superficial partial-thickness burns.**
    Superficial partial-thickness burns (previously *second-degree burns)* are characterized by blanching erythema, pain, and blisters. As blisters arise and rupture, exposed dermis with associated nerve endings for pain, temperature, and light touch make these injuries particularly sensitive. The loss of the covering of dermal papillae results in a glistening wound surface. Edema is typically present. The underlying capillary network remains intact, resulting in hyperemia and brisk capillary refill. Differentiating between deep and superficial partial-thickness burns may not be possible until initial wound care is completed.

12. **What are deep partial-thickness burns?**
    Deep partial-thickness burns (previously more severe *second-degree burns)* extend down to the deep layer of the dermis. Capillary refill is slow or absent, and areas may be erythematous or pale white (nonblanching). Sensation is altered or decreased, and the exposed surface is typically wet with prominent edema. These burns may progress to full-thickness burns in the subsequent hours to days after initial injury.

13. **Describe full-thickness burns.**
    Full-thickness burns (previously *third-degree burns)* penetrate the full thickness of the epidermis and dermis down into the subcutaneous tissue. Capillary networks are cauterized and sensory nerve endings are obliterated, making these burns insensate, nonblanching, and initially dry. Subdermal burns (previously *fourth-degree burns*) involve subcutaneous structures such as muscle, bone, and the interstitial space.

14. **Why are circumferential full-thickness burns important to recognize?**
    Capillary leak and evolving edema of an extremity underneath overlying circumferential eschar can threaten limb perfusion and viability of distal tissues. In extremities with circumferential burns, hourly neurovascular examination is undertaken to ensure adequate perfusion. This includes assessment of temperature changes, capillary refill, evolving paresthesias, and sensation. Emergent escharotomies are performed in patients with circumferential burns and respiratory distress (chest) or a declining neurologic or vascular examination

(extremities). Hand or finger escharotomies are rarely necessary, and should only be considered in consultation with a burn center.

15. **Why, when, and where are thoracic escharotomies done?**
Thoracic circumferential partial- or full-thickness burns can threaten mechanics of ventilation. The physician may be alerted to the early evolution of this complication by worsening lung compliance parameters on the mechanical ventilator. After evaluating for other causes of inability to ventilate (e.g., mucus plugging or kinked or disconnected tubing), thoracic escharotomy is curative and can be performed at the bedside, avoiding unnecessary delays and complications associated with a trip to the operating room. Using bedside electrocautery is the easiest method to perform escharotomies, but a scalpel may also be used.

16. **How does %TBSA impact patient care? How is it calculated?**
Coupled with burn depth, %TBSA drives management decisions, disposition, and impacts survival. Although limitations in physicians' ability to reliably estimate the %TBSA have been demonstrated, it remains an important parameter in patient care. Wallace's Rule of Nines (Fig. 94.1) is one method to calculate %TBSA involved in partial- and full-thickness burns. (Note that percentages differ in children and adults.) A more accurate method for calculating %TBSA being employed at some burn centers utilizes the standardized aid developed by Lund and Browder (Fig. 94.2). Superficial or first-degree burns are not included in the total. Lastly, there is the "palm" rule, where the patient's palm represents approximately 1% of their TBSA. This is helpful in smaller area burn estimation, as physicians often overestimate the size.

17. **How is %TBSA useful in planning fluid resuscitation?**
Immediately after a burn, an inflammatory response causes extravascular fluid shifts in the body, resulting in relative intravascular depletion. The Parkland formula is perhaps the best-known way to calculate the fluid needs of the burn patient proportional to the %TBSA. The total volume required by the patient over the first 24 hours is calculated as:

$$\text{Total fluid in 24 hours} = 4 \text{ mL fluid} \times \text{kg body weight} \times \%\text{TBSA (partial- and full-thickness burns)}$$

Half of this volume is administered over the first 8 hours after the burn; the remainder is administered over the subsequent 16 hours.

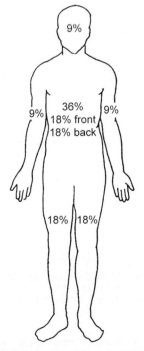

Fig. 94.1 Percentages used in determining extent of burn by Rule of Nines. (From Miller RH. *Textbook of Basic Emergency Medicine.* 2nd ed. St. Louis, MO: Mosby; 1980.)

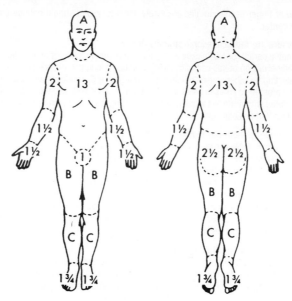

Fig. 94.2 Classic Lund and Bowden chart. The best method for determining percentage of body surface burn is to mark areas of injury on a chart and then compute the total percentage according to patient's age. (From Artz CP, Yarbrough DR 3rd. Burns, including cold, chemical, and electrical injuries. In: Sabiston DC Jr, ed. *Textbook of Surgery*. 11th ed. Philadelphia, PA: Saunders; 1977.)

18. **Calculate a fluid regimen using the Parkland formula in a 70-kg adult suffering 20% TBSA burns.**
    The 24-hour fluid total is 4 mL/kg/%TBSA burned, or:

    $$4\ mL/kg/\% \times 70\ kg \times 20\%, \quad \text{or } 5600\ mL \text{ given over 24 hours.}$$

    Half of this volume is given over the first 8 hours, or 5600 ÷ 2 = 2800 mL over 8 hours, or:

    $$2800 \div 8 = 350\ mL/h\ \text{rate}$$

    The second half is administered over the next 16 hours, or:

    $$2800 \div 16 = 175\ mL/h\ \text{rate}$$

19. **Are there any pitfalls with using the Parkland formula?**
    The Parkland formula may overestimate volume requirements, and can result in over-resuscitation, leading to abdominal compartment syndrome, extremity compartment syndrome, and respiratory failure due to noncardiogenic pulmonary edema in severely burned patients. However, the Parkland formula can be helpful in standardizing care when burn patients are initially evaluated and subsequently transferred to tertiary burn centers.
    The American Burn Life Support program of the American Burn Association recommends the following fluid resuscitation formulas:

    Adult patients: Total fluid in 24 hours = 2–4 mL fluid × kg body weight × %TBSA

    Pediatric patients: Total fluid in 24 hours = 3–4 mL fluid × kg body weight × %TBSA

    Half of the fluid volume is given over the first 8 hours, at which point fluid requirements are recalculated based on urine output (goals of 0.5 mL/kg/h in adults and 1 mL/kg/h in children), to optimize volume status and prevent both over- and under-resuscitation. Patients with electrical or inhalational injury require greater amounts of fluid, and initial fluid resuscitation calculations should favor higher volumes.

20. **What is burn shock?**
    When a patient is given inadequate fluid resuscitation immediately after a burn, increased capillary permeability and insensitive losses combine to rapidly decrease circulating blood volume, threatening tissue perfusion and end-organ function, and resulting in shock. Prompt IV volume resuscitation is essential to prevent burn shock.

As renal failure with oliguria is a common and recognized consequence of under-resuscitation, many protocols focus on maintenance of urine output to gauge adequacy of fluid management. Foley catheters are helpful in accurately measuring urine output. Unless patients can reliably use a urinal or other collection device, a catheter should be placed. Acute adrenal insufficiency can also be an etiology of distributive shock in acutely burned patients, and stress-dose steroids (IV hydrocortisone, 50 mg every 6 hours) should be considered in patients in shock after initial fluid resuscitation.

21. **What are three mechanisms by which smoke inhalation can cause injury?**
    1. Thermal injury to the mouth, tongue, oropharynx, and larynx (i.e., above the glottis)
    2. Particulate and chemical injury to lower airways (i.e., below the glottis)
    3. Metabolic derangements caused by disruption of oxygen kinetics at the cellular level (e.g., CO poisoning)

22. **What are three ways smoke from a fire causes death by asphyxiation?**
    1. Consumption of oxygen by the fire, as well as products of combustion, can lead to asphyxiation. During fire in a closed space, room air oxygen concentration drops from 21% to between 10% and 15%, increasing asphyxiation risk.
    2. CO is an odorless, colorless product of incomplete hydrocarbon combustion that rapidly transits the respiratory epithelium and out-competes oxygen for binding sites on hemoglobin, crippling oxygen delivery in the affected patient.
    3. Cyanide gas is produced in the incomplete combustion of carbon- and nitrogen-containing materials (i.e., wood, plastics, and synthetic polymers). The blood levels of cyanide are often fleeting and unreliable, making the diagnosis difficult. Cellular oxygen utilization is impaired at the electron transport level, and despite normal arterial oxygen tension, patients suffer from tissue anoxia. Lactate levels >8 mmol/L should raise suspicion for the diagnosis.

23. **What should I look for in a patient with CO exposure?**
    Patients with significant CO exposure have nonspecific symptoms, such as nausea, headache, and presyncope, with signs of compensation for cellular hypoxia, such as tachycardia and tachypnea. It is important to note that most pulse oximeters cannot distinguish CO-bound hemoglobin (CO-Hb) from oxyhemoglobin, and even in significant exposure, pulse oximetry readings are normal. Measurements of CO-Hb with co-oximetry typically reveal levels as high as 5% in smokers. Levels in the range of 10%–15% are consistent with CO poisoning. CO poisoning accounts for 80% of smoke inhalation deaths, with most patients dying within the first 24 hours after exposure.

24. **How is CO poisoning treated?**
    Treatment is typically 100% oxygen therapy for hours, with hyperbaric oxygen therapy considered when CO-Hb levels exceed 25% (see Chapter 74).

25. **How do I manage patients with cyanide toxicity?**
    Hydroxycobalamin given intravenously is the recommended treatment (see Chapter 74).

26. **What are characteristics of patients whose burns can be managed in the outpatient setting?**
    - No airway compromise.
    - Wound less than 10% TBSA, so fluid resuscitation is unnecessary.
    - Children must be able to take in adequate fluid by mouth.
    - The patient must have the resources to support an outpatient care plan. This includes adequate pain control, ability to perform dressing changes, access to clean water, and ability to transport to burn follow-up if needed.

27. **What are the elements of an outpatient management plan?**
    The elements of the plan include pain control, wound cleansing, and topical wound care. Educate the patient and caregiver on explicit return precautions, routine burn clinic follow-up visits, and expected long-term course. Patients should receive a recheck with a physician skilled in burn management or in the emergency department (ED). Documentation of this management and education is important. In the era of electronic medical record use, photos utilizing HIPAA compliant software are now emphasized to better share information on the progression of a burn and early recognition of poor healing or signs of burn superinfection.

28. **What about tetanus prophylaxis?**
    Tetanus should be updated for all burn patients, and if uncertainty exists as to the interval since the last tetanus immunization, it is advised that the patient receive a tetanus booster at the time of initial evaluation.

29. **How are children who suffer burns different from adults?**
    Children younger than 2 years have increased morbidity and mortality from burns, and require a modified approach. Resuscitation fluids in children are calculated differently, as noted above.
    In children weighing less than 30 kg, the IV flow rate should be adjusted to maintain slightly more brisk urine output at a rate of 1 mL/kg/h. Children <2 years of age are particularly susceptible to hypoglycemia, as glycogen stores are depleted in a postburn hyperadrenergic state. Careful glucose monitoring is warranted, with a transition to dextrose-containing electrolyte solutions (e.g., normal saline or lactated Ringer's with 5% dextrose) if hypoglycemia develops.

30. **What characteristics of burns suggest nonaccidental trauma?**
    See Chapter 67.

31. **In pediatric patients, what specific concerns should be considered in household electrical injuries?**
    See Chapter 57.

32. **What about the child who bites an electrical cord obtaining a burn at the oral commissure?**
    Injuries at the oral commissure after biting an electrical cord typically require no immediate intervention beyond wound care with topical antibiotics. There is a small risk of lateral erosion into the labial artery in subsequent days that should be anticipated, discussed with caregivers, and prompt a return visit.

33. **What are the special considerations in elderly adults suffering burns?**
    Elderly patients often have diminished mobility, reduced reaction time, and impaired alertness. Physiologic changes with aging, such as atrophic skin, slower epidermal turnover rates, and decreased perfusion, place elderly victims at increased risk for more severe burns, delayed healing, and prolonged recovery. Moreover, the aging of organ systems, such as pulmonary, renal, and cardiovascular systems, threaten the burn patient's ability to compensate and overcome the physiologic insult of the initial injury.

34. **Are there any issues in treating elderly adults who sustain burns?**
    Fluid resuscitation is more difficult than in younger adults, with the typical goal of optimizing cardiac preload resulting in excessive fluid administration in elderly populations. Large increases in mortality rates accompany inhalation injury in this population, and airway management is often required earlier.
    The elderly typically suffer burns in the home from scalding, flame, or both. Solitary living conditions contribute to delay in seeking medical attention and jeopardize the success of an outpatient care plan. Pain management can pose some challenges as underlying renal or liver impairment may limit analgesic choices. Additionally, physicians have been shown to underestimate perceptions of pain in elderly populations, further complicating plans for outpatient analgesia.

35. **What is special about treating facial burns?**
    Avoid silver-containing topical antibiotics (silver sulfadiazine) in treatment of facial wounds out of concern for pigmentation changes with potential negative cosmetic consequences. Triple antibiotic ointments are adequate. Apply to the affected area and leave open to air. Consider corneal injury in any burn involving the face. Examine the eyes early (including fluorescein staining under cobalt light), because facial swelling may quickly preclude thorough evaluation. Pay careful attention to the airway for early signs of involvement, potentially indicating the need for escalation of the patient's care. For auricular and nasal burns, utilize Sulfamylon (mafenide acetate) cream to allow penetration of the cartilage in both areas.

36. **What are general principles in managing patients suffering chemical burns?**
    Patients suffering chemical burns should be considered for transfer to a burn center. Take steps to prevent further patient injury and protect providers. Members of the health care team should wear gloves, gowns, and facial protection while involved in patient care. Garments and jewelry that may contain chemical agents and prolong the damaging effects of exposure must be removed. Continue copious irrigation until the patient is symptom free or transfer is undertaken. Specific chemical exposures, such as hydrofluoric acid, petrol products (gasoline and diesel fuel), or alcohols such as phenol, require special attention and specific management that should be initiated before transfer. If the injury occurs in an industrial setting, obtain the material safety data sheet (MSDS) to identify the exact chemical and important information on treatment.

37. **Is antibiotic prophylaxis indicated in the acutely burned patient?**
    There is no role for systemic antibiotic administration in acute burns. Antibiotics should only be administered to patients with clinical evidence of burn superinfection, which is unlikely until >48 hours after initial injury. Signs of wound infection include purulent drainage from the wound, development of cellulitis surrounding burned areas, or systemic evidence of infection. Another indicator of possible burn cellulitis is increasing pain with dressing changes, or increased pain medication requirements with wound care.

38. **Should silver sulfadiazine be applied to burned areas?**
    Since silver sulfadiazine can increase burn depth, only consider its application in full-thickness burns, as these will definitely need grafting. Avoid silver sulfadiazine application in the acutely burnt patient, allowing burns to declare themselves in 24 hours to differentiate deep partial-thickness burns from full-thickness burns. After initial resuscitation and burn debridement, apply triple antibiotic ointment with petroleum gauze to all burned areas until evaluation by a burn surgeon. This ointment is cheaper and easier to obtain.

Websites
American Burn Association: www.ameriburn.org; accessed January 16, 2019.

BIBLIOGRAPHY

American Burn Association. *Advanced Burn Life Support Provider Manual.* Chicago, IL: American Burn Association; 2011.

Cartotto R, Greenhalgh DG, Cancio C. Burn state of the science: fluid resuscitation. *J Burn Care Res.* 2017;38:e596–e604.

Johnson MR, Richard R. Partial-thickness burns: identification and management. *Adv Skin Wound Care.* 2003;16(4):178–189.

Keck M, Lumenta DB, Andel H, et al. Burn treatment in the elderly. *Burns.* 2009;35(8):1071–1079.

Kim LKP, Martin HCO, Holland AJA. Medical management of paediatric burn injuries: best practice. *J Paediatr Child Health.* 2012;48(4):290–295.

Kupas DF, Miller DD. Out-of-hospital chest escharotomy: a case series and procedure review. *Prehosp Emerg Care.* 2010;14(3):349–354.

Leetch AN, Woolridge D. Emergency department evaluation of child abuse. *Emerg Med Clin North Am.* 2013;31(3):853–873.

Mosier MJ, Lasinski AM, Gamelli RL. Suspected adrenal insufficiency in critically ill burned patients: etomidate-induced or critical illness-related corticosteroid insufficiency? A review of the literature. *J Burn Care Res.* 2015;36(2):272–278.

Nimia HH, Carvalho VF, Isaac C, et al. Comparative study of silver sulfadiazine with other materials for healing and infection prevention in burns: a systematic review and meta-analysis. *Burns.* 2019;45(2):282–292.

Walker PF, Buehner MF, Wood LA, et al. Diagnosis and management of inhalation injury: an updated review. *Crit Care.* 2015;19:351–363.

CHAPTER 95

WOUND MANAGEMENT

Jamal Taha, MD and Maria E. Moreira, MD, FACEP

1. **Why is wound management important?**
   Annually, approximately 12 million traumatic wounds are treated in emergency departments (EDs) across the United States, representing approximately 10% of all ED visits. Patients often reasonably judge a physician's competency based on the functional or cosmetic result of the wound repair and the absence of complications.

2. **What is the difference between functional and cosmetic closure?**
   Functional closure prioritizes maintaining function of the injured body part. A cosmetic repair prioritizes healing with the least amount of scarring.

3. **How do I remember what steps to take when repairing a wound?**
   Use the mnemonic *LACERATE:*
   Look. Evaluate the wound and determine most appropriate closure. Examine for movement, sensation, and pulsation distal to the wound.
   Anesthetize
   Clip and clean. Clipping hair leads to less infection than shaving. Methodical irrigation is the best way to decrease infection risk.
   Equipment/Explore. Have everything needed for repair at the bedside (laceration kit, gloves, suture material, dressing). Explore the wound while putting the extremity through range of motion evaluating for tendon injury or presence of foreign body.
   Repair. Proceed with repair. Debride devitalized tissue if needed.
   Assess results. Reevaluate the wound determining need for additional sutures.
   Tetanus. Give tetanus prophylaxis for dirty or contaminated wounds when the patient has not had a booster in 5 years or for clean wounds within 10 years.
   Educate. Educate the patient on how to care for the wound, signs of infection, and timing of suture removal.

4. **Which factors increase the visibility of scars and compromise wound healing, and how are they minimized?**
   See Table 95.1.

5. **What aspects of history should be obtained in a patient with a traumatic wound?**
   The time, setting, and mechanism of injury are essential to determine whether the wound is contaminated, the possibility of foreign body, or the risk for infection. The patient's current medications, immune status (acquired immunodeficiency syndrome [AIDS], diabetes, chemotherapy), occupation, and handedness (for hand injuries) are important. Tetanus immunization history and allergies to anesthetics, antibiotics, and latex also must be obtained.

6. **What are the most important aspects of the physical examination?**
   Familiarity with underlying anatomy, especially in the regions of the face, neck, hands, and feet, is important. Identify any motor, sensory, and vascular deficits. With extremity injuries, a bloodless field can be obtained by temporarily inflating a sphygmomanometer or placement of a finger tourniquet proximal to the injury. Palpation of the bones adjacent to the site of injury may detect instability or point tenderness from an underlying fracture. Direct inspection and visualization always should be performed through a full range of motion when there is a suspicion of a tendon or joint capsule injury or presence of a foreign body.

7. **What is the most important step I can take to prevent infection?**
   Irrigation with normal saline, generating a pressure of at least 8 psi (by using an 18- or 19-gauge needle and 30-mL syringe) is crucial. While optimal irrigation volume has not been determined, 50–100 mL/cm of wound length serves as a guideline. With gross contamination, copious irrigation should be performed and debridement considered. Tap water is a reasonable alternative to sterile saline for irrigation. Detergents, hydrogen peroxide, and concentrated povidone-iodine should not be used for irrigation because they are toxic to tissues. Exploration; debridement when indicated; hemostasis; and proper repair, dressing, and immobilization are essential adjuncts for proper wound management. Antibiotics have no proven prophylactic benefit in healthy individuals with minor wounds. For heavily contaminated wounds, a mechanical irrigation device should be used to remove all dirt and decrease the bacterial count. A stiff brush, such as a toothbrush, or sharp debridement should be used to remove dirt remaining after irrigation.

Table 95.1 Minimizing Factors that Increase Visibility of Scars

CONTRIBUTING FACTORS	METHODS TO MINIMIZE SCARRING
Direction of wound (e.g., perpendicular to lines of static and dynamic tension)	Layered closure; proper direction in elective incisions of wound
Infection necessitating removal of sutures and debridement, resulting in healing by secondary intention and a wide scar	Proper wound preparation; irrigation and use of delayed closure in contaminated wounds
Wide scar secondary to tension	Layered closure; proper splinting and elevation
Suture marks	Removal of percutaneous sutures within 7 days
Uneven wound edges, resulting in magnification of edges and scar by shadows	Careful, even approximation of wound top layer closure to prevent differential swelling of edges
Inversion of wound edges	Proper placement of simple sutures or use of horizontal mattress sutures
Tattooing secondary to retained dirt or foreign body	Proper wound preparation and debridement
Tissue necrosis	Use of corner sutures on flaps; splinting, and elevation of wounds with marginal circulation or venous return; excise nonviable wound edges before closure
Compromised healing secondary to hematoma	Use of properly conforming dressing and splints
Hyperpigmentation of scar or abraded skin	Use of 15 or greater SPF sunblock for 6–12 months
Superimposition of blood clots between healing wound edges	Proper hemostasis and closure; H_2O_2 swabbing; proper application of compressive dressings
Failure to align anatomic structures properly, such as vermilion border	Meticulous closure and alignment; marking or placement of alignment suture before distortion of wound edges with local anesthesia; use of field block

H_2O_2, Hydrogen peroxide; *SPF,* sun protection factor.
From Markovchick V. Suture materials and mechanical after care. *Emerg Med Clin North Am.* 1992;10(4):673–689.

8. **Which anesthetic agent should be used for local anesthesia?**
   Factors to consider include patient age, medical problems, prior drug reactions, wound size and location, and practice environment in the ED. Lidocaine has been the standard agent used; however, bupivacaine has advantages over lidocaine, related mainly to duration of anesthesia. Patients receiving bupivacaine experience significantly less discomfort during the 6-hour postinfiltration period. Additionally, use of bupivacaine may prevent the need to reanesthetize a wound when repair has been interrupted by the arrival of a higher acuity patient.

9. **What causes the pain of local anesthetic infiltration, and how can it be prevented?**
   Pain is caused by the acidity of the agent and distention of tissue from too-rapid injection with too large a needle directly into the dermis. Minimize pain by injecting slowly, subcutaneously, with a small, 25- or 27-gauge needle, directly through the wound margins. Buffering the anesthetic agent with 1 mL of sodium bicarbonate for every 10 mL of lidocaine also can help reduce pain. Bupivacaine, however, cannot be buffered, because it precipitates as its pH rises. Warming the anesthetic also decreases pain of infiltration.

10. **What is the toxic dosage of lidocaine and bupivacaine?**
    See Table 95. 2. When calculating the dosage of milligrams infiltrated, 1 mL of 1% lidocaine equals 10 mg of lidocaine, and 1 mL of 0.25% bupivacaine equals 2.5 mg of bupivacaine. Use lower maximum dosage limits in patients with chronic illness, the very young or old, or when infiltrating highly vascular areas or mucosa.

11. **Describe the presentation of lidocaine toxicity.**
    Toxicity can occur when the recommended dosage is exceeded or at lower than maximum dosages when infiltrating highly vascular areas or mucous membranes, or in patients at the extremes of age or chronically ill. The main effects are on the central nervous and cardiovascular systems. Central nervous system effects include light-headedness, nystagmus, and sensory disturbances, including visual aura or scotoma, tinnitus, perioral tingling, or a metallic taste in the mouth. Slurred speech, disorientation, muscle twitching, and seizures may follow. Cardiovascular effects include hypotension, bradycardia, and prolonged electrocardiogram (ECG) intervals. In severe toxicity, seizures, coma, and cardiorespiratory arrest can occur.

Table 95.2 Maximum Dose and Duration of Action of Anesthetics

ANESTHETIC	CLASS	MAXIMUM DOSAGE	DURATION
Lidocaine	Amide	4.5 mg/kg (not to exceed 300 mg)	1–2 hours
Lidocaine with epinephrine	Amide	7 mg/kg (not to exceed 500 mg)	2–4 hours
Bupivacaine	Amide	2.5 mg/kg (not to exceed 175 mg)	4–8 hours
Bupivacaine with epinephrine	Amide	3 mg/kg (not to exceed 225 mg)[a]	8–16 hours
Procaine	Ester	8 mg/kg (not to exceed 1 g)	15–45 minutes
Procaine with epinephrine	Ester	10 mg/kg (not to exceed 1 g)	30–60 minutes

[a]Can repeat bupivacaine doses once every 3 hours but should not exceed 400 mg in 24-hour period.

12. **What can I use to anesthetize a patient who is allergic to amide and ester anesthetics?**
    Subdermal diphenhydramine may be injected locally for short-acting analgesia. Prepare a 0.5%–1% solution by diluting 1 mL of 50 mg/mL diphenhydramine into 5–10 mL of saline. The anesthetic effect may take several minutes to become evident. Do not exceed a total dose of 50 mg in adults or 1 mg/kg in children. The patient may become drowsy after the injection.

13. **What are the contraindications to epinephrine as an adjunct to lidocaine and bupivacaine?**
    If there is concern for peripheral vascular compromise to an appendage, epinephrine-containing anesthetics should be avoided. For wounds without underlying vascular compromise, local anesthetics containing epinephrine in a concentration of up to 1:100,000 are safe for repair of most lacerations, including digits. A concentration of up to 1:200,000 is preferred for use on the nose and ears. When used on the scalp and face, the vasoconstriction and resulting hemostasis aid in exploration and repair of the wound and do not increase wound infection.

14. **What is LET?**
    LET is a topical anesthetic consisting of a mixture of lidocaine (4%), epinephrine 1:1,000, and tetracaine (0.5%). It is efficacious for wound anesthesia, has a good margin of safety, and is the topical agent of choice. For optimal effect, it should be placed directly into the wound. Onset of action is 20–30 minutes.

15. **What are the contraindications to LET?**
    An allergy to amide *or* ester anesthetics. Lidocaine is an amide and tetracaine is an ester.

16. **When should regional anesthesia be used?**
    - In wounds that would require large toxic doses of anesthetic
    - When tissue distortion needs to be avoided (e.g., vermillion border)
    - Area where local infiltration is very painful (i.e., plantar surface of foot)

17. **When should procedural sedation be considered?**
    Procedural sedation is a pharmacologic means of lowering the level of consciousness to allow procedures to be performed easily with optimal results (see Chapter 68). Consider its use in patients unable to cooperate with laceration examination and repair.

18. **What is a contaminated wound?**
    Any wound that has a high inoculum of bacteria. Examples are:
    - full-thickness bites
    - wounds of the perineum or axilla with normally high skin flora counts
    - wounds exposed to contaminated water (e.g., ponds, lakes, or coral reefs)

19. **List factors that contribute to wound infection.**
    - Wound age
    - Presence of foreign material
    - Amount of devitalized tissue
    - Presence of bacterial contamination
    - Advanced patient age
    - Ability of the host to mount an adequate immune response

20. **Is a dirty wound the same as a contaminated wound?**
    No. Road rash can appear dirty but has a low bacterial count. In contrast, wounds that occur in a barnyard or are exposed to soil contaminated with fecal material have a high bacterial count and are contaminated.

21. What causes tattooing?
Tattooing is caused by the retention of foreign material and incorporation into the dermis during the healing process. Prevention is through thorough debridement, scrubbing, and irrigation of all dirt and foreign material at the initial encounter. A stiff brush, such as a toothbrush, and soap can assist in removing dirt and asphalt embedded in the dermis.

22. How is road rash managed?
Anesthetize the area with viscous lidocaine and circumferential or field block anesthesia. Remove any foreign bodies with the methods described previously. Consider dressing the wound with silver sulfadiazine, which greatly reduces the pain and may obviate the need for prescription analgesics.

23. When is obtaining a radiograph appropriate?
Radiographs are useful in identifying foreign bodies and fractures. Indications for radiographs include:
- concern for foreign body in wounds penetrating muscle fascia or when entire depth of wound cannot be visualized;
- concern for swallowed teeth or teeth impacted in wound;
- concern for fracture.

24. Which types of foreign bodies are visible on radiographs?
Radiopaque objects (glass, metal, gravel) are visible on radiographs. Typically, glass larger than 2 mm and gravel larger than 1 mm can be visualized. Radiolucent objects including wood, plastics, and some aluminum products are not visualized.

25. What is the role of bedside ultrasound in assessing lacerations?
- More sensitive and specific than a physical examination and local wound exploration in identifying extensor tendon injuries of the thumb and fingers.
- Greater accuracy in diagnosing flexor tendon injuries.
- Helpful in identification and removal of foreign bodies.

26. What is the best method for hair removal?
Clipping or cutting hair with scissors results in lower wound bacterial counts and decreased rates of infection compared to shaving.

27. Define the three different types of wound closure.
- *Primary closure* is closure with sutures, staples, glues, or adhesive tapes within 24 hours of the time of injury.
- *Delayed primary closure* is closure 3–5 days after the injury to decrease the risk of infection.
- *Secondary closure* (healing by secondary intention) is allowing healing by granulation without mechanical approximation of wound margins.

28. Which wounds should be closed primarily?
In healthy patients, primary closure can be performed on any part of the body for up to 18 hours post injury, although the sooner the better and preferably within 8 hours. On the face and scalp, because of increased vascularity of these areas, primary closure can be performed up to 24 hours post injury. However, other considerations for primary repair include the patient's medical history and wound contamination. Patients with contaminated wounds and multiple comorbidities may be better served with delayed closure. The risks and benefits of primary closure should be discussed with the patient.

29. When should delayed primary closure be used?
Consider for all contaminated wounds that are gaping or have significant amounts of tension. It decreases the risk of infection, optimizes cosmesis, and accelerates the healing process.

30. How is a wound prepared for delayed primary closure?
Hemorrhage is controlled and the wound is examined, debrided, and irrigated. Lay a fine layer of mesh gauze in the wound and pack it open. If in 3–5 days there is absence of purulent drainage or wound-margin erythema, the wound is closed in the same fashion as if closed primarily.

31. When should secondary closure be used?
Secondary closure should be used for contaminated wounds that penetrate deeply into tissue and cannot be irrigated adequately. Examples include puncture wounds of the sole of the foot or palm of the hand, and stab wounds that penetrate into subcutaneous tissue and muscle.

32. When are surgical staples indicated?
Staples are appropriate for linear lacerations not involving cosmetically sensitive areas. Staples work best in wounds that are perpendicular to the surface. Stapling techniques include:
- one operator everting both wound edges with forceps while another places staples;
- one wound edge everted with forceps in one hand while stapling with the other hand.

33. **What is surgical glue, and how is it used?**

Surgical glue, 2-octyl cyanoacrylate (DERMABOND), is a polymer used for wound repair. It acts rapidly, polymerizing within 30 seconds at room air and is best for linear lacerations under low tension. The wound is held together manually, and the cyanoacrylate is painted over the wound in three to four coats to ensure adequate closure. Do not apply adhesive within the wound, as it will impede healing. The adhesive sloughs off in 7–10 days. Avoid ointment on the wound as it destroys the adhesive bond.

34. **How do I remove tissue adhesive?**

If the adhesive dries on an undesirable area (e.g., eyelid glued shut), the bond may be loosened with petroleum jelly or antibiotic ointment. Preventative methods include:
- applying a protective covering and petroleum jelly to areas surrounding the wound;
- applying light coats;
- quickly wiping off excess fluid, as adhesives dry in about 15 seconds.

35. **Summarize the advantages and disadvantages of the available techniques for wound closure.**

See Table 95.3.

36. **Which sutures are used for specific locations, how is the wound repaired, and when do I remove the sutures?**

See Table 95.4.

37. **What are some special suturing considerations and techniques?**
- Lip lacerations – place a nonabsorbable suture at the vermillion border lining up the edges precisely for the best cosmetic result. Close the lip with absorbable suture and the skin with nonabsorbable suture.
- Thin fragile skin – place steri-strips parallel to the laceration edge; place stitches through the skin reinforced with steri-strips.
- Simple linear scalp laceration – hair apposition technique – intertwine hair bundles from opposite sides of a laceration in a 360-degree revolution and then secure with a few drops of tissue adhesive.

38. **How are bites treated?**

The approach depends on the age of the bite, animal involved, and location of the injury. Infection risk increases with time from injury to laceration repair. Cat and human bites are more likely to become infected than dog bites and should be left to heal by secondary intention. The exceptions are facial wounds, which require good cosmesis and are less likely to become infected. With dog bites, cosmetic results are improved with primary closure without an increase in infection rate. Repair of most simple dog wounds is recommended except when there is presence of deep puncture wounds, hand or feet involvement, and immunosuppression. (See Chapter 73.) (Fig. 95.1.)

Table 95.3 Advantages and Disadvantages of Wound Closure Techniques

TECHNIQUE	ADVANTAGES	DISADVANTAGES
Sutures	Time-honored method Meticulous closure Greatest tensile strength Lowest dehiscence rate	Removal for nonabsorbable material Anesthesia required Greatest tissue reactivity Slowness of application
Staples	Rapidity of application Low tissue reactivity Low cost	Less meticulous closure than with sutures May interfere with CT and MRI May result in uneven wound edges
Tissue adhesives	Rapidity of application Patient comfort Resistance to bacterial growth No need for removal Sometimes no need for needle stick	Lower tensile strength than sutures Dehiscence over high-tension areas (joints) Wound healing inhibited if placed in the wound High cost
Surgical tapes	Least tissue reactivity Lowest infection rates Rapidity of application Patient comfort Low cost	Lower tensile strength than sutures Highest rate of dehiscence Cannot be used in hairy areas Must remain dry

CT, Computed tomography; *MRI,* magnetic resonance imaging.

From Singer AJ, Hollander JE, Quinn JV. Evaluation and management of traumatic lacerations. *N Engl J Med.*1997;337:1142–1148.

Table 95.4 Use of Sutures for Wound Repair

LOCATION	SUTURE MATERIAL	TECHNIQUE OF CLOSURE AND DRESSING	SUTURE REMOVAL
Scalp	3-0 or 4-0 nylon or polypropylene	Interrupted in galea; single tight layer in scalp; horizontal mattress if bleeding not well controlled by simple sutures	7–10 days
Pinna (ear)	6-0 nylon or 5-0 SA in perichondrium	Close perichondrium with 5-0 SA interrupted; close skin with 6-0 nylon interrupted; stint dressing	4–6 days
Eyebrow	4-0 or 5-0 SA and 6-0 nylon	Layered closure	4–5 days
Eyelid	6-0 nylon or silk	Single layer simple or horizontal mattress	5–6 days
Lip	4-0 silk or SA (mucosa); 5-0 SA (SC, muscle); 6-0 (skin); 4-0 SA	Three layers (mucosa, muscle, skin) if through and through; otherwise, two layers	5-6 days
Oral cavity	4-0 SA	Simple interrupted or horizontal mattress: layered closure if the muscularis of the tongue is involved	7–8 days or allow to dissolve
Face	4-0 or 5-0 SA (SC); 6-0 nylon (skin)	If full-thickness laceration, layered closure desirable	5–6 days
Neck	4-0 SA (SC); 5-0 nylon (skin)	Two-layered closure for best cosmetic results	5–6 days
Trunk	4-0 SA (SC, fat); 4-0 or 5-0 nylon (skin)	Single or layered closure	7–12 days
Extremity	3-0 or 4-0 SA (SC, fat, muscle); 4-0 or 5-0 nylon (skin)	Single or layered closure is adequate, although a layered or running SC closure may give a better cosmetic result; apply a splint if the wound is over a joint	7–14 days
Hands and feet	4-0 or 5-0 nylon	Single-layer closure only with simple or interrupted horizontal mattress suture, at least 5 mm from cut wound edges; horizontal mattress sutures should be used if there is much tension on wound edges; apply splint if wound is over a joint	7–12 days
Nail beds	5-0 SA	Gentle, meticulous placement to obtain even edges. Replace nail under cuticle	Allow to dissolve

SA, Synthetic absorbable sutures such as Vicryl and Dexon; *SC,* subcutaneous.
From Markovchick V. Soft tissue injury and wound repair. In: Reisdorff EJ, Roberts MR, Wiegenstein JG, eds. *Pediatric Emergency Medicine.* Philadelphia: Saunders; 1993:899–908.

39. **What should be included in all follow-up instructions?**
    Include instructions for local wound care, signs of infection, and recommended time of suture removal. Antimicrobial ointment may be applied to decrease the risk of infection except when tissue adhesives are used for closure. Laceration scars are sensitive to ultraviolet radiation and prone to sunburns for up to a year after the initial injury. Sunlight should be avoided, and sunscreen used to help minimize hyperpigmentation and scarring. Inform patients that all wounds will heal with a scar, have a risk of becoming infected, and may have retained foreign material.

40. **How do I remember the direction of the lines of skin tension?**
    You do not. Refer to Figs. 95.2 and 95.3.

41. **Are there any controversies in wound care?**
    The use of prophylactic antibiotics is controversial. In general, their use is not warranted in the normal host. Antibiotics are indicated in patients with soft-tissue wounds who are prone to infective endocarditis. Antibiotics may be

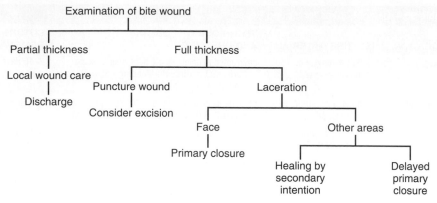

Fig. 95.1 Algorithm for treatment of bites.

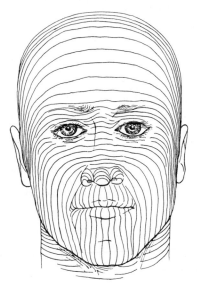

Fig. 95.2 Direction of the lines of skin tension for the face. (From Marx J, Hockberger R, Well R, et al., eds. *Rosen's Emergency Medicine: Concepts and Clinical Practice.* 5th ed. Philadelphia: Mosby; 2002:738.)

indicated when the risk for infection is high, including wounds of the hand and distal foot; contaminated wounds; wounds from human bites extending into the dermis; wounds in which there has been a delay in irrigation and debridement; and wounds that contain fecal material, pus, saliva, or vaginal secretions. Prophylactic antibiotic use should never replace proper wound decontamination.

KEY POINTS: WOUND MANAGEMENT

1. Use a tourniquet, if necessary, on extremities to adequately examine and repair the wound.
2. Irrigation pressure must be at least 8 psi.
3. Wounds may be irrigated with tap water or sterile saline.
4. Local anesthetics with epinephrine of 1:100,000 concentration are safe for use on digits.
5. Most dog bites can be closed primarily. Cat and human bites, except to the face, are left open.

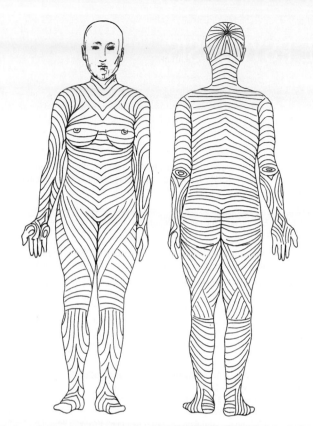

Fig. 95.3 Direction of the lines of skin tension for the body. (From Marx J, Hockberger R, Well R, et al., eds. *Rosen's Emergency Medicine: Concepts and Clinical Practice*. 5th ed. Philadelphia: Mosby; 2002:739.)

BIBLIOGRAPHY

Bansal BC, Wicbc RA, Perkins SD, et al. Tap water for irrigation of lacerations. *Am J Emerg Med*. 2002;20(5):469–472.

Dezfuli B, Taljanovic MS, Melville DM, et al. Accuracy of high-resolution ultrasonography in the detection of extensor tendon lacerations. *Ann Plast Surg*. 2016;76(2):187–192.

Forsch RT. Essentials of skin laceration repair. *Am Fam Physician*. 2008;78(8):945–951.

Forsch RT, Little SH, Williams C. Laceration repair: a practical approach. *Am Fam Physician*. 2017;95(10):628–637.

Howell JM, Chisholm CD. Wound care. *Emerg Med Clin North Am*. 1997;15(2):417–425.

Kennedy SA, Stoll LE, Lauder AS. Human and other mammalian bite injuries of the hand: evaluation and management. *J Am Acad Orthop Surg*. 2015;23(1):47–57.

Moreira ME, Markovchick VJ. Wound management. *Crit Care Nurs Clin North Am*. 2012;24(2):215–237.

Quinn JV, Polevoi SK, Kohn MA. Traumatic lacerations: what are the risks for infection and has the 'golden period' of laceration care disappeared? *Emerg Med J*. 2014;31(2):96–100.

CHAPTER 96

ACUTE PSYCHOSIS

Janetta L. Iwanicki, MD

1. **What is psychosis?**
   Psychosis is a dysfunction of the perception of reality. According to the *Diagnostic and Statistical Manual of Mental Disorders, Fifth Edition (DSM-5),* key features include delusions, hallucinations, and disorganized thinking and speech.

2. **What are delusions?**
   From the *DSM-5* (2013), "delusions are fixed beliefs that are not amenable to change in light of conflicting evidence."

3. **What are hallucinations?**
   "Hallucinations are sensory perceptions without external stimulation" (*DSM-5,* 2013). Hallucinations may occur in any of the five sensory modalities, although auditory hallucinations are most common.

4. **How does a patient in a psychotic state typically appear upon arrival at the emergency department (ED)?**
   Patients in a psychotic state may act strangely, dress bizarrely, respond to hallucinations, harbor false and delusional beliefs, and consistently confuse the reality of events. They are commonly impulsive and in danger of acting on distorted perceptions or delusional ideas, resulting in injury or death. The patient is unable to discriminate whether the stimuli that he or she perceives are internal or external. Thinking and speech are often disorganized and incoherent. Psychomotor behavior may be hypoactive or hyperactive. Emotions can range from apathy and depression to fear and rage.

5. **How should priorities be set when I first encounter a psychotic patient?**
   - Assess the airway, breathing, and circulation (ABCs), if necessary.
   - Observe (quickly assess the patient's impulse control and tendency to physically act out).
   - Control and manage psychotic behavior posing a danger to the patient or others, if necessary.
   - Obtain a history (gather information from everyone who has been involved with the patient).
   - Differentiate between organic and functional causes of psychosis.
   - Do a complete physical examination.
   - Obtain laboratory tests as deemed appropriate.
   - Obtain a psychiatric consultation and disposition.

6. **Why is it important to control psychotic behavior immediately?**
   Patients in a psychotic state have little impulse control, and they cannot distinguish internal from external stimuli. Because of this dysfunction, they should always be considered a potential danger to themselves or to others. The best way to deal with violent behavior is to prevent it. Emergency physicians should recognize patients who are obviously confused, irrational, paranoid, or excited. Any history or comment that suggests violence should be taken seriously. The potential for violence is particularly high in patients who are psychotic secondary to illicit drug use.

7. **Are there behavioral controls that can be used immediately for the psychotic patient?**
   Yes, steps should be taken to avoid confrontation or escalation.
   - *Environmental.* Keep the environment simple and stimulus free, and minimize staff changes.
   - *Interpersonal.* Assume the role of patient advocate, and engage the patient in a calm and self-assured voice. Recognize the patient's right to privacy and dignity.

8. **What options can be exercised if the patient becomes increasingly disorganized, agitated, and violent?**
   See Chapter 98.

9. **How do I obtain a history for a psychotic patient?**
   Because acutely psychotic patients may not be able to provide an adequate history, all available collateral sources for obtaining information must be explored. This may include speaking to emergency medical services (EMS) personnel, family, friends, neighbors, and law enforcement officers, as well as reviewing old medical records. A telephone conversation with caregivers and significant others can also be helpful.

10. **What historical information is important?**
    - *Onset.* Did the behavior change suddenly or gradually?
    - *Longitudinal course.* What was the precipitating event? Is this the first such event? What was the behavior like on previous events?

- *Psychosocial setting.* Obtain information regarding the patient's support system, psychosocial stressors, and psychiatric resources.
- *Previous psychiatric disease.* Determine whether there is organic brain disease, the use or misuse of medication, or a history of illicit drug use.
- What are the current medications, and have they been taken as prescribed?

11. **How should my physical examination be tailored for a psychotic patient?**
    In retrospective reviews, a high percentage of missed organic diagnoses in psychotic patients was because of the lack of complete history and physical examination. Thus a complete and thorough physical examination, including a mental status examination, is imperative. Always note the vital signs and pulse oximetry readings. In most cases, emergency physicians will have built sufficient rapport with patients that they will cooperate with the examination. Tell the patient exactly what you are doing and what you are going to do during the examination. This helps provide structure for the psychotic patient and avoids confusion or misunderstanding.

KEY POINTS: EVALUATION OF THE PSYCHOTIC PATIENT

- Collateral information from friends, family members, EMS providers, etc., may provide crucial details of the patient history.
- Abnormal vital signs or physical examination findings may suggest an organic etiology.
- Prioritize patient and staff safety.

12. **What is the difference between organic and functional psychosis?**
    - Organic psychosis is a reversible or nonreversible dysfunctional mental condition that can be identified as a disturbance in the anatomy, physiology, or biochemistry of the brain (i.e., delirium, dementia, withdrawal states, and intoxications).
    - Functional psychosis is a dysfunctional mental condition identified as schizophrenia, a major affective disorder, or other mental disorders with psychotic features.

13. **Summarize the key points to consider in the differentiation of organic from functional psychosis.**
    See Table 96.1.

14. **List the possible causes of alcohol-related organic psychosis.**
    - Chronic alcoholism
    - Thiamine deficiency (Wernicke encephalopathy)

Table 96.1 *MADFOCS* Mnemonic		
	ORGANIC	**FUNCTIONAL**
Memory deficit	Recently impaired	Remotely impaired
Activity	Hyperactivity and hypoactivity Tremor Ataxia	Repetitive activity Posturing Rocking
Distortions	Visual hallucinations	Auditory hallucinations
Feelings	Emotional lability	Flat affect
Orientation	Disoriented	Oriented
Cognition	Some lucid thoughts Perceives occasionally Attends occasionally Focuses occasionally	No lucid thoughts Unfiltered perceptions Unable to attend Unable to focus
Some other findings	Age >40 Sudden onset Physical examination often abnormal Vital signs may be abnormal Social immodesty Aphasia Consciousness impaired Confabulation	Age <40 Gradual onset Physical examination normal Vital signs usually normal Social modesty Intelligible speech Alert, awake Ambivalence

- Alcohol-dependent withdrawal states
- Alcoholic ketoacidosis or hypoglycemia
- Comorbid psychotic and mood disorder
- Alcohol idiosyncratic intoxication (pathologic intoxication)

15. **Is there a brief, self-limited, and nonorganic psychosis?**
Yes, some individuals may become acutely and briefly psychotic after exposure to an extremely traumatic experience. If such a psychosis lasts for less than 4 weeks, it is termed a *brief psychotic disorder.* Patients with hysterical, borderline, and narcissistic personalities are prone to brief psychotic disorder, and some studies support a genetic vulnerability. Emotional turmoil, confusion, and extremely bizarre behavior and speech are common symptoms on presentation.

16. **Summarize the potentially reversible causes of psychosis.**
DEMENTIA mnemonic:
Drug toxicity
Emotional disorders
Metabolic disorders
Endocrine disorders
Nutritional disorders
Tumors and trauma
Infection
Arteriosclerotic complications

17. **Name the life-threatening causes of acute psychosis.**
WHHHIMP mnemonic:
Wernicke encephalopathy
Hypoxia or hypoperfusion of the central nervous system
Hypoglycemia
Hypertensive encephalopathy
Intracranial hemorrhage
Meningitis/encephalitis
Poisonings

18. **List pharmacologic agents that can cause acute psychosis.**
- Digitalis
- Corticosteroids
- Isoniazid (INH)
- Disulfiram (Antabuse)
- Tricyclics
- Anticonvulsants
- Cimetidine
- Benzodiazepines
- Amphetamines and related drugs
- Antidysrhythmics
- Narcotics
- Barbiturates
- Methyldopa
- Nonsteroidal anti-inflammatory drugs
- Anticancer agents
- Recreational drugs: Alcohol, cocaine, amphetamines, hallucinogens, synthetic cannabinoids

19. **Is laboratory screening necessary in the workup of an acute psychotic patient?**
Patients with established psychiatric diagnoses in the ED with psychiatric chief complaints, benign histories, and normal physical examinations have a low likelihood of clinically significant laboratory findings. Therefore routine laboratory tests are not recommended. If a patient is experiencing his or her first psychotic episode, then laboratory studies are indicated to distinguish functional versus organic psychosis. The following tests are recommended:
- Complete blood count
- Electrolytes, toxicology screens
- Pregnancy test
- Thyroid function tests
- Computed tomography (CT) scan of the brain
    Consider screening for toxic ingestions (e.g., acetaminophen, salicylates) in any patient who expresses suicidal ideation.

20. **Are there any other clinical rules of thumb in the workup of the acute psychotic patient?**
    - Fever and psychosis = meningitis, encephalitis, or sepsis
    - Acute psychosis and alcoholism = Wernicke encephalopathy
    - Headache and psychosis = tumor or intracranial hemorrhage
    - Abdominal pain and psychosis = porphyria
    - Diaphoresis and psychosis = hypoglycemia, delirium tremens, sepsis, sympathomimetic intoxication
    - Autonomic signs and psychosis = toxic or metabolic encephalopathy

21. **When is hospitalization recommended?**
    - If this is the patient's first psychotic episode
    - If the patient is a danger to self or others
    - If the patient is unable to care for himself or herself appropriately
    - If the patient has no social support system
    - If an acute organic psychosis does not clear while the patient is in the ED

22. **How do I treat the acutely psychotic patient in the ED?**
    Treat similarly to treating an acutely agitated patient. See Chapter 98.

KEY POINTS: ACUTE PSYCHOSIS

1. Acute psychosis includes delusions or prominent hallucinations.
2. Use the least restrictive restraint (e.g., isolation, restraints, psychotropic medication).
3. A complete and thorough history and physical examination, including mental status examination, is imperative.
4. Distinguish between organic and functional disorders.

Website

Clinical policy: critical issues in the diagnosis and management of the adult psychiatric patient in the ED: https://www.acep.org/contentassets/04e7623d4991457bbcd9a53a40ba427d/cp-adultpsychiatricpatient-1.pdf; accessed February 15, 2019.

ACKNOWLEDGMENT

The editors gratefully acknowledge the contributions of authors of this chapter in earlier editions.

BIBLIOGRAPHY

American College of Emergency Physicians. Clinical policy for the initial approach to patients presenting with altered mental status. *Ann Emerg Med.* 2017;69:480–498.

American Psychiatric Association. *Diagnostic and Statistical Manual of Mental Disorders.* 5th ed. (DSM-5). Washington, DC: American Psychiatric Association; 2013.

Janiak BD, Atteberry S. Medical clearance of the psychiatric patient in the emergency department. *J Emerg Med.* 2012;43(5):866–870.

Khandanpour N, Hoggard N, Connolly DJ. The role of MRI and CT of the brain in first episodes of psychosis. *Clin Radiol.* 2013;68(3):245–250.

Parmar P, Goolsby CA, Udompanyanan K, et al. Value of mandatory screening studies in emergency department patients cleared for psychiatric admission. *West J Emerg Med.* 2012;13(5):388–393.

Sporer KA, Solares M, Durant EJ, et al. Accuracy of the initial diagnosis among patients with an acutely altered mental status. *Emerg Med J.* 2013;30(3):243–246.

CHAPTER 97

DEPRESSION, SUICIDE, AND POSTTRAUMATIC STRESS DISORDER

Henrik Galust, MD and Carl Bonnett, MD

1. **Why is recognizing depression in the emergency department (ED) important?**
   Patients with depression have a significantly higher risk for suicide attempt, and studies suggest that a significant number of patients who die from suicide visited a health care professional weeks before their death, oftentimes in the ED. Nearly 12 million ED visits occur annually for mental health–related complaints, and of those visits, nearly 600,000 patients are evaluated for suicide attempts. The ED is a critical access point for identifying patients at risk for suicide, providing timely interventions and support, and making referrals for more treatment when warranted.

2. **How is depression classified?**
   According to the American Psychiatric Association's *Diagnostic and Statistical Manual of Mental Disorders, Fifth Edition* (DSM-V), the category of "depressive disorders" includes: major depressive disorder, mood dysregulation disorder, dysthymia, premenstrual dysphoric disorder, substance or medication-induced depression, depressive disorder due to underlying medical condition, and other specified or unspecified depressive disorders. These disorders are unified by their presence of dysphoria (irritable or sad mood).

3. **How is major depression diagnosed?**
   Major depressive disorder, or unipolar depression, is diagnosed through history and examination, ruling out any secondary causes such as substance abuse, underlying medical conditions, or other psychiatric illness. The history must elicit symptoms of either (1) depressed mood or (2) loss of interest or pleasure, with a significant departure from normal functioning for at least 2 weeks, in addition to four or more of the following symptoms occurring nearly every day:
   - Insomnia or hypersomnia
   - Diminished interest or loss of pleasure in most activities
   - Feelings of worthlessness or excessive guilt
   - Fatigue or energy loss
   - Reduced ability to concentrate or make decisions
   - Increase or decrease in appetite or unintentional but significant weight gain or loss
   - Psychomotor agitation or retardation
   - Repetitive thoughts of death, suicidal ideation with or without a plan, or suicide attempt

4. **What is SIG E CAPS?**
   The neurovegetative symptoms of depression can also be easily remembered by Dr. Carey Gross' mnemonic SIG E CAPS, where each letter refers to one of the major diagnostic criteria. One of the symptoms must be depressed mood or loss of interest or pleasure, plus at least four of the following:
   SIG E CAPS
   - **S**leep disturbance
   - **I**nterests/mood
   - **G**uilt
   - **E**nergy
   - **C**oncentration
   - **A**ppetite disturbance
   - **P**sychomotor changes
   - **S**uicidal thinking

5. **Is psychosis ever a feature of depression?**
   Yes. Depression with psychotic features, delusions, or auditory hallucinations represents a severe form of major depression. Patients with this rarer subset of depression are much more likely to experience recurrence, suffer more debilitating symptoms, and have significantly higher mortality rates from suicide compared with patients with nonpsychotic major depression.

6. **What medical conditions might produce symptoms of depression?**
   Various medical, psychiatric or neurologic conditions can cause depression, known as secondary depression. A careful history, physical, and possibly laboratory examination should be performed to rule out any mood disturbances due to underlying medical issues. Some important conditions include:
   - Neurogenic (intracranial neoplasia, cerebrovascular accident, subdural or epidural hematomas, dementia, traumatic brain injury)

- Endocrine (diabetes mellitus, Cushing's syndrome, hypothyroidism, hyperthyroidism, adrenal insufficiency, hypercortisolism)
- Connective tissue disorders (systemic lupus erythematosus)
- Infectious sources (central nervous system [CNS] infection, mononucleosis)

7. **When should clinicians suspect depression in patients with medical complaints?**
Patients may not always admit to symptoms of depression. Consider in patients who present with repeat visitation, nonspecific vague somatic complaints, and the following at-risk populations: patients with chronic pain; those with multiple comorbidities; and those with personal or family history of depression, posttraumatic stress disorder (PTSD), suicide, psychosis, or substance abuse.

8. **What medications or substances of abuse might produce symptoms of depression?**
A myriad of pharmaceuticals and substances of abuse carry the potential to produce symptoms of depression either through intoxication or withdrawal. These include:
- Depressants (alcohol, opiates, benzodiazepines, sedative-hypnotics, barbiturates)
- Antihypertensives (methyldopa, β-blockers)
- Dopamine antagonists (metoclopramide, prochlorperazine, haloperidol)
- Withdrawal from stimulants (amphetamines, cocaine)
- Histamine antagonists (cimetidine, ranitidine)
- Others: systemic steroids, chemotherapeutics, and exposure to heavy metals.

9. **Why should clinicians always inquire about alcohol use when evaluating for depression?**
Alcohol use and abuse is an extremely common comorbid condition with depression:
- Concurrent alcohol use is associated with a dramatic increased risk for suicide.
- Patients cannot be adequately assessed for depression or suicidality if intoxicated.
- Alcohol use can itself cause depression.
- Depression cannot be effectively treated if there is ongoing alcohol abuse.

10. **When should emergency physicians prescribe antidepressants?**
Patients should be informed that antidepressants take 4–6 weeks of consistent use until symptom improvement, and require close monitoring for side effects and dosing adjustments. Therefore treatment of depression is rarely initiated in the ED. If a prescription is written, we recommend a 1- to 2-week supply of medication with a plan for urgent outpatient psychiatric care follow-up.

11. **How is major depression treated?**
Depression is often treated with psychotherapy, pharmacotherapy, or both. Classes of antidepressants used in pharmacotherapy include:
- Selective serotonin reuptake inhibitors (SSRIs) are the most popular and first line in depression treatment given their efficacy, safety, and tolerability – fluoxetine, paroxetine, sertraline, escitalopram.
- Serotonin-norepinephrine reuptake inhibitors (SNRIs) – duloxetine, venlafaxine
- Atypical antidepressants – bupropion, mirtazapine
- Serotonin modulators – trazodone, nefazodone
- Tricyclic antidepressants (TCAs) – amitriptyline, imipramine, nortriptyline
- Monoamine oxidase inhibitors (MAOIs) – tranylcypromine, phenelzine, selegiline

12. **What are some serious or life-threatening side effects of certain antidepressants?**
- Serotonin syndrome, due to serotonin toxicity associated with SSRIs, SNRIs, and serotonin modulators, manifests with a wide range of clinical symptoms and may be life threatening. Onset is usually within 24 hours of any dosage change or initiation of treatment. Diagnosis is made using the Hunter toxicity criteria. Hunter's criteria uses decision rules for patients known to have taken a serotonergic agent and presenting with one of the following: spontaneous clonus; hyperreflexia and tremor; reproducible clonus with agitation or diaphoresis; ocular-type clonus with agitation or diaphoresis; or hypertonia with hyperthermia, ocular-type clonus, or inducible clonus. Treatment consists of stopping the offending agent, supportive care, benzodiazepine, and the antidote cyproheptadine, as needed.
- MAOI use has largely declined in recent years given their potential for lethal drug–drug interactions and dietary interactions – though evidence exists for their continued use in recalcitrant forms of depression or depression with atypical features. Fatal hypertensive crises are known to occur when MAOIs are mixed with foods containing the sympathomimetic tyramine (fermented soy products, wines, beers, aged cheeses). Treatment involves discontinuing the MAOI and avoiding precipitating a hypertensive reaction.
- TCAs can be potentially lethal, and are currently used more commonly as a second- or third-line treatment for depression. Physical findings of TCA toxicity include signs and symptoms of CNS toxicity (altered level of consciousness, delirium, stupor, seizures), cardiac toxicity (sinus tachycardia, hypotension, characteristic QRS widening), and anticholinergic toxicity (hyperthermia, mydriasis, bowel or bladder retention). Treatment involves autonomic support, benzodiazepines for agitation and delirium, and sodium bicarbonate for cardiac toxicity.

13. **How is the disposition of depressed patients managed?**
The ultimate disposition of patients with suspected or confirmed major depression hinges upon the assessment of their safety: whether the patient is a danger to self or others, their level of supportive environment at home or in the community, and any related medical or substance abuse–related issues. Psychiatric evaluation and hospitalization is also warranted for any patient with acute psychotic manifestations, those deemed dangerous to themselves, dangerous to others, or disabled to the extent that they are unable to adequately care for themselves.

14. **What are the different terminologies used in addressing suicide?**
    - Suicide: a fatal act of self-harm with the intention of killing oneself.
    - Suicidal attempt: a nonfatal act of self-harm with the intention of killing oneself.
    - Suicidal threat: a verbal expression of self-harm without the intention of killing oneself.
    - Suicidal ideation: thoughts of killing oneself with or without a plan to do so.
    - Suicidal gesture: an act of self-harm without the intention of killing oneself; intention rather of convincing others that one wishes to die.

15. **What demographic groups are at higher risk for suicide?**
    - Women are $1.2\times$ more likely to attempt suicide; men make more lethal attempts and are $2-4\times$ more likely to die from suicide.
    - Women 45–54 years old and males >65 years old have the highest rates of suicide.
    - Among young US adults, 15–24 years old, suicide is the second leading cause of death.
    - For both men and women, rates of suicide are highest among the Alaskan Native and Indigenous People's populations, followed by non-Hispanics and Whites.
    - Never having been married carries the highest risk of suicide, followed in decreasing magnitude of risk: being widowed, separated, divorced, and married.
    - Access to firearms increases the risk of death from suicide.
    - Additional risk factors include multiple comorbidities, history of drug and alcohol abuse, chronic pain, military experience, members of sexual minorities, history of traumatic brain injury, presence of childhood abuse or neglect, family history of suicide, residents of rural communities, and access to weaponry.

16. **What is the single greatest predictive factor of suicide?**
A prior history of suicide attempt is the single greatest predictive factor of suicide. Patients who continue to express suicidal ideation after an attempt are especially at risk for a subsequent attempt. Previous suicide attempts should always be inquired about as these patients are 100 times more likely to die from suicide than the general public. The risk of completed suicide is much higher in the first year after an attempt, particularly for people >45 years of age.

17. **What factors are protective and decrease the risk of suicide?**
Social support systems, particularly positive family ties, are protective against suicide. Additional protective factors include reliable access to mental and physical health care, feelings of connectedness to community and social institutions (such as religious groups), having effective coping strategies, and parenthood.

18. **What is the initial approach to a suicidal patient in the ED?**
Evaluate and treat any life-threatening conditions (e.g., overdose, poisoning, or trauma). Make the patient to feel comfortable and supported when discussing deeply personal and traumatic events. Approach the patient with empathy and a nonjudgmental tone.

19. **Describe suicide precautions.**
Suicide precautions include the following:
    - Have patients change into hospital attire to facilitate physical examination.
    - Remove potential sources of self-harm such as belts, pills, weapons, etc.
    - Designate a "safe room" that is well-lit, single occupancy, easily accessible, and devoid of objects that may be used for self-injury.
    - Have video monitoring, security personnel, or "sitters" for one-on-one monitoring of patients to prevent attempts at self-harm or leaving before it is deemed safe.

20. **Why is it important to inquire about a specific plan?**
All patients being evaluated for suicide should be asked about any plans regarding suicide. If a plan exists, patients are at increased risk of suicide, particularly if the plan is detailed, violent, or feasible.

21. **Are accidents ever suicide attempts?**
It is important to remember that victims of trauma may have actually attempted suicide. Single-victim accidents, such as a car driven at high speed into a concrete structure, a pedestrian hit by a high-speed vehicle, or a fall from a height, are classic examples of suicide attempts presenting as trauma.

22. **Why is it important to consider type of suicide attempt and likelihood of being rescued in a suicide evaluation?**

In general, a more serious or risky attempt is considered a greater predictor of subsequent attempts. The patient's belief about the lethality of the attempt is at least as important as the physician's assessment of its seriousness.

23. **What is the SAD PERSONS Scale?**

In 1983, Patterson and coworkers used known high-risk characteristics to develop the mnemonic *SAD PERSONS Scale*. The scale was designed to be used by nonpsychiatrists to assess the need for hospitalization in suicidal patients. Hockberger and Rothstein modified the scale to facilitate use in the ED (Table 97.1). A score of ≤5 indicates that a patient probably can be discharged safely. Scores of 6–8 should receive psychiatric consultation; and scores of ≥9 are likely to need psychiatric hospitalization.

24. **In general, which suicidal patients should be hospitalized?**
   - Absolute indications for hospitalization after suicide attempts (involuntarily, if necessary) usually include the following: presence of psychosis; a violent, nearly lethal preplanned attempt; and continued suicidal ideation with definite plans for a repeated attempt.
   - Relative indications include age >45 years old; high risk-to-rescue ratio; serious mental illness; alcoholism; drug addiction; living alone with poor social support; and hopelessness, helplessness, or exhaustion.

KEY POINTS: INDICATIONS FOR SUICIDE PRECAUTIONS AND PSYCHIATRIC CONSULTATION

1. Violent, near-lethal, preplanned attempt
2. Psychotic patient
3. Elderly patient
4. Expression of continued wish to die by suicide

Table 97.1 Modified SAD PERSONS Scale

	MNEMONIC	CHARACTERISTIC	SCORE
S	Sex	Male	1
A	Age	<19 or >45 years	I
D	Depression or hopelessness	Admits to depression or decreased concentration, appetite, sleep, libido	2
P	Previous attempts or psychiatric care	Previous inpatient or outpatient psychiatric care	1
E	Excessive alcohol or drug use	Stigmata of chronic addiction or recent repeated use	1
R	Rational thinking loss	Organic brain syndrome or psychosis	2
S	Separated, widowed, or divorced		1
O	Organized or serious attempt	Well-thought-out plan or life-threatening presentation	2
N	No social supports	No close family, friends, job, or active religious affiliation	1
S	Stated future intent	Determined to repeat attempt or ambivalent	2

Scoring: A positive answer to the presence of depression or hopelessness, lack of rational thought processes, an organized plan or serious suicide attempt, and affirmative or ambivalent statement regarding future intent to commit suicide are each scored 2 points. Each other positive answer is scored 1 point.

SCORE	RISK
<6	Low
6–8	Intermediate
>8	High

Modified from Hockberger RS, Rothstein RJ. Assessment of suicide potential by non-psychiatrists using the SAD PERSONS score. *J Emerg Med.* 1988;6(2):99–107. and Hockberger RS, Smith M. Depression and suicide ideation. In: Wolfson AB, ed. *Clinical Practice of Emergency Medicine.* 4th ed. Philadelphia: Lippincott Williams; 2005.

KEY POINTS: SERIOUS SUICIDE ATTEMPTS

1. Patient thought what they did to commit suicide was likely to kill them.
2. They did it in such a way as to have a low chance of being rescued.
3. They are not talking much about how they are feeling now.
4. They have little social support and are unwilling to accept help.
5. They still want to die.

---

25. **How do suicides among physicians and residents compare to the general population?**

    Nearly 300 physicians die every year as a result of suicide at almost twice the rate of the general population. Studies suggest that, among medical trainees, suicide is the leading cause of death among male residents and is the second leading cause of death among female residents. Medical residents in the earlier years of their training are particularly vulnerable, as most suicides occur during the first 2 years of training. Unfortunately, up to one-third of medical residents report experiencing depression at some point in their training. Beyond how these symptoms affect clinicians on a personal level, they affect the quality of care delivered to patients and are implicated in poorer patient outcomes.

    Websites

    Several excellent tools and resources are available to residents and residency programs aimed at promoting mental health and well-being.

    Crisis and Suicide Prevention
    - https://suicidepreventionlifeline.org
    - https://www.crisistextline.org

    Promoting Physician Wellness
    - https://www.acgme.org/What-We-Do/Initiatives/Physician-Well-Being/Resources/Additional-Resources
    - https://www.acgme.org/Portals/0/PDFs/CLER/CLER_Pathways_V1.1_Digital_Final.pdf
    - https://www.acep.org/how-we-serve/sections/wellness/wellness-resources/#sm.00000palak1ab3fsfxobn06wnu8tx
    - https://www.emra.org/books/emra-wellness-guide/cover/

    Preventing Physician Burnout
    - https://edhub.ama-assn.org/steps-forward/module/2702509
    - https://edhub.ama-assn.org/steps-forward/module/2702511
    - https://www.mededportal.org/publication/10508/
    - http://www.phqscreeners.com/sites/g/files/g10016261/f/201412/PHQ-9_English.pdf

    Coping With Physician Suicide
    - https://www.acgme.org/Portals/0/PDFs/13287_AFSP_After_Suicide_Clinician_Toolkit_Final_2.pdf
    - https://www.acgme.org/Portals/0/PDFs/Webinars/June_21st_Webinar.pdf

    ---

26. **Is there a chance that one of my fellow residents or colleagues might be contemplating suicide?**

    Yes. The psychologist Carl Jung coined the term "The Wounded Healer." Those of us who work in emergency medicine have the privilege of intervening in the lives of others, but we also share with them some of the most horrific trauma imaginable. It is critical to stay very aware of one's coworkers and not be afraid to intervene if you see them showing any of the warning signs described above.

27. **What is Posttraumatic Stress Disorder?**

    PTSD is an anxiety disorder that develops after witnessing or experiencing an event where there was serious threat of death or physical harm or sexual violation. It can be further categorized into simple or complex PTSD. Simple is when symptoms are the result of an isolated event or cluster of events such as combat experience. Complex PTSD refers to symptoms that occur in response to an ongoing trauma, such as the long-term physical abuse of a child.

28. **I know the DSM-V has a really long definition of PTSD, but what are the clinical features of PTSD that I need to know?**

    There are four clusters of symptoms that patients >6 years old require to be diagnosed with PTSD:
    - Reexperiencing the event: recurrent nightmares, thoughts, and memories of the event
    - Alterations in arousal: hypervigilance, anger, always being "on edge"
    - Avoidance: constant desire to avoid people, situations, and other triggers that remind the person of the trauma
    - Negative effects on cognition and mood: diminished interest in life, self-blame, negative beliefs about the world and one's self

29. **What kind of traumatic events can cause PTSD?**

PTSD may be caused by such events as exposure to war as a combatant or civilian, threatened or actual physical assault from sexual violence, torture, incarceration as a prisoner of war, and natural and manmade disasters. The exposure must be actual direct exposure (not indirect through media). The disorder is more severe and long lasting when the traumatic event is caused directly by other human beings or purposely inflicted pain (e.g., torture or sexual violence).

30. **What is meant by intrusive thoughts or events?**

One or more intrusive events may be associated with the original emotional trauma. Such events include memories, dreams, and flashbacks. There may be intense psychological or physiologic reactions to internal or external cues that symbolize the event.

31. **What kinds of avoidance behavior are noted?**

Stimuli associated with the trauma are avoided. This can include avoiding talking about the event and avoiding people or situations that are reminders.

32. **What are negative alterations in cognition and mood associated with PTSD?**

Such features can include memory loss, anger, guilt, loss of interest in previously enjoyed activities, feeling detached from others, or anhedonia.

33. **What kinds of alterations in arousal are noted?**

The patient may experience an intense startle response. Other alterations include irritability or insomnia. Patients may also engage in risky or aggressive behaviors.

34. **What is "trauma informed care?"**

Patients who suffer traumatic events may suffer from long-term mental and physical health effects, impacting the way patients interact with health care systems and their providers. The notion of *trauma informed care* (TIC) encompasses a conceptual and behavioral framework for providers to adopt when caring for patients who may be victims of trauma. The goal of TIC is to better serve this vulnerable patient population by providing exceptional and patient-centered care through establishing trust, rapport, and understanding. TIC emphasizes meaningful changes for providers to raise awareness, prevent retraumatization during patient care, and empowers patients when interacting with health care systems.

35. **Will my patients always check in with a complaint of PTSD?**

Not always. Some patients who are well aware of their condition may very well check in with the desire to have a mental health evaluation. Some patients, however, may present with a constellation of seemingly unrelated symptoms. Important questions in the social history include whether the patient has a history of being involved in the military, law enforcement, or if they have a history of significant psychological trauma.

36. **Will all of my patients be "patients?"**

When it comes to PTSD, some of your most affected "patients" may be your coworkers and emergency medical services (EMS) personnel. The incidence of PTSD is up to 40% in ambulance crews. Prehospital workers are frequently exposed to horrific scenes and interact with many patients who ultimately die during transport to the hospital. This repeated psychological stress, coupled with a cultural propensity in the EMS community to not share one's internal struggles, can lead to coworkers and prehospital providers going down a dark psychological pathway.

37. **I heard someone say that ketamine might actually be helpful for depression and PTSD. Was that just a joke?**

No. There have been multiple studies showing that low-dose intravenous ketamine can be an effective treatment for severe depression, PTSD, and various forms of chronic pain. There is also evidence to suggest that suicidal patients receiving ketamine in the ED may require significantly shorter inpatient psychiatric hospitalizations. This is a relatively new field of study but shows promise as a viable ED treatment.

BIBLIOGRAPHY

American Psychiatric Association. *Diagnostic and Statistical Manual of Mental Disorders.* 5th ed. (DSM-5). Washington, DC: American Psychiatric Association; 2013.

Bobo WV, Vande Voort JL, Croarkin PE, et al. Ketamine for treatment-resistant unipolar and bipolar major depression: critical review and implications for clinical practice. *Depress Anxiety.* 2016;33(8):698–710.

Centers for Disease Control and Prevention. Suicide rates rising across the U.S. Atlanta, Georgia. 2019. https://www.cdc.gov/media/releases/2018/p0607-suicide-prevention.html. Accessed January 4, 2019.

Cuijpers P, Reynolds CF III, Donker T, et al. Personalized treatment of adult depression: medication, psychotherapy, or both? A systematic review. *Depress Anxiety.* 2012;29(10):855–864. doi:10.1002/da.21985.

Haugen PT, Evces M, Weiss DS. Treating posttraumatic stress disorder in first responders: a systematic review. *Clin Psychol Rev.* 2012;32(5):370–380.

King CA, O'Mara RM, Hayward CN, et al. Adolescent suicide risk screening in the emergency department. *Acad Emerg Med.* 2009; 16(11):1234–1241.

Lewis-Schroeder NF, Kieran K, Murphy BL, et al. Conceptualization, assessment, and treatment of traumatic stress in first responders: a review of critical issues. *Harv Rev Psychiatry.* 2018;26(4):216–227.

Mitchell AJ, Vaze A, Rao S. Clinical diagnosis of depression in primary care: a meta-analysis. *Lancet.* 2009;374(9690):609–619. doi:10.1016/S0140-6736(09)60879-5.

Nock MK. Self-injury. *Annu Rev Clin Psychol.* 2010;6:339–363. doi:10.1146/annurev.clinpsy.121208.131258.

Raja S, Hasnain M, Hoersch M, et al. Trauma informed care in medicine: current knowledge and future research directions. *Fam Community Health.* 2015;38(3):216–226. doi:10.1097/FCH.0000000000000071.

Warden S, Spiwak R, Sareen J, et al. The SAD PERSONS scale for suicide risk assessment: a systematic review. *Arch Suicide Res.* 2014;18(4):313–326. doi:10.1080/13811118.2013.824829.

World Health Organization. Preventing suicide: a global imperative, Geneva, Switzerland, 2014, World Health Organization. www.who.int. Accessed January 4, 2019.

CHAPTER 98

MANAGEMENT OF THE VIOLENT PATIENT

Ashley Curry, MD and Scott Simpson, MD, MPH

KEY POINTS: PREVENTING VIOLENCE IN THE ED

1. Recognize and treat agitation early. Acute symptoms confer the highest risk for violence.
2. Attempt verbal de-escalation as an initial intervention for agitated patients.
3. Offer oral medication (consider benzodiazepines or antipsychotics) to aid in de-escalation.
4. Summon staff or security back-up to if concerned about your or the patient's safety.
5. If all the above is ineffective, use physical restraint with or without involuntary medication.

KEY POINTS: GUIDELINES FOR RESTRAINING A VIOLENT PATIENT

1. Ensure staff are adequately trained.
2. Whenever possible, have at least **five** staff present for a restraint episode.
3. Restrain all four limbs.
4. Check patient for injury and proper fitting of restraints.
5. Monitor continuously while in restraints per Joint Commission guidelines.
6. Remove restraints gradually and quickly if feasible to do so.

KEY POINTS: AGITATION IN PEDIATRIC PATIENTS

1. Try their home medication if they already take something for agitation.
2. Use low doses and monitor closely for side effects.
3. Beware of paradoxical reactions to anticholinergic and benzodiazepine medications.

1. **Is violence a problem in the emergency department (ED)?**
   Yes. The ED is often the first place of contact for patients who are agitated or feeling out of control and is one of the most common settings for workplace violence. Over 80% of emergency physicians are verbally threatened at work; almost half have been victims of a physical assault, and most have witnessed an assault. In nearly all cases, assaults and threats were by patients. Despite increase in security measures in hospitals, physicians perceive violence is increasing in hospital settings.

2. **What causes a patient to become violent?**
   Patients become violent for a variety of reasons. Most violence in the ED reflects agitation, a state of hyperactivity and restlessness that may be caused by a number of medical or psychiatric disorders, some of which are listed in Table 98.1. Less frequently, violence is intentionally perpetrated by patients in order to meet their needs or retaliate against providers. Risk factors for such instrumental violence include past violent acts, history of a psychiatric hold for danger to others, past aggressive behavior in the hospital, repeated visits for pain medication, and history of illicit drug use.

3. **What can hospitals do to decrease the risk of violence?**
   Hospitals can decrease the risk of violence by anticipating its occurrence and proactively developing appropriate safety protocols to address the risk of violence. Hospital grounds should be monitored by roving patrol or closed-circuit security cameras. Access to care areas should be controlled. Some hospitals opt to have patients and visitors enter through metal detectors to prevent entrance of weapons into the facility. For patients with a known history of violence, special precautions or care plans can alert staff to the risk of subsequent violent incidents.
   Key personnel should be trained in verbal de-escalation and know how to alert staff and summon additional assistance. Common systems for initiating an alert include use of a code word with other staff, dedicated telephone numbers, and panic alarms. Portable personal alarms allow staff to readily access help in managing violence. Lastly, hospital staff should be educated in the proper application of physical restraints.

Table 98.1 Common Medical Conditions That Manifest as Violent Behavior

Agitation From General Medical Condition
Closed head injury or intracranial hemorrhage
Infection causing encephalitis or meningitis
Encephalopathy (particularly from liver or renal failure)
Exposure to environmental toxins
Metabolic derangement (i.e., hypo/hypernatremia, hypoglycemia, etc.)
Hypoxia
Thyroid disease
Seizure (postictal)
Ingestion or overdose of medications

Agitation From Intoxication/Withdrawal
Alcohol
Recreational drugs (cocaine, MDMA, ketamine, bath salts, inhalants, methamphetamines, GHB)
Medications (opioids, benzodiazepines, barbiturates, baclofen)

Agitation From Psychiatric Disease
Psychotic disorders
Mania
Agitated/irritable depression
Anxiety disorders
Personality disorders

GHB, γ-hydroxybutyrate; *MDMA,* 3,4-methylenedioxymethamphetamine (ecstasy).

4. **How can clinicians preempt a violent episode?**
   - More than history or demography, a patient's risk of violence is most reflected by acute clinical symptoms such as hyperactivity and threatening behaviors. Impending violence is of particular concern among patients exhibiting intoxication, delirium, and challenge to authority.
   - Use of a standardized agitation scale, such as the Behavioural Activity Rating Scale or Richmond Agitation-Sedation Scale, helps staff identify incipient violence and feel safer in their work environment.
   - Offer appropriate anxiolytic medication as indicated, perhaps as prompted by a score on a standardized scale to maintain objectivity.
   - Be alert to any items (on the patient or in the room) that may be used as a weapon.
   - If a patient has a known history of violence, consider placing the patient in an area of the ED with higher monitoring or ready access to security.

5. **What is the initial approach a physician can take to control an agitated or violent patient?**
   Verbal de-escalation is most effective when there is one person designated to try to calm the patient. If there is already a key person in place working effectively to de-escalate the patient, defer to that person and do not intervene. The patient can become overwhelmed or more agitated if multiple people are talking or directing him/her.

   Verbal de-escalation techniques should be initiated as soon as possible. The American Association for Emergency Psychiatry has published guidelines around agitation, including use of verbal de-escalation and voluntary medications (Table 98.2). Use nonconfrontational body language (uncross arms), demonstrate empathy, and offer choices and basic comfort items (food, water, nicotine replacement) to help the patient feel more in control. The offer of oral medications can aid further in de-escalation. A free online video curriculum has demonstrated efficacy in teaching the core skills of verbal de-escalation (see Website box).

6. **What if verbal de-escalation doesn't work?**
   If verbal de-escalation and voluntary medications fail to help the patient regain control, more assertive safety measures may be necessary. As with any emergency event, a leader should be identified. The patient's room should be cleared of movable furniture and objects that might be used as a weapon. Security should be called. In many cases, the presence of security is enough to de-escalate the patient and encourage acceptance of medications. In settings where seclusion is an option, secluding the patient in a room without dangerous implements for a period of reduced stimulation may be effective. If the patient continues to be agitated, physical restraints and involuntarily administered medications may be necessary.

7. **What if the patient has a weapon?**
   - Do not attempt to disarm a patient.
   - Protect yourself, run away, and alert security.
   - If there is an active shooter, run away, hide, or as a last resort, defend yourself.

Table 98.2 De-escalating an Agitated/Violent Patient

10 DOMAINS OF DE-ESCALATION	TIPS
1. Respect personal space	Stay two arm lengths away from agitated patient
2. Do not be provocative	Watch body language, tone, and choice of words
3. Establish verbal contact	Only one person interacts with patient
4. Be concise	Keep wording simple
5. Identify wants and feelings	Ask patient what usually helps when he or she is feeling this way
6. Listen closely to what the patient is saying	Acknowledge that you are listening
7. Agree, or agree to disagree	Agree, when you can
8. Lay down the law and set clear limits	Clearly state unacceptable behaviors (e.g., "screaming is not OK, but crying is")
9. Offer choices and optimism	Offer a choice, but only if a choice is feasible (e.g., "Would you prefer haloperidol or risperidone?")
10. Debrief the patient and staff	It is often helpful to talk about tense situations after the fact

8. How do I restrain a patient?

The team should remain calm and organized when preparing for a restraint episode. Staff members who engage in physical restraint should be trained in the proper methods for placing hands on a patient and proper use of restraints. The number of staff members needed to place restraints varies, depending on a patient's size and physicality, but should ideally never be fewer than five: one person for each limb and one at the head of the patient to provide an ongoing explanation to the patient of what is happening and why. Restraints for violent patients are typically initiated by immobilizing the patient on a bed or gurney and securing all four limbs.

Two-point restraints may be appropriate for some patients with less severe agitation: for instance, a disoriented patient (due to delirium or dementia) who is pulling at intravenous (IV) lines and is not violent. Nonviolent restraints are typically in place only for the purpose of protecting the patient from pulling lines or monitoring equipment and should not be used in the case of violent patients.

The patient should never be restrained in the prone position due to risk of suffocation. Immediately after the restraint, the patient should be examined for any signs of injury and to ensure that restraints are applied appropriately. Restraints need to be snug, but not tight. Each person placing the restraint should check that one finger can move easily between the restraint and the patient's skin. Continue to offer medications orally if indicated. If medication is declined by the patient or unsafe to administer by mouth, proceed with intramuscular (IM) or IV medication.

9. How should restrained patients be monitored?

Patients who are physically restrained need to be continuously monitored by trained staff. Monitoring includes frequent vital sign checks, especially for patients who are sedated. Restraint of the patient does not mean that assessment of the patient stops. It may be necessary to continue to evaluate the patient to identify potential treatable causes of agitation or conditions that require immediate treatment. As a patient calms, the restraints should be reduced, and finally, discontinued.

10. Am I legally allowed to restrain someone?

Yes. Chemical or physical restraint is indicated when patients become imminently dangerous and less restrictive measures have failed. The following should be documented:

- The patient is a danger to themselves or others.
- Less restrictive measures were tried but were not helpful.
- The patient was educated as to why they were placed into restraints or given medication, and indications for removal of restraints.

Courts have routinely held that physicians may administer medications to patients without their consent if they would otherwise present an imminent risk of dangerous behavior. Different jurisdictions and health systems have different training, documentation requirements, and policies around coercive measures such as restraint. All physicians and staff should be familiar with local policies and expectations.

11. **What medications are recommended for emergency treatment of agitation? What doses should I order?**
    The three most common classes of drugs used to treat agitation are benzodiazepines, second-generation antipsychotics, and first-generation antipsychotics. The choice of agent depends on the underlying etiology of agitation. Fig. 98.1 illustrates guidelines for selecting and dosing an initial agent for agitation. In general, oral agents are preferred over IM/IV agents, and there is no difference in efficacy. Ketamine, a dissociative analgesic with an entirely different mechanism, has recently gained popularity in the ED and emergency medical services (EMS) settings for agitated delirium.
    - **Benzodiazepines** are useful in agitation, psychosis, alcohol withdrawal, benzodiazepine withdrawal, and are first-line treatment for some sympathomimetic toxidromes such as cocaine or amphetamine toxicity. Benzodiazepines may also be co-administered with high-potency typical antipsychotics to reduce the risk of dystonia.
    - **Second-generation (atypical) antipsychotics** have replaced first-generation antipsychotics as the antipsychotics of choice in many cases of agitation, particularly agitation due to psychosis or delirium not due to substances. Atypical agents are typically less sedating and have a favorable side-effect profile, with lower instances of extrapyramidal symptoms (EPS) than typical antipsychotics. The pharmacologic profiles of these agents vary: for example, olanzapine is highly sedating but carries a risk of hypotension, whereas ziprasidone is less sedating. When used for acute agitation, antipsychotics are helpful to achieve sedation and acute symptom control; full antipsychotic properties take days to weeks to realize.
    - **First-generation (typical) antipsychotics**, especially haloperidol and droperidol, remain useful in cases of agitation due to a central nervous system (CNS) depressant or as a second line for psychosis or delirium. When using a typical IM antipsychotic such as haloperidol, the clinician should prescribe another medication to protect the patient from EPS by coadministration of an anticholinergic agent (diphenhydramine 25–50 mg IM/IV, benztropine 1 mg IM/IV, or lorazepam 1–2 mg IM/IV).
    - **Ketamine** has become favored by many ED physicians for agitated patients, especially in the prehospital in patients with excited delirium. Ketamine is highly and quickly sedating at current dose recommendations of 4–6 mg/kg IM for agitated delirium. Ketamine is associated with side effects of oversedation, laryngospasm, and need for intubation, particularly when administered in patients who have received other sedatives (e.g., benzodiazepines).

12. **What are the main side effects of these drugs?**
    Benzodiazepines (high risk at high doses or when mixed with a CNS depressant)
    - Respiratory depression
    - Somnolence
    - Hypotension
    - Bradycardia

    Antipsychotics
    - Akathisia: inner feeling of restlessness that can drive agitation. For acute episodes, consider benzodiazepines.
    - Dystonic reactions: severe muscle spasm (e.g., torticollis) that can be treated with diphenhydramine or benztropine.
    - Neuroleptic malignant syndrome (NMS): a rare idiosyncratic reaction characterized by a triad of altered mentation, autonomic instability, and neuromuscular changes; NMS is potentially lethal and requires emergent care.
    - Anticholinergic effects: dry mouth, incontinence and, at high doses, delirium.
    - Hypotension: usually responsive to fluid boluses. Consider use of fall precautions.
    - Lowered seizure threshold: especially important if other medications or recreational drugs are involved.
    - Cardiac arrhythmias and QT prolongation: consider reviewing an electrocardiogram (ECG) if the patient has a cardiac history and hypokalemia, hypomagnesemia, or hypocalcemia, or is receiving IV haloperidol or droperidol.
    - Respiratory depression: use caution when administrating IM olanzapine in the presence of alcohol intoxication or IV/IM benzodiazepines.
    - Death: there is a black box warning on administering these medications for patients with dementia due to an increased risk of death. This warning generally applies to more chronic use, and most cases of death are due to cardiovascular or infectious causes. ED physicians should consider the risks and benefits of these agents and inform patients and family members of administration whenever possible.

    Ketamine
    - Dissociation and hallucinations
    - Hypersalivation
    - Vomiting
    - Oversedation
    - Respiratory depression
    - Hypertension or hypotension
    - Muscle spasms
    - Laryngospasm
    - Emergence reactions

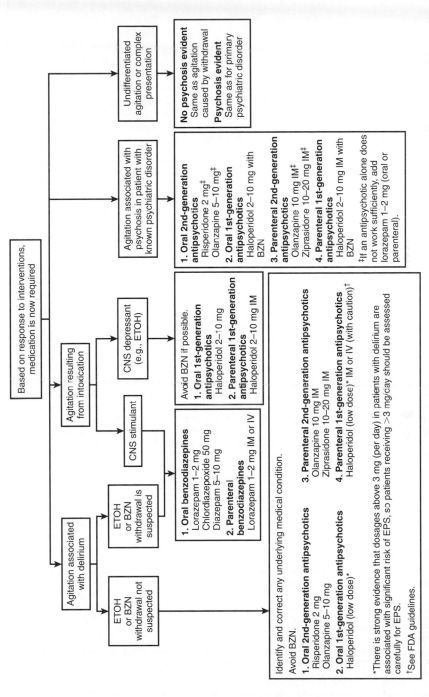

Fig. 98.1 Quick reference for dosing and administration of medications for agitation. *BZN,* Benzod azepine; *CNS,* central nervous system; *EPS,* extrapyramidal symptoms; *ETOH,* ethanol; *FDA,* US Food and Drug Administration; *IM,* intramuscularly; *IV,* intravenously. (From Wilson MP, Pepper D, Currier GW, et al. The psychopharmacology of agitation: consensus statement of the American Association for Emergency Psychiatry Project BETA Psychopharmacology Workgroup. *West J Emerg Med.* 2012;13:26–34. License: http://creativecommns.org/licenses/by-nc/4.0/.)

Table 98.3 Medications for Agitation in Pediatric Patients

MEDICATION	DOSING	WATCH FOR
Diphenhydramine	12.5–50 mg	Paradoxical worsening Sedation Avoid in delirium
Lorazepam	0.5–2 mg	Paradoxical worsening Respiratory depression Sedation
Risperidone Haloperidol Chlorpromazine Olanzapine Droperidol	0.25–1 mg (PO only) 0.5–5 mg PO (1/2 dose if IV) 12.5–50 mg PO (1/2 dose if IM) 2.5–10 mg PO (1/4 dose if IM) 1.25–5 mg IV/IM	Extrapyramidal side effects QT prolongation Sedation

IM, Intramuscular; *IV,* intravenous; *PO,* per os (by mouth).

13. **What about the pediatric patient?**
   As with adult patients, the first step to addressing an agitated child or adolescent is verbal de-escalation. Wherever possible, a child life specialist should be consulted to help calm a child, using developmental and age-appropriate techniques that are nonthreatening. In cases where medication is used, antihistamines, benzodiazepines, and antipsychotics are typically used. In some cases, an alpha-2 agonist (clonidine) is used. Use only antipsychotics that have been tested in multiple randomized controlled trials; overall, the evidence for selecting agents in this population is limited. Again, as with adults, consider the cause of agitation when selecting an agent. Patients who already have a medication prescribed for agitation should be offered a dose in the ED. Patients with attention deficit hyperactivity disorder (ADHD) and autism spectrum disorder are at heightened risk for paradoxical reactions to antihistamines and benzodiazepines, and all children are at greater risk of side effects to medications than adults. Table 98.3 describes options for dosing medications for agitation among pediatric patients.

14. **What should be done after a de-escalation or restraint episode?**
   After any incident of violence, de-escalation, or restraints, immediate debriefing among staff and with the patient is essential. When debriefing with staff, first assure that no one was physically injured in the event. More commonly, injury to staff is psychological rather than physical. Affected staff should be allowed to vent thoughts and feelings related to the event. Use the debriefing period as a time to provide feedback on what went well, and what should be done differently in the future. Connect staff who are injured (emotionally or physically) to appropriate resources to process the event, get appropriate care, and plan for future events and re-entry into the workforce.

> **Website**
> Video seminar on verbal de-escalation: https://youtu.be/musgq94q8GQ.

ACKNOWLEDGMENT

The editors thank Kimberly Nordstrom, MD, Danielle Raeburn, MD, Katherine M. Bakes, MD, and Douglas Ikelheimer, MD, for their contributions to this chapter in previous editions of this text.

BIBLIOGRAPHY

American College of Emergency Physicians. ACEP emergency department violence. September 2018. http://newsroom.acep.org/2009-01-04-emergency-department-violence-fat-sheet. Accessed January 21, 2019.

Behnam M, Tillotson RD, Davis SM, et al. Violence in the emergency department: a national survey of emergency medicine residents and attending physicians. *J Emerg Med.* 2011;40(5):565–579.

Claudius IA, Desai S, Davis E, et al. Case-controlled analysis of patient-based risk factors for assault in the healthcare workplace. *West J Emerg Med.* 2017;18(6):1153–1158.

Gerson R, Malas N, Mroczkowski MM. Crisis in the emergency department: the evaluation and management of acute agitation in children and adolescents. *Child Adolesc Psychiatr Clin N Am.* 2018;27(3):367–386.

Nordstrom K, Zun L, Wilson M, et al. Medical evaluation and triage of the agitated patient: consensus statement of the American Association for Emergency Psychiatry Project Beta Medical Evaluation Workgroup. *West J Emerg Med.* 2012;13(1):3–10.

Richmond JS, Berlin JS, Fishkind AB, et al. Verbal de-escalation of the agitated patient: consensus statement of the American Association for Emergency Psychiatry Project Beta De-escalation Workgroup. *West J Emerg Med.* 2012;13(1):17–25.

Riddell J, Tran A, Bengiamin R, et al. Ketamine as a first-line treatment for severely agitated emergency department patients. *Am J Emerg Med.* 2017;35(7):1000–1004.

Simpson SA, Rylander M. Verbal de-escalation of the agitated patient. May 2017. https://youtu.be/musgq94q8GQ. Accessed January 21, 2019.

Wilson MP, Pepper D, Currier GW, et al. The psychopharmacology of agitation: consensus statement of the American Association for Emergency Psychiatry Project Beta Psychopharmacology Workgroup. *West J Emerg Med.* 2012;13(1):26–34.

CHAPTER 99

INTIMATE PARTNER VIOLENCE

Kari Sampsel, MD, MSc, FRCPC, DipForSci

1. **Is intimate partner violence (IPV) more of a law enforcement issue than a health issue?**
   No, research shows that up to one half of women, and one in eight men, coming to the emergency department (ED) have experienced IPV within their lifetime. The ED is a common first access point for survivors seeking care. Survivors of IPV have higher rates of physical and mental health disorders.

2. **Define IPV**
   Domestic violence, in a broad sense, refers to all violence occurring within a family unit. By this definition, partner abuse, child abuse, and elder abuse are subsets of domestic violence. Violence includes physical actions, such as physical and sexual assault, and nonphysical actions, such as emotional abuse, economic abuse, threats to harm children or destroy property, and prevention of access to health or prenatal care. *IPV* is a more specific and currently accepted term. IPV includes all of the above forms of violence caused by a current or former intimate partner. Most violence survivors state that the nonphysical abuse is more humiliating and distressing to them than physical beatings, and are less likely to be reported to anyone.

3. **What are the risk factors for IPV?**
   IPV occurs in all socioeconomic classes and in all races. Women at greatest risk include those with male partners who abuse alcohol or use drugs; are unemployed; have mental health issues; have a history of pet abuse; or have less than a high school education. The greatest risk occurs when survivors are leaving or have recently left the relationship. Women who are younger than 30 years; who are single, divorced, or separated; have mental health issues; or who abuse drugs or alcohol classically have been viewed as being at increased risk for IPV. It is unclear, however, if some of these risk factors lead to the partner abuse or are a result of living in an abusive situation.

4. **Are men ever survivors of partner abuse?**
   Yes, men do experience partner violence, at a rate of approximately one in eight, including both male and female partners. These are less often physical abuse and more likely to be emotional or verbal abuse. Men may be embarrassed to disclose IPV or think that they will not be believed or worried that they may be the ones arrested if they ask for help. Male IPV is not as lethal compared to women.

5. **If IPV is so common, why have none of my patients experienced it?**
   Many of your patients likely have experienced IPV, but generous estimates find that only 20% of survivors seek help or voluntarily disclose this to their physician. Often, physicians do not know because they do not ask. Current evidence suggests survivors do not feel it is intrusive for their physician to ask about IPV; in fact, they welcome it.

6. **What is the result of a missed diagnosis of IPV?**
   Failure to diagnose IPV may increase the risk of future injury. The risk of homicide increases sixfold on an attempt to leave an abusive relationship. It also furthers the survivor's sense of entrapment and helplessness. Patients may experience a second victimization by being labeled as drug seeking, hysterical, paranoid, or irrational. Patients with multiple repeat visits for the same concern, or chronic conditions without obvious underlying pathology, should be questioned about IPV.

7. **State some of the reasons why physicians choose not to inquire about IPV.**
   The most commonly cited reason is lack of time. Health care providers believe that this issue is too complex and time consuming to deal with, especially in a busy ED. The second most common reason is that they do not know, or do not have the resources, to respond to a disclosure of IPV, and are afraid of making a mistake.

8. **Why are survivors of partner abuse reluctant to disclose the abuse to health care providers, even if asked?**
   Men and women may be embarrassed and humiliated about IPV. There may be cultural or religious beliefs that lead survivors to believe that this is normal or to be expected. They are also commonly told that they deserved the abuse. An abuser might have threatened to harm the survivor, their children, or other loved ones if they disclose to others, or they may believe that no one can help them. They also may be financially or otherwise dependent on the abusive partner.

9. **What are some of the structural and system barriers that might prevent disclosure?**
   Lack of privacy and security are concerns in the ED. Survivors should be interviewed alone, without children or partners present. If necessary, hospital security may be recruited to ensure their safety. Family members or children should not be used as translators when inquiring about abuse. Screening should be done on all patients at risk as part of their health history, with a plan or resources known to the health care provider to respond to a disclosure of IPV.

10. What clues to IPV might be evident in a patient's history?

Historical features suggestive of IPV are very similar to those found in child abuse. Most importantly, a history that is inconsistent with the physical examination findings, delays in seeking care, a changing story over time, or multiple injuries at various stages of healing should raise physician suspicion for IPV. Partner abuse should also be considered in patients with suicidal intentions or attempts, patients who are depressed, patients who have evidence of drug and alcohol abuse, and patients with frequent visits for chronic pain or somatic complaints.

11. What clues may be present on physical examination in a survivor of IPV?

These also overlap heavily with physical signs of child abuse. Common injury patterns include injuries to the face, neck, and throat (especially signs or symptoms of strangulation), ribs, flanks, or buttocks, and defensive wounds to the hands, arms, or back.

KEY POINTS: PHYSICAL EXAMINATION FINDINGS IN IPV

1. Injuries to head, face, and neck (evidence of strangulation)
2. Defensive injuries (hands, arms, and back)
3. Any injury that does not fit with the history
4. Evidence of sexual assault, or frequent, recurrent sexually transmitted infections
5. Injuries in multiple stages of healing

12. How can I increase my recognition of partner abuse?

First, ask about IPV. Any person with an injury should be specifically asked about the circumstances of the injury. Second, raise your level of suspicion in those without injuries, such as mental health, repeat visits, or chronic pain. Remember the clues that might be present in the history or physical examination. If you are considering partner abuse, ask about it.

13. What questions about partner violence can I ask someone without injuries?

- Have you ever been hurt or injured by a partner or ex-partner?
- Are there situations in your relationship where you have felt afraid?
- Has your partner ever hurt you or your children?
- Do you feel safe in your current relationship?
- Do you feel safe at home?
- Is there a partner from a past relationship who is making you feel unsafe now?

14. What about screening all women for IPV? What about screening everyone?

Many medical societies, including the Institute of Medicine, have recommended screening and counseling for interpersonal and domestic violence as part of preventive care. One screening tool is the Partner Violence Screen. This consists of these three questions:

1. Have you been hurt or injured in the past year by anyone? If so, by whom?
2. Do you feel safe in your current relationship?
3. Is there a partner from a previous relationship who is making you feel unsafe now?

This tool is 71% sensitive for detecting IPV. Women who screen positive for IPV are 11 times more likely to experience physical violence in the next 4 months than women who screen negative for IPV. These studies have been done specifically in an adult female population; no evidence currently exists for screening all patients. However, it is important to consider that IPV can occur for anyone, and there are real barriers to disclosure for the adolescent, male, and lesbian, gay, bisexual, transgender, queer, and intersex (LGBTQI+) population.

15. What comments or questions are not recommended when discussing IPV?

- What did you do to them?
- What did you do to deserve this?
- What did you do that made them so mad?
- This has happened before, and you are still with your partner?
- Why didn't you tell anyone?
- You let them do that to you?
- I wouldn't let anyone do that to me.
- Why don't you just leave?

16. What do I do if my patient has an injury caused by their partner?

- Treat their injuries as you would any other traumatic injury.
- Document their history and injuries carefully in the medical records.
- Provide support and empathy; they should be informed that IPV is a common problem, that no one deserves this abuse, and that help is available. Helping survivors access community resources should be a primary goal of ED treatment.

- Inquire about the person's safety and that of their children. Not all survivors want or require shelter placement. Survivors who are experiencing increasingly severe physical injuries or whose abusers have access to firearms are at high risk for severe or lethal injuries. Some of these interventions may be by a social worker or by a domestic violence care program, depending on the clinical setting. To find such a program in your region, consult: https://www.forensicnurses.org/search/custom.asp?id=2100.

17. **Summarize some important points to remember when documenting IPV.**
Document what happened in the patient's own words, including the relationship to the abuser. Record all areas of injuries, bruising, or tenderness; a body map may be helpful. Photographs should only be taken by someone who is trained to follow local legal guidelines for forensic photography; however, it is reasonable to upload images in the medical record to assist in medical documentation of injury. Any treatment and intervention should be documented. In cases in which abuse is highly suspected and the patient is denying abuse, document the reason that you suspect abuse (e.g., the history does not match the physical examination findings).

18. **Do I have any legal responsibilities?**
This varies based on your jurisdiction. In the United States, 45 states have a law that mandates reporting intentionally inflicted injuries; however, these laws vary greatly as to what injuries must be reported. This is not the case in many places internationally, including Canada. Each emergency physician must be familiar with the current reporting requirements in his or her state. The most current review of laws can be found at: www.acf.hhs.gov/sites/default/files/fysb/state_compendium.pdf.

KEY POINTS: WHAT TO DO WITH AN IPV SURVIVOR

1. Treat the injuries as you would any other traumatic injury.
2. Document the history and injuries carefully. (Consider drawing a picture.)
3. Provide support and empathy.
4. Inquire about the patient's safety and that of their children.
5. Refer to community resources or social worker.
6. Notify law enforcement if required in your jurisdiction.

19. **Why are they going home to their abuser, and why don't they just leave?**
Why a survivor does not leave the abusive partner is the wrong question to ask. It implies that the survivor is to blame and that if they would just leave, everything would be okay. IPV survivors are most likely to be killed during the act of leaving, or after they have left their abuser. There are many other valid reasons why people stay in an abusive situation.
They may:
- have no money or job skills;
- have nowhere else to go;
- feel they must stay to protect their children.

20. **What can we do about IPV?**
A more appropriate response to IPV is to ask ourselves how we, as health care providers, might change negative attitudes towards IPV. This begins with health care providers' willingness to ask patients questions and be involved in meeting their needs at that encounter.

ACKNOWLEDGMENT

Debra E. Houry, MD, MPH and Kim M. Feldhaus, MD, were authors on previous editions and developed the initial version.

BIBLIOGRAPHY

Houry D, Kaslow NJ, Kemball RS, et al. Does screening in the emergency department hurt or help victims of intimate partner violence? *Ann Emerg Med.* 2008;51(4):433–442.
Houry D, Rhodes KV, Kemball RS, et al. Differences in female and male victims and perpetrators of partner violence with respect to WEB scores. *J Interpers Violence.* 2008;23(8):1041–1055.
Mathew A, Smith LS, Marsh B, et al. Relationship of intimate partner violence to health status, chronic disease, and screening behaviors. *J Interpers Violence.* 2013;28(12):2581–2592.
Stockl H, Devries K, Rotstein A, et al. The global prevalence of intimate partner homicide: a systematic review. *Lancet.* 2013;382 (9895):859–865.
Tjaden P, Thoennes N. Prevalence and consequences of male-to-female and female-to-male intimate partner violence as measured by the National Violence Against Women Survey. *Violence Against Women.* 2000;6(2):142–161.
Wu V, Huff H, Bhandari M. Pattern of physical injury associated with intimate partner violence in women presenting to the emergency department. *Trauma Violence Abuse.* 2010;11(2):71–82.

EMS MEDICAL OVERSIGHT

Whitney Barrett, MD and Lara D. Rappaport, MD, MPH

CHAPTER 100

KEY POINTS: PHYSICIAN MEDICAL OVERSIGHT OF EMS SYSTEMS

1. EMS physician medical oversight requires ongoing continuing education and quality assurance.
2. EMS physician medical oversight can be direct or indirect.
3. Emergency medical services (EMS) have proven benefit for treatment of cardiac arrest, respiratory distress, and traumatic injury.

1. What is EMS physician medical oversight?

EMS physician medical oversight is defined as the physician supervision of a service, group, or system providing emergency medical services (EMS) care. It provides the means by which physicians give direction and authority to EMS providers to provide emergency medical care outside of the hospital and without a physician being present to ensure that the care provided to ill or injured patients by EMS personnel is appropriate. EMS providers are not independent medical practitioners and therefore must function under the supervision of a licensed physician medical director. The first standardized EMS curriculum was established in 1976 and increased requirements for physician involvement and training of medics.

2. Why is EMS physician medical oversight of prehospital personnel and care important?

EMS physician medical oversight is critical to ensure that medics with appropriate education and training can provide medical care in the out-of-hospital setting safely and effectively. Their safety and effectiveness are a direct reflection of the quality of EMS physician medical oversight and the relationship between providers and the medical director.

3. How is EMS physician medical oversight provided?

There are two types of EMS physician medical oversight, direct and indirect. Direct EMS physician medical oversight is provided at the time prehospital providers are rendering patient care, in-person, by radio, or by telephone contact. Indirect physician medical direction occurs via pre-established protocols and standing orders for common or critical patient presentations. In order to function well, indirect medical direction relies on continuing education of personnel and quality assurance to maintain knowledge of, and ensure appropriate application of, established standards.

4. What type of role is the EMS medical director?

EMS medical directors perform administrative tasks and determine educational priorities. Ultimately responsible for ensuring the provision of clinically sound prehospital medicine, the EMS medical director must first and foremost function as a physician. EMS agency directors or supervisors (usually paramedics themselves) work in conjunction with the medical director on budget, human resources, and administrative policies.

5. Who are the key stakeholders in an EMS system?

The primary stakeholders of an EMS system are the patients. Similar to public health physicians, the EMS medical director has a responsibility to the population as a whole, and must weigh the impact of clinical care decisions for individual patients, as well as those who will next call for care. The other stakeholders in an EMS system are the government and third-party payers, who represent the population and fund components of the system; the hospitals and health care systems; the response agencies; and the personnel who provide EMS response.

6. In what conditions has EMS been demonstrated to have proven benefit?

Prehospital care has demonstrated benefit in multiple broad categories of time-sensitive conditions – cardiac, neurologic, trauma, and respiratory care. EMS is the key determinant in survival from out-of-hospital cardiac arrest, with the most important EMS interventions being defibrillation and high-quality cardiopulmonary resuscitation (CPR) (with minimally interrupted compressions and minimizing perishock pause). Early recognition of patients with ST-elevation myocardial infarction (STEMI) and transportation to appropriate facilities decreases time to definitive intervention. The same is true for acute neurologic problems such as stroke. EMS minimizes death and disability from trauma by rapidly transporting seriously injured patients to trauma centers. Quality EMS care also stabilizes many respiratory issues by providing basic airway management, bronchodilators to patients with reactive airway disease, or noninvasive continuous positive pressure ventilation (CPAP) to patients with chronic obstructive pulmonary disease (COPD) exacerbation or pulmonary edema.

7. **In what other, difficult-to-study ways might EMS be beneficial?**

Some EMS practices are difficult to be studied in a randomized controlled trial, yet are likely to benefit patients. For example, the provision of intravenous (IV) dextrose to the altered hypoglycemic patient is clearly of benefit but rarely studied. Other considerations include providing analgesia to patients in pain, assessing and pronouncing death in the out-of-hospital setting, or recognizing nonaccidental trauma. The prehospital provider performs a key role in gathering data from the scene of the call that often will have a significant influence on the emergency department and hospital course and sometimes in the judicial system.

8. **What are some key controversies in current EMS practice?**

- *The ideal approach to prehospital airway management* remains a major question. In cardiac arrest, it is unclear if passive oxygenation, bag-valve-mask (BVM) ventilation, supraglottic airways, or endotracheal intubation confer a survival advantage. Prehospital endotracheal intubation for trauma or severe respiratory distress has both supporters and detractors. For pediatric patients, most systems recommend BVM or supraglottic airways over prehospital endotracheal intubation. When endotracheal intubation is performed, a growing body of literature supports video laryngoscopy as the preferred technique.
- *The use of long back boards for spinal immobilization* has long been a standard of care in EMS, despite evidence of harm. Alternatives include the use of scoop stretchers, vacuum mattresses, or placement directly on the gurney. In 2013, the National Association of EMS Physicians (NAEMSP) issued a position statement recommending their use only in a small subset of patients. The benefit of cervical collars is also still a question.
- *The use of prehospital epinephrine for adult cardiac arrest* has come into question. At this juncture, there is insufficient evidence to eliminate epinephrine from prehospital protocols, although several studies are trying to address this.
- *The judicious and safe use of lights and sirens* is a topic that has been well-researched recently, with the manner in which EMS providers respond and transport impacting safety of EMS providers, their patients, and the public.

9. **What are the common performance benchmarks of an EMS system?**

There are system-based and patient-focused benchmarks. At a minimum, modern EMS systems should be able to demonstrate timeliness of response to emergent calls and intervention to patients with cardiac arrest, acute coronary syndrome, respiratory distress, and major trauma. Other areas of benchmarking include seizure treatment, stroke management, and treatment of pain.

Patient-centered outcome measures (e.g., neurologically intact survival from cardiac arrest) should be the highest priority. Alternatives include measurement of processes proven to improve outcomes (e.g., minimizing perishock CPR pause, or application of noninvasive CPAP for COPD exacerbation). EMS Compass is a program developed through the National Highway Traffic Safety Administration's (NHTSA's) Office of EMS (http://www.NEMSQA.org) that works to standardize measures and provide resources for EMS quality management and performance improvement programs.

10. **Who are the members of the EMS workforce?**

Prehospital medicine in the United States is practiced by emergency medical responders (EMRs), emergency medical technicians (EMTs), advanced EMTs (AEMTs), and paramedics. Nurses, nurse practitioners, physician assistants, and physicians also provide prehospital care, particularly in aeromedical programs and specialized interfacility transport.

11. **What skills can be performed by prehospital providers at different levels of training?**

EMRs have the least amount of training and may perform basic airway management, including oropharyngeal airways; manually stabilize the cervical spine or extremity fractures; control bleeding; administer a narcotic antagonist (using a unit-dose, premeasured, intranasal or autoinjector device), and apply and use an automated external defibrillator (AED). In addition to the EMR skills, EMTs may place patients on CPAP, assist patients in taking their own prescribed medications, monitor blood glucose, and are trained in the extrication and transportation of patients. Advanced EMTs are permitted to insert supraglottic airways, establish IV access, and provide several key oral, subcutaneous, intramuscular, and IV medications. Paramedics may perform endotracheal intubation and cricothyrotomy, decompress the pleural space, interpret electrocardiograms (ECGs), and provide cardioversion, manual defibrillation, and transcutaneous pacing. Additionally, they have an expanded spectrum of medications they can administer.

Nurses who work in the prehospital setting are primarily involved in critical care and aeromedical transport. Nurse practitioners and physician assistants are relatively rare in the prehospital setting, but perform tasks commensurate with their training in a mobile capacity. Physicians who directly provide routine care in the prehospital setting are usually involved with critical care transports.

12. **How important is physician involvement in education and training for prehospital personnel?**

Physician involvement in the development of educational programs and the delivery of training provides an opportunity to directly interact with and provide guidance to EMS personnel. Having personal knowledge of the skill level of the prehospital providers develops a level of trust in their ability to assess and respond appropriately to most situations they encounter.

13. **What are the different models of EMS systems?**

EMS systems are commonly based with a fire department, third service (separate from police or fire), private entity, or hospital. In the United States, fire department–based systems are most common. In contrast, in many European countries, ambulances are staffed by physicians. Globally, physician extenders staff many ambulances.

14. **What are the strengths and weaknesses of fire department–based EMS?**

Fire department–based systems have the advantage of readiness, the potential to have employees trained both as firefighters and EMS personnel, high job satisfaction, and low attrition. The disadvantages include the cost, fixed location of fire stations, and competing responsibilities of fire suppression and hazardous materials response versus medical care.

15. **What are the strengths and weaknesses of third-service EMS?**

Third-service systems (public safety services separate from fire and police) have the advantage of being able to focus exclusively on EMS in hiring, training, and staffing. Because EMS agencies can bill for their services, they can be more financially self-sufficient than fire department–based agencies. The potential disadvantages include the need to integrate response with other public safety agencies, and the potential for duplication of responses.

16. **What are the strengths and weaknesses of private sector EMS?**

Private sector EMS agencies, similar to third-service agencies, have the advantage of being able to focus exclusively on EMS. In addition, they may be free of municipal hiring restrictions and can bring the benefit of expertise from serving multiple different communities. However, private EMS agencies also have a fiduciary duty to shareholders. This responsibility can make recruitment and retention of EMS personnel more challenging.

17. **What are the strengths and weaknesses of hospital-based EMS?**

Hospital-based systems can bring the resources of a large health care organization to EMS. This can include expertise in quality improvement, purchasing and supply of medications and equipment which can be linked with the hospital, and the ability to follow a patient's care through a system with information technology. However, being tied to a single hospital system can result in a perceived or actual conflict of interest in destination choices, and hospital-based systems can face challenges in integration with other public safety agencies.

18. **What does Pit Crew or High Fidelity CPR consist of?**

This bundle of care model has been shown to improve survival and neurologic outcome:
- Assign clear roles for each rescuer
- Allow minimal compression interruptions
  - Pre-charge the defibrillator while chest compressions continue
  - Count down until shock delivery
  - Have the compressor "hover" over the chest and then immediately resume compressions after the shock
- Use of a metronome or visual feedback for rate and depth of compressions
- Closely monitor respiratory rate to eliminate hyperventilation

BIBLIOGRAPHY

Bass RR, Lawner B, Lee D, et al. Medical oversight of EMS systems. In: Cone DC, ed. *Emergency Medical Services. Clinical Practice and System Oversight*. Vol. 2. Chichester, West Sussex, United Kingdom: John Wiley and Sons; 2015:71–84.

Establishing quality measures for patient care. *EMS Compass*. Available at https://nasemso.org/projects/ems-compass/. Accessed February 15, 2019.

Hopkins CL, Burk C, Moser S, et al. Implementation of pit crew approach and cardiopulmonary resuscitation metrics for out-of-hospital cardiac arrest improves patient survival and neurological outcome. *J Am Heart Assoc*. 2016;5(1):e002892.

Mal S, McLeod S, Iansavichene A, et al. Effect of out-of-hospital noninvasive positive-pressure support ventilation in adult patients with severe respiratory distress: a systematic review and meta-analysis. *Ann Emerg Med*. 2013;63(5):600–601.

Murray B, Kue R. The use of emergency lights and sirens by ambulances and their effect on patient outcomes and public safety: a comprehensive review of the literature. *Prehosp Disaster Med*. 2017;32(2):209–216.

National Highway Traffic Safety Administration. National EMS scope of practice model (prepublication copy) 2018. https://nasemso.org/wp-content/uploads/Prepublication-Display-Copy-2018-National-EMS-Scope-of-Practice-Model-20180929.pdf. Accessed February 15, 2019.

Perkins GD, Ji C, Deikin CD, et al. A randomized trial of epinephrine in out-of-hospital cardiac arrest. *N Engl J Med*. 2018;379(8):711–721.

CHAPTER 101

DISASTER MANAGEMENT

Christopher B. Colwell, MD

1. Define the term disaster.

A disaster is any situation that disrupts normal community function, overwhelms the community's ability to respond to the situation, and threatens the safety or health of the citizens. Simply stated, a disaster is an event where the needs overwhelm the available resources. It is not defined by the size or nature of the event, but rather by the community's ability to respond to it. A car accident with four victims might be enough to overwhelm the available resources in some communities, while in others it may represent a regular occurrence that is easily managed with available resources. Some rural areas may have only one ambulance, a very small number of prehospital personnel with advanced skills, and no local hospital. This could necessitate that emergency medical services (EMS) personnel leave their jurisdiction to transport critically ill patients, thus stripping the community of all EMS resources for ongoing needs.

Disaster: Needs > Resources

2. What is the difference between a mass casualty incident (MCI) and a disaster?

An MCI is an incident that produces a large number of casualties, which generally leads to a medical disaster where patient need exceeds locally available resources. A disaster may imbalance the community's ability to ensure safety of its citizens and may cripple the infrastructure of an area.

3. Are all disasters MCIs?

No, not all disasters are MCIs. For instance, a flood can cause significant damage to homes, communication lines, access to food and other services for a community, and displace many from their homes, but it may not cause a significant number of casualties and thus may not be a true MCI. Disasters may be natural (floods, tsunamis, earthquakes, tornadoes), man-made (plane crash, train crash, industrial explosions, fires, chemical spills, radiation leaks), and terrorist-related (biologic, chemical, explosive, radiologic, or nuclear events).

4. How is an MCI different from a mass gathering?

A mass gathering has been defined as an event of more than 1000 people (although it is sometimes defined as more than 25,000 people) gathered at a specific location, for a specific period of time, and for a specific purpose. Importantly, this creates a situation that may result in a delayed public safety response to medical emergencies by limiting access to patients as a result of the environment, the location, or mere crowd dynamics. Unlike an MCI, which is typically unanticipated and potentially catastrophic (such as the New York Twin Towers collapse of September 11, 2001), the medical response for a mass gathering can be planned, coordinated, and executed to offset a potentially disastrous scenario. However, a mass gathering may become an MCI if circumstances threaten the health and safety of the event patrons (e.g., unusually hot climate and inadequate access to water, causing hundreds of people to suffer from heat-related illnesses).

5. Why is there a need for disaster planning?

The quality of medical care is directly tied to the preparedness and experience of the practitioner, and proficiency of a given medical intervention depends on the frequency of its performance. In a disaster, people are trying to quickly perform what they might not ordinarily do, often in an unfamiliar environment. Therefore it makes sense to regularly plan and exercise the contingencies. No matter how experienced someone is, the level of care, resources, and framework for resource management undergo major alterations during a disaster. The goal of disaster planning is to provide the greatest amount of good for the greatest number of people.

6. Define the all-hazards approach to disaster planning.

To have the right contingencies in place, it is essential to know the potential hazards and threats in a given area. In an all-hazards approach, a review called a *hazard vulnerability analysis,* usually done annually, identifies potential disaster etiologies and sites that could happen in a community, such as a chemical plant explosion, a train crash, or an earthquake. Each event is ranked by likelihood and then by the extent of impact it would have on the ability to provide patient care. Based on this ranking, an agency, hospital, or community can begin to develop emergency plans to deal with the most likely events to ensure that lines of authority are established, appropriate communications occur, and all involved parties understand their roles and responsibilities. A disaster plan ideally should also implement response activities that are as close as possible to normal daily operations.

7. **What are the four phases of a disaster response?**
   1. Activation: initial notification of the incident, establishment of an incident command structure, and response to the incident with attention to scene safety for first responders.
   2. Implementation (response): search and rescue of victims, triage, and initial stabilization and transport of patients.
   3. Mitigation: hazards controlled, treatment provided to patients.
   4. Recovery: responders return to normal operations, restock supplies, and debrief from the event. Displaced persons are sheltered in temporary areas until they can return to their homes.

8. **What is an incident command system (ICS) and what are the benefits of using one?**
   An ICS is a standardized structure that provides command and control of personnel and resources at a disaster or multiagency scene. There are five key functions accomplished through an ICS:
   1. Incident command
   2. Planning
   3. Operations
   4. Logistics and supply
   5. Finance
        Benefits include clarifying chain of command and supervision responsibilities to improve accountability; leveraging interoperable communications systems and plain language to improve communications; providing an orderly, systematic planning process; and fostering cooperation between diverse disciplines and agencies.

9. **What is the National Incident Management System (NIMS)?**
   NIMS, developed by the Department of Homeland Security, standardizes the ICS structure to be used by EMS agencies, fire departments, law enforcement, and hospitals in an effort to enhance response coordination at all levels and for all types of incidents. It is a comprehensive, national approach to incident management that is applicable to all jurisdictional levels and across functional disciplines. It is intended to:
   - be applicable across a full spectrum of potential incidents, hazards, and impacts, regardless of size, location or complexity;
   - improve coordination and cooperation between public and private entities in a variety of incident management activities;
   - provide a common standard for overall incident management.

10. **Does an ICS have to be used for every incident?**
    The ICS is not required for every incident, and some small incidents may be reasonably managed by only one person who performs several functions. However, for large-scale incidents involving multiple local, regional, and, perhaps, even federal agencies, NIMS mandates the use of a formal ICS (Fig. 101.1).

11. **Describe each of the five key functions in an ICS?**
    1. Incident command: conducts and oversees the overall management of the incident response
    2. Planning: determines what is needed to manage the incident
    3. Logistics: obtains and supplies what is needed to manage the incident
    4. Operations: uses what is needed to manage the incident
    5. Finance: pays for it all

12. **What is the weakest link in a response to an incident?**
    The weakest link is nearly always communication. This occurs both in the field and at the hospital, and may be the result of different radio frequencies, overwhelmed cell phone towers, or simply unclear hierarchy and uncertain disaster plans.
        In addition to internal communication of responders, a public information officer should be assigned to communicate with local media, which can inform the community about potential hazards, evacuation routes, and shelters and food access. Reviews of major events that have occurred have consistently identified communication as an area that represents opportunities for improvement.

13. **How does triage occur at a scene?**
    Triage is a French word that means *to sort*. It is the process of assigning degrees of urgency to wounds or illnesses to decide the order of treatment of a large number of patients or casualties. Napoleon's surgeon

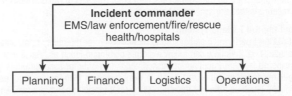

Fig. 101.1 Incident command system (ICS) structure. *EMS,* Emergency medical services.

Dominique Jean Larrey is thought to be the first physician to use triage on a battlefield in the early 1800s to sort out soldiers who could be treated in a nearby hospital and returned to duty. In an MCI, field triage is expanded from solely evaluating an individual patient, to assessing priorities and identifying the sickest patients that should be transported and treated first. Although several systems exist for triaging victims of multicasualty incidents, the basic concept generally identifies four groups of patients:

1. Red (immediate): critical or immediately life-threatening illness or injury (e.g., tension pneumothorax, hypovolemic shock) that have a reasonable chance of survival if treated
2. Yellow (delayed): serious but not immediately life-threatening illness or injury (e.g., most types of fractures)
3. Green (minor): "walking wounded" (e.g., sprains, anxiety attack after witnessing event)
4. Black (dead/dying, or expectant): dead or resource-intensive victims (e.g., 100% total body surface area burn)
   Triage tags or colored tape are used to clearly indicate the categories of patients to assist in rapid reiterative on-scene assessments.

14. How is triage applied in a disaster situation?

It should be assumed that the situation will overwhelm the available resources until there is clear information to the contrary. Therefore, triage will need to occur before definitive treatment or transport until the scene has been assessed and all victims have been identified. In these incidents, the basic philosophy is that the good of the many takes precedence over the good of the few. Ordinarily, we will apply all available resources to the few that need them the most, only turning our attention to others when the sickest have been stabilized. Such an approach assumes resources that may not be available in a disaster situation. Patients falling into the black triage category will not receive the same aggressive treatment they might under other circumstances in order to apply the limited resources to those most likely to benefit from them.

15. Are there any exceptions to this rule of prioritizing patients in the red category over those in the black category?

Yes, in lightning and possibly electrical injuries, where a group of people have been affected, priority will go to those in cardiac arrest because this represents the one situation where a single intervention may immediately change that patient's outcome. Those that are not in cardiac arrest from a lightning strike are generally not in need of immediate medical attention.

16. What triage system is most commonly used in the United States?

Currently, the most common triage system used in the United States is START (simple triage and rapid treatment), which has been widely adopted and is used by organizations such as the Domestic Preparedness branch of the United States Department of Defense. SALT (sort, assess, life-saving interventions, and treat/transport) is similar to the START system but is more comprehensive and adds life-saving techniques to be done during the triage phase. Numerous other triage systems exist, such as JumpSTART for pediatrics, MASS (move, assess, sort, send) triage, Fire Department of New York (FDNY) modified START triage, and the Sacco Triage Method (STM). There is ongoing research to determine which system is the most accurate. Variables such as age (very young or very old), comorbidities, and type of incident (e.g., chemical exposure) may influence the accuracy of currently accepted triage methods.

17. Tell me more about START.

START, developed by the Newport Beach, California Fire Department and Hoag Hospital in 1983 and revised in 1994, is designed to triage a patient in less than 30 seconds. First, those able to ambulate are immediately classified as *walking wounded* and sorted to a separate area (green). Priority is then given to the remaining victims on the ground. The triage officer assesses for breathing and spontaneous respirations. If breathing or circulation is abnormal and the patient is alive (has a pulse), a basic airway maneuver is attempted, such as a jaw thrust or the insertion of an oropharyngeal airway (OPA), and the patient is categorized as *red;* if the patient is not breathing and has no pulse, he or she is triaged into the black category. Assuming normal respirations, perfusion is assessed by radial pulse and capillary refill time (if absent radial pulse and capillary refill >2 seconds, patient is triaged as *red*). Finally, mental status is assessed by the patient's ability to follow commands (if no, triaged to red, and if yes, triaged to yellow). An easy mnemonic used to remember this approach is *RPM: 30, 2, can do,* where *RPM* denotes respirations, perfusion, and mental status, and *30, 2, can do* indicates respiratory rate less than 30, capillary refill less than 2 seconds, and ability to follow commands (Fig. 101.2). Red patients are prioritized first for transport, followed by the yellow patients. Green patients may not actually need an evaluation at the hospital, or may be able to be transported en masse (i.e., a school bus). This sort of rapid assessment allows for maximum use of the limited resources that are available at a disaster scene.

18. Tell me more about the SALT triage system.

Similar to START, SALT first performs a global sorting by assessing for the ability to ambulate. Those who can walk are assessed last. Next, if victims can follow a simple command (such as "Raise your hand if you can hear me"), they are considered less emergent and assessed second. Priority for assessment is given to those not responding, who are then triaged as either *red, black,* or *gray,* based on their injuries and response to immediate life-saving interventions (such as a needle decompression for a tension pneumothorax). An important distinction between the two systems is that SALT triage incorporates a gray color designation for patients who are deemed

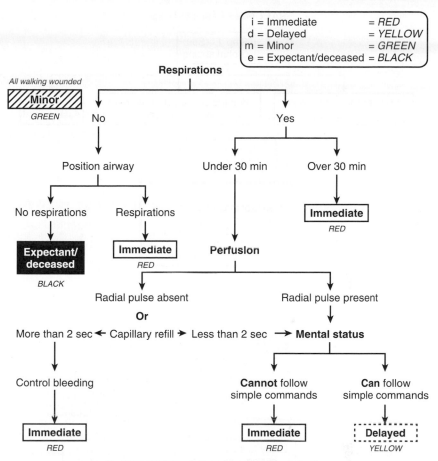

i = Immediate = *RED*
d = Delayed = *YELLOW*
m = Minor = *GREEN*
e = Expectant/deceased = *BLACK*

Fig. 101.2 START (simple triage and rapid treatment) algorithm.

expectant, meaning those who have little likelihood to survive their injuries, even with adequate resources. This also allows for palliative interventions for these patients, so they are not simply left to die (Fig. 101.3).

19. Which one is better, START or SALT?
Studies comparing the START and SALT triage systems have found START easier to learn and use in a real disaster scenario. Some studies have found SALT to be more accurate at classifying patients in the delayed and immediate categories. Notably, both are prone to overtriaging patients (identifying victims as more sick than they really are), which can detrimentally divert limited resources to people who do not truly need them.

20. How does transport occur for victims in an MCI?
On scene, it is important to have open access to ingress and egress routes, so ambulances can quickly and easily transport patients. A coordinated transport plan is essential to prevent the nearest hospital from quickly becoming overwhelmed and turn into the next disaster scene. To distribute patients appropriately and prevent overwhelming any single facility, it is important to ascertain local hospital capabilities (e.g., how many patients they can accommodate, whether they are a trauma center). Red category patients in need of immediate care should be given priority for transport, and ideally sent to a trauma center. Patients with minor injuries or nontraumatic complaints can initially be sent to nontrauma centers. Managing resources may call for acting "outside the box," transporting a patient that might otherwise go to a higher-level trauma center to a lower level or nontrauma center for more basic management.

21. When do patients need to be transported to the hospital emergently (i.e., lights and sirens [L&S])?
The use of warning L&S predates modern EMS systems as a means of improving response to and return from an accident scene. When transporting a patient to a hospital with L&S, there is a well-recognized increased risk of

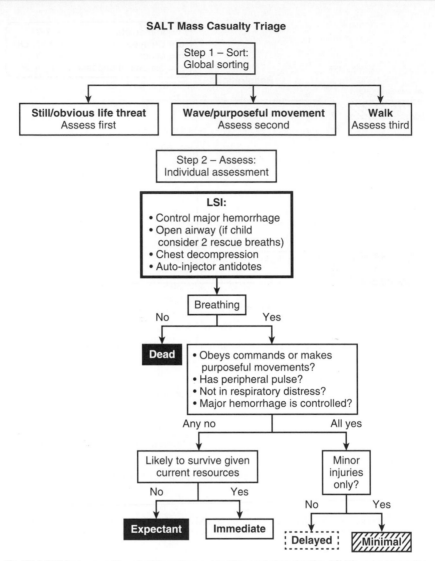

Fig. 101.3 SALT (sort, assess, life-saving interventions, and treat/transport) triage algorithm. *LSI,* Life-saving intervention.

emergency medical vehicle collisions, not only increasing morbidity to those in the ambulance but also to innocent bystanders. Studies have shown that L&S transport to a hospital offers minimal benefit, even for time-critical interventions, offering on average less than 3 minutes faster arrival time over a nonemergent return, even for transports over longer distances. Additionally, patient outcome has not been clearly shown to benefit, bringing into question the utility of this warning system in most scenarios, but particularly in a large-scale disaster or MCI.

22. **What about spinal immobilization for patients?**
Routine spinal immobilization with a cervical collar and backboard for patients with trauma is falling out of favor. There is risk associated with common spinal immobilization practices that are not inconsequential, including increased pain and agitation, increased intracranial pressure (ICP), decreased venous return, respiratory compromise, and the development of pressure sores. Current practice guidelines advocate for the selective use of spinal immobilization, based on the presence of spinal pain and tenderness, symptoms of neurologic compromise (weakness or numbness), altered mentation (including intoxication), or significant distracting injuries. Whereas scoop stretchers and similar devices may facilitate extrication from the scene, particularly in a disaster where terrain may be unstable and difficult to safely navigate, the continued use of a backboard after a patient is on a

gurney and in an ambulance may not be necessary. Spinal precautions can sometimes be maintained by simply securing the patient to the bed and minimizing movement. In an MCI, it may be logistically challenging, if not impossible, to immobilize every injured patient on a backboard with a cervical collar. Although local established protocols should guide standard operational use of spinal immobilization, deviation from protocol may be necessary in a disaster.

23. Can doctors and nurses be helpful on scene for an MCI?
Yes, if they have training and expertise in responding to MCIs and are knowledgeable of and experienced in prehospital medicine and the concept of triage. They should also have a good understanding of local systems and protocols. Physicians at a scene can sometimes be helpful in advising when it is appropriate to deviate from normal procedure and protocols to address unique demands or a particular disaster situation.

24. What is critical incident stress management (CISM)?
CISM helps first responders deal with the emotional aftermath of a disaster. Stress is a normal response to a disaster, which can affect an entire community and an entire country (e.g., shooting at the Harvest Music Festival in Las Vegas in 2017, the Boston marathon bombing of 2013, the Aurora movie theater shooting of 2012, and the terrorist attacks of September 11, 2001). It is not surprising that those on scene are often particularly affected psychologically and perhaps physically. Debriefing is a critically important part of CISM, because it allows all personnel the opportunity to speak openly about their experience in an effort to heal from the event. Debriefing also has the additional benefit of identifying pitfalls of local response and field triage in order to improve future disaster response. EMS systems should have an approach in place to help manage the aftermath of a major event.

KEY POINTS: DISASTER MANAGEMENT

1. Disasters and MCIs occur whenever the needs of an incident exceed the resources available to respond to it.
2. Communication is the most important component to ensuring an efficient and effective response.
3. An ICS can bring order to chaos for a disaster or MCI.

Websites
For more information about the NIMS, ICS, National Preparedness, and Public Health Emergencies, including educational opportunities:
www.fema.gov/nims; accessed February 1, 2019
www.phe.gov/preparedness; accessed February 1, 2019
www.ncbi.nlm.nih.gov; accessed February 1, 2019

BIBLIOGRAPHY

Armstrong JH, Schwartz RB, eds. *Advanced Disaster Life Support Course Manual.* Version 3.0. Chicago: American Medical Association Press; 2011.
Bass RR, Lawner B, Lee D, et al. Medical oversight of EMS systems. In: Cone DC, ed. *Emergency Medical Services. Clinical Practice and System Oversight.* Chichester, West Sussex, United Kingdom: John Wiley and Sons; 2015:71–84.
Carter AJE, Jensen JL, Petrie DA, et al. State of the evidence for emergency medicine services (EMS) care: the evolution and current methodology of the Prehospital Evidence-Based Practice (PEP) program. *Healthc Policy.* 2018;14(1):57–70.
Cross KP, Petry MJ, Cicero MX. A better START for low-acuity victims: data-driven refinement of mass casualty triage. *Prehosp Emerg Care.* 2015;19:272–278.
Fischer PE, Perina DG, Delbridge TR, et al. Spinal motion restriction in the trauma patient – a joint position statement. *Prehosp Emerg Care.* 2018;22(6):659–661.
Gowing JR, Walker KN, Elmer SL, et al. Disaster preparedness among health professionals and support staff: what is effective? An integrative literature review. *Prehosp Disaster Med.* 2017;32(3):321–328.
Isakov A, O'Neal P, Prescott J, et al. Academic-community partnerships for sustainable preparedness and response systems. *Am J Disaster Med.* 2014;9(2):97–106.
Lerner EB, Schwartz RB, Coule PL, et al. Mass casualty triage: an evaluation of the data and development of a proposed national guideline. *Disaster Med Public Health Prep.* 2008;2(suppl 1):25–34.
Millin MG, Brown LH, Craven CK, et al. Evolution of the literature identifying physicians' roles in leadership, clinical development, and practice of the subspecialty of emergency medical services. *Prehosp Disaster Med.* 2011;26(1):49–64.
Miramonti CM, O'Donnell DP, Stevens AC, et al. Mass casualty management. In: Cone DC, ed. *Emergency Medical Services. Clinical Practice and System Oversight.* Chichester, West Sussex, United Kingdom: John Wiley and Sons; 2015:292–302.
Silvestri S, Field A, Mangalat N, et al. Comparison of START and SALT triage methodologies to reference standard definitions and to a field mass casualty simulation. *Am J Disaster Med.* 2017;12(1):27–33.
Watanabe BL, Patterson GS, Kempema JM, et al. Is use of warning lights and sirens associated with increased risk of ambulance crashes? A contemporary analysis using National EMS Information System (NEMSIS) data. *Ann Emerg Med.* 2018;74(1):101–109. doi:10.1016/j.annemergmed.2018.09.032.

CHAPTER 102

PRINCIPLES OF RESPONSE TO WEAPONS OF MASS DESTRUCTION

Caitlin F. Bonney, MD and Edward W. Cetaruk, MD

1. **Why is it important for emergency physicians to be familiar with weapons of mass destruction (WMDs)?**
   Emergency physicians play an integral role in the planning, preparation, and response to not only accidental and natural disasters but also terrorist attacks. A majority of victims (approximately 80%) from these types of mass casualty events typically arrive at health care facilities unannounced, making the response to these events very challenging. Emergency physicians are increasingly being called to take authoritative roles in planning, policy development, and training for mass casualty event response.

2. **How should we prepare for terrorist and mass casualty events?**
   Emergency physicians will be on the front line of any response to mass casualty events (MCEs). Training in MCE response should be integrated into residency training and continued throughout an emergency physician's career via continuing medical education (CME) and hospital MCE exercises. Emergency physicians must maintain a working understanding of chemical, biological, radiological, nuclear, and explosive (CBRNE) weapons, and the ability to effectively respond to an event.

3. **What is the role of hazardous materials (HAZMAT) teams in responding to nuclear, biologic, and chemical (NBC) attacks?**
   HAZMAT teams are highly trained to respond to events that usually occur in relatively confined areas and often with a known substance. HAZMAT teams respond at the site of the event to identify and contain the agent and potentially extract and decontaminate victims. However, terrorist CBRNE attacks will likely occur in population-dense areas to kill and/or contaminate as many people as possible, creating hysteria and fear in the target population. Historically, most patients will self-evacuate from the scene of an attack and present to the closest health care facility where they will require triage, decontamination, and treatment. A biological weapon attack does not lend itself to a traditional HAZMAT or EMS response because a significant amount of time (i.e., the incubation period of the biological agent) will likely have passed between the release of the agent and recognition of the attack. Emergency physicians should be aware of local disaster response agencies and work with them to mobilize the best possible response to an event.

4. **What is unique about a terrorist attack?**
   Terrorists often choose vulnerable targets that are not well protected or pose significant challenges for responders. Hospitals and first responders may be primary or secondary attack targets, specifically to hinder patient care and incident response. Any terrorist attack is, by definition, a crime, and should involve law enforcement. The impact of a terrorist attack extends far beyond the people directly affected. The role of traditional and social media requires strategic communication plans. Terrorists hope to kill or injure as many victims as possible, destroy important structures, and create fear in the greater population.

5. **How should hospitals prepare for terrorist attacks?**
   Hospitals must have plans in place for MCEs using an all-hazards approach. Their response plans should accommodate a large numbers of victims and include partnerships with local agencies. More detailed plans should be made for specific threats (e.g., biologic and chemical weapons). Hospitals must be prepared to manage events independently for at least 72 hours while state and national resources require mobilization. Emergency physicians should be familiar with the incident command system, as they will likely play a significant role in the management of an MCE response. All personnel should be trained in proper use of personal protective equipment (PPE) and decontamination procedures. MCE simulations should be carried out regularly to familiarize staff with the MCE response plan, identify weaknesses, and improve their response.

6. **What makes a good chemical or biologic weapon (in a terrorist's mind)?**
   The ideal weapon would:
   - Create a significant event with high public visibility to sow fear and confusion
   - Create the greatest amount of devastation possible on its intended target
   - Be highly lethal or toxic
   - Be easy to disperse over large areas
   - Be packaged in such a way that it can withstand environmental stressors and the energy transfer during delivery
   - Be relatively easy to obtain
   - Be inexpensive to manufacture and weaponize

7. **What should emergency physicians do to prepare and protect themselves?**

For rapid recognition and treatment of exposed patients, emergency physicians should know the clinical effects of various agents (e.g., chemical weapons and their *toxidromes*; see Chapter 70). Emergency physicians should prioritize the steps needed to protect themselves, emergency department (ED) staff, and the health care facility from inadvertent exposures. The type of PPE needed varies, depending upon the type of agent used in the attack. Emergency physicians should regularly participate in hospital MCE simulations to practice these skills and to identify weaknesses in their response plans.

8. **Describe the levels of PPE.**
   - *Level A.* This suit fully encapsulates the body and prevents water and vapor penetration. Respiratory protection is provided by a self-contained breathing apparatus (SCBA) or supplied air. This level of protection is usually worn for the purpose of rescue, assessing, or mitigating a HAZMAT event, often when the specific agent is unknown and may be immediately dangerous to life and health.
   - *Level B.* Less protective than a level A suit, this is a full-body chemical suit with limited vapor protection. It can be combined with an SCBA or supplied air to increase protection against vapor. This suit is usually worn by responders when the agent has been identified and the exposure levels determined and they are conducting rescue operations or further incident assessment.
   - *Level C.* This is a full-body chemical suit with respiratory protection provided by a powered air-purifying respirator (PAPR). Level C protection is appropriate for hospital personnel involved in decontamination and is the level most likely to be used by medical personnel after a CBRNE incident.
   - *Level D.* This level of PPE provides minimal skin protection and is used when no respiratory protection is required (e.g., street clothing, gloves, standard PPE).

   All levels of PPE require training; levels C and above require specialized training for use. Once a scene is considered safe, personnel must de-escalate to the next lower level of PPE.

9. **What should I know about decontamination?**

Decontamination is a critical aspect of the medical management of CBRNE attacks. The benefits of decontamination are threefold. It protects the patient from continued exposure to residual agent on their clothes or skin, the health care providers from exposure and injury, and the health care facility itself, allowing it to remain open and care for more patients. Patients should be selected for decontamination based on what is known about the exposure. Inhalational CBRNE agent exposures do not require decontamination. Also, patients exposed to biological agents will usually present well after the time of exposure and do not require decontamination.

10. **How is decontamination performed?**

Decontamination is ideally performed at the scene of the exposure, but often occurs when patients arrive to the ED. Every health care facility must have a plan to decontaminate victims, because prior events tell us that most patients will self-present to the ED without prior decontamination. Decontamination should occur outside the health care facility in a preplanned safe, accessible location that can accommodate ambulatory and nonambulatory patients, allows for containment of runoff, if possible, and can be used in all weather conditions. All staff performing decontamination must be trained in decontamination procedures and the proper use of PPE. Contaminated clothing should be removed and safely preserved sealed in plastic bags. Removal of clothing is thought to remove approximately 75%–90% of the contaminant. Decontamination should be done with water (large volume – low pressure), with or without soap. In some cases, the runoff water needs to be contained to prevent contamination of the local water supply and surrounding area. Attempts should be made to keep patients warm during decontamination. Shrapnel suspected to be contaminated should be removed from wounds. Management of acute life-threatening issues (e.g., airway, bleeding) always takes precedence over decontamination for critically ill patients. If possible, and resources allow, treatment (e.g., antidote administration) can be integrated into decontamination procedures.

KEY POINTS: WMDS

1. The most likely WMD to be used by terrorists remains a conventional explosive device (although there are examples of the use of multiple types of weapons in a single incident – e.g., an explosive device followed by the release of a chemical agent). Emergency physicians should be familiar with the management of blast injuries.
2. The ideal terrorist CBRNE weapon is accessible, inexpensive, relatively easy to manufacture and disseminate, and will produce large numbers of casualties.
3. A chemical agent attack will generally be recognized by having a large number of casualties present with similar symptoms over a short time in a relatively small geographic area.
4. Emergency physicians should be familiar with toxidromes that are produced by chemical agents.
5. In the event of a biological agent attack, all patients should be considered to be infectious until a definitive diagnosis of a noncommunicable agent is confirmed.

6. Although possible, terrorist use of a nuclear weapon is unlikely. The most likely radiological incident will be a dirty bomb (RDD, radiological dispersal device) that involves the use of a conventional explosive to disperse radioactive material. Emergency physicians should be familiar with the diagnosis and treatment of radiological victims.
7. Familiarity with PPE, decontamination, and principles of incident command are critical in responding to a CBRNE terrorist attack.

Websites

American Association of Poison Control Centers: https://www.aapcc.org/; accessed February 7, 2019

CDC Terrorism Response: https://www.cdc.gov/niosh/topics/emres/terrorresp.html; accessed February 7, 2019

FEMA: https://www.fema.gov/; accessed February 7, 2019

Hospital Incident Command System. https://emsa.ca.gov/disaster-medical-services-division-hospital-incident-command-system-resources/; accessed February 21, 2021

Strategic National Stockpile: https://www.phe.gov/about/sns/Pages/default.aspx; accessed February 7, 2019

Radiation Emergency Assistance Center/Training Site: https://orise.orau.gov/reacts/; accessed February 7, 2019

BIBLIOGRAPHY

Koenig KL, Boatright CJ, Mancock JA, et al. Health care facilities' "war on terrorism": a deliberate process for recommending personal protective equipment. *Am J Emerg Med.* 2007;25(2):185–195.

Razak S, Hignett S, Barnes J. Emergency department response to chemical, biological, radiological, nuclear, and explosive events: a systematic review. *Prehosp Disaster Med.* 2018;33(5):543–549.

CHAPTER 103

CHEMICAL WEAPONS AND TERRORIST AGENTS

Jonathan Schimmel, MD and Vikhyat S. Bebarta, MD

KEY POINTS

1. Chemical weapon categories include nerve agents, blister agents, nettle agents, blood agents, choking agents, vomiting agents, riot control agents, and incapacitating agents.
2. The mainstay of therapy for nerve agents is atropine, combined with decontamination, pralidoxime, and benzodiazepines (for seizure).

1. **List the characteristics of chemical weapons.**
   - *Volatility* is the tendency of a liquid to evaporate into vapor. Most chemical weapons are liquid at typical atmospheric pressures and temperatures, and are dispersed as fine droplets or vapor after detonation. The more volatile a chemical is, the faster it evaporates. Chlorine, phosgene, and hydrogen cyanide are true gases and so are not described by volatility. Less volatile agents will remain liquids (e.g., venomous agent X [VX], sulfur mustard). All agents except hydrogen cyanide are heavier than air, so they will concentrate in low-lying places.
   - *Persistence* is inversely related to volatility. Persistent chemicals remain on objects and patients longer, with the potential for ongoing exposure.
   - *Toxicity* is an agent's ability to harm a person. For a given concentration of the agent in air and a given exposure duration, agents vary in their degrees of toxicity.
   - *Latency* is the time delay between exposure and manifestation of signs and symptoms. Health care providers must be aware of this principle, because depending on the agent, victims who lack clinical signs or symptoms may still have been exposed and require decontamination and treatment.

2. **What are the different classes of chemical weapons?**
   See Table 103.1.

3. **Describe the pathophysiology and clinical syndrome caused by nerve agents.**
   The pathophysiology of nerve agents is very similar to organophosphate insecticides. Nerve agents inhibit acetylcholinesterase (AChE) at postsynaptic nerve terminals. This prevents the breakdown of acetylcholine, leading to acetylcholine accumulation and overstimulation of muscarinic and nicotinic receptors in the peripheral parasympathetic nervous system and central nervous system (CNS). The cholinergic toxidrome results from that overstimulation. Muscarinic effects include bradycardia, bronchorrhea, salivation, lacrimation, and urination. Nicotinic effects include muscle fasciculations, flaccid weakness/paralysis, hypertension, and tachycardia. The clinical toxidrome is complex, involving many organ systems. Victims typically die by seizures, severe bradycardia, or suffocation through bronchospasm and bronchorrhea.

4. **What is the easiest way to remember the effects of nerve agents?**
   Muscarinic effects can be remembered with the SLUDGE or DUMBBELS mnemonics:
   SLUDGE: **S**alivation, **L**acrimation, **U**rination, **D**efecation, **G**I symptoms, **E**mesis
   DUMBBELS: **D**iarrhea, **U**rination, **M**iosis/muscle weakness, **B**ronchorrhea/**B**radycardia, **E**mesis, **L**acrimation, **S**alivation/ Sweating
   Nicotinic effects can be remembered with the MTWHF mnemonic:
   Mydriasis, **T**achycardia, **W**eakness, **H**ypertension, **F**asciculations
   The patient can have life-threatening bronchorrhea, bradycardia, and bronchospasm (the Killer B's). CNS effects can include seizure, coma, or apnea.

5. **How deadly are nerve agents?**
   All types of nerve agents are rapidly deadly. As an example, the VX dose that kills half of exposed victims (lethal dose 50% or LD_{50}) is 10 mg (skin exposure) for a 70-kg person. This means a drop of VX, only large enough to cover two columns of the Lincoln Memorial on the back of a US penny, is enough to kill half of victims exposed by skin.

Table 103.1 Classes of Chemical Weapons

CLASS	DESCRIPTION	SIGNS AND SYMPTOMS	EXAMPLES AND DESIGNATION
Blister agents/ vesicants	Damage cell components and create blisters on dermal and mucosal surfaces in minutes to hours	Dyspnea, skin pain/vesicles, conjunctivitis, possible severe respiratory compromise	Lewisite Sulfur mustard Nitrogen mustards
Nettle agents	Irritates skin and mucous membranes	Immediate skin erythema, urticaria, pruritis	Phosgene oxime
Blood agents	Absorbed into bloodstream and interferes with aerobic metabolism	Dyspnea, flushed skin, shock	Cyanogen chloride Cyanogen bromide Hydrogen cyanide
Choking/pulmonary agents	Irritate the lining of the lungs and throat, causing edema of mucous membranes	Cough, dyspnea, eye irritation, burning sensation in throat	Chlorine Phosgene
Incapacitating agents	Cause altered cognition or mental status	Altered mental status, anticholinergic syndrome (BZ), opioid toxidrome	3-Quinuclidinyl benzilate (BZ) Fentanyl (aerosolized)
Nerve agents	Inhibit acetylcholinesterase	Cholinergic toxidrome with muscarinic and nicotinic features	Sarin (GB) Soman (GD) Tabun (GA) VX Novichok agents Carbamates
Riot control agents/ tear gas	Very irritating, but largely nonlethal, used for crowd control	Mucous membrane irritation lacrimation, rhinorrhea, cough	Chloroacetophenone Chlorobenzylidene malononitrile Dibenzoxazepine Oleoresin capsicum (pepper spray) Pelargonic acid vanillylamide
Vomiting agents	Irritates eyes, nasal, and respiratory tract; gastrointestinal upset and vomiting	Emesis minutes to hours after exposure	Adamsite

From Centers for Disease Control and Prevention. Emergency preparedness and response: chemical categories. https://emergency.cdc.gov/agent/agentlistchem-category.asp.

6. Is there such a thing as a "nerve gas?"

No, nerve "gas" is a misnomer. Nerve agents are liquid at room temperature, and, due to volatility, a portion evaporates as vapor. To maximize lethality, nerve agents are dispersed as an aerosol of liquid droplets, or by an incendiary device. Chemical weapons that are true gases include chlorine, phosgene, and hydrogen cyanide.

7. What is the treatment for nerve agent toxicity?

Treatment is based on a three-pronged approach.

Atropine is the mainstay of treatment, to counteract the muscarinic effects, dry secretions, and thus improve breathing. High doses of atropine are often needed for organophosphate pesticides. Nerve agents often require less atropine than pesticides, but symptomatic patients still typically require at least several milligrams. Atropine is often started intravenous (IV; if access is established) at 1–2 mg; then the dose is doubled every 5 minutes until adequate control of signs and symptoms.

Oximes reverse the nicotinic effects, such as muscle weakness, of nerve agents. Oximes separate the nerve agent from AChE, allowing for the metabolism of AChE. However, for oximes to be effective, they must be administered before something called "aging" occurs. After nerve agents bind AChE, they develop a permanent covalent bond over time, rendering the enzyme permanently deactivated. This time ranges from 2 minutes for soman to

48 hours for VX. Pralidoxime (also known as 2-PAM) is the only approved oxime in the United States, although other oximes may be used globally. IV pralidoxime is administered slowly at 15 mg/kg, or 1 g in an adult.

Finally, seizures are treated with diazepam and midazolam. If this is unavailable, consider an alternate benzodiazepine.

8. **How are nerve agent antidotes administered?**
   If IV access has been established, then atropine, pralidoxime, and diazepam are administered by that route. All three can also be administered intramuscularly. First responders and service members can also use autoinjectors that contain atropine 2.1 mg + pralidoxime 600 mg in separate chambers. A newer version autoinjector (brand name: DuoDote) contains the same doses, but injects both drugs through the same syringe at the same time for simplification.

9. **How do I decontaminate victims of chemical threat agents?**
   Decontamination of patients should ideally be performed in the prehospital setting. However, hospitals should be prepared to decontaminate outside the emergency department. Hospital staff involved in decontamination should use personal protective equipment. Wet decontamination is the method of choice for liquid or vapor chemical exposure. First remove the victim's clothes and place in sealed bags; then irrigate the patient's skin with soap and copious water. A variety of neutralizing solutions have been suggested for decontamination such as dilute bleach, but most are not used in the hospital setting since they require prolonged contact time (15–20 minutes) and have the potential for causing additional skin injury.

10. **How does cyanide exposure occur, what are common effects of cyanide poisoning, and what are the available therapies?**
    Cyanide may exist in salts (e.g., potassium cyanide [KCN], sodium cyanide [NaCN]), organic nitrile compounds (e.g., acetonitrile), cyanogenic glycosides from plants, or as a gas. Ingested cyanide salts are rapidly lethal at low dose. Acetonitrile is found in artificial nail remover, and ingestion may cause delayed cyanide toxicity as it metabolizes. Cyanogenic glycosides are found in cassava, and in the pits of apricots, peaches, and bitter almonds. They are typically associated with chronic toxicity, but may cause acute toxicity if a large extracted dose is ingested. Hydrogen cyanide gas has been used in battle, and is generated in fires by burning of certain synthetic and natural substances. Cyanide inhibits the utilization of oxygen in the oxidative phosphorylation process and multiple other enzymes, and the patient's course after exposure depends on substance, route, and dose. Acute cyanide toxicity mainly affects the CNS (coma, seizure) and cardiovascular system (shock/tachycardia becomes shock/bradycardia). Laboratory testing shows metabolic acidosis and elevated lactate. The optimal antidotes are either 5 g of IV hydroxocobalamin (vitamin B_{12}) or IV sodium nitrite administered with sodium thiosulfate.

11. **How does chlorine exposure occur, what are common effects of chlorine poisoning, and what are the available therapies?**
    Chlorine is a yellow–green gas, and exposure can occur via swimming pool purification systems, industrial or transport accidents, or military/terrorism exposure. It is also generated by inadvertently mixing sodium hypochlorite (bleach) with hydrochloric acid (HCl). Chlorine is a pulmonary/choking agent and dissolves in mucous membrane water to make HCl. Chlorine has intermediate water solubility, which means symptoms may be delayed up to several hours with irritated mucous membranes, and if severe, individuals may develop acute respiratory distress syndrome. The initial management of chlorine gas exposure is by safely removing the patient from the exposure. Supportive care is the primary therapy with supplemental oxygen, bronchodilators, and mechanical ventilation if needed. Nebulized sodium bicarbonate has been trialed, but evidence is low quality. Some studies support inhaled steroids in moderately ill victims and IV steroids in severe injury, but evidence is weak.

12. **What are vesicant agents, how do they present, and how are they managed?**
    Vesicant agents cause mucosal and dermal irritation with bullae, possible necrosis, and lung and eye injury. The most well-known agent is sulfur mustard, commonly known as mustard gas, which caused extensive morbidity in World War I and has been used again in Syria and other locations in Southwest Asia. Vesicant mechanisms are diverse and not fully clear, but the primary mechanism of mustards is alkylation. The metal chelator dimercaprol (also called British Anti-Lewisite [BAL]) was developed to treat the vesicant Lewisite, which was never used in war or civilian settings. Skin and mucous membrane decontamination is important, even if asymptomatic, given potential latency to symptom onset. Treatment is largely supportive, and newer therapies are being developed to treat lung injury, eye toxicity, systemic inflammation, and skin burns.

13. **What are riot control agents and how are they managed?**
    These agents are intentionally mostly nonlethal and temporarily disable by strongly irritating mucous membranes, skin, and eyes. They are mostly solid at room temperature, and are dispersed as an aerosol with onset in seconds to minutes. Older agents have largely been replaced by oleoresin capsicum (also known known as pepper spray). Risk increases with exposure to high ambient concentrations in an enclosed space for a prolonged period.

Bibliography

Agency for Toxic Substances and Disease Registry. Medical management guidelines for nerve agents: tabun (GA); sarin (GB); soman (GD); and VX. https://www.atsdr.cdc.gov/MHMI/mmg166.pdf. Accessed December 17, 2018.

Anseeuw K, Nicolas D, Guillermo BP, et al. Cyanide poisoning by fire smoke inhalation: a European expert consensus. *Eur J Emerg Med.* 2013;20(1):2–9.

Centers for Disease Control and Prevention. Emergency preparedness and response: chemical categories. https://emergency.cdc.gov/agent/agentlistchem-category.asp. Accessed December 17, 2018.

Ganesan K, Raza SK, Vijayaraghavan R. Chemical warfare agents. *J Pharm Bioallied Sci.* 2010;2(3):166–178.

Newmark J: Nerve agents. *Neurol Clin.* 2005;23(2):623–641.

White CW, Martin JG. Chlorine gas inhalation: human clinical evidence of toxicity and experience in animal models. *Proc Am Thorac Soc.* 2010;7(4):257–263.

CHAPTER 104

BIOLOGICAL WEAPONS OF MASS DESTRUCTION

Caitlin F. Bonney, MD and Edward W. Cetaruk, MD

1. **What is bioterrorism?**
   Bioterrorism is a terrorist attack involving the deliberate release of viruses, bacteria, or biological toxins to cause panic, illness, or death in people, animals, or plants.

2. **How has bioterrorism been used in the past?**
   Biological weapons have been used in warfare since antiquity. In the fourteenth and fifteenth centuries, warring armies would hurl plague-infected corpses over the walls of cities they were attempting to conquer. In 1763, British army officer Jeffrey Amherst ordered the distribution of smallpox-contaminated blankets to Pontiac Native Americans. Accounts exist of biological weapons being used in both World War I and World War II. In 1984, 750 people in Oregon became sick after eating at salad bars in four different local restaurants that were intentionally contaminated with *Salmonella* by the Bhagwan Shree Rajneesh sect. Beginning September 18, 2001, anthrax spores were sent via the US mail system. This attack led to 22 cases of inhalational and cutaneous anthrax, including five fatalities. Many terrorist groups have used or have attempted to acquire biological weapons.

3. **What does a terrorist need to develop a biologic weapon?**
   Preparation of an agent for use as a biological weapon requires (1) acquisition of a highly virulent biological agent, (2) growth of the agent in sufficient quantities, and (3) development of a system to deliver the agent to its target. Information on how to carry out these processes is widely disseminated on the Internet.

4. **How are biologic attacks different from exposure to radiation or chemical agents?**
   A biological weapon attack creates several significant challenges that are different from a radiological or chemical weapon attack. Because of the incubation period between exposure and active infection, the development of clinical symptoms is delayed. The incubation period varies based on several factors such as the organism chosen, its virulence, and inoculum size. Initially, symptoms are often nonspecific, but frequently will include flu-like symptoms such as fever, chills, headache, malaise, respiratory, or gastrointestinal (GI) symptoms. These factors often lead to a significant delay in diagnosis of the infectious agent, significantly impacting the ability to recognize and appropriately respond to a biological weapon attack. Detection of a biological weapon attack depends on passive surveillance (i.e., *incidental* recognition of unusual patterns of disease). Once a biological weapon attack or an outbreak of a novel infection occurs, surveillance becomes active and new cases are actively sought out. A biological weapon attack is rarely apparent when it occurs. Victims will likely disperse from the site of exposure and later present to multiple health care facilities at varied times and geographical locations. A biological weapon attack may become a self-perpetuating event if it involves a communicable agent (e.g., plague, smallpox).

5. **How does the Centers for Disease Control and Prevention (CDC) categorize biologic agents?**
   The CDC prioritizes biologic agents into three categories (A, B, and C), based on the characteristics of the agents, including ease of dissemination and transmission, and ability to create a significant negative impact on public health infrastructure.
   - *Category A*. High-priority agents include organisms that pose a risk to national security because they can be easily disseminated or transmitted from person to person; result in high mortality rates and have the potential for major public health impact; might cause public panic and social disruption; and require special action for public health preparedness. Examples: anthrax *(Bacillus anthracis)*, botulism (*Clostridium botulinum* toxin), smallpox (variola major), viral hemorrhagic fevers (filoviruses [e.g., Ebola, Marburg]).
   - *Category B*. Second highest priority agents include those that are moderately easy to disseminate, generally result in moderate morbidity rates and low mortality rates, and require specific enhancements of the CDC's diagnostic capacity and enhanced disease surveillance. Examples: food safety threats (e.g., *Salmonella* species, *Escherichia coli* O157:H7, *Shigella*), ricin toxin from *Ricinus communis* (castor beans), water safety threats (e.g., *Vibrio cholerae, Cryptosporidium parvum*).
   - *Category C*. Third highest priority agents include emerging pathogens that could be engineered for mass dissemination in the future because of availability, ease of production and dissemination, and potential for high morbidity and mortality rates and major health impact. Examples: emerging infectious diseases such as Nipah virus and hantavirus.

While recognizing agent classes is useful, most victims of a biological weapon attack will present with non-specific symptoms. Initial response to a suspected biological weapon attack should focus on case identification and containment, and treatment of *any* biological agent rather than those on a list of specific biological agents.

6. What are the general descriptive characteristics of biologic agents?
See Table 104.1.

Table 104.1 General Characteristics of Biologic Agents

Infectivity	The ability of an agent to enter, multiply, and survive in a host ID_{50} is the dosage that would infect 50% of an exposed population
Virulence	The relative severity of the disease Different strains of the same agent can cause varying severities of disease
Incubation period	Time between exposure and onset of symptoms
Lethality	The ability of an agent to cause death
Contagiousness	Measured by the number of secondary cases occurring after exposure to the primary case
Mechanisms of transmission	Manner by which the disease is transmitted (i.e., respiratory, blood-borne, vector-borne, food contamination)

From the World Health Organization: Public health response to biological and chemical weapons: WHO guidance (2004). www.who.int/csr/delibepidemics/biochemguide/en/. Accessed January 10, 2019.

7. How are victims of biologic agent exposure decontaminated?
In most cases, victims of a biologic attack will seek treatment when they become clinically ill. This finding indicates that the exposure occurred days earlier, in which case decontamination is not necessary. Only in those instances of recognized contact exposure with the agent or other infectious material is decontamination required. Patients with an exposure to an unknown compound (e.g., white powder in a letter) suspected to be a biological weapon should undergo appropriate decontamination (see Chapter 102). Decontamination personnel must be properly trained and use appropriate procedures and personal protective equipment (PPE) throughout the decontamination process.

8. How should laboratory testing be handled?
Victims of a biological weapon attack will present for health care with nonspecific infectious symptoms usually well before the causative agent is identified. Appropriate supportive medical care and treatment should be started as indicated by the clinical presentation. When a biological weapon attack is suspected, the CDC Laboratory Response Network (LRN) should be activated. The LRN is a network of laboratories developed to respond to biological and chemical threats and other public health emergencies. Activation of the LRN should take place alongside involvement of other public health and law enforcement authorities. Laboratory testing is most useful in confirming diagnosis. Initial management should be based on appropriate medical care and empiric treatment of an unknown infectious disease.

9. What features make anthrax a prototypical biologic attack agent?
Anthrax is accessible, durable in the environment, relatively easy to grow in significant quantity, highly infectious, and highly deadly. *Bacillus anthracis* is an encapsulated, gram-positive, spore-forming bacterium. The spores are highly resistant to environmental factors, allowing them to survive for decades. However, spread of an attack or natural outbreak is limited because anthrax is not transmissible from person to person.

10. What are the features of anthrax infection?
After a biologic attack, anthrax spores enter the lungs, skin, or GI tract. Spores are transported to regional lymph nodes where they germinate and proliferate, causing bacteremia and releasing toxins that cause edema (edema toxin) and hemorrhage and necrosis (lethal toxin). A third toxin that is produced is a protective factor. It acts on the surface of the host cell to allow the other two toxins to enter and become active. Anthrax infection manifests in three clinical forms: inhalational, GI, and cutaneous. The inhalational and cutaneous forms are most likely to be seen after a biologic attack. Cutaneous anthrax begins as a localized lesion with erythema and edema (sometimes marked) that progresses to a painless, necrotic black lesion or ulcer. Inhalational anthrax has an asymptomatic incubation phase of 1–6 days, followed by a brief prodrome with muscles aches, fatigue, and fever. Patients progress to respiratory failure, shock, and death. Fifty percent of cases of inhalational anthrax are accompanied by anthrax meningitis. Multiple clinical forms may be seen after an attack, and patients will present with nonspecific symptoms. Of 10 patients with inhalational anthrax in the 2001 attacks, all had fever, chills, malaise, and fatigue. Most of the patients developed cough, chest discomfort, and dyspnea. Chest radiograph abnormalities were universal, and included widened mediastinum, pleural effusions, air bronchograms, necrotizing pneumonic lesions, or consolidations. Based on experience with the accidental anthrax release and outbreak in

Sverdlovsk, Russia in 1979, we know that most patients develop clinical signs of illness within a week, while some may not become symptomatic for weeks.

11. **What is the treatment for anthrax exposure or infection?**
Anthrax spores may remain in the body for 60 days or more before germination. People who have been exposed to anthrax should take a 60-day course of postexposure antibiotic prophylaxis (e.g., ciprofloxacin or doxycycline). Guidelines are available from the CDC.
   - Patients with inhalational anthrax without evidence of anthrax meningitis should be treated with dual antibiotic therapy (ciprofloxacin plus clindamycin).
   - Patients with suspected, probable, or confirmed anthrax meningitis should be treated with triple antibiotic therapy with good central nervous system penetration (ciprofloxacin plus meropenem plus linezolid).
   - Parenteral combination treatment of systemic anthrax should be provided for at least 2 weeks or until the patient is clinically stable; at that point, the patient may be transitioned to oral monotherapy for prophylaxis against ungerminated spores.
   - Raxibacumab, a novel monoclonal antibody active against anthrax protective antigen, is available from the Strategic National Stockpile (SNS). The CDC recommends that the antitoxin should be administered as an adjunct to IV antimicrobials whenever there is a high level of clinical suspicion for systemic anthrax. However, available doses and resources to administer the 2- to 4-hour infusion may be limited.
   - For cutaneous anthrax, treat with ciprofloxacin or doxycycline.

12. **What is the Strategic National Stockpile?**
The SNS is the United States' national repository of critical medical supplies (e.g., antibiotics, vaccines, chemical antidotes, ventilators) for rapid delivery in the event of a public health threat. The Stockpile is organized for scalable response to public health emergencies and contains enough supplies to respond to multiple large-scale emergencies simultaneously. The SNS includes "Push Packs" of critical supplies prepackaged for immediate transport. They are geographically dispersed for rapid deployment and delivery within 12 hours. Deployment of SNS resources is initiated at the request of a state governor or their designee when a terrorist attack or public health threat is suspected.

13. **What precautions should I take while caring for patients exposed to biologic weapons?**
Most events will not be identified as a biological weapon attack before the first patients present for medical care. Use universal precautions whenever infectious disease is suspected in any patient. PPE and isolation precautions can be modified as appropriate when a specific organism is suspected or identified. Patients infected with a biological agent may require airborne or droplet isolation. Agents such as anthrax and botulism do not undergo person-to-person transmission and do not require special isolation. However, agents such as smallpox and hemorrhagic fevers are highly transmissible and require isolation. All agents should be considered transmissible until identified. Training for all staff on proper use of PPE and isolation precautions should be integrated into the planning phase of a biological weapon attack response.

14. **How will I know if a biological weapon attack has occurred?**
Recognizing a biological weapon attack can be very difficult because there is often no sentinel event to indicate that an attack has occurred. A biological mass casualty event should be suspected when an unusual pattern of an infectious illness occurs, such as an outbreak of an organism not endemic to a particular region or during an unusual time of year, when large numbers of patients present with similar or severe infectious symptoms, or when multiple outbreaks occur simultaneously. Emergency physicians (EPs) should be on the alert for unusual disease patterns (passive surveillance) and alert local and state agencies to initiate investigation (active surveillance).

15. **What should I do if I suspect an attack has occurred?**
Emergency physicians have a major role to play in planning for mass casualty event response and should be involved in the development of response protocols. All EPs should familiarize themselves with their hospitals' internal disaster plans and reporting processes. Early involvement of local and state public health is important for organism identification, case identification and tracking, and epidemiologic follow-up studies. The CDC provides a mechanism to report a suspected biological agent incident, as well as helpful phone numbers that may be needed during the management of an incident. This information can be accessed at the CDC's Emergency Preparedness and Response website located at http://emergency.cdc.gov/ and should be included in emergency response plans.

KEY POINTS: BIOLOGICAL WEAPONS OF MASS DESTRUCTION

1. Biological weapon attacks are used by terrorists to kill or incapacitate a target population, overwhelm health care systems, and sow fear, panic, and confusion.
2. Patients subjected to a biological weapon attack will not show clinical signs and symptoms until some amount of time after the attack (incubation period). Their symptoms may initially be nonspecific and a biological weapon attack may not be apparent at first.

3. Most biological weapon attacks will be recognized by passive surveillance.
4. Once a biological weapon attack is suspected, exposed individuals should be identified and isolated and treated if appropriate (e.g., antibiotic prophylaxis) and local public health and law enforcement agencies should be alerted. Active surveillance should be initiated.
5. Health care workers should practice universal precautions when treating patients with suspected exposure to biological agents.
6. Emergency physicians should be on the lookout for unusual disease patterns or patient presentations that may be the first sign that a biological weapon attack has occurred.

Websites
Biological weapons: http://emergency.cdc.gov/bioterrorism/; accessed January 10, 2019.
Bioterrorism agents: http://emergency.cdc.gov/agent/agentlist-category.asp#catdef; accessed January 10, 2019.
Strategic National Stockpile: https://www.phe.gov/about/sns/Pages/default.aspx; accessed January 10, 2019.
CDC Emergency Preparedness and Response: https://emergency.cdc.gov/bioterrorism/index.asp. Accessed February 7, 2019.
US Army Medical Research Institute of Infectious Diseases: https://www.usamriid.army.mil/, accessed February 7, 2019.
CDC Laboratory Response Network: https://emergency.cdc.gov/lrn/.

BIBLIOGRAPHY

Bozue J, Cote CK, Glass PJ, eds. *Medical aspects of biological warfare.* Washington, DC: Office of the Surgeon General. US Army Medical Department Center and School, Borden Institute; 2018. https://www.cs.amedd.army.mil/Portlet.aspx?ID=66cffe45-c1b8-4453-91e0-9275007fd157. Accessed February 15, 2019.

Withers MR, ed. *USAMRIID's medical management of biological casualties handbook.* 8th ed. Frederick, MD: US Army Medical Research Institute of Infectious Diseases; 2014. https://www.usamriid.army.mil/education/bluebookpdf/USAMRIID%20BlueBook%208th%20 Edition%20-%20Sep%202014.pdf. Accessed February 15, 2019.

CHAPTER 105

RADIATION EMERGENCIES

Keith Baker, MD

1. What are the basic physics of radiation?

In general terms, radiation is energy released from a source and propagated through space. Ionizing radiation carries enough energy to displace electrons from atoms or molecules, thereby ionizing them. Atoms consist of a nucleus of protons and neutrons surrounded by electrons. An element's atomic number reflects its number of protons, while the mass number reflects its number of protons and neutrons. Elements may exist as different isotopes, which have different numbers of neutrons. Some of these isotopes may emit ionizing radiation in the form of particles or electromagnetic energy, and are called radioisotopes. If this ionizing radiation interacts with a biologically important molecule, damage can occur. Protection from ionizing radiation is afforded by shielding, distance, and decreased time of exposure.

2. What are the units of radiation?

See Table 105.1.

Table 105.1 Units of Radiation	
Radiation absorbed dose (rad); Gray (Gy)	Measure of the energy deposited into matter (the body) by ionizing radiation 1 Gy = 100 rad 1 Gy = 1 J/kg The Gy dose is the total amount of energy absorbed per gram of tissue
Radiation equivalent (rem); Sievert (Sv)	Measure of ionizing radiation equivalency 1 Gy (100 rad) of α radiation or neutrons, is more harmful to the body than 1 Gy (100 rad) of β or γ radiation These differences are adjusted for by multiplying by the "K factor," and then expressed as Sv or rem 1 Sv = 100 rem In general, α radiation has K factor of 20, β and γ radiation have K factor of 1, and neutrons have K factor of 5–20 depending on species For α radiation, 1 Gy (100 rad) = 20 Sv (2000 rem) For β and γ radiation, 1 Gy (100 rad) = 1 Sv (100 rem) For neutrons, 1 Gy (100 rad) = 5–20 Sv (500–2000 rem), depending on the species

3. Describe the different types of radiation and their shielding requirements.

See Table 105.2.

Table 105.2 Different Types of Radiation and Shielding Requirements		
RADIATION	**DESCRIPTION**	**SHIELDING**
α-Particles	Consist of two neutrons and two protons that have been ejected from the nucleus of a radioactive atom A doubly charged particle that loses its energy quickly in matter Generally only dangerous if inhaled or swallowed	Stopped by paper
β-Particles	High-energy electrons that are emitted from a nucleus along with an antineutrino Much smaller than α-particles and have only one charge Like α-particles, can cause damage if swallowed or inhaled May also cause cellular damage to unprotected skin Largely found in fallout radiation	Stopped by plastic, glass, or thin metal

Continued on following page

Table 105.2 Different Types of Radiation and Shielding Requirements *(Continued)*

RADIATION	DESCRIPTION	SHIELDING
γ-Rays	Not particles but rather uncharged pulses of very high-energy electromagnetic radiation No mass or charge and only lose energy when they collide with the electron shell of target atoms Easily pass through the human body Potential to cause significant cellular damage	Stopped by concrete, earth, or dense metal, such as lead (however lead aprons generally not thick enough to stop γ-rays)
Neutrons	Uncharged particles emitted during nuclear detonation that could also be seen in the event of a reactor meltdown About the same mass as a proton but no charge Because of lack of charge, interact directly with the nucleus of target atom instead of its electrons Do not react well with material, so they can travel large distances Can cause previously stable atoms to become radioactive	Thick concrete or significant amount of earth

4. **What are the types of radiation injury?**
   - External irradiation: all or a portion of the body is exposed to penetrating radiation from an external source. Significant cellular damage can occur. After exposure, the patient is not radioactive and can be managed like any other patient with no threat to staff.
   - Contamination: radioactive particulate matter released into the environment contaminates the person externally, internally (swallowed or inhaled), or both. Personal protective equipment (PPE) should be worn when treating or decontaminating these patients.
   - Incorporation: the uptake of radioactive material in cells, tissues, or organs. Contamination must first occur for incorporation to occur. Incorporation allows for continued internal exposure and long-term injury and illness.

5. **What are some causes of radiation emergencies?**
   - Accidental exposure: this could occur in a variety of settings, including a health care facility (from material used in nuclear medicine procedures or a radiation source for teletherapy), or from exposure to an abandoned industrial source.
   - Simple radiologic device (also called *environmental exposure*): a radioactive source placed in a public location or within the food or water supply. Although many people would potentially be exposed with this method, very few would likely be significantly contaminated. This type of attack, however, would generate fear and panic.
   - Radiologic dispersal device (RDD): a device designed to disperse radioactive material by using conventional explosives. Also referred to as a *dirty bomb*. Most of the damage results from the actual explosion, with limited dissemination of radioactive material. Exposed or contaminated individuals would be those in close proximity to the blast area.
   - Attack/sabotage/accident of a nuclear reactor: could lead to significant release of radioactive material into the environment.
   - Nuclear bomb: although the most potentially devastating attack, this is the least likely method because there are strict security measures for existing stockpiles, and it is difficult to obtain the money and technology needed to manufacture a new weapon.

6. **Describe the four acute radiation syndromes (ARSs).**
   1. Hematopoietic syndrome: damage to stem cells in the bone marrow results in a reduction in cell lines. Clinical findings include bleeding and infection (due to low platelets and leukocytes). *The threshold for developing this syndrome is whole-body irradiation with 1–2 Gy (100–200 rad).*
   2. Gastrointestinal syndrome: irreversible destruction of the intestinal lining causes severe nausea, vomiting, diarrhea, hemorrhage, and bacterial translocation. The mortality rate is high due to overwhelming sepsis, blood loss, and electrolyte disturbances. *This syndrome occurs after whole-body irradiation with at least 5–6 Gy (500–600 rad).*
   3. Neurovascular syndrome: initial findings include vomiting, fatigue, confusion, ataxia, tachycardia, hypotension, fever, seizures, and coma. Death occurs due to circulatory collapse and increased intracranial pressure. *This syndrome occurs after whole-body irradiation with at least 8–10 Gy (800–1000 rad), with increasingly rapid progression and severity seen as dose increases. This syndrome is nearly uniformly fatal.*
   4. Cutaneous syndrome: can be seen after irradiation of even a small portion of the body, with injury occurring specifically to the area(s) which have been irradiated. Development of injury generally occurs over weeks and can persist for months to years due to poor healing. The following doses refer to dose to a specific area. *At 3–6 Gy (300–600 rad), transient epilation and erythema can occur. Dry desquamation occurs with exposure to 10–15 Gy (1000–1500 rad), wet desquamation with exposure to 15–20 Gy (1500–2000 rad), and ulceration and necrosis with exposure to over 25 Gy (2500 rad). In severe cases death is possible secondary to fluid loss and infection.*

7. **Describe the four stages of ARS.**
   1. Prodromal: symptoms include anorexia, nausea, vomiting, and diarrhea. Symptoms occur minutes to days after the exposure. Generally, the more rapid the onset of symptoms, the greater the radiation dose received by the victim. However this is not always the case, and time to onset of symptoms (or lack of symptoms entirely) should not be used as a stand-alone marker for degree of exposure.
   2. Latent: resolution of symptoms experienced in the initial stage with the patient appearing relatively well. This stage can last from several hours to approximately 2 weeks.
   3. Manifest illness: symptoms will vary depending on radiation dose. See Question 6 on acute radiation syndromes.
   4. Recovery or death: survival is highly unlikely with doses exceeding 10 Gy (1000 rad).

8. **All these numbers are great, but what is the bottom line?**
   - Exposure to 0.5–1.0 Gy is the threshold for prodromal symptoms, but no deaths from acute radiation should occur at this level.
   - Exposure to 3.5–4.5 Gy will be 50% lethal at 60 days if untreated.
   - Exposure to 6.0 Gy is nearly 100% lethal at 60 days if untreated.

9. **How is the absolute lymphocyte count helpful in evaluating ARS?**
   See Table 105.3.

Table 105.3 Role of the Absolute Lymphocyte Count		
MINIMAL LYMPHOCYTE COUNT WITHIN 48 HOURS OF EXPOSURE	**ESTIMATED ABSORBED DOSE (Gy)**	**PROGNOSIS**
1000–3000	0–0.5	Likely no injury
1000–1500	1–2	Significant but good prognosis
500–1000	2–4	Severe, may survive
100–500	4–8	Very severe, likely die
<100	>8	Will almost certainly die

From Koenig KL, Goans RE, Hatchett RJ, et al. Medical treatment of radiological casualties: current concepts. *Ann Emerg Med.* 2005;45: 643–652.

10. **How do I decontaminate a patient who has been exposed to radioactive material?**
    Once the patient is removed from the radiologically hazardous environment, standard PPE is adequate for decontamination personnel (scrubs, masks, gloves, eye protection, and shoe coverings). Decontamination personnel should be equipped with dosimeters to monitor radiation exposure. Decontamination can then be broken down into two components:
    1. Gross decontamination: remove all of the patient's clothes and bag them appropriately. The patient should then wash or be washed with copious amounts of soap and water. Care must be taken to avoid washing contaminated water toward mucous membranes. Care must also be taken to not abrade the skin, because radionuclides can be absorbed through skin abrasions. This process will successfully remove approximately 95% of the contamination.
    2. Secondary decontamination: this is a meticulous process ensuring the patient is fully decontaminated. Eyes, ears, mucous membranes, and wounds are swabbed, and the swabs analyzed for radioactivity. Additionally, these same areas should be copiously irrigated. The patient's eyes should be anesthetized and copiously irrigated. The ears should be checked for perforated tympanic membranes (TMs) and, if intact, irrigated copiously. Dentures should be removed, and the mouth rinsed copiously without swallowing the rinse water. Wounds should be irrigated and covered with waterproof dressings to avoid run-off contamination. The hospital's radiation safety officer should be involved with this process.

11. **What treatment options are available for radiation exposure?**
    A complete primary and secondary survey must be done to ensure that no acute life-threatening issues exist. Life-threatening injuries/medical issues should be addressed prior to decontamination. After appropriate triage and decontamination, supportive care becomes the foundation of treatment. Local cutaneous radiation injury should be approached in the same manner as burns, with involvement of 18% or greater of total body surface area being considered a major burn. Treatment of whole-body irradiation becomes more complicated. Such patients should be considered to be immunocompromised and treated as such. Numerous adjunctive treatments may be useful depending on the clinical picture and degree of exposure, including intravenous fluids, antiemetics, blood products, granulocyte-colony stimulating factor (G-CSF), antibiotics, topical steroids, surgery, and palliative care. Systemic steroids and bone marrow transplant are not generally recommended. Internal decontamination and chelation therapy may be appropriate in certain cases where internal contamination has occurred. There is an excellent overview of these treatments on the Centers for Disease Control and Prevention (CDC) website.

12. When should treatment with potassium iodide (KI) tablets be considered?

After a radiologic or nuclear event, it is possible that radioactive iodine may be released. It may be suspended in the air or contaminate food or water sources, which may be inhaled or ingested. The thyroid gland then absorbs this radioactive iodine, which can lead to irreversible destruction of the gland. KI tablets contain stable (nonradioactive) iodine and, if given before exposure to radioactive iodine, can saturate the thyroid gland. This effectively blocks the thyroid from absorbing the radioactive iodine. The CDC website has an informational sheet about KI tablets, including indications and appropriate dosing. This information can be found at http://emergency.cdc.gov/radiation/ki.asp.

13. What is the most appropriate course of action for a patient with radiologic exposure and associated major trauma or medical issues?

Caring for life-threatening trauma or medical problems always takes precedence over management of the radiologic exposure. Decontamination can and should be delayed in those patients requiring immediate surgical intervention until after the resuscitation and all necessary procedures have been accomplished.

KEY POINTS: RADIATION

1. The absolute lymphocyte count at 48 hours is helpful in predicting the patient's likely outcome. A count less than 1000 indicates a grave prognosis.
2. The four acute radiation syndromes are the hematopoietic syndrome, the gastrointestinal syndrome, the neuro-vascular syndrome, and the cutaneous syndrome.
3. KI is administered to block the thyroid gland from absorbing radioactive iodine after a nuclear event.
4. In general, the more rapid the onset of symptoms such as nausea, vomiting and diarrhea after radiation exposure, the greater the dose of radiation received by the patient. However, this is not always true, and time to onset of these symptoms should not be the only measure used for initial dose assessment.
5. Protection from radiation depends upon appropriate shielding, distance from the source, and minimizing time of exposure.

Websites

KI tablets: https://emergency.cdc.gov/radiation/pdf/ki.pdf; accessed February 16, 2019.

Centers for Disease Control and Prevention: Emergency preparedness and response: radiation emergencies. https://emergency.cdc.gov/radiation/index.asp; accessed February 16, 2019.

Centers for Disease Control and Prevention: Emergency preparedness and response. Acute radiation syndrome: a fact sheet for clinicians. http://emergency.cdc.gov/radiation/arsphysicianfactsheet.asp; accessed February 16, 2019.

BIBLIOGRAPHY

Armed Forces Radiobiology Research Institute. *Medical management of radiologic casualties.* 4th ed. Bethesda, MD; 2013. https://www.usuhs.edu/sites/default/files/media/afrri/pdf/4edmmrchandbook.pdf. Accessed February 16, 2019.

Dainiak N, Gent RN, Carr Z, et al. First global consensus for evidence-based management of the hematopoietic syndrome resulting from exposure to ionizing radiation. *Disaster Med Public Health Prep.* 2011;5(3):202–212.

Hick JL, Bader JL, Coleman CN, et al. Proposed "Exposure And Symptom Triage" (EAST) tool to assess radiation exposure after a nuclear detonation. *Disaster Med Public Health Prep.* 2018;12(3):386–395.

Kyne D. Managing nuclear power plant induced disasters. *J Emerg Manag.* 2015;13(5):417–429.

Ohtsuru A, Tanigawa K, Kumagai A, et al. Nuclear disasters and health: lessons learned, challenges, and proposals. *Lancet.* 2015; 386(9992):489–497.

CHAPTER 106

EXPLOSIVE WEAPONS OF MASS DESTRUCTION

Stephen J. Wolf, MD and Jacob Y. Nacht, MD

1. **With all the other highly effective and lethal terrorist weapons, are people really still using explosives?**

   Absolutely, the widespread use of nuclear, biological, and chemical (NBC) weapons is significantly limited because they are expensive to acquire and difficult to manufacture in an effective dispersal mechanism. Explosive devices are relatively inexpensive, much easier to acquire and assemble, and are increasingly being improvised to create maximal body counts. In 2017, bombing and explosives accounted for almost 50% of the 10,900 terrorist attacks worldwide. In 5025 bombing or explosives incidents, there were more than 12,047 deaths and at least 16,167 injuries. At the Boston Marathon bombing in 2013, 3 people were killed, but more than 250 were injured, with at least 14 victims requiring amputations. The injuries in this event were amplified by nails and ball bearings that were added to the explosive device. Overall, the number of terrorist attacks worldwide has been decreasing since 2014 and bombings and explosives attacks have followed this trend, but still represent the largest single weapon type used, according to the Global Terrorism Database.

2. **Describe the different classes of explosives.**

   Explosives generally belong to one of two categories: low order or high order. Low-order explosives detonate in a process called deflagration, which is a burning process that occurs slower than the speed of sound. Gunpowder is an example of a low-order explosive. High-order explosives detonate faster than the speed of sound, and include such things as dynamite, trinitrotoluene (TNT), ammonium nitrate/fuel oil (ANFO), and C4.

3. **What are the basic physics behind the injuries that explosions cause?**

   The rapid conversion of the solid or liquid explosive material to a gaseous phase creates an immediate and severe rise in atmospheric pressure. After the sudden maximal pressure increase expands outward from the point of detonation, the blast's pressure wave dissipates over time and distance and is followed by a period of low pressure before a return to normal pressures. The overpressure, or maximum pressure, of an explosion only occurs with high-order explosives, is responsible for most of the injuries, and its effect is most notable at air–tissue interfaces. Pressures of 2–5 pounds per square inch (psi) can cause tympanic membrane (TM) rupture, 15 psi is the lung damage threshold, and 30–40 psi is typically considered lethal.

4. **Describe the five blast injury categories.**

   1. Primary: the direct effect produced by contact from the blast shockwave of a high-order explosive with the body. This creates shear and stress forces on tissues. These injuries are much greater when the explosion occurs in a confined space. Typical body systems involved include auditory, pulmonary, gastrointestinal, and ocular.
   2. Secondary: injury produced by impact of primary fragments (pieces of the exploding device or shrapnel) or secondary fragments (fragments from the surrounding environment). Typical injuries include penetrating trauma, amputations, or lacerations, which are usually more common than primary blast injuries.
   3. Tertiary: injuries created when the blast wave propels victims' bodies into objects or large objects strike the body. Typical injuries include crush injuries, closed head injuries, and blunt thoracic and abdominal trauma.
   4. Quaternary: effects include burns, inhalational injury, exposure to toxic substances, and injury from environmental contamination that was created as the result of the explosive device.
   5. Quinary: injuries resulting from additives such as bacteria or radiation (dirty bombs), which may result in a hyperinflammatory response and syndrome.

5. **Is there a quick screening method to triage victims of blast injuries?**

   Otoscopic examination of TM is a quick (but not foolproof) way to assess the severity of blast injury. The TM can be ruptured by an increase in atmospheric pressure as low as 5 psi above normal. If there is no TM rupture, then the chance of hollow-organ injury is significantly lower, but it is not zero. In 17 critically injured patients after the 2004 Madrid train bombing, 13 had ruptured TMs, but 4 did not. If other symptoms, such as shortness of breath, are present, one should suspect additional injuries.

6. **What is blast lung?**

   Blast lung is the significant pulmonary barotrauma caused by exposure to the blast overpressure associated with a high-order explosive detonation. These injuries are significantly more common and severe in closed-space explosions. Mackenzie et al. (2013) defined primary blast lung injury as "radiological and clinical evidence of acute lung injury occurring within 12 hours of exposure and not due to secondary or tertiary injury." The blast wave's impact with the lung causes an immediate autonomic response with subsequent hemorrhage, parenchymal injury, and an inflammatory response. Clinically, this diagnosis is characterized by respiratory difficulty, cough, and hypoxia secondary to poor lung compliance. Presentation may be delayed up to 24–48 hours. In severe injury, patients can develop acute respiratory distress syndrome (ARDS). Plain film radiography will often demonstrate opacification and consolidation secondary to hemorrhage. For those with significant or persistent symptoms a computed tomography (CT) scan should be completed to identify injuries missed on plain film and to further delineate the extent of pulmonary hemorrhage and edema.

Blast lung treatment is principally supportive and is similar to the care for other etiologies of pulmonary contusion. A majority of patients with significant injury will require mechanical ventilation, typically with the same volume-limited parameters used with other ARDS patients. Bronchopleural fistulas, pneumothorax, and air embolism remain as delayed complications of this type of injury. Patients who have normal chest radiographs, normal arterial blood gases, and no complaints that would suggest significant blast lung injury can be considered for discharge after 4–6 hours of observation with strict return precautions for potential delayed symptoms. Therapies to further address the inflammatory response are being investigated currently.

In addition to blast lung, explosions are often associated with fire and smoke production. Inhalation injuries, burns, and exposure to fine dust and contaminants should be considered in the evaluation of patients.

7. What injuries occur to the gastrointestinal system?

Intestinal perforation can occur and is most commonly found in the colon and ileocecal region. Bowel contusion and shearing can lead to wall ischemia and delayed presentation. Patients should be evaluated and resuscitated similar to other causes of blunt abdominal trauma.

8. It seems that explosions could cause significant head injuries. Is this true?

Secondary and tertiary blast injuries to the central nervous system (CNS) include intracranial hemorrhage, cerebral contusion, and parenchymal injury. There is increasing evidence that the primary blast wave can also cause a concussive injury. These injuries can be associated with posttraumatic stress disorder (PTSD). The psychological impact of explosions, especially terrorist incidents, cannot be minimized. These events can be devastating for all those affected and the initial acknowledgment and treatment of this occurs in the emergency department (ED).

9. How common are musculoskeletal injuries?

In recent Middle East combat settings, extremity and musculoskeletal injuries represent approximately 54% of wounds. Two of the most common injuries are traumatic amputations and compartment syndrome. Injuries in this setting are primarily attributed to improvised explosive devices. In the civilian population, events such as the Boston Marathon bombing emphasize the destructive nature of additional shrapnel added to bombs to increase their propensity for injury. Traumatic amputations act as a marker for poor prognosis due to the often-associated additional injuries.

10. Not all explosions are terrorist related. In what other settings might we see these injuries?

According to the Occupational Safety and Health Administration, in 2017 there were 33 incidents reported involving workplace explosions that accounted for 42 fatalities and 14 injuries. Emergency medical services (EMS) providers need to be prepared for explosive-related injuries, regardless of location and perceived exposure to terrorist threats. Other sources of blast injury include fireworks, utility accidents, tire explosions, drug manufacturing mishaps, and industrial accidents.

KEY POINTS

1. Explosions have the potential to cause significant injury at air–tissue interfaces, especially in the auditory, pulmonary, gastrointestinal, and central nervous systems.
2. Presence of significant external injuries should raise the index of concern to screen other systems.
3. Intentional terrorist attacks are not the only potential source of explosive-related injuries.

Websites
National Consortium for the Study of Terrorism and Responses to Terrorism (START); 2018. Global Terrorism Database [Data file]. https://www.start.umd.edu/gtd. Accessed March 3, 2019.
United States Department of Labor. Occupational Health and Safety. Fatality Inspection Data: Work-related Fatalities for Cases Inspected by Federal or State. https://www.osha.gov/dep/fatcat/dep_fatcat.html. Accessed March 3, 2019.

REFERENCE

1. Mackenzie I, Tunnicliffe B, Clasper J, et al. What the intensive care doctor needs to know about blast-related lung injury. *J Intensive Care Soc.* 2013;14(4):303–312.

BIBLIOGRAPHY

Comer JS, Dantowitz A, Chou T, et al. Adjustment among area youth after the Boston Marathon bombing and subsequent manhunt. *Pediatrics.* 2014;134(1):7–14.

Edwards DS, McMenemy L, Stapley SA, et al. 40 years of terrorist bombings - a meta-analysis of the casualty and injury profile. *Injury.* 2016;47(3):646–652.

Scott TE, Kirkman E, Hague M, et al. Primary blast lung injury - a review. *Br J Anaesth.* 2017;118(3):311–316.

CHAPTER 107

TACTICAL MEDICINE

John Knight, MD and Paul R. Hinchey, MD, MBA

1. **What is tactical medicine?**
   Tactical emergency medical support (TEMS) is the close medical support for law enforcement operations and law enforcement officers. TEMS is an extension of emergency medical services (EMS) and emergency medical practice for law enforcement agencies.

2. **What has driven the development of TEMS as an area of practice?**
   Response to active shooter/mass casualty incidents (AS/MCIs), illegal drug and gun trafficking activity, and the service of warrants requires high-risk intervention by law enforcement. The inherent danger of these activities places law enforcement at great risk for traumatic injury and increases the need for specially trained medical personnel. On-scene medical response delivered by providers highly trained in both police tactics and combat care has allowed for more robust, forward-located medical response. Military medical practice has proven that this close point of injury (POI) care increases survival for victims of combat injuries.

3. **How does TEMS influence care?**
   The three most common causes of preventable trauma death in the prehospital environment are uncontrolled extremity hemorrhage, tension pneumothorax, and airway problems. These injuries are time sensitive, and the ability to intervene immediately in a tactical setting has substantially decreased morbidity and mortality.

4. **Provide some specific examples of these incidents.**
   Events such as the Virginia Tech shooting (2007), Boston bombing (2013), and Sutherland Springs Church shooting (2017) show how coordinated law-enforcement and EMS response, using TEMS principles, help reduce morbidity and mortality. Law enforcement and medical personnel can provide near-immediate basic and advanced treatment of hemorrhage control and airway and breathing management.
   The International Association of Fire Fighters (IAFF), Department of Homeland Security, American College of Surgeons, and Hartford Consensus all have language that incorporates the tenets of TEMS into civilian responses for AS/MCI events.

5. **How does practice of this subspecialty fit within emergency medicine?**
   The American Board of Emergency Medicine (ABEM) oversees subspecialties within emergency medicine. In 2013, ABEM issued the first subspecialty certification examination to become board certified in EMS. The increasing sophistication and expanding scope of practice has increased the need for EMS physicians to oversee TEMS programs, and to obtain appropriate levels of combat medicine and law enforcement operational knowledge.

6. **What are the main entities or recognized bodies providing recommendations on the practice and scope of TEMS medicine?**
   The Committee on Tactical Combat Casualty Care (CoTCCC) and Committee for Tactical Emergency Casualty Care (C-TECC) are the two main bodies that provide direction for skills and training for TEMS. The lessons learned from the recent years of US military operations worldwide helped these expert committees identify and develop tactics, techniques, and procedures that have had significant impact in military medicine, civilian emergency medicine, and EMS practice.

7. **What are the goals of TEMS?**
   - Force multiplier – dedicated medical personnel allow law enforcement to remain focused on the mission, and immediate treatment of minor injuries allows law enforcement officers to return to operations.
   - Assess medical threat – analysis and risk assessment to inform placement of TEMS resources for maximal support.
   - Reduce death, injury, and illness among team members, bystanders, victims, and suspects.
   - Provide preventive medicine, monitor environmental effects, and maintain team health to reduce lost work time.
   - Coordinate with receiving facilities for strategic evacuation and definitive care of casualties.
   - Decrease liability through appropriate medical oversight and clinical care of officers, victims, and suspects.
   - Identify and preserve forensic and crime scene evidence that might otherwise be lost or destroyed during clinical care.

8. **In what areas of tactical medicine can emergency physicians have input and participation?**
   Direct oversight of medical training and maintenance of skills is essential to any EMS agency and its providers. TEMS physicians develop protocols, continue education programs, and provide care as tactical medical directors.

9. **What does SWAT stand for?**

   SWAT is an acronym for *special weapons and tactics.*

10. **What is the role of SWAT, and why does it create a need for tactical medicine?**

    SWAT officers are highly trained law enforcement personnel who operate in settings or conditions posing high levels of risk and potential for injury. SWAT teams are called upon to operate in austere environments, in remote areas, and on extended deployments. The increased risk, duration, and occasional remoteness of these operations require immediate access to emergency medical personnel with training in prolonged management of emergent conditions, as well as maintenance of team health, readiness, and overall well-being. EMS providers without specialized training would typically wait at a safe distance and rely on law enforcement to either bring the injured to care or declare the scene safe for EMS entry, resulting in significant delays until medical care can be provided.

11. **What is the difference between cover and concealment?**

    Concealment prevents direct visualization, but does not provide any protection from gunfire or projectiles (e.g., vegetation, walls comprised of drywall, wooden doors). Cover provides both concealment and a barrier (e.g., concrete walls, engine block of a vehicle) to protect from hostile fire. The effectiveness of cover is dependent upon the makeup of the barrier, as well as the nature of the weapon and ammunition being used.

12. **What are the zones of tactical operations, and how are they defined?**

    - *Hot zone.* This area is considered subject to direct hostile action.
    - *Warm zone.* There is a potential for exposure to hostile action and injury, but this threat is not immediate.
    - *Cold zone.* This zone is outside the area of potential hostility, and therefore poses no threat of injury.

13. **What is "barricaded care," or remote patient care?**

    When hostages or casualties cannot be reached by the provider because of exposure to gunfire or a barricaded suspect, a tactical provider may still be able to perform remote assessment and care. Tactical providers can use distant visual assessment techniques (binoculars) or conduct assessment through available communication. Tactical providers can then give instructions to laypersons or the injured to render basic care.

14. **What are the phases of tactical medical care? How are they defined and what care is provided in each phase?**

    - *Care under fire.* Care provided in the hot zone while the victim and provider are still under hostile fire. If imminent danger exists without appropriate security, the initial care is self-aid. When possible, a provider moves the casualty to cover and out of direct fire, and begins immediate control of exsanguinating hemorrhage and evacuation or movement to a casualty collection point (CCP).
    - *Tactical field care.* Care provided in the warm zone where there is no direct hostile fire but the threat still exists. Care in this phase addresses immediate life threats and is the first opportunity to safely address airway management and breathing issues (sucking chest wound, tension pneumothorax). Controlled hemorrhage is rechecked and any major hemorrhage not previously controlled is addressed with the use of additional tourniquets, hemostatic agents, or pressure dressings. The extent of the medical care depends on the security of the environment, equipment available, and timeline to evacuation. If time allows, care may include establishing intravenous (IV) or interosseous (IO) access for volume replacement, analgesia, and prophylactic antibiotics.
    - *Evacuation care.* Care provided in the cold zone where there is no threat of hostility. In a civilian environment, this phase of care is typically provided while on route to definitive care at a level 1 or 2 trauma center. The extent of care depends on the time and distance to care, level of care at the destination, and the means of transport. Care in this phase is like routine civilian trauma care.

15. **What comprises the tactical/military primary assessment, and how does it differ from the traditional primary assessment?**

    Because of the large number of preventable deaths attributed to bleeding, the tactical primary assessment *(XABCDE)* places greater emphasis on early and aggressive hemorrhage control before assessment of airway, breathing, and circulation (ABCs) as follows:

    EXsanguinating hemorrhage
    Airway
    Breathing
    Circulation
    Disability
    Expose

    The military uses a similar model, *MARCH:*

    Massive hemorrhage
    Airway
    Respiratory
    Circulation
    Head injury and **H**ypothermia

16. **How does hemorrhage control in the tactical or combat environment differ from that of civilian care?**
Immediate tourniquet application in all life-threatening extremity hemorrhage is encouraged. Previous algorithms that used tourniquets as a last resort have been disproven. Combat and tactical environments still use direct pressure for compressible wounds, but early placement of a tourniquet for all extremity wounds prevents potential life-threatening hemorrhage. In a controlled environment, the tourniquet may be reassessed for need and efficacy. In addition to tourniquet use, wound packing with hemostatic agents, such as combat gauze, with subsequent direct pressure, has been proven effective at hemorrhage control.

17. **What are desirable features of a tactical/combat tourniquet?**
Tourniquets should be constructed of a wide strap (minimum 1.5 inches wide) to reduce soft-tissue injury, can be self-applied by the injured using one hand, and use a windlass or ratcheting mechanism to generate adequate pressure for hemorrhage control from large vessels.

18. **How can I tell when a tourniquet is appropriately applied?**
A tourniquet should be tight enough to stop hemorrhage and create an extremity that is pulseless. Occasionally, injuries and hemorrhage in larger muscle groups, such as the thigh, may not be controlled with one tourniquet and require the use of a second tourniquet placed adjacent to the first.

19. **In the tactical environment, what are the limitations of using a tourniquet over other hemorrhage control techniques?**
As effective as tourniquets are for extremities, their use is limited in noncompressible areas such as groin or axilla (junctional hemorrhage), thorax, and abdomen. Such junctional or torso injuries require other hemorrhage control techniques (wound packing, junctional compression devices).

20. **What is the maximum time a tourniquet can be left in place without injury or loss of the limb?**
Though it is not known exactly how long any extremity can last without circulation before definite loss of limb, there is general consensus that a tourniquet can be left in place for up to 2 hours with minimal risk of permanent injury. There is some evidence that supports likely amputation after 6 hours due to near-complete muscle damage.

21. **Where should a tourniquet be placed?**
Recommendation for initial tourniquet placement is high on the extremity to expedite decision making under fire. If time allows for identification of the wound, the general guidance is 2 inches above the injury site, not over a joint. If access to definitive care is expected to be delayed, tourniquet placement close to the wound preserves as much limb as possible for future recovery. If utilized, distal placement of a tourniquet over two bones (tibia/fibula and ulna/radius) can make arterial compression more difficult and requires particular attention to efficacy. Regardless of preference, a tourniquet should be tightened until bleeding is stopped, the limb is pulseless, and it should never be applied over a joint.

22. **What are the side effects of failure to adequately tighten a tourniquet?**
If arterial flow is not stopped and a tourniquet has only been applied with enough pressure to prevent venous return, there is a risk of compartment syndrome, potential fasciotomy, and permanent sequelae.

23. **Describe hemostatic agents used in the tactical environment.**
Several products have been developed to aid in clotting as well as dressing wounds using gauze impregnated with various clot-enhancing agents. These products are packed into open, bleeding wounds and have proven to be effective at promoting hemostasis. A newer product has the hemostatic agent embedded in small compressed sponge pellets within a large syringe (XSTAT). With smaller wounds not amenable to wound packing, the syringe can be placed in the wound and the expandable pellets delivered deep into the injury.

24. **What areas of the body are amenable to wound packing in a tactical environment?**
These are primarily the junctional areas, including:
- groin
- buttock
- pelvis/perineum
- axilla
- extremities too proximal for tourniquet placement
- base of neck

25. **Which hemostatic agents are most commonly used?**
- *QuikClot Combat Gauze.* This product is the US military's first choice for hemostatic agents. It uses a nonexothermic mineral compound (kaolin) impregnated in gauze that triggers the intrinsic clotting cascade. Large clots should be quickly evacuated, the source of bleeding identified, and the gauze packed into the wound. To maximize effectiveness, the gauze should be applied directly onto the hemorrhaging vessel(s) and held in place with direct pressure applied for a minimum of 3 minutes to ensure full effect. Saturated combat gauze should be removed and replaced by new gauze with fresh agent.
- *Celox.* A polysaccharide (chitosan) derived from shellfish. When it comes in contact with blood, it forms a gel-like substance that aids in clot formation. It was found to be somewhat less effective than combat gauze, but

has the added benefit of working independently of the clotting cascade. This makes it effective in patients with coagulopathies associated with anticoagulants and hypothermia.
- *HemCon ChitoGauze.* Also a chitosan derivative, it functions in a manner similar to Celox. Like other agents, it is available in a gauze form that facilitates wound packing.

26. **What is the basic airway adjunct of choice in the tactical environment?**
The nasopharyngeal airway (NPA), when used in conjunction with manual airway maneuvers and patient positioning, addresses most airway concerns in the tactical environment.

27. **If basic airway maneuvers fail, what steps should be taken to manage the airway?**
Since airway management generally takes place in tactical field care, a number of options exist. Supraglottic airways (I-Gel, LMA, King LT) may be utilized. Oral or nasal intubation may be considered. Surgical cricothyrotomy uses a minimum of equipment, can be performed quickly, provides a definitive airway, and is generally well-tolerated by the patient once in place. It does not require the use of a laryngoscope, suction, or paralytics, and limits the need for adjuncts to ensure and maintain proper placement.

28. **What is the intervention of choice for managing tension pneumothorax in the field?**
Tension pneumothorax is the second leading cause of preventable death in battlefield settings. Finger or needle thoracostomy using large-bore (10-, 12-, or 14- gauge), long (minimum 3.25 in) over-the-needle catheter is the treatment of choice for decompressing the chest. Smaller gauge or shorter catheters risk failure to evacuate air or enter the chest cavity. A 3.25-inch catheter reached the pleura in 99% of those studied in a military cohort. Typical catheter placement is above the rib in the second intercostal space in the midclavicular line. Ballistic vests or body mass may necessitate a lateral approach at the fourth intercostal space in the mid or anterior axillary line. Finger thoracostomy uses a small incision at the fourth or fifth intercostal space in the midanterior axillary line and pleural penetration above the rib with curved Kelly forceps or a finger to create an opening.

29. **Why is it important to manage a sucking chest wound and what is the device of choice?**
An open pneumothorax (sucking chest wound) interferes with normal pulmonary mechanics. Wounds that are larger than two-thirds of the diameter of the trachea can result in air preferentially being drawn into the thorax through the chest wall defect. These injuries should be managed with an occlusive dressing to prevent air passage through a wound site and restore pulmonary mechanics. The use of commercial devices that incorporate a valve or venting mechanism or taping three sides of an occlusive material have been described as a means of reducing the risk of subsequent tension pneumothorax.

30. **Why is it essential to manage hypothermia in the tactical environment?**
Even mild hypothermia can contribute to coagulopathy, and hypothermia has been independently associated with increased mortality. Hypothermia is common in both combat and civilian trauma victims, with two-thirds of civilian trauma victims arriving at the hospital with hypothermia. Once developed, hypothermia is far more difficult to treat than taking steps to prevent it. Tactical and combat training programs emphasize initiating hypothermia management as soon as possible.

31. **What is the leading cause of combat death?**
Uncontrolled bleeding accounts for nearly 90% of preventable deaths on the battlefield. Nearly 50% of total combat deaths are the result of exsanguinating hemorrhage. Large-vessel injuries in noncompressible areas such as the thorax and abdomen can only be managed at a trauma center. Most preventable deaths are caused by hemorrhage from compressible locations such as junctional and extremity injuries. Increased emphasis on tourniquet and hemostatic use has significantly decreased preventable deaths in the military environment and has started to make an impact in the civilian EMS community.

32. **What are the most common areas of the body injured during combat?**
- Head and neck: 4%–24%
- Thoracic injuries: 4%–15%
- Abdominal injuries: 2%–20%
- Extremity injuries: 50%–75%

33. **Looking into the future.**
- The administration of blood products as the fluid of choice in trauma has been recognized for many years in military combat theaters. Use in the civilian prehospital setting appears to be limited by logistics, but is currently being explored.
- Tranexamic acid (TXA) is an antifibrinolytic agent that prevents clot breakdown and has proven to reduce the need for transfusions in surgery. Though still not officially approved by the US Food and Drug Administration (FDA), it continues to be used off-label in prehospital and combat settings.
- Resuscitative endovascular balloon occlusion of the aorta (REBOA) is an invasive procedure that places an occlusive balloon through the femoral artery into the aorta. The goal is to stop noncompressible bleeding until surgical control can be obtained. The intervention and its efficacy are still being studied. Given the complexity of the procedure, its utility in a tactical environment is in question.

KEY POINTS: TACTICAL MEDICINE

1. Tactical medicine and point of injury emergency care improves victim survival.
2. The most common cause of preventable death after trauma is uncontrolled hemorrhage, particularly from an extremity.
3. There are three zones of tactical operation based upon the likelihood of and potential for threat. The hot zone is subject directly to the threat; the warm zone has the potential for exposure to the threat but it is not immediate; and the cold zone is away from the area of the threat and poses no risk of injury.
4. There are three phases of medical care based upon which zone treatment is being provided in. Care under fire or direct threat care is provided in the hot zone; tactical field care or indirect threat care is provided in the warm zone; and evacuation care is provided in the cold zone.
5. Life-threatening bleeding from an extremity is managed by immediate tourniquet application.

BIBLIOGRAPHY

Callaway DW, Smith EF, Shapiro G, et al. The Committee for Tactical Emergency Care (C-TECC): evolution and application of TCCC guidelines to civilian high threat medicine. *J Spec Oper.* 2011;11:95–100.
Committee for Tactical Combat Casualty Care. TCCC guidelines. *J Spec Oper Med* 2018. https://www.jsomonline.org/TCCC/TCCC-MP%20Curriculum%201708/00%20TCCC-MP%20Guidelines%20180801/TCCC%20Guidelines%20for%20Medical%20%20Personnel%20180801.pdf. Accessed February 18, 2019.
Committee for Tactical Emergency Casualty Care. TECC guidelines; 2015. http://www.c-tecc.org/images/content/TECC_Guidelines_-_JUNE_2015_update.pdf. Accessed February 18, 2019.
Goodwin T, Moore KN, Pasley JD, et al. From the battlefield to main street: tourniquet acceptance, use, and translation from the military to civilian settings. *J Trauma Acute Care Surg.* 2019;87(1S suppl 1):S35–S39.
Jacobs LM, McSwain N, Rotondo M. American College of Surgeons: Improving survival from active shooter events: the Hartford Consensus. *Bull Am Coll Surg.* 2013;98:14–16. http://bulletin.facs.org/2013/06/improving-survival-from-active-shooter-events/. Accessed September 10, 2014.
McEvoy M. Tansexamic acid (TXA): drug whys; June 29, 2015. https://www.ems1.com/ems-products/Ambulance-Disposable-Supplies/articles/2206976-Tranexamic-Acid-TXA-Drug-Whys/.
Morrisey J. Tactical EMS: an overview. EMS1.com; 2013. https://www.ems1.com/ems-education/articles/1482674-Tactical-EMS-An-overview/. Accessed February 18, 2019.
Scerbo MH, Mumm JP, Gates K, et al. Safety and appropriateness of tourniquets in 105 civilians. *Prehosp Emerg Care.* 2016;20:712–722.
Scott Weingart. EMCrit Podcast 133 – The First Prehospital REBOA. *EMCrit Blog.* September 24, 2014. https://emcrit.org/emcrit/emcrit-podcast-133-first-prehospital-reboa/. Accessed February 15, 2019.

INDEX

Page numbers followed by *f* indicate figure, by *t* table, and by *b* box.